D1596468

Neurodegeneration

Neurodegeneration

Edited by

Anthony Schapira, MD, DSc, FRCP, FMedSci
Institute of Neurology, University College London, London, UK

Zbigniew Wszolek, MD
Mayo Clinic, Jacksonville, Florida, USA

Ted M. Dawson, MD, PhD
Johns Hopkins University School of Medicine, Baltimore, Maryland, USA

Nicholas Wood, FRCP, PhD, FMedSci
National Hospital for Neurology and Neurosurgery, Institute of Neurology, London, UK

WILEY Blackwell

This edition first published 2017 © 2017 by John Wiley & Sons Ltd

All rights reserved. No part of this publication may be reproduced, stored in a retrieval system, or transmitted, in any form or by any means, electronic, mechanical, photocopying, recording or otherwise, except as permitted by law. Advice on how to obtain permission to reuse material from this title is available at http://www.wiley.com/go/permissions.

The right of the editors to be identified as the authors of this work has been asserted in accordance with law.

Registered Office(s)
John Wiley & Sons, Inc., 111 River Street, Hoboken, NJ 07030, USA
John Wiley & Sons Ltd, The Atrium, Southern Gate, Chichester, West Sussex, PO19 8SQ, UK

Editorial Office
9600 Garsington Road, Oxford, OX4 2DQ, UK

For details of our global editorial offices, customer services, and more information about Wiley products visit us at www.wiley.com.

Wiley also publishes its books in a variety of electronic formats and by print-on-demand. Some content that appears in standard print versions of this book may not be available in other formats.

Limit of Liability/Disclaimer of Warranty
The contents of this work are intended to further general scientific research, understanding, and discussion only and are not intended and should not be relied upon as recommending or promoting scientific method, diagnosis, or treatment by physicians for any particular patient. In view of ongoing research, equipment modifications, changes in governmental regulations, and the constant flow of information relating to the use of medicines, equipment, and devices, the reader is urged to review and evaluate the information provided in the package insert or instructions for each medicine, equipment, or device for, among other things, any changes in the instructions or indication of usage and for added warnings and precautions. While the publisher and authors have used their best efforts in preparing this work, they make no representations or warranties with respect to the accuracy or completeness of the contents of this work and specifically disclaim all warranties, including without limitation any implied warranties of merchantability or fitness for a particular purpose. No warranty may be created or extended by sales representatives, written sales materials or promotional statements for this work. The fact that an organization, website, or product is referred to in this work as a citation and/ or potential source of further information does not mean that the publisher and authors endorse the information or services the organization, website, or product may provide or recommendations it may make. This work is sold with the understanding that the publisher is not engaged in rendering professional services. The advice and strategies contained herein may not be suitable for your situation. You should consult with a specialist where appropriate. Further, readers should be aware that websites listed in this work may have changed or disappeared between when this work was written and when it is read. Neither the publisher nor authors shall be liable for any loss of profit or any other commercial damages, including but not limited to special, incidental, consequential, or other damages.

Library of Congress Cataloging-in-Publication Data

Names: Schapira, Anthony H. V. (Anthony Henry Vernon), editor. | Wszolek, Zbigniew K., editor. | Dawson, Ted Murray editor. | Wood, N. W. (Nicholas W.), editor.
Title: Neurodegeneration / edited by Anthony Schapira, Zbigniew Wszolek, Ted Dawson, Nicholas Wood.
Other titles: Neurodegeneration (Schapira)
Description: Oxford, UK; Hoboken, NJ: John Wiley & Sons Ltd, 2017. | Includes bibliographical references and index.
Identifiers: LCCN 2016041714 (print) | LCCN 2016043003 (ebook) | ISBN 9780470672686 (cloth : alk. paper) | ISBN 9781118661925 (Adobe PDF) | ISBN 9781118661918 (ePub)
Subjects: | MESH: Neurodegenerative Diseases--physiopathology
Classification: LCC RC355 (print) | LCC RC355 (ebook) | NLM WL 358.5 | DDC 616.8—dc23
LC record available at https://lccn.loc.gov/2016041714

Cover images (top to bottom): © KTSDESIGN/Gettyimages; © KTSDESIGN/SCIENCE PHOTO LIBRARY/Gettyimages; © SEBASTIAN KAULITZKI/Gettyimages; © Mark N Miller, University of California, SF/Gettyimages

Set in 9/11pt Minion Pro by Aptara Inc., New Delhi, India
Printed and bound in Singapore by Markono Print Media Pte Ltd

10 9 8 7 6 5 4 3 2 1

Contents

List of Contributors

Zeshan Ahmed, PhD
Research Fellow,
Department of Molecular Neuroscience,
UCL Institute of Neurology,
London, UK

Craig Blackstone, MD, PhD
Senior Investigator, Cell Biology Section, Neurogenetics Branch,
National Institutes of Neurological Disorders and Stroke,
National Institutes of Health,
Bethesda, Maryland, USA

Erich Peter Bosch, MD
Professor Emeritus of Neurology,
Department of Neurology,
Mayo Clinic Arizona,
Scottsdale, Arizona, USA

Kevin B. Boylan, MD
Associate Professor of Neurology,
Department of Neurology, Mayo Clinic,
Jacksonville, Florida, USA

Jacqueline Chen, PhD
Project Staff,
Department of Neuroscience,
Lerner Research Institute, Cleveland Clinic,
Cleveland, Ohio, USA

H. Brent Clark, MD, PhD
Professor,
Department of Laboratory Medicine and Pathology,
University of Minnesota Medical School,
Minneapolis, Minnesota, USA

Melissa E. Crowder, MD
Research Technician,
Department of Neurology,
Johns Hopkins University School of Medicine,
Baltimore, Maryland, USA

Ruth-Mary deSouza, BSc, MBBS
Neurosurgery trainee and PhD student,
Institute of Neurology,
University College London,
London, UK

Dennis W. Dickson, MD
Robert E. Jacoby Professor of Alzheimer's Research,
Department of Neuroscience, Mayo Clinic,
Jacksonville, Florida, USA

Ranjan Dutta, PhD
Assistant Staff,
Department of Neuroscience,
Lerner Research Institute, Cleveland Clinic,
Cleveland, Ohio, USA

Eric Eggenberger, DO
Professor,
Department of Neurology and Opthalmology,
Michigan State University,
East Lansing, Michigan, USA

Michel Goedert, MD, PhDMRC
Laboratory of Molecular Biology,
Francis Crick Avenue,
Cambridge, UK

Neill R. Graff-Radford, MBBCh, FRCP (Lond)
Professor of Neurology,
Mayo College of Medicine,
Jacksonville, Florida, USA

Salman Haider, BSc (Hons), MBBS, MRCP
Specialty Registrar in Neurology,
London Deanery,
Barking, Havering and
Redbridge University Hospitals NHS Trust,
Essex, UK

Henry Houlden, MD, PhD
Professor of Neurology and Neurogenetics and
MRC Centre for Neuromuscular Diseases,
Department of Molecular Neuroscience,
UCL Institute of Neurology,
Queen Square, London, UK

Barbara Jasinska-Myga, MD, PhD
Assistant Professor of Neurology,
Department of Neurology,
Medical University of Silesia,
Katowice, Poland

Keith A. Josephs, Jr., MD, MST, MSc
Professor of Neurology,
Department of Neurology,
Divisions of Movement Disorders and
Behavioral Neurology, Mayo Clinic Rochester,
Rochester, Minnesota, USA

Qurat ul Ain Khan, MD
Fellow, Mayo College of Medicine,
Jacksonville, Florida, USA

Desmond Kidd, MD, FRCP
Consultant Neurologist,
Department of Clinical Neurosciences and
Head, Department of Neuro-ophthalmology,
Royal Free Hospital, London, and
Honorary Senior Lecturer in Neurology,
University College London,
London, UK

David S. Knopman, MD
Professor of Neurology,
Department of Neurology,
Mayo Clinic Rochester, and Mayo Clinic Alzheimer's
Disease Research Center,
Rochester, Minnesota, USA

Takuya Konno, MD, PhD
Research Fellow,
Department of Neurology,
Mayo Clinic,
Jacksonville, Florida, USA

Pawel P. Liberski, MD, PhD
Professor and Chairman,
Departments of Molecular Pathology and
Neuropathology, Medical University of Lodz,
Lodz, Poland

**Andres M. Lozano, OC, MD, PhD,
FRCSC, FRSC, FCAHS**
University Professor and Dan Family Chairman of Neurosurgery,
Division of Neurosurgery,
University of Toronto,
Toronto Western Hospital,
Toronto, Ontario, Canada

James A. Mastrianni, MD, PhD
Professor of Neurology,
Director, Center for Comprehensive Care and
Research on Memory Disorders,
Department of Neurology, The University of Chicago,
Chicago, Illinois, USA

Mark P. Mattson, PhD
Chief,
Laboratory of Neurosciences,
National Institute on Aging Intramural Research Program,
Baltimore, Maryland, USA

Alisdair McNeill, PhD, MRCP (UK)
Senior Clinical Fellow,
Sheffield Institute of Translational Neuroscience (SITraN), Sheffield,
South Yorkshire, UK

Huw R. Morris, FRCP, PhD
Professor of Clinical Neuroscience,
Department of Clinical Neuroscience,
UCL Institute of Neurology,
London, UK

Daniel L. Murman, MD, MS
Director, Behavioral and Geriatric Neurology Program,
Professor, Department of Neurological Sciences,
University of Nebraska Medical Center,
Omaha, Nebraska, USA

Peter T. Nelson, MD, PhD
Professor of Pathology,
Department of Pathology,
Division of Neuropathology,
University of Kentucky and Sanders-Brown Center on Aging,
Lexington, Kentucky, USA

Janna H. Neltner, MD
Associate Professor of Pathology,
Department of Pathology,
Division of Neuropathology,
University of Kentucky and
Sanders-Brown Center on Aging,
Lexington, Kentucky, USA

Nobuhiko Ohno, MD, PhD
Postdoctoral Fellow,
Department of Neuroscience,
Lerner Research Institute,
Cleveland Clinic,
Cleveland, Ohio, USA

Daniel Ontaneda, MSc, MD
Staff Neurologist,
Mellen Center for Multiple Sclerosis,
Cleveland Clinic,
Cleveland, Ohio, USA

Harry T. Orr, PhD
Professor and Director,
Department of Laboratory Medicine and Pathology and
Institute for Translational Neuroscience,
University of Minnesota Medical School,
Minneapolis, Minnesota, USA

Amelie Pandraud, PhD
Professor of Neurology and Neurogenetics,
MRC Centre for Neuromuscular Diseases,
Department of Molecular Neuroscience,
UCL Institute of Neurology,
Queen Square, London, UK

Marc C. Patterson, MD, FRACP
Professor of Neurology, Pediatrics and Medical Genetics,
Departments of Neurology, Pediatrics and Medical Genetics,
Mayo Clinic Children's Center,
Rochester, Minnesota, USA

Noah J. Pyles
Research Technician,
Department of Neurology,
Johns Hopkins University School of Medicine,
Baltimore, Maryland, USA

Deborah L. Renaud, MD
Neurologist,
Departments of Neurology and Pediatrics,
Mayo Clinic,
Rochester, Minnesota, USA

Mark A. Ross, MD
Professor of Neurology,
Department of Neurology,
Mayo Clinic,
Scottsdale, Arizona, USA

Owen A. Ross, PhD
Associate Professor of Neuroscience,
Department of Neuroscience,
Department of Clinical Genomics,
Mayo Clinic, Jacksonville, Florida, USA

Anna Sailer, MD, PhD
Clinical Fellow,
Department of Neurology,
University Hospital Frankfurt, Frankfurt, Germany

Rodolfo Savica, MD
Assistant Professor of Neurology,
Department of Neurology,
Mayo Clinic Rochester, and
Mayo Clinic Alzheimer's Disease Research Center,
Rochester, Minnesota, USA

Anthony H.V. Schapira, MD, DSc, FRCP, FMedSci
Professor, Institute of Neurology,
University College London,
London, UK

Lucia V. Schottlaender, MD
Research Fellow,
Department of Molecular Neuroscience,
UCL Institute of Neurology,
London, UK

Eric J. Sorenson, MD
Professor of Neurology,
Department of Neurology,
Mayo Clinic,
Rochester, Minnesota, USA

Charlotte J. Sumner, MD
Associate Professor of Neurology and Neuroscience,
Departments of Neurology and Neuroscience,
Johns Hopkins University School of Medicine,
Baltimore, Maryland, USA

Sarah J. Tabrizi, BSc, MBChB, FRCP, PhD, FMedSci
Professor of Clinical Neurology and Consultant Neurologist,
Department of Neurodegenerative Disease,
UCL Institute of Neurology and National Hospital for
Neurology and Neurosurgery,
London, UK

Malcolm Taylor, PhD
Professor of Cancer Genetics, Interim Director,
Institute of Cancer and Genomic Sciences,
University of Birmingham, Edgbaston,
Birmingham, UK

Travis S. Tierney, MD, DPhil
Staff Neurosurgeon,
Division of Neurosurgery,
Nicklaus Children's Hospital,
Miami, Florida, USA

Bruce D. Trapp, PhD
Chair and Professor,
Department of Neuroscience, Lerner Research Institute,
Cleveland Clinic,
Cleveland, Ohio, USA

Christian W. Wider, MD
Chef de Clinique,
Formerly of Department of Clinical Neuroscience,
Lausanne University Hospital (CHUV-UNIL),
Lausanne, Switzerland

Edward Wild, MA, MB, BChir, PhD, MRCP (Neurol)
Principal Research Associate and Consultant Neurologist,
Department of Neurodegenerative Disease,
UCL Institute of Neurology and
National Hospital for Neurology and
Neurosurgery, London, UK

Joseph R. Wooley, MD
Research Technician,
Department of Neurology,
Johns Hopkins University School of Medicine,
Baltimore, Maryland, USA

Zbigniew K. Wszolek, MD
Consultant and Professor of Neurology,
Department of Neurology,
Mayo Clinic,
Jacksonville, Florida, USA

Preface

The study of the function and dysfunction of the human brain and nervous system now constitutes the major focus of the biological sciences. Neurological disorders are often chronic and disabling, associated with a significant reduction in quality of life for patient and caregivers, increased morbidity and dependency, reduced life expectancy and a substantial financial burden on families and state. This pattern is seen with a broad range of neurological diseases, but is exemplified by the neurodegenerative disorders.

The enlarging global population coupled with a rise in life expectancy across the globe has highlighted the imperative of discovering therapies that can prevent the onset, slow or stop the progression of neurodegenerative diseases. While this ambition has been a priority since the first description of disorders such as Alzheimer (AD) or Parkinson (PD) disease, it is only with a clearer understanding of their potential causes that this has become a realistic focus. The advent and application of the molecular neurosciences and neurogenetics to the neurodegenerative diseases have provided the ability to identify often multiple aetiologies and pathogenetic pathways for neuronal dysfunction and death. Huntington disease (HD) is an example where the discovery of the huntingtin triplet repeat and the relationship of its size to clinical features provided invaluable insight into the pathology, selective neurodegeneration and biochemical defects found in HD. However it is only recently that this knowledge has begun to translate into potential treatments. A similar pattern is seen in AD, where the discoveries of amyloid mutations as a cause of familial AD led to the amyloid hypothesis for aetiology and pathogenesis. Again, it is only recently that therapies focussed on the amyloid pathway have come to clinical trial, although with rather uncertain benefits to date. PD has provided a rather more coherent story for the cause and progress of the disease. Studies prior to the application of modern genetics identified mitochondrial dysfunction, protein aggregation and oxidative stress as important features of PD pathogenesis. Subsequently, mutations were discovered in genes encoding proteins participating in these pathways, emphasising the importance of their role in PD. Further genetic and cell biological studies have combined to emphasise the role of lysosomal function and inflammation not only in PD but also in other neurodegenerations. Novel therapies based on these pathways are now emerging for PD and some are in early clinical trial.

HD, AD and PD are but examples of an enormous spectrum of neurodegenerative diseases affecting the central and peripheral nervous systems. It is notable that discoveries in some, e.g. the triplet repeat in HD, provide insight into others, e.g. triplet repeats in the spinocerebellar ataxias. Likewise the identification of mitochondrial dysfunction in PD was followed by evidence for bioenergetics defects in HD and AD. Protein accumulation, misfolding and aggregation, and more recently propagation have become a focus of attention in the neurodegenerative diseases, and a common theme across many of them.

In this text, we have sought to provide the reader with a modern view of the spectrum of neurodegenerative diseases. We have included not only the archetypal neurodegenerations such as AD, PD and HD, but also those disorders that have more recently been identified as distinct at the clinical, pathological and aetiological levels such as multiple system atrophy, progressive supranuclear palsy etc. We have sought to cover the degenerations of spinal cord and peripheral nervous systems, as well as site specific degenerations such as the optic nerve. Axonal loss in multiple sclerosis has been a focus of attention and some now consider that this disease justifies inclusion in the spectrum of neurodegeneration.

Writing and publishing a modern text book has its challenges, as well as its infinite pleasure upon completion. We have sought to be inclusive in providing the reader with an understanding of the range of neurodegenerative diseases, their causes, pathology, clinical expression and possible treatments. The edition is comprehensive, but not intended to be all inclusive. Any omissions are our responsibility and not those of the authors. We thank them for their enthusiasm, diligence and forbearance! We thank the publishers for their help and support in seeing this project through to completion.

Anthony HV Schapira
Zbigniew K Wszolek
Ted M Dawson
Nicholas Wood

Dedication

Christian W. Wider, MD was an Associate Physician at the Department of Neurology and Head of the Neurogenetic Diseases Unit of the Centre hospitalier universitaire vaudois (CHUV) in Lausanne, Switzerland. He completed his three-year Movement Disorders fellowship at the Mayo Clinic Florida in 2009.

Despite his short life he was able to contribute significantly to the research field of clinical genetics of neurodegenerative disorders and dystonia. He was an excellent diagnostician and was loved by his patients.

Dr. Wider died tragically in July 2016. He will be greatly missed by his family, friends, colleagues, and patients.

CHAPTER 1

Pathology of Brain Aging

Janna H. Neltner and Peter T. Nelson

Department of Pathology, Division of Neuropathology, University of Kentucky and Sanders-Brown Center on Aging, Lexington, Kentucky, USA

Introduction

The goal of this chapter is to describe the prevalent pathologic changes that are found in the brains of aged individuals. When comparing older persons' brains with younger persons' brains, it is challenging to distinguish the sequelae of particular diseases from the biological processes linked to "brain aging". What is clear is that there are specific pathological manifestations observed in the brains of elderly individuals and the presence of a subset of those pathologies correlates strongly with the severity of cognitive impairment. Brain aging-linked diseases include neurodegenerative conditions such as Alzheimer's disease (AD), dementia with Lewy bodies (DLB), Parkinson disease dementia (PDD), frontotemporal lobar dementia (FTLD), hippocampal sclerosis of aging (HS-Aging), and others [1–3]. Also strongly implicated in aging-linked cognitive impairment is the heterogeneous group of conditions that manifest as cerebrovascular disease (CVD) pathology. Here we discuss some of the evolving concepts related to the brain changes that are seen in individuals of advanced age, with panels of photomicrographs to depict their appearance from a pathologist's perspective, and a consideration of the linkages between neuropathologic and genetic data. We emphasize that there is increasing awareness of the importance of CVD and HS-Aging pathologies as drivers of cognitive impairment in the "oldest-old".

The need for better understanding of the aging process and human brain pathologies: clinical and epidemiological aspects

Aging is a fundamental property of terrestrial life. Although not considered a disease per se, advanced aging-linked changes can be detrimental to biological fitness. In all cells and organisms that have been observed, there are phenomena characteristic of the mature epoch of life, and multiple mechanisms have been described to explain those phenomena [4, 5]. Senescence near the end of life has been attributed to mitochondrial dysfunction, telomerase activity, free radicals, oxidative stress, and other factors [4, 6–9]. In addition, genes have been described that either stimulate deleterious aging processes or that delay normal aging effects in some organisms (e.g., sirtuins).

Despite the insights that have been gained as described above, the concepts of aging and in particular brain aging are not well defined currently. Two things are certain: (1) aged individuals are going to constitute an ever-greater proportion of the overall population of developed countries in the upcoming decades [3], a demographic fact with far-reaching implications; and (2) advanced human age is accompanied by characteristic medical conditions that affect the central nervous system (CNS) and other tissues [10]. A defining feature of aging is that it is universally linked to the physical time dimension. Median life expectancy in developed countries is approximately 76 years for men and 81 years for women [11]. Here we focus on those individuals that live longer than average, without addressing the problematic question of "when does 'aging' begin?"

The epidemiology of diseases that affect 95-year-olds is not identical to that of 75-year-olds [12]. In extreme old age, human organs develop a combination of vascular pathologies accompanied by weaker regenerative capacity. The background of generalized infirmity, specific high-morbidity diseases, polypharmacy, metabolic and mood disorders, and sleep pattern changes represents a formidable challenge to determining if a specific factor correlates with a specific disease, or contributes to impaired cognitive functioning through other mechanisms [12–15].

This chapter describes some of the prevalent brain pathologies observed in aged persons' brains. These observations help frame a discussion of their relationship with the aging process and with specific brain diseases. A better understanding of these issues will help us to define, diagnose, and treat the distinct conditions linked to cognitive impairment in the elderly as we move past the incorrect perception that "dementia" is linked overwhelmingly to Alzheimer's disease.

Brain pathologies in aging

Neurodegenerative diseases such as AD and DLB are covered in detail in Chapters 9 and 11. We will briefly describe these diseases, focusing on their pathological substrates and definitions. Pathology can provide insights about disease mechanisms when the molecular pathways are modeled in other experimental systems. However, pathological assessments themselves are cross-sectional (generally seen at autopsy) and often relate to the visual manifestation of histochemical or immunohistochemical staining. Here we use photomicrographs to demonstrate the appearances of the various pathological entities linked to brain aging. Our discussion will include two largely under-appreciated brain diseases (HS-Aging and CVD) that are linked to advanced age and which can be correlated with cognitive impairments.

Neurodegeneration, First Edition. Edited by Anthony Schapira, Zbigniew Wszolek, Ted M. Dawson and Nicholas Wood.
© 2017 John Wiley & Sons, Ltd. Published 2017 by John Wiley & Sons, Ltd.

Nonspecific and non-diagnostic pathologies in aging brain

Relative to pristine brains from younger individuals, there are specific alterations that are observed consistently in the aged human brain, some of which are seen in increased abundance in individuals who died with impaired cognition. Our main emphases are on those brain changes that are indicative of a particular disease process and thus are pathologically diagnostic (for example, plaques and tangles in AD). However, there has been substantial focus on less disease-specific brain changes such as synapse loss, myelinopathy, neuroinflammation, glial activation, and the oxidation of proteins, lipids, and nucleic acids [16–19] which are discussed in other chapters of this volume. Some subtypes of those changes may in the future be proven to be specific to "brain aging" or to specific diseases, but more work needs to be performed in those areas. For example, although synaptic pathology is widely considered to be important in AD, and for credible reasons [20, 21], we note that all neurodegenerative diseases that culminate in dementia – without exception – are associated with synapse loss. Thus, loss of synapses is not disease-specific, much less diagnostic of AD. Until a particular, novel synaptic mechanism is universally accepted for AD, the specificity of synapse loss to AD remains unproven. Nor has the direct link between "brain aging" and synapse loss been exactly defined [3]. Further, some brain changes such as Hirano bodies, granulovacuolar degeneration, and cerebral amyloid angiopathy (CAA) are linked with AD [22] but their specificity and correlative impact on cognitive loss have not been firmly established.

An important step forward for neuropathologists is the most recent (2012) revision of the National Institute on Aging–Alzheimer's Association (NIA-AA)_recommendations for the neuropathologic approach to AD diagnoses [1, 23]. These recent consensus guidelines have advanced the field in at least three ways: (1) they removed the necessity of documented ante mortem cognitive impairment so that AD (like any other disease) can be diagnosed using the pathological "gold standard" alone; (2) they provided greater guidance for the diagnoses of non-AD comorbid pathologies such as HS-Aging, DLB, and CVD pathologies; and (3) they provided guidance to pathologists for anatomical regions to sample and stains to employ in the assessment of neurodegenerative diseases.

AD neuropathologic changes: neurofibrillary tangles

Neurofibrillary pathology comprises aberrant, partly insoluble, protease-resistant, hyperphosphorylated tau aggregates – some with paired helical filament appearance by electron microscopy [24] – inside various cellular compartments or extracellular after death of the parent cell. Neurofibrillary tangle (NFT) is the term that describes neurofibrillary pathology found in cell bodies (Figure 1.1A, B). NFTs are not specific for AD [25–27]; indeed, they are found in almost every class of brain disease and are observed universally (yet topographically and quantitatively restricted) in normal aging subjects [28]. NFTs are also found in the brains of individuals who suffered from frontotemporal degeneration with tauopathy (FTD-MAPT), myotonic dystrophy, prion diseases, metabolic diseases, some brain tumors, chronic traumatic encephalopathy, viral encephalitis, and other brain diseases [29–32]. This suggests that NFTs are, at least under some conditions, a secondary response to injury. Yet tau gene (MAPT) mutations can produce clinical dementia with NFTs, which establishes that under some conditions NFTs may be directly linked to the primary or at least proximal neurodegenerative changes [25, 27, 32]. There is no condition with *widespread neocortical NFTs* that lacks cognitive impairment [33, 34].

AD neuropathologic changes: Aβ plaques

In contrast to NFTs, Aβ amyloid plaques (AβPs) are extracellular [35, 36], often roughly spherical structures containing Aβ peptide and other material (Figure 1.1C–F). AβPs may be detected in histological preparations using Congo red, silver stains, and thioflavin-like molecules. Diffuse (or "primitive") AβPs can be visualized using silver stains and anti-Aβ immunostains. AβPs are found in a high proportion of all elderly persons but are not universal [37–39]. A particularly important subtype of AβPs is "neuritic plaques" (NPs), which have also been referred to as "senile plaques", and which are more likely to be associated with cognitive impairment than diffuse AβPs [40–42]. NPs are AβPs that are surrounded by degenerating axons and dendrites that often contain hyperphosphorylated tau aggregates. It is important to note that in elderly individuals, widespread neocortical NFTs are virtually nonexistent without the presence of widespread AβPs, except in the minority of cases with clear-cut tauopathy (e.g., FTD-MAPT). This observation and others (see below) have led researchers to hypothesize that AβP development is "upstream" of neocortical NFTs in AD pathogenesis [43]. Although the clinical–pathological data are complex, it should be stressed that the extant literature does indeed indicate the existence of a specific disease that is characterized by the presence of AβPs and NFTs [34].

Notes on AD pathology in persons past 90 years of age

For a description of the neuropathological hallmarks of AD and how their distributions have been observed in aging, see Table 1.1. Accurate clinical–pathological correlation requires that both components – clinical workup and pathological analyses – are performed optimally; there are potential obstacles to both of these in extremely old individuals for whom clinical assessments are challenging and autopsy rates are generally low. According to many different studies, dementia prevalence in the populations of developed countries is approximately 2% at age 65 and then doubles every five years thereafter [44–46]. Dementia incidence appears to level off after age 90 [46–50] although clinical dementia prevalence probably does keep increasing [51, 52]. In contrast to the increased prevalence of dementia with advanced age (a clinical observation), the appearance of neuritic AβPs and NFTs by pathology seems to level off in older cognitively impaired individuals according to multiple autopsy series [53–56], with the caveat that not all studies agree (discussed in [57, 58]). Further, as previously discussed, there is a greater "background" of hippocampal and brainstem NFTs in chronologically old individuals' brains. These phenomena have been interpreted to indicate a "dissociation" between AD neuropathologic change and cognitive status in extreme old age. However, even in extreme old age, the presence of many neocortical NFTs (Braak neurofibrillary stage VI) correlates with ante mortem cognitive decline [59–61]. Thus, no "dissociation" exists between the AD neuropathologic change and cognitive impairment. The question relates to cognitively impaired individuals of advanced age whose brains lack substantial AD pathology at autopsy. The answer to this question may lie in understanding the many powerful non-AD pathologies that occur beyond the eighth decade of life.

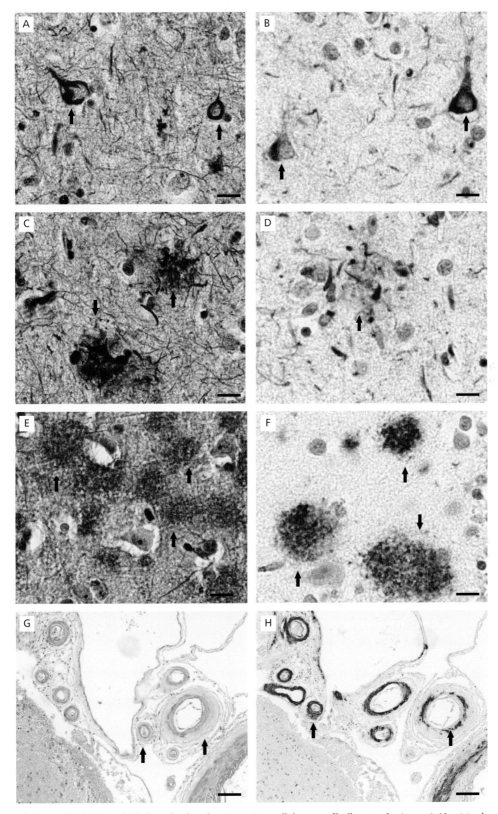

Figure 1.1 Alzheimer's disease (AD). (A) and (B) show the densely staining intracellular neurofibrillary tangles (arrows). Neuritic plaques (B, C, arrows) have a central nidus of amyloid with radiating tau-laden neuritic processes. Diffuse plaques, on the other hand, have only amyloid collections (E, F). Often seen accompanying AD type changes is cerebral amyloid angiopathy, which gives a thickened hyaline appearance to the vessels (G) and stains with amyloid (H). [Scale bar: 10 μm (A–F); 50 μm (G, H). Stains: A, C, E: modified Bielschowsky; B, D: PHF-1 tau immunohistochemistry; F, H: β-AP immunohisto-chemistry; G: H&E.]

Table 1.1 Subtypes and locations of Alzheimer's disease (AD) neuropathologic changes in aging and in different stages of AD.

Human brain condition	Locus coeruleus NFTs	Hippocampal NFTs	Neocortical NFTs	Hippocampal Aβ plaques	Neocortical Aβ plaques
Mid-life without AD or with extremely early AD	+	–	–	–	–
Advanced aging without AD	+/++	+	–	–	–/+
Presumed preclinical AD	++	++	–	–/+	+/++
Presumed early AD	+++	++/+++	+/++	+	++/+++
Late AD without comorbid pathologies	+++	+++	+++	++/+++	+++

Indicator of pathological severity: –, no disease-specific pathology; –/+, scattered or inconsistent pathology; +, low level of pathology; ++, moderate level of pathology; +++, high level of pathology. NFTs, neurofibrillary tangles.

Dementia with Lewy bodies (DLB)

DLB presently can only be diagnosed with certainty at autopsy and there is no known cure; this disease is discussed in greater detail in Chapter 9. The pathology of DLB by definition [62, 63] includes abundant aberrant deposits of α-synuclein (α-SN immunoreactive Lewy bodies and Lewy neurites; see Figure 1.2). Neuropathological data are especially important for cases with mixed pathology, such as AD with concomitant DLB, where precise clinical diagnostic criteria are lacking. Remarkably, some individuals with amyloid precursor protein (APP) gene mutations have early-onset cognitive symptoms with AD+DLB pathology [64, 65]. It is also important to note that "pure" DLB (extensive neocortical Lewy body pathology in individuals lacking AD pathology) is relatively rare and is far more often seen in males than in females, but has a definite cognitive impact [60, 66–69].

HS-aging and pathological TDP-43 inclusions

Hippocampal sclerosis (HS) refers to neuronal cell loss and astrocytosis in subiculum and cornu ammonis (CA) subfields of the hippocampal formation unrelated to AD pathology (Figure 1.3). In contrast to the disease also referred to as "hippocampal sclerosis" that affects younger adults [70], HS in older individuals is associated with significant ante mortem cognitive dysfunction [71, 72] but not necessarily with epilepsy. There is no universally-applied specific nosology for these cases and we use the term "HS-Aging" to refer to the disease with HS pathology in aging individuals [2].

Despite recent progress from many research centers, the specific clinical and pathological features related to HS-Aging have not been definitively characterized. The disease was described decades ago [73, 74], yet researchers and clinicians only recently recognized the high prevalence of HS pathology in aged populations [72, 75–77]. HS-Aging and AD have overlapping clinical and radiographic features related to hippocampal dysfunction and atrophy, so improved clinical identification of HS-Aging patients would enable more specific management of both HS-Aging and AD patients.

In addition to being linked to advanced age, HS-Aging pathology is also associated strongly with aberrant TDP-43 immunohistochemistry [78–80]. In the largest autopsy series of HS-Aging to date, we found that approximately 90% of HS patients had aberrant TDP-43 immunohistochemical staining (Figure 1.3C), in comparison to approximately 10% in older controls irrespective of the presence of other pathologies. TDP-43 is an RNA-binding protein, normally

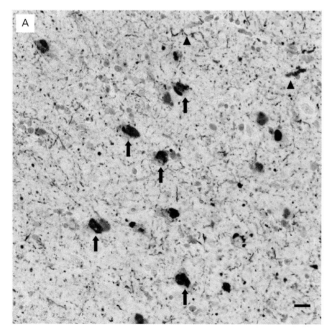
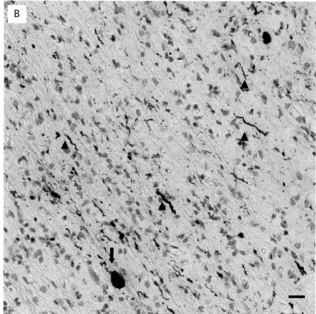

Figure 1.2 α-synucleinopathy in Lewy body disease. The amygdala (A) and olfactory bulb (B), showing both Lewy bodies (arrows) and Lewy neurites (arrowheads). These anatomical locations often harbor some of the earliest α-synucleinopathic changes seen in the brain. [Scale bar: 10 μm; α-synuclein IHC.]

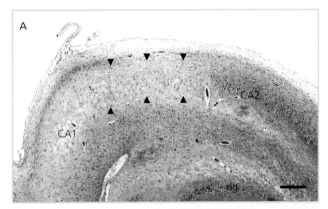

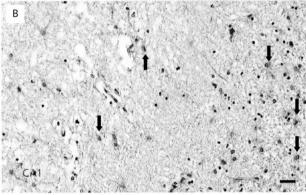

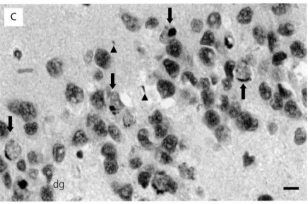

Figure 1.3 Hippocampal sclerosis. (A) A relatively intact CA2 region leading into a markedly sclerotic CA1 region (arrowheads). Examination at higher power (B) shows marked loss of the pyramidal neurons with abundant reactive astrocytes (arrows) and rarefaction of the neuropil. A TDP-43 immunostain (C) shows abnormal dense cytoplasmic localization (arrows) with occasional neuropil threads (arrowheads) in the dentate gyrus (dg). [Scale bar: 0.5 mm (A), 20 μm (B), 10 μm (C).]

localized mainly to the cell nucleus, that is linked pathogenetically with amyotrophic lateral sclerosis (ALS; see Chapter 14) and FTD (see Chapter 12), in addition to HS-Aging. The interface between HS-Aging and TDP-43-positive FTD has not been well defined [81–83]; clearly, HS-Aging cases do not fit neatly into the existing FTD classification [32]. It remains to be seen whether the TDP-43 abnormalities are causally linked with HS-Aging pathology. We did not find a link between HS-Aging and CVD pathology [2]. A speculative hypothesis, dovetailing on the recently described association between TDP-

43 pathology and chronic trauma-induced encephalopathy [84, 85], and the fact that HS-like pathology is observed in some blunt trauma cases [86], is that aberrant TDP-43 with HS pathology in advanced age may reflect physical wear-and-tear.

Whereas the pathological data may be biologically informative, there is a practical need for improved clinical detection of HS-Aging to enable better management of both HS-Aging and AD patients. We found that the neuropsychological profiles of individuals with incipient HS-Aging differed systematically – even in the earliest stages of cognitive decline – relative to individuals who would eventually die with advanced AD pathology [2].

Cerebrovascular disease (CVD) pathology
Although not necessarily considered a "neurodegenerative disease", CVD comprises the most prevalent non-AD pathology in advanced aged brains and is directly relevant to any clinicopathologic study related to dementia among the elderly [3, 61]. The difficulties introduced by this prevalent, multifaceted, and clinically unpredictable disease category in aged individuals have been discussed previously [75, 87–95]; in individuals beyond the age of 90 years, some degree of CVD pathology is practically universal [61, 96–98]. We note the lack of an ideal rubric for CVD clinical–pathological correlation, although the recent NIA-AA criteria attempted to systematize neuropathologic assessment of this complex form of brain injury [23]. Despite its high prevalence and profound impact, researchers tend to under-appreciate the importance of CVD pathology [99–101].

The pathologic findings attributed to CVD are very broad, ranging from lobar hemorrhage/infarction down to mild alterations in small vessel morphology (Figures 1.4, 1.5). Large caliber vessel involvement typically consists of atherosclerosis of the cerebral vessels at various branchpoints around the circle of Willis. While the morphologic changes resemble those of systemic atherosclerotic lesions, severity is usually much less than that seen in the systemic circulation, often falling within the mild category [102]. Blockage of these vessels, by either local disease or emboli from elsewhere, leads to ischemia and, without restoration of blood flow, infarction. Systemic metabolic, toxic, or anoxic insults can also induce pathologies that resemble histomorphologic changes due to disrupted blood flow.

Arguably the most prevalent, and least quantifiable, subtype of CVD pathologies is the small vessel changes noted in the subcortical white matter, deep gray nuclei, and brainstem (Figure 1.5). Thickening of the smaller arterioles and capillaries, due to arteriolosclerosis or lipohyalinosis, is often present. Disruption of the smaller perforating vessels in the subcortical gray matter and brainstem (a process exacerbated by hypertension) can induce lacunar-type infarcts [103]. The Virchow–Robin spaces, normally small slit-like structures hugging the perimeter of the blood vessels, can vary dramatically in size. Pigment-laden macrophages are often seen in the expanded perivascular spaces. The surrounding white matter can take on a ragged, moth-eaten appearance. Corpora amylacea litter the perivascular and subpial parenchyma. These changes, seen both microscopically and to some extent via imaging modalities (where they are known as leukoaraiosis), are found more commonly with increasing age. To date, however, their relative abundance, size, or location cannot be correlated consistently with clinical symptomatology [104, 105].

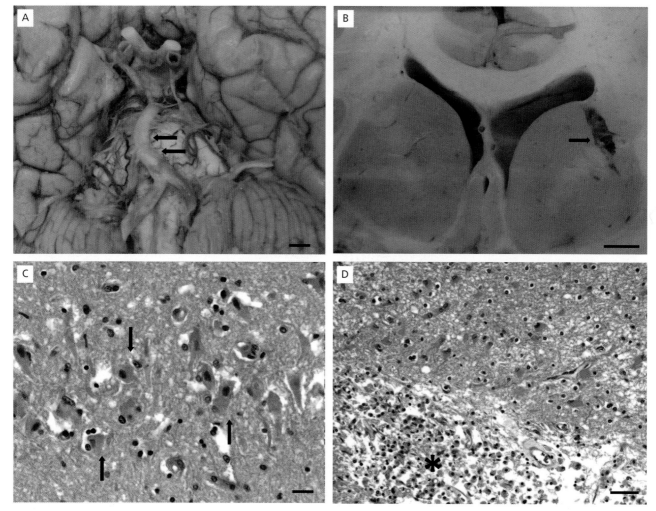

Figure 1.4 Cerebrovascular disease. Atherosclerotic changes may be noted grossly within the basilar artery (arrow) and elsewhere (A). Infarcts that occurred well before death are frequently observed in older patients, particularly within the basal ganglia (B). Microscopically, infarcts can range in appearance from acutely ischemic neurons (C, arrows) in an acute setting, to a macrophage-laden (*) cavity with surrounding gliosis in more chronic lesions (D). [Scale bars: A, B: 1 cm; C, D: 20 μm.]

Genetics and the environment: risk factors and potential therapeutic targets

Human genetics are critically relevant to any discussion of aging and neurodegenerative disease pathology, providing key insights into each. Approximately 70% of a given individual's risk for developing AD pathology is conferred through his or her genetic repertoire [106–108]. Thus genetics is one important place to seek clues as to whether the "aging" phenotype links specifically to AD pathology or to any other prevalent aging-linked brain pathology.

A subset of human genetic aberrations causes well-characterized phenotypes with specific features of advanced human aging in chronologically younger individuals. These diseases are called "progerias" [109, 110]. It has been suggested that progerias provide insights into the pathways that are involved in human aging [111, 112]. Clinical signs and symptoms that may exist even in pre-teens include cognitive impairment, wrinkled skin, atherosclerosis, brittle bones, cataracts, and many other changes, although there is not a single progeria that can be said to definitely cause "accelerated aging".

There is no firm indication that individuals with progerias have any increase in a specific pathology (AD, DLB, HS-Aging, or FTD) linked with brain aging [3]. One non-demented individual with Werner syndrome and apolipoprotein E (APOE) ε4 genotype was reported to have incipient AD-type pathology upon death at age 55 [113]. Otherwise, the link between Werner syndrome (or any other progeria) and AD pathology has been queried and not found to exist [114–116] although some of the progerias do in fact involve cognitive impairment. Mutations of the lamin gene (LMNA) cause a severe autosomal dominant progeria syndrome, muscular dystrophy, and Charcot–Marie–Tooth disease, but not AD [112]. In contrast, gene defects in presenilin-1 (PSEN1) produce early-onset autosomal dominant AD and a wide range of associated neurologic deficits but not a progeria syndrome (see below). Nor is there any firm association between AD and other known aging genes including the sirtuins (for example SIRT1 or SIRT3) although these have been exhaustively analyzed for AD-linked polymorphisms [117]. The dissociation between premature aging-linked genetic aberrations and AD pathology cannot by itself negate the hypothesis that AD is caused by aging mechanisms but it is a pertinent clue because

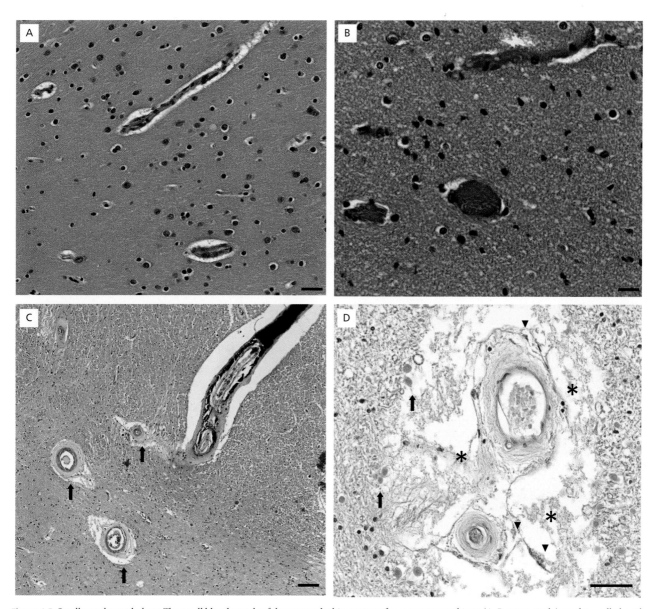

Figure 1.5 Small vessel morphology. The small blood vessels of the gray and white matter of most younger subjects (A, B, respectively) are thin walled, with minimal enlargement of the Virchow–Robin spaces. With age, these vessels often show arteriolosclerosis and lipohyalinosis (short arrows), usually accompanied by a widening of the perivascular spaces (*) with rarefaction of the surrounding white matter, an abundance of corpora amylacea (long arrows), and the presence of pigment-laden macrophages (arrowheads) (C, D). The vessels of the basal ganglia (particularly within the globus pallidus) also frequently undergo extensive mineralization (C). [Scale bars: A, B: 20 μm; C, D: 50 μm.]

there are indeed some genetic factors that strongly contribute to AD pathogenetically.

The highly penetrant human gene loci that alter risk for developing AD are APP, PSEN1, PSEN2, and APOE. None of these genes is known to be directly related to the aging process, nor to aging-related processes such as combating oxidative stress. These AD-affecting genes all influence processing of APP and provide support for the "amyloid cascade hypothesis" [118, 119], in which APP/Aβ dysfunction is a key pathogenetic mechanism in AD. The triplication of APP in the context of Down syndrome can induce AD-like pathology in the human brain as young as 8 years of age [120] with precursor lesions present even during infancy [3]. Even outside of Down syndrome, the focal duplication of the APP gene, and mutations in APP promoter regions that increase APP production, can

cause AD [121, 122]. AD-relevant mutations in the APP gene affect its proteolysis, as do mutations in PSEN1 and PSEN2 [106].

By far the strongest risk factor for late-onset AD is the ε4 variant of the APOE gene [123, 124]. The impact of the APOE ε4 allele in terms of boosting brain Aβ deposition is well established [125–127]. The presence of APOE ε4 alleles correlates with much higher Aβ plaque densities and more extensive cerebral amyloid angiopathy [128, 129]. By contrast with AD, APOE ε4 is not a risk allele for HS-Aging [2, 77]. The strong genetic risk for AD in persons aged 50–80 leads to a survival bias in terms of individuals beyond that age range. Relatively few individuals with APOE ε4 allele (much less with APP or PSEN mutations) survive AD-free past age 90 [130–133]. This survival bias has been discussed previously [3, 134].

There are relatively recently discovered single nucleotide polymorphisms (SNPs) that alter AD risk and these include alleles in CLU, PICALM, and BIN1[135–138] in genome-wide association studies (GWAS). The penetrance of these genes is far weaker (i.e., the effect of the mutation on risk for the disease phenotype is less predictable) in comparison to mutations in APP, PSEN1, PSEN2, or APOE. SNP/GWAS data remain to be fully understood both in normal brain aging and in relation to AD or other brain disease manifestations.

In summary, AD appears to be a predominantly genetic disease that most often manifests in aged individuals but is not inevitable among the "oldest-old" and not necessarily linked to aging mechanisms per se. There are many other genetic diseases (linked to other genetic loci) that manifest late in life with neurodegeneration: trinucleotide repeat diseases, familial prion diseases, familial motor neuron diseases, FTD-MAPT, FTD-TDP, and dozens of other genetic diseases (see for example [139–143]) which also are not necessarily associated with "aging"-linked genes. HS-Aging seems to peak later in the aging spectrum than AD [2] but the genetic substrates of HS-Aging have not been elucidated. Although genetic diseases provide important insights into human aging and senescence, more work remains to be done to understand these complex ideas.

Summary

In the "oldest-old", numerous brain diseases, as defined by histopathologic characteristics, can be correlated with the severity of cognitive impairment [3, 144, 145]. Some of the neurodegenerative diseases (such as AD) appear to be linked with specific genetic changes rather than to "brain aging" per se. But as individuals advance into their ninth decade and beyond, there are many additional contributors to clinical dementia including CVD, HS-Aging, α-synucleinopathies, hematomas, argyrophilic grain disease, neuropsychiatric disorders and their therapies, failure of other organ systems, diabetes, hypertension, chemotherapy, and other side effects linked to medications [71, 81, 146–150]. These diseases are important to consider and inevitably have an impact on clinical trials: since most elderly individuals have comorbid pathologies in their brains, a therapeutic strategy that is effective for a particular disease process may seem to fail because of the presence of other brain diseases in the treated cohort of aged individuals.

References

1. Hyman BT, Phelps CH, Beach TG, Bigio EH, Cairns NJ, Carrillo MC, et al. National Institute on Aging-Alzheimer's Association guidelines for the neuropathologic assessment of Alzheimer's disease. Alzheimers Dement. 2012;8(1):1–13. Epub 2012/01/24.

2. Nelson PT, Schmitt FA, Lin Y, Abner EL, Jicha GA, Patel E, et al. Hippocampal sclerosis in advanced age: clinical and pathological features. Brain. 2011;134(Pt 5):1506–18. Epub 2011/05/21.

3. Nelson PT, Head E, Schmitt FA, Davis PR, Neltner JH, Jicha GA, et al. Alzheimer's disease is not "brain aging": neuropathological, genetic, and epidemiological human studies. Acta Neuropathol. 2011;121(5):571–87. Epub 2011/04/26.

4. Hayflick L. Biological aging is no longer an unsolved problem. Annals of the New York Academy of Sciences. 2007;1100:1–13. Epub 2007/04/27.

5. Holliday R. Understanding ageing. Philos Trans R Soc Lond B Biol Sci. 1997;352(1363):1793–7. Epub 1998/02/14.

6. Harman D. Aging: overview. Ann N Y Acad Sci. 2001;928:1–21. Epub 2002/01/25.

7. Finch CE. The biology of aging in model organisms. Alzheimer Dis Assoc Disord. 2003;17 Suppl 2:S39–41. Epub 2003/06/19.

8. Droge W. Oxidative stress and aging. Adv Exp Med Biol. 2003;543:191–200. Epub 2004/01/10.

9. Kirkwood TB. Systems biology of ageing and longevity. Philos Trans R Soc Lond B Biol Sci. 2011;366(1561):64–70. Epub 2010/12/01.

10. Vaillancourt DE, Newell KM. Changing complexity in human behavior and physiology through aging and disease. Neurobiol Aging. 2002;23(1):1–11. Epub 2002/01/05.

11. CIA World Factbook: Central Intelligence Agency (U.S. Federal Government); 2008.

12. Newman AB, Glynn NW, Taylor CA, Sebastiani P, Perls TT, Mayeux R, et al. Health and function of participants in the Long Life Family Study: A comparison with other cohorts. Aging (Albany NY). 2011;3(1):63–76. Epub 2011/01/25.

13. Jyrkka J, Enlund H, Lavikainen P, Sulkava R, Hartikainen S. Association of polypharmacy with nutritional status, functional ability and cognitive capacity over a three-year period in an elderly population. Pharmacoepidemiol Drug Saf. 2011;20(5):514–22. Epub 2011/02/11.

14. Mayeux R, Reitz C, Brickman AM, Haan MN, Manly JJ, Glymour MM, et al. Operationalizing diagnostic criteria for Alzheimer's disease and other age-related cognitive impairment-Part 1. Alzheimers Dement. 2011;7(1):15–34. Epub 2011/01/25.

15. Rubin EH, Kinscherf DA, Grant EA, Storandt M. The influence of major depression on clinical and psychometric assessment of senile dementia of the Alzheimer type. Am J Psychiatry. 1991;148(9):1164–71. Epub 1991/09/01.

16. Masliah E. Mechanisms of synaptic dysfunction in Alzheimer's disease. Histol Histopathol. 1995;10(2):509–19. Epub 1995/04/01.

17. Scheff SW, Price DA. Synaptic pathology in Alzheimer's disease: a review of ultrastructural studies. Neurobiol Aging. 2003;24(8):1029–46. Epub 2003/12/04.

18. Butterfield DA, Perluigi M, Sultana R. Oxidative stress in Alzheimer's disease brain: new insights from redox proteomics. Eur J Pharmacol. 2006;545(1):39–50. Epub 2006/07/25.

19. Bartzokis G. Age-related myelin breakdown: a developmental model of cognitive decline and Alzheimer's disease. Neurobiol Aging. 2004;25(1):5–18; author reply 49–62. Epub 2003/12/17.

20. Selkoe DJ. Alzheimer's disease is a synaptic failure. Science. 2002;298(5594):789–91. Epub 2002/10/26.

21. Masliah E, Crews L, Hansen L. Synaptic remodeling during aging and in Alzheimer's disease. J Alzheimers Dis. 2006;9(3 Suppl):91–9. Epub 2006/08/18.

22. Duyckaerts C, Delatour B, Potier MC. Classification and basic pathology of Alzheimer disease. Acta Neuropathol. 2009;118(1):5–36. Epub 2009/04/22.

23. Montine TJ, Phelps CH, Beach TG, Bigio EH, Cairns NJ, Dickson DW, et al. National Institute on Aging-Alzheimer's Association guidelines for the neuropathologic assessment of Alzheimer's disease: a practical approach. Acta Neuropathol. 2012;123(1):1–11. Epub 2011/11/22.

24. Terry RD. The fine structure of neurofibrillary tangles in Alzheimer's Disease. J Neuropathol Exp Neurol. 1963;22:629–42. Epub 1963/10/01.

25. Goedert M. Tau protein and neurodegeneration. Semin Cell Dev Biol. 2004;15(1):45–9. Epub 2004/03/24.

26. Arai T, Ikeda K, Akiyama H, Shikamoto Y, Tsuchiya K, Yagishita S, et al. Distinct isoforms of tau aggregated in neurons and glial cells in brains of patients with Pick's disease, corticobasal degeneration and progressive supranuclear palsy. Acta Neuropathol. 2001;101(2):167–73. Epub 2001/03/29.

27. Buee L, Bussiere T, Buee-Scherrer V, Delacourte A, Hof PR. Tau protein isoforms, phosphorylation and role in neurodegenerative disorders. Brain Res Brain Res Rev. 2000;33(1):95–130. Epub 2000/09/01.

28. Bouras C, Hof PR, Giannakopoulos P, Michel JP, Morrison JH. Regional distribution of neurofibrillary tangles and senile plaques in the cerebral cortex of elderly patients: a quantitative evaluation of a one-year autopsy population from a geriatric hospital. Cereb Cortex. 1994;4(2):138–50. Epub 1994/03/01.

29. Bancher C, Leitner H, Jellinger K, Eder H, Setinek U, Fischer P, et al. On the relationship between measles virus and Alzheimer neurofibrillary tangles in subacute sclerosing panencephalitis. Neurobiol Aging. 1996;17(4):527–33. Epub 1996/07/01.

30. Tabaton M, Mandybur TI, Perry G, Onorato M, Autilio-Gambetti L, Gambetti P. The widespread alteration of neurites in Alzheimer's disease may be unrelated to amyloid deposition. Ann Neurol. 1989;26(6):771–8. Epub 1989/12/01.

31. Wang XF, Dong CF, Zhang J, Wan YZ, Li F, Huang YX, et al. Human tau protein forms complex with PrP and some GSS- and fCJD-related PrP mutants possess stronger binding activities with tau in vitro. Mol Cell Biochem. 2008;310(1-2):49–55. Epub 2007/11/27.

32. Cairns NJ, Bigio EH, Mackenzie IR, Neumann M, Lee VM, Hatanpaa KJ, et al. Neuropathologic diagnostic and nosologic criteria for frontotemporal lobar degeneration: consensus of the Consortium for Frontotemporal Lobar Degeneration. Acta Neuropathol. 2007;114(1):5–22.

33. Abner EL, Kryscio RJ, Schmitt FA, Santacruz KS, Jicha GA, Lin Y, et al. "End-stage" neurofibrillary tangle pathology in preclinical Alzheimer's disease: fact or fiction? J Alzheimers Dis. 2011;25(3):445–53. Epub 2011/04/08.

34. Nelson PT, Alafuzoff I, Bigio EH, Bouras C, Braak H, Cairns NJ, et al. Correlation of Alzheimer disease neuropathologic changes with cognitive status: a review of the literature. J Neuropathol Exp Neurol. 2012;71(5):362–81. Epub 2012/04/11.

35. Dickson DW. Neuropathological diagnosis of Alzheimer's disease: a perspective from longitudinal clinicopathological studies. Neurobiol Aging. 1997;18 (4 Suppl):S21–6. Epub 1997/07/01.

36. Selkoe DJ. Biochemistry and molecular biology of amyloid beta-protein and the mechanism of Alzheimer's disease. *Handb Clin Neurol.* 2008;89:245–60. Epub 2008/07/18.

37. Davies L, Wolska B, Hilbich C, Multhaup G, Martins R, Simms G, et al. A4 amyloid protein deposition and the diagnosis of Alzheimer's disease: prevalence in aged brains determined by immunocytochemistry compared with conventional neuropathologic techniques. *Neurology.* 1988;38(11):1688–93.

38. Braak H, Thal DR, Ghebremedhin E, Del Tredici K. Stages of the pathologic process in Alzheimer disease: age categories from 1 to 100 years. *J Neuropathol Exp Neurol.* 2011;70(11):960–9. Epub 2011/10/18.

39. Jicha GA, Abner EL, Schmitt FA, Kryscio RJ, Riley KP, Cooper GE, et al. Preclinical AD Workgroup staging: pathological correlates and potential challenges. *Neurobiol Aging.* 2012;33(3):622. Epub 2011/04/22.

40. Terry RD, Masliah E, Hansen LA. *Structural Basis of the Cognitive Alterations in Alzheimer Disease.* In: TerryRD, KatzmanR, BickKL, editors. Alzheimer Disease. New York: Raven Press; 1994. p. 179–96.

41. Wisniewski HM, Vorbrodt AW, Moretz RC, Lossinsky AS, Grundke-Iqbal I. Pathogenesis of neuritic (senile) and amyloid plaque formation. *Exp Brain Res.* 1982;Suppl 5:3–9. Epub 1982/01/01.

42. Mirra SS. The CERAD neuropathology protocol and consensus recommendations for the postmortem diagnosis of Alzheimer's disease: a commentary. *Neurobiol Aging.* 1997;18(4 Suppl):S91–4.

43. Hardy J, Selkoe DJ. The amyloid hypothesis of Alzheimer's disease: progress and problems on the road to therapeutics. *Science (New York, NY).* 2002;297(5580):353–6.

44. Katzman R, Kawas, C. *The Epidemiology of Dementia and Alzheimer Disease.* In: TerryRD, editor. Alzheimer Disease. New York: Raven Press; 1994. p. 105–22.

45. Gao S, Hendrie HC, Hall KS, Hui S. The relationships between age, sex, and the incidence of dementia and Alzheimer disease: a meta-analysis. *Arch Gen Psychiatry.* 1998;55(9):809–15. Epub 1998/09/15.

46. Kukull WA, Higdon R, Bowen JD, McCormick WC, Teri L, Schellenberg GD, et al. Dementia and Alzheimer disease incidence: a prospective cohort study. *Arch Neurol.* 2002;59(11):1737–46. Epub 2002/11/16.

47. Rocca WA, Cha RH, Waring SC, Kokmen E. Incidence of dementia and Alzheimer's disease: a reanalysis of data from Rochester, Minnesota, 1975–1984. *Am J Epidemiol.* 1998;148(1):51–62. Epub 1998/07/15.

48. Hall CB, Verghese J, Sliwinski M, Chen Z, Katz M, Derby C, et al. Dementia incidence may increase more slowly after age 90: results from the Bronx Aging Study. *Neurology.* 2005;65(6):882–6. Epub 2005/09/28.

49. Rocca WA, Petersen RC, Knopman DS, Hebert LE, Evans DA, Hall KS, et al. Trends in the incidence and prevalence of Alzheimer's disease, dementia, and cognitive impairment in the United States. *Alzheimers Dement.* 2011;7(1):80–93. Epub 2011/01/25.

50. Launer LJ. Counting dementia: There is no one "best" way. *Alzheimers Dement.* 2011;7(1):10–4. Epub 2011/01/25.

51. Corrada MM, Brookmeyer R, Paganini-Hill A, Berlau D, Kawas CH. Dementia incidence continues to increase with age in the oldest old: the 90+ study. *Ann Neurol.* 2010;67(1):114–21. Epub 2010/02/27.

52. Seshadri S, Beiser A, Au R, Wolf PA, Evans DA, Wilson RS, et al. Operationalizing diagnostic criteria for Alzheimer's disease and other age-related cognitive impairment-Part 2. *Alzheimers Dement.* 2011;7(1):35–52. Epub 2011/01/25.

53. Crystal HA, Dickson D, Davies P, Masur D, Grober E, Lipton RB. The relative frequency of "dementia of unknown etiology" increases with age and is nearly 50% in nonagenarians. *Arch Neurol.* 2000;57(5):713–9. Epub 2000/05/18.

54. Haroutunian V, Schnaider-Beeri M, Schmeidler J, Wysocki M, Purohit DP, Perl DP, et al. Role of the neuropathology of Alzheimer disease in dementia in the oldest-old. *Arch Neurol.* 2008;65(9):1211–7. Epub 2008/09/10.

55. Savva GM, Wharton SB, Ince PG, Forster G, Matthews FE, Brayne C. Age, neuropathology, and dementia. *N Engl J Med.* 2009;360(22):2302–9. Epub 2009/05/29.

56. Pathological correlates of late-onset dementia in a multicentre, community-based population in England and Wales. Neuropathology Group of the Medical Research Council Cognitive Function and Ageing Study (MRC CFAS). *Lancet.* 2001;357(9251):169–75. Epub 2001/02/24.

57. Imhof A, Kovari E, von Gunten A, Gold G, Rivara CB, Herrmann FR, et al. Morphological substrates of cognitive decline in nonagenarians and centenarians: A new paradigm? *J Neurol Sci.* 2007;257(1-2):72–9.

58. Jellinger KA, Attems J. Prevalence of dementia disorders in the oldest-old: an autopsy study. *Acta Neuropathol.* 2010;119(4):421–33. Epub 2010/03/06.

59. Dolan D, Troncoso J, Resnick SM, Crain BJ, Zonderman AB, O'Brien RJ. Age, Alzheimer's disease and dementia in the Baltimore Longitudinal Study of Ageing. *Brain.* 2010;133(Pt 8):2225–31. Epub 2010/07/22.

60. Nelson PT, Abner EL, Schmitt FA, Kryscio RJ, Jicha GA, Smith CD, et al. Modeling the association between 43 different clinical and pathological variables and the severity of cognitive impairment in a large autopsy cohort of elderly persons. *Brain Pathol.* 2010;20(1):66–79. Epub 2008/11/22.

61. Nelson PT, Jicha GA, Schmitt FA, Liu H, Davis DG, Mendiondo MS, et al. Clinicopathologic correlations in a large Alzheimer disease center autopsy cohort: neuritic plaques and neurofibrillary tangles "do count" when staging disease severity. *J Neuropathol Exp Neurol.* 2007;66(12):1136–46. Epub 2007/12/20.

62. McKeith I, Mintzer J, Aarsland D, Burn D, Chiu H, Cohen-Mansfield J, et al. Dementia with Lewy bodies. *Lancet Neurol.* 2004;3(1):19–28. Epub 2003/12/25.

63. McKeith IG, Dickson DW, Lowe J, Emre M, O'Brien JT, Feldman H, et al. Diagnosis and management of dementia with Lewy bodies: third report of the DLB Consortium. *Neurology.* 2005;65(12):1863–72. Epub 2005/10/21.

64. Rosenberg CK, Pericak-Vance MA, Saunders AM, Gilbert JR, Gaskell PC, Hulette CM. Lewy body and Alzheimer pathology in a family with the amyloid-beta precursor protein APP717 gene mutation. *Acta Neuropathol.* 2000;100(2):145–52. Epub 2000/08/30.

65. Guyant-Marechal I, Berger E, Laquerriere A, Rovelet-Lecrux A, Viennet G, Frebourg T, et al. Intrafamilial diversity of phenotype associated with app duplication. *Neurology.* 2008;71(23):1925–6. Epub 2008/12/03.

66. Nelson PT, Schmitt FA, Jicha GA, Kryscio RJ, Abner EL, Smith CD, et al. Association between male gender and cortical Lewy body pathology in large autopsy series. *J Neurol.* 2010;257(11):1875–81. Epub 2010/06/22.

67. Nelson PT, Jicha GA, Kryscio RJ, Abner EL, Schmitt FA, Cooper G, et al. Low sensitivity in clinical diagnoses of dementia with Lewy bodies. *J Neurol.* 2010;257(3):359–66. Epub 2009/10/02.

68. Nelson PT, Kryscio RJ, Jicha GA, Abner EL, Schmitt FA, Xu LO, et al. Relative preservation of MMSE scores in autopsy-proven dementia with Lewy bodies. *Neurology.* 2009;73(14):1127–33. Epub 2009/10/07.

69. Gnanalingham KK, Byrne EJ, Thornton A, Sambrook MA, Bannister P. Motor and cognitive function in Lewy body dementia: comparison with Alzheimer's and Parkinson's diseases. *J Neurol Neurosurg Psychiatry.* 1997;62(3):243–52. Epub 1997/03/01.

70. Thom M. Hippocampal sclerosis: progress since Sommer. *Brain Pathol.* 2009;19(4):565–72. Epub 2009/08/03.

71. Corey-Bloom J, Sabbagh MN, Bondi MW, Hansen L, Alford MF, Masliah E, et al. Hippocampal sclerosis contributes to dementia in the elderly. *Neurology.* 1997;48(1):154–60. Epub 1997/01/01.

72. Nelson PT, Abner EL, Schmitt FA, Kryscio RJ, Jicha GA, Smith CD, et al. Modeling the association between 43 different clinical and pathological variables and the severity of cognitive impairment in a large autopsy cohort of elderly persons. *Brain Pathol.* 2010;20(1):66–79. Epub 2008/11/22.

73. Clark AW, White CL, 3rd, Manz HJ, Parhad IM, Curry B, Whitehouse PJ, et al. Primary degenerative dementia without Alzheimer pathology. *Can J Neurol Sci.* 1986;13(4 Suppl):462–70. Epub 1986/11/01.

74. Dickson DW, Davies P, Bevona C, Van Hoeven KH, Factor SM, Grober E, et al. Hippocampal sclerosis: a common pathological feature of dementia in very old (>or = 80 years of age) humans. *Acta Neuropathol.* 1994;88(3):212–21. Epub 1994/01/01.

75. Chui HC, Zarow C, Mack WJ, Ellis WG, Zheng L, Jagust WJ, et al. Cognitive impact of subcortical vascular and Alzheimer's disease pathology. *Ann Neurol.* 2006;60(6):677–87.

76. Zarow C, Sitzer TE, Chui HC. Understanding hippocampal sclerosis in the elderly: epidemiology, characterization, and diagnostic issues. *Curr Neurol Neurosci Rep.* 2008;8(5):363–70. Epub 2008/08/21.

77. Leverenz JB, Agustin CM, Tsuang D, Peskind ER, Edland SD, Nochlin D, et al. Clinical and neuropathological characteristics of hippocampal sclerosis: a community-based study. *Arch Neurol.* 2002;59(7):1099–106. Epub 2002/07/16.

78. Amador-Ortiz C, Lin WL, Ahmed Z, Personett D, Davies P, Duara R, et al. TDP-43 immunoreactivity in hippocampal sclerosis and Alzheimer's disease. *Ann Neurol.* 2007;61(5):435–45. Epub 2007/05/01.

79. Josephs KA, Whitwell JL, Knopman DS, Hu WT, Stroh DA, Baker M, et al. Abnormal TDP-43 immunoreactivity in AD modifies clinicopathologic and radiologic phenotype. *Neurology.* 2008;70(19 Pt 2):1850–7. Epub 2008/04/11.

80. Neumann M, Sampathu DM, Kwong LK, Truax AC, Micsenyi MC, Chou TT, et al. Ubiquitinated TDP-43 in frontotemporal lobar degeneration and amyotrophic lateral sclerosis. *Science (New York, NY).* 2006;314(5796):130–3. Epub 2006/10/07.

81. Amador-Ortiz C, Ahmed Z, Zehr C, Dickson DW. Hippocampal sclerosis dementia differs from hippocampal sclerosis in frontal lobe degeneration. *Acta Neuropathol.* 2007;113(3):245–52.

82. Probst A, Taylor KI, Tolnay M. Hippocampal sclerosis dementia: a reappraisal. *Acta Neuropathol.* 2007;114(4):335–45. Epub 2007/07/20.

83. Hatanpaa KJ, Blass DM, Pletnikova O, Crain BJ, Bigio EH, Hedreen JC, et al. Most cases of dementia with hippocampal sclerosis may represent frontotemporal dementia. *Neurology.* 2004;63(3):538–42. Epub 2004/08/12.

84. McKee AC, Gavett BE, Stern RA, Nowinski CJ, Cantu RC, Kowall NW, et al. TDP-43 proteinopathy and motor neuron disease in chronic traumatic encephalopathy. *J Neuropathol Exp Neurol.* 2010;69(9):918–29. Epub 2010/08/20.

85. King A, Sweeney F, Bodi I, Troakes C, Maekawa S, Al-Sarraj S. Abnormal TDP-43 expression is identified in the neocortex in cases of dementia pugilistica, but is

mainly confined to the limbic system when identified in high and moderate stages of Alzheimer's disease. *Neuropathology*. 2010;30(4):408–19. Epub 2010/01/28.

86. Kotapka MJ, Graham DI, Adams JH, Gennarelli TA. Hippocampal pathology in fatal non-missile human head injury. *Acta Neuropathol*. 1992;83(5):530–4. Epub 1992/01/01.

87. Bowler JV, Munoz DG, Merskey H, Hachinski V. Fallacies in the pathological confirmation of the diagnosis of Alzheimer's disease. *J Neurol Neurosurg Psychiatry*. 1998;64(1):18–24. Epub 1998/01/22.

88. Jellinger KA, Attems J. Neuropathological evaluation of mixed dementia. *J Neurol Sci*. 2007;257(1-2):80–7. Epub 2007/02/28.

89. Schneider JA, Wilson RS, Bienias JL, Evans DA, Bennett DA. Cerebral infarctions and the likelihood of dementia from Alzheimer disease pathology. *Neurology*. 2004;62(7):1148–55.

90. Todorov AB, Go RC, Constantinidis J, Elston RC. Specificity of the clinical diagnosis of dementia. *J Neurol Sci*. 1975;26(1):81–98. Epub 1975/09/01.

91. Jicha GA, Parisi JE, Dickson DW, Johnson K, Cha R, Ivnik RJ, et al. Neuropathologic outcome of mild cognitive impairment following progression to clinical dementia. *Arch Neurol*. 2006;63(5):674–81.

92. Rockwood K. Mixed dementia: Alzheimer's and cerebrovascular disease. *Int Psychogeriatr*. 2003;15 Suppl 1:39–46. Epub 2005/09/30.

93. Kovari E, Gold G, Herrmann FR, Canuto A, Hof PR, Bouras C, et al. Cortical microinfarcts and demyelination affect cognition in cases at high risk for dementia. *Neurology*. 2007;68(12):927–31. Epub 2007/03/21.

94. Jellinger K, Danielczyk W, Fischer P, Gabriel E. Clinicopathological analysis of dementia disorders in the elderly. *J Neurol Sci*. 1990;95(3):239–58. Epub 1990/03/01.

95. Schneider JA, Arvanitakis Z, Bang W, Bennett DA. Mixed brain pathologies account for most dementia cases in community-dwelling older persons. *Neurology*. 2007;69(24):2197–204. Epub 2007/06/15.

96. White L, Petrovitch H, Hardman J, Nelson J, Davis DG, Ross GW, et al. Cerebrovascular pathology and dementia in autopsied Honolulu-Asia Aging Study participants. *Ann N Y Acad Sci*. 2002;977:9–23.

97. White L, Small BJ, Petrovitch H, Ross GW, Masaki K, Abbott RD, et al. Recent clinical-pathologic research on the causes of dementia in late life: update from the Honolulu-Asia Aging Study. *J Geriatr Psychiatry Neurol*. 2005;18(4):224–7. Epub 2005/11/25.

98. Polvikoski TM, van Straaten EC, Barkhof F, Sulkava R, Aronen HJ, Niinisto L, et al. Frontal lobe white matter hyperintensities and neurofibrillary pathology in the oldest old. *Neurology*. 2010;75(23):2071–8. Epub 2010/11/05.

99. Korczyn AD. Mixed dementia – the most common cause of dementia. *Ann N Y Acad Sci*. 2002;977:129–34. Epub 2002/12/14.

100. Thal DR, Ghebremedhin E, Orantes M, Wiestler OD. Vascular pathology in Alzheimer disease: correlation of cerebral amyloid angiopathy and arteriosclerosis/lipohyalinosis with cognitive decline. *J Neuropathol Exp Neurol*. 2003;62(12):1287–301. Epub 2003/12/25.

101. Cordonnier C, van der Flier WM. Brain microbleeds and Alzheimer's disease: innocent observation or key player? Brain. 2011;134(Pt 2):335–44. Epub 2011/01/25.

102. Jellinger KA, Attems J. Neuropathology and general autopsy findings in nondemented aged subjects. *Clin Neuropathol*. 2012;31(2):87–98.

103. Fisher CM. The arterial lesions underlying lacunes. *Acta Neuropathol*. 1968;12(1):1–15. Epub 1968/12/18.

104. Esiri MM, Wilcock GK, Morris JH. Neuropathological assessment of the lesions of significance in vascular dementia. *J Neurol Neurosurg Psychiatry*. 1997;63(6):749–53. Epub 1998/01/07.

105. Gorelick PB, Scuteri A, Black SE, Decarli C, Greenberg SM, Iadecola C, et al. Vascular contributions to cognitive impairment and dementia: a statement for healthcare professionals from the american heart association/american stroke association. *Stroke* 2011;42(9):2672–713. Epub 2011/07/23.

106. Bertram L, Lill CM, Tanzi RE. The genetics of Alzheimer disease: back to the future. *Neuron*. 2010;68(2):270–81. Epub 2010/10/20.

107. Gatz M, Reynolds CA, Fratiglioni L, Johansson B, Mortimer JA, Berg S, et al. Role of genes and environments for explaining Alzheimer disease. *Arch Gen Psychiatry*. 2006;63(2):168–74. Epub 2006/02/08.

108. Wingo TS, Lah JJ, Levey AI, Cutler DJ. Autosomal recessive causes likely in early-onset Alzheimer disease. *Arch Neurol*. 2012;69(1):59–64. Epub 2011/09/14.

109. Kudlow BA, Kennedy BK. Aging: progeria and the lamin connection. *Curr Biol*. 2006;16(16):R652–4. Epub 2006/08/22.

110. Brown WT, Kieras FJ, Houck GE, Jr., Dutkowski R, Jenkins EC. A comparison of adult and childhood progerias: Werner syndrome and Hutchinson-Gilford progeria syndrome. *Adv Exp Med Biol*. 1985;190:229–44. Epub 1985/01/01.

111. Prolla TA. Multiple roads to the aging phenotype: insights from the molecular dissection of progerias through DNA microarray analysis. *Mech Ageing Dev*. 2005;126(4):461–5. Epub 2005/02/22.

112. Burtner CR, Kennedy BK. Progeria syndromes and ageing: what is the connection? Nat Rev Mol Cell Biol. 2010;11(8):567–78. Epub 2010/07/24.

113. Leverenz JB, Yu CE, Schellenberg GD. Aging-associated neuropathology in Werner syndrome. *Acta Neuropathol*. 1998;96(4):421–4. Epub 1998/10/31.

114. Olovnikov AM. Hypothesis: lifespan is regulated by chronomere DNA of the hypothalamus. *J Alzheimers Dis*. 2007;11(2):241–52. Epub 2007/05/25.

115. Martin GM. Genetic modulation of senescent phenotypes in Homo sapiens. *Cell*. 2005;120(4):523–32. Epub 2005/03/01.

116. Martin GM. Genetic modulation of the senescent phenotype in Homo sapiens. *Genome*. 1989;31(1):390–7. Epub 1989/01/01.

117. Albani D, Polito L, Forloni G. Sirtuins as novel targets for Alzheimer's disease and other neurodegenerative disorders: experimental and genetic evidence. *J Alzheimers Dis*. 2010;19(1):11–26. Epub 2010/01/12.

118. Hardy J, Allsop D. Amyloid deposition as the central event in the aetiology of Alzheimer's disease. *Trends Pharmacol Sci*. 1991;12(10):383–8. Epub 1991/10/01.

119. Hardy J. Alzheimer's disease: the amyloid cascade hypothesis: an update and reappraisal. *J Alzheimers Dis*. 2006;9(3 Suppl):151–3.

120. Lemere CA, Blusztajn JK, Yamaguchi H, Wisniewski T, Saido TC, Selkoe DJ. Sequence of deposition of heterogeneous amyloid beta-peptides and APO E in Down syndrome: implications for initial events in amyloid plaque formation. *Neurobiol Dis*. 1996;3(1):16–32. Epub 1996/02/01.

121. Sleegers K, Brouwers N, Gijselinck I, Theuns J, Goossens D, Wauters J, et al. APP duplication is sufficient to cause early onset Alzheimer's dementia with cerebral amyloid angiopathy. *Brain*. 2006;129(Pt 11):2977–83. Epub 2006/08/22.

122. Theuns J, Brouwers N, Engelborghs S, Sleegers K, Bogaerts V, Corsmit E, et al. Promoter mutations that increase amyloid precursor-protein expression are associated with Alzheimer disease. *Am J Hum Genet*. 2006;78(6):936–46. Epub 2006/05/11.

123. Strittmatter WJ, Saunders AM, Schmechel D, Pericak-Vance M, Enghild J, Salvesen GS, et al. Apolipoprotein E: high-avidity binding to beta-amyloid and increased frequency of type 4 allele in late-onset familial Alzheimer disease. *Proc Natl Acad Sci U S A*. 1993;90(5):1977–81. Epub 1993/03/01.

124. Corder EH, Saunders AM, Strittmatter WJ, Schmechel DE, Gaskell PC, Small GW, et al. Gene dose of apolipoprotein E type 4 allele and the risk of Alzheimer's disease in late onset families. *Science* (New York, NY). 1993;261(5123):921–3. Epub 1993/08/13.

125. Lauderback CM, Kanski J, Hackett JM, Maeda N, Kindy MS, Butterfield DA. Apolipoprotein E modulates Alzheimer's Abeta(1-42)-induced oxidative damage to synaptosomes in an allele-specific manner. *Brain Res*. 2002;924(1):90–7. Epub 2002/12/18.

126. Kang DE, Pietrzik CU, Baum L, Chevallier N, Merriam DE, Kounnas MZ, et al. Modulation of amyloid beta-protein clearance and Alzheimer's disease susceptibility by the LDL receptor-related protein pathway. *J Clin Invest*. 2000;106(9):1159–66. Epub 2000/11/09.

127. Biere AL, Ostaszewski B, Zhao H, Gillespie S, Younkin SG, Selkoe DJ. Co-expression of beta-amyloid precursor protein (betaAPP) and apolipoprotein E in cell culture: analysis of betaAPP processing. *Neurobiol Dis*. 1995;2(3):177–87. Epub 1995/06/01.

128. Bennett DA, Wilson RS, Schneider JA, Evans DA, Aggarwal NT, Arnold SE, et al. Apolipoprotein E epsilon4 allele, AD pathology, and the clinical expression of Alzheimer's disease. *Neurology*. 2003;60(2):246–52. Epub 2003/01/29.

129. Rebeck GW, Cho HS, Grabowski TJ, Greenberg SM. The effects of AbetaPP mutations and APOE polymorphisms on cerebral amyloid angiopathy. *Amyloid*. 2001;8 Suppl 1:43–7. Epub 2001/10/26.

130. Myers RH, Schaefer EJ, Wilson PW, D'Agostino R, Ordovas JM, Espino A, et al. Apolipoprotein E epsilon4 association with dementia in a population-based study: The Framingham study. *Neurology*. 1996;46(3):673–7. Epub 1996/03/01.

131. Pertovaara M, Lehtimaki T, Rontu R, Antonen J, Pasternack A, Hurme M. Presence of apolipoprotein E epsilon4 allele predisposes to early onset of primary Sjogren's syndrome. *Rheumatology* (Oxford). 2004;43(12):1484–7. Epub 2004/08/26.

132. Giannattasio C, Poleggi A, Puopolo M, Pocchiari M, Antuono P, Dal Forno G, et al. Survival in Alzheimer's disease is shorter in women carrying heterozygosity at codon 129 of the PRNP gene and no APOE epsilon 4 allele. *Dement Geriatr Cogn Disord*. 2008;25(4):354–8. Epub 2008/03/12.

133. Kulminski AM, Culminskaya I, Ukraintseva SV, Arbeev KG, Arbeeva L, Wu D, et al. Trade-off in the effects of the apolipoprotein E polymorphism on the ages at onset of CVD and cancer influences human lifespan. *Aging Cell*. 2011;10(3):533–41. Epub 2011/02/22.

134. Jicha GA, Parisi JE, Dickson DW, Cha RH, Johnson KA, Smith GE, et al. Age and apoE associations with complex pathologic features in Alzheimer's disease. *J Neurol Sci*. 2008;273(1-2):34–9. Epub 2008/07/26.

135. Jun G, Naj AC, Beecham GW, Wang LS, Buros J, Gallins PJ, et al. Meta-analysis confirms CR1, CLU, and PICALM as alzheimer disease risk loci and reveals interactions with APOE genotypes. *Arch Neurol*. 2010;67(12):1473–84. Epub 2010/08/11.

136. Seshadri S, Fitzpatrick AL, Ikram MA, DeStefano AL, Gudnason V, Boada M, et al. Genome-wide analysis of genetic loci associated with Alzheimer disease. *Jama*. 2010;303(18):1832–40. Epub 2010/05/13.

137. Biffi A, Anderson CD, Desikan RS, Sabuncu M, Cortellini L, Schmansky N, et al. Genetic variation and neuroimaging measures in Alzheimer disease. *Arch Neurol*. 2010;67(6):677–85. Epub 2010/06/19.

138. Belbin O, Carrasquillo MM, Crump M, Culley OJ, Hunter TA, Ma L, et al. Investigation of 15 of the top candidate genes for late-onset Alzheimer's disease. *Hum Genet*. 2011;129(3):273–82. Epub 2010/12/07.

139. Harder A, Jendroska K, Kreuz F, Wirth T, Schafranka C, Karnatz N, et al. Novel twelve-generation kindred of fatal familial insomnia from Germany representing the entire spectrum of disease expression. *Am J Med Genet*. 1999;87(4):311–6. Epub 1999/12/10.

140. Wong K, Sidransky E, Verma A, Mixon T, Sandberg GD, Wakefield LK, et al. Neuropathology provides clues to the pathophysiology of Gaucher disease. *Mol Genet Metab*. 2004;82(3):192–207. Epub 2004/07/06.

141. Ferenci P, Czlonkowska A, Merle U, Ferenc S, Gromadzka G, Yurdaydin C, et al. Late-onset Wilson's disease. *Gastroenterology*. 2007;132(4):1294–8. Epub 2007/04/17.

142. Sedel F, Tourbah A, Fontaine B, Lubetzki C, Baumann N, Saudubray JM, et al. Leukoencephalopathies associated with inborn errors of metabolism in adults. *J Inherit Metab Dis*. 2008;31(3):295–307. Epub 2008/03/18.

143. Adib-Samii P, Brice G, Martin RJ, Markus HS. Clinical spectrum of CADASIL and the effect of cardiovascular risk factors on phenotype: study in 200 consecutively recruited individuals. *Stroke*. 2010;41(4):630–4. Epub 2010/02/20.

144. Brumback-Peltz C, Balasubramanian AB, Corrada MM, Kawas CH. Diagnosing dementia in the oldest-old. *Maturitas*. 2011;70(2):164–8. Epub 2011/08/13.

145. Crystal HA, Dickson DW, Sliwinski MJ, Lipton RB, Grober E, Marks-Nelson H, et al. Pathological markers associated with normal aging and dementia in the elderly. *Ann Neurol*. 1993;34(4):566–73. Epub 1993/10/01.

146. Miller LA, Munoz DG, Finmore M. Hippocampal sclerosis and human memory. *Arch Neurol*. 1993;50(4):391–4. Epub 1993/04/01.

147. Knopman DS, Petersen RC, Cha RH, Edland SD, Rocca WA. Incidence and causes of nondegenerative nonvascular dementia: a population-based study. *Arch Neurol*. 2006;63(2):218–21. Epub 2006/02/16.

148. Erkinjuntti T, Sulkava R, Kovanen J, Palo J. Suspected dementia: evaluation of 323 consecutive referrals. *Acta Neurol Scand*. 1987;76(5):359–64. Epub 1987/11/01.

149. Pao WC, Dickson DW, Crook JE, Finch NA, Rademakers R, Graff-Radford NR. Hippocampal sclerosis in the elderly: genetic and pathologic findings, some mimicking Alzheimer disease clinically. *Alzheimer Dis Assoc Disord*. 2011;25(4):364–8. Epub 2011/02/25.

150. Jagust W. Dementia: finding the signals in the noise. *Lancet Neurol*. 2005;4(1):10–1. Epub 2004/12/29.

CHAPTER 2

Protein Aggregation and Neurodegeneration: Tauopathies and Synucleinopathies

Michel Goedert

MRC Laboratory of Molecular Biology, Cambridge, UK

Introduction

Neurodegenerative diseases such as Alzheimer's disease (AD), Parkinson disease (PD), frontotemporal lobar degeneration (FTLD), amyotrophic lateral sclerosis (ALS), Huntington's disease (HD), and prion diseases are characterized by the progressive dysfunction and death of some nerve cells. The overall clinical picture reflects which nerve cells in the central nervous system are affected. This explains why AD and FTLD are dementing diseases, whereas PD is largely a movement disorder. At present, there are no mechanism-based therapies for these diseases. Where they exist, therapies are at best symptomatic.

Specific protein aggregates constitute the defining neuropathological characteristics of the above diseases. In 1907, Alois Alzheimer in Munich and Oskar Fischer in Prague described neuritic plaques and neurofibrillary tangles [1, 2] in the disease that Emil Kraepelin, Head of the Munich Institute, named after Alzheimer three years later [3]. In 1911, Alzheimer described argyrophilic inclusions in a form of FTLD [4] that was subsequently named Pick disease [5], after Arnold Pick, Head of the Department of Neuropsychiatry at the German University in Prague, where Fischer worked (these inclusions are now called Pick bodies). In 1912, Friedrich Lewy described the inclusions characteristic of PD (Lewy bodies and neurites) in Alzheimer's laboratory in Munich [6]. In the 1960s, electron microscopy showed that these inclusions are made of abnormal filaments [7–9]. Over the past 30 years, a causal connection between inclusion formation and the degenerative process has emerged.

First, the biochemical study of the neuropathological lesions led to the identification of their molecular components. Second, the study of familial forms of AD, FTLD, and PD resulted in the identification of gene defects that cause disease [10, 11]. In most cases, pathogenic mutations led to an overproduction of the amyloidogenic protein or increased its propensity to aggregate. It follows that a toxic property conferred by these mutations causes disease and that a similar toxic property may underlie the sporadic forms of disease.

Neurofibrillary tangles, Pick bodies, and Lewy bodies are intracellular filamentous inclusions. Neurofibrillary tangles and Pick bodies are made of the microtubule-associated protein tau [12–18], whereas Lewy bodies are made of the protein α-synuclein [19]. Mutations in the tau gene (*MAPT*) give rise to an inherited form of frontotemporal dementia and parkinsonism (Figure 2.1) [20–22]. Mutations in the α-synuclein gene (*SNCA*) or an increase in copy number cause dominantly inherited forms of PD and dementia with Lewy bodies (DLB) (Figure 2.2) [23, 24]. Tauopathies and synucleinopathies account for the majority of cases of late-onset neurodegenerative disease.

Amyloids

Some normally soluble proteins can become insoluble and form elongated filaments with a cross-β fiber diffraction pattern [25]. The term amyloid refers to an unbranched protein filament whose repeating substructure consists of β strands that run perpendicular to the filament axis, forming a cross-β sheet of indefinite length [26, 27]. Around 20 amyloid-forming proteins have been identified *in vivo*, many of which are associated with common neurodegenerative diseases [28]. They include β-amyloid (Aβ) and tau in AD, tau in some cases of FTLD, and α-synuclein in PD, DLB, and multiple system atrophy (MSA).

A nucleus consisting of a small number of molecules present at a high enough concentration and with their amyloid-forming segments exposed must form first. Once this nucleus has formed, single molecules can be incorporated at the ends of growing filaments. Amyloid filament formation is thus characterized by a slow nucleation phase, followed by a more rapid growth phase. Filaments can break, which affects their growth kinetics. A full description of amyloid filament formation includes rates of nucleation, growth, and fragmentation, with nucleation being rate-limiting [29].

Atomic structures have been obtained of fibrils made from short peptides of amyloidogenic proteins (so-called "amyloid spines") [30, 31]. They have shown that each β-strand is hydrogen bonded to the strand above and below through its backbone amide groups. When the amino acid side chains also contain amides, as in asparagine and glutamine, those amides form hydrogen bonds with the identical residues in the strands above and below. The amino acid side chains emanating from adjacent β-sheets are tightly interdigitated, like the teeth of a zipper. This region, which is devoid of water, has been called "dry steric zipper".

There is a need to identify the molecular species that are responsible for amyloid-associated cytotoxicity and to discover how these species can cause cell death. It will be important to know if there is a general mechanism of amyloid-associated cytotoxicity or if amyloids assembled from different protein sequences cause cell death through different mechanisms. The challenge of solving these questions lies

Neurodegeneration, First Edition. Edited by Anthony Schapira, Zbigniew Wszolek, Ted M. Dawson and Nicholas Wood.
© 2017 John Wiley & Sons, Ltd. Published 2017 by John Wiley & Sons, Ltd.

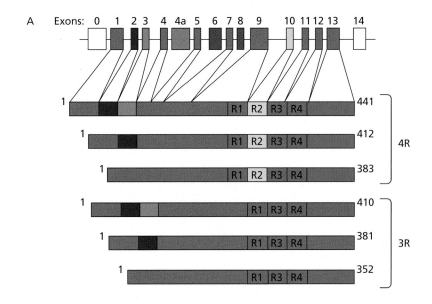

Figure 2.1 Human brain tau isoforms and *MAPT* mutations. (A) *MAPT* and the six tau isoforms expressed in adult human brain. *MAPT* consists of 16 exons (E). Alternative mRNA splicing of E2 (red), E3 (green), and E10 (yellow) gives rise to six tau isoforms (amino acids, 352–441). Constitutively spliced exons (E1, E4, E5, E7, E9, E11, E12, E13) are shown in blue. E0, which is part of the promoter, and E14 are non-coding (white). E6 and E8 (violet) are not transcribed in human brain. E4a (orange) is only expressed in the peripheral nervous system. The repeats (R1–R4) are shown, with three isoforms having four repeats each (4R) and three isoforms having three repeats each (3R). Each repeat is 31 or 32 amino acids in length. Exons and introns are not drawn to scale. (B) Heterozygous missense, deletion, or intronic mutations cause frontotemporal dementia and parkinsonism linked to chromosome 17 (FTDP-17T). (C) Forty-nine coding region mutations in (E) exons 1, 9, 10, 11, 12, and 13 of *MAPT* cause FTDP-17T, as do ten intronic mutations flanking E10.

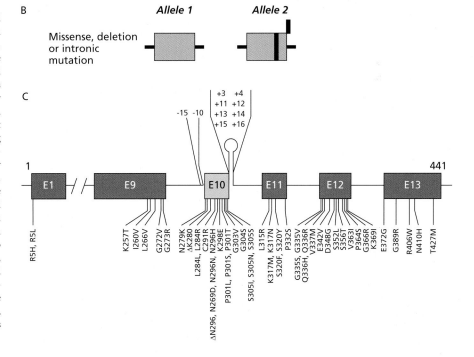

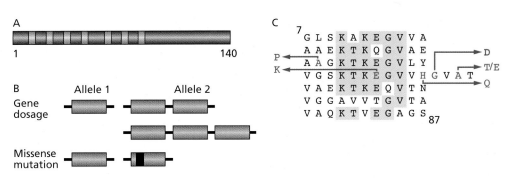

Figure 2.2 Human α-synuclein and its disease-causing mutations. (A) Diagram of the 140 amino acid human α-synuclein protein. The core regions of the seven amino-terminal repeats are shown as blue bars. (B) An increase in gene dosage (duplication or triplication) of the chromosomal region containing *SNCA* or missense mutations in *SNCA* cause dominantly inherited Parkinson disease and dementia with Lewy bodies. (C) The seven repeats (residues 7–87) of human α-synuclein are shown, with the six known disease-causing missense mutations (A30P, E46K, H50Q, G51D, A53E, A53T) indicated in blue text. Amino acids that are identical in at least five of the seven repeats are shaded in blue.

in the low abundance and transient nature of amyloid assembly intermediates, the multitude of species that are formed on- or off-pathway, and the large number of cellular responses to intracellular and extracellular amyloid fibrils and oligomeric species.

Tauopathies

Tau isoforms in human brain and their interactions with microtubules

Tau is a natively unfolded microtubule-associated protein (MAP) that binds to microtubules and is believed to play a role in the assembly of microtubules [10]. It is well established that in nerve cells tau is concentrated in axons, but recent work has also suggested a physiological function in dendrites [32]. Six tau isoforms are expressed in the adult human brain by alternative mRNA splicing from a single gene on chromosome 17q21.31 (Figure 2.1) [33]. They differ by the presence or absence of a 29- or 58-amino acid insert in the amino-terminal half and by the inclusion, or not, of a 31-amino acid repeat encoded by exon 10 of *MAPT* in the carboxy-terminal half of the protein. The exclusion of exon 10 leads to the production of three isoforms, each containing three repeats, and its inclusion to a further three isoforms, each containing four repeats. The repeats and some adjoining sequences constitute the microtubule-binding domains of tau, with four-repeat tau being better at promoting microtubule assembly than tau with three repeats [34]. By nuclear magnetic resonance (NMR) spectroscopy, a fragment consisting of residues S214–E372, which comprises the second half of the proline-rich region and the repeats of tau, binds tightly to taxol-stabilized microtubules [35]. Structural work has also begun to shed light in a more direct manner on the way in which tau and microtubules may interact. Microtubules were assembled with tubulin and tau in the absence of taxol and in the presence of the natural osmolyte trimethylamine *N*-oxide (TMAO). The tau repeats were found to bind to the inner surface of the microtubule, in a region that overlaps with the taxol-binding site of β-tubulin [36]. In this model, part of the proline-rich region provides the link between the amino-terminal projection domain on the outside of the microtubule and the repeat motifs on the inside surface. It may thread through one of the holes between protofilaments. A separate model has been derived from experiments in which tau was bound to preassembled, taxol-stabilized microtubules. Tau was found to bind only to the outer surface of the microtubule, where it localized along the outer ridges of the protofilaments [37]. In a third study, tau bound to a hydrophobic region between tubulin heterodimers, which overlapped with the binding pocket of vinblastine [38].

Similar levels of three- and four-repeat tau isoforms are expressed in adult human cerebral cortex [34]. In developing human brain, only the shortest tau isoform (three repeats and no amino-terminal inserts) is expressed. Although tau is present as multiple forms in vertebrates, isoform ratios are not conserved between species. For instance, tau isoforms with three, four, or five repeats are expressed in adult chicken brain [39], whereas adult rodents express predominantly tau isoforms with four repeats [40].

Similar repeats are found in the otherwise unrelated high-molecular-weight microtubule-associated proteins MAP2 and MAP4. Repeat sequences are conserved throughout evolution, with the genomes of *C. elegans* and *D. melanogaster* each encoding one protein with tau-like repeats [41, 42]. Inactivation of *MAPT* in mice does not cause neurodegeneration, but results in some behavioral changes [43–45].

Tau aggregation

Tau is a natively unfolded protein that assembles into filaments through its tandem repeat region, with the amino-terminal half and the carboxy-terminus forming the "fuzzy coat" of the filament [14, 15, 46]. In some human diseases, including AD, following the death and removal of tangle-bearing cells, filaments made of truncated tau remain in the extracellular space in the form of so-called "ghost tangles" which consist largely of the repeat region of tau. This strongly suggests that the formation of tau aggregates is deleterious. It is supported by experiments showing that the formation of aggregates made of the repeat region of tau induces neurotoxicity in animal models and cultured cells [47–49]. In other human tauopathies, including most cases caused by *MAPT* mutations, filamentous tau aggregates do not accumulate in the extracellular space following the death of nerve cells. The reasons underlying these differences remain to be established. Tau filaments have a cross-β structure characteristic of amyloid filaments [50, 51].

Methods have been developed for assembling tau filaments from purified full-length tau [52–55]. They are based on the interaction of non-phosphorylated tau protein with negatively charged compounds, including sulfated glycosaminoglycans. The binding of heparin leads to the loss of long-range contacts between the amino- and carboxy-termini of tau and between each terminus and the microtubule-binding repeats [56]. The epitopes of aggregation-dependent antibodies Alz50 and MC1 consist of the amino-terminal region and the repeats of tau [57, 58]. It follows that recognition by these antibodies requires intermolecular tau interactions. Heparin induces dimerization of tau [59], with fibrils growing through monomer addition, with no role for heparin in fibril elongation. Synthetic tau filaments resemble those extracted from AD brain, in that they are decorated by antibodies directed against the amino- and carboxy-termini of tau, but not by an antibody against the third repeat [52].

Short amino acid sequences in the second ([275]VQIINK[280]) and third ([306]VQIVYK[311]) repeats are essential for the heparin-induced assembly of tau into filaments [60, 61]. Based on the atomic structure of VQIVYK, an all D-amino acid peptide of six amino acids was designed that blocks the ends of the tau fibril [31]. It inhibited fibril formation by either the VQIVYK peptide or full-length tau. Small molecules that disrupt tau filament formation *in vitro* have also been described [62–64]. However, the mechanisms by which soluble tau protein assembles into insoluble filaments in brain cells remain to be discovered. So far, no anti-tau amyloid compound has been shown to be of therapeutic benefit in humans.

The conformation of tau may influence axonal transport. Studies in squid axoplasm have shown that tau filaments reduced transport through a mechanism involving axonal protein phosphatase-1 and glycogen synthase kinase-3β (GSK3β) [65]. Amino acids 2–18 in tau were necessary and sufficient for the activation of this pathway, suggesting that disease-associated changes in tau conformation lead to increased exposure of the phosphatase-activating domain.

Tau phosphorylation

Abnormal hyperphosphorylation is characteristic of tau inclusions and appears to precede filament assembly and to render tau unable to interact with microtubules [66, 67]. It is common to all diseases with tau filaments. Many phosphorylation sites are known, as are candidate protein kinases and phosphatases [10, 68]. In particular, proline-directed kinases, protein kinases that phosphorylate the KxGS motifs in the repeats, and protein phosphatase 2A (PP2A) have been implicated in the phosphorylation and dephosphorylation of tau protein. It remains to be seen if the abnormal hyperphosphorylation of tau is either necessary or sufficient for filament assembly.

Increased phosphorylation of tau is not always detrimental; it happens reversibly during fetal brain development, hibernation, and hypometabolism [69–72]. It remains to be determined if different mechanisms underlie physiological and pathological tau phosphorylation. In the human diseases, tau may first misfold, which will make it an improved substrate for protein kinases and/or a less good substrate for protein phosphatases. In a more physiological setting, tau may become hyperphosphorylated because of increased protein kinase and/or reduced protein phosphatase activities. Although serine/threonine phosphorylation is a major early characteristic of tau aggregation, other post-translational modifications have also been described in aggregated tau. They include acetylation [73–75], O-GlcNAcylation [76], nitration [77], prolyl isomerization [78, 79], glycation [80, 81], and ubiquitination [82, 83].

Isoform composition of tau filaments

The presence of filamentous deposits made of hyperphosphorylated tau in human brain raises the question why there are multiple tauopathies and not just a single disease. This probably has to do with the fact that different brain regions and distinct cell types are affected in the human tauopathies. These differences between diseases correlate to some extent with the isoform composition of tau filaments. All six brain isoforms are present in the tau filaments of AD [84]. Four-repeat isoforms are characteristic of the tau filaments of progressive supranuclear palsy (PSP), corticobasal degeneration (CBD), and argyrophilic grain disease (AGD) [85–88], whereas three-repeat isoforms characterize the tau filaments of Pick disease [89]. Differences in isoform composition are also reflected in the existence of tau filaments with distinct morphologies [90].

This is reminiscent of mammalian and yeast prions, for which different strains have been described, based on the existence of separate conformers of assembled proteins [91]. Tau isoforms have been reported to have an asymmetric seeding barrier, in that seeds of three-repeat tau could recruit four-repeat tau; however, seeds made of four-repeat tau could not recruit three-repeat tau [92].

Genetics

Human genetics was essential for proving a link between dysfunction of tau and neurodegeneration. In 1994, a dominantly inherited form of FTLD and parkinsonism was linked to chromosome 17q21-22, a region that contains *MAPT* [93], followed by the identification of additional forms of FTLD linked to this region, resulting in the denomination "frontotemporal dementia and parkinsonism linked to chromosome 17" (FTDP-17) for this class of disease [94]. Patients with FTDP-17 had tau inclusions in either nerve cells or in both nerve cells and glial cells. In June 1998, the first mutations in *MAPT* were reported in what is now called FTDP-17T [20–22]. By October 2016, 59 pathogenic *MAPT* mutations had been identified (Figure 2.1). Not all cases of FTDP-17 are caused by mutations in *MAPT*. Since 2006, it has been known that FTDP-17 can be caused by mutations in either *MAPT* or the progranulin gene (*GRN*) [95, 96].

MAPT mutations account for approximately 5% of cases of FTLD and appear to cause disease through a gain of toxic function mechanism [97]. Most mutations are located in exons 9–12 (which encode the repeats) and the introns adjacent to exon 10. They fall into two largely non-overlapping groups: those with a primary effect at the protein level and those influencing the alternative splicing of tau pre-mRNA. Mutations acting at the protein level change or delete single amino acids, thus reducing the ability of tau to interact with microtubules. This partial loss of function may be required for the abnormal aggregation of tau. Some mutations also promote the assembly of tau into filaments. Mutations with a primary effect at

the RNA level are intronic or exonic and increase the alternative mRNA splicing of exon 10. This changes the ratio of three- to four-repeat isoforms, resulting in the relative overproduction of four-repeat tau and the formation of filamentous inclusions made of four-repeat tau.

Known mutations do not directly affect phosphorylation sites, implying that hyperphosphorylation of tau is not the primary event in FTDP-17T. Clinical and neuropathological phenotypes similar or identical to those of Pick disease, PSP, CBD, and AGD have been described. The same mutation can give rise to different clinical syndromes in a single family. Thus, mutation P301S in exon 10 of *MAPT* caused behavioral-variant FTLD in a father and CBD in his son, supporting the view that FTLD and CBD are part of the same disease spectrum [98].

Haplotypes H1 and H2 characterize *MAPT* in populations of European descent. They result from a 900 kb inversion/non-inversion (H1/H2) polymorphism [99]. Because of the suppression of H1/H2 recombination and normal inter-H1 recombination, there are multiple H1 subhaplotypes, but only one major H2 haplotype. Inheritance of the H1 haplotype is a risk factor for PSP, CBD, and PD [100–103]. Of the most common H1 subhaplotypes, H1c is associated with disease risk, which localizes to a regulatory region in intron 0 of *MAPT*. This has been confirmed in a genome-wide association study (GWAS) of PSP, which also implicated proteins involved in vesicle trafficking, white matter function, and the unfolded protein response [104]. The association of H1 with PSP had a stronger odds ratio than that for the *ApoE* ε4/ε4 genotype as a risk locus for AD. It has been reported that the H2 haplotype is associated with increased expression of exon 3 of *MAPT* in gray matter, suggesting that the inclusion of exon 3 may be protective in PSP, CBD, and PD [105]. In addition, reduced expression of 1N4R tau has also been associated with the H2 haplotype [106]. The mechanism underlying this potential protective effect is not known, but could be related to the finding that exon 2- and exon 10-encoded inserts increased the aggregation propensity of tau, whereas the exon 3-encoded insert decreased aggregation [107].

Heterozygous microdeletions at 17q21.31 cause a multisystem disorder of intellectual disability, hypotonia, and distinctive facial features [108–110]. Besides *MAPT*, the deleted region commonly comprises five other genes (corticotropin-releasing hormone receptor 1, intramembrane protease 5, NP 689679.1, NP 787078.1, and KANSL1). Deletions occur on the H2 haplotype through low-copy repeat-mediated, non-allelic homologous recombination. Recent work has conclusively shown that this syndrome is a monogenic disorder caused by haploinsufficiency of *KANSL1*, which encodes the 1105-amino acid long nuclear protein KAT8 regulatory NSL complex subunit 1, a chromatin modifier that influences gene expression through the acetylation of lysine 16 of histone H4 (H4K16) [111, 112]. It follows that a 50% reduction in tau levels is unlikely to have a detrimental effect on brain development.

Animal models of human tauopathies

Mice that express human mutant tau in brain develop filamentous deposits made of hyperphosphorylated tau protein and neurodegeneration [48, 49, 113, 114]. Hyperphosphorylation precedes filament assembly, and additional phosphorylation of soluble tau increases filament formation, suggesting that phosphorylation of tau can promote filament assembly. Deposits of Aβ or Danish amyloid promote filament formation of human mutant tau, demonstrating that extracellular amyloid can drive intraneuronal tau pathology [115–117]. Tau is required for Aβ toxicity in experimental models [118, 119]. In mice lacking *MAPT*, the absence of Aβ toxicity may result from decreased excitotoxicity because of a reduction in the dendritic localization of the tyrosine kinase Fyn that leads to reduced phosphorylation of the NMDA receptor and interaction with postsynaptic density protein-95 (PSD-95) [32, 120]. This suggests that tau has a dendritic function. Separate work in mice has suggested that tau becomes enriched in dendritic spines, where it interferes with neurotransmission when it is abnormally modified and assumes a pathological conformation [121]. In human brain, the presence of hyperphosphorylated tau in spines was not accompanied by dendritic changes. The latter were only observed after the formation of tau aggregates [122]. Filamentous tau deposits also formed in a mouse line expressing all six wild-type human brain tau isoforms in the absence of mouse tau [123].

In rodent brain, adeno-associated virus-mediated expression of human mutant tau led to the formation of filamentous deposits made of hyperphosphorylated tau [124]. In rat brain, virally-mediated expression of wild-type tau also causes aggregation and neurodegeneration [125, 126]. Even though filamentous tau forms in many neurodegenerative diseases, its role in disease pathogenesis remains a subject for debate. In transgenic mice overexpressing human mutant tau in a conditional manner, a dissociation between tangle formation and nerve cell death has been reported [127].

Tau phosphorylation/dephosphorylation has been targeted therapeutically. Lithium chloride, which inhibits the candidate tau kinase GSK3β, improved behavioral deficits and reduced tau pathology in mice transgenic for human mutant P301L tau [128]. Similar effects have been reported when sodium selenate, an activator of PP2A, was used [129]. Increased glycosylation of tau following inhibition of O-GlcNAcase, the enzyme responsible for the hydrolysis of O-linked N-acetylglucosamine, reduced the number of tau inclusions and nerve cell loss in a mouse line transgenic for human mutant P301L tau [130]. This effect appeared to result from a reduction in the aggregation, not the phosphorylation, of tau. Conversely, in a mouse line transgenic for human mutant P301S tau, chronic stress increased tau phosphorylation, inclusion formation, and neurodegeneration in a corticotropin-releasing factor receptor 1-dependent manner [131].

Expression of wild-type and human mutant tau in nerve cells of *D. melanogaster* and *C. elegans* leads to the loss of nerve cells and a reduced lifespan, in the apparent absence of tau filaments [132, 133]. It has been reported that the aggregation of tau is necessary for neurodegeneration in *C. elegans*. In genetic modifier screens, increasing kinase activity enhances tau toxicity, with an increase in phosphatase activity being beneficial [134]. Anti-oxidant defences are also beneficial, with oxidative stress having been linked to abnormal cell cycle activation. The latter is mediated through the target of rapamycin (TOR) in nerve cells of *Drosophila*. In contrast to what has been described in FTDP-17T and mouse models thereof, in invertebrates, tau-induced neurodegeneration involved programmed cell death. As in mice, the neurotoxicity of tau in *Drosophila* was enhanced upon co-expression of Aβ, with oxidative stress, phosphorylation of S262/S356, and activation of DNA repair pathways being involved. In *C. elegans*, loss of a single gene, *sut-2* (suppressor of tau pathology-2), eliminated the toxic effects of human mutant tau, possibly through an increase in autophagic clearance [135].

Synucleinopathies

Three human synucleins

α-Synuclein, β-synuclein, and γ-synuclein range from 127 to 140 amino acids, and are 55–62% identical in sequence, with a similar domain organization [11]. In humans, they are encoded by genes located on chromosomes 4q23 (*SNCA*), 5q35 (*SNCB*), and 10q21 (*SNCC*). Synucleins are only found in vertebrates. More than half of each protein is taken up by six or seven imperfect 11-amino acid repeats with the consensus sequence KTKEGV. This positively charged region is followed by a hydrophobic middle part and a negatively charged carboxy-terminal region. By immunohistochemistry, α- and β-synucleins are abundant and concentrated in nerve terminals, with little staining of nerve cell bodies and dendrites. Ultrastructurally, they are present in close proximity to synaptic vesicles. By contrast, γ-synuclein is found throughout nerve cells.

Synucleins are lipid-binding proteins

For many years, synucleins were thought to have little ordered structure [136]. Recent findings have led to the suggestion that native α-synuclein is a homotetramer with a predominantly α-helical conformation [137]. However, this conclusion is not universally accepted. Monomeric α-synuclein adopts structures rich in α-helical character upon binding to lipid membranes containing acidic phospholipids [138, 139]. This conformation is taken up by amino acids 1–98, with residues 99–140 being unstructured. By NMR spectroscopy, the amino-terminal helical segment of α-synuclein functions as a membrane anchor, its central region determines the affinity for lipid binding, and its carboxy-terminal region is unstructured and only weakly associated with the membrane [140]. α-Synuclein is able to remodel membranes, reminiscent of the behavior of Bin-amphiphysin-Rvs (BAR) proteins [141, 142].

When bound to membranes, α-synuclein has been reported to multimerize and function as a chaperone that promotes the assembly of SNARE complexes [143]. By contrast, other work has reported that α-synuclein inhibits SNARE-mediated vesicle fusion by binding to membranes, without binding SNARE proteins or promoting SNARE complex formation [144].

Synucleins are phosphoproteins, with serine and tyrosine phosphorylation having been observed in transfected cells [145, 146]. It remains to be seen if phosphorylation plays a physiological role in brain. Inactivation of *SNCA* results in mice that are largely normal but do exhibit a reduction in striatal dopamine, suggesting that α-synuclein is a negative regulator of neurotransmitter release [147]. Triple knockout (*SNCA*, *SNCB*, and *SNCC*) mice have an age-dependent neurological impairment and decreased assembly of SNARE complexes, and suffer from premature death [148].

SNCA mutations cause familial PD

In 1997, a missense mutation (A53T) in *SNCA* was found to cause disease in a dominantly inherited form of PD with Lewy body pathology [23]. Five additional missense mutations (A30P, E46K, H50Q, G51D, and A53E) have subsequently been identified in families with PD and DLB (Figure 2.2) [149–155]. All six mutations identified by October 2016 are located in the repeat region of α-synuclein. Overexpression of wild-type α-synuclein has also been identified as a cause of PD and DLB in families with a heterozygous duplication or triplication of the region of chromosome 4 that contains *SNCA* (Figure 2.2) [24, 156, 157]. Moreover, GWAS have shown that sequence variation in the regulatory region of *SNCA* predisposes to idiopathic PD, consistent with the view that even mild overproduction of α-synuclein can be detrimental [158, 159].

Lewy body filaments are made of α-synuclein

The defining pathological hallmark of PD is the presence of abundant Lewy bodies, round inclusions made of aggregated protein, in the cytoplasm of nerve cells [6, 11]. In 1997, Lewy bodies and Lewy neurites from PD and DLB were shown to be immunoreactive for α-synuclein [19]. DLB is characterized by large numbers of Lewy bodies and Lewy neurites in cortical brain areas, in addition to the substantia nigra. Filaments are unbranched, with a length of 200–600 nm and a width of 5–10 nm [160, 161]. The core of the filament extends over 70 amino acids and overlaps with the lipid-binding region of α-synuclein. Filaments have a cross-β structure like other amyloid fibers [162–164]. Only α-synuclein is associated with the filamentous inclusions of Lewy body diseases and α-synuclein-positive structures exceed those stained for ubiquitin, indicating that α-synuclein becomes ubiquitinated after assembly. Hyperphosphorylation at residue S129 is the major post-translational modification of filamentous α-synuclein [165, 166]. G-protein-coupled receptor kinases, casein kinases, and polo-like kinases phosphorylate S129. It remains to be shown unambiguously if phosphorylation at S129 occurs before or after filament assembly. Lewy body pathology is also the defining feature of several rarer diseases, including Lewy body dysphagia and pure autonomic failure. In these diseases, Lewy bodies and Lewy neurites are largely limited to the enteric and peripheral nervous systems [146]. In PD, Lewy body pathology is also present in the enteric and autonomic nervous systems. Incidental Lewy body disease is defined by the presence of small numbers of Lewy bodies and Lewy neurites in the absence of clinical symptoms [167–169]. It is observed in 5–10% of individuals over the age of 60 and may represent a preclinical form of disease.

α-Synuclein-positive neurites appear earlier than Lewy bodies and precede perikaryal immunoreactivity [170]. The neuritic aggregates may be related to an oligomeric form of α-synuclein that has been shown to increase the production of reactive oxygen species, consistent with the view that α-synuclein aggregation accelerates mitochondrial dysfunction [171].

Multiple system atrophy

Glial cytoplasmic inclusions (GCIs, also known as Papp–Lantos inclusions), which are made of filamentous aggregates, are the defining neuropathological feature of MSA [172]. They are found mostly in the cytoplasm and, to a lesser extent, nucleus of oligodendrocytes. Inclusions are also present in some nerve cells. The affected brain regions are mainly the substantia nigra, striatum, locus coeruleus, pontine nuclei, inferior olives, cerebellum, and spinal cord. Typically, nerve cell loss and gliosis are observed. The filamentous GCIs are made of α-synuclein, with the number of α-synuclein-positive structures exceeding that stained for ubiquitin [173–175]. Filament morphologies differ between MSA and Lewy body diseases, suggesting that distinct conformations of assembled α-synuclein can give rise to different neurodegenerative diseases [171]. Sequence variation of *SNCA* is a risk factor for MSA [176, 177]. MSA is a largely sporadic disease, for which a probable neuropathological prodrome has been described [178, 179].

Synthetic α-synuclein filaments

Filaments made from recombinant human α-synuclein have the same appearance as disease filaments [180, 181]. Assembly is nucleation dependent and occurs through the amino-terminal repeats. The negatively charged carboxy-terminal region inhibits assembly. Under the conditions of these experiments, β- and γ-synucleins failed to assemble [162], consistent with their absence from the disease filaments. The aggregation propensity of human α-synuclein is dependent on β-strand contiguity, hydrophilicity, and charge [182]. Assembly assays can be used for the identification of pharmacological modifiers of filament formation. Non-toxic, SDS-stable dimers and oligomers of α-synuclein form in the presence of compounds that inhibit filament formation [183].

Mutations E46K, H50Q, and A53T increase the assembly rates of α-synuclein, whereas mutations A30P, G51D, and A53E reduce filament assembly [184–188]. Mutations A30P, G51D, and A53E also decrease membrane binding when compared to the wild-type protein [187–189]. This may reduce their axonal transport and cause accumulation in nerve cell bodies, resulting in aggregation. Abundant α-synuclein inclusions were present in the brains of patients with mutations A30P, G51D, and A53E in *SNCA* [153–155, 190].

Animal models of human synucleinopathies

Overexpression of wild-type α-synuclein inhibits evoked neurotransmitter release [191]. Mice expressing human mutant α-synuclein in neurons or glial cells develop numerous α-synuclein-positive cell bodies and processes, but filament formation and nerve cell loss are less consistent features [192, 193]. The presence of abundant α-synuclein filaments in brain and spinal cord of mice transgenic for human mutant E46K or A53T α-synuclein has been described [192, 194]. In the E46K line, numerous inclusions of hyperphosphorylated tau were also present. The formation of α-synuclein inclusions correlated with the development of a movement disorder. An increase in phosphatase activity attenuated α-synucleinopathy, suggesting a detrimental role of α-synuclein phosphorylation in the disease process [195]. A major difference with PD was the absence of significant pathology and neurodegeneration in dopaminergic nerve cells of the substantia nigra. This has been achieved in part following the expression of carboxy-terminally truncated human α-synuclein [196]. These mice also exhibited a reduction in the release of dopamine in the striatum. However, a transgenic mouse model that fully recapitulates the behavioral phenotype, neuropathology, and pathophysiology of PD remains to be produced.

A neurotoxin model of α-synuclein pathology has been developed in the rat through the chronic administration of the pesticide rotenone, a high-affinity inhibitor of mitochondrial complex I of the respiratory chain. Although the variability was substantial, some rats developed progressive degeneration of nigrostriatal neurons and Lewy body-like inclusions that were immunoreactive for α-synuclein and ubiquitin [197]. They exhibited bradykinesia, postural instability, and resting tremor. The inhibition of complex I was only partial, suggesting that reactive oxygen species can link mitochondrial dysfunction and α-synuclein aggregation. When overexpressed, α-synuclein can interact with mitochondria. It binds to cardiolipin in the inner mitochondrial membrane, inhibits the activity of complex I, and induces mitochondrial fission [198]. It remains to be seen how these functional effects relate to the pathogenesis of PD. β- and γ-synucleins also promoted the fission of mitochondria.

Adeno-associated and lentiviral vectors have been used to express human wild-type and mutant α-synuclein in the substantia nigra. Lewy body-like inclusions formed and a significant proportion of nerve cells degenerated [199, 200]. The fibrillization of α-synuclein promoted the progressive degeneration of nigral dopaminergic neurons [201]. The aggregation of α-synuclein caused neurodegeneration in these models. However, the underlying mechanisms are less well understood. In transgenic mouse brain, oligomers of α-synuclein have been found in the endoplasmic reticulum. Salubrinal, an anti-endoplasmic reticulum stress compound, delayed the onset of disease [202].

Overexpression of human α-synuclein in *D. melanogaster* results in the formation of filamentous Lewy body-like inclusions, the age-dependent loss of some dopaminergic neurons, and locomotor deficits [203]. Aggregation of α-synuclein is necessary for neurodegeneration, and chaperones modulate these effects [204, 205]. However, there is less agreement as to which molecular species cause neurodegeneration. A prevalent idea is that oligomeric species of α-synuclein are the most neurotoxic. Overexpression of human α-synuclein in *C. elegans* also results in dopaminergic nerve cell loss and motor deficits [206]. Genome-wide screens have identified proteins involved in vesicle transport, lipid metabolism, and protein degradation as modifiers of α-synuclein toxicity, indicating that lipid binding and vesicle transport are important for early toxic events [207].

Experimental transmission of tauopathy and synucleinopathy

Tauopathy can be transmitted experimentally. Injection of brain extracts from human mutant P301S tau-expressing mice (with silver-positive inclusions) into the brain of human wild-type four-repeat tau-expressing mice (without silver-positive inclusions) induced the assembly of wild-type tau into silver-positive inclusions and the spreading of pathology from the sites of injection to neighboring brain regions [208]. The induction of tau pathology was dependent on the presence of insoluble human P301S tau. In parallel, the intercellular transfer of tau inclusions has been described in cell culture [209].

During the process leading to AD, neuronal tau inclusions form first in subcortical regions, from where they appear to spread to the transentorhinal cortex, hippocampal formation, and neocortex (Figure 2.3) [210, 211]. Two studies have shown that aggregated transgenic human mutant tau appears to recruit normal mouse tau into the inclusions [212, 213]. Both groups used an activator transgene that was driving the expression of the tetracycline trans-activator under the entorhinal cortex-specific neuropsin gene promoter, as well as a responder transgene encoding human mutant P301S tau that was only expressed in presence of the tetracycline transactivator (but see also [214]). They described the formation of tau aggregates in the entorhinal cortex, from where they spread to synaptically connected regions of the hippocampus over time.

The spreading of pathology appeared genuine, because laser capture microdissection showed either no expression or greatly reduced expression of human mutant tau outside the entorhinal cortex.

Assembled recombinant tau has also been found to promote the formation of inclusions after injection into the brains of young mice transgenic for human mutant P301S tau, followed by their propagation to distant brain regions [215, 216]. Similar findings were obtained when young mice transgenic for human P301S tau were injected with brain extracts from symptomatic P301S tau mice [217]. Contralateral and anterior/posterior spread of tau pathology was evident in nuclei with strong efferent and afferent connections to the sites of injection, indicating that the spread was dependent on synaptic connections and not on spatial proximity. The intraperitoneal injection of brain extracts from symptomatic mice transgenic for human mutant P301S tau into presymptomatic transgenic mice promoted the formation of tau inclusions in brain, albeit less efficiently than following intracerebral injection [218].

Monomeric tau has been detected in brain interstitial fluid and in cerebrospinal fluid, indicating that it can be released from nerve cells in an activity-dependent manner, despite the lack of a signal sequence [219–221]. It is unclear if tau is released in a free soluble form, if it is packaged into exosomes, or if it travels through nanotubes. It remains to be seen whether the physiological role of monomeric tau is related to the intercellular transfer of tau aggregates.

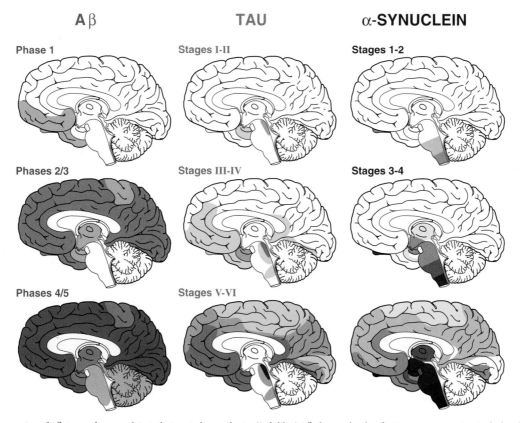

Figure 2.3 Propagation of Aβ, tau, and α-synuclein inclusions in human brain. (Left, blue) Aβ plaques develop first in one or more sites in the basal temporal and orbitofrontal neocortex (phase 1). They are observed later throughout the neocortex, in the hippocampal formation, amygdala, diencephalon, and basal ganglia (phases 2/3). In severe cases of Alzheimer's disease, Aβ plaques are also found in the mesencephalon, lower brainstem, and cerebellar cortex (phases 4/5). (Middle, green) Tau inclusions develop in subcortical areas, as well as in the transentorhinal and entorhinal regions (stages I and II). This is followed by the presence of tau inclusions in the hippocampal formation and some parts of the neocortex (stages III and IV), followed by large parts of the neocortex (stages V and VI). (Right, red) α-Synuclein-positive Lewy pathology ascends from the brainstem. The first inclusions are present in the olfactory bulb and the dorsal motor nucleus of the vagal and glossopharyngeal nerves of the medulla oblongata (stages 1 and 2). From the brainstem, the pathology appears to spread through the pons to the midbrain and basal forebrain (stages 3 and 4), followed by the neocortex (stages 5 and 6). This figure is based on the work of Braak and colleagues [210, 211, 245]. Reproduced with permission of Springer and Elsevier.

In vitro studies have shown that filaments made from recombinant tau and filaments from the brains of AD patients are taken up by cells through macropinocytosis and induce the aggregation of cytoplasmic tau [222]. Internalization of aggregated tau depended on the presence of sulfated glycosaminoglycans on the cell surface [223], similar to what has been described for some viruses [224]. Aggregated tau is released into the extracellular space, but the underlying mechanisms remain to be identified.

Neuronal and glial tau inclusions formed following the intracerebral injection of brain homogenates from humans with pathologically confirmed tauopathies into mice transgenic for wild-type human tau [225]. They were present after the injection of brain homogenates from cases of AD, tangle-only dementia, PSP, CBD, AGD, and Pick disease. Lesions reminiscent of human cases were observed following injection of AGD, PSP, and CBD brain extracts, the inclusions of which are made of four-repeat tau. The transgenic line used for injection expresses a single isoform of wild-type four-repeat human tau. Moreover, filamentous tau pathology propagated over time to neighboring brain regions, with the exception of Pick disease extracts, for which induced tau inclusions remained confined to the injected areas. These findings are compatible with the view that different tau strains exist that are capable of inducing distinct tauopathies.

These findings were confirmed and extended by work showing that morphologically distinct seeded aggregates made of four-repeat tau formed in HEK293 cells and behaved like strains [226]. Aggregate morphologies were distinct following injection into the hippocampus of young mice transgenic for human mutant P301S tau, from where they could be serially passaged. When HEK293 cells expressing four-repeat tau were seeded with tau aggregates from these brains, inclusions formed that were identical to those present to begin with.

The finding that Lewy bodies are present in grafted fetal brain cells a decade or more after transplantation into the striatum of PD patients suggested transmissibility of α-synuclein pathology [227–229]. Lewy pathology developed in the grafts, consistent with the spread of α-synuclein seeds from the diseased host tissues to the grafts, followed by nucleated assembly. In the grafts, up to 5% of dopaminergic neurons contained Lewy bodies, similar to the proportion of Lewy body-bearing neurons in the substantia nigra from PD patients. It has been estimated that nerve cells with Lewy bodies may die within 6 months of inclusion formation, with Lewy bodies and nerve cell loss reaching a steady state [230].

The acceleration of endogenous α-synuclein aggregation has been described in the brains of young, presymptomatic mice, in conjunction with an earlier onset of symptoms, following the intracerebral injection of brain tissues from older, symptomatic mice [231, 232]. The injection of brain homogenates from patients with MSA into heterozygous mice transgenic for human mutant A53T α-synuclein, which do not develop α-synuclein inclusions or neurodegeneration, induced neuronal inclusions and neurodegeneration [233, 234]. Moreover, following the intrastriatal injection of murine α-synuclein filaments into wild-type mice, a time- and connectivity-dependent spread of Lewy pathology and loss of nigral dopaminergic neurons were observed [235]. Similarly, the intranigral injection of murine and human α-synuclein filaments into wild-type mice resulted in the formation of Lewy pathology and neurodegeneration [236]. Long-term *in vivo* imaging showed that aggregated recombinant α-synuclein could seed the ordered assembly of expressed α-synuclein [237]. Inclusion-bearing neurons degenerated, demonstrating that inclusion formation was linked to cellular toxicity. The intramuscular injection of assembled recombinant α-synuclein

into presymptomatic mice transgenic for human mutant A53T α-synuclein promoted the formation of α-synuclein inclusions in brain, indicating the existence of mechanisms by which α-synuclein aggregates can be transported from muscle to brain [238].

Extracellular aggregates of α-synuclein, in both fibrillar and oligomeric forms, enter neuronal cells by receptor-mediated endocytosis and move through the endosomal pathway, to be degraded by lysosomes [239]. The recruitment of soluble α-synuclein depended on the presence of an amyloidogenic sequence [240]. Neuronal cells release α-synuclein through non-classical endocytosis; this is increased by stress and may require the misfolding of α-synuclein [241, 242]. Some of the released protein is present in exosomes [243]. In a compartmentalized culture system, α-synuclein aggregates traveled in both anterograde and retrograde directions [244].

During the process leading to PD, the first α-synuclein-positive structures in the brain form in the dorsal motor nucleus of the glossopharyngeal and vagal nerves, the intermediate reticular zone, the olfactory bulb, and the anterior olfactory nucleus (Figure 2.3) [245]. The pathology ascends from vulnerable regions in the medulla oblongata to the pontine tegmentum, midbrain, basal forebrain, and cerebral cortex. α-Synuclein deposits may even form earlier in the enteric and peripheral nervous systems, suggesting that Lewy body diseases may originate outside the central nervous system. Incidental Lewy body disease may be at one end of the spectrum, with DLB at the other end, and with Lewy body dysphagia, pure autonomic failure, and PD in-between.

Morphological differences between α-synuclein filaments have been described in human diseases [174]. The same was true when recombinantly expressed human wild-type α-synuclein was assembled into filaments *in vitro*, resulting in strain-like properties, as evidenced by different levels of toxicity, seeding, and propagation [246, 247]. Tau inclusions have also been described in some synucleinopathies [248–250] and earlier work had shown that α-synuclein can nucleate tau aggregation [251]. Experimentally, some α-synuclein fibrils seeded tau assembly, whereas others only seeded α-synuclein aggregation [252]. Both strains of aggregated α-synuclein exhibited different properties upon proteinase K digestion. They resembled prion strains in terms of their different structures, different seeding properties, and heritability of phenotypic traits.

Work over the past few years has led to the development of a unifying the theory of the mechanism of neurodegeneration. Following an initiating misfolding event, the prion-like replication and intercellular transfer of pathology may provide a mechanism for the rapid propagation of protein inclusions through the nervous system. A stochastic misfolding event may be the primary cause, with the subsequent influence of more deterministic processes. This notwithstanding, the early misfolding of a given disease protein appears to be non-random at the level of brain regions, suggesting that selective neuronal vulnerability may also play an important role. The existence of a variety of dementing and movement disorders with tau and α-synuclein deposits suggests the existence of distinct tau prion strains and α-synuclein prion strains.

Additional therapeutic implications

Much has been learned about the mechanisms underlying human tauopathies and synucleinopathies, and relevant animal models have been generated. Aggregation of tau and α-synuclein is at the heart of the neurodegenerative process. Consequently, work aimed at reducing aggregation is central for the development of mechanism-based therapies. As aggregation is concentration dependent, safe reduction in the levels of soluble tau and α-synuclein is an important therapeutic objective.

A reduction in tau might be achieved through antisense or RNA interference approaches [253], or through decreased expression [254]. As described previously, a partial reduction of tau is well tolerated. Soluble tau is degraded by the ubiquitin-proteasome system, with the carboxy-terminus of heat shock protein 70-interacting protein (CHIP) and heat shock protein 90 playing important roles [255–257].

An increase in the degradation of tau aggregates is a complementary approach. Aggregates are probably not accessible to the ubiquitin-proteasome system, but may be degraded by the autophagy/lysosome system. Activation of autophagy by trehalose has led to a reduction in tau aggregation and neurodegeneration in mice transgenic for human mutant P301S tau [258].

The mechanisms that regulate the expression of α-synuclein in vivo are poorly understood. More is known about its clearance. Monoubiquitination promotes the degradation of α-synuclein by the proteasome, with SIAH-2 and USP9X playing key roles [259, 260]. The autophagy/lysosome system was initially believed to be involved only in the clearance of aggregated α-synuclein, but it now appears that degradation by the lysosome may also contribute to the turnover of soluble forms of the protein [261, 262]. Treatment with α-synuclein small interfering RNA rescued total and aggregated α-synuclein levels in mouse brain [263]. Moreover, boosting the degradation of α-synuclein has also been shown to be effective [264, 265].

Degradation of tau can be enhanced through activation of the immune system [266]. This is especially relevant, given the spreading of tau pathology [267]. Immunization targeting phosphorylated tau reduced tau inclusions and nerve cell dysfunction. Similar findings have been reported in mouse models of synucleinopathies [268].

Acknowledgments

MG is an Honorary Professor in the Department of Clinical Neurosciences, University of Cambridge. He is supported by the UK Medical Research Council (MC_U105184291) and the EU Joint Programme – Neurodegenerative Disease Research.

References

1. Alzheimer A. Über eine eigenartige Erkrankung der Hirnrinde. *Allg. Z. Psychiat.* 1907; 64: 146–148.
2. Fischer O. Miliare Nekrosen mit drusigen Wucherungen der Neurofibrillen, eine regelmässige Veränderung der Hirnrinde bei seniler Demenz. *Monatsschr Psychiat Neurol* 1907; 22: 361–372.
3. Kraepelin E. Psychiatrie. Ein Lehrbuch für Studierende und Ärzte, 8. Auflage, Band II: Klinische Psychiatrie. Barth, Leipzig, 1910.
4. Alzheimer A. Über eigenartige Krankheitsfälle des späteren Alters. *Z ges Neurol Psychiat* 1911; 4: 356–385.
5. Pick A. Über die Beziehungen der senilen Hirnatrophie zur Aphasie. *Prager Med Wochenschr* 1892; 17: 165–167.
6. Lewy F. Paralysis agitans. I. Pathologische Anatomie. *In: Handbuch der Neurologie* Vol. 3 (eds M Lewandowsky and G Abelsdorff), pp. 920–933. Springer, Berlin, 1912.
7. Kidd M. Paired helical filaments in electron microscopy of Alzheimer's disease. *Nature* 1963; 197: 192–193.
8. Terry RD, Gonatas NK, Weiss M. Ultrastructural studies in Alzheimer's presenile dementia. *Am J Pathol* 1964; 44: 269–297.
9. Duffy PE and Tennyson VM. Phase and electron microscopic observations of Lewy bodies and melanin granules in the substantia nigra and locus coeruleus in Parkinson's disease. *J Neuropathol Exp Neurol* 1965; 24: 398–414.
10. Spillantini MG, Goedert M. Tau pathology and neurodegeneration. *Lancet Neurol* 2013; 12: 609–622.
11. Goedert M, Spillantini MG, Del Tredici K et al. 100 years of Lewy pathology. *Nature Rev Neurol* 2013; 9: 13–24.
12. Brion JP, Passareiro H, Nunez J et al. Mise en évidence immunologique de la protéine tau au niveau des lésions de dégénérescence neurofibrillaire de la maladie d'Alzheimer. *Arch Biol* 1985; 95: 229–235.
13. Grundke-Iqbal I, Iqbal K, Tung YC et al. Abnormal phosphorylation of the microtubule-associated protein tau in Alzheimer cytoskeletal pathology. *Proc Natl Acad Sci USA* 1986; 83: 4913–4917.
14. Goedert M, Wischik CM, Crowther RA et al. Cloning and sequencing of the cDNA encoding a core protein of the paired helical filament of Alzheimer disease: identification as the microtubule-associated protein tau. *Proc Natl Acad Sci USA* 1988; 85: 4051–4055.
15. Wischik CM, Novak M, Thogersen HC et al. Isolation of a fragment of tau derived from the core of the paired helical filament of Alzheimer disease. *Proc Natl Acad Sci USA* 1988; 85: 4506–4510.
16. Kondo J, Honda T, Mori H et al. The carboxyl third of tau is tightly bound to paired helical filaments. *Neuron* 1988; 1: 827–834.
17. Lee VMY, Balin BJ, Otvos L et al. A68: a major subunit of paired helical filaments and derivatized forms of normal tau. *Science* 1991; 251: 675–678.
18. Pollock NJ, Mirra SS, Binder LI et al. Filamentous aggregates in Pick's disease, progressive supranuclear palsy, and Alzheimer's disease share antigenic determinants with microtubule-associated protein tau. *Lancet* 1986; II: 1211.
19. Spillantini MG, Schmidt ML, Lee VMY et al. α-Synuclein in Lewy bodies. *Nature* 1997; 388: 839–840.
20. Poorkaj P, Bird TD, Wijsman E et al. Tau is a candidate gene for chromosome 17 frontotemporal dementia. *Ann Neurol* 1998; 43: 815–825.
21. Hutton M, Lendon CL, Rizzu P et al. Association of missense and 5'-splice site mutations in *tau* with the inherited dementia FTDP-17. *Nature* 1998; 393: 702–705.
22. Spillantini MG, Murrell JR, Goedert M et al. Mutation in the tau gene in familial multiple system tauopathy with presenile dementia. *Proc Natl Acad Sci USA* 1998; 95: 7737–7741.
23. Polymeropoulos MHC, Leroy E, Ide SE et al. Mutation in the alpha-synuclein gene identified in families with Parkinson's disease. *Science* 1997; 276: 2045–2047.
24. Singleton AB, Farrer M, Johnson J et al. alpha-Synuclein locus triplication causes Parkinson's disease. *Science* 2003; 302: 841.
25. Astbury WT, Dickinson S, Bailey K. The X-ray interpretation of denaturation and the structure of the seed globulins. *Biochem J* 1935; 29: 2351–2360.
26. Cohen AS, Calkins E. Electron microscopic observations on a fibrous component in amyloid of diverse origins. *Nature* 1959; 183: 1202–1203.
27. Eanes ED, Glenner GG. X-ray diffraction studies on amyloid filaments. *J Histochem Cytochem* 1968; 16: 673–677.
28. Eisenberg D, Jucker M. The amyloid state of proteins in human diseases. *Cell* 2012; 148: 1188–1203.
29. Knowles TPJ, Vendruscolo M, Dobson CM. The amyloid state and its association with protein misfolding diseases. *Nat Rev Mol Cell Biol* 2014; 15: 384–396.
30. Sawaya MR, Sambashivan S, Nelson R et al. Atomic structures of amyloid cross-β spines reveal varied steric zippers. *Nature* 2007; 447: 453–457.
31. Sievers SA, Karanicolas J, Chang HW et al. Structure-based design of non-natural amino-acid inhibitors of amyloid fibril formation. *Nature* 2011; 475: 96–100.
32. Ittner LM, Ke YD, Delerue F et al. Dendritic function of tau mediates amyloid-beta toxicity in Alzheimer's disease mouse models. *Cell* 2010; 142: 387–397.
33. Goedert M, Spillantini MG, Jakes R et al. Multiple isoforms of human microtubule-associated protein tau: Sequences and localization in neurofibrillary tangles of Alzheimer's disease. *Neuron* 1989; 3: 519–526.
34. Goedert M, Jakes R. Expression of separate isoforms of human tau protein: Correlation with the tau pattern in brain and effects on tubulin polymerization. *EMBO J* 1990; 9: 4225–4230.
35. Fauquant C, Redeker V, Landrieu I et al. Systematic identification of tubulin-interacting fragmenmts of the microtubule-associated protein tau leads to a highly efficient promoter of microtubule assembly. *J Biol Chem* 2011; 286: 33358–33368.
36. Kar S, Fan J, Smith MJ. Repeat motifs of tau bind to the insides of microtubules in the absence of taxol. *EMBO J* 2003; 22: 70–77.
37. Al-Bassam J, Ozer RS, Safer D et al. MAP2 and tau bind longitudinally along the outer ridges of microtubule protofilaments. *J Cell Biol* 2002; 157: 1187–1195.
38. Kadavath H, Höfele RV, Biernat J et al. Tau stabilizes microtubules by binding at the interface between tubulin heterodimers. *Proc Natl Acad Sci USA* 2015; 112: 7501–7506.
39. Yoshida H, Goedert M. Molecular cloning and functional characterization of chicken brain tau: Isoforms with up to five tandem repeats. *Biochemistry* 2002; 41: 15203–15211.
40. Götz J, Probst A, Spillantini MG et al. Somatodendritic localisation and hyperphosphorylation of tau protein in transgenic mice expressing the longest human brain tau isoform. *EMBO J* 1995; 14: 1304–1313.
41. Goedert M, Baur CP, Ahringer J et al. PTL-1, a microtubule-associated protein with tau-like repeats from the nematode *Caenorhabditis elegans*. *J Cell Sci* 1996; 109: 2661–2672.

42. Heidary G, Fortini ME. Identification and characterization of the *Drosophila* tau homolog. *Mech Dev* 2001; 108: 171–178.

43. Harada A, Oguchi K, Okabe S et al. Altered microtubule organization in small-calibre axons of mice lacking tau protein. *Nature* 1994; 369: 488–491.

44. Ikegami S, Harada A, Hirokawa N. Muscle weakness, hyperactivity, and impairment in fear conditioning in tau-deficient mice. *Neurosci Lett* 2000; 279: 129–132.

45. Kimura T, Whitcomb DJ, Jo J et al. Microtubule-associated protein tau is essential for long-term depression in the hippocampus. *Phil Trans R Soc B* 2014; 369: 20130144.

46. Wegmann S, Medalsy ID, Mandelkow E et al. The fuzzy coat of pathological human tau fibrils is a two-layered polyelectrolyte brush. *Proc Natl Acad Sci USA* 2013; 110: E313-E321.

47. Khlistunova I, Biernat J, Wang Y et al. Inducible expression of tau repeat domain in cell models of tauopathy. Aggregation is toxic to cells but can be reversed by inhibitor drugs. *J Biol Chem* 2006; 281: 1205–1214.

48. Lewis J, McGowan E, Rockwood J et al. Neurofibrillary tangles, amyotrophy and progressive motor disturbance in mice expressing mutant (P301L) tau protein. *Nat Genet* 2000; 25: 402–405.

49. Allen B, Ingram E, Takao M et al. Abundant tau filaments and nonapoptotic neurodegeneration in transgenic mice expressing human P301S tau protein. *J Neurosci* 2002; 22: 9340–9351.

50. Berriman J, Serpell LC, Oberg KA et al. Tau filaments from human brain and from *in vitro* assembly of recombinant protein show cross-β structure. *Proc Natl Acad Sci USA* 2003; 100: 9034–9038.

51. Daebel V, Chinnathambi S, Biernat J et al. β-Sheet core of tau paired helical filaments revealed by solid-state NMR. *J Am Chem Soc* 2012; 134: 13982–13989.

52. Goedert M, Jakes R, Spillantini MG et al. Assembly of microtubule-associated protein tau into Alzheimer-like filaments induced by sulphated glycosaminoglycans. *Nature* 1996; 383: 550–553.

53. Pérez M, Valpuesta JM, Medina M et al. Polymerization of tau into filaments in the presence of heparin: the minimal sequence required for tau-tau interactions. *J Neurochem* 1996; 67: 1183–1190.

54. Kampers T, Friedhoff P, Biernat J et al. RNA stimulates aggregation of microtubule-associated protein tau into Alzheimer-like paired helical filaments. *FEBS Lett* 1996; 399: 344–349.

55. Wilson DM, Binder LI. Free fatty acids stimulate the polymerization of tau and amyloid beta peptides. *Am J Pathol* 1997; 150: 2181–2195.

56. Elbaum-Garfinkle S, Rhoades E. Identification of an aggregation-prone structure of tau. *J Am Chem Soc* 2012; 134: 16607–16613.

57. Carmel G, Mager EM, Binder LI et al. The structural basis of monoclonal antibody Alz50's selectivity for Alzheimer's disease pathology. *J Biol Chem* 1996; 20: 32789–32795.

58. Jicha GA, Bowser R, Kazam IG et al. Alz-50 and MC-1, a new monoclonal antibody raised to paired helical filaments, recognize conformational epitopes on recombinant tau. *J Neurosci Res* 1997; 48: 128–132.

59. Ramachandran G, Udgaonkar JB. Mechanistic studies unravel the complexity inherent in tau aggregation leading to Alzheimer's disease and the tauopathies. *Biochemistry* 2013; 52: 4107–4126.

60. Von Bergen M, Friedhoff P, Biernat J et al. Assembly of tau protein into Alzheimer paired helical filaments depends on a local sequence motif [(306)VQIVYK(311)] forming beta structure. *Proc Natl Acad Sci USA* 2000; 97: 5129–5134.

61. Von Bergen M, Barghorn S, Li L et al. Mutations of tau protein in frontotemporal dementia promote aggregation of paired helical filaments by enhancing local β-structure. *J Biol Chem* 2001; 276: 48165–48174.

62. Taniguchi S, Suzuki N, Masuda M et al. Inhibition of heparin-induced tau filament formation by phenothiazines, polyphenols and porphyrins. *J Biol Chem* 2005; 280: 7614–7623.

63. Crowe A, Huang W, Ballatore C et al. Identification of aminothienopyridazine inhibitors of tau assembly by quantitative high-throughput screening. *Biochemistry* 2009; 48: 7732–7745.

64. Bulic B, Pickhardt M, Mandelkow W. Progress and developments in tau aggregation inhibitors for Alzheimer disease. *J Med Chem* 2013; 56: 4135–4155.

65. Kanaan NM, Morfini GA, LaPointe NE et al. Pathogenic forms of tau inhibit kinesin-dependent axonal transport through a mechanism involving activation of axonal phosphotransferases. *J Neurosci* 2011; 31: 9858–9868.

66. Bramblett GT, Goedert M, Jakes R et al. Abnormal tau phosphorylation at Ser396 in Alzheimer's disease recapitulates development and contributes to reduced microtubule binding. *Neuron* 1993; 10: 1089–1099.

67. Yoshida H, Ihara Y. Tau in paired helical filaments is functionally distinct from fetal tau: assembly incompetence of paired helical filament-tau. *J Neurochem* 1993; 61: 1183–1186.

68. Hanger DP, Anderton BH, Noble W. Tau phosphorylation: the therapeutic challenge for neurodegenerative disease. *Trends Mol Med* 2009; 15: 112–119.

69. Goedert M, Jakes R, Crowther RA et al. The abnormal phosphorylation of tau protein at Ser202 in Alzheimer disease recapitulates phosphorylation during development. *Proc Natl Acad Sci USA* 1993; 90: 5066–5070.

70. Arendt T, Stieler J, Strijkstra AM et al. Reversible paired helical filament-like phosphorylation of tau is an adaptive process associated with neuronal plasticity in hibernating animals. *J Neurosci* 2003; 23: 6972–6981.

71. Arendt T, Bullmann T. Neuronal plasticity in hibernation and the proposed role of the microtubule-associated protein tau as a "master switch" regulating synaptic gain in neuronal networks. *Am J Physiol* 2013; 305: R478–R489.

72. Planel E, Miyasaka T, Launey T et al. Alterations in glucose metabolism induce hypothermia leading to tau hyperphosphorylation through differential inhibition of kinase and phosphatase activities: Implications for Alzheimer's disease. *J Neurosci* 2004; 24: 2401–2411.

73. Min SW, Cho SH, Zghou Y et al. Actetylation of tau inhibits its degradation and contributes to tauopathy. *Neuron* 2010; 67: 953–966.

74. Cohen TJ, Guo JL, Hurtado D et al. The acetylation of tau inhibits its function and promotes pathological tau aggregation. *Nat Commun* 2011; 2: 252.

75. Irwin DJ, Cohen TJ, Grossman M et al. Acetylated tau, a novel pathological signature in Alzheimer's disease and other tauopathies. *Brain* 2012; 135: 807–818.

76. Arnold CS, Johnson GVW, Cole RN et al. The microtubule-associated protein tau is extensively modified with O-linked N-acetylglucosamine. *J Biol Chem* 1996; 271: 28741–28744.

77. Reynolds MR, Reyes JF, Fu Y et al. Tau nitration occurs at tyrosine 29 in the fibrillar lesions of Alzheimer's disease and other tauopathies. *J Neurosci* 2006; 26: 10636–10645.

78. Lu PJ, Wulf G, Zhou XZ et al. The prolyl isomerase Pin1 restores the function of Alzheimer-associated phosphorylated tau protein. *Nature* 1999; 399: 784–788.

79. Nakamura K, Greenwood A, Binder LI et al. Proline isomer-specific antibodies reveal the early pathogenic tau conformation in Alzheimer's disesase. *Cell* 2012; 149: 232–244.

80. Smith MA, Taneda S, Richey PL et al. Advanced Maillard reaction end products are associated with Alzheimer disease pathology. *Proc Natl Acad Sci USA* 1994; 91: 5710–5714.

81. Ledesma MD, Bonay P, Colaco C et al. Analysis of microtubule-associated protein tau glycation in paired helical filaments. *J Biol Chem* 1994; 269: 21614–21619.

82. Mori H, Kondo J, Ihara Y. Ubiquitin is a component of paired helical filaments in Alzheimer's disease. *Science* 1987; 235: 1641–1644.

83. Cripps D, Thomas SN, Jeng Y et al. Alzheimer disease-specific conformation of hyperphosphorylated paired helical filament-tau is polyubiquitinated through Lys-48, Lys-11 and Lys-6 ubiquitin conjugation. *J Biol Chem* 2006; 281: 10825–10831.

84. Goedert M, Spillantini MG, Cairns NJ et al. Tau proteins of Alzheimer paired helical filaments: Abnormal phosphorylation of all six brain isoforms. *Neuron* 1992; 8: 159–168.

85. Flament S, Delacourte A, Verny M et al. Abnormal tau proteins in progressive supranuclear palsy. Similarities and differences with the neurofibrillary degeneration of the Alzheimer type. *Acta Neuropathol* 1991; 81: 591–596.

86. Spillantini MG, Goedert M, Crowther RA et al. Familial multiple system tauopathy with presenile dementia: a disease with abundant neuronal and glial tau filaments. *Proc Natl Acad Sci USA* 1997; 94: 4113–4118.

87. Ksiezak-Reding H, Morgan K, Mattiace LA et al. Ultrastructure and biochemical composition of paired helical filaments in corticobasal degeneration. *Am J Pathol* 1994; 145: 1496–1508.

88. Tolnay M, Sergeant N, Ghestem A et al. Argyrophilic grain disease and Alzheimer's disease are distinguished by their different distribution of tau protein isoforms. *Acta Neuropathol* 2002; 104: 425–434.

89. Delacourte A, Robitaille Y, Sergeant N et al. Specific pathological tau protein variants characterize Pick's disease. *J Neuropathol Exp Neurol* 1996; 55: 159–168.

90. Crowther RA, Goedert M. Abnormal tau-containing filaments in neurodegenerative diseases. *J Struct Biol* 2000; 130: 271–279.

91. Prusiner SB. Biology and genetics of prions causing neurodegeneration. *Annu Rev Genet* 2013; 47: 601–623.

92. Dinkel PD, Siddiqua A, Huynh H et al. Variations in filament conformation dictate seeding barrier between three- and four-repeat tau. *Biochemistry* 2011; 50: 4330–4336.

93. Wilhelmsen KC, Lynch T, Pavlou E et al. Localization of disinhibition-dementia-parkinsonism-amyotrophy complex to 17q21-22. *Am J Hum Genet* 1994; 55: 1159–1165.

94. Foster NL, Wilhelmsen K, Sima AA et al. Frontotemporal dementia and parkinsonism linked to chromosome 17: a consensus conference. *Ann Neurol* 1997; 41: 706–715.

95. Baker M, Mackenzie IR, Pickering-Brown SM et al. Mutations in progranulin cause tau-negative frontotemporal dementia linked to chromosome 17. *Nature* 2006; 442: 916–919.

96. Cruts M, Gijselinck I, Van der Zee et al. Null mutations in progranulin cause ubiquitin-positive frontotemporal dementia linked to chromosome 17q21. *Nature* 2006; 442: 920–924.

97. Goedert M, Ghetti B, Spillantini MG. Frontotemporal dementia. Implications for understanding Alzheimer disease. *Cold Spring Harb Perspect Med* 2012; 2: a006254.

98. Bugiani O, Murrell JR, Giaccone G et al. Frontotemporal dementia and cortico-basal degeneration in a family with a P301S mutation in *Tau*. *J Neuropathol Exp Neurol* 1999; 58: 667–677.

99. Stefansson H, Helgason A, Thorleifsson G et al. A common inversion under selection in Europeans. *Nat Genet* 2005; 37: 129–137.

100. Conrad C, Andreadis A, Trojanowski JQ et al. Genetic evidence for the involvement of tau in progressive supranuclear palsy. *Ann Neurol* 1997; 41: 277–281.

101. Baker M, Litvan I, Houlden H et al. Association of an extended haplotype in the tau gene with progressive supranuclear palsy. *Hum Mol Genet* 1999; 8: 711–715.

102. Houlden H, Baker M, Morris HR et al. Corticobasal degeneration and progressive supranuclear palsy share a common haplotype. *Neurology* 2001; 56: 1702–1706.

103. Pastor P, Ezquerra M, Munoz E et al. Significant association between the tau gene A0/A0 genotype and Parkinson's disease. *Ann Neurol* 2000; 47: 242–245.

104. Höglinger GU, Melhem NM, Dickson DW et al. Identification of common variants influencing risk of the tauopathy progressive supranuclear palsy. *Nat Genet* 2011; 43: 699–705.

105. Caffrey TM, Joachim C, Wade-Martins R. Haplotype-specific expression of the N-terminal exons 2 and 3 at the human *MAPT* locus. *Neurobiol Aging* 2008; 29: 1923–1929.

106. Valenca GT, Srivastava GP, Oliveiro-Filho J, et al. The role of *MAPT* haplotype H2 and isoform 1N/4R in parkinsonism of older adults. *PLoS ONE* 2016; 11: e0157452.

107. Zhong Q, Congdon EE, Nagaraja HN et al. Tau isoform composition influences rate and extent of filament formation. *J Biol Chem* 2012; 287: 20711–20719.

108. Koolen DA, Vissers LELM, Pfundt R et al. A new chromosome 17q21.31 microdeletion syndrome associated with a common inversion polymorphism. *Nat Genet* 2006; 38: 999–1001.

109. Sharp AJ, Hansen S, Selzer RR et al. Discovery of previously unidentified genomic disorders from the duplication architecture of the human genome. *Nat Genet* 2006; 68: 812–814.

110. Shaw-Smith C, Pittman AM, Willatt L et al. Microdeletion encompassing *MAPT* at chromosome 17q21.3 is associated with developmental delay and learning disability. *Nat Genet* 2006; 38: 1032–1037.

111. Zollino M, Orteschi D, Murdolo M et al. Mutations in *KANSL1* cause the 17q21.31 microdeletion syndrome phenotype. *Nat Genet* 2012; 44: 636–638.

112. Koolen DA, Kramer JM, Neveling K et al. Mutations in the chromatin modifier gene *KANSL1* cause the 17q21.31 microdeletion syndrome. *Nat Genet* 2012; 44: 639–641.

113. Götz J, Chen F, Barmettler R et al. Tau filament formation in transgenic mice expressing P301L tau. *J Biol Chem* 2001; 276: 529–534.

114. Yoshiyama Y, Higuchi M, Zhang B et al. Synapse loss and microglial activation precede tangles in a P301S tauopathy mouse model. *Neuron* 2007; 53: 337–351.

115. Lewis J, Dickson DW, Lin WL et al. Enhanced neurofibrillary degeneration in transgenic mice expressing mutant tau and APP. *Science* 2001; 293: 1487–1491.

116. Bolmont T, Clavaguera F, Meyer-Luehmann M et al. Induction of tau pathology by intracerebral infusion of amyloid-beta-containing brain extract and by amyloid-beta deposition in APP x Tau transgenic mice. *Am J Pathol* 2007; 171: 2012–2020.

117. Coomaraswamy J, Kilger E, Wölfing H et al. Modeling familial Danish dementia in mice supports the concept of the amyloid hypothesis of Alzheimer's disease. *Proc Natl Acad Sci USA* 2010; 107: 7969–7674.

118. Roberson ED, Scearce-Levie K, Palop JJ et al. Reducing endogenous tau ameliorates amyloid-β-induced deficits in an Alzheimer's disease model. *Science* 2007; 316: 750–754.

119. Huang Y, Mucke L. Alzheimer mechanisms and therapeutic strategies. *Cell* 2012; 148: 1204–1222.

120. Larson M, Sherman MW, Amar F et al. The complex PrP^C-Fyn couples human oligomeric Aβ with pathological tau changes in Alzheimer's disease. *J Neurosci* 2012; 32: 16857–16871.

121. Hoover BR, Reed MN, Su J et al. Tau mislocalization to dendritic spines mediates synaptic dysfunction independently of neurodegeneration. *Neuron* 2010; 68: 1067–1081.

122. Merino-Serrais P, Benavides-Piccione R, Blazquez-Llorca L et al. The influence of phospho-tau on dendritic spines of cortical pyramidal neurons in patients with Alzheimer's disease. *Brain* 2013; 136: 1913–1928.

123. Andorfer C, Kress Y, Espinoza M et al. Hyperphosphorylation and aggregation of tau in mice expressing normal human tau isoforms. *J Neurochem* 2003; 86: 582–590.

124. Siman R, Loin YG, Malthankar-Phatak G et al. A rapid gene delivery-based mouse model for early-stage Alzheimer disease-type tauopathy. *J Neuropathol Exp Neurol* 2013; 72: 1062–1071.

125. Klein RL, Dayton RD, Diaczynsky CG et al. Pronounced microgliosis and neurodegeneration in aged rats after tau gene transfer. *Neurobiol Aging* 2010; 31: 2091–2102.

126. Caillierez R, Bégard S, Lécolle K et al. Lentiviral delivery of the human wild-type tau protein mediates a slow and progressive neurodegenerative tau pathology in the rat brain. *Mol Ther* 2013; 21: 1358–1368.

127. SantaCruz K, Lewis J, Spires T et al. Tau suppression in a neurodegenerative mouse model improves memory function. *Science* 2005; 309: 476–481.

128. Noble W, Planel E, Zehr C et al. Inhibition of glycogen synthase kinase-3 by lithium correlates with reduced tauopathy and degeneration *in vivo*. *Proc Natl Acad Sci USA* 2005; 102: 6900–6905.

129. Van Eersel J, Ke YD, Liu X et al. Sodium selenate mitigates tau pathology, neurodegeneration, and functional deficits in Alzheimer's disease models. *Proc Natl Acad Sci USA* 2010; 107: 13888–13893.

130. Yuzwa SA, Shan X, Macauley MS et al. Increasing O-GlcNAc slows neurodegeneration and stabilizes tau against aggregation. *Nat Chem Biol* 2012; 8: 393–399.

131. Carroll JC, Iba M, Bangasser DA et al. Chronic stress exacerbates tau pathology, neurodegeneration, and cognitive performance through a corticotrophin-releasing factor receptor-dependent mechanism in a transgenic mouse model of tauopathy. *J Neurosci* 2011; 5: 14436–14449.

132. Wittmann CW, Wszolek MF, Shulman JH et al. Tauopathy in *Drosophila*: Neurodegeneration without neurofibrillary tangles. *Science* 2001; 293: 711–714.

133. Kraemer BC, Zhang B, Leverenz JB et al. Neurodegeneration and defective neurotransmission in a *Caenorhabditis elegans* model of tauopathy. *Proc Natl Acad Sci USA* 2003; 100: 9980–9985.

134. Feany MB. New approaches to the pathology and genetics of neurodegeneration. *Am J Pathol* 2010; 176: 2058–2066.

135. Guthrie CR, Schellenberg GD, Kraemer BC. SUT-2 potentiates tau-induced neurotoxicity in *Caenorhabditis elegans*. *Hum Mol Genet* 2009; 18: 1825–1838.

136. Weinreb PH, Zhen W, Poon AW et al. NACP, a protein implicated in Alzheimer's disease and learning, is natively unfolded. *Biochemistry* 1996; 35: 13709–13715.

137. Bartels T, Choi JG, Selkoe DJ. α-Synuclein occurs physiologically as a helically folded tetramer that resists aggregation. *Nature* 2011; 477: 107–110.

138. Davidson WS, Jonas A, Clayton DF et al. Stabilization of α-synuclein secondary structure upon binding to synthetic membranes. *J Biol Chem* 1998; 273: 9443–9449.

139. Eliezer D, Kutluay E, Bussell R et al. Conformational properties of alpha-synuclein in its free and lipid-associated states. *J Mol Biol* 2001; 307: 1061–1073.

140. Fusco G, De Simone A, Gopinath T et al. Direct observation of the three regions in α-synuclein that determine its membrane-bound behaviour. *Nat Commun* 2014; 5: 3827.

141. Jao CC, Der-Sarkissian A, Chen J et al. Structure of membrane-bound alpha-synuclein studied by site-directed spin labelling. *Proc Natl Acad Sci USA* 2004; 101: 8331–8336.

142. Varkey J, Isas JM, Mizuno N et al. Membrane curvature induction and tubulation are common features of synucleins and apolipoproteins. *J Biol Chem* 2010; 285: 32486–32493.

143. Burré J, Sharma M, Südhof TC. α-Synuclein assembles into higher-order multimers upon membrane binding to promote SNARE complex formation. *Proc Natl Acad Sci USA* 2014; 111: E4274–E4283.

144. DeWitt DC, Rhoades E. α-Synuclein can inhibit SNARE-mediated vesicle fusion through direct interactions with lipid bilayers. *Biochemistry* 2013; 52: 2385–2387.

145. Okochi M, Walter J, Koyama A et al. Constitutive phosphorylation of the Parkinson's disease-associated alpha-synuclein. *J Biol Chem* 2000; 275: 390–397.

146. Goedert M. Alpha-synuclein and neurodegenerative diseases. *Nat Rev Neurosci* 2001; 2: 492–501.

147. Abeliovich A, Schmitz Y, Farinas I et al. Mice lacking α-synuclein display functional deficits in the nigrostriatal dopamine system. *Neuron* 2000; 25: 239–252.

148. Greten-Harrison B, Polydoro M, Morimoto-Tomita M et al. αβγ-Synuclein triple knockout mice reveal age-dependent neuronal dysfunction. *Proc Natl Acad Sci USA* 2010; 107: 19573–19578.

149. Krüger R, Kuhn W, Müller T et al. Ala30Pro mutation in the gene encoding alpha-synuclein in Parkinson's disease. *Nat Genet* 1998; 18: 106–108.

150. Zarranz JJ, Alegre J, Gómez-Esteban JC et al. The new mutation, E46K, of alpha-synuclein causes Parkinson and Lewy body dementia. *Ann Neurol* 2004; 55: 164–173.

151. Proukakis C, Dudzik CG, Brier T et al. A novel α-synuclein missense mutation in Parkinson disease. *Neurology* 2013; 80: 1062–1064.

152. Appel-Cresswell S, Vilarino-Guell C, Encarnacion M et al. Alpha-synuclein p.H50Q, a novel pathogenic mutation for Parkinson's disease. *Mov Disord* 2013; 28: 811–813.

153. Kiely AP, Asi YT, Kara E et al. α-Synucleinopathy associated with G51D *SNCA* mutation: a link between Parkinson's disease and multiple system atrophy? *Acta Neuropathol* 2013; 125: 753–769.

154. Lesage S, Anheim M, Letournel F et al. G51D α-synuclein mutation causes a novel parkinsonian-pyramidal syndrome. *Ann Neurol* 2013; 73: 459–471.

155. Pasanen P, Myllykangas L, Siitonen M et al. A novel α-synuclein mutation A53E associated with atypical multiple system atrophy and Parkinson's disease-type pathology. *Neurobiol Aging* 20140; 35: 2180.e1–2180.e5.

156. Chartier-Harlin MC, Kachergus J, Roumier C et al. α-Synuclein locus duplication as a cause of familial Parkinson's disease. *Lancet* 2004; 364: 1167–1169.

157. Ibanez P, Bonnet AM, Débarges B et al. Causal relation between α-synuclein gene duplication and familial Parkinson's disease. *Lancet* 2004; 364: 1169–1171.

158. Satake W, Nakabayashi Y, Mizuta I et al. Genome-wide association study identifies common variants at four loci as genetic risk factors for Parkinson's disease. *Nat Genet* 2009; 41: 1303–1307.

159. Simón-Sanchez J, Schulte C, Bras JM et al. Genome-wide association study reveals genetic risk underlying Parkinson's disease. *Nat Genet* 2009; 41: 1308–1312.

160. Spillantini MG, Crowther RA, Jakes R et al. α-Synuclein in filamentous inclusions of Lewy bodies from Parkinson's disease and dementia with Lewy bodies. *Proc Natl Acad Sci USA* 1998; 95: 6469–6473.

161. Baba M, Nakajo S, Tu PH et al. Aggregation of α-synuclein in Lewy bodies of sporadic Parkinson's disease and dementia with Lewy bodies. *Am J Pathol* 1998; 152: 879–884.

162. Serpell LC, Berriman J, Jakes R et al. Fiber diffraction of synthetic α-synuclein filaments shows amyloid-like cross-β conformation. *Proc Natl Acad Sci USA* 2000; 97: 4897–4902.

163. Rodriguez JA, Ivanova MI, Sawaya MR et al. Structure of the toxic core of α-synuclein from invisible crystals. *Nature* 2015; 525: 486–490.

164. Tuttle MD, Comellas G, Nieuwkoop AJ et al. Solid-state NMR structure of a pathogenic fibril of full-length human α-synuclein. *Nat Struct Mol Biol* 2016; 23: 409–415.

165. Fujiwara H, Hasegawa M, Dohmae N et al. α-Synuclein is phosphorylated in synucleinopathy lesions. *Nat Cell Biol* 2002; 4: 160–164.

166. Anderson JP, Walker DE, Goldstein JM et al. Phosphorylation of Ser-129 is the dominant pathological modification of α-synuclein in familial and sporadic Lewy body disease. *J Biol Chem* 2006; 281: 29739–29752.

167. Fearnley JM, Lees AJ. Ageing and Parkinson's disease: Substantia nigra regional selectivity. *Brain* 1991; 114: 2283–2301.

168. Dickson DW, Fujishiro H, Delledonne A et al. Evidence that incidental Lewy body disease is presymptomatic Parkinson's disease. *Acta Neuropathol* 2008; 115: 437–444.

169. Beach TG, Adler CH, Sue LI et al. Reduced striatal tyrosine hydroxylase in incidental Lewy body disease. *Acta Neuropathol* 2008; 115: 445–451.

170. Kanazawa T, Adachi E, Orino S et al. Pale neurites, premature α-synuclein aggregates with centripetal extension from axon collaterals. *Brain Pathol* 2012; 22: 67–78.

171. Cremades N, Cohen SIA, Deas E et al. Direct observation of the interconversion of normal and toxic forms of α-synuclein. *Cell* 2012; 149: 1048–1059.

172. Papp MI, Kahn JE, Lantos PL. Glial cytoplasmic inclusions in the CNS of patients with multiple system atrophy. *J Neurol Sci* 1989; 94: 79–100.

173. Wakabayashi K, Yoshimoto M, Tsuji S et al. α-Synuclein immunoreactivity in glial cytoplasmic inclusions in multiple system atrophy. *Neurosci Lett* 1998; 249: 180–182.

174. Spillantini MG, Crowther RA, Jakes R et al. Filamentous α-synuclein inclusions link multiple system atrophy with Parkinson's disease and dementia with Lewy bodies. *Neurosci Lett* 1998; 251: 205–208.

175. Tu PH, Galvin JE, Baba M et al. Glial cytoplasmic inclusions in white matter oligodendrocytes of multiple system atrophy brains contain insoluble α-synuclein. *Ann Neurol* 1998; 44: 415–422.

176. Scholz SW, Houlden H, Schulte C et al. *SNCA* variants are associated with increased risk for multiple system atrophy. *Ann Neurol* 2009; 65: 610–614.

177. Al-Chalabi A, Dürr A, Wood NW et al. Genetic variants of the α-synuclein gene *SNCA* are associated with multiple system atrophy. *PLoS ONE* 2009; 4: e7114.

178. Parkkinen L, Hartikainen P, Alazuloff I. Abundant glial alpha-synuclein pathology in a case without overt clinical symptoms. *Clin Neuropathol* 2007; 26: 276–283.

179. Fujishiro H, Ahn TM, Frigerio R et al. Glial cytoplasmic inclusions in neurologically normal elderly: prodromal multiple system atrophy? *Acta Neuropathol* 2008; 116: 269–275.

180. Conway KA, Harper JD, Lansbury PT. Accelerated *in vitro* fibril formation by a mutant α-synuclein linked to early-onset Parkinson disease. *Nat Med* 1998; 4: 1318–1320.

181. Crowther RA, Jakes R, Spillantini MG et al. Synthetic filaments assembled from C-terminally truncated α-synuclein. *FEBS Lett* 1998; 436: 309–312.

182. Zibaee S, Jakes R, Fraser G et al. Sequence determinants for amyloid fibrillogenesis of human α-synuclein. *J Mol Biol* 2007; 374: 454–464.

183. Masuda M, Suzuki N, Taniguchi S et al. Small molecule inhibitors of α-synuclein filament assembly. *Biochemistry* 2006; 45: 6085–6094.

184. Conway KA, Lee SJ, Rochet JC et al. Acceleration of oligomerization, not fibrillization, is a shared property of both α-synuclein mutations linked to early-onset Parkinson's disease: Implications for pathogenesis and therapy. *Proc Natl Acad Sci USA* 2000; 97: 571–576.

185. Choi W, Zibaee S, Jakes R et al. Mutation E46K increases phospholipid binding and assembly into filaments of human α-synuclein. *FEBS Lett* 2004; 576: 363–368.

186. Ghosh D, Mondal M, Mohite GM et al. The Parkinson's disease-associated H50Q mutation accelerates α-synuclein aggregation *in vitro*. *Biochemistry* 2013; 52: 6925–6927.

187. Rutherford NJ, Moore BD, Golde TE et al. Divergent effects of the H50Q and G51D *SNCA* mutations on the aggregation of α-synuclein. *J Neurochem* 2014; 131: 859–867.

188. Ghosh D, Sahay S, Ranjan P et al. The newly discovered Parkinson's disease associated Finnish mutation (A53E) attenuates α-synuclein aggregation and membrane binding. *Biochemistry* 2014; 53: 6419–6421.

189. Jensen PH, Nielsen MH, Jakes R et al. Binding of α-synuclein to rat brain vesicles abolished by familial Parkinson's disease mutation. *J Biol Chem* 1998; 273: 26292–26294.

190. Seidel K, Schöls L, Nuber S et al. First appraisal of brain pathology owing to A30P mutant alpha-synuclein. *Ann Neurol* 2010; 67: 684–689.

191. Nemani VM, Lu W, Berge V et al. Increased expression of alpha-synuclein reduces neurotransmitter release by inhibiting synaptic vesicle recycling after endocytosis. *Neuron* 2010; 65: 66–79.

192. Giasson BI, Duda JE, Quinn SM et al. Neuronal α-synucleinopathy with severe movement disorder in mice expressing A53T α-synuclein. *Neuron* 2002; 34: 521–533.

193. Yazawa I, Giasson BI, Sasaki R et al. Mouse model of multiple system atrophy α-synuclein expression in oligodendrocytes causes glial and neuronal degeneration. *Neuron* 2005; 45: 847–859.

194. Emmer KL, Waxman EA, Covey JP et al. E46K human α-synuclein transgenic mice develop Lewy-like and tau pathology associated with age-dependent, detrimental motor impairment. *J Biol Chem* 2011; 286: 35104–35118.

195. Lee KW, Chen W, Junn E et al. Enhanced phosphatase activity attenuates α-synucleinopathy in a mouse model. *J Neurosci* 2011; 31: 6963–6971.

196. Garcia-Reitböck P, Anichtchik O, Bellucci A et al. SNARE protein redistribution and synaptic failure in a transgenic mouse model of Parkinson's disease. *Brain* 2010; 133: 2032–2044.

197. Betarbet R, Sherer TB, MacKenzie G et al. Chronic systemic pesticide exposure reproduces features of Parkinson's disease. *Nat Neurosci* 2000; 3: 1301–1306.

198. Nakamura K, Nermani VM, Azarbal F et al. Direct membrane association drives mitochondrial fission by the Parkinson disease-associated protein alpha-synuclein. *J Biol Chem* 2011; 286: 20710–20726.

199. Kirik D, Rosenblad C, Burger C et al. Parkinson-like neurodegeneration induced by targeted overexpression of α-synuclein in the nigrostriatal system. *J Neurosci* 2002; 22: 2780–2791.

200. Lo Bianco C, Ridet JL, Schneider BL et al. α-Synucleinopathy and selective dopaminergic neuron loss in a rat lentiviral-based model of Parkinson's disease. *Proc Natl Acad Sci USA* 2002; 99: 10813–10818.

201. Trachtenberg G, Garrido M, Tereshchemko Y et al. Aggregation of α-synuclein promotes progressive *in vivo* neurotoxicity in adult rat dopaminergic neurons. *Acta Neuropathol* 2012; 123: 671–683.

202. Colla E, Coune P, Liu Y et al. Endoplasmic reticulum stress is important for the manifestations of α-synucleinopathy *in vivo*. *J Neurosci* 2012; 342: 3306–3320.

203. Feany MB, Bender WW. A *Drosophila* model of Parkinson's disease. *Nature* 2000; 404: 394–398.

204. Auluck PK, Chan HY, Trojanowski JQ et al. Chaperone suppression of α-synuclein toxicity in a *Drosophila* model for Parkinson's disease. *Science* 2002; 295: 865–898.

205. Périquet M, Fulga T, Myllykangas L et al. Aggregated α-synuclein mediates dopaminergic neurotoxicity *in vivo*. *J Neurosci* 2007; 27: 3338–3346.

206. Lakso M, Vartiainen S, Moilanen AM et al. Dopaminergic neuronal loss and motor deficits in *Caenorhabditis elegans* overexpressing human α-synuclein. *J Neurochem* 2003; 86: 165–172.

207. Kuwahara T, Koyama A, Koyama S et al. A systematic RNAi screen reveals involvement of endocytic pathway in neuronal dysfunction in α-synuclein transgenic *C. elegans*. *Hum Mol Genet* 2008; 17: 2997–3009.

208. Clavaguera F, Bolmont T, Crowther RA et al. Transmission and spreading of tauopathy in transgenic mouse brain. *Nat Cell Biol* 2009; 11: 909–913.

209. Frost B, Jacks RL, Diamond MI. Propagation of tau misfolding from the outside to the inside of a cell. *J Biol Chem* 2009; 284: 12845–12852.

210. Braak H, Braak E. Neuropathological staging of Alzheimer-related changes. *Acta Neuropathol* 1991; 82: 239–259.

211. Braak H, Del Tredici K. The pathological process underlying Alzheimer's disease under thirty. *Acta Neuropathol* 2011; 121: 171–181.

212. Liou L, Drouet V, Wu JW et al. Trans-synaptic spread of tau pathology in vivo. *PLoS ONE* 2012; 7: e3102.

213. De Calignon A, Polydoro M, Suarez-Calvet M et al. Propagation of tau pathology as a model of early Alzheimer's disease. *Neuron* 2012; 73: 685–697.

214. Yetman MJ, Lillehaug S, Bjaalie JG et al. Transgene expression in the Nop-tTA driver line is not inherently restricted to the entorhinal cortex. *Brain Struct Funct* 2016; 221: 2231–2249.

215. Guo JL, Lee VMY. Seeding of normal tau by pathological tau conformers drives pathogenesis of Alzheimer-like tangles. *J Biol Chem* 2011; 286: 15317–15331.

216. Clavaguera F, Lavenir I, Falcon B et al. "Prion-like" template misfolding in tauopathies. *Brain Pathol* 2013; 23: 342–349.

217. Ahmed Z, Cooper J, Murray TK et al. A novel in vivo model of tau propagation with rapid and progressive neurofibrillary tangle pathology: the pattern of spread is determined by connectivity, not proximity. *Acta Neuropathol* 2012; 127: 667–683.

218. Clavaguera F, Hench J, Lavenir I et al. Peripheral administration of tau aggregates triggers intracerebral tauopathy in transgenic mice. *Acta Neuropathol* 2014; 127: 299–301.

219. Yamada K, Cirrito JR, Steward FR et al. In vivo microdialysis reveals age-dependent decrease of brain interstitial fluid tau levels in P301S human tau transgenic mice. *J Neurosci* 2011; 31: 13110–13117.

220. Pooler AM, Phillips EC, Lau DH et al. Physiological release of endogenous tau is stimulated by neuronal activity. *EMBO Rep* 2013; 14: 389–394.

221. Yamada K, Holth JK, Liao F et al. Neuronal activity regulates extracellular tau in vivo. *J Exp Med* 2014; 211: 387–394.

222. Kfoury N, Holmes BB, Jiang H et al. Transcellular propagation of tau aggregation by fibrillar species. *J Biol Chem* 2012; 287: 19440–19451.

223. Holmes BB, DeVos SL, Kfoury et al. Heparan sulphate proteoglycans mediate internalization and propagation of specific proteopathic seeds. *Proc Natl Acad Sci USA* 2013; 110: E3138–E3147.

224. Summerford C, Samulski RG. Membrane-associated heparan sulphate proteoglycan is a receptor for adeno-associated virus type 2 virions. *J Virol* 1998; 72: 1438–1445.

225. Clavaguera F, Akatsu H, Fraser G et al. Brain homogenates from human tauopathies induce tau inclusions in mouse brain. *Proc Natl Acad Sci USA* 2013; 110: 9535–9540.

226. Sanders DW, Kaufman SK, DeVos SL et al. Distinct tau prion strains propagate in cells and mice and define different tauopathies. *Neuron* 2014; 82: 1271–1288.

227. Li JY, Englund E, Holton Jl et al. Lewy bodies in grafted neurons in subjects with Parkinson's disease suggest host-to-graft disease propagation. *Nat Med* 2008; 14: 501–503.

228. Kordower JH, Chu Y, Hauser RA et al. Lewy body-like pathology in long-term embryonic transplants in Parkinson's disease. *Nat Med* 2008; 14: 504–506.

229. Li W, Englund E, Widner H et al. Extensive graft-derived dopaminergic innervation is maintained 24 years after transplantation in the degenerating parkinsonian brain. *Proc Natl Acad Sci USA* 2016; 113: 6544–6549.

230. Greffard S, Verny M, Bonnet AM et al. A stable proportion of Lewy body bearing neurons in the substantia nigra suggests a model in which the Lewy body causes neuronal death. *Neurobiol Aging* 2010; 31: 99–103.

231. Mougenot AL, Nicot S, Bencsik A et al. Prion-like acceleration of a synucleinopathy in a transgenic mouse model. *Neurobiol Aging* 2012; 33: 2225–2228.

232. Luk KC, Kehm VM, Zhang B et al. Intracerebral inoculation of pathological α-synuclein initiates a rapidly progressive neurodegenerative α-synucleinopathy in mice. *J Exp Med* 2012; 209: 975–986.

233. Watts JC, Giles K, Oehler A et al. Transmission of multiple system atrophy prions to transgenic mice. *Proc Natl Acad Sci USA* 2013; 110: 19555–19560.

234. Prusiner SB, Woerman AL, Mordes DA et al. Evidence for α-synuclein prions causing multiple system atrophy in humans with parkinsonism. *Proc Natl Acad Sci USA* 2015; 112: E5308–E5317.

235. Luk KC, Kehm V, Carroll J et al. Pathological α-synuclein transmission initiates Parkinson-like neurodegeneration in nontransgenic mice. *Science* 2012; 338: 949–953.

236. Masuda-Suzukake M, Nonaka T, Hosokawa M et al. Prion-like spreading of pathological α-synuclein in brain. *Brain* 2013; 136: 1128–1138.

237. Osterberg VR, Spinelli KJ, Weston LJ et al. Progressive aggregation of α-synuclein and selective degeneration of Lewy inclusion-bearing neurons in a mouse model of parkinsonism. *Cell Rep* 2015; 10: 1252–1260.

238. Sacino AN, Brooks M, Thomas MA et al. Intramuscular injection of α-synuclein induces CNS α-synuclein pathology and a rapid-onset motor phenotype in transgenic mice. *Proc Natl Acad Sci USA* 2014; 111: 10732–10737.

239. Lee HJ, Suk JE, Bae EJ et al. Assembly-dependent endocytosis and clearance of extracellular α-synuclein. *Int J Biochem Cell Biol* 2008; 40: 1835–1849.

240. Luk KC, Song C, O'Brien P et al. Exogenous α-synuclein fibrils seed the formation of Lewy body-like intracellular inclusions in cultured cells. *Proc Natl Acad Sci USA* 2009; 106: 20051–20056.

241. Jang A, Lee HJ, Suk JE et al. Non-classical exocytosis of α-synuclein is sensitive to folding states and promoted under stress conditions. *J Neurochem* 2010; 113: 1263–1274.

242. Lee HJ, Bae EJ, Lee SJ. Extracellular α-synuclein – a novel and crucial factor in Lewy body diseases. *Nat Rev Neurol* 2014; 10: 92–98.

243. Danzer KM, Haasen D, Karow AR et al. Different species of α-synuclein oligomers induce calcium influx and seeding. *J Neurosci* 2007; 27: 9220–9232.

244. Volpicelli-Daley LA, Luk KC, Patel TP et al. Exogenous alpha-synuclein fibrils induce Lewy body pathology leading to synaptic dysfunction and neuron death. *Neuron* 2011; 72: 57–71.

245. Braak H, Del Tredici K, Rüb U et al. Staging of brain pathology related to sporadic Parkinson's disease. *Neurobiol Aging* 2003; 24: 197–211.

246. Heise H, Hoyer W, Becker S et al. Molecular-level secondary structure, polymorphism, and dynamics of full-length α-synuclein fibrils studied by solid-state NMR. *Proc Natl Acad Sci USA* 2005; 102: 15871–15876.

247. Peelaerts W, Bousset L, Van der Perren A et al. α-Synuclein strains cause distinct synucleinopathies after local and systemic administration. *Nature* 2015; 522: 340–344.

248. Gwinn-Hardy K, Mehta NS, Farrer M et al. Distinctive neuropathology revealed by α-synuclein antibodies in hereditary parkinsonism and dementia linked to chromosome 4p. *Acta Neuropathol* 2000; 99: 663–672.

249. Duda JE, Giasson BI, Mabon ME et al. Concurrence of α-synuclein and tau brain pathology in the Contursi kindred. *Acta Neuropathol* 2002; 104: 7–11.

250. Greenbaum EA, Graves CL, Mishizen-Eberz AJ et al. The E46K mutation in alpha-synuclein increases amyloid fibril formation. *J Biol Chem* 2005; 280: 7800–7807.

251. Giasson BI, Forman MS, Higuchi M et al. Initiation and synergistic fibrillization of tau and alpha-synuclein. *Science* 2003; 300: 636–640.

252. Guo JL, Covell DJ, Daniels JP et al. Distinct α-synuclein strains differentially promote tau inclusions in neurons. *Cell* 2013; 154: 103–117.

253. DeVos SL, Gocharoff DK, Chen G et al. Antisense reduction of tau in adult mice protects against seizures. *J Neurosci* 2013; 33: 12887–12897.

254. Evans CG, Jinwal UK, Makley LN et al. Identification of dihydropyridines that reduce cellular tau levels. *Chem Commun* 2011; 47: 529–531.

255. David DC, Layfield R, Serpell LC et al. Proteasomal degradation of tau protein. *J Neurochem* 2002; 83: 176–185.

256. Petrucelli L, Dickson D, Kehoe K et al. CHIP and Hsp70 regulate tau ubiquitination, degradation and aggregation. *Hum Mol Genet* 2004; 13: 703–714.

257. Luo W, Dou F, Roudina A et al. Roles of heat shock protein 90 in maintaining and facilitating the neurodegenerative phenotype in tauopathies. *Proc Natl Acad Sci USA* 2007; 104: 9511–9516.

258. Schaeffer V, Lavenir I, Ozcelik S et al. Stimulation of autophagy reduces neurodegeneration in a mouse model of human tauopathy. *Brain* 2012; 135: 2169–2178.

259. Liani E, Eyal A, Avraham E et al. Ubiquitylation of synphilin-1 and alpha-synuclein by SIAH and its presence in cellular inclusions and Lewy bodies imply a role in Parkinson's disease. *Proc Natl Acad Sci USA* 2004; 101: 5500–5505.

260. Rott R, Szsargel R, Haskin J et al. α-Synuclein fate is determined by USP9X-regulated monoubiquitination. *Proc Natl Acad Sci USA* 2011; 108: 18666–18671.

261. Mak SK, McCormack AL, Manning-Bog AB et al. Lysosomal degradation of alpha-synuclein in vivo. *J Biol Chem* 2010; 285: 13621–13629.

262. Tofaris GK, Kim HT, Hourez R et al. Ubiquitin ligase Nedd4 promotes alpha-synuclein degradation by the endosomal-lysosomal pathway. *Proc Natl Acad Sci USA* 2011; 108: 17004–17009.

263. Cooper JM, Wiklander O, Nordin JZ et al. Systemic exosomal siRNA delivery reduced alpha-synuclein aggregates in brains of transgenic mice. *Mov Disord* 2014; 29: 1476–1485.

264. Decressac M, Mattson B, Weikop P et al. TFEB-mediated autophagy rescues midbrain dopamine neurons from α-synuclein toxicity. *Proc Natl Acad Sci USA* 2013; 110: E1817–E1826.

265. Spencer B, Potkar R, Trejo M et al. Beclin 1 gene transfer activates autophagy and ameliorates the neurodegenerative pathology in alpha-synuclein models of Parkinson's and Lewy body diseases. *J Neurosci* 2009; 29: 13578–13588.

266. Herrmann A, Spires-Jones T. Clearing the way for tau immunotherapy in Alzheimer's disease. *J Neurochem* 2015; 143: 1–4.

267. Goedert M, Falcon B, Clavaguera F et al. Prion-like mechanisms in the pathogenesis of tauopathies and synucleinopathies. *Curr Neurol Neurosci Rep* 2014; 14: 495.

268. Schapira AHV, Olanow CW, Greenamyre JT et al. Slowing of neurodegeneration in Parkinson's disease and Huntington's disease: future therapeutic perspectives. *Lancet* 2014; 384: 545–555.

CHAPTER 3

Prion Degeneration

James A. Mastrianni

Department of Neurology, Center for Comprehensive Care and Research on Memory Disorders, The University of Chicago, Chicago, Illinois, USA

Clinical definition and epidemiology

Prion diseases are invariably fatal neurodegenerative diseases that result from the accumulation of a misfolded isoform (PrP^{Sc}) of the normal (cellular) form of the prion protein (PrP^C). There are three modes of occurrence associated with prion disease: (i) 90% are spontaneous with unknown risk factors; (ii) roughly 10% are familial, resulting from one of several mutations of the PrP gene (*PRNP*); and (iii) less than 1% occur through horizontal transmission of disease via exposure to prions, the infectious units of prion disease. Prion disease occurs throughout the world with a yearly incidence of one per million. There is no obvious gender preference. Historically, the highest incidence of prion disease may have been localized to the highlands of New Guinea, where cannibalistic rituals acted as the medium by which a prion disease known as kuru was transmitted.

Spectrum of clinical phenotype

Prion disease is best described as a family of diseases with variable but overlapping clinical and histopathological phenotypes. The core features most associated with prion diseases are progressive cognitive decline, ataxia, often with pyramidal and extrapyramidal involvement, and myoclonic jerks. Prior to the recognition that PrP was the common thread that linked these diseases, the two most common disease subtypes, Creutzfeldt–Jakob disease (CJD) and Gerstmann–Sträussler–Scheinker disease (GSS), were described and subsequently defined by their clinicopathological profiles. Once the molecular basis of disease was recognized, histopathologic phenotypes revealed new clinical phenotypes that extended beyond these classic diseases. Currently, there are four major subtypes of prion disease that are defined specifically by their histopathologic profile, although each is associated with a "classic" clinical phenotype, based on the most common presentation observed. The predominant clinical feature at onset, age at onset, and rate of disease progression are helpful guides for distinguishing the different subtypes. In addition to CJD and GSS, fatal insomnia (FI) and variant CJD (vCJD) make up the major phenotypes currently observed. Kuru is a prion disease transmitted through the practice of cannibalism in the Fore tribe located in the highlands of New Guinea. It is largely of historical interest and will not be highlighted here. Recently, an additional phenotype has been described, labeled variably protease-sensitive prion disease (VPSPr). CJD and FI have sporadic (s) and familial (f) occurrences, whereas GSS has been identified only in people who carry a mutation in the *PRNP* gene. Based on the histopathology of VPSPr, it has been suggested this is a sporadic form of GSS, although the clinical phenotype is not classic for that subtype. Genetic forms of prion disease typically present earlier in life and progress at a slower pace than sporadic forms. In rare cases, GSS may run a 20-year course. Acquired forms of prion disease include iatrogenic CJD (iCJD), which results from exposure to prion-contaminated biologicals (growth hormone, gonadotropic hormone, dura mater grafts, etc.) or instruments (most notably depth electrodes), and vCJD, caused by consumption of food or products contaminated with bovine spongiform encephalopathy (BSE), the cause of "mad cow disease". The major subtypes are described here and distinguishing characteristics are summarized in Table 3.1.

Sporadic Creutzfeldt–Jakob disease (sCJD)

sCJD is the most common prion disease and therefore the best characterized. It has a median age at onset of roughly 68 years, but ranges from the twenties to early nineties. In 90% of cases, disease progresses to death within 1 year of onset, although most cases lead to death within 4–6 months. The "classic triad" of disease includes rapidly progressive dementia, ataxia, and myoclonus. At onset, the vast majority of patients display cognitive impairment, manifest as confusion, concentration difficulties, and memory impairment that progresses to dementia. Gait, or truncal, ataxia, but also unilateral or bilateral appendicular ataxia typically follows the cognitive problems. However, in approximately 25–30% of patients, ataxia is the first symptom of disease [1]. Roughly 10% develop visual obscurations and distortions as the initial symptoms, labeled as the Heidenhain variant of CJD. Differences in presentation of sCJD appear to be determined, at least in part, by the *PRNP* genotype at codon 129, a common polymorphic site that plays a role in disease risk and phenotype (see subsection Genetics). Spontaneous myoclonus, affecting a single limb or multiple limbs, or stimulus-induced myoclonus, particularly startle myoclonus, is observed in roughly two-thirds of patients. The latter is characterized by the synchronous flexion of all limbs and the neck induced by tactile stimulation, a noise (hand clap), turning the lights on, or even someone walking into the room. In addition to these core symptoms, a variety of neurologic features have been reported, including, but not limited to, weakness, rigidity, bradykinesia, tremor, alien hand syndrome, focal sensory or motor loss, aphasia, visual distortions or field cuts, and chorea. At end-stage, akinetic mutism is typical, although myoclonic jerks may persist.

Neurodegeneration, First Edition. Edited by Anthony Schapira, Zbigniew Wszolek, Ted M. Dawson and Nicholas Wood.
© 2017 John Wiley & Sons, Ltd. Published 2017 by John Wiley & Sons, Ltd.

Table 3.1 Phenotypes of current human prion diseases.

Prion disease subtype	Primary presentation	Age at onset (range)	Duration	Pathology	Associated studies
1. Sporadic					
a. sCJD	Dementia, ataxia, myoclonus	~65 years (17–91), rare under 40	~4–6 months for most, rarely up to 15 months	Generalized gray matter SD[a] and gliosis	CSF + in 50–70% (tau, 14-3-3) EEG + in 50–70% (periodic) MRI (DWI) + in >90%
b. SFI	Insomnia, dysautonomia, ataxia, dementia	~45±10 years	~12–14 months	Gliosis and neuronal loss within thalamus and inferior olive	PET shows hypometabolism of thalami, EEG normal or slow
c. VPSPr	Often aphasia, extrapyramidal features, frontal lobe features	~67±10 years	30±21 months	Moderate SD and punctate PrP plaques	EEG and MRI are not helpful
2. Familial					
a. fCJD	As in sCJD	<55 years (20s–80s)[b]	~1–5 years, some 4–6 months	As in sCJD	PRNP mutation
b. GSS	Ataxia, then dementia, some with primary cognitive or frontal lobe syndrome	<55 years (20s–60s)[b]	~2–6 years, some >10 years	PrP-amyloid plaques, gliosis, some SD	CSF typically negative, EEG normal or slow, MRI (DWI) not well studied
c. FFI	As in SFI	As in SFI	As in SFI	As in SFI	As in SFI PRNP genotype – D178N/129M
3. Acquired					
a. iCJD	Progressive cerebellar syndrome with hGH, CJD-like presentation with depth electrodes, corneal transplants, and dural grafts	Incubation period: ~12 years (hGH) ~1 year (cornea/ electrodes) ~7 years (dura)	~15 months (hGH) ~7 months (dura)	hGH – cerebellar atrophy, extensive SD, some with punctate PrP plaques Central inoculation – resembles sCJD pathology/some dura-related show "florid plaques" similar to vCJD	EEG slow in hGH, periodic in others MRI (DWI) not well studied, but (+) in small study of dura recipients CSF markers less helpful
b. vCJD	Depression, apathy, later dementia and ataxia	~median 26 years (range 12–74)	~14 months (range 6–84)	Florid plaques and diffuse SD	CSF negative EEG normal or slow MRI – "pulvinar sign" Tonsillar biopsy + PrPres

[a] SD.

[b] Mutation-dependent variability.

CSF, cerebrospinal fluid; DWI, diffusion weighted imaging; EEG, electroencephalography; fCJD, familial Creutzfeldt–Jakob disease; FFI, familial fatal insomnia; GSS, Gerstmann–Sträussler–Scheinker disease; hGH, human growth hormone; iCJD, iatrogenic Creutzfeldt–Jakob disease; MRI, magnetic resonance imaging; PrP, prion protein; sCJD, sporadic Creutzfeldt–Jakob disease; SD, spongiform degeneration; SFI, sporadic fatal insomnia; vCJD, variant Creutzfeldt–Jakob disease; VPSPr, variably protease-sensitive prion disease.

Familial Creutzfeldt–Jakob disease (fCJD)

Several mutations of the PRNP gene are associated with fCJD (Table 3.2). Single amino acid substitutions constitute the majority of mutations, although a minority result from the insertion of one or more octapeptide repeat segments between codons 51 and 90 (see subsection Genetics). The clinical phenotype of fCJD overlaps with that of sCJD; however genetic forms typically present with an earlier age at onset (<55 years) and have a longer duration of disease (~1–3 years). In the vast majority, a family history can be identified, while in some, such as the Val180Ile mutation, which is typically associated with late-onset disease [2], and Glu200Lys mutation, which presents in young and older individuals, the premature death of carriers from unrelated causes may mask a family history [3]. Genotype–phenotype correlations are observed with some mutations, although the occurrence of many is too small to confirm a consistent phenotype, while analysis of the more common mutations, such as Asp178Asn and Glu200Lys, often reveals a marked variability in clinical phenotype [4]. However, the consistent feature among these is the histopathology, which is similar to that of sCJD, as described in the section Prion-related histopathologies.

Table 3.2 Mutations and polymorphisms of PRNP

Phenotype	Substitutions	Truncations/insertions	Octapeptide repeat insertions (base pair #)	Octapeptide repeat deletions (base pair #)
fCJD	G114V, R148H, D178N-129V, V180I, T183A, H187R[a], T188A, T188K, E196K, E200K, V203I, R208H, V210I, E211Q, M232R, P238S	None	1(24), 2(48), 4(96), 5(120), 6(144), 7(168)	2(24)
GSS	P102L, P105L/T/S, A117V, G131V, A133V, F198S, D202N, Q212P, Q217R, Y218N, M232T	Y145*[b], Q160*, Y163*, Y226*, Q227*, 8-aa insert(129/130)[c]	8(192)[d], 9(216), [7(168)][e]	–
FFI	D178N-129M	–	–	–
Polymorphisms	M129V, N171S, E219K	–	—–	1(24)

Letter coding is as follows: *, stop codon; A, alanine; D, aspartate; E, glutamate; F, phenylalanine; G, glycine; H, histidine; I, isoleucine; K, lysine; L, leucine; M, methionine; N, asparagine; P, proline; Q, glutamine; R, arginine; S, serine; T, threonine; V, valine; Y, tyrosine.

[a] Atypical phenotype – early psychiatric symptoms with or without dementia and histology shows "curly PrP deposits".

[b] Associated with vascular PrP amyloid (congophilic angiopathy).

[c] A 24-bp insertion coding for LGGLGGYV between residue 129 and 130.

[d] Huntington disease like-1 (HDL-1) reported with an 8-OPRI case.

[e] Atypical case (linked to 129V, while other 7-OPRIs linked to M129).

Iatrogenic Creutzfeldt–Jakob disease (iCJD)

The exposure of humans to biologicals (human growth hormone, gonadotropic hormone), tissues (dura mater, corneas), or instruments (brain electrodes, surgical instruments) contaminated with prions has been linked to the development of iCJD. The largest number of cases came from human growth hormone extracts, reported from the UK, France, the Netherlands, and the USA [5–9], and dura mater transplants [10]. In general, iCJD is more often associated with the onset of cerebellar ataxia than dementia. Studies that may be positive in sCJD, such as periodic sharp wave complexes (PSWCs) on the EEG, are often not present in iCJD [11–16].

Variant Creutzfeldt–Jakob disease (vCJD)

This subtype was first recognized in 1995 in a teenager who initially developed behavioral problems and subsequently displayed ataxia and progressive encephalopathy [17]. A brain biopsy showed features of CJD in addition to PrP amyloid plaque deposits, a histopathology that had not previously been seen. Several cases followed in other teenagers and young adults [18–20] and these were collectively reported as a "new variant" of CJD [21], based not only on the atypical pathology but also on the presence of a characteristic but previously unrecognized western blot pattern of protease-resistant PrP^{Sc} (see section Protease-resistant PrP^{Sc} and PrP^{Sc} typing). vCJD has been reported in about 200 patients throughout the world, with the greatest number of cases in the UK (173) and France (25). Three cases have been reported in the USA, although two emigrated from the UK not long before they manifested disease, and the third, who is thought to have been exposed as a child, emigrated from Saudi Arabia in 2005. Compared with sCJD, vCJD more often presents with psychiatric features, particularly apathy and depression, in addition to painful dysesthesias. Teens and young adults (ages 17–42 years) are primarily affected and the course of disease is slightly greater than one year.

Early work indicated that vCJD was detectable in the peripheral lymphoreticular system, raising a concern about transmission through blood transfusions. Because of this, the American Red Cross prohibits blood donations from individuals who spent an aggregate of 3 months in the UK between 1980 and 1996 or who have received blood transfusions in any UK country from 1980 to the present time. In addition, all blood donations are leukodepleted in the UK, as the white cells appear to be a reservoir of prions in vCJD. Secondary infection with vCJD from transfusion has been reported in five instances. Four cases occurred following transfusion of non-leukocyte-depleted blood from asymptomatic donors who subsequently died of vCJD [22–25]. Of these four cases, three were symptomatic with vCJD. The two remaining asymptomatic cases were discovered through post mortem examination of organs of individuals who died without neurological symptoms. PrP^{Sc} was detected in the appendix of one case who received blood from a person who developed signs of vCJD 18 months after donating [23], while the other case was a hemophiliac who received only plasma-derived blood products and had PrP^{res} detected in the spleen [25], raising concern about the safety of plasma products.

Gerstmann–Sträussler–Scheinker disease (GSS)

The classic expression of GSS, as originally described by Gerstmann [26, 27], includes ataxia of gait and/or dysarthria as the most prominent features, followed by pyramidal and extrapyramidal signs and symptoms, with dementia occurring late in the disease. Several variations in the presentation have been reported, including those that present with cognitive impairment suggestive of Alzheimer's disease, or with behavioral features suggesting frontotemporal lobar dementia (FTLD). In others, spastic paraparesis or an isolated movement disorder may mark the onset of disease. Duration is typically between 2 and 7 years, although cases extending beyond 10 years have been reported. GSS-related mutations of *PRNP* include amino acid substitutions, a single insertion of 8 amino acids (LGGLGGYV) between residue 129 and 130 [28], octapeptide repeat insertions (OPRIs), and early stop sequences that result in truncated PrP molecules (Table 3.2).

Fatal insomnia (FI)

Fatal insomnia was originally described in a pedigree with several occurrences of a disease heralded by progressive and intractable insomnia leading to death within approximately 1 year [29]. Although not initially considered a prion disease, it was eventually linked to the Asp178Asn mutation of *PRNP* [30]. Importantly, it was recognized that this mutation must be allelic with Met coding at codon 129 for the FI phenotype, whereas those cases that carried the same dominant Asp178Asn mutation, but with Val at 129, displayed a clinical and histopathological phenotype most consistent with fCJD [31]. A clinical, pathological, and transmissible phenocopy of FI was subsequently recognized in a patient who lacked the gene defect, supporting a spontaneous misfolding of PrP into the PrP^{Sc} conformation linked to FFI or, possibly, the generation of a somatic mutation of *PRNP* in the central nervous system [32]. A handful of cases of sporadic FI (SFI) have been reported [33].

The typical presentation of either sporadic (SFI) or familial (FFI) FI includes intractable insomnia, often in isolation for several months, at which time the patient may develop autonomic dysfunction (excessive lacrimation, hypertension, and hidrosis), ataxia, and variable pyramidal and extrapyramidal signs and symptoms, with relatively spared cognitive function (mainly attention, vigilance, and subcortical network impairment) until later in the course. Phenotypic heterogeneity has been reported [34] and, in some cases, it is important to recognize that the insomnia is not always the most prominent feature. Age at disease onset ranges from 36 to 62 years (average 51 years) and time to death is generally 1–2 years (range 8–72 months) [35].

Variably protease-sensitive prion disease (VPSPr)

In 2008, 11 cases of prion disease that lacked obvious protease-resistant PrP^{Sc}, but displayed punctate extracellular PrP plaque-like deposits in several cortical brain regions, were described [36]. Initially recognized only in individuals with the 129VV genotype, this disease subtype has since been described in individuals with the 129MV genotype and rarely in 129MM individuals [37]. Protease resistance is lowest in the 129VV cases and greatest in 129MM cases. The pattern of PK-resistant PrP differs from typical sCJD, with smaller fragments of around 7 and 16 kDa bands, similar to those seen in GSS. Common features of clinical disease included aphasia, ataxia, and parkinsonian signs. In 129VV cases, frontal lobe-like features, including impulsivity, euphoria, or apathy, are prominent. As of this writing, transmissibility of VPSPr has not been demonstrated.

Pathology/pathophysiology of prion diseases

Prion-related histopathologies

Sporadic and familial CJD is characterized by the presence of diffuse spongiform degeneration (i.e., vacuolation) within the cerebral neocortex, molecular layer of the cerebellar cortex, and deep gray matter nuclei. Astrocytic gliosis is consistently present (Figure 3.1). The vacuoles, which vary in size from 5 to 100 μm, represent focal swellings of axonal and dendritic neuronal processes associated with the loss of synaptic organelles and accumulation of abnormal membranes [38–40]. Ultrastructural features of autophagy have also been reported in CJD [41].

GSS is linked to the presence of extracellular deposits of amyloid composed of PrP. PrP stained are labeled by Congo Red or thioflavin S. The multicentric plaque, which is most characteristic, appears as a central amyloid core surrounded by smaller PrP amyloid satellites (Figure 3.1), although other morphologies, from punctate to diffuse deposits, may be present. Plaque deposits appear to be composed of peptide fragments of 7 and/or 11–14 kDa, which have been amino- and carboxy-terminally clipped and span residues of 58–150 and 81–150 of the mutant alleles [42].

The pathology of FFI and SFI is generally limited to gliosis and neuronal dropout within the anterior and dorsal medial nuclei of the thalamus, and the inferior olivary nucleus, with only minimal spongiform degeneration detected. Cases of longer duration tend to display greater levels of spongiform degeneration, especially evident within temporal lobes [35].

The presence of florid plaques comprised of a PrP-amyloid core surrounded by a halo of spongiform degeneration is the pathognomonic feature of vCJD. The plaques can be found throughout the cerebral cortex, especially within the occipital lobe, and also within the molecular layer of the cerebellum [43]. Spongiform degeneration is also prominent, especially within the caudate and putamen, in addition to scattered, sometimes prominent astrocytic gliosis [43] (Figure 3.1).

In the small number of VPSPr cases thus far reported, the pathology is characterized by moderate spongiform degeneration of the cerebral and cerebellar cortex, in addition to the presence of punctate and target-like PrP amyloid [37].

Protease-resistant PrP^{Sc} and PrP^{Sc} typing

PrP^{Sc} is characterized by a relative resistance to proteinase K (PK) compared with PrP^{C}, which is highly sensitive to PK. When incubated in PK, the first 67 amino acids of PrP^{Sc} are cleaved at approximately residue 90, leaving a protease-resistant core of PrP90–230, also known as PrP27–30, based on its migration rate following gel electrophoresis. As the glycosylation sites at residues 181 and 197 are contained within the PK-resistant core, three protein bands

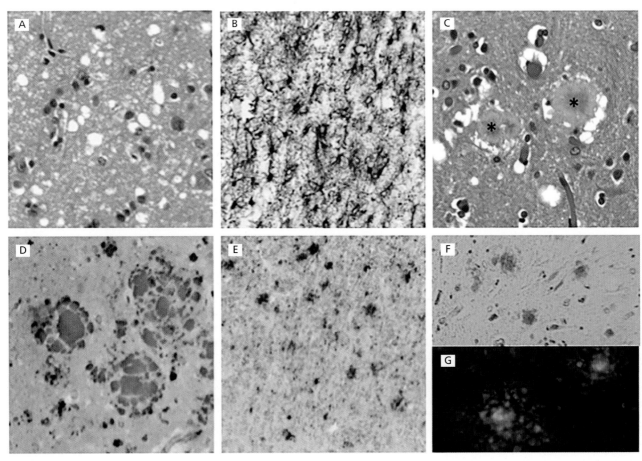

Figure 3.1 Histopathologies associated with prion disease. (A) Spongiform degeneration (SD) in a hematoxylin and eosin (H&E) stained section of frontal cortex from a case of sCJD. SD is the predominant pathology of sCJD, iCJD, and vCJD. It is present in GSS at relatively low levels and is minimally detected in FI. (B) Gliosis, detected by glial fibrillary acidic protein (GFAP) antibody, in frontal cortex from a case of sCJD. Gliosis is a common feature of all prion diseases. In sFI and FFI, gliosis and neuronal dropout is most prominent within anteroventral and mediodorsal thalamic nuclei. (C) Florid plaques in the frontal cortex of an H&E stained section from a case of vCJD (courtesy of James Ironside, University of Edinburgh). Note the central amyloid core surrounded by SD, resembling a daisy (asterisk). (D–G) PrP amyloid deposits from GSS. Immunohistochemical staining with anti-PrP antibody in (D) and (E) shows multicentric type plaques (D) and punctate PrP accumulations (E). PrP plaques are Congo Red positive (F) and they bind Thioflavin S (G), confirming they are true amyloid.

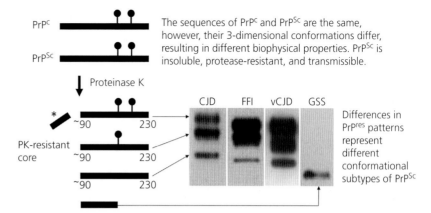

Figure 3.2 Protease resistance of PrP^Sc from the principal prion disease subtypes. Proteinase K cleaves the first ~67 amino acids (*) of PrP^Sc, leaving a PK-resistant core of amino acids 90–231 (PrP^res). In most prion diseases, three protease-resistant bands are observed, reflecting the un-, mono-, and di-glycosylated fractions. In most GSS cases, cleavage of the C-terminal end also occurs, leaving only unglycosylated fragments that are smaller, typically ~7–14 kDa.

can be visualized on the western blot (Figure 3.2). In brain samples from sporadic, familial, and variant CJD, PrP^Sc is generally easily detectable and highly resistant to PK, whereas that derived from GSS and VPSPr is more sensitive. In sporadic and familial FI, PK-resistant PrP^Sc (also labeled PrP^res) is present, but often restricted to the thalamus or brainstem. The efficiency with which prion disease is transmitted to appropriate experimental hosts such as transgenic mice expressing human PrP or non-human primates, appears to correlate well with the presence of PrP^res; thus, CJD is easily transmissible to transgenic mice that express human PrP, whereas GSS and, at the time of this writing, VPSPr, are less or not transmissible.

The banding pattern of PrP^res displayed on a western blot varies among the different subtypes (Figure 3.2), which supports the concept that different conformational subtypes of PrP^Sc underlie the differences in phenotype among these diseases. This is best exemplified by SFI, in which the PrP^res compares well with the genetic form of FI, both of which differ from typical CJD. In most cases of GSS, an amino- and carboxy-terminal truncation leads to the presence of a 7 or 14 kDa PrP^res fragment, suggesting a common underlying conformation.

Within the major subtype of sCJD, different conformations of PrP^res exist, which appear to be determined by the genotype of the polymorphic codon 129 [44]. Two major PrP^Sc types are designated, based only on the migration rate of the unglycosylated fraction of PrP^res: type 1 runs at about 21 kDa and type 2 runs at about 19 kDa. Based on this property, five subtypes of sCJD have been recognized, including, in order of prevalence, sCJDMM1, sCJDVV2, sCJDMV2, sCJDMM2, and sCJDVV1. These subtypes generally correlate with different clinical and histopathologic features, based primarily on the initial onset of either rapidly progressive dementia or ataxia, and by differences in distribution and size of the vacuoles (see [45] for review). Of note, although a single PrP^Sc type may predominate within the brain of each case, a significant proportion of cases may carry both type 1 and type 2 conformations within their brain. With the occurrence of vCJD, a new molecular type of PrP^Sc emerged, primarily distinguished by its prominent diglycosylated fraction compared to sCJD PrP^Sc types, which tend to have a more prominent monoglycosylated fraction [46].

In addition to these major PrP^Sc types associated with CJD, several "atypical" patterns that lack the diglycosylated band have been reported in genetic and non-genetic forms of prion disease [47–50].

Prion propagation
Prion propagation occurs via a template-assisted interaction of PrP^Sc with PrP^C, leading to the generation of new PrP^Sc (Figure 3.3). Experimental transmission of human prion disease to non-human

primates [51] and transgenic mice that express human PrP is well documented [52]. More recently, the bank vole has been shown to be susceptible to human prions, although in general a species barrier exists between human prions and other rodents typically used in prion bioassays [53]. As mentioned above, the greater the level of PrP^res, the greater the efficiency of transmission, in general. Thus, all forms of CJD are readily transmissible, whereas GSS, with its reduced level of PrP^res, is more difficult to transmit to potentially receptive animal hosts. Prion propagation has also been modeled *in vitro*, using a method known as the protein misfolding conversion assay (PMCA), which involves mixing a small amount of prion-infected sample with homogenized normal brain, the latter providing PrP^C substrate. This mixture is subjected to alternating cycles of sonication and incubation that are designed to disrupt prion fibrils, generating unbound PrP^Sc molecules that can interact more efficiently with PrP^C, resulting in more efficient amplification of PrP^Sc [54].

Support for the hypothesis that prion propagation occurs via a template-assisted process comes from experimental transmission studies and some PMCA work that shows that the conformation of PrP^Sc is transferable to receptive PrP^C or hosts expressing receptive PrP^C molecules [55–57]. In general, transmission is more efficient between homologous PrP^Sc and PrP^C molecules. Conformational adaptation of the PrP^C may factor into the susceptibility of passage between species with differing PrP sequences [55, 58]. Specific alterations in sequence at key sites may limit the efficacy of formation of a PrP^Sc–PrP^C complex, resulting in a reduced rate of transmission. A key example is the common polymorphism at codon 129. It has been well documented that transgenic mice expressing human PrP with residue 129 that differs from the human prions with which it is inoculated have a significantly longer survival than mice inoculated with prions carrying the same sequence at residue 129 [59, 60].

Prion pathogenesis
Until recent years, much of the focus has been on understanding the nature of PrP^Sc generation and propagation. Thus, the basis for neurotoxicity in prion disease is still largely unknown. Apoptotic cell death is evident in the brains of experimental rodent models, humans, and animals with prion disease, in addition to cell culture models of prion toxicity [61–65]. Interestingly, PrP^C has been shown to possess anti-apoptotic effects [66, 67], supporting the idea that this function is lost when PrP^C acquires the PrP^Sc conformation. The ultrastructural features of autophagy have also been recognized in naturally-occurring prion diseases in animals and humans, although whether this represents a response to prion neurotoxicity or contributes to it has not been fully addressed [68, 69].

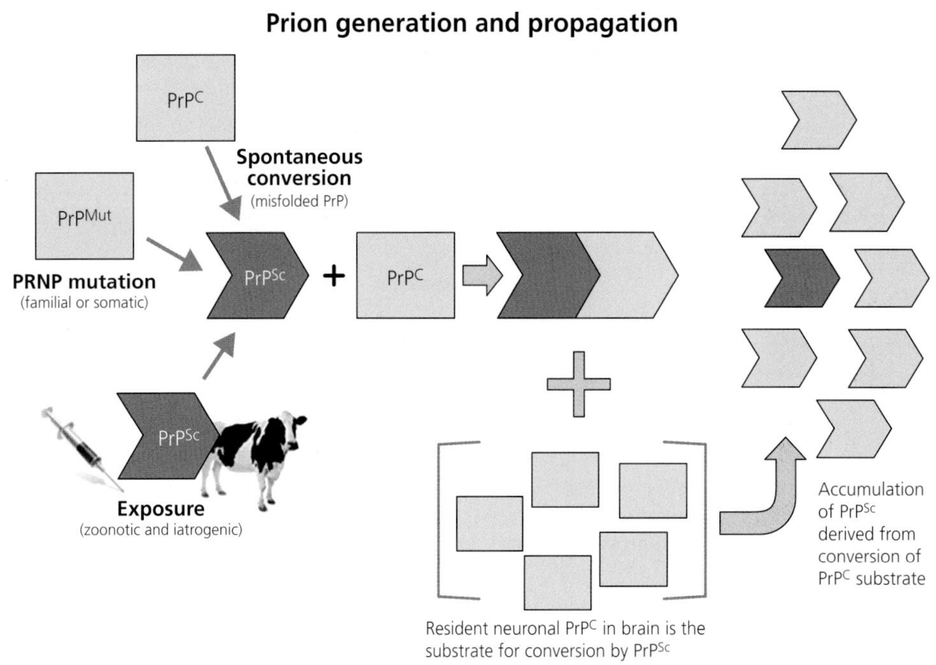

Prion generation and propagation

Figure 3.3 Generation of PrP^Sc occurs by spontaneous conversion of PrP^C, a mutation of PRNP that predisposes the misfolding of PrP^Sc, or by introduction of prions from an exogenous source. Once present within the CNS, PrP^Sc propagates in an autocatalytic process by associating with and templating its conformation onto resident PrP^C, thereby accumulating PrP^Sc. Thus, neuronal stores of PrP^C provide the substrate that is converted to PrP^Sc from a single infectious unit (dark shaded unit). This process has led to the consideration of two major concepts of prion-related neurodegeneration: a loss of function of PrP^C versus a toxic gain of function of PrP^Sc.

Two principal theories of prion pathogenesis were initially posited: (i) that the accumulation of misfolded isoforms of PrP induces cellular toxicity; and (ii) that the reduction of PrP^C that results from its conversion to PrP^Sc leads to the loss of a necessary cellular function. The normal function of PrP^C is as yet unknown, however several reports have suggested a variety of diverse possible functions including, but not limited to: synapse formation and function [70, 71], a role in signaling pathways [72–74], binding and delivery of copper to cells [75], antioxidant activity, and anti-apoptotic function against Bax mediated cell death [76, 77]. More recently, PrP^C has been proposed to be a receptor for amyloid-β oligomers and a mediator of neurotoxicity in Alzheimer's disease [78], in addition to suppressing beta-secretase cleavage of amyloid precursor protein (APP) [79]. PrP knockout mice [80, 81] and adult mice in which Prnp ablation is induced [82] do not develop prion disease symptoms and as such have not supported the loss of function theory, whereas animal models overexpressing mutated PrP, even those lacking wild-type PrP, develop prion pathologies that overlap with those seen in humans [83–87] and therefore support the toxic gain of function hypothesis. As with Alzheimer's disease and other neurotoxic aggregated proteins, the toxic species of prion disease is suggested to be soluble oligomers. Recent work suggests that the most highly infectious and toxic species is an oligomer of approximately 14–28 PrP molecules [88].

Transgenic mice that express PrP lacking its GPI anchor (i.e., PrP[GPI–]) have provided important insight into the nature of prion pathogenesis [89]. When PrP(GPI–) expressing mice that lack PrP^C (i.e., ablated background) are inoculated with scrapie they generate extracellular PrP plaques but display no clinical disease nor is neuronal death observed. However, when PrP(GPI–) is expressed in the presence of PrP^C, neurotoxicity occurs. These

and other data have led to speculation that PrP^C functions as a signaling molecule, a hypothesis supported by a study that found that an antibody that cross-links PrP^C led to rapid neuronal apoptosis in hippocampus [73]. Another possible mechanism for prion pathogenesis is via altered membrane topology or trafficking [90–92]. Although the vast majority of PrP^C is properly oriented and anchored on the extracellular membrane surface, a small percentage may inappropriately orient with the carboxy-terminal end within the endoplasmic reticulum (ER) lumen (^CtmPrP) and this fraction has been shown to be increased in disease states and in some familial mutations. Finally, neurotoxicity has been demonstrated in a mouse model that expresses PrP lacking the peptide sequences for the GPI anchor and ER entry signal, resulting in the accumulation of PrP in the cytosol [91]. Although ER-associated degradation (ERAD) has been postulated as a mechanism for the generation of cytosolic PrP (cyPrP), others suggest that PrP reaches the cytosol and is subject to proteasomal degradation because of inefficient translocation into the ER [93]. Controversy also exists as to whether cyPrP accumulates to a significant extent in cytosol during disease, as its degradation by the proteasome is highly efficient [93]. It has also been reported that cyPrP may insert into lipid membranes of ER, plasmalemma, and endocytic vesicles as another possible mechanism of cellular disruption and death and as a way to explain the normally low levels of detection [94].

Genetics

Approximately 10% of all cases of prion disease can be attributed to an autosomal dominant mutation of the prion protein gene (PRNP). PRNP is located on the short arm of chromosome 20 (20pter-p12). A single exon encodes the 253 amino acid protein. Mutations of the gene include: (i) single base pair alterations resulting in single amino acid substitutions, found in association with fCJD and GSS; (ii) early stop sequence mutations, resulting in a truncated molecule, found only in cases of GSS; and (iii) insertions or deletions of the octapeptide repeat segment [Pro-(His/Gln)-Gly-Gly-Gly-(-/Trp)-Gly-Gln] that is normally repeated five times between residues 51 and 90, resulting in an extended or shortened protein. From one to nine, but not three, octapeptide repeat insertions (OPRIs) or the deletion of two octapeptide repeats (2-OPRD), have been associated with either fCJD or GSS (Table 3.2). In general, the shorter OPRIs and 2-OPRD typically produce a CJD phenotype while the longer OPRIs produce a GSS phenotype (Table 3.2). All mutations are autosomal dominant and penetrance is nearly 100%. Genetic prion disease typically presents earlier in life than non-genetic cases, mostly prior to age 55, and has a longer duration of 3–7 and up to 10 or more years. A small number of mutations, such as Glu200Lys and Val210Ile, display variable penetrance with disease onset occurring in early or late life. In these cases, mutation carriers may develop symptoms before the carrier parent. These mutations also tend to produce a more rapid onset and progression of short duration, typical of sCJD. Thus, the early death of the parent of a patient with prion disease should raise concern for genetic prion disease, despite an early or late age at onset and a clear family history. Further support for genetic testing of all cases of prion disease comes from carriers of the Val180Ile mutation, who typically present in the seventh and eighth decade and often lack a positive family history. Genotype–phenotype correlations are generally consistent with respect to the major subtypes of disease and the mutations with which they are associated (Table 3.2), although it should be noted that there is marked clinical variability among individuals carrying the same mutation, even those reported within a single pedigree.

The polymorphic codon 129 of PRNP is of central importance to both genetic and sporadic prion disease. Homozygosity for either methionine (M) or valine (V), the two possible substitutions at this position, is observed in roughly 50% of the normal population but in over 80% of sCJD cases. Homozygosity is also over-represented in iCJD, and all but one individual affected by vCJD following primary exposure had the 129MM genotype [95]. In sCJD, the codon 129 genotype appears to influence the phenotype such that 129MM is more often associated with the classic presentation of rapidly progressive dementia, while 129MV and 129VV is more likely to be associated to an ataxic presentation [96]. The most striking role of the polymorphic codon 129 is to determine the phenotype of FFI. When the D178N mutation is allelic with 129V, the phenotype is fCJD, but when allelic with 129M, the FI phenotype is observed [31]. The finding that the protease-resistant fragment of PrP^{Sc} in these two states differs, as does that in sCJD with different coding at 129, supports the idea that the conformation of PrP^{Sc} is determined, at least in part, by the sequence at residue 129 and this, in turn, affects the phenotype of disease.

Other key polymorphisms include Glu219Lys, Asn171Ser, and Gly127Val. Glu219Lys is present in approximately 6% of the Japanese population, but was not found in a small series of Japanese with sCJD, suggesting that it affords protection against CJD. This has been supported by studies in cultured cells and transgenic mice where PrP-Glu219Lys is shown to act as a dominant-negative inhibitor of scrapie transmission when co-expressed with wild-type PrP [97]. The Asn171Ser polymorphism was recently reported to modify the phenotype of a family carrying the Asp178Asn/129V genotype [98]. The Gly127Val polymorphism was recently identified in a small group of healthy individuals in the region of New Guinea where kuru was prevalent, supporting the notion that this rare polymorphism confers protection against prion infection [99].

Environment

The vast majority of cases occur spontaneously, as a sporadic or genetic form of prion disease; however acquired forms of prion disease do exist, as exemplified by iCJD, described earlier in this chapter. Iatrogenic CJD (iCJD) has been reported as a result of exposure to prion-contaminated tissues or surgical instruments previously used in individuals with prion disease. At the time of writing, these include 3 corneal transplants, approximately 160 growth hormone cases, approximately 5 from gonadotropic hormone, approximately 135 dura mater grafts, and approximately 6 from neurosurgical instruments, including brain electrodes used for seizure mapping [8, 100–104]. Because of the resistant nature of prions to typical modes of sterilization, autoclaving instruments at routine times and temperatures is not sufficient for prion decontamination [105].

Prion diseases are not limited to humans. Scrapie, a naturally occurring transmissible spongiform encephalopathy (TSE) of sheep, has long been recognized. The observation that scrapie occurred in multiple sheep within a flock suggested its transmissible nature, which was eventually proven when healthy sheep succumbed to scrapie following inoculation with brain homogenate from scrapie-sick sheep [106–108]. Although a link between scrapie and human prion disease has never been made, the occurrence of bovine spongiform encephalopathy (BSE) in the late 1990s underscored the potential for zoonotic prion disease to develop into a public health threat for humans. Consumption of beef contaminated with BSE was linked to a new strain of CJD termed variant CJD (vCJD) in the UK and Europe. Approximately 200 individuals worldwide have thus far developed vCJD, the incidence of which peaked in 2000, with 28 cases reported in the UK. In 2011, 5 cases were reported. Individuals homozygous for methionine at codon 129 (129MM) have been nearly exclusively affected. Whether a second wave of vCJD will occur in less susceptible 129MV or 129VV individuals remains a question and concern.

In the USA, a naturally occurring disease of cervids, known as chronic wasting disease of deer and elk (CWD), was first reported in 1967 in a wildlife research facility in northern Colorado and then in free-ranging deer and elk in northeastern Colorado and southeastern Wyoming [109]. CWD has since spread throughout the USA and Canada and has been detected as far east as Virginia and New York. This natural spread has led to work that supports the shedding of CWD prions into the environment from decomposing carcasses of affected animals, or from feces, urine, and saliva of living animals [110–112]. Low titers of CWD prions have been reported in soil and water samples of endemic areas [113]. Direct evidence for CWD transmission to humans has not been demonstrated by intense surveillance studies to identify new strains of CJD, and transgenic mice that express human prion protein have not demonstrated sensitivity to CWD prions, suggesting a substantial species barrier to humans [114], although *in vitro* amplification assays suggest the potential is present [58].

Clinical prodrome and biomarkers

The rarity and rapid progression of prion diseases in general makes early detection difficult. However, in hindsight, many patients report mild neurological disturbances, including vertigo, fatigue, impaired sleep, headaches, or other vague symptoms that precede the obvious onset of disease by a year or more [115]. Known biomarkers for sCJD include a characteristic pattern of restricted diffusion on brain MRI, 1–2 Hz periodic sharp wave complexes (PSWCs) on the EEG, and elevated 14-3-3 and/or tau protein in cerebrospinal fluid (CSF). Neuron-specific enolase may also be increased in the CSF. FI is uniquely associated with a focal reduction of ^{18}FDG uptake by positron emission tomography (PET). These markers are used in the diagnostic workup of prion disease, as described in more detail in the next section.

Examination and investigations (including imaging)

A comprehensive history and neurological exam that includes an assessment of cognitive function, either using brief standardized assessments such as Folstein's Mini Mental State Exam (MMSE) or the Montreal Cognitive Assessment (MoCA) battery, should be performed in all cases. Depending on the subtype of disease, the approach may differ. For instance, sCJD, because of its progressive course, may warrant hospitalization to rule out CNS infection or an inflammatory process. In general, when a prion disease is considered, the most helpful studies include brain MRI, especially diffusion-weighted images (DWI), EEG, and CSF analysis. None of these studies is individually diagnostic, but when combined with a comprehensive workup to rule out other conditions that may masquerade as prion disease, they provide increased assurance of the diagnosis.

Magnetic resonance imaging (MRI)

DWI of the brain commonly shows hyperintensities of the cortical ribbon and/or basal ganglia (caudate and putamen) in sCJD. These findings are much less common in genetic forms of prion disease, although they have been reported with some *PRNP* mutations [116–118]. In vCJD, the pulvinar of the thalamus is more likely to exhibit hyperintensities with proton density imaging (PDI) or DWI. This marker has not been well studied in GSS, FFI, or SFI.

Electroencephalogram (EEG)

Periodic sharp wave complexes (PSWCs) at a frequency of 0.5–2 per second are seen in approximately 65% of sCJD cases, but they are much less common or absent in other subtypes. Some mutations associated with a faster course of progression than typical fCJD, such as E200K and V210I, are more likely to show periodic discharges. This relationship is also evident in sCJD, such that more slowly progressive cases have a lower likelihood to exhibit PSWCs. The EEG in FI displays diffuse slowing rather than PSWCs [119].

Cerebrospinal fluid (CSF)

A mild increase in total protein (~10% above normal), a high level of tau protein (>1200 pg/mL), neuron-specific enolase (NSE), and/or 14-3-3 protein support the diagnosis of prion disease. However, these proteins only represent dying neurons and are not specific to prion disease. False positive elevations in 14-3-3 have been reported with herpes encephalitis, acute stroke, and other neurological conditions that result in rapid neuronal cell death. In addition, in some case series, 14-3-3 was reported to be negative in nearly half of all cases [120]. Normal CSF cell count and glucose levels are the norm.

A significant leukocytosis within CSF strongly argues against a prion disease diagnosis.

Positron emission tomography (PET)

^{18}FDG uptake has been studied in prion disease but it does not have a consistent pattern except in FI, where a reduction in metabolic activity in the thalamus is a characteristic feature. Single photon emission tomography may be a substitute for this study.

Other tests

Because prion disease is a diagnosis of exclusion, a comprehensive battery of blood tests should rule out the possibility of infectious, inflammatory, toxic/metabolic, malignant, and paraneoplastic conditions. Thus, in addition to the typical panel of blood tests for evaluations of dementia (complete blood count, comprehensive medical panel, thyroid-stimulating hormone, vitamin B_{12}, and in endemic areas, rapid plasma reagin), the following should also be sent: liver function panel that includes ammonia, C-reactive protein (CRP), copper and ceruloplasmin, heavy metal screen, serum and urine protein electrophoresis, and a connective tissue disease workup (erythrocyte sedimentation rate, CRP, anti-nuclear antibodies, rheumatoid factor, anti-dsDNA, anti-SS-A, anti-SS-B, c-ANCA, and p-ANCA antibodies), a full paraneoplastic panel including anti-GAD65 antibody, anti-Ma and anti-Ta antibodies, and anti-NMDA receptor antibodies, Lyme antibodies, and HIV. To rule out Hashimoto's encephalopathy, a steroid-responsive condition that can masquerade as CJD, anti-thyroglobulin and anti-thyroperoxidase antibodies should also be sent, regardless of a euthyroid state. CSF testing should include cell count, protein, IgG synthesis, oligoclonal bands, polymerase chain reaction (PCR) for *T. whipplei*, herpes simplex virus, Lyme, and appropriate cultures for other pathogens.

Additional studies

An overnight polysomnogram may be useful for detecting a reduction in total sleep time in the early stages of FI.

Diagnosis and prognosis

The clinical diagnosis of prion disease is often difficult. Because of its rarity and because the early symptoms may be nonspecific, the diagnosis is often delayed. Specific criteria for sCJD and vCJD were established by the World Health Organization (WHO) and later modified and expanded to include fCJD and iCJD (Table 3.3). The diagnosis of prion disease subtypes is based largely on the clinical presentation, as described above, and the exclusion of other conditions. A positive mutation within the *PRNP* gene assists to confirm a familial prion disease. The differential diagnosis is extensive and includes other neurodegenerative diseases such as dementia with Lewy bodies, Huntington's disease, Alzheimer's disease, spinocerebellar ataxia (SCA), and all frontotemporal lobar dementias (FTLDs). In addition to these conditions, autoimmune causes such as Hashimoto's encephalopathy, as noted above, CNS vasculitis, limbic encephalitis, and other paraneoplastic syndromes have been mistaken for prion disease. Finally, other toxic/metabolic and infectious etiologies, such as heavy metal toxicity and CNS viral infections, may be initially misdiagnosed as prion disease. Prognosis for all prion diseases is poor, although the rate of progression varies, depending on the specific subtype of prion disease, as described above. All subtypes are invariably fatal.

Table 3.3 Diagnostic criteria of prion disease.

I. Sporadic CJD

A. Definite:

Histopathological presence of spongiform degeneration (vacuolation) and gliosis, and/or western blot presence of protease-resistant PrP. Note, this is the histopathology for CJD, not for other prion subtypes (see below).

B. Probable:

Rapidly progressive dementia; *and* at least two of the following:
  i. Myoclonus
  ii. Visual or cerebellar signs
  iii. Pyramidal/extrapyramidal signs
  iv. Akinetic mutism
and a positive result from at least one of the following:
  a. Periodic EEG
  b. Positive CSF 14-3-3 (or extremely elevated tau protein >1200–1500 pg/mL*) in patients with disease under 2 years duration
  c. MRI of brain with high signal abnormalities in basal ganglia (or cortical ribbon) by diffusion weighted imaging (DWI) or fluid attenuated inversion recovery (FLAIR)
and the absence of:
  Routine investigations indicating an alternative diagnosis
(* author's additional modifications – tau levels may be greater than 3000 pg/mL)

C. Possible:

Progressive dementia *and* at least two of the following features:
  i. Myoclonus
  ii. Visual or cerebellar signs
  iii. Pyramidal/extrapyramidal signs
  iv. Akinetic mutism
and the absence of a positive result for any of the three tests described for Probable
  CJD (a–c, above)
and duration of illness less than 2 years
and without routine investigations indicating an alternative diagnosis

II. Iatrogenic CJD

Progressive cerebellar syndrome in a recipient of human cadaveric-derived pituitary hormone; or sporadic CJD with a recognized exposure risk, e.g., antecedent neurosurgery with dura mater implantation.

III. Familial CJD

Definite or probable CJD plus definite or probable CJD in a first degree relative, and/or neuropsychiatric disorder plus disease-specific *PRNP* gene mutation.

IV. Variant Creutzfeldt–Jakob disease (vCJD)

A. Definite:

Neuropathologic examination of brain tissue shows:
  i. Widespread florid plaques.
  ii. Extensive spongiform degeneration and immunohistochemical detection of prion protein deposits throughout the cerebellum and cerebrum.

B. Probable:
  a. Current age or age at death <55 years
  b. Progressive neuropsychiatric disorder for more than 6 months
  c. At least four of the following five symptoms:
    1. Early psychiatric symptoms (depression, anxiety, apathy withdrawal, delusions)
    2. Persistent painful sensory symptoms (including both frank pain and/or unpleasant dysesthesia)
    3. Ataxia
    4. Myoclonus, chorea or dystonia
    5. Dementia
  d. EEG does not show the typical appearances of sporadic CJD or no EEG has been performed
  e. Routine investigations do not suggest an alternative diagnosis
  f. Symmetrical high signal in the posterior thalamus (pulvinar) on a MRI brain scan
  g. No history of potential iatrogenic exposure

Note: A positive tonsil biopsy for PrP[pres], combined with criteria a, e, and g above also constitutes a diagnosis of Probable vCJD.

Treatment options (including comorbid conditions)

Medical

There are no available therapies for prion disease. Medical management for comorbid features of disease involves the use of antiepileptic drugs for seizures that may develop, and clonazepam for myoclonus. Supportive devices for gait imbalance, if that is an early symptom of disease, should be provided, in addition to consultation with physical and occupational therapy. If psychotic symptoms of delusions or hallucinations develop, atypical anti-psychotics (quetiapine, olanzapine, risperidone) in low doses with upward titration until symptoms improve, should be considered.

Some agents with potential therapeutic effect have been tested in humans with prion disease. Most notable of these is quinacrine, an anti-malarial that showed promise in an *in vitro* model of mouse neuroblastoma cells chronically infected with prions [121]. Clinical trials conducted in 107 subjects with various forms of CJD in the UK, 32 patients with primarily sCJD in France, and a similar number of sCJD patients from the USA failed to demonstrate a clinical benefit [122–124]. Another drug that has received considerable attention is pentosan polysulfate (PPS), a polysulfated amine that has been proposed to sequester prions from other interacting proteins. PPS modestly delayed death in rodents infected with prions [125, 126], and, in a series of small and anecdotal studies, it was reported to extend the course of sCJD in some individuals but not others [127–129]. Because it poorly penetrates the blood–brain barrier, PPS must be delivered intracerebroventricularly. A noteworthy anecdotal report describes a young man with vCJD treated with intraventricular PPS, beginning 19 months after his initial symptoms, who showed a prolonged survival of 51 months at the time of the report [127, 130]. Because the median duration of vCJD was 13 months (range 6–39), this was considered significant. Whether the prolonged duration was his natural course or a result of the PPS could not be determined. Interestingly, another study found PPS to inhibit the amplification of PrP^{Sc} *in vitro*, using PMCA [131]. Two other drugs have been applied to human prion disease: flupirtine, a non-opioid analgesic, and doxycycline, a tetracycline antibiotic. Flupirtine was found to exhibit anti-apoptotic effects in an in vitro assay of prion toxicity [132], which led to a clinical trial in 28 patients with sporadic and genetic CJD that showed no benefit in survival [133]. Doxycycline prolonged survival in a rodent model of scrapie and reduced PrP^{Sc} generation *in vitro* (see [134] for review). A trial of doxycycline in 44 sCJD and 7 genetic CJD cases was reported to significantly prolong survival with a median of 292 days (range 162–635 days) compared with historical controls of 167 days (range 33–1448 days) [135]. Additional studies with doxycycline are in progress. Finally, data in cell culture and rodent models of prion disease provide some support that autophagy inducers might be beneficial in prion disease [136–138].

In addition to the above agents, anti-PrP antibody therapy, designed to block the interaction of PrP^{Sc} with PrP^{C} [139–141], is being explored, as is the attractive approach of RNA inhibition (RNAi) to knock down PrP^{C} expression, thereby reducing the total PrP^{C} substrate for conversion to PrP^{Sc} [142]. While these have only been studied *in vitro* or in rodent models of prion disease, they are promising strategies for human application.

Surgical

There is no indication for surgery in a patient diagnosed with prion disease. In the past, brain biopsies were occasionally performed on patients with an unclear diagnosis, but their use is now limited, in light of the cumbersome preparation and decontamination procedures required in the operating room.

Social

The tumultuous course of prion disease is devastating for the patient and the family. As such, a social worker should be involved as soon as a diagnosis is made, to assist with ensuring that the patient will have adequate support at home and/or help the transition to palliative care or hospice, in addition to assisting the family with any other social issues. In the USA, post mortem examination should be made in all cases, with referral of cases to the National Prion Surveillance Center at Case Western University, for disease confirmation, *PRNP* genetic testing, and PrP^{Sc} typing.

Future developments

Despite the unusual nature of prion disease, the future goals are similar to those of other neurodegenerative diseases. At the basic level, the normal function of PrP still needs to be clarified, as does the pathogenic process that underlies disease. On the clinical front, more sensitive and specific tests to allow earlier diagnosis and detection of prions are a focus of interest and need. Because prion disease is transmissible, tests that detect prions in biologicals, foods, and wild game are also under intense investigation. PMCA technology

has seen widespread application and promise with respect to this area of study. An extension of this technique, known as real-time quaking-induced conversion (RTQuIC), has been shown to be very highly specific and sensitive for detecting prions within CSF [143]. Therapy for prion disease is especially needed, but clinical trials are extremely challenging because of the rarity of disease and the rapid progression of most cases. Successful studies in transgenic models of disease are likely to provide the best approach for screening potentially useful therapies.

References

1. Gomori, A.J., et al., The ataxic form of Creutzfeldt-Jakob disease. *Arch. Neurol.*, 1973. 29: p. 318–323.
2. Yamada, M., et al., [Prion disease surveillance in Japan: analysis of 1,241 patients]. Rinsho shinkeigaku = Clinical neurology, 2009. 49(11): p. 939–942.
3. Spudich, S., et al., Complete penetrance of Creutzfeldt-Jakob disease in Libyan Jews carrying the E200K mutation in the prion protein gene. *Mol. Med.*, 1995. 1: p. 607–613.
4. Kovacs, G.G., et al., Mutations of the prion protein gene phenotypic spectrum. *J. Neurol.*, 2002. 249(11): p. 1567–1582.
5. Anderson, J.R., C.M.C. Allen, and R.O. Weller, Creutzfeldt-Jakob disease following human pituitary-derived growth hormone administration [Abstr.]. *Neuropathol. Appl. Neurobiol.*, 1990. 16: p. 543.
6. Billette de Villemeur, T., et al., *Creutzfeldt-Jakob disease in children treated with growth hormone. Lancet*, 1991. 337: p. 864–865.
7. Billette de Villemeur, T., et al., Iatrogenic Creutzfeldt-Jakob disease in three growth hormone recipients: a neuropathological study. *Neuropathol. Appl. Neurobiol.*, 1994. 20: p. 111–117.
8. Brown, P., et al., Potential epidemic of Creutzfeldt-Jakob disease from human growth hormone therapy. *N. Engl. J. Med.*, 1985. 313: p. 728–731.
9. Gibbs, C.J., Jr., et al., Creutzfeldt-Jakob disease infectivity of growth hormone derived from human pituitary glands. *N. Engl. J. Med.*, 1993. 328: p. 358–359.
10. Creutzfeldt-Jakob disease associated with cadaveric dura mater grafts – Japan, January 1979-May 1996. *MMWR. Morb. Mortal. Wkly Rep.*, 1997. 46(45): p. 1066–1069.
11. Brown, P., M.A. Preece, and R.G. Will, "Friendly fire" in medicine: hormones, homografts, and Creutzfeldt-Jakob disease. *Lancet*, 1992. 340: p. 24–27.
12. Otto, D., Jacob-Creutzfeldt disease associated with cadaveric dura. *J. Neurosurg.*, 1987. 67: p. 149.
13. Thadani, V., et al., Creutzfeldt-Jakob disease probably acquired from a cadaveric dura mater graft. *Case report. J. Neurosurg.*, 1988. 69: p. 766–769.
14. Nisbet, T.J., I. MacDonaldson, and S.N. Bishara, Creutzfeldt-Jakob disease in a second patient who received a cadaveric dura mater graft. *J. Am. Med. Assoc.*, 1989. 261: p. 1118.
15. Masullo, C., et al., Transmission of Creutzfeldt-Jakob disease by dural cadaveric graft. *J. Neurosurg.*, 1989. 71: p. 954.
16. Willison, H.J., A.N. Gale, and J.E. McLaughlin, Creutzfeldt-Jakob disease following cadaveric dura mater graft. *J. Neurol. Neurosurg. Psychiatry*, 1991. 54: p. 940.
17. Bateman, D., et al., Sporadic Creutzfeldt-Jakob disease in a 18-year-old in the UK (Lett.). *Lancet*, 1995. 346: p. 1155–1156.
18. Britton, T.C., et al., Sporadic Creutzfeldt-Jakob disease in a 16-year-old in the UK (Lett.). *Lancet*, 1995. 346: p. 1155.
19. Chazot, G., et al., New variant of Creutzfeldt-Jakob disease in a 26-year-old French man. *Lancet*, 1996. 347: p. 1181.
20. Kopp, N., et al., Creutzfeldt-Jakob disease in a 52-year-old woman with florid plaques. *Lancet*, 1996. 348: p. 1239–1240.
21. Will, R.G., et al., A new variant of Creutzfeldt-Jakob disease in the UK. *Lancet*, 1996. 347: p. 921–925.
22. Llewelyn, C.A., et al., Possible transmission of variant Creutzfeldt-Jakob disease by blood transfusion. *Lancet*, 2004. 363(9407): p. 417–421.
23. Peden, A.H., et al., Preclinical vCJD after blood transfusion in a PRNP codon 129 heterozygous patient. *Lancet*, 2004. 364(9433): p. 527–529.
24. Wroe, S.J., et al., Clinical presentation and pre-mortem diagnosis of variant Creutzfeldt-Jakob disease associated with blood transfusion: a case report. *Lancet*, 2006. 368(9552): p. 2061–2067.
25. Peden, A., et al., Variant CJD infection in the spleen of a neurologically asymptomatic UK adult patient with haemophilia. *Haemophilia*, 2010. 16(2): p. 296–304.
26. Gerstmann, J., Über ein noch nicht beschriebenes Reflex-phanomen bei einer Erkrankung des zerebellaren Systems. Wien. *Med. Wochenschr.*, 1928. 78: p. 906–908.

27. Gerstmann, J., E. Sträussler, and I. Scheinker, Über eine eigenartige hereditär-familiäre Erkrankung des Zentralnervensystems zugleich ein Beitrag zur frage des vorzeitigen lokalen Alterns. *Z. Neurol.*, 1936. 154: p. 736–762.

28. Hinnell, C., et al., Gerstmann-Straussler-Scheinker disease due to a novel prion protein gene mutation. *Neurology*, 2011. 76(5): p. 485–487.

29. Lugaresi, E., et al., Fatal familial insomnia and dysautonomia with selective degeneration of thalamic nuclei. *N. Engl. J. Med.*, 1986. 315: p. 997–1003.

30. Petersen, R.B., et al., Analysis of the prion protein gene in thalamic dementia. *Neurology*, 1992. 42: p. 1859–1863.

31. Goldfarb, L.G., et al., Fatal familial insomnia and familial Creutzfeldt-Jakob disease: disease phenotype determined by a DNA polymorphism. *Science*, 1992. 258: p. 806–808.

32. Mastrianni, J.A., et al., Prion protein conformation in a patient with sporadic fatal insomnia. *N. Engl. J. Med.*, 1999. 340(21): p. 1630–1638.

33. Parchi, P., et al., A subtype of sporadic prion disease mimicking fatal familial insomnia. *Neurology*, 1999. 52(9): p. 1757–1763.

34. McLean, C.A., et al., The D178N (cis-129M) "fatal familial insomnia" mutation associated with diverse clinicopathologic phenotypes in an Australian kindred. *Neurology*, 1997. 49: p. 552–558.

35. Montagna, P., et al., Familial and sporadic fatal insomnia. *Lancet Neurol.*, 2003. 2(3): p. 167–176.

36. Gambetti, P., et al., A novel human disease with abnormal prion protein sensitive to protease. *Ann. Neurol.*, 2008. 63(6): p. 697–708.

37. Zou, W.Q., et al., Variably protease-sensitive prionopathy: a new sporadic disease of the prion protein. *Ann. Neurol.*, 2010. 68(2): p. 162–172.

38. Beck, E., et al., The pathogenesis of transmissible spongiform encephalopathy – an ultrastructural study. *Brain*, 1982. 105: p. 755–786.

39. Chou, S.M., et al., Transmission and scanning electron microscopy of spongiform change in Creutzfeldt-Jakob disease. *Brain*, 1980. 103: p. 885–904.

40. Lampert, P.W., D.C. Gajdusek, and C.J. Gibbs, Jr., Subacute spongiform virus encephalopathies. Scrapie, kuru and Creutzfeldt-Jakob disease: a review. *Am. J. Pathol.*, 1972. 68: p. 626–652.

41. Liberski, P.P., D.C. Gajdusek, and P. Brown, How do neurons degenerate in prion diseases or transmissible spongiform encephalopathies (TSEs): neuronal autophagy revisited. *Acta Neurobiol. Exp. (Wars.)*, 2002. 62(3): p. 141–147.

42. Ghetti, B., et al., Hereditary prion protein amyloidoses. *Clin. Lab. Med.*, 2003. 23(1): p. 65–85, viii.

43. Ironside, J.W., et al., Neuropathology of variant Creutzfeldt-Jakob disease. *Acta Neurobiol. Exp. (Wars.)*, 2002. 62(3): p. 175–182.

44. Parchi, P., et al., Typing prion isoforms (Lett.). *Nature*, 1997. 386: p. 232–233.

45. Gambetti, P., et al., Sporadic and familial CJD: classification and characterisation. *Br. Med. Bull.*, 2003. 66: p. 213–239.

46. Wadsworth, J.D., et al., Molecular and clinical classification of human prion disease. *Br. Med. Bull.*, 2003. 66: p. 241–254.

47. Tunnell, E., et al., A novel PRNP-P105S mutation associated with atypical prion disease and a rare PrPSc conformation. *Neurology*, 2008. 71(18): p. 1431–1438.

48. Zanusso, G., et al., Novel prion protein conformation and glycotype in Creutzfeldt-Jakob disease. *Arch. Neurol.*, 2007. 64(4): p. 595–599.

49. Chasseigneaux, S., et al., V180I mutation of the prion protein gene associated with atypical PrPSc glycosylation. *Neurosci. Lett.*, 2006. 408(3): p. 165–169.

50. Grasbon-Frodl, E., et al., Loss of glycosylation associated with the T183A mutation in human prion disease. *Acta Neuropathol. (Berl.)*, 2004. 108(6): p. 476–484.

51. Brown, P., et al., Human spongiform encephalopathy: the National Institutes of Health series of 300 cases of experimentally transmitted disease. *Ann. Neurol.*, 1994. 35: p. 513–529.

52. Telling, G.C., et al., Transmission of Creutzfeldt-Jakob disease from humans to transgenic mice expressing chimeric human-mouse prion protein. *Proc. Natl. Acad. Sci. USA*, 1994. 91: p. 9936–9940.

53. Nonno, R., et al., Efficient transmission and characterization of Creutzfeldt-Jakob disease strains in bank voles. *PLoS Pathog.*, 2006. 2(2): p. e12.

54. Soto, C., G.P. Saborio, and L. Anderes, Cyclic amplification of protein misfolding: application to prion-related disorders and beyond. *Trends Neurosci.*, 2002. 25(8): p. 390–394.

55. Castilla, J., et al., Crossing the species barrier by PrP(Sc) replication in vitro generates unique infectious prions. *Cell*, 2008. 134(5): p. 757–768.

56. Meyerett, C., et al., In vitro strain adaptation of CWD prions by serial protein misfolding cyclic amplification. *Virology*, 2008. 382(2): p. 267–276.

57. Jones, M., et al., The application of in vitro cell-free conversion systems to human prion diseases. *Acta Neuropathol.*, 2011. 121(1): p. 135–143.

58. Barria, M.A., et al., Generation of a new form of human PrP(Sc) in vitro by inter-species transmission from cervid prions. *J. Biol. Chem.*, 2011. 286(9): p. 7490–7495.

59. Wadsworth, J.D., et al., Human prion protein with valine 129 prevents expression of variant CJD phenotype. *Science*, 2004. 306(5702): p. 1793–1796.

60. Mallik, S., et al., Live cell fluorescence resonance energy transfer predicts an altered molecular association of heterologous PrPSc with PrPC. *J. Biol. Chem.*, 2010. 285(12): p. 8967–8975.

61. Dorandeu, A., et al., Neuronal apoptosis in fatal familial insomnia. *Brain Pathol.*, 1998. 8(3): p. 531–537.

62. Fairbairn, D.W., et al., Detection of apoptosis induced DNA cleavage in scrapie-infected sheep brain. *FEMS Microbiol. Lett.*, 1994. 115: p. 341–346.

63. Gray, F., et al., Neuronal apoptosis in creutzfeldt-jakob disease. *J. Neuropathol. Exp. Neurol.*, 1999. 58(4): p. 321–328.

64. Hetz, C., et al., Caspase-12 and endoplasmic reticulum stress mediate neurotoxicity of pathological prion protein. *EMBO J.*, 2003. 22(20): p. 5435–5445.

65. Kristiansen, M., et al., Disease-related prion protein forms aggresomes in neuronal cells leading to caspase activation and apoptosis. *J. Biol. Chem.*, 2005. 280(46): p. 38851–38861.

66. Bounhar, Y., et al., Prion protein protects human neurons against Bax-mediated apoptosis. *J. Biol. Chem.*, 2001. 276(42): p. 39145–39149.

67. Chiarini, L.B., et al., Cellular prion protein transduces neuroprotective signals. *EMBO J.*, 2002. 21(13): p. 3317–3326.

68. Sikorska, B., et al., Autophagy is a part of ultrastructural synaptic pathology in Creutzfeldt-Jakob disease: a brain biopsy study. *Int. J. Biochem. Cell Biol.*, 2004. 36(12): p. 2563–2573.

69. Liberski, P.P., et al., Cell death and autophagy in prion diseases (transmissible spongiform encephalopathies). *Folia Neuropathol.*, 2008. 46(1): p. 1–25.

70. Kanaani, J., et al., Recombinant prion protein induces rapid polarization and development of synapses in embryonic rat hippocampal neurons in vitro. *J. Neurochem.*, 2005. 95(5): p. 1373–1386.

71. Collinge, J., et al., Prion protein is necessary for normal synaptic function. *Nature*, 1994. 370: p. 295–297.

72. Spielhaupter, C. and H.M. Schatzl, PrPC directly interacts with proteins involved in signaling pathways. *J. Biol. Chem.*, 2001. 276(48): p. 44604–44612.

73. Solforosi, L., et al., Cross-linking cellular prion protein triggers neuronal apoptosis in vivo. *Science*, 2004. 303(5663): p. 1514–1516.

74. Mouillet-Richard, S., et al., Signal transduction through prion protein. *Science*, 2000. 289(5486): p. 1925–1928.

75. Brown, D.R., et al., The cellular prion protein binds copper in vivo. *Nature*, 1997. 390: p. 684–687.

76. Roucou, X., et al., Cytosolic prion protein is not toxic and protects against Bax-mediated cell death in human primary neurons. *J. Biol. Chem.*, 2003. 278(42): p. 40877–40881.

77. Roucou, X. and A.C. LeBlanc, Cellular prion protein neuroprotective function: implications in prion diseases. *J. Mol. Med.*, 2005. 83(1): p. 3–11.

78. Lauren, J., et al., Cellular prion protein mediates impairment of synaptic plasticity by amyloid-beta oligomers. *Nature*, 2009. 457(7233): p. 1128–1132.

79. Parkin, E.T., et al., Cellular prion protein regulates beta-secretase cleavage of the Alzheimer's amyloid precursor protein. *Proc. Natl. Acad. Sci. U S A*, 2007. 104(26): p. 11062–11067.

80. Büeler, H., et al., Mice devoid of PrP are resistant to scrapie. *Cell*, 1993. 73: p. 1339–1347.

81. Manson, J.C., et al., 129/Ola mice carrying a null mutation in PrP that abolishes mRNA production are developmentally normal. *Mol. Neurobiol.*, 1994. 8: p. 121–127.

82. Mallucci, G.R., et al., Post-natal knockout of prion protein alters hippocampal CA1 properties, but does not result in neurodegeneration. *EMBO J.*, 2002. 21(3): p. 202–210.

83. Hsiao, K., et al., Spontaneous neurodegeneration in transgenic mice with prion protein codon 101 proline->leucine substitution. *Ann. N.Y. Acad. Sci.*, 1991. 640: p. 166–170.

84. Jackson, W.S., et al., Spontaneous generation of prion infectivity in fatal familial insomnia knockin mice. *Neuron*, 2009. 63(4): p. 438–450.

85. Yang, W., et al., A new transgenic mouse model of Gerstmann-Straussler-Scheinker syndrome caused by the A117V mutation of PRNP. *J. Neurosci.*, 2009. 29(32): p. 10072–10080.

86. Chiesa, R., et al., Neurological illness in transgenic mice expressing a prion protein with an insertional mutation. *Neuron*, 1998. 21(6): p. 1339–1351.

87. Dossena, S., et al., Mutant prion protein expression causes motor and memory deficits and abnormal sleep patterns in a transgenic mouse model. *Neuron*, 2008. 60(4): p. 598–609.

88. Silveira, J.R., et al., The most infectious prion protein particles. *Nature*, 2005. 437(7056): p. 257–261.

89. Chesebro, B., et al., Anchorless prion protein results in infectious amyloid disease without clinical scrapie. *Science*, 2005. 308(5727): p. 1435–1439.

90. Hegde, R.S., et al., A transmembrane form of the prion protein in neurodegenerative disease. *Science*, 1998. 279: p. 827–834.

91. Ma, J., R. Wollmann, and S. Lindquist, Neurotoxicity and neurodegeneration when PrP accumulates in the cytosol. *Science*, 2002. 298(5599): p. 1781–1785.

92. Stewart, R.S., et al., Neurodegenerative illness in transgenic mice expressing a transmembrane form of the prion protein. *J. Neurosci.*, 2005. 25(13): p. 3469–3477.

93. Rane, N.S., J.L. Yonkovich, and R.S. Hegde, Protection from cytosolic prion protein toxicity by modulation of protein translocation. *EMBO J.*, 2004. 23(23): p. 4550–4559.

94. Wang, X., et al., The interaction between cytoplasmic prion protein and the hydrophobic lipid core of membrane correlates with neurotoxicity. *J. Biol. Chem.*, 2006. 281(19): p. 13559–13565.

95. Collee, J.G., R. Bradley, and P.P. Liberski, Variant CJD (vCJD) and bovine spongiform encephalopathy (BSE): 10 and 20 years on: part 2. *Folia Neuropathol.*, 2006. 44(2): p. 102–110.

96. Parchi, P., et al., Molecular basis of phenotypic variability in sporadic Creutzfeldt-Jakob disease. *Ann. Neurol.*, 1996. 39: p. 767–778.

97. Perrier, V., et al., Dominant-negative inhibition of prion replication in transgenic mice. *Proc. Natl. Acad. Sci. U S A*, 2002. 99(20): p. 13079–13084.

98. Appleby, B.S., et al., D178N, 129Val and N171S, 129Val genotype in a family with Creutzfeldt-Jakob disease. *Dement. Geriatr. Cogn. Disord.*, 2010. 30(5): p. 424–431.

99. Mead, S., et al., A novel protective prion protein variant that colocalizes with kuru exposure. *N. Engl J. Med.*, 2009. 361(21): p. 2056–2065.

100. Bernoulli, C., et al., Danger of accidental person-to-person transmission of Creutzfeldt-Jakob disease by surgery. *Lancet*, 1977. 1(8009): p. 478–479.

101. Davanipour, Z., et al., Possible modes of transmission of Creutzfeldt-Jakob disease. *N. Engl. J. Med.*, 1984. 311: p. 1582–1583.

102. Buchanan, C.R., M.A. Preece, and R.D.G. Milner, Mortality, neoplasia and Creutzfeldt-Jakob disease in patients treated with pituitary growth hormone in the United Kingdom. *Br. Med. J.*, 1991. 302: p. 824–828.

103. Fradkin, J.E., et al., Creutzfeldt-Jakob disease in pituitary growth hormone recipients in the United States. *JAMA*, 1991. 265: p. 880–884.

104. Healy, D.L. and J. Evans, Creutzfeldt-Jakob disease after pituitary gonadotrophins. *Br. J. Med.*, 1993. 307: p. 517–518.

105. Dickinson, A.G. and D.M. Taylor, Resistance of scrapie agent to decontamination. *N. Engl. J. Med.*, 1978. 299: p. 1413–1414.

106. Brotherston, J.G., et al., Spread of scrapie by contact to goats and sheep. *J. Comp. Pathol.*, 1968. 78: p. 9–17.

107. Dickinson, A.G. and J.T. Stamp, Experimental scrapie in Cheviot and Suffolk sheep. *J. Comp. Pathol.*, 1969. 79: p. 23–26.

108. Hadlow, W.J., et al., *Natural infection of sheep with scrapie virus, in Slow Transmissible Diseases of the Nervous System*, Vol. 2, S.B.Prusiner and W.J.Hadlow, Editors. 1979, Academic Press: New York. p. 3–12.

109. Williams, E.S. and S. Young, Chronic wasting disease of captive mule deer: a spongiform encephalopathy. *J. Wildl. Dis.*, 1980. 16: p. 89–98.

110. Angers, R.C., et al., Prions in skeletal muscles of deer with chronic wasting disease. *Science*, 2006. 311(5764): p. 1117.

111. Pulford, B., et al., Detection of PrP CWD in feces from naturally exposed Rocky Mountain elk (Cervus elaphus nelsoni) using protein misfolding cyclic amplification. *J. Wildlife Dis.*, 2012. 48(2): p. 425–434.

112. Haley, N.J., et al., Detection of CWD prions in urine and saliva of deer by transgenic mouse bioassay. *PloS one*, 2009. 4(3): p. e4848.

113. Nichols, T.A., et al., Detection of protease-resistant cervid prion protein in water from a CWD-endemic area. *Prion*, 2009. 3(3): p. 171–183.

114. Kong, Q., et al., Chronic wasting disease of elk: transmissibility to humans examined by transgenic mouse models. *J. Neurosci.*, 2005. 25(35): p. 7944–7949.

115. Brown, P., et al., Creutzfeldt-Jakob disease: clinical analysis of a consecutive series of 230 neuropathologically verified cases. Ann. Neurol., 1986. 20: p. 597–602.

116. Iwaski, Y., et al., [Clinicopathological characteristics of Creutzfeldt-Jakob disease with a PrP V180I mutation and M129V polymorphism on different alleles]. *Rinsho Shinkeigaku*, 1999. 39(8): p. 800–806.

117. Breithaupt, M., et al., Magnetic resonance imaging in E200K and V210I mutations of the prion protein gene. *Alzheimer Dis. Assoc. Disord.*, 2012. 27(1): p. 87–90.

118. Irisawa, M., et al., A case of Gerstmann-Straussler-Scheinker syndrome. *Magn. Reson. Med. Sci.*, 2007. 6(1): p. 53–57.

119. Gambetti, P., et al., Fatal familial insomnia and familial Creutzfeldt-Jakob disease: clinical, pathological and molecular features. *Brain Pathol.*, 1995. 5: p. 43–51.

120. Geschwind, M.D., et al., Challenging the clinical utility of the 14-3-3 protein for the diagnosis of sporadic Creutzfeldt-Jakob disease. *Arch. Neurol.*, 2003. 60(6): p. 813–816.

121. Korth, C., et al., Acridine and phenothiazine derivatives as pharmacotherapeutics for prion disease. *Proc. Natl. Acad. Sci. U S A*, 2001. 98(17): p. 9836–9841.

122. Collinge, J., et al., Safety and efficacy of quinacrine in human prion disease (PRION-1 study): a patient-preference trial. *Lancet Neurol.*, 2009. 8(4): p. 334–344.

123. Haik, S., et al., Compassionate use of quinacrine in Creutzfeldt-Jakob disease fails to show significant effects. *Neurology*, 2004. 63(12): p. 2413–2415.

124. Geschwind, M.D., Clinical trials for prion disease: difficult challenges, but hope for the future. *Lancet Neurol.*, 2009. 8(4): p. 304–306.

125. Ehlers, B. and H. Diringer, Dextran sulphate 500 delays and prevents mouse scrapie by impairment of agent replication in spleen. *J. Gen. Virol.*, 1984. 65: p. 1325–1330.

126. Doh-ura, K., et al., Treatment of transmissible spongiform encephalopathy by intraventricular drug infusion in animal models. *J. Virol.*, 2004. 78(10): p. 4999–5006.

127. Parry, A., et al., Long term survival in a patient with variant Creutzfeldt-Jakob disease treated with intraventricular pentosan polysulphate. *J. Neurol., Neurosurg. Psychiatry*, 2007. 78(7): p. 733–734.

128. Terada, T., et al., Less protease-resistant PrP in a patient with sporadic CJD treated with intraventricular pentosan polysulphate. *Acta Neurol. Scand*, 2010. 121(2): p. 127–130.

129. Bone, I., et al., Intraventricular pentosan polysulphate in human prion diseases: an observational study in the UK. *Eur. J. Neurol.*, 2008. 15(5): p. 458–464.

130. Todd, N.V., et al., Cerebroventricular infusion of pentosan polysulphate in human variant Creutzfeldt-Jakob disease. *J. Infect.*, 2005. 50(5): p. 394–396.

131. Yokoyama, T., et al., Heparin enhances the cell-protein misfolding cyclic amplification efficiency of variant Creutzfeldt-Jakob disease. *Neurosci. Lett.*, 2011. 498(2): p. 119–123.

132. Perovic, S., et al., Effect of flupirtine on Bcl-2 and glutathione level in neuronal cells treated in vitro with the prion protein fragment (PrP106-126). *Exp. Neurol.*, 1997. 147(2): p. 518–524.

133. Otto, M., et al., Efficacy of flupirtine on cognitive function in patients with CJD: A double-blind study. *Neurology*, 2004. 62(5): p. 714–718.

134. Forloni, G., et al., Tetracyclines and prion infectivity. *Infect. Disord. Drug Targets*, 2009. 9(1): p. 23–30.

135. Zerr, I., Therapeutic trials in human transmissible spongiform encephalo-pathies: recent advances and problems to address. *Infect. Disord. Drug Targets*, 2009. 9(1): p. 92–99.

136. Aguib, Y., et al., Autophagy induction by trehalose counteracts cellular prion infection. *Autophagy*, 2009. 5(3): p. 361–369.

137. Heiseke, A., et al., Lithium induces clearance of protease resistant prion protein in prion-infected cells by induction of autophagy. *J. Neurochem.*, 2009. 109(1): p. 25–34.

138. Sarkar, S. and D.C. Rubinsztein, Small molecule enhancers of autophagy for neurodegenerative diseases. *Mol. Biosyst.*, 2008. 4(9): p. 895–901.

139. Pankiewicz, J., et al., Clearance and prevention of prion infection in cell culture by anti-PrP antibodies. *Eur. J. Neurosci.*, 2006. 23(10): p. 2635–2647.

140. White, A.R., et al., Monoclonal antibodies inhibit prion replication and delay the development of prion disease. *Nature*, 2003. 422(6927): p. 80–83.

141. Shimizu, Y., et al., A novel anti-prion protein monoclonal antibody and its single-chain fragment variable derivative with ability to inhibit abnormal prion protein accumulation in cultured cells. *Microbiol. Immunol.*, 2010. 54(2): p. 112–121.

142. White, M.D. and G.R. Mallucci, RNAi for the treatment of prion disease: a window for intervention in neurodegeneration? CNS Neurol. *Disord. Drug Targets*, 2009. 8(5): p. 342–352.

143. Atarashi, R., et al., Real-time quaking-induced conversion: A highly sensitive assay for prion detection. *Prion*, 2011. 5(3): p. 150–153.

CHAPTER 4

Excitotoxicity

Mark P. Mattson

Laboratory of Neurosciences, National Institute on Aging Intramural Research Program, Baltimore, Maryland, USA

Clinical definition and epidemiology

Excitotoxicity is not a clinical diagnosis; instead it is a mechanism of neuronal degeneration believed to occur in a broad range of neurological disorders that involve the degeneration and death of neurons. Excitotoxicity can be defined as degeneration of neurons that occurs as the result of excessive activation of excitatory receptors, most commonly ionotropic glutamate receptors [1]. Ionotropic glutamate receptors include 2-amino-3-(5-methyl-3-oxo-1,2- oxazol-4-yl)propanoic acid (AMPA) and kainate receptors which flux mostly Na^+, and N-methyl-D-aspartate (NMDA) receptors which flux large amounts of Ca^{2+} [2] (Figure 4.1). Severe epileptic seizures can cause excitotoxic neuronal damage as the result of uncontrolled release of glutamate from presynaptic terminals, a "pure" form of excitotoxicity [3]. However, research during the past three decades has provided considerable evidence that physiological levels of glutamate receptor activation can contribute to neuronal degeneration when the nervous system suffers from a severe acute insult or a chronic neurodegenerative disorder.

Numerous studies of animal models have demonstrated the importance of glutamate receptor activation/excitotoxicity in the death of neurons in severe epileptic seizures, as well as the death of many neurons in focal ischemic stroke and global cerebral ischemia (cardiac arrest). Antagonists of AMPA and NMDA receptors can reduce the extent of brain damage and improve functional outcome in such animal models but, when tested in human patients, failed to improve the outcome [4, 5]. Similarly, positive effects of γ-aminobutyric acid (GABA) receptor agonists in preclinical studies were followed by clinical trials that revealed no benefits in stroke patients [5]. With regard to traumatic brain and spinal cord injury, animal models suggest a role for excitotoxicity in the neurodegenerative process, but clinical trials of glutamate receptor antagonists have not been positive [6, 7].

Four major neurodegenerative disorders in descending order of prevalence are Alzheimer's disease (AD), Parkinson disease (PD), Huntington's disease (HD), and amyotrophic lateral sclerosis (ALS). Evidence from studies of experimental models of these disorders, and some epidemiological and clinical data, point to the involvement of an excitatory imbalance and glutamate receptor-mediated cellular Ca^{2+} overload in the disease processes. The aging process is itself an important factor that sets the stage for the neuronal dysfunction and death in AD, PD, HD, and ALS [8]. The reasons that specific populations of neurons are selectively vulnerable in these four disorders (hippocampal and frontal cortical neurons in AD; brainstem autonomic neurons and midbrain dopaminergic neurons in PD; striatal medium spiny neurons in HD; and motor neurons in ALS) have not been established. However, there is evidence that disease-related processes in those neurons render them vulnerable to excitotoxicity. Thus, AD amyloid β-peptide (Aβ) increases the vulnerability of human cortical neurons to excitotoxicity [9], mitochondrial toxins used in PD models caused selective excitotoxic death of dopaminergic neurons [10], mutant huntingtin protein that causes HD renders neurons vulnerable to NMDA receptor-mediated excitotoxicity [11], and evidence from the research of Rothstein suggests that impaired glial glutamate transport contributes to excitotoxic death of motor neurons in ALS [12].

Spectrum of clinical phenotype

Epileptic seizures are a clinical manifestation of excessive unbridled activation of glutamate receptors. If severe and not controlled by drugs or diet, seizure-related excitotoxicity can occur, resulting in a range of behavioral abnormalities. The symptoms depend upon which brain region and neuronal circuits are included in the epileptic focus, and upon the relative vulnerability of neurons to excitotoxicity. For example, among the different types of neurons in the hippocampus, the CA1 neurons are particularly vulnerable to being damaged and killed by epileptic seizures, whereas dentate gyrus granule neurons are highly resistant to excitotoxicity [13]. Damage to hippocampal pyramidal neurons and entorhinal cortex neurons caused by seizures can result in cognitive deficits in patients with epilepsy [14], while damage to the amygdala can cause impaired control of emotion resulting in outbursts of anger, crying, etc. [15].

A sudden onset of amnesia or loss of motor control can be caused by exposures to excitotoxic neurotoxins. Three striking examples include cases in which more than one person in the same location developed symptoms similar to AD, PD, or HD. In 1987, scores of people developed severe memory impairment within a few days to weeks after eating at the same restaurant. Investigations identified the cause as domoic acid, a potent agonist of the kainate type of glutamate receptor, which was present in high amounts in shellfish served at the restaurant [16]. Kainic acid is another potent kainate receptor agonist that has been widely used to induce seizures and selective damage to hippocampal neurons in animal models of epilepsy (Figure 4.2). A second example is that of a group of illicit drug users in California

Neurodegeneration, First Edition. Edited by Anthony Schapira, Zbigniew Wszolek, Ted M. Dawson and Nicholas Wood.
© 2017 John Wiley & Sons, Ltd. Published 2017 by John Wiley & Sons, Ltd.

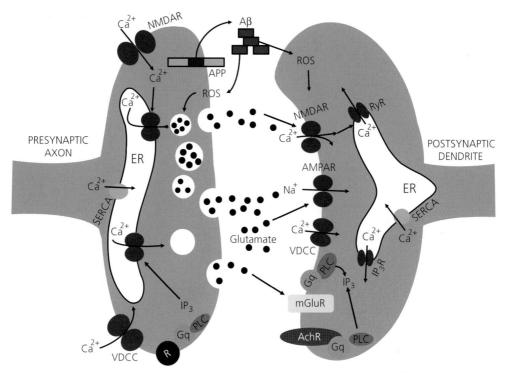

Figure 4.1 The early synaptic events in excitotoxicity: activation of glutamate receptors and Ca^{2+} influx. Depolarization of the plasma membrane in the presynaptic terminal (left) results in calcium influx through voltage-dependent Ca^{2+} channels (VDCC) which triggers fusion of synaptic vesicles with the membrane and release of glutamate into the extracellular milieu of the synapse. Ca^{2+} may also be released from the endoplasmic reticulum (ER) through either inositol triphosphate (IP_3) receptors or Ca^{2+}-activated ryanodine receptors. The ER also contributes to restoration of resting cytosolic Ca^{2+} levels by pumping Ca^{2+} into the ER via the sarco-endoplasmic reticulum Ca^{2+} ATPase (SERCA). Glutamate activates postsynaptic AMPA receptors (AMPAR) resulting in Na^+ influx and membrane depolarization. The membrane depolarization then activates VDCC and NMDA receptors (NMDAR) resulting in Ca^{2+} influx. In addition, Ca^{2+} release from the ER can be triggered by activation of metabotropic glutamate receptors (mGluR) and acetylcholine receptors (AchR). The vulnerability of synapses to excitotoxicity can be increased by the amyloid β-peptide (Aβ) which is generated from the amyloid precursor protein (APP), thought to be concentrated in presynaptic terminals. Aβ promotes excitotoxicity by inducing the production of reactive oxygen species (ROS). Gq, GTP-binding protein q; PLC, phospholipase C. Source: Kapogiannis 2011 [111]. Reproduced with permission of Elsevier.

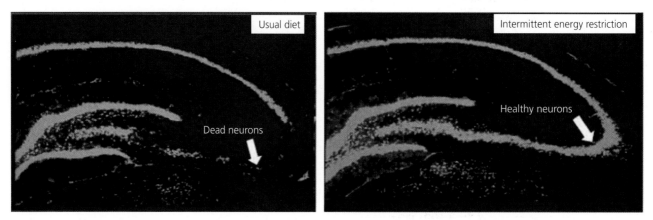

Figure 4.2 Intermittent dietary energy restriction protects hippocampal neurons against excitotoxin-induced death. These images are adapted from a study in which young adult rats were maintained for 3 months on either the usual ad libitum diet or an alternate day fasting (intermittent energy restriction) diet [70]. The excitotoxin kainic acid was then injected into the hippocampus and several days later the learning and memory performance of the rats was tested. The rats were then euthanized and coronal brain sections were stained with a dye (cresyl violet) that selectively stains neurons. The upper image shows the hippocampus of one of the rats in the usual diet group and the lower image shows the hippocampus of one of the rats in the intermittent energy restriction group. The neurons are yellow. Note that most of the neurons in region CA3 were killed by the excitotoxin in the rat in the control diet group, whereas most of the CA3 neurons in the rat in the energy restriction group withstood the excitotoxic challenge.

who rapidly developed PD-like symptoms as the result of unwittingly injecting themselves with1-methyl-4-phenyl-1,2,5,6-tetrahydropyridine (MPTP) [17]. Subsequent research showed that a metabolite of MPTP called MPP⁺ is selectively transported into dopaminergic neurons where it impairs mitochondrial complex I and renders neurons vulnerable to excitotoxicity [18]. A third example originated in China where numerous individuals developed HD-like symptoms after consuming sugar cane; the cause was a toxin called 3-nitropropionic acid (3NP) produced by fungus growing in the sugar cane [19]. 3NP was subsequently shown to cause selective excitotoxic degeneration of medium spiny neurons in the striatum, the same neurons most vulnerable in HD [20]. Thus, domoic acid, MPTP, and 3NP can cause neurological symptoms similar to those of AD, PD, and HD, respectively. These and related neurotoxins are widely used in animal models where, as in humans, they cause selective excitotoxic degeneration and associated neurochemical and behavioral deficits.

A most interesting, but as yet unsolved, mysterious neurodegenerative disorder confined to several South Pacific islands near Guam includes symptoms and neuropathological features of ALS, PD, and AD [21]. Degeneration of motor neurons, substantia nigra dopaminergic neurons, and hippocampal and cortical neurons occurs in a progressive manner in affected individuals when they are in their fifth and sixth decades of life. There is no discernible genetic basis for this Guam syndrome, and the absence of the disorder in Guamanian natives who moved to the United States and those who changed their diets on the islands strongly suggests an environmental/dietary cause. An excitotoxin(s) present in the seeds of the cycad plant, a food staple of the natives, has been implicated but not proven to be the cause [21].

Some evidence suggests that some instances of common sporadic forms of neurodegenerative disorders are caused by an environmental excitotoxin or an agent that renders neurons vulnerable to excitotoxicity. Exposure to pesticides, manmade or naturally occurring, continues to be considered as a risk factor for PD. Epidemiological studies have reported a statistically significant, albeit small, elevated risk for PD in workers in the farming and chemical industries [22]. The pesticide rotenone, which has been widely used by gardeners, when administered to rodents can cause PD-like pathology and symptoms albeit only when administered in relatively high amounts [23].

A major theme of this chapter is that there is an excitotoxic component to the degeneration of neurons that occurs in a range of acute and chronic neurodegenerative conditions. The clinical manifestations of such excitotoxic damage are exactly those that define the disorder, be it stroke, traumatic injury, AD, PD, HD, or ALS. While most of the evidence comes from studies of experimental models, there is also clinical evidence of an excitotoxic imbalance in some of these disorders. For example, AD patients often develop seizures early in the disease process, possibly because of a process called homeostatic disinhibition [24]. As the disease progresses there is an overall reduction in glutamate levels in the most affected brain regions (e.g., hippocampus), which may result from the death of glutamatergic neurons [25]. The concentration of glutamate in the cerebrospinal fluid of ALS patients is significantly elevated compared to age-matched control subjects [26], suggesting an abnormal (excitotoxic) elevation of extracellular glutamate levels in this disorder. Finally, the only two drugs that can significantly slow the progression of neurodegenerative disorders, albeit modestly, are the NMDA receptor antagonist memantine for AD patients [27] and riluzole for ALS patients [28]. Thus, there is a rationale to pursue the development of novel interventions aimed at protecting neurons against excitotoxicity in a broad range of neurodegenerative conditions.

Pathology/pathophysiology specific to the disease

The morphological and biochemical features of excitotoxic degeneration of neurons have been extensively studied and reviewed [1, 29, 30]. Excitotoxic neuronal death can manifest in two distinct forms, necrosis and apoptosis. Necrosis is characterized by rapid swelling of the cell and intracellular organelles accompanied by disruption of membrane integrity and cell lysis. Excitotoxic necrosis is largely the result of an uptake of water secondary to Na⁺ influx and cellular energy (ATP and NAD⁺) depletion (Figure 4.3). Because glutamate receptors are concentrated in postsynaptic regions of dendrites, the dendrites will typically swell and degenerate, followed by the cell body and the axon. The axon may remain intact for some time (many hours) after the rest of the neuron is "dead" because it lacks glutamate receptors [31]. Neurons undergoing glutamate receptor-mediated apoptosis exhibit a reduction in the size of the cell body and nuclear chromatic condensation and fragmentation, with retention of plasma membrane and organellar integrity. Cellular energy levels are typically maintained, albeit at a reduced level, until late in the cell death process. Neurites degenerate much

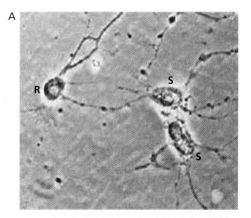

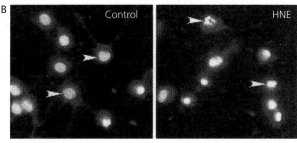

Figure 4.3 Excitotoxic necrosis and apoptosis are morphologically distinct forms of neuronal death(A) Phase contrast images showing three neurons in a dissociated hippocampal cell culture that had been exposed to a high concentration of glutamate. Two of the neurons were sensitive to excitotoxic necrosis (S), while the other neuron was resistant (R). Note that the two vulnerable neurons exhibit cell and nuclear swelling, and neurite degeneration whereas the resistant neuron does not exhibit these morphological features. Adapted from Kruman et al. 1997 [112]. (B) Rat hippocampal neurons in cultures that had been exposed either to vehicle (control) or 4-hydroxynonenal (HNE), an aldehydic product of membrane lipid peroxidation that is known to increase the vulnerability of neurons to excitotoxicity. The neurons were stained with a fluorescent DNA-binding dye (Hoechst dye). Note that the nuclear DNA in the control neurons is distributed uniformly throughout the nucleus, whereas the nuclear chromatin in the HNE-treated neurons exhibits condensation and fragmentation. Adapted from Mattson et al. 1989 [113].

more slowly than occurs in necrosis. Typically, acute insults such as an ischemic stroke or traumatic brain injury result in rapid (minutes to hours) necrosis of neurons in the most severely affected brain region, and delayed (many hours to days or weeks) apoptotic death of neurons in the surrounding less severely affected regions.

Glutamate receptor activation is, by definition, the trigger of excitotoxic damage to neurons. Both the intensity and duration of glutamate receptor activation can determine whether or not excitotoxicity occurs. Importantly, the threshold level of glutamate receptor activation that can trigger excitotoxic damage is influenced by many different factors including the level of activation of other neurotransmitter receptors on the same neuron, cellular energy availability, the presence of neurotrophic factors, and oxidative stress. For example, activation of inhibitory GABA receptors or neurotrophic factor receptors can raise the excitotoxic threshold, whereas oxidative stress and reduced glucose transport into neurons can lower the threshold [30–32].

There are at least four different types of glutamate receptors, all of which are mostly concentrated in the postsynaptic plasma membrane, although some glutamate receptors are located extrasynaptically. In addition, some of the glutamate receptors are expressed in astrocytes and oligodendrocytes. AMPA, kainate, and NMDA receptors are all multi-subunit (heteromeric) ion channels [33]. AMPA and kainate receptor flux mainly Na^+ into the cell, resulting in membrane depolarization, although there is a form of AMPA receptor that lacks the GluR2 subunit and is highly permeable to Ca^{2+}. NMDA receptors include an NR1 subunit and either an NR2A or NR2B subunit, and when activated by glutamate flux high amounts of Ca^{2+}. Opening of the NMDA receptor channel requires membrane depolarization, which is normally triggered by AMPA receptor activation. In most pathological conditions where excitotoxicity is believed to occur (seizures, cerebral ischemia, trauma, Alzheimer's disease, Parkinson disease, Huntington's disease, and ALS), activation of AMPA and NMDA receptors is implicated in neuronal degeneration and death [34–36].

In contrast to the ionotropic receptors, if and to what extent metabotropic receptors (mGluRs) contribute to excitotoxic processes remains to be established [37]. Activation of mGluRs results in Ca^{2+} release from the endoplasmic reticulum (ER), which might potentiate excitotoxic Ca^{2+} overload. On the other hand, Ca^{2+} release from the ER may activate adaptive cellular stress responses including the production of neuroprotective protein chaperones [38]. In addition, mGluRs also activate protein kinase C which can up-regulate the expression of genes encoding proteins that promote neuronal survival. Moreover, there are five mGluRs, some of which have been reported to promote excitotoxicity while others protect neurons against excitotoxicity.

Sodium and calcium influx are the immediate events resulting from glutamate receptor activation that, in turn, initiate excitotoxic neuronal injury. If AMPA/kainate receptors are activated at very high levels for a time period of many minutes to an hour or more, the Na^+ influx through both the receptor channels and voltage-gated Na^+ channels may overwhelm the capability of the plasma membrane Na^+/K^+-ATPase to expel the Na^+ from the cell. As a result the neuron will swell and its plasma membrane can rupture (i.e., excitotoxic necrosis). Neurons are particularly prone to excitotoxic necrosis when their ATP levels are depleted, as may occur in ischemia or trauma. Sodium influx may also play a necessary role in NMDA receptor-mediated excitotoxic apoptosis, because of the requirement of membrane depolarization for Ca^{2+} influx through the NMDA receptor channel.

Calcium influx is believed to play a pivotal role in the excitotoxic neuronal degeneration that occurs in AD, PD, HD, and ALS. There is reason to believe that antagonists of NMDA receptors and voltage-dependent Ca^{2+} channels have the potential to protect the neurons in each of the latter disorders [39–42]. Ca^{2+} activates, directly or indirectly, multiple enzymes involved in excitotoxic cell death including calpains [43], caspases [44], and oxidases [45]. In addition, Ca^{2+} uptake by mitochondria can increase the production of reactive oxygen species (ROS) and can impair ATP production [32]. The usual concentration of Ca^{2+} in neurons under resting conditions is approximately 100 nM, and in response to normal synaptic activation of glutamate receptors the local dendritic Ca^{2+} concentration can increase more than 10-fold, but then rapidly returns to the basal level within seconds. However, excitotoxicity occurs when the Ca^{2+} concentration is elevated for prolonged time periods, even if the magnitude is considerably less than that which occurs locally during synaptic activation (e.g., 300 nM). Four major mechanisms for the rapid removal of Ca^{2+} from the cytoplasm are the plasma membrane Ca^{2+}-ATPase, the plasma membrane Na^+/Ca^{2+} exchanger, the ER Ca^{2+}-ATPase, and Ca^{2+}-binding proteins such as calbindin and parvalbumin [46]. Dysfunction of one or more of these Ca^{2+}-lowering systems may render neurons vulnerable to excitotoxicity.

Oxidative stress is another contributory factor in excitotoxicity, particularly the slower non-necrotic forms of glutamate receptor-mediated cell death. A major source of ROS in neurons is mitochondria wherein superoxide is generated during the process of oxidative phosphorylation, mostly at electron transport chain complexes I and III [47]. Superoxide is normally rapidly converted to hydrogen peroxide in a reaction catalyzed by superoxide dismutases located in the mitochondria (SOD2) and cytoplasm (SOD1). Hydrogen peroxide, in turn, can be converted to water via the activities of catalase and glutathione peroxidase. However, even very low amounts of Fe^{2+} or Cu^+ can act upon hydrogen peroxide to cause the production of hydroxyl radical which is highly reactive and "attacks" double-bonds in membrane fatty acids to initiate a self-propagating process called lipid peroxidation [48]. Another major source of oxidative stress during the excitotoxic process is the enzyme nitric oxide synthase, which is activated by Ca^{2+} resulting in the production of the free radical nitric oxide. Nitric oxide can damage cellular proteins by first interacting with superoxide resulting in the generation of peroxynitrite which, in turn, directly reacts with tyrosine residues in proteins resulting in protein nitration [49]. Free radicals also damage DNA; if this damage is sufficiently extensive it can trigger apoptosis mediated by the "tumor suppressor" protein p53 [30].

In contrast to the weak evidence for the involvement of exposure to an environmental excitotoxin as a major cause of AD, PD, and ALS, there is strong evidence that cellular and molecular changes that occur during aging, including oxidative stress, endanger neurons by promoting an excitotoxic imbalance. An illustrative example focuses on membrane-associated oxidative stress and lipid peroxidation that increases in neurons during normal aging and is exacerbated in AD, PD, and ALS. In AD, amyloid β-peptide self-aggregates and during this process can initiate membrane lipid peroxidation resulting in the generation of the aldehyde 4-hydroxynonenal [40]. In a process called the Michael addition, 4-hydroxynonenal covalently modifies proteins on cysteine, lysine, and histidine residues. The function of several proteins relevant to excitotoxicity has been shown to be modified and impaired by 4-hydroxynonenal including the plasma membrane Na^+/K^+- and Ca^{2+}-ATPases [50], the neuronal glucose transporter GLUT3 [51], and a glutamate transporter in astrocytes [52]. Neurons can be protected against excitotoxic injury by some antioxidants, including SOD2 and glutathione, suggesting a potential for enhancement of antioxidant defenses in neurological disorders that involve excitotoxicity.

Genetics

Because excitotoxicity is a mechanism of neuronal degeneration and not a disease per se, the genetics of excitotoxicity can be defined as the inheritance of genes that increase (or decrease) the vulnerability of neurons to excitotoxicity. At one end of the spectrum is epilepsy, which can be considered a (largely) excitotoxic disorder. Considerable progress has been made in identifying genetic aberrancies that cause inherited forms of epilepsy. Some cases of dominantly inherited epilepsies (e.g., generalized epilepsy with febrile seizures, and Dravet syndrome) are caused by mutations in genes encoding subunits of voltage-gated Na^+ channels [53]. Other inherited epilepsies appear to result from reduced activity in GABAergic neurons. GABA receptor mutations can cause inherited epilepsies [54] including a missense mutation (R43Q) of the $\gamma2$ subunit of the GABA-A receptor which is linked to an inherited generalized epilepsy [55]. Deletion of the GABA-A receptor gene has been linked to Angelman syndrome, a disorder characterized by ataxia, seizures, and cognitive deficits [56]. Mutations in Cl^- channels, K^+ channels, and the K^+/Cl^- cotransporter can also cause syndromes that include seizures as a prominent symptom [56]. Other mutations have been identified in proteins not previously associated with the regulation of neuronal excitability including leucine-rich glioma inactivated 1 which causes autosomal dominant partial epilepsy with auditory features [57].

Beyond epilepsy, the case could be made that mutations that cause other neurological disorders involving neuronal degeneration increase the vulnerability of neurons to excitotoxicity. Mutations in the β-amyloid precursor protein (APP) and presenilin-1 (PS1) cause rare inherited forms of early-onset familial AD [58]. APP and PS1 mutations result in an alteration of the enzymatic cleavage of APP such that increased amounts of a neurotoxic form of amyloid β-peptide ($A\beta$) are produced. $A\beta$ self-aggregates to form oligomers, and during this process of aggregation $A\beta$ generates ROS (hydrogen peroxide) and (in the presence of Fe^{2+} or Cu^+) hydroxyl radical. In this way, $A\beta$ induces membrane lipid peroxidation and impairs the function of ion-motive ATPases and glutamate transporters, thereby rendering neurons vulnerable to excitotoxicity [9, 40]. In addition to increasing $A\beta$ production, PS1 mutations can render neurons vulnerable to excitotoxicity by increasing the accumulation of Ca^{2+} in the endoplasmic reticulum [59, 60].

Inherited forms of PD can be caused by mutations in α-synuclein, PINK1, Parkin, DJ-1, or LRRK2. Studies of cultured cells and mice expressing these PD mutations suggest a common pathogenic action involving mitochondrial impairment, increased oxidative stress, and intracellular accumulation of α-synuclein [61]. Inasmuch as cellular energy deficits, oxidative stress, and proteotoxic stress can increase the vulnerability of neurons to excitotoxicity [32, 40, 62], mutations that cause PD likely sensitize neurons to excitotoxic damage. Trinucleotide (CAG) repeats in the huntingtin gene result in pathogenic polyglutamine repeats in huntingtin that cause HD. By mechanisms not yet understood, mutant huntingtin renders medium spiny neurons in the striatum vulnerable to excitotoxic degeneration [63]. The genetics of ALS are also consistent with a role for disease-causing mutations adversely affecting the ability of motor neurons to cope with excitotoxic stress. Thus, ALS mutations in Cu/Zn-SOD result in increased oxidative stress and perturbed Ca^{2+} handling in motor

neurons that increase their vulnerability to excitotoxicity [64]. Cu/Zn-SOD mutations may also impair glutamate transport in astrocytes [65]. Finally, mutations in tau that cause frontotemporal dementia (FTD) may promote excitotoxicity by altering voltage-gated Ca^{2+} channels [66], and loss-of-function mutations in progranulin that can cause FTD may eliminate a neurotrophic function of progranulin [67]. Thus, there are many genetic factors that can promote excitotoxicity, particularly when neurons experience the adversities of aging or a pro-excitotoxic environment (see Environment).

Environment

Cases of excitotoxic neuronal degeneration caused by exposure to an environmental toxin are very rare and, as yet, there is no convincing evidence that exposure to lower amounts of such toxins causes more common cases of neurodegenerative disorders. Instead, two environmental factors that may influence neuronal vulnerability to excitotoxic degeneration are diet (particularly energy intake) and exercise. Perhaps the first evidence that diet can modify excitotoxicity was back in around 400 BC when Greek physicians such as Erasistratus found that seizures could be reduced by fasting. Much more recently, in the early 1920s, Dr. Wilder at the Mayo Clinic found that seizures can in many cases be controlled by a diet high in fat and low in carbohydrates and protein [68]; this type of diet is believed effective because it increases the level of fatty acids (ketone bodies) available to neurons. Fasting also elevates levels of ketone bodies, suggesting that a ketogenic diet and fasting may share a common excitoprotective mechanism of action [69].

Studies of animals have shown that dietary energy restriction (limited daily feeding or intermittent fasting) can protect neurons against excitotoxic damage in experimental models of severe epileptic seizures [70, 71] (Figure 4.2), stroke [72], AD [73], PD [74, 75], and HD [70, 76]. Intermittent energy restriction can also improve the outcome of traumatic spinal cord injury [77] and traumatic brain injury [78]. Recent findings have provided evidence that dietary energy restriction, particularly intermittent fasting, can protect neurons against excitotoxicity by inducing a mild adaptive cellular stress response [79]. Neurotrophic factors such as BDNF and FGF2, protein chaperones such as HSP70 and GRP78, and antioxidant enzymes such as HO-1 are among the anti-excitotoxic proteins upregulated in neurons in mice maintained on an alternate day fasting diet [72]. A set of adaptive stress response proteins that overlaps with those up-regulated by energy restriction is also up-regulated in response to exercise and cognitive stimulation (Table 4.1).

Epidemiological studies and interventional trials in humans have shown that regular exercise throughout life is beneficial for brain health in general and may protect against multiple neurodegenerative disorders [80–82]. Compared to their more sedentary control counterparts, rodents that exercise on running wheels exhibit improved functional outcomes in experimental models of epileptic seizures [83], AD [84], PD [85], and stroke [86]. Exercise enhances synaptic plasticity and stimulates neurogenesis in the hippocampus, both of which have been associated with improved learning and memory, particularly spatial learning and pattern separation [87, 88]. Exercise can also induce the expression of vascular endothelial growth factor, which promotes the growth of cerebral blood vessels and enhances cerebral blood flow [89, 90].

Collectively, the available evidence suggests that lack of exercise, excessive energy intake, and diets high in trans fatty acids

Table 4.1 Modification of expression of proteins involved in excitoprotective cellular stress adaptation, as affected by energy restriction, exercise, and cognitive stimulation.

Protein	Energy restriction	Exercise	Cognitive challenges
Secreted			
BDNF	++	+++	+++
GDNF	++	++	++
VEGF	?	++	++
Membrane			
PMRS enzymes	++	?	?
Glucose transporter	++	++	?
NMDA receptors	+/−	+	++
AMPA receptors	+/−	+	++
Cytoplasm			
HSP-70	++	+	?
HO-1	++	?	?
Mitochondria			
SOD2	?	+	?
Endoplasmic reticulum			
GRP-78	++	++	?
Nucleus			
APE-1	?	++	?
SIRT1	++	++	
PGC-1α	?	++	?

AMPA, 2-amino-3-(5-methyl-3-oxo-1,2- oxazol-4-yl)propanoic acid; APE-1, apurinic/apyrimidinic endonuclease 1; BDNF, brain-derived neurotrophic factor; GDNF, glial cell line-derived neurotrophic factor; GRP-78, glucose regulated protein 78; HO-1, heme oxygenase 1; HSP-70, heat-shock protein 70; NMDA, N-methyl-D-aspartate; PGC-1α, peroxisome proliferator-activated receptor γ co-activator 1α; PMRS, plasma membrane redox system; SIRT1, sirtuin 1; SOD2, mitochondrial Mn-superoxide dismutase; VEGF, vascular endothelial cell growth factor.

and simple sugars promote an excitotoxic environment. Because all of these environmental factors are modifiable, major healthcare efforts should focus on mitigating these risks. Medical school curricula should include an emphasis on preventative medicine with new approaches for prescribing diet and lifestyle interventions, and follow-up to enhance compliance.

Diagnostic considerations in excitotoxicity

There are currently no specific diagnostic tests for excitotoxicity per se. Instead, disorders that involve excitotoxicity are diagnosed based upon the established criteria for those disorders.

Treatment approaches

Because epilepsy is the result of neuronal hyperexcitability and uncontrolled activation of glutamatergic synapses, the treatments for epilepsy can be considered anti-excitotoxic. While all anti-epileptic drugs inhibit neuronal network activity, the molecular mechanisms of action differ amongst the drugs [91]. The mechanisms of action include: inhibition of voltage-gated Na+ channels (e.g., phenytoin, brivaracetam, and eslicarbazepine acetate); activation of GABA receptors/Cl− channels (diazepam and stiripentol); inhibition of presynaptic voltage-gated ion channels (e.g., pregabalin); and inhibition of NMDA receptors (e.g., remacemide). There is also a potential for anti-excitotoxic agents to retard the neurodegenerative process in age-related neurodegenerative disorders. As evidence, the NMDA receptor open channel blocker memantine demonstrated an ability to slow the progression of AD [92]. In addition, riluzole (an agent that reduces extracellular glutamate levels) extends the survival of ALS patients [28]. Preclinical findings

further support disease-modifying actions of anti-excitotoxic drugs including the K+ channel opener diazoxide in animal models of stroke [93] and AD [94], and the anticonvulsant valproate in animal models of AD [95] and ALS [96, 97].

An alternative to drugs that block a specific early event in the excitotoxic cascade (glutamate release, glutamate receptor activation, or Ca^{2+} influx) is to engage adaptive cellular stress responses so as to help neurons restore cellular ion and energy homeostasis. Dietary interventions are a viable approach for reducing neuronal damage and functional impairment in acute neurodegenerative conditions and for delaying or eliminating the onset of multiple age-related neurodegenerative disorders. Dietary energy restriction and a ketogenic diet can be effective treatments for seizures [69, 70], and energy restriction is neuroprotective in animal models of traumatic brain and spinal cord injury [77, 78], ischemic stroke [72, 98], AD [73, 99, 100], PD [74, 75], and HD [76].

Pharmacological approaches for excitoprotection that target cellular energy metabolism have proven effective in animal models and have, in some cases, moved to clinical trials in humans. One example involves analogs of glucagon-like peptide 1 (GLP-1), a peptide released into the blood from intestinal epithelial cells in response to food intake. GLP-1 is a 30 amino acid peptide that increases the sensitivity to insulin of muscle and liver cells. However, GLP-1 is normally cleaved by a protease called DPP-IV and has a half-life in the blood of a few minutes. A long-lasting, protease-resistant analog of GLP-1 called exendin-4 was developed for the treatment of type 2 diabetes and is now widely prescribed under the name Byetta [101]. Exendin-4 enters the brain and binds to GLP-1 receptors widely expressed in neurons, resulting in generation of the second messenger cyclic AMP. Numerous studies have demonstrated neuroprotective actions of exendin-4 in animal models of neurodegenerative conditions that involve excitotoxicity including: direct exposure to excitotoxins [102], HD [103], stroke [104], PD [104], AD [105, 106], and ALS [107]. Clinical trials of GLP-1 analogs in AD and PD patients are currently in progress. Another approach to enhance neuronal bioenergetics includes creatine supplementation, which has proven effective in reducing neuronal damage in models of stroke [108], traumatic brain injury [109], and HD and PD [110].

Future developments

A major goal of future research on excitotoxicity should be to understand how neurons can be protected without compromising their functionality. Because glutamate is the major excitatory neurotransmitter, glutamate receptor antagonists will have side effects. Drugs that enhance K+ channel activity, inhibit presynaptic Ca^{2+} channels, or enhance GABAergic transmission can protect neurons against excitotoxicity, although side effects will occur as well. In contrast, approaches that counteract the conditions that render neurons vulnerable to excitotoxicity may enable optimal function of the nervous system. These include improving cellular calcium handling, enhancing cellular bioenergetics, and up-regulating antioxidant defenses. This can be accomplished by dietary energy restriction and exercise, although implementing such an approach in the general population remains problematic. Finally, because excitotoxicity is in most cases a downstream consequence of an underlying chronic disease, therapeutic approaches that target early pivotal events in the disease process (e.g., Aβ accumulation in AD or mitochondrial impairment in PD) will preclude excitotoxicity (Figure 4.4).

Ischemic stroke	Trauma	Alzheimer's disease	Parkinson disease
Oxygen deprivation Glucose deprivation Oxidative stress	Cellular damage Ion dyshomeostasis Oxidative stress	Aging/oxidative damage Altered APP processing Aβ aggregation Impaired stress adaptation Membrane-associated ROS	Aging/oxidative damage Mitochondrial impairment α-Synuclein accumulation Impaired stress adaptation

EXCITO-TOXICITY

Ischemic stroke	Trauma	Alzheimer's disease	Parkinson disease
Membrane depolarization Calcium dysregulation Synaptic dysfunction ATP and NAD depletion	Calcium dysregulation Mitochondrial impairment ATP and NAD depletion	Synaptic dysfunction Calcium dysregulation Tau aggregation Mitochondrial impairment DNA damage	Synaptic dysfunction Calcium dysregulation DNA damage
Necrosis or apoptosis	Necrosis or apoptosis	Neuron death	Neuronal death

Figure 4.4 Examples of cellular alterations leading to excitotoxicity in acute (stroke and trauma) and chronic (Alzheimer's and Parkinson diseases) disorders. The conditions shown in red font are early and pivotal events in the neurodegenerative cascade upstream of excitotoxicity.

Acknowledgment

This work was supported by the Intramural Research Program of the National Institute on Aging.

References

1. Lau A, Tymianski M. (2010) Glutamate receptors, neurotoxicity and neurodegeneration. *Pflugers Arch.* 460, 525–542.
2. Lodge D. (2009) The history of the pharmacology and cloning of ionotropic glutamate receptors and the development of idiosyncratic nomenclature. *Neuropharmacology* 56, 6–21.
3. Meldrum B. (1991) Excitotoxicity and epileptic brain damage. *Epilepsy Res.* 10, 55–61.
4. Boxer PA, Cordon JJ, Mann ME, Rodolosi LC, Vartanian MG, Rock DM, Taylor CP, Marcoux FW. (1990) Comparison of phenytoin with noncompetitive N-methyl-D-aspartate antagonists in a model of focal brain ischemia in rat. *Stroke* 21;III47–51.
5. Ginsberg MD. (2008) Neuroprotection for ischemic stroke: past, present and future. *Neuropharmacology* 55, 363–389.
6. Ikonomidou C, Turski L. (2002) Why did NMDA receptor antagonists fail clinical trials for stroke and traumatic brain injury? *Lancet Neurol.* 1, 383–386.
7. Park E, Velumian AA, Fehlings MG. (2004) The role of excitotoxicity in secondary mechanisms of spinal cord injury: a review with an emphasis on the implications for white matter degeneration. *J Neurotrauma* 21, 754–774.
8. Mattson MP, Magnus T. (2006) Ageing and neuronal vulnerability. *Nat Rev Neurosci.* 7, 278–294.
9. Mattson MP, Cheng B, Davis D, Bryant K, Lieberburg I, Rydel RE. (1992) beta-Amyloid peptides destabilize calcium homeostasis and render human cortical neurons vulnerable to excitotoxicity. *J Neurosci.* 12, 376–389.
10. Henchcliffe C, Beal MF. (2008) Mitochondrial biology and oxidative stress in Parkinson disease pathogenesis. *Nat Clin Pract Neurol.* 4, 600–609.
11. Okamoto, S., Pouladi, M.A., Talantova, M., Yao, D., Xia, P., Ehrnhoefer, D.E., Zaidi, R., Clemente, A., Kaul, M., Graham, R.K., et al. (2009). Balance between synaptic versus extrasynaptic NMDA receptor activity influences inclusions and neurotoxicity of mutant huntingtin. *Nat. Med.* 15, 1407–1413.
12. Rothstein JD. (2009) Current hypotheses for the underlying biology of amyotrophic lateral sclerosis. *Ann Neurol.* 65, S3–9.
13. Meldrum BS. (2002) Concept of activity-induced cell death in epilepsy: historical and contemporary perspectives. *Prog Brain Res.* 135, 3–11.
14. Schwarcz R, Witter MP. (2002) Memory impairment in temporal lobe epilepsy: the role of entorhinal lesions. *Epilepsy Res.* 50, 161–177.
15. Aroniadou-Anderjaska V, Fritsch B, Qashu F, Braga MF. (2008) Pathology and pathophysiology of the amygdala in epileptogenesis and epilepsy. *Epilepsy Res.* 78, 102–116.
16. Jeffery B, Barlow T, Moizer K, Paul S, Boyle C. (2004) Amnesic shellfish poison. *Food Chem Toxicol.* 42, 545–557.
17. Langston JW, Ballard P, Tetrud JW, Irwin I. (1983) Chronic Parkinsonism in humans due to a product of meperidine-analog synthesis. *Science* 219, 979–980.
18. Storch A, Hwang YI, Gearhart DA, Beach JW, Neafsey EJ, Collins MA, Schwarz J. (2004) Dopamine transporter-mediated cytotoxicity of beta-carbolinium derivatives related to Parkinson's disease: relationship to transporter-dependent uptake. *J Neurochem.* 89, 685–694.
19. Liu X, Luo X, Hu W. (1992) Studies on the epidemiology and etiology of moldy sugarcane poisoning in China. *Biomed Environ Sci.* 5, 161–177.
20. Beal MF, Brouillet E, Jenkins BG, Ferrante RJ, Kowall NW, Miller JM, Storey E, Srivastava R, Rosen BR, Hyman BT. (1993) Neurochemical and histologic characterization of striatal excitotoxic lesions produced by the mitochondrial toxin 3-nitropropionic acid. *J Neurosci.* 13, 4181–4192.
21. Cox PA, Sacks OW. (2002) Cycad neurotoxins, consumption of flying foxes, and ALS-PDC disease in Guam. *Neurology* 58, 956–959.
22. Hatcher JM, Pennell KD, Miller GW. (2008) Parkinson's disease and pesticides: a toxicological perspective. *Trends Pharmacol Sci.* 29, 322–329.
23. Betarbet R, Sherer TB, MacKenzie G, Garcia-Osuna M, Panov AV, Greenamyre JT. (2000) Chronic systemic pesticide exposure reproduces features of Parkinson's disease. *Nat Neurosci.* 3, 1301–1306.
24. Gleichmann M, Chow VW, Mattson MP. (2011) Homeostatic disinhibition in the aging brain and Alzheimer's disease. *J Alzheimers Dis.* 24, 15–24.
25. Rupsingh R, Borrie M, Smith M, Wells JL, Bartha R. (2011) Reduced hippocampal glutamate in Alzheimer disease. *Neurobiol Aging.* 32, 802–810.
26. Rothstein JD, Tsai G, Kuncl RW, Clawson L, Cornblath DR, Drachman DB, Pestronk A, Stauch BL, Coyle JT. (1990) Abnormal excitatory amino acid metabolism in amyotrophic lateral sclerosis. *Ann Neurol.* 28, 18–25.
27. Tampi RR, van Dyck CH. (2007) Memantine: efficacy and safety in mild-to-severe Alzheimer's disease. *Neuropsychiatr Dis Treat.* 3, 245–258.
28. Cheah BC, Vucic S, Krishnan AV, Kiernan MC. (2010) Riluzole, neuroprotection and amyotrophic lateral sclerosis. *Curr Med Chem.* 17, 1942–1999.
29. Leist M, Nicotera P. (1998) Apoptosis, excitotoxicity, and neuropathology. *Exp Cell Res.* 239, 183–201.
30. Mattson MP. (2003) Excitotoxic and excitoprotective mechanisms: abundant targets for the prevention and treatment of neurodegenerative disorders. *Neuromolecular Med.* 3, 65–94.
31. Mattson MP, Kater SB. (1989) Excitatory and inhibitory neurotransmitters in the generation and degeneration of hippocampal neuroarchitecture. *Brain Res.* 478, 337–348.
32. Nicholls DG. (2008) Oxidative stress and energy crises in neuronal dysfunction. *Ann N Y Acad Sci.* 1147, 53–60.
33. Traynelis SF, Wollmuth LP, McBain CJ, Menniti FS, Vance KM, Ogden KK, Hansen KB, Yuan H, Myers SJ, Dingledine R. (2010) Glutamate receptor ion channels: structure, regulation, and function. *Pharmacol Rev.* 62, 405–496.
34. Lipton SA. (2004) Paradigm shift in NMDA receptor antagonist drug development: molecular mechanism of uncompetitive inhibition by memantine in the treatment of Alzheimer's disease and other neurologic disorders. *J Alzheimers Dis.* 6, S61–74.
35. Milnerwood AJ, Raymond LA. (2010) Early synaptic pathophysiology in neurodegeneration: insights from Huntington's disease. *Trends Neurosci.* 33, 513–523.
36. Kalia LV, Kalia SK, Salter MW. (2008) NMDA receptors in clinical neurology: excitatory times ahead. *Lancet Neurol.* 7, 742–755.
37. Lea PM 4th, Faden AI. (2003) Modulation of metabotropic glutamate receptors as potential treatment for acute and chronic neurodegenerative disorders. *Drug News Perspect.* 16, 513–522.
38. Berridge MJ. (2002) The endoplasmic reticulum: a multifunctional signaling organelle. *Cell Calcium* 32, 235–249.

39. Rodnitzky RL. (1999) Can calcium antagonists provide a neuroprotective effect in Parkinson's disease? *Drugs* 57, 845–849.

40. Mattson MP. (2004) Pathways towards and away from Alzheimer's disease. *Nature* 430, 631–639.

41. Appel SH, Beers D, Smith RG, Wilson JE. (2000) Altered calcium homeostasis in ALS as a target for therapy. *Amyotroph Lateral Scler Other Motor Neuron Disord.* 1 Suppl 4, 27–32.

42. Mattson MP. (2007) Calcium and neurodegeneration. *Aging Cell* 6, 337–350.

43. Doshi S, Lynch DR. (2009) Calpain and the glutamatergic synapse. *Front Biosci (Schol Ed).* 1, 466–476.

44. Glazner GW, Chan SL, Lu C, Mattson MP. (2000) Caspase-mediated degradation of AMPA receptor subunits: a mechanism for preventing excitotoxic necrosis and ensuring apoptosis. *J Neurosci.* 20, 3641–3649.

45. Szydlowska K, Tymianski M. (2010) Calcium, ischemia and excitotoxicity. *Cell Calcium* 47, 122–129.

46. Schwaller B. (2010) Cytosolic Ca_{2+} buffers. *(2010) Cold Spring Harb Perspect Biol.* 2(11), a004051.

47. Mattson MP, Gleichmann M, Cheng A. (2008) Mitochondria in neuroplasticity and neurological disorders. *Neuron* 60, 748–766.

48. Mattson MP. (2009) Roles of the lipid peroxidation product 4-hydroxynonenal in obesity, the metabolic syndrome, and associated vascular and neurodegenerative disorders. *Exp Gerontol.* 44, 625–633.

49. Guix FX, Uribesalgo I, Coma M, Muñoz FJ. (2005) The physiology and pathophysiology of nitric oxide in the brain. *Prog Neurobiol.* 76, 126–152.

50. Mark RJ, Lovell MA, Markesbery WR, Uchida K, Mattson MP. (1997) A role for 4-hydroxynonenal, an aldehydic product of lipid peroxidation, in disruption of ion homeostasis and neuronal death induced by amyloid beta-peptide. *J Neurochem.* 68, 255–264.

51. Mark RJ, Pang Z, Geddes JW, Uchida K, Mattson MP. (1997) Amyloid beta-peptide impairs glucose transport in hippocampal and cortical neurons: involvement of membrane lipid peroxidation. *J Neurosci.* 17, 1046–1054.

52. Blanc EM, Keller JN, Fernandez S, Mattson MP. (1998) 4-hydroxynonenal, a lipid peroxidation product, impairs glutamate transport in cortical astrocytes. *Glia* 22, 149–160.

53. Escayg A, Goldin AL. (2010) Sodium channel SCN1A and epilepsy: mutations and mechanisms. *Epilepsia* 51, 1650–1658.

54. Kang JQ, Macdonald RL. (2009) Making sense of nonsense GABA(A) receptor mutations associated with genetic epilepsies. *Trends Mol Med.* 15, 430–438.

55. Fedi M, Berkovic SF, Macdonell RA, Curatolo JM, Marini C, Reutens DC. (2008) Intracortical hyperexcitability in humans with a GABAA receptor mutation. *Cereb Cortex* 18, 664–669.

56. Galanopoulou AS. (2010) Mutations affecting GABAergic signaling in seizures and epilepsy. *Pflugers Arch.* 460, 505–523.

57. Fukata Y, Lovero KL, Iwanaga T, Watanabe A, Yokoi N, Tabuchi K, Shigemoto R, Nicoll RA, Fukata M. (2010) Disruption of LGI1-linked synaptic complex causes abnormal synaptic transmission and epilepsy. *Proc Natl Acad Sci U S A.* 107, 3799–3804.

58. St George-Hyslop PH. (2000) Molecular genetics of Alzheimer's disease. *Biol Psychiatry.* 47, 183–199.

59. Guo Q, Fu W, Sopher BL, Miller MW, Ware CB, Martin GM, Mattson MP. (1999) Increased vulnerability of hippocampal neurons to excitotoxic necrosis in presenilin-1 mutant knock-in mice. *Nat Med.* 5, 101–106.

60. Guo Q, Sebastian L, Sopher BL, Miller MW, Glazner GW, Ware CB, Martin GM, Mattson MP. (1999) Neurotrophic factors [activity-dependent neurotrophic factor (ADNF) and basic fibroblast growth factor (bFGF)] interrupt excitotoxic neurodegenerative cascades promoted by a PS1 mutation. *Proc Natl Acad Sci USA.* 96, 4125–4130.

61. Cookson MR, Bandmann O. (2010) Parkinson's disease: insights from pathways. *Hum Mol Genet.* 19, R21–27.

62. Olanow CW. (2007) The pathogenesis of cell death in Parkinson's disease – 2007. *Mov Disord.* 22 (Suppl 17), S335–342.

63. Heng MY, Detloff PJ, Wang PL, Tsien JZ, Albin RL. (2009) In vivo evidence for NMDA receptor-mediated excitotoxicity in a murine genetic model of Huntington disease. *J Neurosci.* 29, 3200–3205.

64. Kruman II, Pedersen WA, Springer JE, Mattson MP. (1999) ALS-linked Cu/Zn-SOD mutation increases vulnerability of motor neurons to excitotoxicity by a mechanism involving increased oxidative stress and perturbed calcium homeostasis. *Exp Neurol.* 160, 28–39.

65. Ilieva H, Polymenidou M, Cleveland DW. (2009) Non-cell autonomous toxicity in neurodegenerative disorders: ALS and beyond. *J Cell Biol.* 187, 761–772.

66. Furukawa K, Wang Y, Yao PJ, Fu W, Mattson MP, Itoyama Y, Onodera H, D'Souza I, Poorkaj PH, Bird TD, Schellenberg GD. (2003) Alteration in calcium channel properties is responsible for the neurotoxic action of a familial frontotemporal dementia tau mutation. *J Neurochem.* 87, 427–436.

67. Xu J, Xilouri M, Bruban J, Shioi J, Shao Z, Papazoglou I, Vekrellis K, Robakis NK. (2011) Extracellular progranulin protects cortical neurons from toxic insults by activating survival signaling. *Neurobiol Aging.* 32, 2326. e5–16.

68. Wilder RM (1921) The effect of ketonemia on the course of epilepsy. *Mayo Clin Bull.* 2, 307.

69. Maalouf M, Rho JM, Mattson MP. (2009) The neuroprotective properties of calorie restriction, the ketogenic diet, and ketone bodies. *Brain Res Rev.* 59, 293–315.

70. Bruce-Keller AJ, Umberger G, McFall R, Mattson MP. (1999) Food restriction reduces brain damage and improves behavioral outcome following excitotoxic and metabolic insults. *Ann Neurol.* 45, 8–15.

71. Qiu G, Spangler EL, Wan R, Miller M, Mattson MP, So KF, Cabo RD, Zou S, Ingram DK. (2012) Neuroprotection provided by dietary restriction in rats is further enhanced by reducing glucocortocoids. *Neurobiol Aging.* 33, 2398–2410.

72. Arumugam TV, Phillips TM, Cheng A, Morrell CH, Mattson MP, Wan R. (2010) Age and energy intake interact to modify cell stress pathways and stroke outcome. *Ann Neurol.* 67, 41–52.

73. Halagappa VK, Guo Z, Pearson M, Matsuoka Y, Cutler RG, Laferla FM, Mattson MP. (2007) Intermittent fasting and caloric restriction ameliorate age-related behavioral deficits in the triple-transgenic mouse model of Alzheimer's disease. *Neurobiol Dis.* 26, 212–220.

74. Duan W, Mattson MP. (1999) Dietary restriction and 2-deoxyglucose administration improve behavioral outcome and reduce degeneration of dopaminergic neurons in models of Parkinson's disease. *J Neurosci Res.* 57, 195–206.

75. Maswood N, Young J, Tilmont E, Zhang Z, Gash DM, Gerhardt GA, Grondin R, Roth GS, Mattson J, Lane MA, Carson RE, Cohen RM, Mouton PR, Quigley C, Mattson MP, Ingram DK. (2004) Caloric restriction increases neurotrophic factor levels and attenuates neurochemical and behavioral deficits in a primate model of Parkinson's disease. *Proc Natl Acad Sci U S A.* 101, 18171–18176.

76. Duan W, Guo Z, Jiang H, Ware M, Li XJ, Mattson MP. (2003) Dietary restriction normalizes glucose metabolism and BDNF levels, slows disease progression, and increases survival in huntingtin mutant mice. *Proc Natl Acad Sci U S A.* 100, 2911–2916.

77. Plunet WT, Streijger F, Lam CK, Lee JH, Liu J, Tetzlaff W. (2008) Dietary restriction started after spinal cord injury improves functional recovery. *Exp Neurol.* 213, 28–35.

78. Rich NJ, Van Landingham JW, Figueiroa S, Seth R, Corniola RS, Levenson CW. (2010) Chronic caloric restriction reduces tissue damage and improves spatial memory in a rat model of traumatic brain injury. *J Neurosci Res.* 88, 2933–2939.

79. Stranahan AM, Mattson MP. (2012) Recruiting adaptive cellular stress responses for successful brain ageing. *Nat Rev Neurosci.* 13, 209–216.

80. Kramer AF, Erickson KI. (2007) Capitalizing on cortical plasticity: influence of physical activity on cognition and brain function. *Trends Cogn Sci.* 11, 342–348.

81. Geda YE, Roberts RO, Knopman DS, Christianson TJ, Pankratz VS, Ivnik RJ, Boeve BF, Tangalos EG, Petersen RC, Rocca WA. (2010) Physical exercise, aging, and mild cognitive impairment: a population-based study. *Arch Neurol.* 67, 80–86.

82. Ahlskog JE. (2011) Does vigorous exercise have a neuroprotective effect in Parkinson disease? *Neurology* 77, 288–294.

83. Gobbo OL, O'Mara SM. (2005) Exercise, but not environmental enrichment, improves learning after kainic acid-induced hippocampal neurodegeneration in association with an increase in brain-derived neurotrophic factor. *Behav Brain Res.* 159, 21–26.

84. Parachikova A, Nichol KE, Cotman CW. (2008) Short-term exercise in aged Tg2576 mice alters neuroinflammation and improves cognition. *Neurobiol Dis.* 30, 121–129.

85. Tillerson JL, Caudle WM, Reverón ME, Miller GW. (2003) Exercise induces behavioral recovery and attenuates neurochemical deficits in rodent models of Parkinson's disease. *Neuroscience* 119, 899–911.

86. Endres M, Gertz K, Lindauer U, Katchanov J, Schultze J, Schröck H, Nickenig G, Kuschinsky W, Dirnagl U, Laufs U. (2003) Mechanisms of stroke protection by physical activity. *Ann Neurol.* 54, 582–590.

87. Creer DJ, Romberg C, Saksida LM, van Praag H, Bussey TJ. (2010) Running enhances spatial pattern separation in mice. *Proc Natl Acad Sci USA.* 107, 2367–2372.

88. Lazarov O, Mattson MP, Peterson DA, Pimplikar SW, van Praag H. (2010) When neurogenesis encounters aging and disease. *Trends Neurosci.* 33, 569–579.

89. Fabel K, Fabel K, Tam B, Kaufer D, Baiker A, Simmons N, Kuo CJ, Palmer TD. (2003) VEGF is necessary for exercise-induced adult hippocampal neurogenesis. *Eur J Neurosci.* 18, 2803–2812.

90. Van der Borght K, Kóbor-Nyakas DE, Klauke K, Eggen BJ, Nyakas C, Van der Zee EA, Meerlo P. (2009) Physical exercise leads to rapid adaptations in hippocampal vasculature: temporal dynamics and relationship to cell proliferation and neurogenesis. *Hippocampus* 19, 928–936.

91. Brodie MJ. (2010) Antiepileptic drug therapy the story so far. *Seizure* 19, 650–655.

92. Bullock R. (2006) Efficacy and safety of memantine in moderate-to-severe Alzheimer disease: the evidence to date. *Alzheimer Dis Assoc Disord*. 20, 23–29.

93. Liu D, Lu C, Wan R, Auyeung WW, Mattson MP. (2002) Activation of mitochondrial ATP-dependent potassium channels protects neurons against ischemia-induced death by a mechanism involving suppression of Bax translocation and cytochrome c release. *J Cereb Blood Flow Metab*. 22, 431–443.

94. Qing H, He G, Ly PT, Fox CJ, Staufenbiel M, Cai F, Zhang Z, Wei S, Sun X, Chen CH, Zhou W, Wang K, Song W. (2008) Valproic acid inhibits Abeta production, neuritic plaque formation, and behavioral deficits in Alzheimer's disease mouse models. *J Exp Med*. 205, 2781–2789.

95. Sugai F, Yamamoto Y, Miyaguchi K, Zhou Z, Sumi H, Hamasaki T, Goto M, Sakoda S. (2004) Benefit of valproic acid in suppressing disease progression of ALS model mice. *Eur J Neurosci*. 20, 3179–3183.

96. Rouaux C, Panteleeva I, René F, Gonzalez de Aguilar JL, Echaniz-Laguna A, Dupuis L, Menger Y, Boutillier AL, Loeffler JP. (2007) Sodium valproate exerts neuroprotective effects in vivo through CREB-binding protein-dependent mechanisms but does not improve survival in an amyotrophic lateral sclerosis mouse model. *J Neurosci*. 27, 5535–5545.

97. Feng HL, Leng Y, Ma CH, Zhang J, Ren M, Chuang DM. (2008) Combined lithium and valproate treatment delays disease onset, reduces neurological deficits and prolongs survival in an amyotrophic lateral sclerosis mouse model. *Neuroscience* 155, 567–572.

98. Yu ZF, Mattson MP (1999) Dietary restriction and 2-deoxyglucose administration reduce focal ischemic brain damage and improve behavioral outcome: evidence for a preconditioning mechanism. *J Neurosci Res*. 57, 830–839.

99. Wang J, Ho L, Qin W, Rocher AB, Seror I, Humala N, Maniar K, Dolios G, Wang R, Hof PR, Pasinetti GM. (2005) Caloric restriction attenuates beta-amyloid neuropathology in a mouse model of Alzheimer's disease. *FASEB J*. 19, 659–661.

100. Patel NV, Gordon MN, Connor KE, Good RA, Engelman RW, Mason J, Morgan DG, Morgan TE, Finch CE. (2005) Caloric restriction attenuates Abeta-deposition in Alzheimer transgenic models. *Neurobiol Aging*. 26, 995–1000.

101. Kim W, Egan JM. (2008) The role of incretins in glucose homeostasis and diabetes treatment. *Pharmacol Rev*. 60, 470–512.

102. Perry T, Haughey NJ, Mattson MP, Egan JM, Greig NH (2002) Protection and reversal of excitotoxic neuronal damage by glucagon-like peptide-1 and exendin-4. *J Pharmacol Exp Ther*. 302, 881–888.

103. Martin B, Golden E, Carlson OD, Pistell P, Zhou J, Kim W, Frank BP, Thomas S, Chadwick WA, Greig NH, Bates GP, Sathasivam K, Bernier M, Maudsley S, Mattson MP, Egan JM. (2009) Exendin-4 improves glycemic control, ameliorates brain and pancreatic pathologies, and extends survival in a mouse model of Huntington's disease. *Diabetes* 58, 318–328.

104. Li Y, Perry T, Kindy MS, Harvey BK, Tweedie D, Holloway HW, Powers K, Shen H, Egan JM, Sambamurti K, Brossi A, Lahiri DK, Mattson MP, Hoffer BJ, Wang Y, Greig NH. (2009) GLP-1 receptor stimulation preserves primary cortical and dopaminergic neurons in cellular and rodent models of stroke and Parkinsonism. *Proc Natl Acad Sci U S A*. 106, 1285–1290.

105. Li Y, Duffy KB, Ottinger MA, Ray B, Bailey JA, Holloway HW, Tweedie D, Perry T, Mattson MP, Kapogiannis D, Sambamurti K, Lahiri DK, Greig NH. (2010) GLP-1 receptor stimulation reduces amyloid-beta peptide accumulation and cytotoxicity in cellular and animal models of Alzheimer's disease. *J Alzheimers Dis*. 19, 1205–1219.

106. Wang XH, Li L, Hölscher C, Pan YF, Chen XR, Qi JS. (2010) Val8-glucagon-like peptide-1 protects against Aβ1-40-induced impairment of hippocampal late-phase long-term potentiation and spatial learning in rats. *Neuroscience* 170, 1239–1248.

107. Li Y, Chigurupati S, Holloway HW, Mughal M, Tweedie D, Bruestle DA, Mattson MP, Wang Y, Harvey BK, Ray B, Lahiri DK, Greig NH. (2012) Exendin-4 ameliorates motor neuron degeneration in cellular and animal models of amyotrophic lateral sclerosis. *PLoS One*. 7(2):e32008.

108. Perasso L, Spallarossa P, Gandolfo C, Ruggeri P, Balestrino M. (2013) Therapeutic use of creatine in brain or heart ischemia: available data and future perspectives. *Med Res Rev*. 33, 336–363.

109. Sullivan PG, Geiger JD, Mattson MP, Scheff SW. (2000) Dietary supplement creatine protects against traumatic brain injury. *Ann Neurol*. 48, 723–729.

110. Adhihetty PJ, Beal MF. (2008) Creatine and its potential therapeutic value for targeting cellular energy impairment in neurodegenerative diseases. *Neuromolecular Med*. 10, 275–290.

111. Kapogiannis D, Mattson MP. (2011) Disrupted energy metabolism and neuronal circuit dysfunction in cognitive impairment and Alzheimer's disease. *Lancet Neurol*. 10, 187–198.

112. Kruman I, Bruce-Keller AJ, Bredesen D, Waeg G, Mattson MP. (1997) Evidence that 4-hydroxynonenal mediates oxidative stress-induced neuronal apoptosis. *J Neurosci*. 17, 5089–5100.

113. Mattson MP, Guthrie PB, Hayes BC, Kater SB. (1989) Roles for mitotic history in the generation and degeneration of hippocampal neuroarchitecture. *J Neurosci*. 9, 1223–1232.

CHAPTER 5

Etiology and Pathogenesis of Parkinson Disease

Ruth-Mary deSouza and Anthony H.V. Schapira

Institute of Neurology, University College London, London, UK

Introduction

Although Parkinson disease (PD) is characterized by dopaminergic cell death in the substantia nigra, it is recognized as significantly more than just a motor disorder and has widespread pathology and consequences remote from the basal ganglia. Non-motor and neuropsychological abnormalities may be detected from its prodromal stages onwards [1, 2]. PD is the second most common neurodegenerative disease (Alzheimer's being the most common) and has a significant impact on biopsychosocial functioning, quality of life, carer burden, and overall healthcare costs. Despite advances in medical and surgical therapies, the etiology and pathogenesis of PD remain incompletely defined. Important abnormalities have been identified at the genetic, cellular, and molecular levels using experimental PD models and clinical studies. How such factors evolve and interact to precipitate PD and perpetuate its progression is as yet unknown. The focus of this review is to discuss the major groups of factors that have been implicated in the etiopathogenesis of PD and how these may overlap. The factors are considered individually and evidence highlighting their interplay in the development of PD is also considered.

Experimental models for studying PD

Animal models of PD are usually classified as pharmacological or genetic. More recently human cell culture models have been developed. Pharmacological models involve neurotoxins administered systemically or directly into the basal ganglia. Two of the most common toxins are 6-hydroxydopamine (6-OHDA) and 1-methyl-4-phenyl-1,2,3,6-tetrahydropyridine (MPTP) used in rodent and primate models. These toxins are specific to the dopaminergic neurons of the striatonigral pathway and result in motor features of PD but do not produce all the clinical, biochemical, and pathological features of the disease. Other agents toxic to the dopamine system include paraquat, rotenone, and reserpine.

MPTP toxicity was first encountered in the 1970s when a series of heroin users, after injecting a contaminated batch of the drug, developed acute-onset levodopa-responsive parkinsonian features [3]. MPTP lesioning can be acute or chronic, unilateral or bilateral, and systemic or intracarotid [4]. Tailoring of the MPTP regimen based on clinical response led to primate models that can be used for translational studies simulating clinical trials [5]. Disadvantages of the MPTP model are poor replication of global progression

and non-motor features, necrotic cell death, and no expression of α-synuclein aggregates [6]. 6-OHDA, unlike MPTP, does not cross the blood–brain barrier (BBB) and requires stereotactic injection of the striatonigral neuronal field, usually done unilaterally. 6-OHDA lesioning can be done in stages to simulate a more chronic process. The 6-OHDA model produces more localized damage than the MPTP model, with extra-striatal involvement rarely seen. Non-motor and non-dopaminergic features of PD are poorly produced and α-synuclein aggregates are seldom found – so Parkinson-like motor features are produced but not PD. A number of drugs that have been reported as neuroprotective in animal neurotoxic models have not translated into clinical effectiveness.

Transgenic models of PD are primarily rodent models that are engineered to replicate common genetic findings in human PD patients. α-Synuclein is an important, albeit rare, genetic association of PD [7]. The importance of α-synuclein lies in its aggregation and propagation in PD brains, and its presence as the major component of Lewy bodies [8, 9]. Other genetic models include LRRK2, GBA, DJ-1, PINK1, parkin, and ATP13A2 [10]. Genetic models variably show the characteristic features of PD, synuclein aggregates, striatonigral cell death, apoptosis, and global involvement of neuronal networks. Despite the fact that α-synuclein knock out mice demonstrate motor impairment, it has been observed that disproportionately little actual striatonigral dopaminergic neuronal degeneration occurs [11]. The α-synuclein model however demonstrates non-motor aspects of PD such as cognitive impairment, autonomic dysfunction, and colonic hypomotility [12, 13]. A useful feature of the α-synuclein models is that they demonstrate features of early, prodromal PD, such as olfactory abnormalities [14], which can be used to study the role of intervention in early PD. Fusion models of a toxic insult to a genetic PD model are also used to simulate the situation of a putative environmental insult in a genetically predisposed subject [15].

Stem cell culture models are more recent than toxic and genetic models. They involve *in vitro* generation of a cell population from a chosen cell line. Cell culture of dopaminergic neurons can arise from animal lines, humans with PD, non-PD human cell lines, and human stem cells including pluripotent lines. Advantages of induced human pluripotent stem cells are that they can be reprogrammed into dopaminergic cells, can be taken from patients with genetic forms of PD, are potentially amenable to high-throughput genetic sequencing, can be cultured into the specific subtype of dopaminergic neurons most susceptible to PD (A9 region), and can

Neurodegeneration, First Edition. Edited by Anthony Schapira, Zbigniew Wszolek, Ted M. Dawson and Nicholas Wood.
© 2017 John Wiley & Sons, Ltd. Published 2017 by John Wiley & Sons, Ltd.

be used to study drug delivery. A limitation of stem cell culture is the study of their interaction with associated cells such as microglia and immune system cells that are thought to be important in the pathogenesis of PD.

Genetics and the development of PD

Genetic aspects of PD can be considered in terms of familial forms of PD with a Mendelian inheritance pattern or the sporadic occurrence of PD risk alleles. Familial monogenetic cases account for approximately 10–15% of PD. Polygenetic associations with PD are also described and refer to the presence of multiple alleles that are known to raise the risk of the disease. Autosomal dominant (AD) forms of PD include mutations in the leucine-rich repeat kinase 2 (LRRK2) and α-synuclein (SNCA) genes. These forms of the disease have relatively high penetrance [16]. SNCA codes for α-synuclein, a protein that is of unknown function but which forms the basis of pathological aggregates. Inherited PD has been associated with mutations or replications of the SNCA gene, and sporadic PD is strongly associated with abnormalities at the SNCA gene locus and with variants that lead to its overexpression. α-Synuclein pathology arises when this normally monomeric protein misfolds and aggregates into sheets, producing characteristic Lewy bodies. Mutations of LRRK2 are seen in familial PD (autosomal dominant transmission) as well as sporadic PD. Reports of the prevalence of this mutation vary; it is most common in those of Ashkenazi or Berber descent, but generally accounts for 5% of familial PD and up to 0.5–1.0% of sporadic disease. LRRK2 mutations are also associated with malignancies such as melanoma and breast cancer. The function of the LRRK2 protein is unknown, although it is implicated in autophagy, lymphocyte function, and intracellular "housekeeping". Genes such as parkin, LRRK2, DJ-1, and PINK are important in regulating normal mitochondrial function. Mitochondrial dysfunction is heavily implicated in the pathogenesis of PD and is discussed later in the chapter.

Autosomal recessive forms of PD include homozygous (or compound heterozygous) mutations in PINK1, parkin, and DJ-1 [17–19]. Mutations of these genes are present in both familial and sporadic cases of PD, although more frequently seen in the former. Mutations in parkin are the most common, being found in approximately 15% of familial PD cases, and PINK1 in around 8%. DJ-1 mutations are very rare. The mechanism of PD related to parkin, PINK, and DJ-1 is believed to be induction of mitochondrial dysfunction. Parkin is of particular interest since Lewy bodies do not develop in this form of PD, suggesting a different pathomechanism induced by this gene and highlighting the prominent role of the mitochondria. An atypical PD course, with earlier disease onset, pyramidal features, dystonia eye signs, and early cognitive involvement, can be seen in autosomal recessive forms associated with ATP13A2, PLA2G6, and FBXO7.

Glucocerebrosidase (GBA) codes for a lysosomal hydrolase. GBA homozygous mutations are found in the autosomal recessive glycogen storage disorder, Gaucher disease. Heterozygous carriers of GBA mutations have a higher incidence of PD, which develops at an earlier age and is associated with a higher incidence of cognitive features than non-GBA PD. The mechanism of GBA-induced PD is not believed to be solely via lysosomal dysfunction and aberrant autophagy. There is evidence to suggest that a heterozygous mutation of GBA leads to α-synuclein aggregation. This highlights the potential for interaction between different genetic mechanisms that

increase the risk of PD. It is possible that these interact in an additive or a synergistic manner, but further research is required into the effects of gene interactions in development of PD. How GBA mutations translate into phenotypic PD is incompletely understood but a number of mechanisms including vesicle transport processes and endoplasmic reticular stress are thought to contribute [20, 21]. Specific features of PD, such as cognitive decline, are associated with genetic abnormalities. Dementia is prominently associated with mutations in GBA and in microtubule-associated tau protein (MATP), the latter also being found in cortical dementias with tau accumulation, leading to the possibility of some shared genetic aspects of dementia and PD [22].

Outside the clear Mendelian PD cases, the ability to perform genome-wide (GWA) studies has led to the discovery of a number of high-risk alleles that are associated with PD rather than directly causative. A recent meta-analysis of GWA studies involving more than 13,000 PD patients has identified over 28 variant genes at 24 loci that increase the risk of PD singly and in combination [23]. Genetic PD risk has ethnic variations. Clinically, genetic testing is not routinely performed for all PD cases if there is a negative family history, and GWA is mainly limited to research at present. Different genetic forms of PD demonstrate particular phenotypic features, for example early cognitive involvement in the GBA patients, dementia in the α-synuclein patients, and higher risk of treatment-related motor complications in the parkin patients.

The role of micro-RNAs (miRNA) in PD pathogenesis has come under investigation in recent years. miRNA are endogenous short non-coding sequences that exert powerful effects on multiple post-transcriptional genes [24]. Studies on human PD post mortem brains have used miRNA analysis to show that compared to matched controls, in early PD, mir-34b/c depletion in cells is associated with reduced parkin and DJ-1 expression. Reduced parkin and DJ-1 are known to induce mitochondrial dysfunction, a putative mechanism for PD [25]. mir-7 and mir-153 are involved in post-transcriptional regulation of α-synuclein. mir-7 and mir-153 deficiency leads to excess α-synuclein production, and overexpression of mir-7 and mir-153 reduces α-synuclein expression by almost 50% [26]. miRNA-mediated regulation of other PD associated genes such as LRRK2 has been described.

Epigenetics, changes in the function of genes in response to dynamic environmental stimuli without a change in their coding sequence, have been implicated in neurodegenerative disease [27]. Epigenetic changes increase with age, and age is the single biggest risk factor for PD. Epigenetic mechanisms include DNA methylation, RNA silencing, and histone modification [28, 29]. miRNA are well described to be susceptible to epigenetic changes in central nervous system (CNS) pathologies, although little is understood about specific epigenetic miRNA changes in PD. Although the genetic contributions identified only account for a small proportion of the etiopathogenesis of PD, it is the interactions of genetic susceptibility with other pathogenic factors that are of current interest. There is a role for examining neurodegeneration in the same way as neuro-oncological models, where a genetic susceptibility combined with a burden of environmental and endogenous insults stimulates carcinogenesis, maintained by epigenetic defences within the tumor.

In summary, the known genetic contributions to PD pathogenesis include autosomal dominant or Mendelian genes, high-risk alleles, micro-RNAs, and modifiable epigenetic changes. Somatic mutations and age-related mutations of mitochondrial DNA have been described [30, 31] and somatic mutations hypothesized [32].

Mitochondria

The role of mitochondria in PD was reported by Schapira and colleagues in 1989 and subsequently [33–35]. Mitochondria generate ATP via an enzyme-dependent electrochemical gradient with four complexes. They are also involved in apoptosis [36]. The production of ATP generates reactive oxygen species (ROS), so-called "free radicals" that are normally "neutralized" by enzymes such as superoxide dismutase and catalase. Factors stimulating ROS overproduction and/or impaired clearance may include iron deposition and disturbed calcium homeostasis. Accumulation of ROS has been shown to cause cellular damage, apoptosis, immune reactivity, and inflammation. Striatal dopaminergic neurons are reported to be more sensitive than cortical neurons to the destructive effects of ROS. ROS-mediated destruction of dopaminergic striatal neurons has been described in PD with defects in complex I and complex III of the electron transport chain [33–35]. Mitochondrial dysfunction in PD has been demonstrated outside the basal ganglia such in as the frontal lobes and indeed outside the CNS in sites such as enteric neurons, platelets, and fibroblasts [37–40]; it has also been described in pre-clinical PD. Cortical and striatal mitochondrial DNA changes are described in PD although whether they are causative or reactive to ROS is not fully understood. The relationship between mitochondria-driven neuronal destruction in PD and mitochondrial DNA changes is further complicated by the relationship between mitochondrial function and genetic forms of PD. Elevated α-synuclein and mitochondrial dysfunction are known to coexist in PD models [41]. Studies have shown that the presence of α-synuclein mutations impairs mitochondrial function and magnifies the destructive effect of mitochondrial toxins on dopaminergic neurons, whilst α-synuclein-negative models are less susceptible to mitochondrial toxins [42–44]. Parkin, LRRK2, DJ-1, and PINK are found in mitochondrial DNA and are associated with regulation of normal mitochondrial function [45]. The up- and down-regulation of these genes in certain studies can impair mitochondrial function and in others is reported to be protective by reducing ROS production and neuronal death. In summary, the evidence suggests that mitochondrial dysfunction can lead to striatonigral cell death and may interact in a destructive and in a protective manner with genes known to be associated with PD.

Mitochondria have recently been a focus of interest to enhance function and cell survival in PD. A potential strategy to reverse mitochondrial bioenergetic dysfunction is through the regulation of mitochondrial protein transcription and biogenesis. Peroxisome proliferator-activated receptor γ (PPARγ) coactivator-1α (PGC-1α) regulates mitochondrial activity and with SIRT1 enhances transcriptional factors for mitochondrial biogenesis. SIRT1 is one of a family of sirtuins, known to catalyze NAD+-dependent protein deacetylation, yielding nicotinamide and O-acetyl-ADP-ribose which regulate longevity, apoptosis, and DNA repair[46]. SIRT1 interacts directly with PGC-1α to increase its activity and lead to the induction of gene transcription. Activation of PPARγ transactivates target genes with the support of PGC-1α. Drugs that activate PPARγ include rosiglitazone, pioglitazone, and troglitazone – drugs designed for the treatment of diabetes mellitus but limited and in some cases withdrawn due to toxicity concerns. Resveratrol (RSV) is a natural polyphenolic compound found in the skin of grapes and has been shown significantly to increase SIRT1 and PGC-1α activities and increase mitochondrial biogenesis [47]. RSV and bezafibrate, another PGC-1α agonist, have demonstrated protective properties in animal models of PD [48, 49].

Attention has recently been drawn to glucagon-like peptide 1 (GLP-1), which originates in the L-cells of the intestine. GLP-1 and the longer half-life GLP-1-like peptide exendin-4 (EX-4) have been used for type 2 diabetes. GLP-1 and EX-4 promote cellular growth, reduce apoptosis, and may be anti-inflammatory, although the precise mode(s) of action remain uncertain [50, 51]. An open-label randomized study of exendin (exenatide) in PD (Clinical trials.gov Identifier NCT01174810) has been completed and showed benefit in an open-label study [52].

An alternative strategy to enhance mitochondrial function via transcription has come through the observation that Engrailed proteins can ameliorate the toxic effects of MPTP-induced dopaminergic cell death *in vivo* [53]. *Engrailed 1* and *2* are homeobox genes important in neural development, but are expressed throughout life in mesencephalic dopamine neurons. They appear to function by acting as cytosolic regulators of mRNA translation of mitochondrial proteins. Engrailed-deficient mice have dopaminergic degeneration, most severe in the pars compacta and ventral tegmental area [54]. There are reports of Engrailed-1 polymorphisms being associated with an increased risk for PD [55]. Expression of exogenous Engrailed 1 and 2 protects against MPTP toxicity in mice by enhancing the translation of two mitochondrial complex I subunits (Ndufs1 and 3) and increasing the activity of this respiratory chain protein [53]. Similar protection was seen against 6-hydroxydopamine and the A30P *SNCA* mutation. Thus, Engrailed or similar complex I regulators may be valid targets for future development in PD neuroprotection.

A different and perhaps even complementary strategy to increase mitochondrial biogenesis in PD is to enhance destruction of defective mitochondria. Mitochondrial fission–fusion helps maintain the mitochondrial pool and the removal of defective mitochondria by autophagy (mitophagy) [56–58]. Parkin and PINK1 proteins have recently been identified as playing an important role in the mitophagy pathway [59–61]. A fall in mitochondrial potential may be triggered by a number of factors including a decrease in oxidative phosphorylation or oxidant stress. Lowered membrane potential decreases the processing of PINK1 and results in the accumulation of full-length protein on the outer membrane, which in turn acts as a signal for parkin recruitment to mitochondria [62]. Parkin translocates from the cytosol to the mitochondrion in response to a fall in mitochondrial membrane potential [63]. Parkin and PINK1 involvement in mitophagy includes the ubiquitination of MFN 1 and 2 by parkin [64]. HtrA2 is thought to participate in mitochondrial turnover and has also been identified as a phosphorylation target of PINK1 [65]. Importantly, it now appears that mutations of parkin or PINK1 that cause PD interfere with mitophagy efficiency and result in accumulation of defective mitochondria [64]. This can be reversed by up-regulation of parkin or PINK1 with the removal of defective mitochondria. The recent demonstration of abnormal expression of autophagy proteins in PD brain has further highlighted the importance of degradation pathways in the pathogenesis of this disease [66, 67]. Up-regulation of the translation inhibitor 4E-BP ameliorates the effects of PINK1/parkin mutants in *Drosophila*, and rapamycin, a drug that activates 4E-BP and autophagy, is protective in these mutants [68].

Neuroinflammation, immunity, and the widespread Lewy body pathology in PD

Inflammation is a cellular and immune response to an insult that aims to restore normal tissue structure and function. Evidence of neuroinflammation in PD started to emerge in the 1980s, with reports of HLA-DR-positive microglia in post mortem studies of PD patients [69]. Activated microglia are known to release cytokines and chemokines, which in turn transform the inflammatory response into an inflammatory cascade. Neuroinflammation generated by an endotoxic lipopolysaccharide (LPS) model of PD has been shown to be associated with striatonigral dopaminergic neuronal death [70]. Inflammation in PD models is not confined to the basal ganglia; it has been seen in the midbrain and cortical regions. No single mechanism has been found to precipitate the inflammation, but there is evidence that protein misfolding as a result of mutations such as those of α-synuclein leads to microglial activation and the release of inflammatory mediators [71]. Loss of dopaminergic neurons is accelerated in α-synuclein-positive rodents when an inflammatory insult is applied. Administration of inflammatory mediators in neuronal cell cultures appears to up-regulate α-synuclein expression, suggesting that the processes are synergistic. Parkin and PINK mutations increased the vulnerability of dopaminergic neurons when subjected to inflammation and also increased mitochondrial sensitivity to calcium [72]. Inflammatory mediators are also believed to weaken the BBB and to promote ROS formation, suggesting interaction with mitochondrial pathways [73].

In humans, positron emission tomography (PET) based studies have demonstrated microglial activity in human PD, in early and late stages of the disease [74]. Studies in humans with PD have shown different levels, subtype proportions, and functional activity of cytokines and T cells in the cerebrospinal fluid, peripheral blood, and striatal regions compared with patients without PD. Studies examining the role of the innate and adaptive immune responses in early PD have shown both systems to be activated in PD and associated with production of inflammatory mediators. The role of inflammation outside the CNS has been considered too as there is evidence suggesting a role for enteric and olfactory inflammation in the early stages of PD, and PD has a well-described association with autoimmune diseases.

Braak et al. found that in human post mortem PD brains, Lewy bodies were located in particular locations that correlated with the clinical stage of the disease. The Braak hypothesis suggests that the early PD disease process may begin in the olfactory and enteric systems and travels retrogradely, possibly via the vagus towards the brainstem before propagating to the basal ganglia and beyond [75]. The large number of CNS and peripheral sites found to be involved in PD is certainly suggestive of a global neurodegenerative process. These sites are summarized by Surmeier and Sulzer in their 2013 review and include all divisions of the autonomic nervous system, enteric neurons, noradrenergic neurons of the heart and skin, hypothalamus, brainstem, Meynert's nucleus, amygdala, hippocampus, and other regions [76].

What initiates this diverse process and the mechanism by which peripheral neural pathology travels to the CNS in Braak's hypothesis is incompletely defined but there is work suggesting that α-synuclein plays a prominent role and the conduit may be the autonomic nervous system (see also Prion-like mechanism of α-synuclein spread). α-Synuclein has been shown to be able to transfer from cell to cell and along axons. In a series of studies, Pan-Montojo et al. have demonstrated that administering rotenone into the guts of mice generated ROS and induced enteric neurons to express high levels of α-synuclein and aggregates of the misfolded protein, eventually detectable in the CNS and associated with PD-like features, dopaminergic neuronal destruction, and CNS α-synuclein expression. In a subsequent study in the same model,

sectioning the parasympathetic and sympathetic nerves halted disease progression and α-synuclein transport [77, 78]. *In vivo* studies have demonstrated cell to cell transfer of α-synuclein, perhaps via prion-like transfer mechanisms [79]. Assuming the Braak hypothesis does contribute to the pathogenesis of PD, the index insult to the olfactory and enteric systems is yet to be determined, or alternatively may represent a stochastic event. Numerous environmental agents and viruses have been reported to be associated with PD (but not causative). Whether these agents, when in contact with peripheral neurons, set up a cellular response and precipitate the events in the Braak hypothesis is under investigation.

Activated microglia are known to express MHC2 in the basal ganglia and cortex in PD, whilst MHC is barely detectable in glial cells of individuals without PD. MHC2 is responsible for activating T cells and cascading the immune response. PD is associated with some MHC2 polypeptide coding abnormalities although no single MCH2 locus is consistently implicated. SNCA, LRRK2, and parkin genes all have close interactions with cells of the immune system, the genes being coded within the immune cells and regulating their function. Lymphocytes from PD patients show increased ROS and apoptotic markers than those from controls, tying the immune–inflammatory component of PD in with the genetic and mitochondrial aspects of PD. In summary, neuroinflammation and an immune response seem to be present in all stages of PD, to be a self-perpetuating cascade, and to interact with other putative mechanisms of PD (genetic, toxic) to amplify and perpetuate neurodegeneration.

Prion-like mechanism of α-synuclein spread

Prion diseases are characterized by the spread of pathological proteinaceous particles at intracellular, intercellular, tissue, and organism levels. There is *in vitro* and *in vivo* animal and human evidence that α-synuclein can spread between neurons. The first of this evidence came from post mortem studies on PD patients who had received fetal mesencephalic dopaminergic neuronal grafts into their putamen or caudate nuclei in the 1990s. α-Synuclein deposits were detected in the transplanted cells of patients who had the transplant more than 10 years previously [80]. At the intracellular level, studies that labeled preformed α-synuclein fibrils (pathological) have demonstrated that these fibrils recruit further normal, endogenous intracellular α-synuclein into the pathological aggregate. At the intercellular level, *in vitro* and *in vivo* studies confirm that normal neuronal stem cells, when transplanted into an environment of α-synuclein overexpression, also start to develop α-synuclein fibrils [81]. The mechanisms for intercellular transfer ("seeding") may include endosomal-mediated transfer and tunneling nanotubes between cells. This finding challenges the assumption that in PD the pathology affects multiple neurons simultaneously – the pathology may start in a few cells and then propagate by "template recruitment" of other cells [82]. Recent evidence, however, shows that α-synuclein is not solely an intracellular protein; it can exist in the extracellular space, which could imply complex intercellular transportation mechanisms [83]. Once transported into a "virgin" neuron, the α-synuclein begins to aggregate; it then may be released from a dying cell and taken up by another cell to propagate the pathological process [84]. α-Synuclein monomers, oligomers, and aggregates have all been shown to be able to be transported by endocytosis and exocytosis [85]. Considering tissue level, the Braak hypothesis proposes that α-synuclein aggregates self-propagate along axons between autonomic, peripheral, and central neurons. Evidence for a prion-like mechanism in the Braak theory includes studies that demonstrate that axonal transection does not prevent neuronal transmission of α-synuclein [81]. Further support for tissue level transmission of pathological α-synuclein comes from a mouse study in which transgenic mice were injected with intramuscular α-synuclein preformed fibrils and subsequently demonstrated neuronal synuclein fibrils [86]. Recasens and Dehay outline some of the key unanswered questions concerning the prion-like spread of α-synuclein in PD [87]. These include any differences between α-synuclein that spreads and that which is toxic, co-factors in spread, immune response, and the role of glia in this process.

Environmental risk factors

When addressing PD and environmental factors, it is important to consider environmental agents in terms of risk level rather than direct causation as there is no evidence that any single substance is directly responsible for the disease itself (not the same as parkinsonian features as caused by MPTP). Pesticides such as paraquat, organochlorine 2,4-dichlorophenoxyacetic acid (2,4-D), and permethrin are associated, although not necessarily consistently, in epidemiological studies with increased risk of PD. Other factors implicated in PD etiology include farming and rural living. Tanner et al. suggest that the common factor to pesticides that are associated with PD is induction of mitochondrial complex I dysfunction. This risk is amplified in individuals lacking the enzymes to degrade these chemicals [88]. Traumatic brain injury (TBI) is a risk factor for PD [89]. Postulated mechanisms of delayed neurodegeneration after TBI include inflammatory response to injury and a disrupted BBB allowing passage of environmental agents. The effect of TBI is amplified by the presence of a long Rep1 variant in the α-synuclein gene [90]. These findings highlight the gene–environment balance, in that an environmental insult in a genetically susceptible host may lead to disease. Some animal studies demonstrate that toxin-induced dopaminergic neuron destruction is greater in mice with overexpression of α-synuclein and parkin deficiency versus wild-type mice [91]. Other genes (LRRK2) increase α-synuclein levels after a toxic insult but this actually results in less dopaminergic neuronal destruction than in wild types, indicating a potentially protective role for α-synuclein, at least initially. Epigenetic changes may also modulate the effect of environmental insults [29]. This balance between α-synuclein being protective in some situations and destructive in others is complex and not fully understood – it is likely to involve cross-talk between genetic, inflammatory, and immune responses. In conclusion, environmental factors are implicated in the etiology of PD, especially in susceptible hosts, but are only one part of the pathomechanism [92]. At this stage, attaching a "weighting" to the contribution of particular environmental agents to PD risk is not possible, but may become so over time with long-term observational studies.

Recurrent themes

Reviewing the evidence surrounding the etiopathogenesis of PD, a few key themes recur, which can be considered in terms of initiation and perpetuation of the disease. These include the role of α-synuclein, mitochondrial dysfunction, genetic changes, inflammation and immunity, and transmission of neurodegeneration. The interaction of these factors appears important in the progression from initial insult

to clinical PD in susceptible individuals such as those with high-risk PD alleles. The initial insult, if there is one, remains unknown. It may be that, similar to cancer biology, PD occurs as the result of a multi-hit hypothesis, where a number of factors accumulate in a susceptible individual to create and maintain a disease process.

References

1. Postuma RB, Aarsland D, Barone P, Burn DJ, Hawkes CH, Oertel W, Ziemssen T. Identifying prodromal Parkinson's disease: pre-motor disorders in Parkinson's disease. *Mov Disord* 2012; 27: 617–26.
2. Chaudhuri KR, Healy DG, Schapira AH. Non-motor symptoms of Parkinson's disease: diagnosis and management. *Lancet Neurol* 2006; 5: 235–45.
3. Davis GC, Williams AC, Markey SP, Ebert MH, Caine ED, Reichert CM, Kopin IJ. Chronic Parkinsonism secondary to intravenous injection of meperidine analogues. *Psychiatry Res* 1979; 1: 249–54.
4. Jakowec MW, Petzinger GM. 1-methyl-4-phenyl-1,2,3,6-tetrahydropyridine-lesioned model of parkinson's disease, with emphasis on mice and nonhuman primates. *Comp Med* 2004; 54: 497–513.
5. Potts LF, Wu H, Singh A, Marcilla I, Luquin MR, Papa SM. Modeling Parkinson's disease in monkeys for translational studies, a critical analysis. *Exp Neurol* 2014; 256: 133–43.
6. McDowell KA, Shin D, Roos KP, Chesselet MF. Sleep dysfunction and EEG alterations in mice overexpressing alpha-synuclein. *J Parkinsons Dis* 2014; 4: 531–9.
7. Mullin S, Schapira A. The genetics of Parkinson's disease. *Br Med Bull* 2015; 114: 39–52.
8. Spillantini MG, Schmidt ML, Lee VM, Trojanowski JQ, Jakes R, Goedert M. Alpha-synuclein in Lewy bodies. *Nature* 1997; 388: 839–40.
9. Ibanez P, Bonnet AM, Debarges B, Lohmann E, Tison F, Pollak P, Agid Y, Durr A, Brice A. Causal relation between alpha-synuclein gene duplication and familial Parkinson's disease. *Lancet* 2004; 364: 1169–71.
10. Crabtree DM, Zhang J. Genetically engineered mouse models of Parkinson's disease. *Brain Res Bull* 2012; 88: 13–32.
11. Giraldez-Perez R, Antolin-Vallespin M, Munoz M, Sanchez-Capelo A. Models of alpha-synuclein aggregation in Parkinson's disease. *Acta Neuropathol Commun* 2014; 2: 176.
12. Kudo T, Loh DH, Truong D, Wu Y, Colwell CS. Circadian dysfunction in a mouse model of Parkinson's disease. *Exp Neurol* 2011; 232: 66–75.
13. Wang L, Fleming SM, Chesselet MF, Tache Y. Abnormal colonic motility in mice overexpressing human wild-type alpha-synuclein. *Neuroreport* 2008; 19: 873–6.
14. Fleming SM, Tetreault NA, Mulligan CK, Hutson CB, Masliah E, Chesselet MF. Olfactory deficits in mice overexpressing human wildtype alpha-synuclein. *Eur J Neurosci* 2008; 28: 247–56.
15. Manning-Bog AB, Langston JW. Model fusion, the next phase in developing animal models for Parkinson's. *Neurotox Res* 2007; 11: 219–40.
16. Healy DG, Falchi M, O'Sullivan SS, Bonifati V, Durr A, Bressman S, Brice A, Aasly J, Zabetian CP, Goldwurm S, Ferreira JJ, Tolosa E, Kay DM, Klein C, Williams DR, Marras C, Lang AE, Wszolek ZK, Berciano J, Schapira AH, Lynch T, Bhatia KP, Gasser T, Lees AJ, Wood NW. Phenotype, genotype, and worldwide genetic penetrance of LRRK2-associated Parkinson's disease: a case-control study. *Lancet Neurol* 2008; 7: 583–90.
17. Lucking CB, Durr A, Bonifati V, Vaughan J, De Michele G, Gasser T, Harhangi BS, Meco G, Denefle P, Wood NW, Agid Y, Brice A. Association between early-onset Parkinson's disease and mutations in the parkin gene. *N Engl J Med* 2000; 342: 1560–7.
18. Bonifati V, Rohe CF, Breedveld GJ, Fabrizio E, De Mari M, Tassorelli C, Tavella A, Marconi R, Nicholl DJ, Chien HF, Fincati E, Abbruzzese G, Marini P, De Gaetano A, Horstink MW, Maat-Kievit JA, Sampaio C, Antonini A, Stocchi F, Montagna P, Toni V, Guidi M, Dalla LA, Tinazzi M, De Pandis F, Fabbrini G, Goldwurm S, de Klein A, Barbosa E, Lopiano L, Martignoni E, Lamberti P, Vanacore N, Meco G, Oostra BA. Early-onset parkinsonism associated with PINK1 mutations: frequency, genotypes, and phenotypes. *Neurology* 2005; 65: 87–95.
19. Djarmati A, Hedrich K, Svetel M, Schafer N, Juric V, Vukosavic S, Hering R, Riess O, Romac S, Klein C, Kostic V. Detection of Parkin (PARK2) and DJ1 (PARK7) mutations in early-onset Parkinson disease: Parkin mutation frequency depends on ethnic origin of patients. *Hum Mutat* 2004; 23: 525.
20. Beavan MS, Schapira AH. Glucocerebrosidase mutations and the pathogenesis of Parkinson disease. *Ann Med* 2013; 45: 511–21.
21. Schapira AH. Glucocerebrosidase and Parkinson disease: Recent advances. *Mol Cell Neurosci* 2015; 66: 37–42.
22. Mollenhauer B, Rochester L, Chen-Plotkin A, Brooks D. What can biomarkers tell us about cognition in Parkinson's disease? *Mov Disord* 2014; 29: 622–33.

23. Nalls MA, Pankratz N, Lill CM, Do CB, Hernandez DG, Saad M, DeStefano AL, Kara E, Bras J, Sharma M, Schulte C, Keller MF, Arepalli S, Letson C, Edsall C, Stefansson H, Liu X, Pliner H, Lee JH, Cheng R, Ikram MA, Ioannidis JP, Hadjigeorgiou GM, Bis JC, Martinez M, Perlmutter JS, Goate A, Marder K, Fiske B, Sutherland M, Xiromerisiou G, Myers RH, Clark LN, Stefansson K, Hardy JA, Heutink P, Chen H, Wood NW, Houlden H, Payami H, Brice A, Scott WK, Gasser T, Bertram L, Eriksson N, Foroud T, Singleton AB. Large-scale meta-analysis of genome-wide association data identifies six new risk loci for Parkinson's disease. *Nat Genet* 2014; 46: 989–93.

24. Lewis BP, Burge CB, Bartel DP. Conserved seed pairing, often flanked by adenosines, indicates that thousands of human genes are microRNA targets. *Cell* 2005; 120: 15–20.

25. Minones-Moyano E, Porta S, Escaramis G, Rabionet R, Iraola S, Kagerbauer B, Espinosa-Parrilla Y, Ferrer I, Estivill X, Marti E. MicroRNA profiling of Parkinson's disease brains identifies early downregulation of miR-34b/c which modulate mitochondrial function. *Hum Mol Genet* 2011; 20: 3067–78.

26. Doxakis E. Post-transcriptional regulation of alpha-synuclein expression by mir-7 and mir-153. *J Biol Chem* 2010; 285: 12726–34.

27. Egger G, Liang G, Aparicio A, Jones PA. Epigenetics in human disease and prospects for epigenetic therapy. *Nature* 2004; 429: 457–63.

28. Varela MA, Roberts TC, Wood MJ. Epigenetics and ncRNAs in brain function and disease: mechanisms and prospects for therapy. *Neurotherapeutics* 2013; 10: 621–31.

29. Ammal KN, Tarannum S, Thomas B. Epigenetic landscape of Parkinson's disease: emerging role in disease mechanisms and therapeutic modalities. *Neurotherapeutics* 2013; 10: 698–708.

30. Reeve AK, Krishnan KJ, Elson JL, Morris CM, Bender A, Lightowlers RN, Turnbull DM. Nature of mitochondrial DNA deletions in substantia nigra neurons. *Am J Hum Genet* 2008; 82: 228–35.

31. Kraytsberg Y, Kudryavtseva E, McKee AC, Geula C, Kowall NW, Khrapko K. Mitochondrial DNA deletions are abundant and cause functional impairment in aged human substantia nigra neurons. *Nat Genet* 2006; 38: 518–20.

32. Proukakis C, Houlden H, Schapira AH. Somatic alpha-synuclein mutations in Parkinson's disease: hypothesis and preliminary data. *Mov Disord* 2013; 28: 705–12.

33. Schapira AH, Cooper JM, Dexter D, Jenner P, Clark JB, Marsden CD. Mitochondrial complex I deficiency in Parkinson's disease. *Lancet* 1989; 1: 1269.

34. Schapira AH, Cooper JM, Morgan-Hughes JA, Landon DN, Clark JB. Mitochondrial myopathy with a defect of mitochondrial-protein transport. *N Engl J Med* 1990; 323: 37–42.

35. Schapira AH, Cooper JM, Dexter D, Clark JB, Jenner P, Marsden CD. Mitochondrial complex I deficiency in Parkinson's disease. *J Neurochem* 1990; 54: 823–7.

36. Schapira AH. Mitochondrial disease. *Lancet* 2006; 368: 70–82.

37. Krige D, Carroll MT, Cooper JM, Marsden CD, Schapira AH. Platelet mitochondrial function in Parkinson's disease. The Royal Kings and Queens Parkinson Disease Research Group. *Ann Neurol* 1992; 32: 782–8.

38. van der Merwe C, Loos B, Swart C, Kinnear C, Henning F, van der Merwe L, Pillay K, Muller N, Zaharie D, Engelbrecht L, Carr J, Bardien S. Mitochondrial impairment observed in fibroblasts from South African Parkinson's disease patients with parkin mutations. *Biochem Biophys Res Commun* 2014; 447: 334–40.

39. Thomas RR, Keeney PM, Bennett JP. Impaired complex-I mitochondrial biogenesis in Parkinson disease frontal cortex. *J Parkinsons Dis* 2012; 2: 67–76.

40. Braidy N, Gai WP, Xu YH, Sachdev P, Guillemin GJ, Jiang XM, Ballard JW, Horan MP, Fang ZM, Chong BH, Chan DK. Alpha-synuclein transmission and mitochondrial toxicity in primary human foetal enteric neurons in vitro. *Neurotox Res* 2014; 25: 170–82.

41. Mullin S, Schapira A. alpha-Synuclein and mitochondrial dysfunction in Parkinson's disease. *Mol Neurobiol* 2013; 47: 587–97.

42. Chinta SJ, Mallajosyula JK, Rane A, Andersen JK. Mitochondrial alpha-synuclein accumulation impairs complex I function in dopaminergic neurons and results in increased mitophagy in vivo. *Neurosci Lett* 2010; 486: 235–9.

43. Klivenyi P, Siwek D, Gardian G, Yang L, Starkov A, Cleren C, Ferrante RJ, Kowall NW, Abeliovich A, Beal MF. Mice lacking alpha-synuclein are resistant to mitochondrial toxins. *Neurobiol Dis* 2006; 21: 541–8.

44. Fountaine TM, Venda LL, Warrick N, Christian HC, Brundin P, Channon KM, Wade-Martins R. The effect of alpha-synuclein knockdown on MPP+ toxicity in models of human neurons. *Eur J Neurosci* 2008; 28: 2459–73.

45. Schapira AH. Mitochondria in the aetiology and pathogenesis of Parkinson's disease. *Lancet Neurol* 2008; 7: 97–109.

46. Blander G, Guarente L. The Sir2 family of protein deacetylases. *Annu Rev Biochem* 2004; 73: 417–35.

47. Howitz KT, Bitterman KJ, Cohen HY, Lamming DW, Lavu S, Wood JG, Zipkin RE, Chung P, Kisielewski A, Zhang LL, Scherer B, Sinclair DA. Small molecule activators of sirtuins extend Saccharomyces cerevisiae lifespan. *Nature* 2003; 425: 191–6.

48. Khan MM, Ahmad A, Ishrat T, Khan MB, Hoda MN, Khuwaja G, Raza SS, Khan A, Javed H, Vaibhav K, Islam F. Resveratrol attenuates 6-hydroxydopamine-induced oxidative damage and dopamine depletion in rat model of Parkinson's disease. *Brain Res* 2010; 1328: 139–51.

49. Jin F, Wu Q, Lu YF, Gong QH, Shi JS. Neuroprotective effect of resveratrol on 6-OHDA-induced Parkinson's disease in rats. *Eur J Pharmacol* 2008; 600: 78–82.

50. Harkavyi A, Whitton PS. Glucagon-like peptide 1 receptor stimulation as a means of neuroprotection. *Br J Pharmacol* 2010; 159: 495–501.

51. Aviles-Olmos I, Limousin P, Lees A, Foltynie T. Parkinson's disease, insulin resistance and novel agents of neuroprotection. *Brain* 2013; 136: 374–84.

52. Aviles-Olmos I, Dickson J, Kefalopoulou Z, Djamshidian A, Ell P, Soderlund T, Whitton P, Wyse R, Isaacs T, Lees A, Limousin P, Foltynie T. Exenatide and the treatment of patients with Parkinson's disease. *J Clin Invest* 2013; 123: 2730–6.

53. Alvarez-Fischer D, Fuchs J, Castagner F, Stettler O, Massiani-Beaudoin O, Moya KL, Bouillot C, Oertel WH, Lombes A, Faigle W, Joshi RL, Hartmann A, Prochiantz A. Engrailed protects mouse midbrain dopaminergic neurons against mitochondrial complex I insults. *Nat Neurosci* 2011; 14: 1260–6.

54. Sonnier L, Le Pen G, Hartmann A, Bizot JC, Trovero F, Krebs MO, Prochiantz A. Progressive loss of dopaminergic neurons in the ventral midbrain of adult mice heterozygote for Engrailed1. *J Neurosci* 2007; 27: 1063–71.

55. Haubenberger D, Reinthaler E, Mueller JC, Pirker W, Katzenschlager R, Froehlich R, Bruecke T, Daniel G, Auff E, Zimprich A. Association of transcription factor polymorphisms PITX3 and EN1 with Parkinson's disease. *Neurobiol Aging* 2011; 32: 302–7.

56. Dagda RK, Chu CT. Mitochondrial quality control: insights on how Parkinson's disease related genes PINK1, parkin, and Omi/HtrA2 interact to maintain mitochondrial homeostasis. *J Bioenerg Biomembr* 2009; 41: 473–9.

57. Chan DC. Mitochondria: dynamic organelles in disease, aging, and development. *Cell* 2006; 125: 1241–52.

58. Chen H, Chan DC. Mitochondrial dynamics – fusion, fission, movement, and mitophagy – in neurodegenerative diseases. *Hum Mol Genet* 2009; 18: R169–R176.

59. Poole AC, Thomas RE, Andrews LA, McBride HM, Whitworth AJ, Pallanck LJ. The PINK1/Parkin pathway regulates mitochondrial morphology. *Proc Natl Acad Sci U S A* 2008; 105: 1638–43.

60. Deng H, Dodson MW, Huang H, Guo M. The Parkinson's disease genes pink1 and parkin promote mitochondrial fission and/or inhibit fusion in Drosophila. *Proc Natl Acad Sci U S A* 2008; 105: 14503–8.

61. Ashrafi G, Schwarz TL. The pathways of mitophagy for quality control and clearance of mitochondria. *Cell Death Differ* 2013; 20: 31–42.

62. Matsuda N, Sato S, Shiba K, Okatsu K, Saisho K, Gautier CA, Sou YS, Saiki S, Kawajiri S, Sato F, Kimura M, Komatsu M, Hattori N, Tanaka K. PINK1 stabilized by mitochondrial depolarization recruits Parkin to damaged mitochondria and activates latent Parkin for mitophagy. *J Cell Biol* 2010; 189: 211–21.

63. Narendra D, Tanaka A, Suen DF, Youle RJ. Parkin is recruited selectively to impaired mitochondria and promotes their autophagy. *J Cell Biol* 2008; 183: 795–803.

64. Gegg ME, Cooper JM, Chau KY, Rojo M, Schapira AH, Taanman JW. Mitofusin 1 and mitofusin 2 are ubiquitinated in a PINK1/parkin-dependent manner upon induction of mitophagy. *Hum Mol Genet* 2010; 19: 4861–70.

65. Plun-Favreau H, Klupsch K, Moisoi N, Gandhi S, Kjaer S, Frith D, Harvey K, Deas E, Harvey RJ, McDonald N, Wood NW, Martins LM, Downward J. The mitochondrial protease HtrA2 is recruited by Parkinson's disease-associated kinase PINK1. *Nat Cell Biol* 2007; 9: 1243–52.

66. Alvarez-Erviti L, Rodriguez-Oroz MC, Cooper JM, Caballero C, Ferrer I, Obeso JA, Schapira AH. Chaperone-mediated autophagy markers in Parkinson disease brains. *Arch Neurol* 2010; 67: 1464–72.

67. Chu Y, Dodiya H, Aebischer P, Olanow CW, Kordower JH. Alterations in lysosomal and proteasomal markers in Parkinson's disease: relationship to alpha-synuclein inclusions. *Neurobiol Dis* 2009; 35: 385–98.

68. Tain LS, Mortiboys H, Tao RN, Ziviani E, Bandmann O, Whitworth AJ. Rapamycin activation of 4E-BP prevents parkinsonian dopaminergic neuron loss. *Nat Neurosci* 2009; 12: 1129–35.

69. McGeer PL, Itagaki S, Akiyama H, McGeer EG. Rate of cell death in parkinsonism indicates active neuropathological process. *Ann Neurol* 1988; 24: 574–6.

70. Castano A, Herrera AJ, Cano J, Machado A. The degenerative effect of a single intranigral injection of LPS on the dopaminergic system is prevented by dexamethasone, and not mimicked by rh-TNF-alpha, IL-1beta and IFN-gamma. *J Neurochem* 2002; 81: 150–7.

71. Su X, Maguire-Zeiss KA, Giuliano R, Prifti L, Venkatesh K, Federoff HJ. Synuclein activates microglia in a model of Parkinson's disease. *Neurobiol Aging* 2008; 29: 1690–701.

72. Akundi RS, Huang Z, Eason J, Pandya JD, Zhi L, Cass WA, Sullivan PG, Bueler H. Increased mitochondrial calcium sensitivity and abnormal expression of innate immunity genes precede dopaminergic defects in Pink1-deficient mice. *PLoS One* 2011; 6: e16038.

73. Lukiw WJ, Bjattacharjee S, Zhao Y, Pogue AI, Percy ME. Generation of reactive oxygen species (ROS) and pro-inflammatory signaling in human brain cells in primary culture. *J Alzheimers Dis Parkinsonism* 2012; Suppl 2: 001.

74. Gerhard A, Pavese N, Hotton G, Turkheimer F, Es M, Hammers A, Eggert K, Oertel W, Banati RB, Brooks DJ. In vivo imaging of microglial activation with [11C](R)-PK11195 PET in idiopathic Parkinson's disease. *Neurobiol Dis* 2006; 21: 404–12.

75. Braak H, Rub U, Gai WP, Del Tredici K. Idiopathic Parkinson's disease: possible routes by which vulnerable neuronal types may be subject to neuroinvasion by an unknown pathogen. *J Neural Transm* 2003; 110: 517–36.

76. Surmeier DJ, Sulzer D. The pathology roadmap in Parkinson disease. *Prion* 2013; 7: 85–91.

77. Pan-Montojo F, Anichtchik O, Dening Y, Knels L, Pursche S, Jung R, Jackson S, Gille G, Spillantini MG, Reichmann H, Funk RH. Progression of Parkinson's disease pathology is reproduced by intragastric administration of rotenone in mice. *PLoS One* 2010; 5: e8762.

78. Pan-Montojo F, Schwarz M, Winkler C, Arnhold M, O'Sullivan GA, Pal A, Said J, Marsico G, Verbavatz JM, Rodrigo-Angulo M, Gille G, Funk RH, Reichmann H. Environmental toxins trigger PD-like progression via increased alpha-synuclein release from enteric neurons in mice. *Sci Rep* 2012; 2: 898.

79. Angot E, Steiner JA, Lema Tome CM, Ekstrom P, Mattsson B, Bjorklund A, Brundin P. Alpha-synuclein cell-to-cell transfer and seeding in grafted dopaminergic neurons in vivo. *PLoS One* 2012; 7: e39465.

80. Kordower JH, Chu Y, Hauser RA, Freeman TB, Olanow CW. Lewy body-like pathology in long-term embryonic nigral transplants in Parkinson's disease. *Nat Med* 2008; 14: 504–6.

81. Chauhan A, Jeans AF. Is Parkinson's disease truly a prion-like disorder? An appraisal of current evidence. *Neurol Res Int* 2015; 2015: 345285.

82. Goedert M, Falcon B, Clavaguera F, Tolnay M. Prion-like mechanisms in the pathogenesis of tauopathies and synucleinopathies. *Curr Neurol Neurosci Rep* 2014; 14: 495.

83. Oueslati A, Ximerakis M, Vekrellis K. Protein transmission, seeding and degradation: key steps for alpha-synuclein prion-like propagation. *Exp Neurobiol* 2014; 23: 324–36.

84. Brundin P, Li JY, Holton JL, Lindvall O, Revesz T. Research in motion: the enigma of Parkinson's disease pathology spread. *Nat Rev Neurosci* 2008; 9: 741–5.

85. Hansen C, Angot E, Bergstrom AL, Steiner JA, Pieri L, Paul G, Outeiro TF, Melki R, Kallunki P, Fog K, Li JY, Brundin P. alpha-Synuclein propagates from mouse brain to grafted dopaminergic neurons and seeds aggregation in cultured human cells. *J Clin Invest* 2011; 121: 715–25.

86. Sacino AN, Brooks M, Thomas MA, McKinney AB, Lee S, Regenhardt RW, McGarvey NH, Ayers JI, Notterpek L, Borchelt DR, Golde TE, Giasson BI. Intramuscular injection of alpha-synuclein induces CNS alpha-synuclein pathology and a rapid-onset motor phenotype in transgenic mice. *Proc Natl Acad Sci U S A* 2014; 111: 10732–7.

87. Recasens A, Dehay B. Alpha-synuclein spreading in Parkinson's disease. *Front Neuroanat* 2014; 8: 159.

88. Tanner CM, Goldman SM, Ross GW, Grate SJ. The disease intersection of susceptibility and exposure: chemical exposures and neurodegenerative disease risk. *Alzheimers Dement* 2014; 10: S213–S225.

89. Perry DC, Sturm VE, Peterson MJ, Pieper CF, Bullock T, Boeve BF, Miller BL, Guskiewicz KM, Berger MS, Kramer JH, Welsh-Bohmer KA. Association of traumatic brain injury with subsequent neurological and psychiatric disease: a meta-analysis. *J Neurosurg* 2015; 1-16.

90. Goldman SM, Kamel F, Ross GW, Jewell SA, Bhudhikanok GS, Umbach D, Marras C, Hauser RA, Jankovic J, Factor SA, Bressman S, Lyons KE, Meng C, Korell M, Roucoux DF, Hoppin JA, Sandler DP, Langston JW, Tanner CM. Head injury, alpha-synuclein Rep1, and Parkinson's disease. *Ann Neurol* 2012; 71: 40–8.

91. Frank-Cannon TC, Tran T, Ruhn KA, Martinez TN, Hong J, Marvin M, Hartley M, Trevino I, O'Brien DE, Casey B, Goldberg MS, Tansey MG. Parkin deficiency increases vulnerability to inflammation-related nigral degeneration. *J Neurosci* 2008; 28: 10825–34.

92. Pan-Montojo F, Reichmann H. Considerations on the role of environmental toxins in idiopathic Parkinson's disease pathophysiology. *Transl Neurodegener* 2014; 3: 10.

CHAPTER 6

Parkinson Disease: Treatment Options – Surgical Therapy

Travis S. Tierney[1] and Andres M. Lozano[2]

[1] Division of Neurosurgery, Nicklaus Children's Hospital, Miami, Florida, USA
[2] Division of Neurosurgery, University of Toronto and Toronto Western Hospital, Toronto, Ontario, Canada

Introduction

Contemporary neuromodulation in the form of deep brain stimulation (DBS) offers, at least in theory, the potential to treat the full symptomatic spectrum of Parkinson disease (PD) including dopamine-induced, dopamine-responsive, and certain dopamine-non-responsive features. Chronic high-frequency stimulation of the pallidum and subthalamic nucleus has become the most common treatment for advanced PD with an estimated 8000 to 10,000 patients worldwide undergoing these procedures yearly. In this chapter we review standard and emerging surgical targets, common patient selection criteria, and efficacy data for three key targets: the subthalamic nucleus (STN), the internal segment of the globus pallidus (GPi), and the pedunculopontine nucleus (PPN). Although ablative surgery including pallidotomy [1] and subthalamotomy [2] is still used in selective cases and in certain countries, safety concerns (particularly if surgery is performed bilaterally) have limited their use and further discussion of these options will be brief. Despite the appreciation that surgery can improve both drug-induced and primary disease symptoms, no surgical intervention has yet been shown to slow ongoing neurodegeneration in patients with PD. Experimental neurorestoration strategies including transplantation and gene therapy offer the hope of modifying disease progression and some of these more promising ongoing efforts are highlighted towards the end of this section.

Standard surgical targets for Parkinson disease: the pallidum and subthalamic nucleus

Clinical interest in surgery for PD gained significant momentum as the drug-induced motor and non-motor side-effects of prolonged levodopa therapy (e.g., dyskinesia, motor fluctuations, and psychiatric disorders) began to become widely recognized [3, 4]. The first effective surgical treatment for some of these problems came with revival of Leksell's posteroventral pallidotomy [1], followed shortly by the application of chronic high-frequency stimulation of the pallidum [5] and subthalamic nucleus [6, 7]. Each of these surgical interventions controls not only the cardinal motor manifestations of PD but also drug-induced motor side effects of levodopa including motor fluctuations and dyskinesias, now the most common

modern indication for surgery [8]. In 2002, the US Food and Drug Administration (FDA) approved both subthalamic (STN) and globus pallidus (GPi) deep brain stimulation (DBS) for the treatment of PD. Since then over 80,000 patients have been treated [9]. Over the same interval, the number of patients undergoing pallidotomy has declined [10], but as discussed below, this ablative procedure continues to be a useful alternative to DBS for some patients.

A number of observational studies have documented the sustained motor benefits of STN [11–14] and GPi [15–19] DBS for PD. Reductions in drug-induced dyskinesia range from 50 to 90% and are accompanied by improvements in unified Parkinson disease rating scale (UPDRS) motor scores that are superior (Class 1 evidence) to optimal medication regimens alone [20–22]. Two Class 1 trials have directly compared outcomes between the STN and GPi targets [23, 24] and found that GPi stimulation may be slightly more effective in reducing the dyskinesia, but that overall beneficial effects on motor performance did not significantly differ between surgical arms. The antidyskinetic effect of STN stimulation often occurs in the context of a concomitant decrease in postoperative dopaminergic medication, whereas pallidal stimulation alleviates dyskinesia without significant dose reductions [25]. Indeed, surgically-resistant off-medication symptoms such as bradykinesia and axial instability usually prohibit significant dose reductions following pallidal stimulation. On the other hand, cognitive decline [26–28] and adverse psychiatric outcomes including depression and suicide [24, 29, 30] have more often been shown to occur following STN DBS. However, it is unclear if these complications arise from off-target stimulation of limbic circuitry located within the ventromedial STN, occur as a result of medication withdrawal, or are linked to some other as yet unknown factor. Preoperative vulnerability to deterioration in cognition and mood may be revealed by neurocognitive testing, which should be undertaken prior to any surgical consideration [21, 31, 32].

Like pallidal DBS, pallidotomy is an effective surgical intervention for controlling the primary motor manifestations of PD as well as drug-induced motor side effects of chronic levodopa therapy [33]. However, because bilateral lesions carry a significantly higher risk of a permanent dysarthria, motor weakness, and pseudobulbar cognitive impairment [34–36], surgery to place a single lesion contralateral to the most affected side is usually performed. When axial symptoms are severe, staged bilateral lesions are sometimes considered

Neurodegeneration, First Edition. Edited by Anthony Schapira, Zbigniew Wszolek, Ted M. Dawson and Nicholas Wood.
© 2017 John Wiley & Sons, Ltd. Published 2017 by John Wiley & Sons, Ltd.

to reduce the risk of cognitive complications from simultaneous bilateral lesions (York et al., 2008). While several high-level studies have documented durable long-term effects of pallidotomy in controlling both primary motor symptoms [37–39] and dyskinesia [40, 41], a randomized controlled trial that directly compared unilateral pallidotomy to bilateral STN DBS [42] showed that bilateral stimulation (vs unilateral pallidotomy) was more effective in controlling off-medication motor symptoms at one year (reduction in UPDRS motor subscores of 32% vs 53%, respectively); this benefit was maintained at 4 years (27% for pallidotomy vs 46% for STN DBS) [43]. Despite the potential inherent advantage of bilateral surgery for stimulation, unilateral pallidotomy was *not* shown to be inferior to DBS surgery in ameliorating drug-induced motor complications where control in both groups on the Clinical Dyskinesia Rating Scale at short- and long-term follow-up was excellent. These Class 1 comparative data most strongly suggest to us that while unilateral pallidotomy may be slight less effective in controlling the primary motor manifestations of PD compared with bilateral DBS, it can still be considered a durable option for advanced patients who experience significant drug-induced motor complications. In special circumstances, creation of a permanent lesion might even be preferable to placement of chronic implants. For example, pallidotomy may be offered to patients living in remote areas with difficult access to specialized centers for postoperative programming, to those unable to tolerate any form of general anesthesia for tunneling of lead extensions, or in cases of recurrent DBS hardware infections where conversion to a lesion using the implanted DBS electrode is possible [44].

Patient selection

The ideal surgical candidate with PD has maintained a clear response to levodopa [45, 46], but has begun to suffer motor fluctuations and dyskinesia despite an optimal oral regimen [47]. When patients do not exhibit a significant reduction (>30%) on the UPDRS motor subscale to a formal levodopa challenge [48], alternative diagnoses should be considered because atypical forms of parkinsonism have been shown to respond less well or not at all to surgery [49]. Although there are insufficient data to establish firm cutoffs for patient age, disease duration, or disease severity, some evidence suggests that greater benefit occurs for younger patients [50, 51] with shorter disease durations [52], and that older patients may be more prone to surgery-related hemorrhage [53, 54]. Cognitive impairment frequently accompanies advanced PD [55]. Because of the potential increased risk of stimulation-induced deterioration, the presence of dementia is usually an exclusionary criterion, especially for STN surgery, [32, 56]. Indications for pallidotomy do not differ significantly from those for stimulation but, as discussed above, certain patients who are unable or unwilling to undergo hardware placement may still be considered candidates for unilateral pallidotomy.

Emerging targets for Parkinson disease: the pedunculopontine area

Debilitating levodopa-non-responsive symptoms that include disorders of cognition, mood, gait and posture, sleep, and autonomic regulation are increasingly being recognized as major drivers of disability and decreased quality of life in patients with advanced PD [57, 58]. Over time, nearly all patients develop these impairments despite standard medical and surgical care [59]. For example, long-term longitudinal studies show that the incidence of dementia

is 50% at 10 years and 83% at 20 years. Ten years after the diagnosis of PD, approximately 50% of patients are falling frequently, and at 20 years many of these patients have suffered a fracture as a consequence of falling [55]. Because gait impairment and postural instability associated with advanced PD underlie significant mortality and morbidity, there has been a great deal of renewed interest in understanding the pathophysiology of gait [60]. This has led directly to the examination of a novel target for DBS in the area of the pontomesencephalic junction [61].

The anatomical locations of midbrain locomotor regions were first identified in pioneering work in cats, and in bipedal animals these areas are thought to correspond to the region of the cholinergic pedunculopontine nucleus complex [62, 63]. A number of groups have now begun to implant electrodes into this region in humans (Figure 6.1) with the hope of ameliorating some of the gait disturbances associated with advanced PD [64–67]. A paper by Moro et al. [68] documents sustained reduction in falls and freezing through the first postoperative year in six patients with advanced PD who received a unilateral pedunculopontine stimulator (Table 6.1). Approximately 100 patients worldwide have now undergone similar therapy in open trials. Long-term controlled studies will be required to address a number of outstanding issues including the precise target of electrical stimulation within the pedunculopontine region, selection of best responders, and durability of the intervention. A number of other novel neuromodulatory targets have been investigated in patients with PD, including the motor cortex [69], dorsal spinal columns [70], and cerebellum [71], with limited improvements in motor behavior.

Experimental surgery for Parkinson disease: some potential future directions

Major innovations in surgery for PD are aimed at slowing or stopping ongoing neurodegeneration. So far, clear evidence for any form of neuroprotection in humans with PD has been elusive, but many promising strategies are being pursued. For example, early clinical trials that directly infused the putative neurotrophic peptide glial-derived neurotrophic factor (GDNF) were quite promising [72, 73], but fell short when tested in a double-blind fashion [74, 75]. Improvements in catheter design and distribution along with better formulation of the delivered compounds may yet yield true neuroprotective benefits. A number of interesting preclinical studies using adeno-associated virus to deliver glutamic acid *decarboxylase* genes to the subthalamic nucleus have shown reversal of parkinsonian behavior in rodent and primate models [76, 77]. In preliminary clinical trials, this approach has been shown to be safe and modestly efficacious compared with sham controls [78, 79]. Other experiments using gene therapy to modulate dopamine metabolism with either single or multiple genes are also being examined [80, 81]. Another study of neurotrophic gene therapy utilizing an AAV2-neurturin construct with double-blind delivery to the putamen and substantia nigra was well tolerated, but did not yield significant clinical benefit [82]. In other gene therapy-related work, it is possible to combine gene therapy with light stimulation using the technique of optogenetics [83–85]. In these experiments, neurons are transfected with light-sensitive channels that allow movement of positively or negatively charged ions across the plasma membrane causing excitation or inhibition of neural elements [86]. This technique has so far only been used in preclinical experiments on animals [87], but it is possible that the technology may be adapted for humans, where the

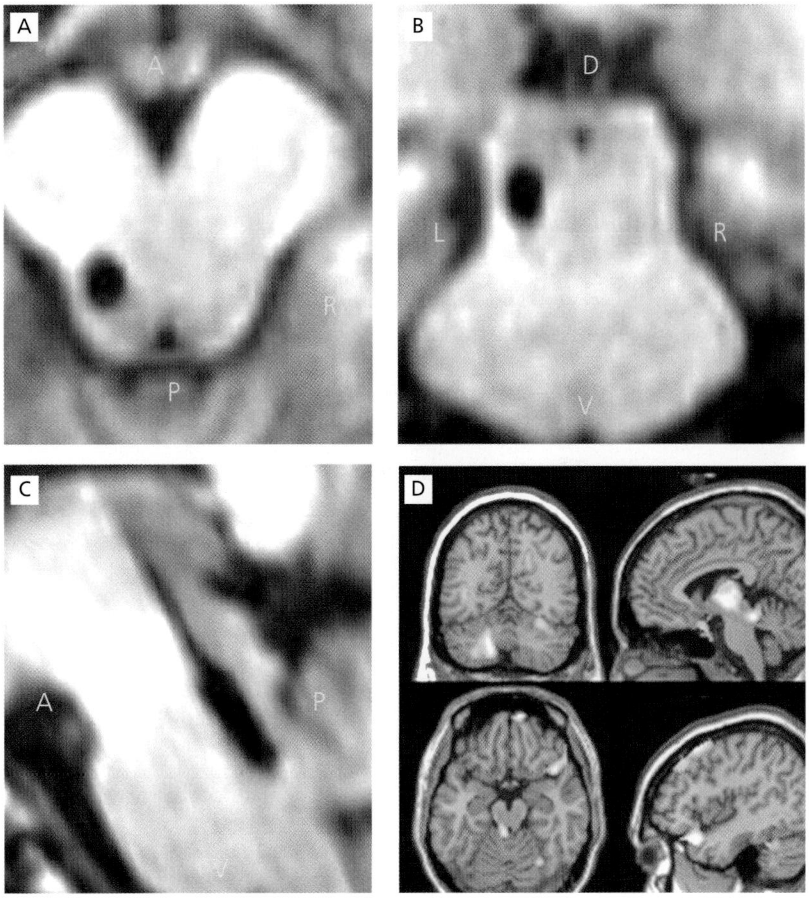

Figure 6.1 T1-weighted axial (A), coronal (B), and sagittal (C) MR images showing the location of a deep brain electrode within the pedunculopontine nucleus complex (PPN) in a patient with postural instability associated with advanced PD. The small red dot in each panel marks the location of the active electrode. A, anterior; P, posterior; L, left; R, right; D, dorsal; V, ventral. (Source: Moro et al. [68]. Reproduced with permission of Oxford University Press.) (D) Areas of increased blood flow during PPN DBS as measured by [^{15}O] H$_2$O uptake on PET: bilaterally in the thalamus and cerebellum and in the ipsilateral ventral midbrain around the PPN. At the cortical level, significant clusters were found in the contralateral dorsolateral prefrontal cortex (BA 8/9 and 10), caudal anterior cingulate cortex extending to the posterior cingulate cortex (BA 24 and BA 23/30), the orbitofrontal cortex (BA 11), the superior and middle temporal gyrus (BA 38 and 21), and ipsilateral occipital cortex (BA 19) (Source: Ballanger et al. 2009 [89]. Reproduced with permission of John Wiley & Sons, Inc.)

Table 6.1 Effects of unilateral PPN DBS on UPDRS part II subscores (falling and freezing) after 3 and 12 months of stimulation.

Patient no.	UPDRS-II item 13 (falling)			UPDRS-II item 14 (freezing)		
	Pre-op	3 months	12 months	Pre-op	3 months	12 months
1	4	0	0	3	0	1
2	2	0	1	3	0	3
3	3	2	2	2	2	2
4	3	1	2	2	1	2
5	3	1	0	3	1	2
6	2	2	0	3	2	2
Mean	2.8	0.9	0.8	3.0	1.0	2.0
(SD)	(0.7)	(0.8)	(0.9)	(1.0)	(0.9)	(1.0)
P value*		0.04	0.02		0.04	0.10

* Compared to baseline. UPDRS, unified Parkinson disease rating scale. Adapted from Moro et al., 2010 [68].

primary advantage would be to enhance stimulation specificity by limiting off-target effects caused by the spread of electrical excitability often seen with standard DBS [88].

Summary

Several effective surgical options are currently available to treat a wide spectrum of parkinsonian symptoms. Among the most well studied interventions are deep brain stimulation and ablative lesions of the pallidum and high-frequency stimulation of the subthalamic nucleus.

These are the only two DBS targets approved by the FDA for PD. In addition to treating the motor side effects of chronic levodopa, both targets have been shown to have superior efficacy compared with standard oral medication alone in ameliorating the cardinal motor symptoms of PD. Other surgical approaches are being developed to treat dopamine-non-responsive symptoms including stimulation of the PPN to improve gait and posture. The future of surgery for PD is aimed at more than merely symptomatic therapy. Hopefully, with advances in direct infusion delivery and gene therapy, the possibility of durable neuroprotection will soon be realized.

References

1. Laitinen, L. V., Bergenheim, A. T. and Hariz, M. I. (1992) Leksell's posteroventral pallidotomy in the treatment of Parkinson's disease. *J Neurosurg* 76, 53–61.
2. Alvarez, L., Macias, R., Lopez, G., Alvarez, E., Pavon, N., Rodriguez-Oroz, M. C., Juncos, J. L., Maragoto, C., Guridi, J., Litvan, I., Tolosa, E. S., Koller, W., Vitek, J., DeLong, M. R. and Obeso, J. A. (2005) Bilateral subthalamotomy in Parkinson's disease: initial and long-term response. *Brain* 128, 570–83.
3. Benabid, A. L., Chabardes, S., Torres, N., Piallat, B., Krack, P., Fraix, V. and Pollak, P. (2009) Functional neurosurgery for movement disorders: a historical perspective. *Prog Brain Res* 175, 379–91.
4. Marsden, C. D. and Parkes, J. D. (1976) "On-off" effects in patients with Parkinson's disease on chronic levodopa therapy. *Lancet* 1, 292–6.
5. Siegfried, J. and Lippitz, B. (1994) Bilateral chronic electrostimulation of ventroposterolateral pallidum: a new therapeutic approach for alleviating all parkinsonian symptoms. *Neurosurgery* 35, 1126–9; discussion 1129-30.
6. Benabid, A. L., Pollak, P., Gross, C., Hoffmann, D., Benazzouz, A., Gao, D. M., Laurent, A., Gentil, M. and Perret, J. (1994) Acute and long-term effects of subthalamic nucleus stimulation in Parkinson's disease. *Stereotact Funct Neurosurg* 62, 76–84.

7. Pollak, P., Benabid, A. L., Gross, C., Gao, D. M., Laurent, A., Benazzouz, A., Hoffmann, D., Gentil, M. and Perret, J. (1993) [Effects of the stimulation of the subthalamic nucleus in Parkinson disease]. *Rev Neurol (Paris)* 149, 175–6.

8. Sankar, T. and Lozano, A. M. (2011) Surgical approach to l-dopa-induced dyskinesias. *Int Rev Neurobiol* 98, 151–71.

9. Medtronic (2016) Products and Procedures. Vol. 2016. http://professional.medtronic.com/pt/neuro/dbs-md/prod/#.V9svXPkrJD8 [accessed on 30 September 2016]

10. Gross, R. E. (2008) What happened to posteroventral pallidotomy for Parkinson's disease and dystonia? *Neurotherapeutics* 5, 281–93.

11. Kleiner-Fisman, G., Fisman, D. N., Sime, E., Saint-Cyr, J. A., Lozano, A. M. and Lang, A. E. (2003) Long-term follow up of bilateral deep brain stimulation of the subthalamic nucleus in patients with advanced Parkinson disease. *J Neurosurg* 99, 489–95.

12. Krack, P., Batir, A., Van Blercom, N., Chabardes, S., Fraix, V., Ardouin, C., Koudsie, A., Limousin, P. D., Benazzouz, A., LeBas, J. F., Benabid, A. L. and Pollak, P. (2003) Five-year follow-up of bilateral stimulation of the subthalamic nucleus in advanced Parkinson's disease. *N Engl J Med* 349, 1925–34.

13. Pahwa, R., Wilkinson, S. B., Overman, J. and Lyons, K. E. (2003) Bilateral subthalamic stimulation in patients with Parkinson disease: long-term follow up. *J Neurosurg* 99, 71–7.

14. Schupbach, W. M., Chastan, N., Welter, M. L., Houeto, J. L., Mesnage, V., Bonnet, A. M., Czernecki, V., Maltete, D., Hartmann, A., Mallet, L., Pidoux, B., Dormont, D., Navarro, S., Cornu, P., Mallet, A. and Agid, Y. (2005) Stimulation of the subthalamic nucleus in Parkinson's disease: a 5 year follow up. *J Neurol Neurosurg Psychiatry* 76, 1640–4.

15. Ghika, J., Villemure, J. G., Fankhauser, H., Favre, J., Assal, G. and Ghika-Schmid, F. (1998) Efficiency and safety of bilateral contemporaneous pallidal stimulation (deep brain stimulation) in levodopa-responsive patients with Parkinson's disease with severe motor fluctuations: a 2-year follow-up review. *J Neurosurg* 89, 713–8.

16. Lyons, K. E., Wilkinson, S. B., Troster, A. I. and Pahwa, R. (2002) Long-term efficacy of globus pallidus stimulation for the treatment of Parkinson's disease. *Stereotact Funct Neurosurg* 79, 214–20.

17. Moro, E., Lozano, A. M., Pollak, P., Agid, Y., Rehncrona, S., Volkmann, J., Kulisevsky, J., Obeso, J. A., Albanese, A., Hariz, M. I., Quinn, N. P., Speelman, J. D., Benabid, A. L., Fraix, V., Mendes, A., Welter, M. L., Houeto, J. L., Cornu, P., Dormont, D., Tornqvist, A. L., Ekberg, R., Schnitzler, A., Timmermann, L., Wojtecki, L., Gironell, A., Rodriguez-Oroz, M. C., Guridi, J., Bentivoglio, A. R., Contarino, M. F., Romito, L., Scerrati, M., Janssens, M. and Lang, A. E. (2010) Long-term results of a multicenter study on subthalamic and pallidal stimulation in Parkinson's disease. *Mov Disord* 25, 578–86.

18. Rodriguez-Oroz, M. C., Obeso, J. A., Lang, A. E., Houeto, J. L., Pollak, P., Rehncrona, S., Kulisevsky, J., Albanese, A., Volkmann, J., Hariz, M. I., Quinn, N. P., Speelman, J. D., Guridi, J., Zamarbide, I., Gironell, A., Molet, J., Pascual-Sedano, B., Pidoux, B., Bonnet, A. M., Agid, Y., Xie, J., Benabid, A. L., Lozano, A. M., Saint-Cyr, J., Romito, L., Contarino, M. F., Scerrati, M., Fraix, V. and Van Blercom, N. (2005) Bilateral deep brain stimulation in Parkinson's disease: a multicentre study with 4 years follow-up. *Brain* 128, 2240–9.

19. Volkmann, J., Allert, N., Voges, J., Sturm, V., Schnitzler, A. and Freund, H. J. (2004) Long-term results of bilateral pallidal stimulation in Parkinson's disease. *Ann Neurol* 55, 871–5.

20. Deuschl, G., Schade-Brittinger, C., Krack, P., Volkmann, J., Schafer, H., Botzel, K., Daniels, C., Deutschlander, A., Dillmann, U., Eisner, W., Gruber, D., Hamel, W., Herzog, J., Hilker, R., Klebe, S., Kloss, M., Koy, J., Krause, M., Kupsch, A., Lorenz, D., Lorenzl, S., Mehdorn, H. M., Moringlane, J. R., Oertel, W., Pinsker, M. O., Reichmann, H., Reuss, A., Schneider, G. H., Schnitzler, A., Steude, U., Sturm, V., Timmermann, L., Tronnier, V., Trottenberg, T., Wojtecki, L., Wolf, E., Poewe, W. and Voges, J. (2006) A randomized trial of deep-brain stimulation for Parkinson's disease. *N Engl J Med* 355, 896–908.

21. Weaver, F. M., Follett, K., Stern, M., Hur, K., Harris, C., Marks, W. J., Jr., Rothlind, J., Sagher, O., Reda, D., Moy, C. S., Pahwa, R., Burchiel, K., Hogarth, P., Lai, E. C., Duda, J. E., Holloway, K., Samii, A., Horn, S., Bronstein, J., Stoner, G., Heemskerk, J. and Huang, G. D. (2009) Bilateral deep brain stimulation vs best medical therapy for patients with advanced Parkinson disease: a randomized controlled trial. *Jama* 301, 63–73.

22. Williams, A., Gill, S., Varma, T., Jenkinson, C., Quinn, N., Mitchell, R., Scott, R., Ives, N., Rick, C., Daniels, J., Patel, S. and Wheatley, K. (2010) Deep brain stimulation plus best medical therapy versus best medical therapy alone for advanced Parkinson's disease (PD SURG trial): a randomised, open-label trial. *Lancet Neurol* 9, 581–91.

23. Anderson, V. C., Burchiel, K. J., Hogarth, P., Favre, J. and Hammerstad, J. P. (2005) Pallidal vs subthalamic nucleus deep brain stimulation in Parkinson disease. *Arch Neurol* 62, 554–60.

24. Follett, K. A., Weaver, F. M., Stern, M., Hur, K., Harris, C. L., Luo, P., Marks, W. J., Jr., Rothlind, J., Sagher, O., Moy, C., Pahwa, R., Burchiel, K., Hogarth, P.,

Lai, E. C., Duda, J. E., Holloway, K., Samii, A., Horn, S., Bronstein, J. M., Stoner, G., Starr, P. A., Simpson, R., Baltuch, G., De Salles, A., Huang, G. D. and Reda, D. J. (2010) Pallidal versus subthalamic deep-brain stimulation for Parkinson's disease. *N Engl J Med* 362, 2077–91.

25. Guridi, J., Obeso, J. A., Rodriguez-Oroz, M. C., Lozano, A. A. and Manrique, M. (2008) L-dopa-induced dyskinesia and stereotactic surgery for Parkinson's disease. *Neurosurgery* 62, 311–23; discussion 323-5.

26. Parsons, T. D., Rogers, S. A., Braaten, A. J., Woods, S. P. and Troster, A. I. (2006) Cognitive sequelae of subthalamic nucleus deep brain stimulation in Parkinson's disease: a meta-analysis. *Lancet Neurol* 5, 578–88.

27. York, M. K., Dulay, M., Macias, A., Levin, H. S., Grossman, R., Simpson, R. and Jankovic, J. (2008) Cognitive declines following bilateral subthalamic nucleus deep brain stimulation for the treatment of Parkinson's disease. *J Neurol Neurosurg Psychiatry* 79, 789–95.

28. Zangaglia, R., Pacchetti, C., Pasotti, C., Mancini, F., Servello, D., Sinforiani, E., Cristina, S., Sassi, M. and Nappi, G. (2009) Deep brain stimulation and cognitive functions in Parkinson's disease: A three-year controlled study. *Mov Disord* 24, 1621–8.

29. Strutt, A. M., Simpson, R., Jankovic, J. and York, M. K. (2012) Changes in cognitive-emotional and physiological symptoms of depression following STN-DBS for the treatment of Parkinson's disease. *Eur J Neurol* 19, 121–7.

30. Voon, V., Krack, P., Lang, A. E., Lozano, A. M., Dujardin, K., Schupbach, M., D'Ambrosia, J., Thobois, S., Tamma, F., Herzog, J., Speelman, J. D., Samanta, J., Kubu, C., Rossignol, H., Poon, Y. Y., Saint-Cyr, J. A., Ardouin, C. and Moro, E. (2008) A multicentre study on suicide outcomes following subthalamic stimulation for Parkinson's disease. *Brain* 131, 2720–8.

31. Okun, M. S., Fernandez, H. H., Wu, S. S., Kirsch-Darrow, L., Bowers, D., Bova, F., Suelter, M., Jacobson, C. E. 4th, Wang, X., Gordon, C. W., Jr., Zeilman, P., Romrell, J., Martin, P., Ward, H., Rodriguez, R. L. and Foote, K. D. (2009) Cognition and mood in Parkinson's disease in subthalamic nucleus versus globus pallidus interna deep brain stimulation: the COMPARE trial. *Ann Neurol* 65, 586–95.

32. Saint-Cyr, J. A., Trepanier, L. L., Kumar, R., Lozano, A. M. and Lang, A. E. (2000) Neuropsychological consequences of chronic bilateral stimulation of the subthalamic nucleus in Parkinson's disease. *Brain* 123 (Pt 10), 2091–108.

33. Alkhani, A. and Lozano, A. M. (2001) Pallidotomy for parkinson disease: a review of contemporary literature. *J Neurosurg* 94, 43–9.

34. de Bie, R. M., de Haan, R. J., Schuurman, P. R., Esselink, R. A., Bosch, D. A. and Speelman, J. D. (2002) Morbidity and mortality following pallidotomy in Parkinson's disease: a systematic review. *Neurology* 58, 1008–12.

35. Hariz, M. I. and De Salles, A. A. (1997) The side-effects and complications of posteroventral pallidotomy. *Acta Neurochir Suppl* 68, 42–8.

36. Parkin, S. G., Gregory, R. P., Scott, R., Bain, P., Silburn, P., Hall, B., Boyle, R., Joint, C. and Aziz, T. Z. (2002) Unilateral and bilateral pallidotomy for idiopathic Parkinson's disease: a case series of 115 patients. *Mov Disord* 17, 682–92.

37. de Bie, R. M., de Haan, R. J., Nijssen, P. C., Rutgers, A. W., Beute, G. N., Bosch, D. A., Haaxma, R., Schmand, B., Schuurman, P. R., Staal, M. J. and Speelman, J. D. (1999) Unilateral pallidotomy in Parkinson's disease: a randomised, single-blind, multicentre trial. *Lancet* 354, 1665–9.

38. Fine, J., Duff, J., Chen, R., Chir, B., Hutchison, W., Lozano, A. M. and Lang, A. E. (2000) Long-term follow-up of unilateral pallidotomy in advanced Parkinson's disease. *N Engl J Med* 342, 1708–14.

39. Vitek, J. L., Bakay, R. A., Freeman, A., Evatt, M., Green, J., McDonald, W., Haber, M., Barnhart, H., Wahlay, N., Triche, S., Mewes, K., Chockkan, V., Zhang, J. Y. and DeLong, M. R. (2003) Randomized trial of pallidotomy versus medical therapy for Parkinson's disease. *Ann Neurol* 53, 558–69.

40. Hariz, M. I. and Bergenheim, A. T. (2001) A 10-year follow-up review of patients who underwent Leksell's posteroventral pallidotomy for Parkinson disease. *J Neurosurg* 94, 552–8.

41. Kleiner-Fisman, G., Lozano, A., Moro, E., Poon, Y. Y. and Lang, A. E. (2010) Long-term effect of unilateral pallidotomy on levodopa-induced dyskinesia. *Mov Disord* 25, 1496–8.

42. Esselink, R. A., de Bie, R. M., de Haan, R. J., Steur, E. N., Beute, G. N., Portman, A. T., Schuurman, P. R., Bosch, D. A. and Speelman, J. D. (2006) Unilateral pallidotomy versus bilateral subthalamic nucleus stimulation in Parkinson's disease: one year follow-up of a randomised observer-blind multi centre trial. *Acta Neurochir (Wien)* 148, 1247–55; discussion 1255.

43. Esselink, R. A., de Bie, R. M., de Haan, R. J., Lenders, M. W., Nijssen, P. C., van Laar, T., Schuurman, P. R., Bosch, D. A. and Speelman, J. D. (2009) Long-term superiority of subthalamic nucleus stimulation over pallidotomy in Parkinson disease. *Neurology* 73, 151–3.

44. Oh, M. Y., Hodaie, M., Kim, S. H., Alkhani, A., Lang, A. E. and Lozano, A. M. (2001) Deep brain stimulator electrodes used for lesioning: proof of principle. *Neurosurgery* 49, 363-7; discussion 367–9.

45. Charles, P. D., Van Blercom, N., Krack, P., Lee, S. L., Xie, J., Besson, G., Benabid, A. L. and Pollak, P. (2002) Predictors of effective bilateral subthalamic nucleus stimulation for PD. *Neurology* 59, 932–4.

46. Kleiner-Fisman, G., Herzog, J., Fisman, D. N., Tamma, F., Lyons, K. E., Pahwa, R., Lang, A. E. and Deuschl, G. (2006) Subthalamic nucleus deep brain stimulation: summary and meta-analysis of outcomes. *Mov Disord* 21 Suppl 14, S290–304.

47. Follett, K. A. (2004) Comparison of pallidal and subthalamic deep brain stimulation for the treatment of levodopa-induced dyskinesias. *Neurosurg Focus* 17, E3.

48. Welter, M. L., Houeto, J. L., Tezenas du Montcel, S., Mesnage, V., Bonnet, A. M., Pillon, B., Arnulf, I., Pidoux, B., Dormont, D., Cornu, P. and Agid, Y. (2002) Clinical predictive factors of subthalamic stimulation in Parkinson's disease. *Brain* 125, 575–83.

49. Shih, L. C. and Tarsy, D. (2007) Deep brain stimulation for the treatment of atypical parkinsonism. *Mov Disord* 22, 2149–55.

50. Derost, P. P., Ouchchane, L., Morand, D., Ulla, M., Llorca, P. M., Barget, M., Debilly, B., Lemaire, J. J. and Durif, F. (2007) Is DBS-STN appropriate to treat severe Parkinson disease in an elderly population? *Neurology* 68, 1345–55.

51. Ory-Magne, F., Brefel-Courbon, C., Simonetta-Moreau, M., Fabre, N., Lotterie, J. A., Chaynes, P., Berry, I., Lazorthes, Y. and Rascol, O. (2007) Does ageing influence deep brain stimulation outcomes in Parkinson's disease? *Mov Disord* 22, 1457–63.

52. Schupbach, W. M., Maltete, D., Houeto, J. L., du Montcel, S. T., Mallet, L., Welter, M. L., Gargiulo, M., Behar, C., Bonnet, A. M., Czernecki, V., Pidoux, B., Navarro, S., Dormont, D., Cornu, P. and Agid, Y. (2007) Neurosurgery at an earlier stage of Parkinson disease: a randomized, controlled trial. *Neurology* 68, 267–71.

53. Sansur, C. A., Frysinger, R. C., Pouratian, N., Fu, K. M., Bittl, M., Oskouian, R. J., Laws, E. R. and Elias, W. J. (2007) Incidence of symptomatic hemorrhage after stereotactic electrode placement. *J Neurosurg* 107, 998–1003.

54. Zrinzo, L., Foltynie, T., Limousin, P. and Hariz, M. I. (2011) Reducing hemorrhagic complications in functional neurosurgery: a large case series and systematic literature review. *J Neurosurg*.

55. Hely, M. A., Reid, W. G., Adena, M. A., Halliday, G. M. and Morris, J. G. (2008) The Sydney multicenter study of Parkinson's disease: the inevitability of dementia at 20 years. *Mov Disord* 23, 837–44.

56. Aybek, S., Gronchi-Perrin, A., Berney, A., Chiuve, S. C., Villemure, J. G., Burkhard, P. R. and Vingerhoets, F. J. (2007) Long-term cognitive profile and incidence of dementia after STN-DBS in Parkinson's disease. *Mov Disord* 22, 974–81.

57. Aarsland, D., Marsh, L. and Schrag, A. (2009) Neuropsychiatric symptoms in Parkinson's disease. *Mov Disord* 24, 2175–86.

58. Soh, S. E., Morris, M. E. and McGinley, J. L. (2011) Determinants of health-related quality of life in Parkinson's disease: a systematic review. *Parkinsonism Relat Disord* 17, 1–9.

59. Merola, A., Zibetti, M., Angrisano, S., Rizzi, L., Ricchi, V., Artusi, C. A., Lanotte, M., Rizzone, M. G. and Lopiano, L. (2011) Parkinson's disease progression at 30 years: a study of subthalamic deep brain-stimulated patients. *Brain* 134, 2074–84.

60. Morris, M. E., Iansek, R. and Galna, B. (2008) Gait festination and freezing in Parkinson's disease: pathogenesis and rehabilitation. *Mov Disord* 23 Suppl 2, S451–60.

61. Tierney, T. S., Sankar, T. and Lozano, A. M. (2011) Deep brain stimulation emerging indications. *Prog Brain Res* 194C, 83–95.

62. Karachi, C., Grabli, D., Bernard, F. A., Tande, D., Wattiez, N., Belaid, H., Bardinet, E., Prigent, A., Nothacker, H. P., Hunot, S., Hartmann, A., Lehericy, S., Hirsch, E. C. and Francois, C. (2010) Cholinergic mesencephalic neurons are involved in gait and postural disorders in Parkinson disease. *J Clin Invest* 120, 2745–54.

63. Pahapill, P. A. and Lozano, A. M. (2000) The pedunculopontine nucleus and Parkinson's disease. *Brain* 123 (Pt 9), 1767–83.

64. Ferraye, M. U., Debu, B., Fraix, V., Goetz, L., Ardouin, C., Yelnik, J., Henry-Lagrange, C., Seigneuret, E., Piallat, B., Krack, P., Le Bas, J. F., Benabid, A. L., Chabardes, S. and Pollak, P. (2010) Effects of pedunculopontine nucleus area stimulation on gait disorders in Parkinson's disease. *Brain* 133, 205–14.

65. Mazzone, P., Sposato, S., Insola, A., Dilazzaro, V. and Scarnati, E. (2008) Stereotactic surgery of nucleus tegmenti pedunculopontine [corrected]. *Br J Neurosurg* 22 Suppl 1, S33–40.

66. Pereira, E. A., Muthusamy, K. A., De Pennington, N., Joint, C. A. and Aziz, T. Z. (2008) Deep brain stimulation of the pedunculopontine nucleus in Parkinson's disease. Preliminary experience at Oxford. *Br J Neurosurg* 22 Suppl 1, S41–4.

67. Stefani, A., Lozano, A. M., Peppe, A., Stanzione, P., Galati, S., Tropepi, D., Pierantozzi, M., Brusa, L., Scarnati, E. and Mazzone, P. (2007) Bilateral deep brain stimulation of the pedunculopontine and subthalamic nuclei in severe Parkinson's disease. *Brain* 130, 1596–607.

68. Moro, E., Hamani, C., Poon, Y. Y., Al-Khairallah, T., Dostrovsky, J. O., Hutchison, W. D. and Lozano, A. M. (2010) Unilateral pedunculopontine stimulation improves falls in Parkinson's disease. *Brain* 133, 215–24.

69. Moro, E., Schwalb, J. M., Piboolnurak, P., Poon, Y. Y., Hamani, C., Hung, S. W., Arenovich, T., Lang, A. E., Chen, R. and Lozano, A. M. (2011) Unilateral subdural motor cortex stimulation improves essential tremor but not Parkinson's disease. *Brain* 134, 2096–105.

70. Thevathasan, W., Mazzone, P., Jha, A., Djamshidian, A., Dileone, M., Di Lazzaro, V. and Brown, P. (2010) Spinal cord stimulation failed to relieve akinesia or restore locomotion in Parkinson disease. *Neurology* 74, 1325–7.

71. Ni, Z., Pinto, A. D., Lang, A. E. and Chen, R. (2010) Involvement of the cerebellothalamocortical pathway in Parkinson disease. *Ann Neurol* 68, 816–24.

72. Gill, S. S., Patel, N. K., Hotton, G. R., O'Sullivan, K., McCarter, R., Bunnage, M., Brooks, D. J., Svendsen, C. N. and Heywood, P. (2003) Direct brain infusion of glial cell line-derived neurotrophic factor in Parkinson disease. *Nat Med* 9, 589–95.

73. Slevin, J. T., Gerhardt, G. A., Smith, C. D., Gash, D. M., Kryscio, R. and Young, B. (2005) Improvement of bilateral motor functions in patients with Parkinson disease through the unilateral intraputaminal infusion of glial cell line-derived neurotrophic factor. *J Neurosurg* 102, 216–22.

74. Lang, A. E., Langston, J. W., Stoessl, A. J., Brodsky, M., Brooks, D. J., Dhawan, V., Elias, W. J., Lozano, A. M., Moro, E., Nutt, J. G., Stacy, M., Turner, D. and Wooten, G. F. (2006) GDNF in treatment of Parkinson's disease: response to editorial. *Lancet Neurol* 5, 200–2.

75. Nutt, J. G., Burchiel, K. J., Comella, C. L., Jankovic, J., Lang, A. E., Laws, E. R., Jr., Lozano, A. M., Penn, R. D., Simpson, R. K., Jr., Stacy, M. and Wooten, G. F. (2003) Randomized, double-blind trial of glial cell line-derived neurotrophic factor (GDNF) in PD. *Neurology* 60, 69–73.

76. During, M. J., Kaplitt, M. G., Stern, M. B. and Eidelberg, D. (2001) Subthalamic GAD gene transfer in Parkinson disease patients who are candidates for deep brain stimulation. *Hum Gene Ther* 12, 1589–91.

77. Emborg, M. E., Carbon, M., Holden, J. E., During, M. J., Ma, Y., Tang, C., Moirano, J., Fitzsimons, H., Roitberg, B. Z., Tuccar, E., Roberts, A., Kaplitt, M. G. and Eidelberg, D. (2007) Subthalamic glutamic acid decarboxylase gene therapy: changes in motor function and cortical metabolism. *J Cereb Blood Flow Metab* 27, 501–9.

78. Kaplitt, M. G., Feigin, A., Tang, C., Fitzsimons, H. L., Mattis, P., Lawlor, P. A., Bland, R. J., Young, D., Strybing, K., Eidelberg, D. and During, M. J. (2007) Safety and tolerability of gene therapy with an adeno-associated virus (AAV) borne GAD gene for Parkinson's disease: an open label, phase I trial. *Lancet* 369, 2097–105.

79. LeWitt, P. A., Rezai, A. R., Leehey, M. A., Ojemann, S. G., Flaherty, A. W., Eskandar, E. N., Kostyk, S. K., Thomas, K., Sarkar, A., Siddiqui, M. S., Tatter, S. B., Schwalb, J. M., Poston, K. L., Henderson, J. M., Kurlan, R. M., Richard, I. H., Van Meter, L., Sapan, C. V., During, M. J., Kaplitt, M. G. and Feigin, A. (2011) AAV2-GAD gene therapy for advanced Parkinson's disease: a double-blind, sham-surgery controlled, randomised trial. *Lancet Neurol* 10, 309–19.

80. Christine, C. W., Starr, P. A., Larson, P. S., Eberling, J. L., Jagust, W. J., Hawkins, R. A., VanBrocklin, H. F., Wright, J. F., Bankiewicz, K. S. and Aminoff, M. J. (2009) Safety and tolerability of putaminal AADC gene therapy for Parkinson disease. *Neurology* 73, 1662–9.

81. Eberling, J. L., Jagust, W. J., Christine, C. W., Starr, P., Larson, P., Bankiewicz, K. S. and Aminoff, M. J. (2008) Results from a phase I safety trial of hAADC gene therapy for Parkinson disease. *Neurology* 70, 1980–3.

82. Warren Olanow, C., Bartus, R. T., Baumann, T. L., Factor, S., Boulis, N., Stacy, M., Turner, D. A., Marks, W., Larson, P., Starr, P. A., Jankovic, J., Simpson, R., Watts, R., Guthrie, B., Poston, K., Henderson, J.M., Stern, M., Baltuch, G., Goetz, C. G., Herzog, C., Kordower, J. H., Alterman, R., Lozano, A. M., Lang, A. E. (2015) Gene delivery of neurturin to putamen and substantia nigra in Parkinson disease: A double-blind, randomized, controlled trial. *Ann Neurol* 78, 248–57.

83. Boyden, E. S., Zhang, F., Bamberg, E., Nagel, G. and Deisseroth, K. (2005) Millisecond-timescale, genetically targeted optical control of neural activity. *Nat Neurosci* 8, 1263–8.

84. Nagel, G., Ollig, D., Fuhrmann, M., Kateriya, S., Musti, A. M., Bamberg, E. and Hegemann, P. (2002) Channelrhodopsin-1: a light-gated proton channel in green algae. *Science* 296, 2395–8.

85. Zhang, F., Gradinaru, V., Adamantidis, A. R., Durand, R., Airan, R. D., de Lecea, L. and Deisseroth, K. (2010) Optogenetic interrogation of neural circuits: technology for probing mammalian brain structures. *Nat Protoc* 5, 439–56.

86. Han, X. and Boyden, E. S. (2007) Multiple-color optical activation, silencing, and desynchronization of neural activity, with single-spike temporal resolution. *PLoS One* 2, e299.

87. Aravanis, A. M., Wang, L. P., Zhang, F., Meltzer, L. A., Mogri, M. Z., Schneider, M. B. and Deisseroth, K. (2007) An optical neural interface: in vivo control of rodent motor cortex with integrated fiberoptic and optogenetic technology. *J Neural Eng* 4, S143–56.

88. Gradinaru, V., Mogri, M., Thompson, K. R., Henderson, J. M. and Deisseroth, K. (2009) Optical deconstruction of parkinsonian neural circuitry. *Science* 324, 354–9.

89. Ballanger, B., Lozano, A. M., Moro, E., van Eimeren, T., Hamani, C., Chen, R., Cilia, R., Houle, S., Poon, Y. Y., Lang, A. E., Strafella, A. P. (2009) Cerebral blood flow changes induced by pedunculopontine nucleus stimulation in patients with advanced Parkinson's disease: A [^{15}O] H$_2$O PET study. *Hum Brain Mapp* 30, 3901–9.

CHAPTER 7

Multiple System Atrophy: Clinical, Genetics, and Neuropathology

Lucia V. Schottlaender[1], Anna Sailer[1], Zeshan Ahmed[1], Dennis W. Dickson[2], Henry Houlden[1], and Owen A. Ross[2]

[1]Department of Molecular Neuroscience, UCL Institute of Neurology, London, UK
[2]Department of Neuroscience, Mayo Clinic, Jacksonville, Florida, USA

History and definition

The term multiple system atrophy (MSA) was first introduced by Graham and Oppenheimer in 1969 [1], joining together three diseases that until then had been considered distinct entities: olivopontocerebellar atrophy [2], Shy–Drager syndrome [3], and striatonigral degeneration [4]. In 1989, the clinical phenotype of MSA was unified and the first clinical diagnostic criteria proposed [5] (Tables 7.1 and 7.2). In the same year, Papp and Lantos permanently consolidated these three disorders after discovering glial argyrophilic cytoplasmic inclusions (GCIs) as the pathological hallmark of the disease [6]. In 1999 the main component of GCIs was identified as misfolded, hyperphosphorylated, fibrillar α-synuclein [7]. These findings have classified MSA as an α-synucleinopathy, neuropathologically linked to other synucleinopathies such as idiopathic Parkinson disease (iPD) and dementia with Lewy bodies (DLB) [8–10].

MSA is a sporadic progressive neurodegenerative disease and a distinct clinicopathological entity. Clinically, MSA is characterized by a variable combination of autonomic dysfunction, parkinsonism (P), and cerebellar ataxia and pyramidal signs (C), and may change its clinical emphasis as it evolves [5]. Patients can be designated MSA-P or MSA-C according to the predominant parkinsonian or cerebellar clinical feature [11]. Often the designation MSA-mixed is used when cerebellar and parkinsonian signs equally occur at presentation. Pathologically, MSA consists of positive α-synuclein GCIs in the basal ganglia, cerebellum, pons, inferior olivary nuclei, and spinal cord accompanied by neurodegeneration and gliosis [8].

Epidemiology

Although MSA is a rare disease it may account for up to 10% of cases with primary parkinsonism [12, 13] and up to 34% of these MSA cases may remain misdiagnosed until autopsy [13]. MSA is often misdiagnosed as PD with autonomic features or as progressive supranuclear palsy (PSP) or corticobasal degeneration (CBD). The first and longest up-to-date prospective study on the incidence of MSA was conducted in Minnesota and lasted for 15 years. An incidence of 0.6 cases per 100,000 person-years for the overall population and of 3 per 100,000 when considering the population above 50 years of age was reported [14]. More recently, age-adjusted incidence rates of 0.11/100,000 for MSA in a population-based study in Russia [15] and 2.4/100,000 for MSA-P in a population-based study in Sweden were published [16]. Age-adjusted prevalence was 1.86/100,000 and 4.4/100,000 in Gironde, France [17, 18], and London, UK [19], respectively. Other studies may show similar or even higher prevalence rates but are mostly focused on PD and only mention incidental MSA or atypical parkinsonism (AiPD) cases [20].

Regarding gender distribution, it was historically believed that males were more frequently affected than women (male : female): 1.9:1 [21], 2:1 [5, 16, 17, 19, 22], 1.2:1 [13], 1.3:1 [15, 23, 24] and 1.4:1 [25]; however, some groups found that MSA was more frequent in women 1:3 [19], 1:1.2 [26]. Finally, an equal gender distribution has been reported by the European MSA study group and almost equal gender distribution by the German Competence Network on PD [27, 28]. Mean age of onset is between 54 and 67 years (range 31–85) [17, 18, 24, 26–30]. Mean age at diagnosis has been estimated in two prospective studies at 62 and 72 years [15, 16]. The mean age at death was 60.3 years (range 37–84 years) in a meta-analysis including 203 pathologically proven cases [24], and 64.7 (±9 years) in a retrospective series of 83 definite MSA cases [26].

The two types of MSA, MSA-P and MSA-C, show a different distribution within populations. The final analysis of the European MSA Registry that included 19 centers in 10 countries (nine European and Israel) reported 68% MSA-P and 32% MSA-C [28]. The North American MSA study group determined a similar clinical predominance of 60% MSA-P and 13% MSA-C. The remaining 27% was classified as mixed type [31]. Two retrospective studies in Japan have reported frequencies for MSA-P of 33% and 16% and MSA-C 67% and 84% [23, 25]. Surprisingly, in a large Korean retrospective series, the predominant variant of MSA was similar to that of western populations: 55% of cases were classified as MSA-P, 28% as MSA-C, and 17% as mixed type [30].

Spectrum of clinical phenotype

The core features of MSA are parkinsonism, cerebellar syndrome, and autonomic dysfunction; pyramidal signs are also not uncommon in patients with MSA.

Neurodegeneration, First Edition. Edited by Anthony Schapira, Zbigniew Wszolek, Ted M. Dawson and Nicholas Wood.
© 2017 John Wiley & Sons, Ltd. Published 2017 by John Wiley & Sons, Ltd.

Table 7.1 Diagnostic criteria of MSA.

Definite MSA	Neuropathological findings of widespread and abundant CNS α-synuclein-positive glial cytoplasmic inclusions in association with neurodegenerative changes in striatonigral or olivopontocerebellar structures
Probable MSA	A sporadic, progressive, adult (>30y) onset disease characterized by: • Autonomic failure involving urinary incontinence (inability to control the release of urine from the bladder, with erectile dysfunction in males) or an orthostatic decrease of blood pressure within 3 minutes of standing from a previous 3 minute interval in the recumbent position by at least 30 mmHg systolic or 15 mmHg diastolic and • Poorly levodopa responsive parkinsonism (bradykinesia with rigidity, tremor, or postural instability) or • A cerebellar syndrome (gait ataxia with cerebellar dysarthria, limb ataxia, or cerebellar oculomotor dysfunction)

Possible MSA	A sporadic, progressive, adult (>30y) onset disease characterized by:
	• Parkinsonism (bradykinesia with rigidity, tremor, or postural instability) or
	• A cerebellar syndrome (gait ataxia with cerebellar dysarthria, limb ataxia, or cerebellar oculomotor dysfunction) and
	• At least one feature suggesting autonomic dysfunction (otherwise unexplained urinary urgency, frequency, or incomplete bladder emptying, erectile dysfunction in males, or significant orthostatic blood pressure decline that does not meet the level required in probable MSA) and
	• At least one of the following additional features:
	  – Possible MSA-P or MSA-C
	    • Babinski sign with hyperreflexia
	    • Stridor
	  – Possible MSA-P
	    • Rapidly progressive parkinsonism
	    • Poor response to levodopa
	    • Postural instability within 3 years of motor onset
	    • Gait ataxia, cerebellar dysarthria, limb ataxia, or cerebellar oculomotor dysfunction
	    • Dysphagia within 5 years of motor onset
	    • Atrophy on MRI of putamen, middle cerebellar peduncle, pons, or cerebellum
	    • Hypometabolism on FDG-PET in putamen, brainstem, or cerebellum
	  – Possible MSA-C
	    • Parkinsonism (bradykinesia and rigidity)
	    • Atrophy on MRI of putamen, middle cerebellar peduncle, or pons
	    • Hypometabolism on FDG-PET in putamen
	    • Presynaptic nigrostriatal dopaminergic denervation on SPECT or PET

Source: Gilman et al. 2008 [32]. Reproduced with permission of Wolters Kluwer Health, Inc.
FDG-PET, fluorodeoxyglucose-positron emission tomography; MRI, magnetic resonance imaging; MSA-C, MSA with cerebellar features; MSA-P, MSA with predominant parkinsonism; PET, positron emission tomography; SPECT, single photon emission computed tomography.

Table 7.2 Features supporting (red flags) and not supporting a diagnosis of MSA.

Supporting features	Non-supporting features
• Orofacial dystonia • Disproportionate antecollis • Camptocornia (severe anterior flexion of the spine) and/or Pisa syndrome (severe lateral flexion of the spine) • Contractures of hands or feet • Inspiratory sighs • Severe dysphonia • Severe dysarthria • New or increased snoring • Cold hands and feet • Pathologic laughter or crying • Jerky, myoclonic postural/action tremor	• Classic pill-rolling rest tremor • Clinically significant neuropathy • Hallucinations not induced by drugs • Onset after age 75 years • Family history of ataxia or parkinsonism • Dementia (on DSM-IV) • White matter lesions suggesting multiple sclerosis

Source: Gilman et al. 2008 [32]. Reproduced with permission of Wolters Kluwer Health, Inc.

Motor disturbances

The initial motor disturbance in 203 pathologically proven MSA cases was parkinsonism in 58% of cases and cerebellar ataxia in 29% [24].

Parkinsonism

Parkinsonism is defined by the presence of bradykinesia and rigidity, accompanied by an impairment of postural stability and tremor [13]. MSA patients often present with a predominantly akinetic–rigid form of parkinsonism. Postural instability occurs earlier and progresses more rapidly than in iPD [32]. Tremor is rarer and usually presents as an irregular postural/action tremor, often incorporating myoclonus [21, 32]. The classical pill-rolling tremor seen in PD is found in less than 10% of definite MSA cases [13, 24].

Although levodopa response is a red flag for the clinical diagnosis of MSA, efficacy of levodopa treatment has been reported in 28–65% of definite MSA cases [13, 24, 33–36]. A 51% symptom improvement due to levodopa was found in clinical MSA cases by the German Competence Network on PD [27]. In addition, deterioration of mobility after levodopa withdrawal, despite a lack of prior evident benefit, can occur in MSA [21, 33]. Unfortunately, levodopa responsiveness persists for several years in only approximately 10% of cases [21]. A trial of 1 g of levodopa (with a peripheral decarboxylase inhibitor) per day for at least 3 months (if tolerated) should be made in every MSA case before defining unresponsiveness [32]. Moreover, levodopa responsiveness should be demonstrated by objective evidence such as an improvement of 30% or more on the unified multiple system atrophy rating scale (UMSARS) [32, 37].

Dystonia

Many patients with MSA present with dystonia. The most common sign of dystonia is antecollis; other features seen in MSA are torticollis, focal limb dystonia, axial dystonia, and orofacial dystonia [24, 38]. Antecollis is present in up to 12% of pathologically confirmed cases [13, 24, 39]. It is characterized by a forward flexion and anterior shift of the neck without weakness of residual neck extension [40].

Cerebellar syndrome

Progressive gait ataxia is the most common cerebellar feature of MSA. It is often accompanied by cerebellar dysarthria and oculomotor dysfunction; limb ataxia is less prominent [32].

Oculomotor dysfunction

Early oculomotor abnormalities in MSA may include square-wave jerks, jerky pursuit, and dysmetric saccades. Other eye signs are nystagmus and limitation of up- and down-gaze [13, 21, 32]. Moreover, excessive square-wave jerks, mild hypometria of saccades, impaired vestibulo-ocular reflex, and spontaneous or positioning downbeat nystagmus have been suggested as diagnostic clues of MSA [41]. In contrast, the presence of slow saccades or moderate to severe gaze restriction suggests a diagnosis other than MSA, usually PSP [41].

Dysarthria

Dysarthria is present in most cases of MSA and denotes a combination of hypophonic, monotonous parkinsonian dysarthria together with cerebellar quivering, high-pitched, strained, slurred and scanning speech [13, 21].

Pyramidal signs

Pyramidal signs are also a frequent feature of MSA. An extensor plantar response can be seen in up to 41% of cases and hyperreflexia in 46% [21, 28]. However, these findings are usually isolated, spasticity is present only in 10% of cases, and paresis is unreported [21, 24].

Non-motor symptoms

Non-motor symptoms (urinary problems, erectile dysfunction [ED], syncope, REM sleep behavior disorder, stridor, fecal incontinence, constipation, and sudomotor disturbances) occurring before any motor disorder are present in 31% of MSA cases [42]. Gastrointestinal symptoms, pain, urinary symptoms, orthostatic hypotension (OH), sleep disturbances, fatigue, attention and memory impairment, and psychiatric disorders were present in more than half of MSA cases in an observational multicenter study in Italy [43].

Autonomic dysfunction

Symptomatic dysautonomia was present in 99% of patients in the final analysis of the European MSA Registry, and autonomic dysfunction was the most frequent feature of MSA [26]. Autonomic failure typically comprises urogenital dysfunction and orthostatic hypotension [44]. MSA patients can present with syncope, micturition dysfunction (urinary urge incontinence, urgency, retention, hesitancy, double micturition, persistent daytime frequency, nocturia), fecal incontinence, and ED [13, 21]. Importantly, MSA usually begins with bladder dysfunction in females, and with ED in males [45]. Although early ED is nearly universal in men with MSA, it is an unspecific sign [46]. The most common gastrointestinal symptom seen in MSA is constipation, which can be severe. Fecal incontinence can also occur [42]. In addition, skin vasomotor disturbances are present in MSA, and anhidrosis is a frequent finding [47].

Sensory problems

Sensory symptoms and signs are rare and unspecific. Moreover, it is difficult to separate them from comorbidities in wheelchair-bound and bedridden patients [21].

Dysphagia

Dysphagia is a frequent feature in MSA patients and accounts for high morbidity [13]. Some degree of dysphagia has been recently reported in a prospective cohort in France in 64.1% of MSA cases [48]. Severe dysphagia was found in 32% of cases in a post mortem study [26].

Respiratory and sleep problems

Obstructive and central sleep apnea and laryngeal stridor are some of the breathing problems that affect MSA patients. Stridor occurs in a large proportion of MSA patients [49]. Importantly, obstructive sleep apnea can also cause sudden death [21, 42]. Nearly all patients with MSA have some form of sleep disruption. REM sleep behavior disorder (RBD) represents the most common clinical and polysomnographic finding in MSA [49]. RBD-related symptoms and neurophysiologic features are qualitatively similar in MSA and iPD [50]. Other sleep disorders in MSA are sleep apnea, excessive daytime sleepiness, insomnia, and restless leg syndrome [28, 51].

Cognitive problems and psychiatric disturbances

Cognitive impairment has been largely considered unrelated to MSA and the diagnostic criteria regard dementia as a non-supportive feature [32]. However, a prospective cohort of 372 patients with MSA showed a 20% impairment in the Mattis Dementia Rating Scale and 32% in the Frontal Assessment Battery [52]. Further, MSA-P patients seem to show more severe and widespread cognitive dysfunctions than MSA-C patients [53]. Depression and anxiety are present in MSA in approximately 40% of cases [28, 54].

Olfaction

Mild hyposmia was found in clinical MSA cases [55–58], but a retrospective analysis of 4 definite MSA cases showed normal olfaction in all of them [59]. If this finding was to be confirmed and replicated it could potentially help in differentiating MSA from iPD.

Apraxia

It has been thought for years that apraxia was not a feature of MSA [60, 61]. However, there is a recent report suggesting presence of ideomotor and ideational apraxia in MSA, and to a higher degree than in iPD [62]. Also, apraxia of eye lid opening with blepharospasm has been observed in Korea [63].

Pathology/pathophysiology specific to the disease

Pathology

Pathologically, depending on the anatomic brain regions of predominant neuronal loss, MSA is classified into two variants: olivopontocerebellar atrophy (OPCA) and striatonigral degeneration (SND), which correspond to the clinical subtypes of MSA-C and MSA-P respectively. Macroscopically, the overall weight of an MSA brain is usually not altered. Atrophy of the cerebellum, middle cerebellar peduncle, and pontine base is seen in OPCA cases and atrophy and dark discoloration of the putamen, more pronounced posteriorly, are seen in SND cases [64]. Histopathologically, neuronal loss, gliosis, myelin pallor, and axonal degeneration are consistent findings in MSA (Figure 7.1). Neuronal loss is more severe in the substantia nigra, dorsolateral zone of the caudal putamen, locus

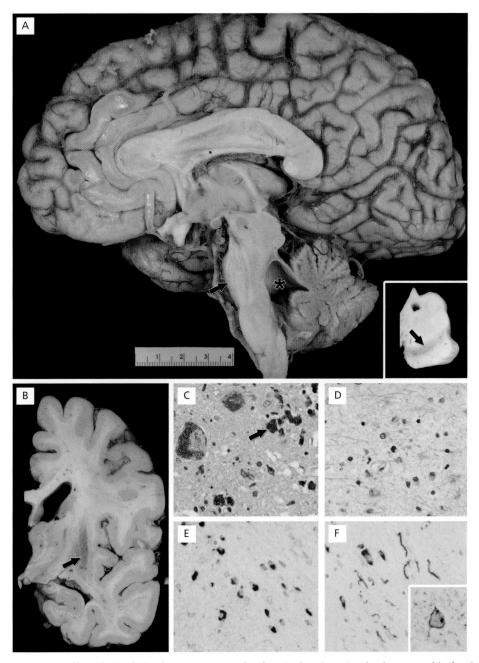

Figure 7.1 (A) Macroscopic image of hemi-brain of MSA showing severe atrophy of pontine base (arrow) with enlargement of the fourth ventricle (asterisk), but unremarkable supratentorial structures. Inset lower right shows a transverse section of midbrain with severe neuromelanin pigment loss in the substantia nigra (arrow). (B) Coronal section of brain at the level of the mammillothalamic tract shows brown discoloration and atrophy (arrow) of the posterior putamen. (C) Hematoxylin & eosin stained section of substantia nigra shows neuronal loss with neuromelanin pigment-laden macrophages (arrow). (D) Hematoxylin & eosin stained section of cerebellar white matter shows severe myelinated fiber loss and gliosis. (E) Immunohistochemistry for α-synuclein shows many glial cytoplasmic inclusions (GCIs) in the pontine base. (F) Immunohistochemistry for α-synuclein shows GCIs as well as neuronal thread-like processes in the pontine base. Inset shows a neuronal cytoplasmic inclusion in the inferior olivary nucleus. All images are from a 71-year-old African American man with MSA. All microscopic images are originally 400×.

coeruleus, vermis, cerebellar hemisphere, inferior olivary nucleus, intermediolateral cell column, and Onuf's nucleus [24, 65]. In addition, neuronal loss is also present in the motor and supplementary motor cortex of MSA brains [66, 67]. White matter tracts associated with striatonigral and olivopontocerebellar regions, such as the external capsule, striato-pallidal fibers, transverse pontine fibers, and cerebellar white matter, have a significant reduction in myelin staining [6, 64]. Moreover, reactive astrocytes [68] and activated microglia are common and important histological findings, and even the degree of astrogliosis has been found to parallel the severity of neurodegeneration [64, 65].

The neuropathological hallmark of MSA is the presence of α-synuclein immunoreactive GCIs or Papp–Lantos inclusions (Figure 7.1) which occur in oligodendrocytes (Figure 7.2) [64].

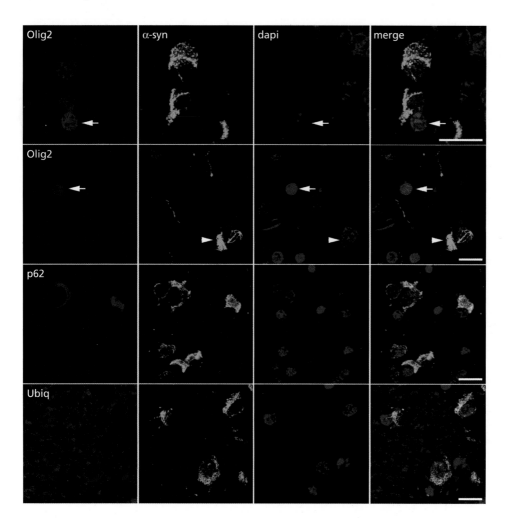

Figure 7.2 Confocal microscopy together with double immunofluorescence staining using antibodies to an oligodendroglia-specific marker (Olig2) and α-synuclein (α-syn) confirm that GCIs occur in oligodendrocytes; arrows indicate oligodendrocytes without GCIs, and arrowheads show an α-synuclein-positive neuronal inclusion, with cytoplasmic and nuclear elements. A subset of α-synuclein-positive GCIs are detected by p62 immunoreactivity, but the co-localization (yellow) of these two markers is not complete. GCIs are also weakly positive for ubiquitin-specific antibodies (Ubiq), which are not as specific and can have a low and diffuse pattern of staining. Sections were counterstained with DAPI (blue). Scale bars 15 μm [64].

The main component of GCIs is misfolded, fibrillar, hyperphosphorylated α-synuclein [9, 10]. However, a growing list of proteins such as ubiquitin (Figure 7.2) and leucine-rich repeat kinase 2 (LRRK2) have been reported in GCIs, indicating that they are a highly complex proteinaceous aggregate [64, 69]. Interestingly, the frequency of positive α-synuclein GCIs correlates significantly with the severity of neuronal loss and disease duration [65]. In addition, GCIs are rarely if ever observed in normal individuals lacking the clinical manifestations of a movement disorder [70]. Besides GCIs, there are other α-synuclein immunoreactive inclusions in MSA, found in oligodendroglial nuclei, neuronal nuclei (NNIs), neuronal cytoplasm (NCIs), and neuronal processes of some of the grey nuclei [70] (Figure 7.2). As a pathological variant of MSA, minimal change MSA has been described in two cases with unusual age of onset (<40 years) that pathologically presented with widespread GCIs and neuronal loss restricted to the substantia nigra and locus coeruleus [71]. Table 7.3 summarizes clinicopathological correlations in MSA.

Pathophysiology

Alpha-synuclein aggregates seem to play a fundamental role in MSA pathogenesis. However, the origin of the α-synuclein deposited in GCIs is not yet understood [44]. Alpha-synuclein expression is absent in oligodendrocytes of normal brains [72] and α-synuclein mRNA is not expressed in oligodendrocytes of MSA brains or

Table 7.3 Clinicopathological correlations of MSA.

Clinical features	Site of MSA pathology
• Cognitive impairment	• Unknown. (Could be frontal cortex 64])
• Akinesia, rigidity, dystonia, no response to levodopa, dysexecutive syndrome	• Striatum [65]
• Ataxia, oculomotor disorders, dysarthria	• Olivopontocerebellar system [65]
• REM sleep behavior disorder, postural instability	• Pedunculopontine nucleus [165]
• Stridor	• Nucleus ambiguus [166] (could be dystonia as well [167])
• Cardiovagal failure	• Ventrolateral nucleus ambiguus [167]
• Central sleep apnea	• Raphe and arcuate nucleus [165]
• Orthostatic hypotension	• Catecholaminergic rostral ventrolateral medulla nuclei, intermediolateral columns of the thoracolumbar cord [164, 167]
• Bladder, rectal, and sexual dysfunction	• Onuf's and inferior intermediolateral sacral nuclei, pontine micturition center [164]
• Gastrointestinal problems	• Unknown
• Dysphagia	• Unknown

normal controls [73], suggesting that its accumulation is ectopic. One hypothesis postulates that oligodendrocytes might be unable to degrade α-synuclein or even that the accumulation of α-synuclein may overcome the ability to be degraded by oligodendrocytes [44].

Early myelin alterations in MSA brains have been demonstrated by the presence of altered myelin basic protein and p25alpha (tubulin polymerization-promoting protein, TPPP) [44, 74]. p25alpha co-localizes with α-synuclein-positive GCIs and is abnormally accumulated in MSA oligodendrocytes [44, 75–78]. p25alpha is redistributed from myelin to the cell soma preceding α-synuclein aggregations, and this is accompanied by an increase in cell body size, suggesting that p25alpha might play a role in early events during the formation of GCIs [74, 78]. Most of these findings have strengthened the hypothesis that MSA is a primary oligodendrogliopathy with GCI accumulation causing oligodendroglia–myelin degeneration [74].

Microglial activation seems to play an important role in MSA pathogenesis through neuroinflammatory mechanisms; in mouse models, microgliosis is a severe and consistent feature [79]. It is unknown if such neuroinflammation is a primary event leading to cell loss or if it is a secondary response to cell loss [64]. In a mouse model of MSA with overexpression of human α-synuclein in oligodendrocytes, it was suggested that microglial activation was an early event and correlated with neuronal loss. Moreover, microglial numbers and activation were suppressed with minocycline, an important finding that if replicated could lead to neuroprotective therapeutic strategies [80].

However, there are also accumulations of fibrillar α-synuclein in neurons, and these seem to be relevant to the disease process. NNIs might also develop early in the disease process in pontine nuclei and inferior olives as shown in MSA brains [81–83]. Based on these findings and in similarities with other synucleinopathies, two coexisting degenerative processes in MSA have been proposed: GCI-linked oligodendropathy with secondary neurodegeneration, and neuronal α-synucleinopathy associated with aggregation formation [83]. Nevertheless, considering minimal change MSA, where GCIs are widespread and neuronal loss is confined to striatonigral or olivopontocerebellar systems, and given that NNIs and NCIs show no spatial correlation with GCI distribution, a primary pathological event in glial cells seems to be more likely [44, 74].

Environmental risk factors

The role of environmental risk factors in MSA pathogenesis is unclear. It has been proposed that exposure to metal dusts/fumes, plastic monomers and additives, organic solvents, and pesticides could increase the risk of MSA [84], as well as an occupational history of farming [85]. However, this has been recently questioned by two case-control studies from France and Korea [86, 87]. Although statistical significance has not been reached, smoking has been suggested to be a protective factor for MSA, as in iPD [17, 85, 88], but this has been also questioned by a case-control study in France [87]. This same study has also shown complex results concerning the role of anti-inflammatory drugs in MSA. Although the researchers did not find a significant association between risk of MSA and anti-inflammatory drug consumption, there was a strong dose–risk relation between increased aspirin intake and decreased risk of MSA [88]. The total iron levels were elevated in the basal ganglia, particularly in the substantia nigra and the striatum, of brains of confirmed MSA cases. Nevertheless, the role of this accumulation in the pathogenesis of MSA remains unknown [89–91].

Genetics

Only a handful of patients have ever reported a family history of MSA, and therefore inherited forms of the disease are rare [92–94].

Although other genetic disorders can manifest signs that overlap or mimic MSA, the role of genetic factors in susceptibility to MSA itself remains controversial. For example, genomic multiplication of the α-synuclein locus (SNCA) has been observed to cause parkinsonism, dementia, and autonomic dysfunction, consistent with the MSA phenotype [95, 96]. However, no pathogenic mutation has yet been found in MSA; direct sequencing of the exons of the SNCA gene in 11 pathologically confirmed MSA cases did not reveal any coding variants [97]. The identification of SNCA multiplication families demonstrates that overexpression of the α-synuclein protein can result in parkinsonism with autonomic dysfunction similar to MSA [95]. A patient with parkinsonism and early autonomic dysfunction who received a diagnosis of "probable MSA" was later found to harbor an SNCA duplication [98]. This case would suggest that overexpression of the SNCA gene resulting in increased levels of α-synuclein protein can lead to autonomic dysfunction and a clinical presentation of MSA. Although this hypothesis is supported by increased levels of the α-synuclein protein in MSA blood plasma, two other studies show no differential SNCA mRNA expression pattern in brain samples of patients with MSA in comparison to controls [99–101].

In 2006, work by the European MSA study group (EMSA-SG) using haplotype-tagging single nucleotide polymorphisms (SNPs) of the SNCA gene did not observe an association with risk of MSA [102]. However, Scholz and colleagues reported recessive association of an SNP (rs111931074) in the 3′ untranslated region (UTR) of the SNCA gene which increases the risk for MSA by approximately 6-fold in a subset of pathologically confirmed cases [103]. This association was independently confirmed in a second pathological MSA series [104]. A third study has also suggested that variants across the SNCA locus increase disease risk [105]; it is also worth noting that the earlier EMSA-SG study did not contain the SNP rs111931074. A study has also nominated a common variation at the MAPT (H1-haplotype) gene as a risk for MSA and it has been recently reported that glial tau pathology is also present in MSA cases, supporting a role for the aberrant expression of the MAPT gene [106, 107]. This finding supports the notion that a genetic overlap with PD/parkinsonism exists and may promote the study of other PD-related genes in MSA. Efforts for the first unbiased genome-wide association study in MSA are ongoing and require a massive collaborative approach. A number of candidate gene association studies have been performed investigating various cellular pathways including oxidative stress and inflammation; for a comprehensive review of candidate gene studies see Stemberger et al., 2011 [108].

The use of next-generation sequencing approaches (exome, whole-genome, and transcriptome) in pathology-confirmed MSA cases may help resolve the underlying genetic basis of what appears to be a complex multigenic disorder. Recently, the first whole-genome sequencing study in a proband from a Japanese family with MSA nominated recessive mutations in the COQ2 gene to be the cause of the disease phenotype [109]. A number of other small families were identified and a common substitution was associated with an increased risk of disease. The COQ2 mutations are predicted to result in a loss-of-function which subsequently leads to a COQ10 deficiency [109]. A number of follow-up studies have not yet been able to replicate the findings and therefore the nomination of COQ2 as the first causative gene for MSA remains equivocal [110–113]. Identifying genes that cause, or influence risk to, MSA will nominate new therapeutic intervention strategies and direct functional *in vitro* and *in vivo* studies.

Investigations

When a clinical diagnosis of MSA is suspected and other mimics such as a tumor and paraneoplastic phenomenon have been excluded, imaging, autonomic function tests, and uroneurology are important to help support a diagnosis of MSA [114]. Bladder function assessment often detects early abnormalities consistent with neurogenic dysfunction. Urodynamic tests frequently indicate detrusor hyperreflexia and abnormal urethral sphincter function followed later in disease progression by increased residual urine volume as detected by ultrasound. Cardiovascular autonomic dysfunction in MSA can be investigated by either a standing blood pressure test, or by tilt-table testing [8]. Imaging of cardiac innervation with single-photon emission computed tomography (SPECT) and [123I]metaiodobenzylguanidine (MIBG) and with positron emission tomography (PET) and [18F]fluorodopa has shown preserved sympathetic postganglionic neurons in MSA, in contrast to iPD [32, 115]. However, some denervation has been reported in MSA [116] and more recently severe cardiac denervation was reported in MSA using PET and [11C]hydroxyepinephrine [117]. MRI demonstration of putaminal, pontine, and middle cerebellar peduncle atrophy is helpful in both MSA-P and MSA-C [118]. Posterior putaminal hypointensity, hyperintense lateral putaminal rim, hot cross bun sign, and middle cerebellar peduncle hyperintensity on T2-weighted images can also be helpful in MSA [32] (Figure 7.3). Unfortunately, although the hot cross bun sign and the slit-like void signal are features of MSA, they are nonspecific findings [119]. Striatal or brainstem hypometabolism demonstrated by functional imaging with PET [18F]fluorodeoxyglucose can also aid diagnosis [32, 120]. In a patient with cerebellar ataxia and absence of parkinsonian features, evidence of nigrostriatal dopaminergic denervation from functional imaging may point to the diagnosis of MSA-C [121] and in a patient with parkinsonian features unaccompanied by ataxia, findings of cerebellar hypometabolism can orientate diagnosis towards MSA-P [32]. Finally, the consensus criteria have defined neuroimaging pointers that can aid MSA diagnosis in possible cases (Tables 7.1 and 7.4) [32].

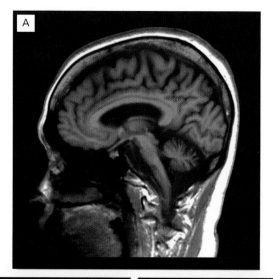

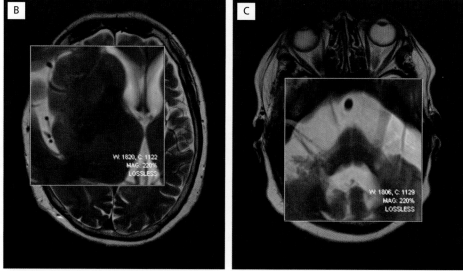

Figure 7.3 (A) Sagittal T1-weighted MRI showing generalized volume loss and marked cerebellar and brainstem atrophy. Note flattening of the pons. (B) Axial T2-weighted MRI demonstrating a right lateral hyperintense putaminal rim. (C) Axial T2-weighted MRI exemplifying a hot cross bun sign in the pons. These images are from a 61-year-old Caucasian female with MSA.

Table 7.4 Structural and functional imaging in MSA.

Structural imaging in MSA*	
• Conventional MRI at 1.5T	MSA cases may show low putamen, middle cerebellar peduncle (MCP), and brainstem signals and atrophy, and a hyperintense rim on T2 but these features, while supportive (especially vs iPD), are not present in all cases and not specific vs other AiPDs
• MRI-based quantitative assessment of atrophy of different brain structures including MRI-based planimetry and volumetry	Quantitative MR measures of atrophy of different brain structures may help to distinguish MSA from iPD (decreased MCP width in MSA; decreased putaminal volume in MSA-P) and PSP (decreased ratio of the area of the midbrain to the area of pons in patients with PSP), but neither of these specific studies has been reproduced
• Diffusion weighted imaging (DWI)	DWI looks promising for separating atypical from typical iPD showing increased diffusivity in the putamen. However, PSP patients can also show increased putaminal diffusivity. The finding of increased diffusivity in the MCP in patients with MSA vs PSP has to be reproduced by others
• Transcranial sonography (TCS)	TCS may be helpful in supporting a diagnosis of MSA as midbrain hyperechogenicity is usually absent, while 90% of iPD cases show altered nigral signal. Separation between MSA and PSP patients is suboptimal for both substantia nigra and lentiform hyperechogenicity. Importantly, at least 10% of the population have a temporal bone window insufficient for an adequate brain parenchyma sonographic analysis
Functional imaging in MSA	
• Presynaptic dopaminergic imaging	Imaging presynaptic dopaminergic function with PET or SPECT reliably separates parkinsonian from non-parkinsonian conditions but does not allow discrimination of MSA from other parkinsonian conditions
• Postsynaptic dopaminergic imaging	MSA cases show reduced putamen dopamine D2 receptor binding, whereas this is normal or elevated in iPD. However, the iPD and MSA ranges overlap and one-third of MSA cases show normal D2 availability
• FDG-PET	FDG-PET can be helpful for discriminating typical from atypical iPD, particularly when combined with computer-assisted statistical parametric mapping which increases the sensitivity relative to visual analysis from 80% to 95%. MSA cases show striatal, brainstem, and cerebellar hypometabolism while putamen metabolism is elevated and frontotemporal metabolism reduced in iPD
• Imaging cardiac sympathetic innervation	Most iPD cases show reduced myocardial sympathetic innervation with MIBG SPECT or ^{18}F-dopamine PET, whereas this is not seen in MSA or PSP; however, early iPD may show normal cardiac sympathetic innervation and MSA may show reduced cardiac sympathetic innervation

*Importantly, structural imaging was scarcely used in patients with MSA-C. It seems that signal changes at 1.5T and atrophy in different brainstem regions (especially MCP and pons) on conventional MRI and reduced brainstem volume on MR-volumetry may help to differentiate patients with MSA-C from patients with idiopathic cerebellar ataxia with extracerebellar presentation not corresponding to MSA-C.
AiPD, atypical parkinsonism; FDG-PET, fluorodeoxyglucose-positron emission tomography; iPD, idiopathic Parkinson disease; MIBG SPECT, [123I]-metaiodobenzylguanidine single photon emission computed tomography; PSP, progressive supranuclear palsy.
Source: Brooks & Seppi 2009 [119]. Reproduced with permission of John Wiley & Sons, Inc.

Diagnosis and prognosis

Diagnosis

Definite diagnosis of MSA requires pathology. However, great efforts have been made to approach an accurate diagnosis in living patients. Clinical diagnostic criteria were first proposed by Quinn in 1989 [5] and divided MSA into three categories: possible, probable, and definite. In 1998, the first consensus criteria were published and the subdivision of MSA into MSA-P and MSA-C was introduced [11, 122]. The second consensus criteria were proposed in 2008 [32]. Definite cases have pathologically confirmed CNS α-synuclein-positive GCIs with neurodegenerative changes in striatonigral or olivopontocerebellar structures. Probable MSA cases have progressive adult-onset autonomic abnormalities, poorly levodopa-responsive parkinsonism, or cerebellar ataxia, whereas possible cases have progressive adult-onset disease including parkinsonism or cerebellar ataxia and at least one feature suggesting autonomic dysfunction plus one other feature that may be a clinical or a neuroimaging abnormality (Table 7.1). In addition, the consensus conference pointed out supporting and non-supporting features useful to differentiate MSA cases from other diseases (Table 7.2) [32].

In a retrospective validation exercise on 59 MSA clinical cases, of which 51 were pathologically confirmed MSA cases and the remaining were false-positive cases diagnosed as iPD ($n = 6$), PSP ($n = 1$), and cerebrovascular disease ($n = 1$), sensitivity and positive predictive values (PPV) were estimated. In the patients' first clinic visit, sensitivity was 41% for possible cases and 18% for probable cases, and PPV was 95% and 100% respectively. Regarding the last clinic visit before pathological confirmation, sensitivity of possible cases was 92% and probable 63%, and PPV 89% and 91% [123]. These results are similar to the previous studies on the first consensus criteria and Quinn's

criteria [124, 125] and overall they show a high PPV but a low sensitivity. However, this was a retrospective study and did not consider complementary studies that are included in the latest consensus criteria. Furthermore, for research purposes, disease onset is defined as the initial presentation of any motor or autonomic features, as defined in the criteria for possible MSA, with the exception of male ED, which appears to be unspecific [32]. Finally, whereas most MSA patients present with one predominant motor feature and can be classified as MSA-P or MSA-C, this may change over time, and with disease progression considerable overlap of signs and symptoms occurs. According to the consensus statement of MSA, the classification of mixed-type MSA is not recommended [32].

Differential diagnosis

The most common diagnostic pitfall is that MSA-P patients are confused with iPD. This can account for up to 55% of misdiagnosed MSA-P. PSP and CBD are the next differentials to be considered [126]. Moreover, cases of DLB can present with prominent autonomic features and could be confused with MSA-P [127]. When approaching an MSA-C case one should always consider the dominantly inherited spinocerebellar ataxias 1, 2, 3, 6, or 7, even in the absence of a family history [32]. About 24% of cases with late-onset cerebellar ataxia will turn out to have confirmed MSA [128]. Likewise, fragile X tremor/ataxia syndrome and primary progressive multiple sclerosis need to be ruled out [126]. Furthermore, in patients with an aggressive clinical course of cerebellar syndrome, even in the absence of malaise, a paraneoplastic disorder should be investigated [32]. Finally, cerebrovascular diseases may mimic MSA and can be ruled out with imaging [126]. Although less likely, cases of amyotrophic lateral sclerosis can also be misdiagnosed as MSA [52].

Prognosis

MSA-P has a much faster disease progression when compared to iPD [31], and the UMSARS shows an annual decline in these patients [129]. Reported median survival times are from 6.2 to 10 years (range 0.5–24) [5, 13, 21–23, 29, 30] and mean disease duration from 3.2 to 7.9 years (range 1–17) [17–19, 26, 27, 86]. Median times from onset to walking aid, wheelchair requirement, and bedridden state in MSA patients are 3, 5, and 8 years respectively [23]. Early autonomic failure, older age at onset [21, 23, 29], a shorter interval from disease onset to reaching the first clinical milestone, and not being admitted to residential care have been reported as independent factors predicting shorter disease duration in a study that included 83 MSA pathologically confirmed cases [26]. In addition, a study on 230 Japanese patients found that evolution from initial symptoms to MSA within 3 years strongly predicted an aggressive course and a shorter survival [23]. When ED is included in initial symptoms, female gender appears to affect survival [21], and disease duration [26] whereas when ED is not included there is no significant association [23]. Clinical phenotype (MSA-C vs MSA-P) does not seem to influence survival [23, 44]. Early development of autonomic failure in a study that analyzed 49 consecutive patients with pathologically confirmed MSA was shown to be an independent predictor factor for rapid disease progression and shorter survival in MSA [130]. This was also confirmed by O'Sullivan and colleagues in a post mortem study [26]. Stridor onset can also play a role in predicting poor prognosis in MSA [131]. Among causes of death in MSA patients, the most common are nocturnal sudden death, sudden death (cardiopulmonary arrest), urinary infections, infectious pneumonia, aspiration pneumonia, and wasting syndrome [132–134]. It is of note that causes of death in MSA are usually secondary to disease-related events [132].

The natural history of MSA has been studied by the "Neuroprotection and Natural History in Parkinson Plus Syndromes (NNIPPS) study", reporting a 43% death rate during 3 years of follow-up. Moreover the study provides data on the progression of disability in MSA patients and is important since it provides information useful for comparison of outcome measures in present and future therapeutic trials [31].

Treatment options

In the EMSA-SG final analysis of the European MSA registry, which enrolled 437 MSA patients from 19 centers in 10 countries, the management of MSA was inconsistent and different between centers. Only 36% of patients with dysautonomia and 82% with Parkinsonism received pharmacological treatment [28].

Non-medical treatment

Physiotherapy is very important in helping patients with balance and maintaining mobility, preventing contractures, and improving functional abilities. Speech therapy is essential for communication purposes and improving swallowing, especially when patients have stridor and often need a speech aid such as a LiteWriter™. Occupational therapy ameliorates motor impairment and quality of life [135–137] and should always be offered to patients with MSA. Patients may also require psychology input as this disorder is terminal; counseling improves quality of life.

Medical and surgical treatment

Motor impairment, autonomic dysfunction, and depression are associated with a poor health-related quality of life in MSA; hence therapeutic management should target these features [135, 138]. Moreover, breathing problems can be a cause of sudden death in MSA patients and therefore they should be given appropriate consideration [134]. Although there have been isolated reports on beneficial effects of deep brain stimulation (DBS) in MSA [139, 140], harmful adverse effects [141–143] and poor and time-limited effectiveness [144] are described as well. Experts concur that DBS is currently not recommended for MSA patients [8, 135, 145]. For specific symptomatic management see Table 7.5.

Neuroprotection

Over the last 20 years, thanks to the creation of International MSA networks (European MSA study group [146], the Japanese MSA consortium, the North American MSA study group [147] and the Chinese MSA study group) a number of clinical trials have been performed. Moreover, the implementation of the UMSARS also facilitates the unification of outcome measures.

- Placebo-controlled trials with human growth hormone (GH) [148], riluzole [149, 150], minocycline [151], and estrogen [152] have failed to show significant disease-modifying properties. However, it should be noted that the trial with GH showed a trend to a smaller increase in the Unified Parkinson disease rating scale (UPDRS) and UMSARS scores over time as well as in OH and cardiovascular variability [148]. Further trials are needed to confirm these results.
- Clinical trials with fluoxetine (NCT01146548), intravenous immunoglobulin (NCT00750867), rifampicin (rifampin; NCT01287221), and rasagiline (NCT00977665) targeting neuroprotection in MSA are ongoing.
- Moreover, erythropoietin has been shown to be neuroprotective in a mouse model of MSA. Both motor deficits and striatonigral pathology were reduced [153]. Further studies are needed to consider erythropoietin as a target for clinical studies.

Future and experimental developments

Anti-inflammatory approaches

As MSA pathophysiology accounts for important inflammatory processes and a strong dose–risk relation between increased aspirin intake and decreased risk of MSA [87] has been reported, some therapeutic attempts have been made. As mentioned previously, a clinical trial with minocycline showed negative results [151]. However, results on myeloperoxidase inhibition in a transgenic mouse model showed that this inhibition could reduce motor impairment and be protective against neurodegeneration [154]. These results require replication.

Neurotransplantation

Evidence in double toxin–double lesion mouse models of MSA has raised the possibility of restoring levodopa responsiveness in MSA-P by striatal allografting [155, 156]. However, the role of host α-synuclein pathology on grafts and of pro-inflammatory responses on host striatum and its effects on functional outcomes and graft survival is currently under study [157].

Mesenchymal autologous stem cell therapy

An open and unblinded study that consecutively injected intra-arterial and intravenous autologous mesenchymal stem cells in 29 MSA patients showed feasibility and safety over a 12-month follow-up period. The authors reported delayed progression of

Table 7.5 Symptomatic management of MSA. Adapted from Wenning & Stefanova 2009 [44] and Flabeau et al. 2010 [135].

Non-medical treatment		
Should be offered to all MSA patients		• Physiotherapy • Occupational therapy • Speech therapy • Psychotherapy
Medical treatment		
In the absence of efficacious neuroprotective or preventive treatment, MSA management is mainly symptomatic and based on experts' experience		
Movement disorders	– Parkinsonism	• First choice: levodopa (up to 1000 mg/day, if tolerated and necessary) with domperidone to prevent nausea and vomiting. It should be noted that levodopa can cause worsening of OH, hypersexuality, delirium, and dyskinesias • Second choice: dopamine agonists (iPD titration schemes) • Third choice: amantadine (100 mg t.i.d.)
	– Dystonia	• Botulinum toxin injection in oro-facial (caution in antecollis because of risk of severe dysphagia) and in limb dystonia [168]
Cerebellar ataxia		• No drug therapy available
Autonomic symptoms	– Orthostatic hypotension	• First choice: non-pharmacological strategies: elastic support stockings or tights, high-salt diet, frequent small meals, head-up tilt of the bed at night, ingestion of water [169, 170] • If needed: add midodrine (2.5–30 mg t.i.d.) or fludrocortisone (0.1–0.3 mg) at night [171–173] • If needed: add or L-threo-DOPS (100 mg t.i.d.) [174, 175] • If needed: replace midodrine with ephedrine (15–45 mg t.i.d.) or L-threo-DOPS (100 mg t.i.d.) • Consider desmopressin once daily (to avoid water intoxication) before bedtime
	– Urinary failure – postvoid residue <100 mL	• Anticholinergics for detrusor hyperactivity [trospium chloride (20 mg b.i.d. or 15 mg t.i.d.), oxybutynin (2.5–5 mg b.i.d. to t.i.d.), tolterodine (2 mg b.i.d.)]. Especial attention should be paid to central side effects with anticholinergic drugs • Alpha-adrenergic antagonists for urethral hypertony (prazosin or tamsulosin). Be careful with exacerbation of OH • Alternative treatment can be intra-detrusor or urethral sphincter botulinum toxin injection
	– Urinary failure – postvoid residue >100 mL (patients usually reach this volume in the second year after disease onset) [176]	• All patients should try clean intermittent self-catheterization (CISC) [177] • In the advanced stages of MSA urethral or suprapubic permanent catheterization may become necessary • A last option for MSA patients who do not tolerate CISC is urinary surgery
	– Erectile dysfunction	• First choice: sildenafil (50–100 mg) [178]. Be careful with worsening of OH • Other options may be oral yohimbine (2.5–5 mg) or intracavernosal injection of papaverine
	– Constipation	• High fluid and fiber intake, laxatives
Other treatments	– Breathing problems	• CPAP (for prominent stridor and sleep apnea) • Tracheostomy (in case of life-threatening and/or daytime stridor or abnormal vocal cord mobility on laryngoscopy)
	– Swallowing and nutritional problems	• PEG when necessary
	– Drooling	• Botulinum toxin for sialorrhea
	– Depression	• Serotonin reuptake inhibitors. Paroxetine was found to produce motor improvement [179] and could be a last choice to consider • Psychotherapy
	– REM sleep behavior disorder	• Clonazepam

CPAP, continuous positive airway pressure; OH, orthostatic hypotension; PEG, percutaneous endoscopic gastrostomy.

neurological deficits with achievement of functional improvement measured by UMSARS and PET scan [158]. However, the design of the study, the possibility of confounding effects, and the lack of pre-clinical experimental evidence on underlying mechanisms of action mean that these results should be interpreted with caution [159]. A double-blind placebo-controlled, randomized clinical trial with autologous mesenchymal stem cells is on-going (NCT00911365).

Conclusions

In 1989, Niall Quinn in his article "Multiple system atrophy – the nature of the beast" ended by saying: "We desperately need better diagnosis of MSA if we are to seek the cause, and hence a preventive

or retardant treatment, for this terrible affliction. In the meantime, we need to draw on all our skills and compassion to help and comfort those who are struck by the disease" [5].

Unfortunately, despite the important efforts and remarkable progress that have been made in the last 25 years in understanding MSA, treatment approaches have not changed much from those times. Evidently MSA needs more attention and more work before we can offer patients disease-modifying therapies and improve disease prognosis.

The authors conclude that the way forward with MSA research should be to enroll patients in specialized clinics joining national and international databases and registries. Utilization of the UMSARS and sharing of imaging and psychometry data is very useful. Research through DNA and brain banks, and serum and CSF biomarkers protocols, are essential for MSA diagnosis. As we enter the era of individualized/precision medicine, the collection of comprehensive clinical datasets and the use of robust unbiased genomic approaches will be critical. Genetic variation, both protective and risk, will drive disease susceptibility and inform prognosis and therapeutic intervention strategies. We are beginning to get a better understanding of the heritability and genomic architecture of MSA with the recent publication of the first genome-wide association study [160–162]. Although no signal reached a strict statistical level of significance, a number of interesting candidates, including the previously discussed *MAPT* gene, were nominated [163, 164]. The challenge moving forward will be to use these genetic insights to resolve the underlying etiology and heterogeneity of MSA, to generate better model systems for drug development and therapeutics.

References

1. Graham JG, Oppenheimer DR. Orthostatic hypotension and nicotine sensitivity in a case of multiple system atrophy. *Journal of Neurology, Neurosurgery, and Psychiatry*. 1969;32(1):28–34.
2. Dejerine J, Thomas AA. L'atrophie olivo-ponto-cerebelleuse. *Nouvelle Iconographie de la Salpêtrière*. 1900(13):330–70.
3. Shy GM, Drager GA. A neurological syndrome associated with orthostatic hypotension: a clinical-pathologic study. *Archives of Neurology*. 1960;2:511–27.
4. Adams R, Van Bogaert L, Van der Eecken H. [Nigro-striate and cerebello-nigro-striate degeneration. *(Clinical uniqueness and pathological variability of presenile degeneration of the extrapyramidal rigidity type]. Psychiatria et Neurologia*. 1961;142:219–59.
5. Quinn N. Multiple system atrophy – the nature of the beast. *Journal of Neurology, Neurosurgery, and Psychiatry*. 1989;Suppl:78–89.
6. Papp MI, Kahn JE, Lantos PL. Glial cytoplasmic inclusions in the CNS of patients with multiple system atrophy (striatonigral degeneration, olivopontocerebellar atrophy and Shy-Drager syndrome). *Journal of the Neurological Sciences*. 1989;94(1-3):79–100.
7. Dickson DW, Liu W, Hardy J, Farrer M, Mehta N, Uitti R, et al. Widespread alterations of alpha-synuclein in multiple system atrophy. *The American Journal of Pathology*. 1999;155(4):1241–51.
8. Stefanova N, Bücke P, Duerr S, Wenning GK. Multiple system atrophy: an update. *Lancet Neurology*. 2009;8(12):1172–8.
9. Spillantini MG, Crowther RA, Jakes R, Cairns NJ, Lantos PL, Goedert M. Filamentous alpha-synuclein inclusions link multiple system atrophy with Parkinson's disease and dementia with Lewy bodies. *Neuroscience Letters*. 1998;251(3):205–8.
10. Wakabayashi K, Yoshimoto M, Tsuji S, Takahashi H. Alpha-synuclein immunoreactivity in glial cytoplasmic inclusions in multiple system atrophy. *Neuroscience Letters*. 1998;249(2-3):180–2.
11. Gilman S, Low PA, Quinn N, Albanese A, Ben-Shlomo Y, Fowler CJ, et al. Consensus statement on the diagnosis of multiple system atrophy. *Journal of the Autonomic Nervous System*. 1998;74(2-3):189–92.
12. Hughes AJ, Daniel SE, Kilford L, Lees AJ. Accuracy of clinical diagnosis of idiopathic Parkinson's disease: a clinico-pathological study of 100 cases. *Journal of Neurology, Neurosurgery, and Psychiatry*. 1992;55(3):181–4.
13. Wenning GK, Ben-Shlomo Y, Magalhães M, Daniel SE, Quinn NP. Clinicopathological study of 35 cases of multiple system atrophy. *Journal of Neurology, Neurosurgery, and Psychiatry*. 1995;58(2):160–6.
14. Bower JH, Maraganore DM, McDonnell SK, Rocca WA. Incidence of progressive supranuclear palsy and multiple system atrophy in Olmsted County, *Minnesota, 1976 to 1990. Neurology*. 1997;49(5):1284–8.
15. Winter Y, Bezdolnyy Y, Katunina E, Avakjan G, Reese JP, Klotsche J, et al. Incidence of Parkinson's disease and atypical parkinsonism: Russian population-based study. *Movement Disorders: Official Journal of the Movement Disorder Society*. 2010;25(3):349–56.
16. Linder J, Stenlund H, Forsgren L. Incidence of Parkinson's disease and parkinsonism in northern Sweden: a population-based study. *Movement Disorders: Official Journal of the Movement Disorder Society*. 2010;25(3):341–8.
17. Chrysostome V, Tison F, Yekhlef F, Sourgen C, Baldi I, Dartigues JF. Epidemiology of multiple system atrophy: a prevalence and pilot risk factor study in Aquitaine, France. *Neuroepidemiology*. 2004;23(4):201–8.
18. Tison F, Yekhlef F, Chrysostome V, Sourgen C. Prevalence of multiple system atrophy. *Lancet*. 2000;355(9202):495–6.
19. Schrag A, Ben-Shlomo Y, Quinn NP. Prevalence of progressive supranuclear palsy and multiple system atrophy: a cross-sectional study. *Lancet*. 1999;354(9192):1771–5.
20. Wermuth L, Bech S, Petersen MS, Joensen P, Weihe P, Grandjean P. Prevalence and incidence of Parkinson's disease in The Faroe Islands. *Acta Neurologica Scandinavica*. 2008;118(2):126–31.
21. Wenning GK, Ben Shlomo Y, Magalhães M, Daniel SE, Quinn NP. Clinical features and natural history of multiple system atrophy. *An analysis of 100 cases. Brain: A Journal of Neurology*. 1994;117 (Pt 4):835–45.
22. Schrag A, Wenning GK, Quinn N, Ben-Shlomo Y. Survival in multiple system atrophy. *Movement Disorders: Official Journal of the Movement Disorder Society*. 2008;23(2):294–6.
23. Watanabe H, Saito Y, Terao S, Ando T, Kachi T, Mukai E, et al. Progression and prognosis in multiple system atrophy: an analysis of 230 Japanese patients. *Brain: A Journal of Neurology*. 2002;125(Pt 5):1070–83.
24. Wenning GK, Tison F, Ben Shlomo Y, Daniel SE, Quinn NP. Multiple system atrophy: a review of 203 pathologically proven cases. *Movement Disorders: Official Journal of the Movement Disorder Society*. 1997;12(2):133–47.
25. Yabe I, Soma H, Takei A, Fujiki N, Yanagihara T, Sasaki H. MSA-C is the predominant clinical phenotype of MSA in Japan: analysis of 142 patients with probable MSA. *Journal of the Neurological Sciences*. 2006;249(2):115–21.
26. O'Sullivan SS, Massey LA, Williams DR, Silveira-Moriyama L, Kempster PA, Holton JL, et al. Clinical outcomes of progressive supranuclear palsy and multiple system atrophy. *Brain: A Journal of Neurology*. 2008;131(Pt 5):1362–72.
27. Wüllner U, Schmitz-Hübsch T, Abele M, Antony G, Bauer P, Eggert K. Features of probable multiple system atrophy patients identified among 4770 patients with parkinsonism enrolled in the multicentre registry of the German Competence Network on Parkinson's disease. *Journal of Neural Transmission (Vienna, Austria: 1996)*. 2007;114(9):1161–5.
28. Köllensperger M, Geser F, Ndayisaba J-P, Boesch S, Seppi K, Ostergaard K, et al. Presentation, diagnosis, and management of multiple system atrophy in Europe: final analysis of the European multiple system atrophy registry. *Movement Disorders: Official Journal of the Movement Disorder Society*. 2010;25(15):2604–12.
29. Ben-Shlomo Y, Wenning GK, Tison F, Quinn NP. Survival of patients with pathologically proven multiple system atrophy: a meta-analysis. *Neurology*. 1997;48(2):384–93.
30. Kim H-J, Jeon BS, Lee J-Y, Yun JY. Survival of Korean patients with multiple system atrophy. *Movement Disorders: Official Journal of the Movement Disorder Society*. 2011;26(5):909–12.
31. May S, Gilman S, Sowell BB, Thomas RG, Stern MB, Colcher A, et al. Potential outcome measures and trial design issues for multiple system atrophy. *Movement Disorders: Official Journal of the Movement Disorder Society*. 2007;22(16):2371–7.
32. Gilman S, Wenning GK, Low PA, Brooks DJ, Mathias CJ, Trojanowski JQ, et al. Second consensus statement on the diagnosis of multiple system atrophy. *Neurology*. 2008;71(9):670–6.
33. Hughes AJ, Colosimo C, Kleedorfer B, Daniel SE, Lees AJ. The dopaminergic response in multiple system atrophy. *Journal of Neurology, Neurosurgery, and Psychiatry*. 1992;55(11):1009–13.
34. Colosimo C, Albanese A, Hughes AJ, de Bruin VM, Lees AJ. Some specific clinical features differentiate multiple system atrophy (striatonigral variety) from Parkinson's disease. *Archives of Neurology*. 1995;52(3):294–8.
35. Fearnley JM, Lees AJ. Striatonigral degeneration. *A clinicopathological study. Brain: A Journal of Neurology*. 1990;113 (Pt 6):1823–42.
36. Rajput AH, Rozdilsky B, Rajput A, Ang L. Levodopa efficacy and pathological basis of Parkinson syndrome. *Clinical Neuropharmacology*. 1990;13(6):553–8.
37. Wenning GK, Tison F, Seppi K, Sampaio C, Diem A, Yekhlef F, et al. Development and validation of the Unified Multiple System Atrophy Rating Scale (UMSARS). *Movement Disorders: Official Journal of the Movement Disorder Society*. 2004;19(12):1391–402.
38. Boesch SM, Wenning GK, Ransmayr G, Poewe W. Dystonia in multiple system atrophy. *Journal of Neurology, Neurosurgery, and Psychiatry*. 2002;72(3):300–3.
39. Quinn N. Disproportionate antecollis in multiple system atrophy. *Lancet*. 1989;1(8642):844.
40. van de Warrenburg BPC, Cordivari C, Ryan AM, Phadke R, Holton JL, Bhatia KP, et al. The phenomenon of disproportionate antecollis in Parkinson's disease and multiple system atrophy. *Movement Disorders: Official Journal of the Movement Disorder Society*. 2007;22(16):2325–31.
41. Anderson T, Luxon L, Quinn N, Daniel S, Marsden CD, Bronstein A. Oculomotor function in multiple system atrophy: clinical and laboratory features in 30 patients. *Movement Disorders: Official Journal of the Movement Disorder Society*. 2008;23(7):977–84.

42. Colosimo C. Nonmotor presentations of multiple system atrophy. *Nature Reviews Neurology*. 2011;7(5):295–8.

43. Colosimo C, Morgante L, Antonini A, Barone P, Avarello TP, Bottacchi E, et al. Non-motor symptoms in atypical and secondary parkinsonism: the PRIAMO study. *Journal of Neurology*. 2010;257(1):5–14.

44. Wenning GK, Stefanova N. Recent developments in multiple system atrophy. *Journal of Neurology*. 2009;256(11):1791–808.

45. Kirchhof K, Apostolidis AN, Mathias CJ, Fowler CJ. Erectile and urinary dysfunction may be the presenting features in patients with multiple system atrophy: a retrospective study. *International Journal of Impotence Research*. 2003;15(4):293–8.

46. Wenning GK, Krismer F, Poewe W. New insights into atypical parkinsonism. *Current Opinion in Neurology*. 2011;24(4):331–8.

47. Donadio V, Nolano M, Elam M, Montagna P, Provitera V, Bugiardini E, et al. Anhidrosis in multiple system atrophy: a preganglionic sudomotor dysfunction? Movement Disorders: Official Journal of the Movement Disorder Society. 2008;23(6):885–8.

48. Fernagut P-O, Vital A, Canron M-H, Tison F, Meissner WG. Ambiguous mechanisms of dysphagia in multiple system atrophy. *Brain: A Journal of Neurology*. 2012:135(Pt 2):e205.

49. Plazzi G, Corsini R, Provini F, Pierangeli G, Martinelli P, Montagna P, et al. REM sleep behavior disorders in multiple system atrophy. *Neurology*. 1997;48(4):1094–7.

50. Iranzo A, Santamaría J, Rye DB, Valldeoriola F, Martí MJ, Muñoz E, et al. Characteristics of idiopathic REM sleep behavior disorder and that associated with MSA and PD. *Neurology*. 2005;65(2):247–52.

51. Moreno-López C, Santamaría J, Salamero M, Del Sorbo F, Albanese A, Pellecchia MT, et al. Excessive daytime sleepiness in multiple system atrophy (SLEEMSA study). *Archives of Neurology*. 2011;68(2):223–30.

52. Brown RG, Lacomblez L, Landwehrmeyer BG, Bak T, Uttner I, Dubois B, et al. Cognitive impairment in patients with multiple system atrophy and progressive supranuclear palsy. *Brain: A Journal of Neurology*. 2010;133(Pt 8):2382–93.

53. Kawai Y, Suenaga M, Takeda A, Ito M, Watanabe H, Tanaka F, et al. Cognitive impairments in multiple system atrophy: MSA-C vs MSA-P. *Neurology*. 2008;70(16 Pt 2):1390–6.

54. Schrag A, Sheikh S, Quinn NP, Lees AJ, Selai C, Mathias C, et al. A comparison of depression, anxiety, and health status in patients with progressive supranuclear palsy and multiple system atrophy. *Movement Disorders: Official Journal of the Movement Disorder Society*. 2010;25(8):1077–81.

55. Abele M, Riet A, Hummel T, Klockgether T, Wüllner U. Olfactory dysfunction in cerebellar ataxia and multiple system atrophy. *Journal of Neurology*. 2003;250(12):1453–5.

56. Nee LE, Scott J, Polinsky RJ. Olfactory dysfunction in the Shy-Drager syndrome. *Clinical Autonomic Research: Official Journal of the Clinical Autonomic Research Society*. 1993;3(4):281–2.

57. Silveira-Moriyama L, Mathias C, Mason L, Best C, Quinn NP, Lees AJ. Hyposmia in pure autonomic failure. *Neurology*. 2009;72(19):1677–81.

58. Wenning GK, Shephard B, Hawkes C, Petruckevitch A, Lees A, Quinn N. Olfactory function in atypical parkinsonian syndromes. *Acta Neurologica Scandinavica*. 1995;91(4):247–50.

59. Glass PG, Lees AJ, Mathias C, Mason L, Best C, Williams DR, et al. Olfaction in pathologically proven patients with multiple system atrophy. *Movement Disorders: Official Journal of the Movement Disorder Society*. 2012;27(2):327–8.

60. Leiguarda RC, Pramstaller PP, Merello M, Starkstein S, Lees AJ, Marsden CD. Apraxia in Parkinson's disease, progressive supranuclear palsy, multiple system atrophy and neuroleptic-induced parkinsonism. *Brain: A Journal of Neurology*. 1997;120 (Pt 1):75–90.

61. Ozsancak C, Auzou P, Dujardin K, Quinn N, Destée A. Orofacial apraxia in corticobasal degeneration, progressive supranuclear palsy, multiple system atrophy and Parkinson's disease. *Journal of Neurology*. 2004;251(11):1317–23.

62. Uluduz D, Ertürk O, Kenangil G, Ozekmekçi S, Ertan S, Apaydin H, et al. Apraxia in Parkinson's disease and multiple system atrophy. *European Journal of Neurology: The Official Journal of the European Federation of Neurological Societies*. 2010;17(3):413–8.

63. Yoon WT, Chung EJ, Lee SH, Kim BJ, Lee WY. Clinical analysis of blepharospasm and apraxia of eyelid opening in patients with parkinsonism. *Journal of Clinical Neurology (Seoul, Korea)*. 2005;1(2):159–65.

64. Ahmed Z, Asi YT, Sailer A, Lees AJ, Houlden H, Revesz T, et al. Review: The neuropathology, pathophysiology and genetics of multiple system atrophy. *Neuropathology and Applied Neurobiology*. 2012;38(1):4–24.

65. Ozawa T, Paviour D, Quinn NP, Josephs KA, Sangha H, Kilford L, et al. The spectrum of pathological involvement of the striatonigral and olivopontocerebellar systems in multiple system atrophy: clinicopathological correlations. *Brain: A Journal of Neurology*. 2004;127(Pt 12):2657–71.

66. Spargo E, Papp MI, Lantos PL. Decrease in neuronal density in the cerebral cortex in multiple system atrophy. *European Journal of Neurology*. 1996;3(5):450–6.

67. Tsuchiya K, Ozawa E, Haga C, Watabiki S, Ikeda M, Sano M, et al. Constant involvement of the Betz cells and pyramidal tract in multiple system atrophy: a clinicopathological study of seven autopsy cases. *Acta Neuropathologica*. 2000;99(6):628–36.

68. Song YJC, Halliday GM, Holton JL, Lashley T, O'Sullivan SS, McCann H, et al. Degeneration in different parkinsonian syndromes relates to astrocyte type and astrocyte protein expression. *Journal of Neuropathology and Experimental Neurology*. 2009;68(10):1073–83.

69. Jellinger KA, Lantos PL. Papp-Lantos inclusions and the pathogenesis of multiple system atrophy: an update. *Acta Neuropathologica*. 2010;119(6):657–67.

70. Trojanowski JQ, Revesz T. Proposed neuropathological criteria for the post mortem diagnosis of multiple system atrophy. *Neuropathology and Applied Neurobiology*. 2007;33(6):615–20.

71. Wenning GK, Quinn N, Magalhães M, Mathias C, Daniel SE. "Minimal change" multiple system atrophy. *Movement Disorders: Official Journal of the Movement Disorder Society*. 1994;9(2):161–6.

72. Solano SM, Miller DW, Augood SJ, Young AB, Penney JB, Jr. Expression of alpha-synuclein, parkin, and ubiquitin carboxy-terminal hydrolase L1 mRNA in human brain: genes associated with familial Parkinson's disease. *Annals of Neurology*. 2000;47(2):201–10.

73. Miller DW, Johnson JM, Solano SM, Hollingsworth ZR, Standaert DG, Young AB. Absence of alpha-synuclein mRNA expression in normal and multiple system atrophy oligodendroglia. *Journal of Neural Transmission (Vienna, Austria: 1996)*. 2005;112(12):1613–24.

74. Wenning GK, Stefanova N, Jellinger KA, Poewe W, Schlossmacher MG. Multiple system atrophy: a primary oligodendrogliopathy. *Annals of Neurology*. 2008;64(3):239–46.

75. Jellinger KA. P25alpha immunoreactivity in multiple system atrophy and Parkinson disease. *Acta Neuropathologica*. 2006;112(1):112.

76. Kovács GG, Gelpi E, Lehotzky A, Höftberger R, Erdei A, Budka H, et al. The brain-specific protein TPPP/p25 in pathological protein deposits of neurodegenerative diseases. *Acta Neuropathologica*. 2007;113(2):153–61.

77. Lindersson E, Lundvig D, Petersen C, Madsen P, Nyengaard JR, Højrup P, et al. p25alpha Stimulates alpha-synuclein aggregation and is co-localized with aggregated alpha-synuclein in alpha-synucleinopathies. *The Journal of Biological Chemistry*. 2005;280(7):5703–15.

78. Song YJC, Lundvig DMS, Huang Y, Gai WP, Blumbergs PC, Højrup P, et al. p25alpha relocalizes in oligodendroglia from myelin to cytoplasmic inclusions in multiple system atrophy. *The American Journal of Pathology*. 2007;171(4):1291–303.

79. Stefanova N, Tison F, Reindl M, Poewe W, Wenning GK. Animal models of multiple system atrophy. *Trends in Neurosciences*. 2005;28(9):501–6.

80. Stefanova N, Reindl M, Neumann M, Kahle PJ, Poewe W, Wenning GK. Microglial activation mediates neurodegeneration related to oligodendroglial alpha-synucleinopathy: implications for multiple system atrophy. *Movement Disorders: Official Journal of the Movement Disorder Society*. 2007;22(15):2196–203.

81. Wakabayashi K, Mori F, Nishie M, Oyama Y, Kurihara A, Yoshimoto M, et al. An autopsy case of early ("minimal change") olivopontocerebellar atrophy (multiple system atrophy-cerebellar). *Acta Neuropathologica*. 2005;110(2):185–90.

82. Yoshida M. Multiple system atrophy: alpha-synuclein and neuronal degeneration. *Neuropathology: Official Journal of the Japanese Society of Neuropathology*. 2007;27(5):484–93.

83. Nishie M, Mori F, Yoshimoto M, Takahashi H, Wakabayashi K. A quantitative investigation of neuronal cytoplasmic and intranuclear inclusions in the pontine and inferior olivary nuclei in multiple system atrophy. *Neuropathology and Applied Neurobiology*. 2004;30(5):546–54.

84. Nee LE, Gomez MR, Dambrosia J, Bale S, Eldridge R, Polinsky RJ. Environmental-occupational risk factors and familial associations in multiple system atrophy: a preliminary investigation. *Clinical Autonomic Research: Official Journal of the Clinical Autonomic Research Society*. 1991;1(1):9–13.

85. Vanacore N, Bonifati V, Fabbrini G, Colosimo C, De Michele G, Marconi R, et al. Case-control study of multiple system atrophy. *Movement Disorders: Official Journal of the Movement Disorder Society*. 2005;20(2):158–63.

86. Seo J-H, Yong SW, Song SK, Lee JE, Sohn YH, Lee PH. A case-control study of multiple system atrophy in Korean patients. *Movement Disorders: Official Journal of the Movement Disorder Society*. 2010;25(12):1953–9.

87. Vidal J-S, Vidailhet M, Elbaz A, Derkinderen P, Tzourio C, Alpérovitch A. Risk factors of multiple system atrophy: a case-control study in French patients. *Movement Disorders: Official Journal of the Movement Disorder Society*. 2008;23(6):797–803.

88. Vanacore N, Bonifati V, Fabbrini G, Colosimo C, Marconi R, Nicholl D, et al. Smoking habits in multiple system atrophy and progressive supranuclear palsy. European Study Group on Atypical Parkinsonisms. *Neurology*. 2000;54(1):114–9.

89. Berg D, Hochstrasser H. Iron metabolism in Parkinsonian syndromes. *Movement Disorders: Official Journal of the Movement Disorder Society.* 2006;21(9):1299–310.

90. Dexter DT, Carayon A, Javoy-Agid F, Agid Y, Wells FR, Daniel SE, et al. Alterations in the levels of iron, ferritin and other trace metals in Parkinson's disease and other neurodegenerative diseases affecting the basal ganglia. *Brain: A Journal of Neurology.* 1991;114 (Pt 4):1953–75.

91. Dexter DT, Jenner P, Schapira AH, Marsden CD. Alterations in levels of iron, ferritin, and other trace metals in neurodegenerative diseases affecting the basal ganglia. The Royal Kings and Queens Parkinson's Disease Research Group. *Annals of Neurology.* 1992;32 Suppl:S94–100.

92. Hara K, Momose Y, Tokiguchi S, Shimohata M, Terajima K, Onodera O, et al. Multiplex families with multiple system atrophy. *Archives of Neurology.* 2007;64(4):545–51.

93. Hohler AD, Singh VJ. Probable hereditary multiple system atrophy-autonomic (MSA-A) in a family in the United States. *Journal of Clinical Neuroscience.* 2012;19(3):479–80.

94. Wullner U, Schmitt I, Kammal M, Kretzschmar HA, Neumann M. Definite multiple system atrophy in a German family. *Journal of Neurology Neurosurgery and Psychiatry.* 2009;80(4):449–50.

95. Ross OA, Braithwaite AT, Skipper LM, Kachergus J, Hulihan MM, Middleton FA, et al. Genomic investigation of alpha-synuclein multiplication and parkinsonism. *Annals of Neurology.* 2008;63(6):743–50.

96. Singleton AB, Farrer M, Johnson J, Singleton A, Hague S, Kachergus J, et al. alpha-Synuclein locus triplication causes Parkinson's disease. *Science.* 2003;302(5646):841.

97. Ozawa T, Takano H, Onodera O, Kobayashi H, Ikeuchi T, Koide R, et al. No mutation in the entire coding region of the alpha-synuclein gene in pathologically confirmed cases of multiple system atrophy. *Neuroscience Letters* 1999;270(2):110–2.

98. Fuchs J, Nilsson C, Kachergus J, Munz M, Larsson EM, Schule B, et al. Phenotypic variation in a large Swedish pedigree due to SNCA duplication and triplication. *Neurology.* 2007;68(12):916–22.

99. Lee PH, Lee G, Park HJ, Bang OY, Joo IS, Huh K. The plasma alpha-synuclein levels in patients with Parkinson's disease and multiple system atrophy. *Journal of Neural Transmission.* 2006;113(10):1435–9.

100. Ozawa T, Okuizumi K, Ikeuchi T, Wakabayashi K, Takahashi H, Tsuji S. Analysis of the expression level of alpha-synuclein mRNA using postmortem brain samples from pathologically confirmed cases of multiple system atrophy. *Acta Neuropathologica.* 2001;102(2):188–90.

101. Vogt IR, Lees AJ, Evert BO, Klockgether T, Bonin M, Wullner U. Transcriptional changes in multiple system atrophy and Parkinson's disease putamen. *Experimental Neurology.* 2006;199(2):465–78.

102. Ozawa T, Healy DG, Abou-Sleiman PM, Ahmadi KR, Quinn N, Lees AJ, et al. The alpha-synuclein gene in multiple system atrophy. *Journal of Neurology Neurosurgery and Psychiatry.* 2006;77(4):464–7.

103. Scholz SW, Houlden H, Schulte C, Sharma M, Li A, Berg D, et al. SNCA variants are associated with increased risk for multiple system atrophy. *Annals of Neurology.* 2009;65(5):610–4.

104. Ross OA, Vilarino-Guell C, Wszolek ZK, Farrer MJ, Dickson DW. Reply to: SNCA variants are associated with increased risk of multiple system atrophy. *Annals of Neurology.* 2010;67(3):414–5.

105. Al-Chalabi A, Durr A, Wood NW, Parkinson MH, Camuzat A, Hulot JS, et al. Genetic variants of the alpha-synuclein gene SNCA are associated with multiple system atrophy. *PLoS One.* 2009;4(9):e7114.

106. Nagaishi M, Yokoo H, Nakazato Y. Tau-positive glial cytoplasmic granules in multiple system atrophy. *Neuropathology.* 2011;31(3):299–305.

107. Vilarino-Guell C, Soto-Ortolaza AI, Rajput A, Mash DC, Papapetropoulos S, Pahwa R, et al. MAPT H1 haplotype is a risk factor for essential tremor and multiple system atrophy. *Neurology.* 2011;76(7):670–2.

108. Stemberger S, Scholz SW, Singleton AB, Wenning GK. Genetic players in multiple system atrophy: unfolding the nature of the beast. *Neurobiology of Aging.* 2011;32(10):1924 e5–14.

109. Mutations in COQ2 in familial and sporadic multiple-system atrophy. The New England Journal of Medicine. *[Multicenter Study Research Support, Non-U.S. Gov't].* 2013;369(3):233–44.

110. Mitsui J, Tsuji S. Mutant COQ2 in multiple-system atrophy. *The New England Journal of Medicine. [Comment Letter].* 2014;371(1):82–3.

111. Quinzii CM, Hirano M, DiMauro S. Mutant COQ2 in multiple-system atrophy. *The New England Journal of Medicine. [Comment Letter].* 2014;371(1):81–2.

112. Schottlaender LV, Houlden H. Mutant COQ2 in multiple-system atrophy. *The New England Journal of Medicine. [Comment Letter].* 2014;371(1):81.

113. Sharma M, Wenning G, Kruger R. Mutant COQ2 in multiple-system atrophy. *The New England Journal of Medicine. [Comment Letter].* 2014;371(1):80–1.

114. Seppi K, Poewe W. Brain magnetic resonance imaging techniques in the diagnosis of parkinsonian syndromes. *Neuroimaging Clinics of North America.* 2010;20(1):29–55.

115. Courbon F, Brefel-Courbon C, Thalamas C, Alibelli M-J, Berry I, Montastruc J-L, et al. Cardiac MIBG scintigraphy is a sensitive tool for detecting cardiac sympathetic denervation in Parkinson's disease. *Movement Disorders: Official Journal of the Movement Disorder Society.* 2003;18(8):890–7.

116. Nagayama H, Hamamoto M, Ueda M, Nagashima J, Katayama Y. Reliability of MIBG myocardial scintigraphy in the diagnosis of Parkinson's disease. *Journal of Neurology, Neurosurgery, and Psychiatry.* 2005;76(2):249–51.

117. Raffel DM, Koeppe RA, Little R, Wang C-N, Liu S, Junck L, et al. PET measurement of cardiac and nigrostriatal denervation in Parkinsonian syndromes. *Journal of Nuclear Medicine: Official Publication, Society of Nuclear Medicine.* 2006;47(11):1769–77.

118. Seppi K, Schocke MFH, Wenning GK, Poewe W. How to diagnose MSA early: the role of magnetic resonance imaging. *Journal of Neural Transmission (Vienna, Austria: 1996).* 2005;112(12):1625–34.

119. Brooks DJ, Seppi K. Proposed neuroimaging criteria for the diagnosis of multiple system atrophy. *Movement Disorders: Official Journal of the Movement Disorder Society.* 2009;24(7):949–64.

120. Gilman S. Functional imaging with positron emission tomography in multiple system atrophy. *Journal of Neural Transmission (Vienna, Austria: 1996).* 2005;112(12):1647–55.

121. Gilman S, Koeppe RA, Junck L, Little R, Kluin KJ, Heumann M, et al. Decreased striatal monoaminergic terminals in multiple system atrophy detected with positron emission tomography. *Annals of Neurology.* 1999;45(6):769–17.

122. Gilman S, Low PA, Quinn N, Albanese A, Ben-Shlomo Y, Fowler CJ, et al. Consensus statement on the diagnosis of multiple system atrophy. *Journal of the Neurological Sciences.* 1999;163(1):94–8.

123. Osaki Y, Ben-Shlomo Y, Lees AJ, Wenning GK, Quinn NP. A validation exercise on the new consensus criteria for multiple system atrophy. *Movement Disorders: Official Journal of the Movement Disorder Society.* 2009;24(15):2272–6.

124. Colosimo C, Vanacore N, Bonifati V, Fabbrini G, Rum A, De Michele G, et al. Clinical diagnosis of multiple system atrophy: level of agreement between Quinn's criteria and the consensus conference guidelines. *Acta Neurologica Scandinavica.* 2001;103(4):261–4.

125. Osaki Y, Wenning GK, Daniel SE, Hughes A, Lees AJ, Mathias CJ, et al. Do published criteria improve clinical diagnostic accuracy in multiple system atrophy? *Neurology.* 2002;59(10):1486–91.

126. Quinn NP. How to diagnose multiple system atrophy. *Movement Disorders: Official Journal of the Movement Disorder Society.* 2005;20 Suppl 12:S5–S10.

127. Horimoto Y, Matsumoto M, Akatsu H, Ikari H, Kojima K, Yamamoto T, et al. Autonomic dysfunctions in dementia with Lewy bodies. *Journal of Neurology.* 2003;250(5):530–3.

128. Gilman S, Little R, Johanns J, Heumann M, Kluin KJ, Junck L, et al. Evolution of sporadic olivopontocerebellar atrophy into multiple system atrophy. *Neurology.* 2000;55(4):527–32.

129. Geser F, Wenning GK, Seppi K, Stampfer-Kountchev M, Scherfler C, Sawires M, et al. Progression of multiple system atrophy (MSA): a prospective natural history study by the European MSA Study Group (EMSA SG). *Movement Disorders: Official Journal of the Movement Disorder Society.* 2006;21(2):179–86.

130. Tada M, Onodera O, Tada M, Ozawa T, Piao Y-S, Kakita A, et al. Early development of autonomic dysfunction may predict poor prognosis in patients with multiple system atrophy. *Archives of Neurology.* 2007;64(2):256–60.

131. Silber MH, Levine S. Stridor and death in multiple system atrophy. *Movement Disorders: Official Journal of the Movement Disorder Society.* 2000;15(4):699–704.

132. Papapetropoulos S, Tuchman A, Laufer D, Papatsoris AG, Papapetropoulos N, Mash DC. Causes of death in multiple system atrophy. *Journal of Neurology, Neurosurgery, and Psychiatry.* 2007;78(3):327–9.

133. Shimohata T, Ozawa T, Nakayama H, Tomita M, Shinoda H, Nishizawa M. Frequency of nocturnal sudden death in patients with multiple system atrophy. *Journal of Neurology.* 2008;255(10):1483–5.

134. Tada M, Kakita A, Toyoshima Y, Onodera O, Ozawa T, Morita T, et al. Depletion of medullary serotonergic neurons in patients with multiple system atrophy who succumbed to sudden death. *Brain: A Journal of Neurology.* 2009;132(Pt 7):1810–9.

135. Flabeau O, Meissner WG, Tison F. Multiple system atrophy: current and future approaches to management. *Therapeutic Advances in Neurological Disorders.* 2010;3(4):249–63.

136. Jain S, Dawson J, Quinn NP, Playford ED. Occupational therapy in multiple system atrophy: a pilot randomized controlled trial. *Movement Disorders: Official Journal of the Movement Disorder Society.* 2004;19(11):1360–4.

137. Wedge F. The impact of resistance training on balance and functional ability of a patient with multiple system atrophy. *Journal of Geriatric Physical Therapy (2001).* 2008;31(2):79–83.

138. Winter Y, Spottke AE, Stamelou M, Cabanel N, Eggert K, Höglinger GU, et al. Health-related quality of life in multiple system atrophy and progressive supranuclear palsy. *Neuro-Degenerative Diseases.* 2011;8(6):438–46.

139. Ullman M, Vedam-Mai V, Resnick AS, Yachnis AT, McFarland NR, Merritt S, et al. Deep brain stimulation response in pathologically confirmed cases of multiple system atrophy. *Parkinsonism & Related Disorders.* 2012;18(1):86–8

140. Visser-Vandewalle V, Temel Y, Colle H, van der Linden C. Bilateral high-frequency stimulation of the subthalamic nucleus in patients with multiple system atrophy–parkinsonism. *Report of four cases. Journal of Neurosurgery.* 2003;98(4):882–7.

141. Lambrecq V, Krim E, Meissner W, Guehl D, Tison F. [Deep-brain stimulation of the internal pallidum in multiple system atrophy]. *Revue Neurologique.* 2008;164(4):398–402.

142. Santens P, Patrick S, Vonck K, Kristl V, De Letter M, Miet DL, et al. Deep brain stimulation of the internal pallidum in multiple system atrophy. *Parkinsonism & Related Disorders.* 2006;12(3):181–3.

143. Tarsy D, Apetauerova D, Ryan P, Norregaard T. Adverse effects of subthalamic nucleus DBS in a patient with multiple system atrophy. *Neurology.* 2003;61(2):247–9.

144. Talmant V, Esposito P, Stilhart B, Mohr M, Tranchant C. [Subthalamic stimulation in a patient with multiple system atrophy: a clinicopathological report]. *Revue Neurologique.* 2006;162(3):363–70.

145. Shih LC, Tarsy D. Deep brain stimulation for the treatment of atypical parkinsonism. *Movement Disorders: Official Journal of the Movement Disorder Society.* 2007;22(15):2149–55.

146. Geser F, Seppi K, Stampfer-Kountchev M, Köllensperger M, Diem A, Ndayisaba JP, et al. The European Multiple System Atrophy-Study Group (EMSA-SG). *Journal of Neural Transmission (Vienna, Austria: 1996).* 2005;112(12):1677–86.

147. Gilman S, May SJ, Shults CW, Tanner CM, Kukull W, Lee VM-Y, et al. The North American Multiple System Atrophy Study Group. *Journal of Neural Transmission (Vienna, Austria: 1996).* 2005;112(12):1687–94.

148. Holmberg B, Johansson J-O, Poewe W, Wenning G, Quinn NP, Mathias C, et al. Safety and tolerability of growth hormone therapy in multiple system atrophy: a double-blind, placebo-controlled study. *Movement Disorders: Official Journal of the Movement Disorder Society.* 2007;22(8):1138–44.

149. Bensimon G, Ludolph A, Agid Y, Vidailhet M, Payan C, Leigh PN. Riluzole treatment, survival and diagnostic criteria in Parkinson plus disorders: the NNIPPS study. *Brain: A Journal of Neurology.* 2009;132(Pt 1):156–71.

150. Seppi K, Peralta C, Diem-Zangerl A, Puschban Z, Mueller J, Poewe W, et al. Placebo-controlled trial of riluzole in multiple system atrophy. *European Journal of Neurology: The Official Journal of the European Federation of Neurological Societies.* 2006;13(10):1146–8.

151. Dodel R, Spottke A, Gerhard A, Reuss A, Reinecker S, Schimke N, et al. Minocycline 1-year therapy in multiple-system-atrophy: effect on clinical symptoms and [(11)C] (R)-PK11195 PET (MEMSA-trial). *Movement Disorders: Official Journal of the Movement Disorder Society.* 2010;25(1):97–107.

152. Heo J-H, Lee S-T, Chu K, Kim M. The efficacy of combined estrogen and buspirone treatment in olivopontocerebellar atrophy. *Journal of the Neurological Sciences.* 2008;271(1-2):87–90.

153. Köllensperger M, Krismer F, Pallua A, Stefanova N, Poewe W, Wenning GK. Erythropoietin is neuroprotective in a transgenic mouse model of multiple system atrophy. *Movement Disorders: Official Journal of the Movement Disorder Society.* 2011;26(3):507–15.

154. Stefanova N, Georgievska B, Eriksson H, Poewe W, Wenning GK. Myeloperoxidase inhibition ameliorates multiple system atrophy-like degeneration in a transgenic mouse model. *Neurotoxicity Research.* 2012;21(4):393–404.

155. Köllensperger M, Stefanova N, Pallua A, Puschban Z, Dechant G, Hainzer M, et al. Striatal transplantation in a rodent model of multiple system atrophy: effects on L-Dopa response. *Journal of Neuroscience Research.* 2009;87(7):1679–85.

156. Puschban Z, Stefanova N, Petersén A, Winkler C, Brundin P, Poewe W, et al. Evidence for dopaminergic re-innervation by embryonic allografts in an optimized rat model of the Parkinsonian variant of multiple system atrophy. *Brain Research Bulletin.* 2005;68(1-2):54–8.

157. Stefanova N, Hainzer M, Stemberger S, Couillard-Després S, Aigner L, Poewe W, et al. Striatal transplantation for multiple system atrophy – are grafts affected by alpha-synucleinopathy? *Experimental Neurology.* 2009;219(1):368–71.

158. Lee PH, Kim JW, Bang OY, Ahn YH, Joo IS, Huh K. Autologous mesenchymal stem cell therapy delays the progression of neurological deficits in patients with multiple system atrophy. *Clinical Pharmacology and Therapeutics.* 2008;83(5):723–30.

159. Quinn N, Barker RA, Wenning GK. Are trials of intravascular infusions of autologous mesenchymal stem cells in patients with multiple system atrophy currently justified, and are they effective? *Clinical Pharmacology and Therapeutics.* 2008;83(5):663–5.

160. Federoff M, Price TR, Sailer A, et al. Genome-wide estimate of the heritability of multiple system atrophy. *Parkinsonism & Related Disorders.* 2016;22:35–41.

161. Federoff M, Schottlaender LV, Houlden H, Singleton A. Multiple system atrophy: the application of genetics in understanding etiology. *Clinical autonomic research: official journal of the Clinical Autonomic Research Society* 2015;25:19–36.

162. Sailer A, Scholz SW, Nalls MA, et al. A genome-wide association study in multiple system atrophy. *Neurology.* 2016;87(15):1591–1598.

163. Labbe C, Heckman MG, Lorenzo-Betancor O et al. *MAPT haplotype diversity in multiple system atrophy. Parkinsonism & Related Disorders.* 2016;30:40–45.

164. Benarroch EE. Brainstem in multiple system atrophy: clinicopathological correlations. *Cellular and Molecular Neurobiology.* 2003;23(4-5):519–26.

165. Benarroch EE. Brainstem respiratory control: substrates of respiratory failure of multiple system atrophy. *Movement Disorders: Official Journal of the Movement Disorder Society.* 2007;22(2):155–61.

166. Benarroch EE, Schmeichel AM, Sandroni P, Low PA, Parisi JE. Involvement of vagal autonomic nuclei in multiple system atrophy and Lewy body disease. *Neurology.* 2006;66(3):378–83.

167. Oppenheimer DR. Lateral horn cells in progressive autonomic failure. *Journal of the Neurological Sciences.* 1980;46(3):393–404.

168. Müller J, Wenning GK, Wissel J, Seppi K, Poewe W. Botulinum toxin treatment in atypical parkinsonian disorders associated with disabling focal dystonia. *Journal of Neurology.* 2002;249(3):300–4.

169. Freeman R. Clinical practice. *Neurogenic orthostatic hypotension. The New England Journal of Medicine.* 2008;358(6):615–24.

170. Low PA, Singer W. Management of neurogenic orthostatic hypotension: an update. *Lancet Neurology.* 2008;7(5):451–8.

171. Jankovic J, Gilden JL, Hiner BC, Kaufmann H, Brown DC, Coghlan CH, et al. Neurogenic orthostatic hypotension: a double-blind, placebo-controlled study with midodrine. *The American Journal of Medicine.* 1993;95(1):38–48.

172. Low PA, Gilden JL, Freeman R, Sheng KN, McElligott MA. Efficacy of midodrine vs placebo in neurogenic orthostatic hypotension. A randomized, double-blind multicenter study. Midodrine Study Group. *JAMA: The Journal of the American Medical Association.* 1997;277(13):1046–51.

173. Wright RA, Kaufmann HC, Perera R, Opfer-Gehrking TL, McElligott MA, Sheng KN, et al. A double-blind, dose-response study of midodrine in neurogenic orthostatic hypotension. *Neurology.* 1998;51(1):120–4.

174. Kaufmann H, Saadia D, Voustianiouk A, Goldstein DS, Holmes C, Yahr MD, et al. Norepinephrine precursor therapy in neurogenic orthostatic hypotension. *Circulation.* 2003;108(6):724–8.

175. Mathias CJ. L-dihydroxyphenylserine (Droxidopa) in the treatment of orthostatic hypotension: the European experience. *Clinical Autonomic Research: Official Journal of the Clinical Autonomic Research Society.* 2008;18 Suppl 1:25–9.

176. Ito T, Sakakibara R, Yasuda K, Yamamoto T, Uchiyama T, Liu Z, et al. Incomplete emptying and urinary retention in multiple-system atrophy: when does it occur and how do we manage it? Movement Disorders: Official Journal of the Movement Disorder Society. 2006;21(6):816–23.

177. Fowler CJ, O'Malley KJ. Investigation and management of neurogenic bladder dysfunction. *Journal of Neurology, Neurosurgery, and Psychiatry.* 2003;74 Suppl 4:iv27–iv31.

178. Hussain IF, Brady CM, Swinn MJ, Mathias CJ, Fowler CJ. Treatment of erectile dysfunction with sildenafil citrate (Viagra) in parkinsonism due to Parkinson's disease or multiple system atrophy with observations on orthostatic hypotension. *Journal of Neurology, Neurosurgery, and Psychiatry.* 2001;71(3):371–4.

179. Friess E, Kuempfel T, Modell S, Winkelmann J, Holsboer F, Ising M, et al. Paroxetine treatment improves motor symptoms in patients with multiple system atrophy. *Parkinsonism & Related Disorders.* 2006;12(7):432–7.

CHAPTER 8

Progressive Supranuclear Palsy

Huw R. Morris

Department of Clinical Neuroscience, UCL Institute of Neurology, London, UK

Introduction

Progressive supranuclear palsy (PSP) is now used both as a patho-logical and clinicopathological term. Pathologically, PSP involves neurofibrillary degeneration with a specific pattern of neuronal and glial tau deposition, and it has become clear that pathologi-cally defined PSP can have a wide range of clinical presentations, overlapping with other neurodegenerative conditions [1]. Clini-cally, PSP can be diagnosed with guidance from formal opera-tional research diagnostic criteria (most commonly the National Institute for Neurological Disorders-Society for Progressive Supranuclear Palsy – NINDS-SPSP, or the Natural History, Neuro-protection and Biology of Parkinson's Plus Syndromes – NNIPPS criteria) [2, 3]. Over the last 10 years there has been a detailed description of the diverse clinical presentations of PSP pathology, relating to large series of pathological material collected by centers with a special interest in PSP. Currently, it is difficult to determine the relative importance of the different clinical manifestations of PSP pathology because of a lack of large community-based clin-icopathological studies that encompass diverse clinical presenta-tions. The clinical PSP syndrome, now known as PSP-Richardson's syndrome (PSP-RS), has a high predictive value for PSP pathol-ogy, although occasionally other conditions can masquerade as PSP-RS [4, 5]. Significant advances have been made in genetics and molecular pathology. Our understanding of the interplay of genetic factors and the identification of the best targets for thera-peutic intervention is incomplete, but significant progress has been made in this area. There are now several clinical rating scales that can be used to track the progression of PSP, and several bio-markers have been evaluated in both diagnostic and longitudinal disease progression studies.

Clinical definition and epidemiology

The term PSP-RS was defined to distinguish the classical clini-cal features of PSP from alternative clinical presentations of PSP pathology, as discussed below [6]. This conforms to the clinical–pathological syndrome described by Steele, Richardson, and Olszewksi in 1963 and 1964 and to the NINDS-SPSP operational criteria defined in 1996 [2, 7, 8]. In recent years, clinical epide-miological work has been carried out on patients meeting criteria for PSP-RS using the NINDS-SPSP criteria, and the prevalence of other forms of neurofibrillary tangle parkinsonism and atypical

clinical presentations of PSP pathology is at present unknown. The core features of PSP (PSP-RS) were defined by Steele, Richard-son, and Olszewski as involving "defects of ocular gaze, spasticity of facial muscles with dysarthria and sometimes dysphagia" and "extensor rigidity of the neck with head retraction and dementia" [7]. The eye movement disorder particularly involved downward gaze, and facial spasticity was described with a staring expression, open mouth, and brisk jaw and facial jerks. The dementia was mild with personality change and impaired intellectual ability. Patho-logically, these early cases had neurofibrillary tangle degeneration with granulovacuolar degeneration particularly involving the palli-dum, red nucleus, and subthalamic nucleus with similar changes in substantia nigra, locus coeruleus, and cerebellar dentate nucleus. The NINDS-SPSP clinical diagnostic criteria stipulated that clini-cally probable PSP involved a vertical supranuclear palsy, with gait imbalance and falls in the first year of symptoms, with clinically possible PSP involving either a vertical supranuclear gaze palsy or slowing of vertical saccadic eye movements with gait imbalance and falls in the first year of symptoms [2, 9]. Additionally, the crite-ria applied to patients with a progressive condition occurring over the age of 40, with appropriate exclusion criteria. A 2003 review reported that falls in the first year of symptoms could be amended to falls or the tendency to fall in the first year of symptoms. The NINDS-SPSP clinically probable criteria have been reported to have a high specificity (100%) but a lower sensitivity (50–62%) [9]. Amendments have been suggested which may increase the sensi-tivity of the NINDS-SPSP diagnostic criteria. The NNIPPS criteria for the diagnosis of PSP stipulate a supranuclear ophthalmoplegia with falls or postural instability in the first three years of symptoms and have a sensitivity of 95% and a specificity of 84%, within a study of both multiple system atrophy (MSA) and PSP [3]. It can be difficult to date the onset of neurodegenerative conditions, and insidious symptoms in the early phases of the disease may cause difficulty in meeting diagnostic criteria.

Many of the clinical features of PSP have been studied in detail. A clinical cohort study reported that symptoms relating to mobility or balance are most common, followed by cognitive problems and bulbar dysfunction in 15%. Tremor, not usually considered to be a core feature of PSP, can occur in 13% of patients [10]. Particularly important for some patients in early disease is the insidious person-ality, behavioral, and cognitive change reported by Richardson in the earliest descriptions of the disease. A large Dutch study carried

Neurodegeneration, First Edition. Edited by Anthony Schapira, Zbigniew Wszolek, Ted M. Dawson and Nicholas Wood.
© 2017 John Wiley & Sons, Ltd. Published 2017 by John Wiley & Sons, Ltd.

out by Donker Kaat and colleagues showed that 20% of PSP patients had predominant cognitive or behavioral features, and some of these patients were misdiagnosed as having behavioral variant frontotemporal dementia (bvFTD) [11]. PSP is the prototypic subcortical dementia, characterized by slowing of thought processes, apathy, and difficulty in manipulating knowledge [12]. The NNIPPS study prospectively assessed cognitive function in 311 PSP patients. They found that 57% of PSP patients had significant cognitive impairment, and that this correlated with greater age and clinical severity [13]. In the early stages of the disease approximately half of all PSP patients had cognitive impairment [13]. The predominant feature of the cognitive profile of PSP was impaired verbal fluency, consistent with a frontal executive disorder, but there were also less marked deficits in memory, attention, conceptualization, and visuospatial function. bvFTD involves impairment of emotion recognition, and this has also been described in PSP, with impairment particularly related to the perception of negative emotions [14]. The cognitive features of PSP have traditionally been thought to relate to frontal cortical pathology and to the disruption of frontostriatal circuits, but a recent detailed psychological–pathological study indicated that executive dysfunction in PSP correlated with the amount of tau deposition in both the superior frontal gyrus and the parietal supra-marginal gyrus [15].

Eye movement abnormalities are a hallmark feature of PSP and the abnormalities evolve through the disease course. PSP patients develop slowing of vertical saccades, with preserved saccadic latency and prominent square-wave jerks [16]. Initially, there is slowing of vertical saccades but as the disease progresses there is limitation of vertical saccades and then complete failure of up- and down-gaze, often with preservation of horizontal eye movements [16]. Full eye movements can be generated using the doll's head maneuver through the early and mid-stages of the disease but in end-stage disease there may be complete loss of eye movements, including those generated by the vestibulo-ocular reflex. Impaired vertical saccades have been related to degeneration of the rostral interstitial nucleus of the medial longitudinal fasciculus [17]. Many patients with PSP develop retrocollis and abnormalities of neck posture when turning, and these abnormalities have been linked to degeneration of the interstitial nucleus of Cajal, together with impaired re-setting head movements [18, 19]. PSP patients have a marked loss of spontaneous blinking with a slowing of the blink rate to around 6 blinks per minute as compared to 22 blinks per minute in normal control subjects [20]. PSP involves blepharospasm in the middle to late disease stages, and involuntary eye closure can lead to significant functional disability. It is also associated with eyelid retraction, levator inhibition, also known as apraxia of eye-opening, and supranuclear palsy of eye closure, also known as apraxia of eye closure [21, 22].

The most prominent feature is usually gait disturbance with frequent falls, and often patients sustain injuries during falls, which have a major effect on morbidity and quality of life. Patients with early-stage PSP usually have a staggering or lurching gait with large steps, contrasting with the gait disorder of Parkinson disease (PD). As the disease progresses they develop an uncontrolled descent when sitting, and have difficulty in standing from a seated position without assistance. They then need assistance when standing and eventually usually become wheelchair dependent. A clinical milestones study has demonstrated that on average PSP-RS patients develop frequent falls within 3 years of disease onset, and become wheelchair dependent 5 years into the disease course [23]. The development of the gait and balance disorder is multifactorial:

important factors include down-gaze palsy, extensor posturing of the neck, and impaired vestibular reflexes. A recent study has shown that the balance disorder in PSP is correlated with decreased thalamic metabolism, thought to relate to degeneration of pedunculopontine and lateral tegmental cholinergic innervation of the thalamus in PSP [24, 25].

PSP is often characterized as a parkinsonian or a Parkinson plus condition, and there is profound slowness of movement and response, but bradykinesia in PSP is different to that in PD. In PD repeated finger taps, and other movements, show a progressive reduction in speed and amplitude, whereas in PSP there is a marked reduction in the amplitude of finger taps with concomitant micrographia, without a progressive decrement [26]. Some patients have fast, small finger taps. The micrographia of PSP may relate to the degree of involvement of the globus pallidus with lack of compensatory cerebellar input [26].

Early studies of the prevalence of PSP were based on varied clinical diagnostic criteria and in some cases PSP patients were identified within studies assessing PD and parkinsonism. Studies from Italy, the United States, and the Faroe Islands identified a PSP prevalence of between 1.4 and 4.7/100,000 [27–29]. Two UK-based studies, from the North-West of England and London, using comprehensive case ascertainment in primary care, produced very similar prevalence estimates for PSP at 6.4 and 6.5/100,000 [30, 31]. A study from Japan identified a very similar prevalence rate to the UK at 5.8/100,000, with an increased rate in men as compared to women, although this did not reach statistical significance [32]. The study based in the North-West of England demonstrated the increased level of case ascertainment achieved with community-based ascertainment, as compared to regional and national specialist studies. The incidence of PSP is difficult to establish because of the rarity of the condition, and many of the studies of incidence either pre-date the publication of the NINDS-SPSP criteria, report PSP incidence within a cohort of patients evaluated for parkinsonism, or calculate incidence based on prevalence data. Studies within PD incidence studies are likely to underestimate the incidence of PSP, since some patients may be receiving treatment for primary balance or ophthalmologic disorders, particularly in the early stages of the disease. Estimates of the incidence of PSP range from 0.1/100,000/year to 1.1/100,000/year, both from direct incidence studies and extrapolated from prevalence data [33, 34]. The large UK national cohort identified a median age at onset for PSP of 66 (range 41–83) years with no significant differences between male and female prevalence rates. A large cohort of over 1000 pathologically verified PSP cases was assembled for a genome-wide association study (GWAS) and the mean age of onset for PSP in this study was 68 years, with 55% male subjects. The median survival for PSP patients is between 5 and 7 years; features indicating rapid progression, for example the development of swallowing problems in the first two years of disease, are associated with a worse prognosis [10]. About two-thirds of PSP patients die from respiratory related causes and there is a higher death rate in the winter months [35]. PSP is under-recorded on death certificates, and frequently respiratory disease is listed as a cause of death without any reference to the underlying neurodegenerative problem [36, 37].

Misdiagnosis and delay in diagnosis is a major problem. In the North-West of England community study 41% of PSP patients had an initial incorrect diagnosis such as PD, cerebrovascular disease, or normal pressure hydrocephalus before the eventual correct diagnosis of PSP [31].

Spectrum of the clinical phenotype

Two comprehensive reviews have addressed the clinical diversity associated with PSP pathology [1, 38]. In the landmark Queen Square Brain Bank study of Williams and colleagues, 68% of patients with a post mortem diagnosis of PSP fell into a clinically typical PSP group, which the researchers named PSP-Richardson's syndrome (PSP-RS). The majority of the remainder of the cases had atypical clinical features and were categorized as PSP-parkinsonism (PSP-P) [6]. PSP-P may involve a partial response to levodopa, tremor, asymmetry, and dystonia but unlike Lewy body disorders it is not associated with levodopa-induced dyskinesias or visual hallucinations [6, 39]. Although a gait and balance disorder is not an early feature of PSP-P, this emerges in time with 60% of patients developing frequent falls 6 years after disease onset and 50% becoming wheelchair dependent within 9 years [23]. PSP-P progresses less rapidly than PSP-RS, with a mean disease duration of 12 years as compared to 6 years for PSP-RS in the Queen Square Brain Bank study [23]. It appears that PSP-P is initially similar to PD, but then involves an early loss of levodopa response with the development of a gait and balance disorder. Further prospective studies will be needed in unselected parkinsonism cohorts to evaluate the frequency and clinical course of PSP-P. PSP pathology is also associated with other clinical syndromes. One percent of patients archived in the Queen Square Brain Bank were defined as having pure akinesia with gait freezing (PAGF), and the vast majority of these cases had PSP pathology. PAGF involves a primary gait disorder, often with micrographia and relatively little upper limb bradykinesia and stiffness [40].

A variety of cortical syndromes can be associated with PSP pathology including behavioral variant FTD (PSP-bvFTD), primary lateral sclerosis (PSP-PLS), corticobasal syndrome (PSP-CBS), and progressive apraxia of speech (PSP-AOS) [1, 38, 41–45]. PSP pathology can therefore be associated with brainstem predominant clinical syndromes (PSP-P, PSP-PAGF), PSP-RS with both brainstem and cortical disease, and cortical predominant syndromes (PSP-bvFTD, PSP-CBS, and PSP-AOS) [38]. As expected, these clinical variants are associated with variation in topographic and molecular pathology, although clinicopathological correlation studies have usually been based on small numbers of selected cases. In terms of brainstem predominant syndromes there is a further variant of PSP pathology known as pallido-nigro-luysian atrophy, associated with the formation of axonal spheroids in the globus pallidus and substantia nigra, which has been particularly associated with PAGF [46].

In terms of heterogeneity within the clinical rubric of PSP-RS, this has been related principally to neuropsychology. Schofield and colleagues have described variant clinical features in PSP patients including language difficulties relating to pathology in Broca's area, and visuospatial impairment related to pathology in the supramarginal gyrus [15]. Clearly there may be an overlap between cases of PSP-RS with defined neuropsychological deficits beyond frontal executive dysfunction, and the cortical variants of PSP described in the previous paragraph.

Pathology

Histopathology

A variety of macroscopic pathological changes are seen at autopsy and with the development of increasingly precise neuroimaging these are likely to become increasingly important in diagnosis and in tracking disease progression in life. There is atrophy of the brainstem, particularly the midbrain tectum, pons, and superior cerebellar peduncle [47]. The substantia nigra is depigmented, with atrophy and discoloration of the subthalamic nucleus. There is enlargement of the cerebral aqueduct and third ventricle.

Microscopically, PSP is characterized by the formation of tau-containing neurofibrillary tangles which can be visualized with silver staining, such as Gallyas stains, or with immunocytochemistry using antibodies that recognize phosphorylated tau. Neurofibrillary degeneration affects multiple brain areas and is usually most pronounced in the subthalamic nucleus, substantia nigra, and globus pallidus [7, 48]. The involvement of the substantia nigra shows a different pattern to PD. In PD there is particular involvement of the ventro-lateral tier of the substantia nigra pars compacta, whereas in PSP there is involvement of the dorsal and ventro-medial parts together with involvement of the substantia nigra pars reticulata [49]. There is less severe involvement of the thalamus and striatum, and variable involvement of the cortex. Multiple areas of the brainstem are affected including the midbrain tectum and tegmentum and pontine and medullary tegmentum [48]. The cerebellar dentate nucleus undergoes grumose (grainy) degeneration with dentate neurons surrounded by degenerating presynaptic terminals. Specific glial pathology is seen in PSP, with tau-positive tufted astrocytes seen particularly in the putamen and cortex, so that there is a distinct distribution of neuronal and glial tau pathology (Figure 8.1). In addition to tufted astrocytes, oligodendroglial coiled bodies are frequent, with tau-positive threads common in the diencephalon and brainstem. The glial pathology of PSP contrasts with the glial pathology of corticobasal degeneration (CBD), in which oligodendroglial coiled bodies are less frequent and threads are predominantly seen in glial white matter [38, 47]. Additionally CBD pathology does not display prominent tufted astrocytes but instead astrocytic plaques, with the accumulation of tau in more distal astrocytic processes [50].

The number of diverse clinical and pathological forms of PSP and the relative rarity of the disease make it difficult to define a pathological staging system. However, an important study from the Banner Sun Health Research Institute described a series of elderly individuals with incidental PSP pathology and compared the findings to patients with clinical typical PSP [51]. Over 6% of neurologically unaffected elderly individuals recruited to the brain and body donation program had PSP-type neuropathology. The most significant differences between incidental and clinical PSP cases related to Gallyas-positive pathology, gliosis, and neuronal loss in the putamen, globus pallidus, and subthalamic nucleus, confirming that these areas are the most severely affected and most relevant to clinically defined PSP [51].

There are clinical and pathological overlaps between PSP and post-encephalitic parkinsonism, the parkinsonism dementia complex of Guam, FTD with parkinsonism linked to chromosome 17 with *MAPT* mutations (FTDP-17T), post-traumatic parkinsonism, and a variant of PSP identified on the island of Guadeloupe. Many of these conditions involve axial parkinsonism, a prominent gait and balance disorder, and a supranuclear gaze palsy with prominent tau neurofibrillary degeneration [52, 53]. However, there are differences in the molecular pathology and probable etiology as outlined below.

Molecular pathology

The tau (*MAPT*) gene encodes the microtubule binding protein tau, which is alternatively spliced to form six different isoforms varying in the presence of exons 2, 3, and 10 [54, 55]. Exon 10 encodes

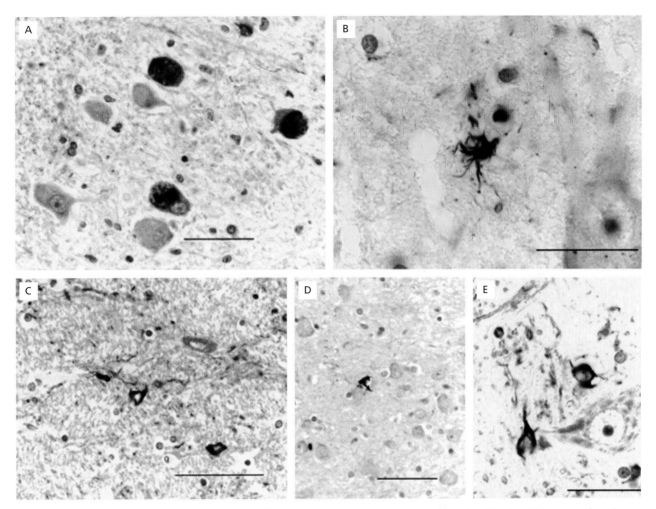

Figure 8.1 Histopathology of progressive supranuclear palsy.(A) Anti-tau antibody staining intraneuronal "globose" tangles within neurons from the peri-aqueductal gray area of the midbrain. (B) Anti-tau antibody staining "coiled" inclusions within oligodendroglia from white matter in brainstem. (C) Gallyas silver stain demonstrating an astrocyte with "tufted" morphology. (D) Gallyas silver stain demonstrating a thorny astrocyte from white matter in brainstem. (E) Gallyas stain demonstrating two intraglial inclusions adjacent to a neuron. Courtesy of Dr. Jim Neal, Department of Pathology, University Hospital of Wales, Cardiff, UK.

a potential fourth microtubule binding domain, so that tau iso-forms containing exon 10 are known as four-repeat tau (4R tau) and those without exon 10 are known as three-repeat tau (3R tau). In normal human brain there is a 1:1 ratio of 3R to 4R tau. PSP is defined pathologically by the neuronal and glial deposition of insoluble phosphorylated tau, recognized by antibodies specific for phosphorylated tau such as AT8 [56]. At the electron microscopic level the tau deposits consist predominantly of straight filaments with a 15 nm diameter. Western blot analysis of insoluble tau in Alzheimer's disease brain identifies three major hyperphosphorylated bands at 60, 64, and 68 kDa. In PSP only two bands are seen, at 64 and 68 kDa, and dephosphorylation analysis indicates that this protein is made up almost exclusively of 4R tau [57–60]. More recently, specific antibodies have been developed that recognize either 4R or 3R tau and confirm that PSP pathology is comprised primarily of 4R tau [61]. There is regional variation in tau isoform deposition in PSP. Work carried out by Luk and colleagues, using a 3R/4R sandwich enzyme-linked immunosorbent assay (ELISA), showed that frontal cortex and caudate had increased levels of 4R tau as compared with occipital cortex, an area free of PSP pathology [62].

A further study looked at 3R and 4R MAPT RNA using reverse transcription polymerase chain reaction (rtPCR), and soluble and insoluble 3R and 4R tau protein using specific 3R and 4R anti-bodies [63]. Analysis of the caudate nucleus, specifically affected by PSP pathology, confirmed an increase in both 4R *MAPT* RNA and 4R tau protein with a 4R:3R ratio of 3–4:1. Importantly, insoluble tau isolated by high-speed centrifugation from PSP caudate nucleus consisted almost exclusively of 4R tau protein. The predominant pathological expression of 4R tau immediately suggests a link to some forms of FTDP-17T. In FTDP-17T there are both coding and non-coding autosomal dominant mutations in *MAPT* which lead to an autosomal dominant tauopathy with both FTD and parkin-sonism. Most mutations are located in the microtubule domains encoded by exons 9, 10, 11, and 12. The non-coding mutations are clustered around the alternatively spliced exon 10 intron/exon junction or within exonic splice enhancer elements, and affect exon 10 splicing [64, 65]. For example, the commonest *MAPT* mutation identified in FTDP-17T families in the UK is the *MAPT* exon 10+16 mutation [64, 66, 67]. This disease leads to extensive neuronal and glial deposition of 4R tau protein. The mutation does not affect the amino acid sequence of tau but alters the 4R:3R ratio from 1:1 to between 2 and 4:1 [68]. The similarity between *MAPT* splicing and tau isoform deposition in FTDP-17T and PSP suggests that there may be an overlap in the molecular pathogenesis.

Tau and neurodegeneration in PSP

Although coding and splicing mutations in *MAPT* are pathogenic and there is extensive tau deposition in FTDP-17T and PSP, the link between tau and neurodegeneration is not completely understood. Coding mutations in *MAPT* are thought to lead to a loss of microtubule binding, potentially leading to an increase in free tau, which may form toxic fibrils. Mutant tau has generally been shown to form insoluble fibrils more readily than wild-type tau [69, 70]. However, these factors are unlikely to be directly important in PSP, where the tau has normal sequence. The earliest pathogenic mechanism in PSP and in FTDP-17 with splice mutations appears to be alteration in the tau 4R:3R ratio. The reasons for the toxicity of an increased 4R:3R ratio are unknown but there are several possible mechanisms, which may act in concert: (i) 4R tau is more prone to aggregation than 3R tau and this may lead to the formation of toxic species [70], and (ii) 4R tau binds to microtubules more avidly than 3R tau so that an increase in 4R tau may lead to an interruption in the normal turnover and plasticity of microtubules [71, 72]. Post-translational modification of tau may also be important either as a primary mechanism or as a consequence of abnormalities in intracellular tau. Abnormal phosphorylation of tau occurs in both Alzheimer's disease (AD) and PSP. Phosphorylation of tau leads to a reduction in microtubule binding, which can be regained on dephosphorylation [73]. Recently, other forms of post-translational modification have been identified which may be relevant to the pathogenesis of PSP and related disorders. Tau in PSP is acetylated at a lysine residue (K280) and this also impairs microtubule binding and increases the likelihood of fibrillization [74].

The identification of Lewy body like structures in transplanted fetal neurons in PD has increased the interest in the possibility of cell to cell transmission in neurodegenerative disease neuropathology, in a "prion-like" fashion [75]. Recently, it has been shown that tau pathology can be transmitted from transgenic mice expressing the P301L mutant tau, to mice expressing wild-type human tau by direct injection, with spreading and propagation of fibrillar tau pathology [76]. This may represent a further mechanism by which the 4R:3R tau ratio is important in that 4R tau can seed the formation of fibrils with 4R but not 3R tau, meaning that a mixture of 4R:3R tau may be relatively resistant to the propagation of abnormal tau pathology [77].

Genetics

A number of small studies have described an increased familial recurrence risk in PSP, and there are some reported autosomal dominant PSP families, although PSP is not generally considered a familial disease [78, 79]. Some patients with FTDP-17T have very similar clinical phenotypes to PSP, which possibly confounds some studies. In general, families with FTDP-17T have bvFTD or progressive non-fluent aphasia, although some patients may have a very prominent PD-like presentation [80]. However, a series of specific *MAPT* mutations have been described as causing a PSP-like phenotype with a prominent early gait and balance disorder and a supranuclear gaze palsy. These mutations include MAPT R5L, exon 10+3, exon+16, N279K, L284R, DelN296, P301L, G303V, and S305S [80–82]. These changes include a series of mutations that affect the 4R:3R tau RNA and protein ratio. The clinical and

molecular pathological overlap between PSP and FTDP-17 helps to corroborate the link between the pathogenesis of these conditions. However, in some of these families gaze palsy and gait disturbance are late features and it is not clear how many of these families would meet NINDS-SPSP criteria for PSP. Epidemiological studies of PSP looking at multiple possible risk factors have produced inconsistent results on the relative risk. A large Dutch study showed an excess of a positive family history of dementia and particularly parkinsonism in the relatives of patients with PSP, and in 14% of cases there seemed to be a clear autosomal dominant family history [79]. Only one of these families carried a *MAPT* gene mutation (P301L), suggesting that there may be an autosomal dominant cause of PSP which is separate to FTDP-17T. This is corroborated by reports of linkage in a large PSP kindred to chromosome 1q31.1, although no further families have been linked to this region and the causative gene mutation has not been identified [83].

A significant amount of work has been carried out looking at non-Mendelian genetic susceptibility to PSP, and an increasing amount is known about this area. In 1997 Conrad and colleagues reported an association between a microsatellite marker in *MAPT* and PSP, and this finding was widely replicated in Caucasian samples in relatively small sample sets [84, 85]. Baker and colleagues showed that the associated A0 allele occurred on an extended MAPT haplotype known as the H1 haplotype which accounted for 93% of PSP haplotypes as compared to 78% of control haplotypes [86]. The haplotype was originally described as a 100 kb haplotype spanning MAPT, but it has subsequently been identified as part of a large 900 kb inversion on chromosome 17q21 [87, 88]. The inversion is likely to have originated in Africa, with the most recent common ancestor dated to between 14,000 and 108,000 years ago [88]. The H2 haplotype is now associated with European ancestry and it becomes progressively less common in admixed populations. The H2 haplotype frequency is 20–29% in a range of populations from the Orkneys to the Middle East with an H2 haplotype frequency of <1% in South American, South African, and Asian populations [89]. Theoretically this should mean that PSP is more common in Asian populations but this has not been corroborated by epidemiological studies to date [32]. The H1 haplotype is also associated with other 4R tauopathies including CBD and argyrophilic grain disease, but not 3R tauopathies such as Pick's disease [90–92].

Pittman and colleagues have further refined the association between MAPT and PSP, and shown that there are separate association signals at the tau locus [93]. The primary association between MAPT and PSP relates to the H1/H2 haplotypes, defined by a series of single nucleotide polymorphisms (SNPs) and an insertion/deletion polymorphism. The H2 haplotype occurs on 21% of control chromosomes as compared to 6% of PSP chromosomes. There is also a distinct H1 sub-haplotype designated H1c which is a risk factor for PSP and occurs on 11% of control chromosomes and 23% of PSP chromosomes [94]. The links between the MAPT susceptibility alleles and the development of disease remain uncertain, however there is evidence supporting both an increased level of tau expression and an increase in the expression of 4R-containing tau isoforms [95–97].

A large GWAS of genetic susceptibility to PSP was completed by Höglinger and colleagues, allowing a hypothesis-free approach to genetic variants that increase the risk of PSP [98]. The first study phase included 1114 pathologically confirmed PSP cases and 3816 controls, and the replication stage included 1051 clinically and pathologically diagnosed cases. Four loci were strongly associated with the risk of developing PSP, assigned to the STX6, EIF2AK3, MOBP, and MAPT genes, all reaching significance levels of $<5 \times 10^{-8}$. At the MAPT locus following controlling for the H1 haplotype, by conditional analysis on the rs8070723 allele, there was a residual association effect conferred by the rs242557 allele. This finding effectively corroborates the findings of Pittman and colleagues with respect to two association signals present at MAPT, relating to both the H1/H2 haplotypes defined by rs8070723 and the H1c haplotype, tagged by rs242557.

The association of three novel genes with PSP is an exciting finding which provides new insights into the pathogenesis of the disease. Two of the proteins are implicated in protein quality control mechanisms and one in the structure of brainstem white matter. *STX6* encodes syntaxin-6, a SNARE class protein localized to the *trans*-Golgi network and endoplasmic reticulum (ER). It is thought to have a role in vesicle formation and in targeting abnormal proteins for lysosomal degradation [98]. It has previously been shown to have a role in regulating the levels of the cell surface cystic fibrosis transmembrane conductance regulator [99]. Eukaryotic translation initiation factor 2 α kinase 3 (*EIF2AK3*), also known as PKR-like endoplasmic reticulum kinase (PERK), is a component of the ER unfolded protein response (UPR). Autosomal recessive mutations in *EIF2AK3* lead to a rare infantile condition (Wolcott–Rallison syndrome) characterized by diabetes and skeletal dysplasia [100]. PERK is activated when unfolded proteins accumulate in the ER and phosphorylates EIF-2α leading to suppression of protein translation. This stress response is thought to facilitate the clearance of abnormal proteins. *MOBP* encodes the oligodendrocyte protein MOBP, which is highly expressed in the white matter of the pons, medulla, cerebellum, and midbrain, implicating for the first time a primary abnormality of white matter in the pathogenesis of PSP.

Environment

There is no definitive evidence on the role of environmental factors in the pathogenesis of PSP. Two small retrospective studies have been carried out including 50 and 79 PSP patients. Possible associations were reported with living in sparsely populated areas and meat consumption, but these have not been replicated [101, 102]. It is clear that there are likely to be environmental risk factors for other related tauopathies such as repetitive head injury in boxers with post-traumatic parkinsonism, and exposure to tropical plants, specifically neurotoxic alkaloids, in atypical parkinsonism on Guadeloupe, but it is not clear whether these risk factors are relevant to patients with PSP [53].

Clinical prodrome and biomarkers

The commonest prodromal symptoms in PSP relate to relatively nonspecific symptoms such as personality or behavioral change. The frequency of PSP means that it is difficult to establish a PSP prodrome in epidemiologically representative cohorts.

A crucial part of the development of new treatments in PSP will be the ability to track longitudinal change in PSP using clinical rating scales or para-clinical biomarkers. A number of scales/biomarkers have been studied in PSP as an adjunct to diagnosis and as a possible aid in the assessment of disease progression. Scales used for Parkinson disease, such as the unified Parkinson disease rating scale (UPDRS) do not capture the specific deficits of PSP. The PSP rating scale (PSP-RS) was developed as a longitudinal scale by Golbe and colleagues to evaluate PSP with a 100-point scale including domains relating to daily activities, behavior, bulbar, ocular motor, and limb motor function [103]. The PSP-RS performs well in tracking disease with a mean increase of 11.3 (±11 points) per year [103]. PSP-RS

scores are a good predictor of disease progression and mortality, with subjects having a PSP-RS of >70 having a 47% 1-year survival. A more recent study that combined serial imaging with serial measures of the PSP-RS reported an even more rapid decline in PSP-RS over time, with an 18-point increase in the PSP-RS over a 12-month period [104]. A specific PSP quality of life scale has been developed (PSP-QoL) with excellent psychometric properties which correlates with disease severity and progression but data on longitudinal progression have not yet been reported [105]. MRI may identify the macroscopic pathological features of PSP and is important in helping to rule out alternative diagnoses [106, 107]. The identified features include the "hummingbird" sign, related to midbrain atrophy with tapering of the midbrain on sagittal MR images, and the "morning glory flower" sign with a concave appearance of the midbrain tegmentum on axial images. About 75% of PSP cases can be diagnosed using MR imaging, blind to the clinical diagnosis [107]. Useful imaging features relate to midbrain atrophy. Two studies have looked at longitudinal changes in volumetric brain imaging over time and report a progressive loss of total brain volume and specific progressive atrophy in thalamus, midbrain, and superior cerebellar peduncle [104, 108, 109]. These studies suggest that progressive MRI volumetric measures could be used as a surrogate marker, which would enable short-term PSP treatment trials with smaller numbers of patients [104, 109]. CSF biomarkers have been studied principally as an adjunct to diagnosis, and there are reports of an increase in CSF tau levels in CBD as compared to PSP. Borroni and colleagues have identified a reduction in a truncated tau species in PSP cerebrospinal fluid (CSF), but this has not been replicated [110–113]. It is likely that, with increasing sophistication both in measuring different tau isoforms and their post-translational modification, there will be more specific and sensitive CSF biomarkers for PSP CSF. Ideally, we would be able to validate future therapeutic approaches to PSP using changes in CSF tau biochemistry.

Examination and investigations

The examination of a suspected PSP patient will include the usual assessment of tone, rigidity, bradykinesia, tremor, and gait used in the movement disorders clinic. However, there are parts of the examination that are worth emphasizing as being particularly important in the diagnosis and differential diagnosis of PSP. Traditionally PSP is described as a Parkinson plus condition although in movement disorders practice CBD, multiple system atrophy, cortical Lewy body disease, and frontal gait disorders due to vascular disease are the most relevant differential diagnoses [5]. A clinical assessment of patients suspected to have PSP should involve: (i) cognitive assessment including evaluation for the presence of frontal lobe features, specifically the examination of initial letter verbal fluency; (ii) careful assessment of eyelid and ocular motility, including a bedside assessment of saccadic latency and velocity; (iii) specific assessment of neck rigidity in addition to the normal assessment of limb tone; (iv) evaluation of gait, balance, and posture including standing and sitting, step size, and tendency to fall; and (v) assessment of bradykinesia looking for the small-amplitude finger taps characteristically seen in PSP [114]. The condition most commonly confused with PSP is CBD so the presence of ocular apraxia (with delay in initiation of normal velocity saccades), cortical sensory loss (assessed with graphesthesia, joint position sense, and stereognosis), clinically significant asymmetry, and dystonia should be carefully assessed. Having said this, some of these features may occur in patients with pathologically confirmed PSP, but not typical PSP-RS, so the distinction between these conditions may not be straightforward. Pragmatically, patients should be clinically defined as having either a PSP-RS phenotype or a corticobasal syndrome phenotype. Other conditions reported to cause vertical supranuclear gaze palsies and/or mimic PSP include midbrain tumors, neurosyphilis, Creutzfeldt–Jakob disease, some spinocerebellar ataxias, particularly SCA7, Whipple's disease, and cerebral autosomal dominant arteriopathy with subcortical infarcts and leukoencephalopathy (CADASIL) [115–118]. Appropriate imaging, genetic tests, and CSF analysis may be necessary to exclude these conditions. MR imaging may provide support for the diagnosis of PSP with midbrain and superior cerebellar peduncle atrophy but a reportedly normal MRI scan does not exclude the diagnosis of PSP. As indicated above, MR imaging shows promise as a biomarker for tracking the progression of PSP. The different pattern of involvement of nigro-striatal pathways in PSP leads to a different pattern in dopaminergic denervation using functional imaging. PSP cases have greater denervation of the caudate, and more symmetric denervation using dopaminergic imaging, than do PD cases where there is relatively selective involvement of the posterior putamen [119]. Fluorodeoxyglucose positron emission tomography (FDG-PET) can be used to map differences in regional metabolism in PSP. PSP cases with a classical gait and balance disorder (PSP-RS) have marked thalamic hypometabolism, consistent with the hypothesis that cholinergic denervation of the thalamus is associated with a gait and balance disorder in PSP [24].

Diagnosis and prognosis

The diagnosis of PSP is clinical based on appropriate clinical features and the exclusion of alternative diagnoses. At the moment functional, structural, and CSF biomarkers are not included as adjuncts to clinical diagnosis, aside from excluding alternative diseases, but it is likely that this situation will change in the future.

The NINDS-SPSP research diagnostic criteria are a valuable guide to diagnosis but in movement disorders clinics many physicians will make a clinical diagnosis of PSP in patients who have a delayed gait and balance disorder and who do not meet the strict NINDS-PSP diagnostic criteria. This approach is supported by the existence of late gait and balance disorders in PSP-P, the sensitivity and specificity of the NNIPPS clinical diagnostic criteria, and the reports of a prodromal cognitive-behavioral syndrome in some patients, before the development of a gait and balance disorder. PSP is an inexorably progressive condition with a median survival of 7 years. The progression of the disease as measured by the PSP-RS and by the emergence of clinical milestones is associated with a reduced life expectancy.

Treatments

The mainstay of treatment in PSP is the provision of appropriate support and social care, and the avoidance of complications associated with dysphagia and immobility. Many patients develop weight loss, respiratory infections, and aspiration pneumonia together with injuries and complications related to fractures and falls; many of these complications can be avoided with good multi-disciplinary care. Many clinicians suggest a trial of levodopa and/or amantadine, but although there are anecdotal and retrospective reports of effectiveness there is no randomized controlled trial evidence

of their value [120]. Local botulinum toxin injections can be used to treat eyelid disorders in PSP, which for some patients can cause significant functional disability. There have been relatively few trials of disease-modifying therapy in PSP. The NNIPPS study was successful in recruiting and randomizing 362 PSP patients from across Europe, and produced a wealth of data on the clinical features and natural history of this condition, which are referred to throughout this chapter [3]. However, treatment with riluzole did not alter the natural history of PSP in this trial. Approximately 50% of the PSP patients recruited died over the 3-year follow-up period of the NNIPPS study, confirming the malignant natural history of this condition. Many patients and their families benefit from information and support from patient organizations such as CurePSP and the PSP Association and these charities also provide the opportunity to meet with other patients and families affected by this condition. The patient advocacy organizations emphasize the importance of review by occupational therapists, physiotherapists speech and language therapists, and dieticians with experience of PSP and the appropriate expertise to provide therapeutic interventions. As the condition progresses dysphagia becomes increasingly important and nearly all patients will need advice on appropriate diet and strategies to maintain nutrition and avoid respiratory tract infections. Some patients opt to have percutaneous gastrostomy (PEG) feeding and this seems to improve quality of life. Increasingly, palliative care teams are involved in providing symptom control and respite care for patients with PSP and their families.

Future developments

The clinical nosology of PSP is becoming increasingly complex and there are clinical overlaps both with other tauopathies and with other disorders that can cause related clinical syndromes. For example, TDP43-positive neuropathology and Alzheimer's disease can cause corticobasal syndromes (CBS) so within the rubric of CBS come CBD, PSP-CBS, CBS with TDP43-positive neuropathology, and CBS with AD neuropathology. Prospective clinical studies involving the use of standardized clinical data collection will become important in developing the most accurate clinical picture of these disorders. It is likely that CSF analysis and imaging will become increasingly useful in defining the neuropathology. For example, PET-based amyloid imaging and CSF amyloid and tau analysis might be useful in defining CBS due to AD.

The publication of the GWAS study in PSP has raised the possibility that primary abnormalities in the heat shock/translation inhibition response and the clearance of misfolded proteins may have a central role in PSP pathogenesis. It will be important to establish whether these pathways have any specificity for tau-related pathology. Similarly an important next step is to discover whether there is any relationship between the cellular susceptibility to PSP and the expression of MOBP.

The overlap between tau pathology in PSP and AD combined with the lack of success of anti-amyloid therapies in AD to date has increased the interest in the development of anti-tau therapies in PSP and related conditions. The major areas in the development of tau therapies have been summarized in a number of reviews [70, 121, 122]. Potential therapeutic approaches include the use of: (i) microtubule stabilizing agents; (ii) tau kinase inhibitors or phosphatase enhancers; (iii) anti-tau aggregation therapy; (iv) tau aggregate clearance agents; and (v) agents that improve mitochondrial function. Most interest has focused on the use of tau kinase inhibitors, based on the loss of microtubule binding and possible increased tau aggregation related to phosphorylation at serine/threonine-proline sites across tau protein. Administration of lithium, a GSK-3 inhibitor, to transgenic tau P301L mutant mice led to a reduction in tau hyperphosphorylation, neurofibrillary tangle formation, and axonal degeneration [123]. However, within the NINDS study of lithium in PSP patients the primary endpoint of patient tolerability was not reached as only 1 of 14 patients was able to tolerate a full 28-week course of lithium (www .clinicaltrials.gov). There are further trials which have studied the potential therapeutic effect of further tau kinase inhibitors including sodium valproate and tideglusib (www.clinicaltrials.gov). These relatively small studies recruited 28 patients and 146 patients respectively and neither has shown a disease-modifying effect of these agents [124, 125]. Stabilization of microtubules is an attractive potential therapy for PSP. A number of taxol-related compounds which stabilize microtubules, such as paclitaxel, are in clinical use as chemotherapeutic agents, however the use of these drugs is likely to be limited by side effects such as neutropenia and polyneuropathy. The octapeptide NAP (davunetide) has microtubule-stabilizing effects and leads to a reduction in tau phosphorylation. Use of davunetide in a double transgenic tau mouse model leads to an improvement in cognitive function and a decrease in tau phosphorylation and the formation of insoluble tau. A large randomized controlled trial of davunetide in PSP has not demonstrated a benefit from davunetide treatment [126]. Tau degradation can occur through the ubiquitin proteasome system or through macroautophagy. Chaperones are important in the direction of abnormal proteins for proteasomal degradation and the HSP70/carboxy terminus of HSP70-interacting protein (HSP/CHIP70) complex appears to be important in regulating tau degradation [127]. Inhibition of HSP90 leads to chaperone induction and increased activity of the HSP70/CHIP complex and represents a further potential avenue for tau therapeutics. Recently, there has been increased interest in macroautophagy, which may be an important route for degradation of abnormal large tau aggregates; positive preclinical studies have been carried out with rapamycin, which is a potent inducer of macroautophagy [128]. Methylthioninium chloride is an inhibitor of tau aggregation which may be helpful in PSP, and this is currently under evaluation as a therapy for Alzheimer's disease [129]. A further potentially important therapeutic area is mitochondrial function. Patients with PSP have evidence of complex 1 deficiency on analysis of cybrids derived from patient platelets [130]. A small randomized trial of coenzyme Q10 has shown positive results in PSP patients and further larger scale trials are ongoing [131].

Conclusions

There has been a dramatic increase in our knowledge of PSP over the last 10 years, related to clinicopathological studies, the identification of *MAPT* mutations, large-scale collaborative GWAS studies, and an increasing interest in tau therapeutics. There are an increasing number of therapeutic trials in progress for PSP, particularly focusing on disease-modifying therapies, and this has led to optimism that new disease-modifying therapies can be developed. In parallel it will be important to develop and improve support and care for PSP patients and their families.

Acknowledgement

Professor Huw Morris is supported by the PSP Association and CBD Solutions.

References

1. Williams DR, Lees AJ. Progressive supranuclear palsy: clinicopathological concepts and diagnostic challenges. *The Lancet Neurology*. 2009 Mar;8(3):270–9.
2. Litvan I, Agid Y, Calne D, Campbell G, Dubois B, Duvoisin R, et al. Clinical research criteria for the diagnosis of progressive supranuclear palsy (Steele-Richardson-Olszewski syndrome): report of the NINDS-SPSP international workshop. *Neurology*. 1996 Jul;47(1):1–9.
3. Bensimon G, Ludolph A, Agid Y, Vidailhet M, Payan C, Leigh PN. Riluzole treatment, survival and diagnostic criteria in Parkinson plus disorders: the NNIPPS study. *Brain : a journal of neurology*. 2009 Jan;132(Pt 1):156–71.
4. Hughes AJ, Daniel SE, Ben-Shlomo Y, Lees AJ. The accuracy of diagnosis of parkinsonian syndromes in a specialist movement disorder service. *Brain : a journal of neurology*. 2002 Apr;125(Pt 4):861–70.
5. Josephs KA, Dickson DW. Diagnostic accuracy of progressive supranuclear palsy in the Society for Progressive Supranuclear Palsy brain bank. *Movement disorders : official journal of the Movement Disorder Society*. 2003 Sep;18(9):1018–26.
6. Williams DR, de Silva R, Paviour DC, Pittman A, Watt HC, Kilford L, et al. Characteristics of two distinct clinical phenotypes in pathologically proven progressive supranuclear palsy: Richardson's syndrome and PSP-parkinsonism. *Brain : a journal of neurology*. 2005 Jun;128(Pt 6):1247–58.
7. Richardson JC, Steele J, Olszewski J. Supranuclear ophthalmoplegia, pseudobulbar palsy, nuchal dystonia and dementia. A clinical report on eight cases of "heterogenous system degeneration". *Transactions of the American Neurological Association*. 1963 Jan;88:25–9.
8. Steele JC, Richardson JC, Olszewski J. Progressive supranuclear palsy. A heterogeneous degeneration involving the brain stem, basal ganglia and cerebellum with vertical gaze and pseudobulbar palsy, nuchal dystonia and dementia. *Archives of neurology*. 1964 Apr;10:333–59.
9. Litvan I, Bhatia KP, Burn DJ, Goetz CG, Lang AE, McKeith I, et al. SIC task force appraisal of clinical diagnostic criteria for parkinsonian disorders. *Movement Disorders*. 2003;18(5):467–86.
10. Nath U, Ben-Shlomo Y, Thomson RG, Lees AJ, Burn DJ. Clinical features and natural history of progressive supranuclear palsy: A clinical cohort study. *Neurology*. 2003 Mar 25;60(6):910–6.
11. Donker Kaat L, Boon AJ, Kamphorst W, Ravid R, Duivenvoorden HJ, van Swieten JC. Frontal presentation in progressive supranuclear palsy. *Neurology*. 2007 Aug 21; 69(8):723–9.
12. Albert ML, Feldman RG, Willis AL. The "subcortical dementia" of progressive supranuclear palsy. *Journal of neurology, neurosurgery, and psychiatry*. 1974 Feb;37(2):121–30.
13. Brown RG, Lacomblez L, Landwehrmeyer BG, Bak T, Uttner I, Dubois B, et al. Cognitive impairment in patients with multiple system atrophy and progressive supranuclear palsy. *Brain : a journal of neurology*. 2010 Jun;133(Pt 8):2382–93.
14. Ghosh BCP, Rowe JB, Calder AJ, Hodges JR, Bak TH. Emotion recognition in progressive supranuclear palsy. *Journal of neurology, neurosurgery, and psychiatry*. 2009 Oct;80(10):1143–5.
15. Schofield EC, Hodges JR, Bak TH, Xuereb JH, Halliday GM. The relationship between clinical and pathological variables in Richardson's syndrome. *Journal of neurology*. 2012 Mar;259(3):482–90.
16. Rivaud-Péchoux S, Vidailhet M, Gallouedec G, Litvan I, Gaymard B, Pierrot-Deseilligny C. Longitudinal ocular motor study in corticobasal degeneration and progressive supranuclear palsy. *Neurology*. 2000 Mar 14;54(5):1029–32.
17. Chen AL, Riley DE, King SA, Joshi AC, Serra A, Liao K, et al. The disturbance of gaze in progressive supranuclear palsy: implications for pathogenesis. *Frontiers in neurology*. 2010 Jan;1:1–19.
18. Murdin L, Bronstein AM. Head deviation in progressive supranuclear palsy: enhanced vestibulo-collic reflex or loss of resetting head movements? Journal of neurology. 2009 Jul;256(7):1143–5.
19. Juncos JL, Hirsch EC, Malessa S, Duyckaerts C, Hersh LB, Agid Y. Mesencephalic cholinergic nuclei in progressive supranuclear palsy. *Neurology*. 1991 Jan;41(1):25–30.
20. Bologna M, Agostino R, Gregori B, Belvisi D, Ottaviani D, Colosimo C, et al. Voluntary, spontaneous and reflex blinking in patients with clinically probable progressive supranuclear palsy. *Brain : a journal of neurology*. 2009 Feb;132 (Pt 2):502–10.
21. Yoon WT, Chung EJ, Lee SH, Kim BJ, Lee WY. Clinical analysis of blepharospasm and apraxia of eyelid opening in patients with parkinsonism. *Journal of clinical neurology (Seoul, Korea)*. 2005 Oct;1(2):159–65.
22. Friedman DI, Jankovic J, McCrary JA. Neuro-ophthalmic findings in progressive supranuclear palsy. *Journal of clinical neuro-ophthalmology*. 1992 Jun;12(2):104–9.
23. O'Sullivan SS, Massey LA, Williams DR, Silveira-Moriyama L, Kempster PA, Holton JL, et al. Clinical outcomes of progressive supranuclear palsy and multiple system atrophy. *Brain : a journal of neurology*. 2008 May;131(Pt 5):1362–72.

24. Srulijes K, Reimold M, Liscic RM, Bauer S, Dietzel E, Liepelt-Scarfone I, et al. Fluorodeoxyglucose positron emission tomography in Richardson's syndrome and progressive supranuclear palsy-parkinsonism. *Movement disorders : official journal of the Movement Disorder Society.* 2012 Jan;27(1):151–5.

25. Hirano S, Shinotoh H, Shimada H, Aotsuka A, Tanaka N, Ota T, et al. Cholinergic imaging in corticobasal syndrome, progressive supranuclear palsy and frontotemporal dementia. *Brain : a journal of neurology.* 2010 Jul;133(Pt 7):2058–68.

26. Ling H, Massey LA, Lees AJ, Brown P, Day BL. Hypokinesia without decrement distinguishes progressive supranuclear palsy from Parkinson's disease. *Brain : a journal of neurology.* 2012 Apr;135(Pt 4):1141–53.

27. Wermuth L, Joensen P, Bünger N, Jeune B. High prevalence of Parkinson's disease in the Faroe Islands. *Neurology.* 1997 Aug;49(2):426–32.

28. Golbe LI, Davis PH, Schoenberg BS, Duvoisin RC. Prevalence and natural history of progressive supranuclear palsy. *Neurology.* 1988 Jul;38(7):1031–4.

29. Chiò A, Magnani C, Schiffer D. Prevalence of Parkinson's disease in Northwestern Italy: comparison of tracer methodology and clinical ascertainment of cases. *Movement disorders : official journal of the Movement Disorder Society.* 1998 May;13(3):400–5.

30. Schrag A, Ben-Shlomo Y, Quinn NP. Prevalence of progressive supranuclear palsy and multiple system atrophy: a cross-sectional study. *Lancet.* 1999 Nov 20;354(9192):1771–5.

31. Nath U, Ben-Shlomo Y, Thomson RG, Morris HR, Wood NW, Lees AJ, et al. The prevalence of progressive supranuclear palsy (Steele-Richardson-Olszewski syndrome) in the UK. *Brain.* 2001 Jul;124(Part 7):1438–49.

32. Kawashima M, Miyake M, Kusumi M, Adachi Y, Nakashima K. Prevalence of progressive supranuclear palsy in Yonago, Japan. *Movement disorders : official journal of the Movement Disorder Society.* 2004 Oct;19(10):1239–40.

33. Winter Y, Bezdolnyy Y, Katunina E, Avakjan G, Reese JP, Klotsche J, et al. Incidence of Parkinson's disease and atypical parkinsonism: Russian population-based study. *Movement disorders : official journal of the Movement Disorder Society.* 2010 Feb 15;25(3):349–56.

34. Bower JH, Maraganore DM, McDonnell SK, Rocca WA. Incidence of progressive supranuclear palsy and multiple system atrophy in Olmsted County, Minnesota, 1976 to 1990. *Neurology.* 1997 Nov;49(5):1284–8.

35. Papapetropoulos S, Singer C, McCorquodale D, Gonzalez J, Mash DC. Cause, seasonality of death and co-morbidities in progressive supranuclear palsy (PSP). *Parkinsonism & related disorders.* 2005 Nov;11(7):459–63.

36. Nath U, Thomson R, Wood R, Ben-Shlomo Y, Lees A, Rooney C, et al. Population based mortality and quality of death certification in progressive supranuclear palsy (Steele-Richardson-Olszewski syndrome). *Journal of neurology, neurosurgery, and psychiatry.* 2005 Apr;76(4):498–502.

37. Maxwell R, Wells C, Verne J. Under-reporting of progressive supranuclear palsy. *Lancet.* 2010 Dec 18;376(9758):2072.

38. Dickson DW, Ahmed Z, Algom AA, Tsuboi Y, Josephs KA. Neuropathology of variants of progressive supranuclear palsy. *Current opinion in neurology.* 2010 Aug;23(4):394–400.

39. Williams DR, Lees AJ. What features improve the accuracy of the clinical diagnosis of progressive supranuclear palsy-parkinsonism (PSP-P)? *Movement disorders : official journal of the Movement Disorder Society.* 2010 Feb 15;25(3):357–62.

40. Williams DR, Holton JL, Strand K, Revesz T, Lees AJ. Pure akinesia with gait freezing: a third clinical phenotype of progressive supranuclear palsy. *Movement disorders : official journal of the Movement Disorder Society.* 2007 Nov 15;22(15):2235–41.

41. Hassan A, Parisi JE, Josephs KA. Autopsy-proven progressive supranuclear palsy presenting as behavioral variant frontotemporal dementia. *Neurocase.* 2012;18(6):478–88.

42. Josephs KA, Boeve BF, Duffy JR, Smith GE, Knopman DS, Parisi JE, et al. Atypical progressive supranuclear palsy underlying progressive apraxia of speech and nonfluent aphasia. *Neurocase.* 2005 Aug;11(4):283–96.

43. Josephs KA, Katsuse O, Beccano-Kelly DA, Lin W-L, Uitti RJ, Fujino Y, et al. Atypical progressive supranuclear palsy with corticospinal tract degeneration. *Journal of neuropathology and experimental neurology.* 2006 Apr;65(4):396–405.

44. Josephs K a, Duffy JR. Apraxia of speech and nonfluent aphasia: a new clinical marker for corticobasal degeneration and progressive supranuclear palsy. *Current opinion in neurology.* 2008 Dec;21(6):688–92.

45. Papapetropoulos S, Scaravilli T, Morris H, An SF, Henderson DC, Quinn NP, et al. Young onset limb spasticity with PSP-like brain and spinal cord NFT-tau pathology. *Neurology.* 2005 Feb;64(4):731–3.

46. Ahmed Z, Josephs KA, Gonzalez J, Delledonne A, Dickson DW. Clinical and neuropathologic features of progressive supranuclear palsy with severe pallido-nigro-luysial degeneration and axonal dystrophy. *Brain.* 2008;131(Pt 2):460–72.

47. Dickson DW, Rademakers R, Hutton ML. Progressive supranuclear palsy: pathology and genetics. *Brain pathology (Zurich, Switzerland).* 2007 Jan;17(1):74–82.

48. Hauw JJ, Daniel SE, Dickson D, Horoupian DS, Jellinger K, Lantos PL, et al. Preliminary NINDS neuropathologic criteria for Steele-Richardson-Olszewski syndrome (progressive supranuclear palsy). *Neurology.* 1994 Nov;44(11):2015–9.

49. Hardman CD, Halliday GM, McRitchie DA, Cartwright HR, Morris JG. Progressive supranuclear palsy affects both the substantia nigra pars compacta and reticulata. *Experimental neurology.* 1997 Mar;144(1):183–92.

50. Komori T. Tau-positive glial inclusions in progressive supranuclear palsy, corticobasal degeneration and Pick's disease. *Brain pathology (Zurich, Switzerland).* 1999 Oct;9(4):663–79.

51. Evidente VGH, Adler CH, Sabbagh MN, Connor DJ, Hentz JG, Caviness JN, et al. Neuropathological findings of PSP in the elderly without clinical PSP: possible incidental PSP? Parkinsonism & related disorders. 2011 Jun;17(5):365–71.

52. Morris HR, Lees AJ, Wood NW. Neurofibrillary tangle parkinsonian disorders – Tau pathology and tau genetics. *Movement disorders.* 1999 Sep;14(5):731–6.

53. Geddes JF, Hughes AJ, Lees AJ, Daniel SE. Pathological overlap in cases of parkinsonism associated with neurofibrillary tangles. A study of recent cases of postencephalitic parkinsonism and comparison with progressive supranuclear palsy and Guamanian parkinsonism-dementia complex. *Brain : a journal of neurology.* 1993 Feb;116(Pt 1):281–302.

54. Andreadis A, Brown WM, Kosik KS. Structure and novel exons of the human tau gene. *Biochemistry.* 1992 Nov 3;31(43):10626–33.

55. Goedert M, Spillantini MG, Jakes R, Rutherford D, Crowther RA. Multiple isoforms of human microtubule-associated protein tau: sequences and localization in neurofibrillary tangles of Alzheimer's disease. *Neuron.* 1989 Oct;3(4):519–26.

56. Schmidt ML, Huang R, Martin JA, Henley J, Mawal-Dewan M, Hurtig HI, et al. Neurofibrillary tangles in progressive supranuclear palsy contain the same tau epitopes identified in Alzheimer's disease PHFtau. *Journal of neuropathology and experimental neurology.* 1996 May;55(5):534–9.

57. Flament S, Delacourte A, Verny M, Hauw JJ, Javoy-Agid F. Abnormal Tau proteins in progressive supranuclear palsy. Similarities and differences with the neurofibrillary degeneration of the Alzheimer type. *Acta neuropathologica.* 1991 Jan;81(6):591–6.

58. Buée L, Bussière T, Buée-Scherrer V, Delacourte A, Hof PR. Tau protein isoforms, phosphorylation and role in neurodegenerative disorders. *Brain Research Reviews.* 2000 Aug;33(1):95–130.

59. Feany MB, Dickson DW. Neurodegenerative disorders with extensive tau pathology: a comparative study and review. *Annals of neurology.* 1996 Aug;40(2):139–48.

60. Spillantini MG, Goedert M. Tau protein pathology in neurodegenerative diseases. *Trends in neurosciences.* 1998 Oct;21(10):428–33.

61. de Silva R, Lashley T, Gibb G, Hanger D, Hope A, Reid A, et al. Pathological inclusion bodies in tauopathies contain distinct complements of tau with three or four microtubule-binding repeat domains as demonstrated by new specific monoclonal antibodies. *Neuropathology and applied neurobiology.* 2003 Jun;29(3):288–302.

62. Luk C, Giovannoni G, Williams DR, Lees AJ, Silva RD. Development of a sensitive ELISA for quantification of three- and four-repeat tau isoforms in tauopathies. *Journal of Neuroscience Methods.* 2009;180:34–42.

63. Luk C, Vandrovcova J, Malzer E, Lees A, de Silva R. Brain tau isoform mRNA and protein correlation in PSP brain. *Translational Neuroscience.* 2010 Oct 12;1(1):30–6.

64. Hutton M, Lendon CL, Rizzu P, Baker M, Froelich S, Houlden H, et al. Association of missense and 5'-splice-site mutations in tau with the inherited dementia FTDP-17. *Nature.* 1998 Jun 18;393(6686):702–5.

65. D'Souza I, Poorkaj P, Hong M, Nochlin D, Lee VM, Bird TD, et al. Missense and silent tau gene mutations cause frontotemporal dementia with parkinsonism-chromosome 17 type, by affecting multiple alternative RNA splicing regulatory elements. *Proceedings of the National Academy of Sciences of the United States of America.* 1999 May 11;96(10):5598–603.

66. Pickering-Brown S, Baker M, Bird T, Trojanowski J, Lee V, Morris H, et al. Evidence of a founder effect in families with frontotemporal dementia that Harbor the tau+16 splice mutation. *American journal of medical genetics part B-Neuropsychiatric genetics.* 2004 Feb;125B(1):79–82.

67. Morris HR, Perez-Tur J, Janssen JC, Brown J, Lees AJ, Wood NW, et al. Mutation in the tau exon 10 splice site region in familiar frontotemporal dementia. *Annals of neurology.* 1999 Feb;45(2):270–1.

68. Grover A, Houlden H, Baker M, Adamson J, Lewis J, Prihar G, et al. 5' splice site mutations in tau associated with the inherited dementia FTDP-17 affect a stem-loop structure that regulates alternative splicing of exon 10. *The Journal of biological chemistry.* 1999 May 21;274(21):15134–43.

69. Goedert M, Ghetti B, Spillantini MG. Frontotemporal dementia: implications for understanding Alzheimer disease. *Cold Spring Harbor perspectives in medicine.* 2012 Feb;2(2):a006254.

70. Lee VM, Brunden KR, Hutton M, Trojanowski JQ. Developing therapeutic approaches to tau, selected kinases, and related neuronal protein targets. *Cold Spring Harbor perspectives in medicine.* 2011 Sept;1(1):a006437

71. Panda D, Samuel JC, Massie M, Feinstein SC, Wilson L. Differential regulation of microtubule dynamics by three- and four-repeat tau: implications for the onset of neurodegenerative disease. *Proceedings of the National Academy of Sciences of the United States of America.* 2003 Aug 5;100(16):9548–53.

72. Goedert M, Jakes R. Expression of separate isoforms of human tau protein: correlation with the tau pattern in brain and effects on tubulin polymerization. *The EMBO journal.* 1990 Dec;9(13):4225–30.

73. Bramblett GT, Goedert M, Jakes R, Merrick SE, Trojanowski JQ, Lee VM. Abnormal tau phosphorylation at Ser396 in Alzheimer's disease recapitulates development and contributes to reduced microtubule binding. *Neuron.* 1993 Jun;10(6):1089–99.

74. Cohen TJ, Guo JL, Hurtado DE, Kwong LK, Mills IP, Trojanowski JQ, et al. The acetylation of tau inhibits its function and promotes pathological tau aggregation. *Nature communications.* 2011 Jan;2:252.

75. Li J-Y, Englund E, Holton JL, Soulet D, Hagell P, Lees AJ, et al. Lewy bodies in grafted neurons in subjects with Parkinson's disease suggest host-to-graft disease propagation. *Nature medicine.* 2008 May;14(5):501–3.

76. Clavaguera F, Bolmont T, Crowther RA, Abramowski D, Frank S, Probst A, et al. Transmission and spreading of tauopathy in transgenic mouse brain. *Nature cell biology.* 2009 Jul;11(7):909–13.

77. Nonaka T, Watanabe ST, Iwatsubo T, Hasegawa M. Seeded aggregation and toxicity of {alpha}-synuclein and tau: cellular models of neurodegenerative diseases. *The Journal of biological chemistry.* 2010 Nov 5;285(45):34885–98.

78. Rojo A, Pernaute RS, Fontan A, Ruiz PG, Honnorat J, Lynch T, et al. Clinical genetics of familial progressive supranuclear palsy. *Brain.* 1999 Jul;122(Part 7):1233–45.

79. Donker Kaat L, Boon AJW, Azmani A, Kamphorst W, Breteler MMB, Anar B, et al. Familial aggregation of parkinsonism in progressive supranuclear palsy. *Neurology.* 2009 Jul 14;73(2):98–105.

80. Wszolek ZK, Tsuboi Y, Ghetti B, Pickering-Brown S, Baba Y, Cheshire WP. Frontotemporal dementia and parkinsonism linked to chromosome 17 (FTDP-17). *Orphanet journal of rare diseases.* 2006 Jan;1:30.

81. Rohrer JD, Paviour D, Vandrovcova J, Hodges J, de Silva R, Rossor MN. Novel L284R MAPT mutation in a family with an autosomal dominant progressive supranuclear palsy syndrome. *Neuro-degenerative diseases.* 2011 Jan;8(3):149–52.

82. Morris HR, Osaki Y, Holton J, Lees AJ, Wood NW, Revesz T, et al. Tau exon 10 +16 mutation FTDP-17 presenting clinically as sporadic young onset PSP. *Neurology.* 2003 Jul;61(1):102–4.

83. Ros R, Gómez Garre P, Hirano M, Tai YF, Ampuero I, Vidal L, et al. Genetic linkage of autosomal dominant progressive supranuclear palsy to 1q31.1. *Annals of neurology.* 2005 May;57(5):634–41.

84. Conrad C, Andreadis A, Trojanowski JQ, Dickson DW, Kang D, Chen X, et al. Genetic evidence for the involvement of tau in progressive supranuclear palsy. *Annals of neurology.* 1997 Feb;41(2):277–81.

85. Morris HR, Janssen JC, Bandmann O, Daniel SE, Rossor MN, Lees AJ, et al. The tau gene A0 polymorphism in progressive supranuclear palsy and related neurodegenerative diseases. *Journal of neurology neurosurgery and psychiatry.* 1999 May;66(5):665–7.

86. Baker M, Litvan I, Houlden H, Adamson J, Dickson D, Perez-Tur J, et al. Association of an extended haplotype in the tau gene with progressive supranuclear palsy. *Human molecular genetics.* 1999 Apr;8(4):711–5.

87. Stefansson H, Helgason A, Thorleifsson G, Steinthorsdottir V, Masson G, Barnard J, et al. A common inversion under selection in Europeans. *Nature genetics.* 2005 Feb;37(2):129–37.

88. Donnelly MP, Paschou P, Grigorenko E, Gurwitz D, Mehdi SQ, Kajuna SLB, et al. The distribution and most recent common ancestor of the 17q21 inversion in humans. *American journal of human genetics.* 2010 Feb 12;86(2):161–71.

89. Evans W, Fung HC, Steele J, Eerola J, Tienari P, Pittman A, et al. The tau H2 haplotype is almost exclusively Caucasian in origin. *Neuroscience letters.* 2004 Oct;369(3):183–5.

90. Morris HR, Baker M, Yasojima K, Houlden H, Khan MN, Wood NW, et al. Analysis of tau haplotypes in Pick's disease. *Neurology.* 2002 Aug;59(3):443–5.

91. Houlden H, Baker M, Morris HR, MacDonald N, Pickering-Brown S, Adamson J, et al. Corticobasal degeneration and progressive supranuclear palsy share a common tau haplotype. *Neurology.* 2001 Jun 26;56(12):1702–6.

92. Togo T, Sahara N, Yen S-H, Cookson N, Ishizawa T, Hutton M, et al. Argyrophilic grain disease is a sporadic 4-repeat tauopathy. *Journal of neuropathology and experimental neurology.* 2002 Jun;61(6):547–56.

93. Pittman AM, Myers AJ, Abou-Sleiman P, Fung HC, Kaleem M, Marlowe L, et al. Linkage disequilibrium fine mapping and haplotype association analysis of the tau gene in progressive supranuclear palsy and corticobasal degeneration. *Journal of medical genetics.* 2005 Nov;42(11):837–46.

94. Pittman AM, Myers AJ, Abou-sleiman P, Fung HC, Marlowe L, Duckworth J, et al. Linkage disequilibrium fine-mapping and haplotype association analysis of the tau gene in progressive supranuclear palsy and corticobasal degeneration. *Journal of medical genetics.* 2005 Nov;42(11):837–46.

95. Myers AJ, Pittman AM, Zhao AS, Rohrer K, Kaleem M, Marlowe L, et al. The MAPT H1c risk haplotype is associated with increased expression of tau and especially of 4 repeat containing transcripts. *Neurobiology of disease.* 2007 Mar;25(3):561–70.

96. Caffrey TM, Joachim C, Paracchini S, Esiri MM, Wade-Martins R. Haplotype-specific expression of exon 10 at the human MAPT locus. *Human molecular genetics.* 2006 Dec 15;15(24):3529–37.

97. Rademakers R, Melquist S, Cruts M, Theuns J, Del-Favero J, Poorkaj P, et al. High-density SNP haplotyping suggests altered regulation of tau gene expression in progressive supranuclear palsy. *Human molecular genetics.* 2005 Nov 1; 14(21):3281–92.

98. Höglinger GU, Melhem NM, Dickson DW, Sleiman PMA, Wang L-S, Klei L, et al. Identification of common variants influencing risk of the tauopathy progressive supranuclear palsy. *Nature genetics.* 2011 Jan 19;43(7):699–705.

99. Cheng J, Cebotaru V, Cebotaru L, Guggino WB. Syntaxin 6 and CAL mediate the degradation of the cystic fibrosis transmembrane conductance regulator. *Molecular biology of the cell.* 2010 Apr 1;21(7):1178–87.

100. Julier C, Nicolino M. Wolcott-Rallison syndrome. *Orphanet journal of rare diseases.* 2010 Jan;5:29.

101. Vidal J-S, Vidailhet M, Derkinderen P, de Gaillarbois TD, Tzourio C, Alpérovitch A. Risk factors for progressive supranuclear palsy: a case-control study in France. *Journal of neurology, neurosurgery, and psychiatry.* 2009 Nov;80(11):1271–4.

102. Davis PH, Golbe LI, Duvoisin RC, Schoenberg BS. Risk factors for progressive supranuclear palsy. *Neurology.* 1988 Oct;38(10):1546–52.

103. Golbe LI, Ohman-Strickland PA. A clinical rating scale for progressive supranuclear palsy. *Brain : a journal of neurology.* 2007 Jun;130(Pt 6):1552–65.

104. Whitwell JL, Xu J, Mandrekar JN, Gunter JL, Jack CR, Josephs KA. Rates of brain atrophy and clinical decline over 6 and 12-month intervals in PSP: Determining sample size for treatment trials. *Parkinsonism & related disorders.* 2012 Mar;18(3):252–6.

105. Schrag A, Selai C, Quinn N, Lees A, Litvan I, Lang A, et al. Measuring quality of life in PSP: the PSP-QoL. *Neurology.* 2006 Jul 11;67(1):39–44.

106. Schrag A, Good CD, Miszkiel K, Morris HR, Mathias CJ, Lees AJ, et al. Differentiation of atypical parkinsonian syndromes with routine MRI. *Neurology.* 2000 Feb;54(3):697–702.

107. Massey LA, Micallef C, Paviour DC, O'Sullivan SS, Ling H, Williams DR, et al. Conventional magnetic resonance imaging in confirmed progressive supranuclear palsy and multiple system atrophy. *Movement Disorders.* 2012 Dec;27(14):1754–62.

108. Paviour DC, Price SL, Jahanshahi M, Lees AJ, Fox NC. Longitudinal MRI in progressive supranuclear palsy and multiple system atrophy: rates and regions of atrophy. *Brain : a journal of neurology.* 2006 Apr;129(Pt 4):1040–9.

109. Paviour DC, Price SL, Lees AJ, Fox NC. MRI derived brain atrophy in PSP and MSA-P. Determining sample size to detect treatment effects. *Journal of neurology.* 2007 Apr;254(4):478–81.

110. Borroni B, Gardoni F, Parnetti L, Magno L, Malinverno M, Saggese E, et al. Pattern of Tau forms in CSF is altered in progressive supranuclear palsy. *Neurobiology of aging.* 2009 Jan;30(1):34–40.

111. Borroni B, Malinverno M, Gardoni F, Alberici A, Parnetti L, Premi E, et al. Tau forms in CSF as a reliable biomarker for progressive supranuclear palsy. *Neurology.* 2008 Nov;71(22):1796–803.

112. Kuiperij HB, Verbeek MM. Diagnosis of progressive supranuclear palsy: can measurement of tau forms help? Neurobiology of aging. 2012 Jan;33(1):204. e17–8.

113. Keck V. *The Search for a Cause: An Anthropological Perspective of a Neurological Disease in Guam, Micronesia.* Mangilao: University of Guam, Micronesian Area Research Center; 2011.

114. Bak TH, Crawford LM, Hearn VC, Mathuranath PS, Hodges JR. Subcortical dementia revisited: similarities and differences in cognitive function between progressive supranuclear palsy (PSP), corticobasal degeneration (CBD) and multiple system atrophy (MSA). *Neurocase.* 2005 Aug;11(4):268–73.

115. Enevoldson TP, Sanders MD, Harding AE. Autosomal dominant cerebellar ataxia with pigmentary macular dystrophy. A clinical and genetic study of eight families. *Brain : a journal of neurology.* 1994 Jun;117(Pt 3):445–60.

116. Josephs KA, Tsuboi Y, Dickson DW. Creutzfeldt-Jakob disease presenting as progressive supranuclear palsy. *European journal of neurology : the official journal of the European Federation of Neurological Societies.* 2004 May;11(5):343–6.

117. Van Gerpen JA, Ahlskog JE, Petty GW. Progressive supranuclear palsy phenotype secondary to CADASIL. *Parkinsonism & related disorders*. 2003 Aug;9(6):367–9.

118. Josephs KA, Ishizawa T, Tsuboi Y, Cookson N, Dickson DW. A clinicopathological study of vascular progressive supranuclear palsy: a multi-infarct disorder presenting as progressive supranuclear palsy. *Archives of neurology*. 2002 Oct;59(10):1597–601.

119. Brooks DJ, Ibanez V, Sawle GV, Quinn N, Lees AJ, Mathias CJ, et al. Differing patterns of striatal 18F-dopa uptake in Parkinson's disease, multiple system atrophy, and progressive supranuclear palsy. *Annals of neurology*. 1990 Oct;28(4):547–55.

120. Nieforth KA, Golbe LI. Retrospective study of drug response in 87 patients with progressive supranuclear palsy. *Clinical neuropharmacology*. 1993 Aug;16(4):338–46.

121. Schneider A, Mandelkow E. Tau-based treatment strategies in neurodegenerative diseases. *Neurotherapeutics : the journal of the American Society for Experimental NeuroTherapeutics*. 2008 Jul;5(3):443–57.

122. Stamelou M, de Silva R, Arias-Carrión O, Boura E, Höllerhage M, Oertel WH, et al. Rational therapeutic approaches to progressive supranuclear palsy. *Brain : a journal of neurology*. 2010 Jun;133(Pt 6):1578–90.

123. Noble W, Planel E, Zehr C, Olm V, Meyerson J, Suleman F, et al. Inhibition of glycogen synthase kinase-3 by lithium correlates with reduced tauopathy and degeneration in vivo. *Proceedings of the National Academy of Sciences of the United States of America*. 2005 May 10;102(19):6990–5.

124. Tolosa E, Litvan I, Höglinger GU, Burn D, Lees A, Andrés M V, et al. A phase 2 trial of the GSK-3 inhibitor tideglusib in progressive supranuclear palsy. *Movement disorders : official journal of the Movement Disorder Society*. 2014 Apr;29(4):470–8.

125. Leclair-Visonneau L, Rouaud T, Debilly B, Durif F, Houeto J-L, Kreisler A, et al. Randomized placebo-controlled trial of sodium valproate in progressive supranuclear palsy. *Clinical neurology and neurosurgery*. 2016 Jul;146:35–9.

126. Boxer AL, Lang AE, Grossman M, Knopman DS, Miller BL, Schneider LS, et al. Davunetide in patients with progressive supranuclear palsy: a randomised, double-blind, placebo-controlled phase 2/3 trial. *Lancet Neurol*. 2014 Jul;13(7):676–85.

127. Dickey C a, Dunmore J, Lu B, Wang J-W, Lee WC, Kamal A, et al. HSP induction mediates selective clearance of tau phosphorylated at proline-directed Ser/Thr sites but not KXGS (MARK) sites. *FASEB journal : official publication of the Federation of American Societies for Experimental Biology*. 2006 Apr;20(6):753–5.

128. Berger Z, Ravikumar B, Menzies FM, Oroz LG, Underwood BR, Pangalos MN, et al. Rapamycin alleviates toxicity of different aggregate-prone proteins. *Human molecular genetics*. 2006 Feb 1;15(3):433–42.

129. Wischik CM, Bentham P, Wischik DJ, Seng KM. O3-04-07: Tau aggregation inhibitor (TAI) therapy with rember™ arrests disease progression in mild and moderate Alzheimer's disease over 50 weeks. *Alzheimer's and Dementia*. 2008 Jul;4(4):T167.

130. Swerdlow RH, Golbe LI, Parks JK, Cassarino DS, Binder DR, Grawey AE, et al. Mitochondrial dysfunction in cybrid lines expressing mitochondrial genes from patients with progressive supranuclear palsy. *Journal of neurochemistry*. 2000 Oct;75(4):1681–4.

131. Stamelou M, Reuss A, Pilatus U, Magerkurth J, Niklowitz P, Eggert KM, et al. Short-term effects of coenzyme Q10 in progressive supranuclear palsy: a randomized, placebo-controlled trial. *Movement disorders : official journal of the Movement Disorder Society*. 2008 May;23(7):942–9.

CHAPTER 9
Dementia with Lewy Bodies

Rodolfo Savica and David S. Knopman

Department of Neurology, Mayo Clinic Rochester, and Mayo Clinic Alzheimer's Disease Research Center, Rochester, Minnesota, USA

Clinical definition

Dementia with Lewy bodies (DLB) is a clinicopathological entity. Clinically, it is a neurodegenerative disorder characterized by the insidious onset and gradual progression of cognitive impairment, a movement disorder similar to Parkinson disease (PD), and alterations in the normal control of sleep and wakefulness (Figure 9.1). It has clinical and pathological characteristics that may overlap with other neurodegenerative diseases including Alzheimer's disease (AD), PD, progressive supranuclear palsy, corticobasal degeneration, vascular dementia, and frontotemporal degeneration (FTD). Its onset is almost always insidious. The diagnosis of DLB derives from the clinical history and examination. The current diagnostic criteria are those from a 2005 consensus conference [1] (Table 9.1).

Pathologically, DLB is one of the Lewy body diseases. Lewy bodies are the hallmark of PD, Parkinson disease dementia (PDD), and multiple system atrophy as well as DLB. Lewy bodies are cytoplasmic inclusions consisting of the protein α-synuclein. In 1961 Okazaki et al. reported two male patients affected with dementia and parkinsonism. Autopsy showed Lewy bodies in the cerebral cortex [2]. In 1984 Kosaka et al. described the typical distribution of the Lewy body in the cerebral cortex; thus, their observations represent the time point at which the current usage of the term DLB originated [3]. In the 1990s, the eponymous name of the pathological lesion of PD, the Lewy body, was first used as a name for the clinicopathological conditions that included typical PD without dementia, and two disorders with dementia: PDD and DLB.

The consensus criteria drew an important distinction between DLB and PDD based on the temporal sequence of symptoms. In clinical practice DLB should be diagnosed when dementia occurs before or concurrently with parkinsonism. PDD should be diagnosed only when dementia occurs more than one year after the onset of parkinsonism. This "12-month rule" is somewhat arbitrary. Either in clinical or research settings, it is not always possible to identify clearly the time of onset of one symptom. However, the distinction between PDD and DLB may roughly map onto the spectrum of less to more coexistent Alzheimer pathology accompanying the Lewy body pathology, as well as topography of Lewy body distribution.

Epidemiology

DLB is the second most common type of degenerative dementia in older people, accounting for 10–15% of the cases that come to autopsy [4–6]. In population studies of people older than 65 the prevalence of DLB ranged from 0.1% [7] to 2.0% [8]. The prevalence of DLB in dementia varies between 2.8% [9] and 30.5% [8] in the different studies using the same clinical criteria. The prevalence of DLB rises with age. When the study population is older than 70 or 75 years of age, the prevalence of DLB has ranged as high as 5.0% [10] of the general population to 21.9% [10] among demented individuals. Higher prevalence has been reported in studies conducted in Europe compared to Japan [9], including a prevalence among dementia patients of 30.5% in North London, England [8], and 21.9% in Finland [10]. Projections of prevalence of dementias by 2030 and 2050 indicate that the prevalence of DLB will increase 131% by 2050 [11] in the USA and Europe. Such projections have obvious imprecision, but the point is that with an aging population future caseloads for DLB will only rise.

The Cache County Study (Cache County Utah) estimated an incidence rate of 0.1% of DLB cases per year in people older than 65 years of age, corresponding to a 3.2% rate of incident cases of DLB of the cases of dementia [12]. In a study conducted in Olmsted County, Minnesota, the incidence of DLB was estimated to be 3.5/100,000 person-years. Incidence increased with age and was higher in men than in women, especially after 60 years of age [13]. In the same study, the incidence of PDD was 2.5/100,000 person-years overall and increased with age, similarly in men and women (2.3 vs 2.7). The incidence of DLB and PDD combined was 5.9 overall and was higher in men than in women. A meta-analysis reported that there was a difference in the incidence of DLB according to the different population settings: 4.2% of all diagnosed dementias in the community, but 7.5% in secondary care. Overall the incidence of DLB was 3.8% of newly diagnosed cases of dementia. Notably, it seemed clear that there was an increased incidence of DLB when using the revised consensus criteria as compared to the earlier consensus criteria [14].

Considering the difficulties in diagnosis and in case identification, there are no studies in the literature, that we are aware of, that have explored the role of risk or protective factors in the development of DLB. However, it is possible that the findings of PD may apply to some extent to DLB, considering the clinical resemblance between these two diseases and the sharing of a common hallmark, the deposition of α-synuclein.

The frequency of Lewy body pathology at autopsy may be considerably higher than the prevalence of the clinical disorder The Honolulu Study of Aging, which is a population-based study, showed that about 12.2% of the brains examined of normal men older than

Neurodegeneration, First Edition. Edited by Anthony Schapira, Zbigniew Wszolek, Ted M. Dawson and Nicholas Wood.
© 2017 John Wiley & Sons, Ltd. Published 2017 by John Wiley & Sons, Ltd.

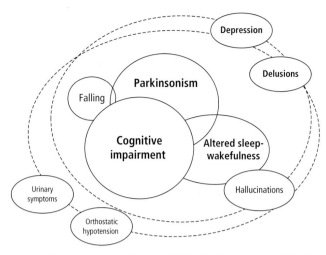

Figure 9.1 The overlapping features of DLB. The Venn diagram highlights the core features of the clinical presentation of DLB, as well as some of the features that frequently occur simultaneously.

Table 9.1 Criteria for the clinical diagnosis of dementia with Lewy bodies (DLB).

1 **Central feature** (essential for a diagnosis of possible or probable DLB)
  • Dementia defined as progressive cognitive decline of sufficient magnitude to interfere with normal social or occupational function
  • Prominent or persistent memory impairment may not necessarily occur in the early stages but is usually evident with progression
  • Deficits on tests of attention, executive function, and visuospatial ability may be especially prominent
2 **Core features** (two core features are sufficient for a diagnosis of probable DLB, one for possible DLB)
  • Fluctuating cognition with pronounced variations in attention and alertness
  • Recurrent visual hallucinations that are typically well formed and detailed
  • Spontaneous features of parkinsonism
3 **Suggestive features** (if one or more of these is present in the presence of one or more core features, a diagnosis of probable DLB can be made. In the absence of any core features, one or more suggestive features is sufficient for possible DLB. Probable DLB should not be diagnosed on the basis of suggestive features alone.)
  • REM sleep behavior disorder
  • Severe neuroleptic sensitivity
  • Low dopamine transporter uptake in basal ganglia demonstrated by SPECT or PET imaging
4 **Supportive features** (commonly present, not proven to have diagnostic specificity)
  • Repeated falls and syncope
  • Transient, unexplained loss of consciousness
  • Severe autonomic dysfunction, e.g., orthostatic hypotension, urinary incontinence
  • Hallucinations in other modalities
  • Systematized delusions
  • Depression
  • Relative preservation of medial temporal lobe structures on CT/MRI scan
  • Generalized low uptake on SPECT/PET perfusion scan with reduced occipital activity
  • Abnormal (low uptake) MIBG myocardial scintigraphy
  • Prominent slow wave activity on EEG with temporal lobe transient sharp waves
5 A diagnosis of DLB is *less likely*
  • In the presence of cerebrovascular disease evident as focal neurologic signs or on brain imaging
  • In the presence of any other physical illness or brain disorder sufficient to account in part or in total for the clinical picture
  • If parkinsonism only appears for the first time at a stage of severe dementia
6 **Temporal sequence** of symptoms
  DLB should be diagnosed when dementia occurs before or concurrently with parkinsonism (if it is present). The term Parkinson disease dementia (PDD) should be used to describe dementia that occurs in the context of well-established Parkinson disease

Source: McKeith et al. 2005 [1]. Reproduced with permission of Wolters Kluwer Health, Inc.

60 years of age had Lewy body pathology [15]. These findings have been confirmed by other authors [16]. Thus, Lewy body pathology may exist in an asymptomatic or preclinical form, but the lag between the appearance of preclinical Lewy body pathology and the eventual appearance of clinical manifestations is not known.

Spectrum of clinical phenotypes of DLB

The clinical criteria for DLB proposed in the 2005 Consensus conference [1] have as their cornerstones a cognitive disorder and parkinsonism. The syndromic overlap between DLB, PD, mild cognitive impairment, and dementia due to AD can cause difficulties in the identification and in the treatment of DLB.

DLB is, by definition, a dementing illness. Patients with DLB typically exhibit mental slowing and loss of mental agility. Executive dysfunction and visuospatial dysfunction are the most prominent cognitive deficits, with impairments in learning and short-term memory loss more variable [17, 18]. Thus, whereas the deficits in mental agility and executive dysfunction are more prominent, the intensity of the memory deficits is typically less in DLB compared to AD dementia. Cognitive fluctuations may be recurrent with pronounced variations in alertness and attention; however, they may not always be present [1]. Cognitive fluctuations represent the intersection of the disorder of the control of attention and concentration with the disorder of maintenance of wakefulness.

Parkinsonism is the other cornerstone of the DLB phenotype, and most, although not all DLB patients exhibit one or motor symptoms. Falling is a common initial manifestation of the motor disorder. It may have a multifactorial basis: DLB patients may have a parkinsonian-type postural instability, orthostatic hypotension, poor judgment, and impaired spatial cognition. Rigidity, bradykinesia, and gait instability dominate the presentation of DLB [19]. These features are of obvious value for differentiating DLB from AD dementia [20]. Rest tremor does not seem to be consistently associated with DLB, although a more symmetric postural tremor is relatively common. The presence of myoclonus is associated with the diagnosis of DLB [21]; however, it occurs in some patients with AD dementia.

A less than optimal response to levodopa and less perceived need to treat parkinsonism are also important characteristics that support the diagnosis of DLB [21, 22]. However, many patients with DLB with parkinsonism may have benefits from treatment with levodopa, even if the improvement is not totally satisfactory [22].

Complex, well-formed visual hallucinations may be present in the early stages of the disease and are particularly characteristic of DLB [23]. Visual hallucinations are far more common than auditory ones, although the latter occasionally occur. Apathy is very common, and combines with the sleep disorders, depression, and loss of executive function to disable the patient with DLB to a greater extent than any individual feature might predict. Other psychiatric symptoms such as delusions and depression may also be present in the disease [24]. Psychosis and dementia may precede the other symptoms of DLB [25]. In some patients, the neuropsychiatric symptoms – especially the visual hallucinations or depression – dominate the clinical presentation.

The other major symptom complex within the DLB spectrum is a disorder of sleep and wakefulness. A history of rapid eye movement sleep behavior disorder (RBD) may be the first symptom of DLB, preceding other symptoms by decades [26–28]. RBD appears to be specific for synucleinopathies as its occurrence is almost entirely limited to DLB, PD with or without dementia, and multiple system atrophy (MSA). Adding RBD as a core feature to the diagnostic formulation for DLB improves sensitivity [29]. Independent of RBD, patients with DLB often exhibit excessive daytime sleepiness. For some patients, the tendency to wish to sleep up to 20 hours per day is the major determinant of impaired quality of life in the disease.

DLB may also present with autonomic disturbances; thus MSA should be taken in consideration in the differential diagnosis as well [30]. While urinary disturbances tend to occur later in the other dementing disorders, urinary incontinence may anticipate the cognitive decline in DLB [31].

Anosmia is common in DLB though rarely a prominent complaint [32]. Anosmia has been proposed as a diagnostic test for DLB; however, the symptom is common in the elderly for a variety of non-neurological reasons and therefore, is not specific for DLB.

The diverse manifestations of DLB present in a similarly diverse way. The cognitive disorder, the parkinsonism, or the disorder of maintenance of normal sleep and wakefulness may each dominate the presentation and be joined by a few or most of the other symptom types (Figure 9.1).

Pathology and pathophysiology

Alpha-synuclein, a 140 amino acid cytosolic protein, is the key pathogenic protein in DLB [33]. It is encoded by a gene on chromosome 4 [1] and seems to be localized specifically in presynaptic terminals

[34]. The function of α-synuclein is not totally understood; however, it seems to play a role in synaptic vesicle production. When aggregated it is insoluble, depositing in the brain and becoming the main component of the fibrils constituting Lewy bodies [35]. The mechanism underlying the dysregulation of α-synuclein and the subsequent development of Lewy bodies is still unknown. It is possible that there is an up-regulation of normal α-synuclein production due to changes in mRNA expression. It is also possible that the presence of Lewy bodies in the brain is a normal response of the neurons to toxic fibrils that have been formed by dysfunctional proteosomes [24].

The core pathological changes in DLB are Lewy bodies, Lewy neurites, and variable levels of AD pathology (Figure 9.2). Use of α-synuclein immunohistochemistry is the key to the histopathological diagnosis of DLB. According to the staging of Lewy body pathology proposed by Braak et al. [36], Lewy bodies initially develop in the brainstem and then may involve more rostral structures, following an ascending pattern of distribution. The common locations for Lewy bodies and Lewy neurites are the brainstem (substantia nigra and locus coeruleus), limbic structures and basal forebrain (amygdala, nucleus basalis, transentorhinal cortex, and cingulate gyrus), and neocortex (frontal, temporal, and parietal). The consensus group formulated a neuropathological diagnostic scheme for DLB (Table 9.2) [1].

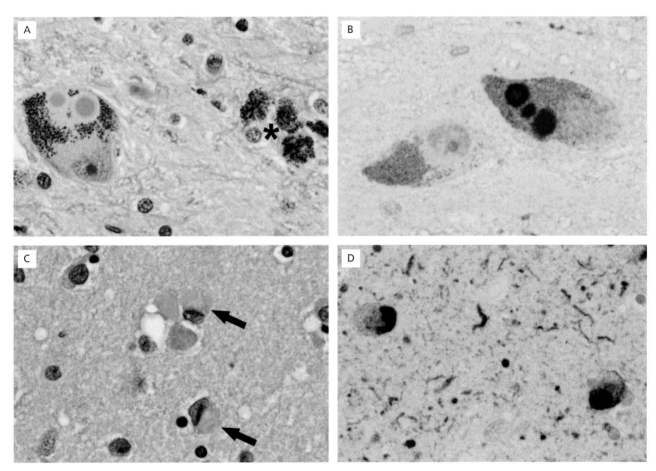

Figure 9.2 Neuropathological features of DLB. (A, B) Brainstem type Lewy bodies (asterisk in A shows extraneuronal neuromelanin in macrophages); (C, D) cortical type Lewy bodies (arrows). (A, C) Hematoxylin and eosin; (B, D) α-synuclein immunohistochemistry. Courtesy of Dennis Dickson MD, Mayo Clinic Jacksonville.

Table 9.2 The neuropathological diagnosis of DLB. The table depicts the neuropathological certainty of the DLB diagnosis.

	Alzheimer type pathology		
	NIA Low Braak Stage 0–2	NIA Intermediate Braak Stages 3–4	NIA High Braak Stages 5–6
None	Low	Low	Low
Brainstem	Low	Low	Low
Limbic	High	Intermediate	Low
Diffuse	High	High	Intermediate (Br 5) Low (Br 6)

Source: McKeith et al. 2005 [1]. Reproduced with permission of Wolters Kluwer Health, Inc.

The initial appearance of Lewy body pathology in brainstem structures that are involved in the control of sleep and wakefulness [36] explains why RBD may occur many years before the diagnosis of synucleinopathies [27, 37]. The sequential appearance of parkinsonism in the PDD phenotype also fits with the Braak scheme. However, the early appearance of dementia seems to suggest that cortical involvement might sometimes occur earlier than the Braak staging system would predict.

There have been variable reports on the relationship of the number of Lewy bodies to the severity of clinical symptoms, some reporting weak relationships [38, 39] and others a stronger one [40, 41]. The presence of Lewy bodies in the temporal lobes is related to the generation of complex hallucinations [42]. Ultimately, synaptic loss and not Lewy bodies is the key correlate of cognitive impairment [43].

AD pathology frequently coexists with Lewy body pathology. The variable presence of AD pathology contributes to the difficulty in defining the relationship between burden of Lewy pathology and cognitive impairment [44]. The number of the neurofibrillary tangles correlates with the clinical features to some extent. In fact, patients with many neurofibrillary tangles, corresponding to a higher Braak AD stage, are more likely to have a clinical pattern resembling AD dementia, while patients with lower Braak AD stages seem to have more the clinical features of DLB [45, 46].

Many older patients may have more than one neurodegenerative syndrome [44, 47, 48]. In individual patients who come to autopsy, clinical–pathological correlations may seem more uncertain than when data from carefully selected case series are considered. Perhaps the key point is that one pathological process should not be viewed in isolation. Whether additively or multiplicatively, the greater the number of pathological processes that are operative, the greater the cognitive impairment. The combination of AD pathology and Lewy body pathology is highly likely to be associated with dementia.

Genetics

In general, there appears to be only a very small genetic contribution to the etiology of DLB. Mutations in the α-synuclein gene were found in two kindreds with familial parkinsonism associated with Lewy body pathology [49, 50]. Mutations of α-synuclein have been reported in sporadic cases of DLB; in particular, a mutation of A53T α-synuclein has been described in the USA [51]. The E46K mutation was identified in a Spanish family with autosomal dominant DLB [52]. A triplication of the α-synuclein gene was reported, causing different phenotypes from PD to DLB within one large family [53]. Moreover, some studies showed a possible familial predisposition to develop DLB. In particular, DLB and the core features

of DLB seem to aggregate in families. Siblings of subjects with clinically diagnosed DLB are at increased risk of DLB and visual hallucinations [54].

Mutations in other genes may produce a phenotype resembling DLB. In patients with mutations in the *MAPT* gene on chromosome 17, phenotypic features of parkinsonism and cognitive impairment that resemble DLB may be seen, but the underlying pathology is that of a tauopathy. The tau protein is not a main component of Lewy bodies [55]. The H1 haplotype of the *MAPT* gene appears to be associated with an increased risk of dementia in persons with PD [56]. The DLB phenotype has been observed in some families with *PGRN* mutations [57]. There are a number of other dominantly inherited parkinsonian disorders associated with other rare gene mutations in *PARK2* (parkin), *PARK7* (DJ-1), *PARK6* (PINK1), and *PARK8* (LRRK2) [58]. Clinical phenotypes in these latter familial disorders typically do not match that of DLB.

Environmental factors

Environmental risk factors have been considered to play a role in neurodegenerative disorders and they have been extensively studied in many of them. Numerous studies have been associated with PD and AD but limited information is available for DLB. No study, so far, has explored the risk or protective factors for DLB. The reasons should be clear. The relatively low prevalence and the need for expert diagnosis make traditional population-based epidemiological investigations very challenging. The phenotypic heterogeneity adds to the complexity. Case-control studies that use prevalent cases from memory or movement disorder clinics are likely to be subject to various biases that make conclusions uncertain.

Biomarkers

As of 2016, it is not possible to diagnose DLB or Lewy body diseases in general in an asymptomatic state except by diagnosing RBD by history or by formal sleep studies. The early diagnosis of a complicated disease such as DLB has obvious importance for establishing the prognosis and for planning long-term management. For these reasons, the search for specific biomarkers of DLB is a focus of current research.

Several biomarkers have been studied for the early identification of DLB. Cerebrospinal fluid (CSF) levels of α-synuclein have been a recent focus. Low levels of α-synuclein have been reported in the CSF of patients with PD as compared with controls [59]; however, α-synuclein levels seem to be elevated in DLB, AD, and vascular dementia [60]. Reduced levels of a particular α-synuclein immunoreactivity band differentiated DLB from controls [61], but more work is needed to understand how CSF α-synuclein levels can be used to differentiate DLB from other dementias, or how to use it in early diagnosis. At the time of this writing, measurement of CSF α-synuclein cannot be considered a viable biomarker for DLB.

Another possible target in CSF may be DJ-1 (*PARK7*) that has been recently identified in patients with DLB. It may serve as a surrogate for protein misfolding or oxidative stress damage [60]. Although promising, DJ-1 in CSF has been studied only in PD and not in DLB.

A novel biomarker of future interest is the glucocerebrosidase (*GBA*) gene located on chromosome 1q21. Mutations of the *GBA* gene are characteristic of the lysosomal storage disease Gaucher disease, an autosomal recessive disorder. GBA mutations have been proven to be common in patients with PD [62–65], perhaps as many as 10% [65]. One study found that β-glucocerebrosidase activity was selectively reduced in DLB, consistent with alterations in the expression of the *GBA* gene [66].

Although some other biomarkers have been studied in the CSF, their potential for identification of DLB is less certain. Inflammatory cytokines have been studied in neurodegenerative disorders but their role as biomarkers of DLB is still unclear. For example, the interleukins Il-1a, Il-1b, and TNF-α have been associated with an increased risk of AD [67] and of PD [68], but these findings were not investigated in DLB.

Biomarkers for AD may also be useful for indicating a second pathophysiological process in the setting of a clinical diagnosis of DLB. If markers such as total tau, 181-phosphorylated tau, and β-amyloid-42 were abnormal in a manner typical of AD pathophysiology [69], it would be likely that an AD pathophysiological process was present along with Lewy body pathophysiology.

Structural neuroimaging and functional neuroimaging may also have a role as biomarkers for the pathophysiology of DLB. Structural magnetic resonance imaging (MRI) does not demonstrate a unique signature of DLB [70], but it provides much information about alternative pathophysiologies. For example, the medial temporal areas seem to be relatively preserved in DLB as compared with AD [71, 72]. On the other hand, newer MR techniques appear promising. Functional connectivity imaging using MR has shown altered connectivity patterns in the precuneus and posterior cingulate areas in clinically diagnosed DLB compared to AD dementia [73].

Because dopaminergic deficiency in the striatum is an expected feature of DLB, single photon emission computed tomography (SPECT) measurements of dopaminergic function are an attractive imaging biomarker for DLB. Dopamine transporter SPECT using the tracer [123]I-2 beta-carbomethoxy-3 beta-(4-iodophenyl)-N-(3-fluoropropyl) nortopane (FP-CIT) has recently been approved in the USA for the diagnosis of PD [74] (Figure 9.3).

Using positron emission tomography (PET), striatal dopamine uptake can be measured with the tracer [18F]fluoro-dopa. It can show a decrease in both caudate and putamen in DLB as compared with AD and controls [75]. PET imaging can also be used with [18F]-fluorodeoxyglucose (FDG) for the diagnosis of DLB. The advantage of FDG-PET imaging is that it can aid more broadly in the differential diagnosis of a dementing illness by providing information about AD and behavior variant frontotemporal dementia. DLB cases have been reported to have the same pattern of hypometabolism as AD,

with involvement of the medial temporal lobes [76], but DLB cases have a primary involvement of the occipital areas with a possible hypometabolism evident in the striatum [77, 78] (Figure 9.4).

Post mortem neurochemical studies have demonstrated that there is a severe cholinergic deficit in DLB [79]. Therefore, reduced cholinergic activity has been considered a potential biomarker of DLB. Although the measurement can be complicated, a PET study using N-^{11}C-methyl-4-piperidyl compared the mapping of cholinergic activity in DLB, PDD, and normal subjects. One study showed a marked reduction of cholinergic activity in the medial occipital cortex in DLB and PDD [80].

Pittsburgh Compound B (PIB) PET imaging for brain β-amyloidosis has had a major impact on the study of dementing illness. Abnormal amyloid imaging is specific and sensitive for the diagnosis of the underlying pathophysiology of AD. In the context of the diagnosis of DLB, the value of amyloid PET imaging with PIB or its ^{18}F analogs is comparable to that of CSF AD biomarkers: it provides evidence for the presence of AD pathophysiology that would represent a second process if DLB were suspected clinically. A large proportion of DLB cases have levels of PIB retention in the range seen in patients with typical AD [70, 81]. Tau PET imaging has also been applied to DLB. Typically, some cases of DLB show some accumulation of tau PET tracer. [82]

Cardiac ^{123}I-meta-iodobenzylguanidine (^{123}I-MIBG) has been used to investigate DLB based on the rationale that autonomic dysfunction occurs in DLB but very rarely in other degenerative or cerebrovascular dementias. Several studies have demonstrated that ^{123}I-MIBG can differentiate DLB from other dementias [84–86] with a diagnostic accuracy of 95% (sensitivity 94%, specificity 96%) [85]. However, other studies find 123I-MIBG imaging to have about the same accuracy as other biomarkers. [83]

Testing of autonomic function using various measures of cardiovascular and hemodynamic regulation can be used to establish dysfunction in the central autonomic nervous system [87]. While autonomic testing cannot establish a diagnosis of DLB, autonomic dysfunction is common in DLB and often becomes a management issue.

Sleep studies may be useful in DLB, first to establish the presence of RBD or other disturbances of sleep, and second to begin the process of managing disturbances of sleep and wakefulness [28]. Demonstration of RBD in asymptomatic persons may be the only way at present to diagnose DLB in asymptomatic persons [27, 88, 89]. Sometimes the history of dream enactment behavior is so

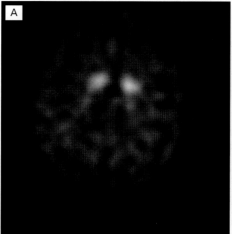 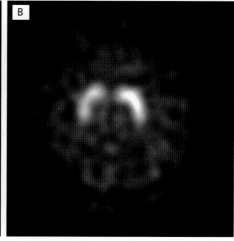

Figure 9.3 Dopamine transporter imaging in DLB using ^{123}I-FP-CIT SPECT. The image in the left panel (A) shows reduced levels of dopamine transporter in a patient with mild DLB. The panel on the right (B) shows a normal pattern of tracer uptake in the striatum of a patient with AD dementia. Courtesy of Bradley Boeve MD and Val Lowe MD, Mayo Clinic Rochester.

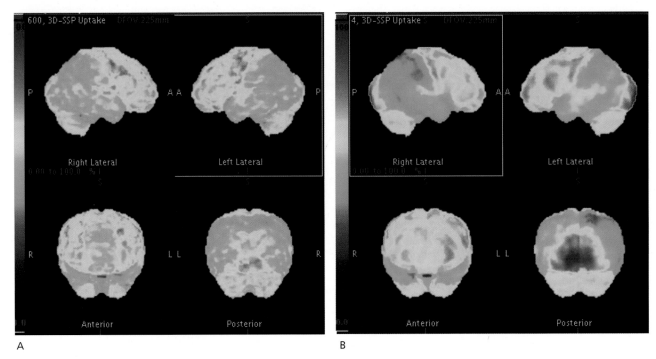

Figure 9.4 ^{18}F-FDG-PET imaging in DLB. The Z-score maps from the 3-dimensional statistical surface projection mapping of the regional metabolic rate of glucose uptake using the pons as internal reference in two patients, one with DLB (A) and one with AD dementia (B). Note the hypometabolism in the parietal, temporal, and occipital lobes. Although both the DLB and the AD dementia patient have temporal and parietal hypometabolism, occipital lobe metabolism is reduced in the DLB but not in the AD dementia patient. Source: Ferman et al. 2004 [20]. Reproduced with permission of Wolters Kluwer Health, Inc.

obvious that polysomnographic studies performed in a sleep laboratory are not needed to make a clinical diagnosis of probable RBD. In more subtle cases, formal sleep studies are needed. The polysomnographic diagnosis of RBD requires the observation of rapid eye movement sleep without atonia with or without dream enactment behavior during rapid eye movement sleep [90].

Diagnosis

A series of consensus conferences [1, 91, 92] have progressively refined the diagnostic criteria for LBD. In the revised criteria of the DLB Consortium [1] (Table 9.1) that are now currently used, the central feature necessary for the diagnosis of possible or probable LBD is the presence of dementia, defined as a progressive cognitive decline with a persistent or prominent memory impairment that worsens over time. Deficits in attention, executive function, and visuospatial ability may be especially prominent. Two of the following core features are sufficient for the diagnosis of probable LBD, but only one for possible DLB: fluctuating cognition, recurrent visual hallucinations, features of parkinsonism. Suggestive features are RBD, neuroleptic sensitivity, and low dopamine transporter uptake in basal ganglia as demonstrated by SPECT and PET imaging. The presence of one or more suggestive features together with one core feature is considered sufficient for a diagnosis of probable DLB. One or more suggestive features are sufficient for possible DLB. A clinical–pathological analysis showed that the consensus criteria for DLB were reasonably sensitive (85%) and specific (73%) [29].

The diagnosis of DLB is challenging, but there may be some features that are unique to DLB compared to other dementias. The diagnosis of DLB is strongly suggested when more than one of the following occurs in the setting of a dementing illness: fluctuating cognitive symptoms [93, 94], visual hallucinations, a long history of RBD [29], and autonomic dysfunction [24].

The diagnosis of DLB is fundamentally a clinical one. It requires a detailed history from the patient and a knowledgeable informant. In addition to obtaining a full and complete picture of the patient's daily functioning, there are numerous related topics that must be explored. These include symptoms of depression, the presence of hallucinations, and other psychotic symptoms. Gait, balance, and history of falling are also essential parts of the history. Particular attention must be paid to the evaluation of cognitive fluctuations and alterations in the control of sleep and wakefulness. Specific queries about excessive daytime sleepiness and nighttime RBD are essential. Because disturbances of central autonomic functioning also accompany DLB, a detailed history regarding bowel and bladder function is necessary. Symptoms of orthostatic hypotension must also be sought.

The diagnosis also requires a cognitive assessment. At the least, a standardized, reliable, brief cognitive assessment (i.e., a bedside mental status examination) must be performed. In patients with mild cognitive changes, more detailed neuropsychological testing should be performed [1, 91]. Brief cognitive assessments lack the precision to evaluate learning and memory, visuospatial functioning, and executive functioning in a way that may be needed to establish the diagnosis of a cognitive profile consistent with DLB.

DLB has a distinctive, although not entirely specific, neuropsychological pattern that differentiates it from other neurodegenerative diseases [17, 20]. The neuropsychological pattern of DLB involves dysfunction in attentional, executive, and visuospatial domains. In contrast, in early AD dementia, the most common neuropsychological deficits are in the episodic memory domains. Executive function, verbal memory, and visuospatial memory tend to be more severely impaired in DLB than in PDD [95–97], most of which might be explained by overall severity of the cognitive deficits rather than by differences in regional involvement by pathology in the two disorders. Although neuropsychological testing may help to differentiate DLB from AD or PDD, these three entities may share many of the same neuropsychological features.

The motoric features of DLB are somewhat nonspecific, including impaired postural stability, rigidity, bradykinesia, and masked facies [19]. These symptoms and signs may be seen in typical PD, as well as in corticobasal syndrome and progressive supranuclear palsy.

The differential diagnosis of suspected DLB can be very broad because of the simultaneous presence of a cognitive disorder and a movement disorder. Any disorder that can cause dementia must be considered. The most common would be AD dementia, dementia due to cerebrovascular disease, behavior variant frontotemporal dementia, corticobasal syndrome, and progressive supranuclear palsy. Multiple system atrophy would also be a consideration except for the prominent dementia that is part of DLB. A primary psychiatric diagnosis such as late-life psychosis might also occasionally be plausible. Other causes of fluctuating cognition such as systemic diseases, acute infections, or drug intoxication should also be excluded. The slow and insidious time course of DLB almost always allows it to be distinguished from Creutzfeldt–Jakob disease. All three clinical features of normal pressure hydrocephalus – dementia, gait disorder, urinary urgency – are very common in DLB. The absence of ventricular enlargement out of proportion to the degree of sulcal widening is the main point of distinction between normal pressure hydrocephalus and DLB.

As discussed in the section on biomarkers, there is no specific laboratory test that is considered to be comparable to the clinical diagnosis. Structural MRI is probably warranted as part of the initial evaluation of a patient with suspected DLB to rule out other diseases. In addition, functional studies can provide additional clues to the diagnosis.

Prognosis

The prognosis for DLB is that of inexorable progression. Some studies have claimed that the rate of cognitive decline in DLB is faster than that of AD dementia [98], but others have failed to find such a difference [99]. In rare patients with DLB there may be rapid symptoms progression to death within 1–2 years [100]. Most patients survive longer. Survival studies in DLB showed that the average survival after the diagnosis was about the same as for patients with typical AD dementia [101], but there is much variability from patient to patient. The age at onset and the presence of other comorbidities may have a substantial impact on survival in DLB.

Treatment options and management

After an accurate diagnosis of DLB has been made, the next step is to prioritize the management of the main symptoms of the patient. It is up to the patient and caregiver, in partnership with the physician, to prioritize the patient's problems. Because an essential feature of DLB is the multiplicity of symptoms, they must be prioritized in order to develop a rational plan for treatment. The most bothersome and relevant complaints for the patient and the caregiver should be

Table 9.3 Symptoms in DLB, their pharmacological management, and complications.

Symptom	Pharmacologic intervention	Possible complications of the therapy
Gait disorder	Levodopa or dopaminergic agonists	Hallucinations and delusions Exacerbation of postural hypotension
Cognitive disorder	Cholinomimetic drugs	Unpleasant dreams Urinary urgency Postural hypotension
Dream enactment behavior	Melatonin Clonazepam	Daytime drowsiness Worsening balance if awakened at night
Excessive daytime sleepiness	Modafinil	Increased irritability
Urinary urgency	Anticholinergics	Increased confusion
Orthostatic hypotension	Midodrine	None relevant
Depression	Various new generation antidepressants	Sedation, worsening gait difficulty, increased confusion

at the top of the list. In contrast, the more easily treatable problems might not necessarily be priorities for the patient and family. For example, even if a gait disorder happened to be present and amenable to dopaminergic therapies, other symptoms may be of greater importance in the daily life of the patient and spouse. Because only one medication should be manipulated at a time, it is important to operate in a stepwise approach, asking the patient and the caregiver to rank the symptoms and complaints in order to understand which ones are the most relevant for their daily life. Table 9.3 lists some of the major symptoms, their pharmacological management, and the complications of the pharmacological treatments.

There are many pharmacological options for treating the extrapyramidal features, neuropsychiatric and cognitive complaints, autonomic dysfunction, and sleep disorders of DLB [24, 102]. Carbidopa/levodopa is still the mainstay of treatment for PD [103] and may be very useful for DLB. However, the benefits of therapy are less obvious than in PD [102]. In a patient with predominant extrapyramidal features such as tremor, bradykinesia, rigidity, and gait disturbance, a trial with levodopa (up to 900 mg/day) is warranted. However, levodopa is associated with a series of adverse effects that may increase some of the symptoms of DLB. For example, levodopa can exacerbate postural hypotension that may be present. In addition, it is possible that levodopa increases the severity and the frequency of hallucinations when present [103]. If benefits from levodopa justify continuation of the therapy, adjustment of the dosage may be necessary. When there is an exacerbation of hallucinations, however, a decision to use an antipsychotic simultaneously with levodopa must be considered. Fortunately, patients with DLB treated with levodopa tend not have severe dyskinesias as compared with patients with PD [100]. Dopaminergic agonists in the treatment of extrapyramidal symptoms of DLB are not considered as first line, because the risks of hallucination, memory complaints, and sleep abnormalities that are associated with this class of medications are greater than with levodopa [103].

Cholinesterase inhibitors should be considered for the symptoms of the dementia. Unfortunately, as in the case of AD dementia, the role of these medications is palliative and not disease modifying. They do not have any role in delaying the progression of the underlying biological disease. Cholinesterase inhibitors must be titrated up to the usual dosage used for AD. However, even based on limited experience, it seems that cholinesterase inhibitors are more effective in DLB as compared with AD [104]. The use of these drugs may improve the fluctuations of cognition, visual hallucinations, apathy, and sleep disorders of patients with DLB [105], although it should be acknowledged that clinical trial evidence for such an assertion is limited to one trial [106]. On the other hand, cholinesterase inhibitors are not only associated with the typical adverse events reported in AD such as nausea but they can also cause postural hypotension, urinary frequency, and hyper-salivation in subjects with DLB [107]. Because DLB patients often have autonomic disturbances that affect bladder control, the cholinomimetic effects on the bladder may produce unacceptable urinary incontinence.

Hallucinations can be challenging to treat in DLB, but success is feasible. First, the clinician must be certain that secondary causes such as infection, high temperature, or drug intoxication have been excluded. When considering antipsychotic medications to treat hallucinations, their inevitable risk for side effects must be seriously weighed against the consequences of the hallucinations themselves. The question of impact of the hallucinations on daily life should be a prime determinant on whether to treat them or not. If hallucinations are present but do not frighten the patient or lead to disruptive behavior, consideration might be given to not treating with an antipsychotic drug. The choice of an antipsychotic medication is not trivial. All of the first generation antipsychotics have been associated with unacceptable levels of side effects such as worsening of parkinsonism in 50% of patients. They are also associated with increased mortality. Adverse events with most of the second generation antipsychotics are also unacceptable [104, 108]. If agitation needs to be treated, quetiapine, in our experience, is the most suitable antipsychotic for DLB patients [105]. Quetiapine, while sedating, does not cause extrapyramidal side effects [103]. Low doses of quetiapine (25 mg) may be sufficient to treat the hallucinations; however, sometimes much higher doses are needed. It is important to obtain electrocardiographic evaluations before starting this medication because a known complication of antipsychotic drugs is prolongation of the QT interval [109].

Sleep disturbances such as RBD must also be addressed for therapeutic interventions. If the RBD is infrequent enough, or mild enough, no treatment may be needed. However, if the behaviors are frequent or significantly disrupt the sleep of the spouse, RBD should be treated. Melatonin may be a reasonable first approach. It is often effective in doses of 3–12 mg. If melatonin is ineffective, then clonazepam may be considered [88].

Excessive daytime sleepiness is sometimes a major factor in poor quality of life for patient and spouse. If improvement of nighttime sleep hygiene does not improve daytime alertness, the use of drugs such as modafinil or armodafinil could be considered [110].

Depression is a common symptom in DLB. Generally speaking, several of the selective serotonin reuptake inhibitors are modestly effective and well tolerated in DLB patients. Anti-depressants that may cause orthostatic hypotension should be avoided.

Non-pharmacological treatment needs to be tailored to the individual and his or her family, based on the needs of the patient and the skills and weaknesses of the primary caregiver. Social engagement and physical activity are helpful strategies to improve cognition and to avoid personal isolation. While we have generally referred to the primary caregiver as spouse, in many instances it might be an adult child. In addition to trying to improve the quality of life for the patients through manipulation of medications and the environment, improvement in quality of life for the caregiver is also critical to success.

Future development

DLB is a complex disorder that still requires to be completely understood. However we hope that it will be better elucidated in coming years. There is a growing knowledge of synucleinopathies and the possible treatment. A better understanding of specific early biomarkers of DLB will further contribute to provide information on the early phase of the disease. The early diagnosis of DLB will help to develop treatment that can modify and delay the progression of the disease. In addition, the identification of the different clinical phenotypes will be needed to differentiate and individualize the treatment. The pathological similarity between PD, AD, and DLB will be important for DLB patients because when new disease-modifying drugs finally become available for PD or AD, such drugs will be used in DLB.

Funding: DSK was supported by NIH grants P50 AG16574 and U01 AG06786, and the Robert H. and Clarice Smith and Abigail Van Buren Alzheimer's Disease Research Program of the Mayo Foundation.
Disclosures: Dr. Knopman serves on a Data SafetyMonitoring Board for Lundbeck Pharmaceuticals and for the DIAN study, and is an investigator in clinical trials sponsored by TauRx, Biogen, and Lilly Pharmaceuticals. Dr. Savica has no disclosures.

References

1. McKeith IG, Dickson DW, Lowe J, et al. Diagnosis and management of dementia with Lewy bodies: third report of the DLB Consortium. *Neurology* 2005;65:1863–72.
2. Okazaki H, Lipkin LE, Aronson SM. Diffuse intracytoplasmic ganglionic inclusions (Lewy type) associated with progressive dementia and quadriparesis in flexion. *J Neuropathol Exp Neurol* 1961;20:237–44.
3. Kosaka K, Yoshimura M, Ikeda K, Budka H. Diffuse type of Lewy body disease: progressive dementia with abundant cortical Lewy bodies and senile changes of varying degree – a new disease? *Clin Neuropathol* 1984;3:185–92.
4. Knopman D, Parisi JE, Boeve BF, et al. Vascular dementia in a population-based autopsy study. *Arch Neurol* 2003;60:569–76.
5. Lim A, Tsuang D, Kukull W, et al. Clinico-neuropathological correlation of Alzheimer's disease in a community-based case series. *J Am Geriatr Soc* 1999;47:564–9.
6. Holmes C, Cairns N, Lantos P, Mann A. Validity of current clinical criteria for Alzheimer's disease, vascular dementia and dementia with Lewy bodies. *Br J Psychiatry* 1999;174:45–50.
7. de Silva HA, Gunatilake SB, Smith AD. Prevalence of dementia in a semi-urban population in Sri Lanka: report from a regional survey. *Int J Geriatr Psychiatry* 2003;18:711–5.
8. Stevens T, Livingston G, Kitchen G, et al. Islington study of dementia subtypes in the community. *Br J Psychiatry* 2002;180:270–6.
9. Yamada T, Hattori H, Miura A, Tanabe M, Yamori Y. Prevalence of Alzheimer's disease, vascular dementia and dementia with Lewy bodies in a Japanese population. *Psychiatry Clin Neurosci* 2001;55:21–5.
10. Rahkonen T, Eloniemi-Sulkava U, Rissanen S, et al. Dementia with Lewy bodies according to the consensus criteria in a general population aged 75 years or older. *J Neurol Neurosurg Psychiatry* 2003;74:720–4.
11. Bach JP, Ziegler U, Deuschl G, Dodel R, Doblhammer-Reiter G. Projected numbers of people with movement disorders in the years 2030 and 2050. *Mov Disord* 2011;26:2286–90.
12. Miech RA, Breitner JC, Zandi PP, et al. Incidence of AD may decline in the early 90s for men, later for women: The Cache County study. *Neurology* 2002;58:209–18.
13. Savica R, Grossardt BR, Bower JH, Ahlskog JE, Rocca WA. Incidence and pathology of synucleinopathies and tauopathies related to parkinsonism. *JAMA Neurol* 2013;70:859–66.
14. Hogan DB, Fiest KM, Roberts JI, et al. The prevalence and incidence of dementia with Lewy bodies: a systematic review. *Can J Neurol Sci* 2016;43 Suppl 1:S83–95.
15. Abbott RD, Ross GW, Petrovitch H, et al. Bowel movement frequency in late-life and incidental Lewy bodies. *Mov Disord* 2007;22:1581–6.
16. Frigerio R, Fujishiro H, Ahn TB, et al. Incidental Lewy body disease: Do some cases represent a preclinical stage of dementia with Lewy bodies? *Neurobiol Aging* 2009;32:857–63.
17. Ferman TJ, Smith GE, Boeve BF, et al. Neuropsychological differentiation of dementia with Lewy bodies from normal aging and Alzheimer's disease. *Clin Neuropsychol* 2006;20:623–36.

18. Tiraboschi P, Salmon DP, Hansen LA, et al. What best differentiates Lewy body from Alzheimer's disease in early-stage dementia? *Brain* 2006;129:729–35.

19. Burn DJ, Rowan EN, Minett T, et al. Extrapyramidal features in Parkinson's disease with and without dementia and dementia with Lewy bodies: A cross-sectional comparative study. *Mov Disord* 2003;18:884–9.

20. Ferman TJ, Smith GE, Boeve BF, et al. DLB fluctuations: specific features that reliably differentiate DLB from AD and normal aging. *Neurology* 2004;62:181–7.

21. Louis ED, Klatka LA, Liu Y, Fahn S. Comparison of extrapyramidal features in 31 pathologically confirmed cases of diffuse Lewy body disease and 34 pathologically confirmed cases of Parkinson's disease. *Neurology* 1997;48:376–80.

22. Bonelli SB, Ransmayr G, Steffelbauer M, et al. L-dopa responsiveness in dementia with Lewy bodies, Parkinson disease with and without dementia. *Neurology* 2004;63:376–8.

23. Manford M, Andermann F. Complex visual hallucinations. Clinical and neurobiological insights. *Brain* 1998;121 (Pt 10):1819–40.

24. McKeith I, Mintzer J, Aarsland D, et al. Dementia with Lewy bodies. *Lancet Neurol* 2004;3:19–28.

25. Burkhardt CR, Filley CM, Kleinschmidt-DeMasters BK, et al. Diffuse Lewy body disease and progressive dementia. *Neurology* 1988;38:1520–8.

26. Boeve BF, Silber MH, Parisi JE, et al. Synucleinopathy pathology and REM sleep behavior disorder plus dementia or parkinsonism. *Neurology* 2003;61:40–5.

27. Claassen DO, Josephs KA, Ahlskog JE, et al. REM sleep behavior disorder preceding other aspects of synucleinopathies by up to half a century. *Neurology* 2010;75:494–9.

28. Boeve BF, Silber MH, Ferman TJ. REM sleep behavior disorder in Parkinson's disease and dementia with Lewy bodies. *J Geriatr Psychiatry Neurol* 2004;17:146–57.

29. Ferman TJ, Boeve BF, Smith GE, et al. Inclusion of RBD improves the diagnostic classification of dementia with Lewy bodies. *Neurology* 2011;77:875–82.

30. Thaisetthawatkul P, Boeve BF, Benarroch EE, et al. Autonomic dysfunction in dementia with Lewy bodies. *Neurology* 2004;62:1804–9.

31. Del-Ser T, Munoz DG, Hachinski V. Temporal pattern of cognitive decline and incontinence is different in Alzheimer's disease and diffuse Lewy body disease. *Neurology* 1996;46:682–6.

32. Olichney JM, Murphy C, Hofstetter CR, et al. Anosmia is very common in the Lewy body variant of Alzheimer's disease. *J Neurol Neurosurg Psychiatry* 2005;76:1342–7.

33. Tong J, Wong H, Guttman M, et al. Brain alpha-synuclein accumulation in multiple system atrophy, Parkinson's disease and progressive supranuclear palsy: a comparative investigation. *Brain* 2010;133:172–88.

34. Lee HJ, Patel S, Lee SJ. Intravesicular localization and exocytosis of alpha-synuclein and its aggregates. *J Neurosci* 2005;25:6016–24.

35. Luis CA, Barker WW, Gajaraj K, et al. Sensitivity and specificity of three clinical criteria for dementia with Lewy bodies in an autopsy-verified sample. *Int J Geriatr Psychiatry* 1999;14:526–33.

36. Braak H, Ghebremedhin E, Rub U, Bratzke H, Del Tredici K. Stages in the development of Parkinson's disease-related pathology. *Cell Tissue Res* 2004;318:121–34.

37. Boeve BF, Silber MH, Saper CB, et al. Pathophysiology of REM sleep behaviour disorder and relevance to neurodegenerative disease. *Brain* 2007;130:2770–88.

38. Harding AJ, Halliday GM. Cortical Lewy body pathology in the diagnosis of dementia. *Acta Neuropathol* 2001;102:355–63.

39. Gomez-Tortosa E, Newell K, Irizarry MC, et al. Clinical and quantitative pathologic correlates of dementia with Lewy bodies. *Neurology* 1999;53:1284–91.

40. Samuel W, Galasko D, Masliah E, Hansen LA. Neocortical Lewy body counts correlate with dementia in the Lewy body variant of Alzheimer's disease. *J Neuropathol Exp Neurol* 1996;55:44–52.

41. Kovari E, Gold G, Herrmann FR, et al. Lewy body densities in the entorhinal and anterior cingulate cortex predict cognitive deficits in Parkinson's disease. *Acta Neuropathol* 2003;106:83–8.

42. Harding AJ, Broe GA, Halliday GM. Visual hallucinations in Lewy body disease relate to Lewy bodies in the temporal lobe. *Brain* 2002;125:391–403.

43. Masliah E, Rockenstein E, Veinbergs I, et al. Dopaminergic loss and inclusion body formation in alpha-synuclein mice: implications for neurodegenerative disorders. *Science* 2000;287:1265–9.

44. Jellinger KA, Attems J. Prevalence and impact of vascular and Alzheimer pathologies in Lewy body disease. *Acta Neuropathol* 2008;115:427–36.

45. Lippa CF, McKeith I. Dementia with Lewy bodies: improving diagnostic criteria. *Neurology* 2003;60:1571–2.

46. Merdes AR, Hansen LA, Jeste DV, et al. Influence of Alzheimer pathology on clinical diagnostic accuracy in dementia with Lewy bodies. *Neurology* 2003;60:1586–90.

47. Fotuhi M, Hachinski V, Whitehouse PJ. Changing perspectives regarding late-life dementia. *Nat Rev Neurol* 2009;5:649–58.

48. Piguet O, Halliday GM, Creasey H, Broe GA, Kril JJ. Frontotemporal dementia and dementia with Lewy bodies in a case-control study of Alzheimer's disease. *Int Psychogeriatr* 2009;21:688–95.

49. Polymeropoulos MH, Lavedan C, Leroy E, et al. Mutation in the alpha-synuclein gene identified in families with Parkinson's disease. *Science* 1997;276:2045–7.

50. Kruger R, Kuhn W, Muller T, et al. Ala30Pro mutation in the gene encoding alpha-synuclein in Parkinson's disease. *Nat Genet* 1998;18:106–8.

51. Yamaguchi K, Cochran EJ, Murrell JR, et al. Abundant neuritic inclusions and microvacuolar changes in a case of diffuse Lewy body disease with the A53T mutation in the alpha-synuclein gene. *Acta Neuropathol* 2005;110:298–305.

52. Zarranz JJ, Alegre J, Gomez-Esteban JC, et al. The new mutation, E46K, of alpha-synuclein causes Parkinson and Lewy body dementia. *Ann Neurol* 2004;55:164–73.

53. Singleton AB, Farrer M, Johnson J, et al. alpha-Synuclein locus triplication causes Parkinson's disease. *Science* 2003;302:841.

54. Nervi A, Reitz C, Tang MX, et al. Familial aggregation of dementia with Lewy bodies. *Arch Neurol* 2011;68:90–3.

55. Goedert M, Ghetti B, Spillantini MG. Tau gene mutations in frontotemporal dementia and parkinsonism linked to chromosome 17 (FTDP-17). Their relevance for understanding the neurogenerative process. *Ann N Y Acad Sci* 2000;920:74–83.

56. Seto-Salvia N, Clarimon J, Pagonabarraga J, et al. Dementia risk in Parkinson disease: disentangling the role of MAPT haplotypes. *Arch Neurol* 2011;68:359–64.

57. Kelley BJ, Haidar W, Boeve BF, et al. Prominent phenotypic variability associated with mutations in Progranulin. *Neurobiol Aging* 2009;30:739–51.

58. Sundal C, Fujioka S, Uitti RJ, Wszolek ZK. Autosomal dominant Parkinson's disease. *Parkinsonism Relat Disord* 2012;18 Suppl 1:S7–S10.

59. Mukaetova-Ladinska EB, Milne J, Andras A, et al. Alpha- and gamma-synuclein proteins are present in cerebrospinal fluid and are increased in aged subjects with neurodegenerative and vascular changes. *Dement Geriatr Cogn Disord* 2008;26:32–42.

60. Hong Z, Shi M, Chung KA, et al. DJ-1 and alpha-synuclein in human cerebrospinal fluid as biomarkers of Parkinson's disease. *Brain* 2010;133:713–26.

61. Ballard C, Jones EL, Londos E, et al. Alpha-synuclein antibodies recognize a protein present at lower levels in the CSF of patients with dementia with Lewy bodies. *Int Psychogeriatr* 2010;22:321–7.

62. Tayebi N, Walker J, Stubblefield B, et al. Gaucher disease with parkinsonian manifestations: does glucocerebrosidase deficiency contribute to a vulnerability to parkinsonism? *Mol Genet Metab* 2003;79:104–9.

63. Aharon-Peretz J, Badarny S, Rosenbaum H, Gershoni-Baruch R. Mutations in the glucocerebrosidase gene and Parkinson disease: phenotype-genotype correlation. *Neurology* 2005;65:1460–1.

64. Neumann J, Bras J, Deas E, et al. Glucocerebrosidase mutations in clinical and pathologically proven Parkinson's disease. *Brain* 2009;132:1783–94.

65. Seto-Salvia N, Pagonabarraga J, Houlden H, et al. Glucocerebrosidase mutations confer a greater risk of dementia during Parkinson's disease course. *Mov Disord* 2012;27:393–9.

66. Parnetti L, Balducci C, Pierguidi L, et al. Cerebrospinal fluid beta-glucocerebrosidase activity is reduced in dementia with Lewy bodies. *Neurobiol Dis* 2009;34:484–6.

67. Ho GJ, Drego R, Hakimian E, Masliah E. Mechanisms of cell signaling and inflammation in Alzheimer's disease. *Curr Drug Targets Inflamm Allergy* 2005;4:247–56.

68. Wahner AD, Sinsheimer JS, Bronstein JM, Ritz B. Inflammatory cytokine gene polymorphisms and increased risk of Parkinson disease. *Arch Neurol* 2007;64:836–40.

69. Shaw LM, Vanderstichele H, Knapik-Czajka M, et al. Cerebrospinal fluid biomarker signature in Alzheimer's disease neuroimaging initiative subjects. *Ann Neurol* 2009;65:403–13.

70. Kantarci K, Lowe VJ, Boeve BF, et al. Multimodality imaging characteristics of dementia with Lewy bodies. *Neurobiol Aging* 2012;33:2091–105.

71. Sabattoli F, Boccardi M, Galluzzi S, et al. Hippocampal shape differences in dementia with Lewy bodies. *Neuroimage* 2008;41:699–705.

72. Firbank MJ, Blamire AM, Krishnan MS, et al. Diffusion tensor imaging in dementia with Lewy bodies and Alzheimer's disease. *Psychiatry Res* 2007;155:135–45.

73. Galvin JE, Price JL, Yan Z, Morris JC, Sheline YI. Resting bold fMRI differentiates dementia with Lewy bodies vs Alzheimer disease. *Neurology* 2011;76:1797–803.

74. McKeith I, O'Brien J, Walker Z, et al. Sensitivity and specificity of dopamine transporter imaging with 123I-FP-CIT SPECT in dementia with Lewy bodies: a phase III, multicentre study. *Lancet Neurol* 2007;6:305–13.

75. Hu XS, Okamura N, Arai H, et al. 18F-fluorodopa PET study of striatal dopamine uptake in the diagnosis of dementia with Lewy bodies. *Neurology* 2000;55:1575–7.

76. Ishii K, Soma T, Kono AK, et al. Comparison of regional brain volume and glucose metabolism between patients with mild dementia with lewy bodies and those with mild Alzheimer's disease. *J Nucl Med* 2007;48:704–11.

77. Mosconi L, Tsui WH, Herholz K, et al. Multicenter standardized 18F-FDG PET diagnosis of mild cognitive impairment, Alzheimer's disease, and other dementias. *J Nucl Med* 2008;49:390–8.

78. Teune LK, Bartels AL, de Jong BM, et al. Typical cerebral metabolic patterns in neurodegenerative brain diseases. *Mov Disord* 2010;25:2395–404.

79. Lippa CF, Smith TW, Perry E. Dementia with Lewy bodies: choline acetyltransferase parallels nucleus basalis pathology. *J Neural Transm* 1999;106:525–35.

80. Shimada H, Hirano S, Shinotoh H, et al. Mapping of brain acetylcholinesterase alterations in Lewy body disease by PET. *Neurology* 2009;73:273–8.

81. Gomperts SN, Rentz DM, Moran E, et al. Imaging amyloid deposition in Lewy body diseases. *Neurology* 2008;71:903–10.

82. Gomperts SN, Locascio JJ, Makaretz SJ, et al. Tau Positron Emission Tomographic Imaging in the Lewy Body Diseases. *JAMA Neurol* 2016;73:1334–41.

83. Tiraboschi P, Corso A, Guerra UP, et al. (123) I-2beta-carbomethoxy-3beta-(4-iodophenyl)-N-(3-fluoropropyl) nortropane single photon emission computed tomography and (123) I-metaiodobenzylguanidine myocardial scintigraphy in differentiating dementia with lewy bodies from other dementias: A comparative study. *Ann Neurol* 2016;80:368–78.

84. Wada-Isoe K, Kitayama M, Nakaso K, Nakashima K. Diagnostic markers for diagnosing dementia with Lewy bodies: CSF and MIBG cardiac scintigraphy study. *J Neurol Sci* 2007;260:33–7.

85. Estorch M, Camacho V, Paredes P, et al. Cardiac (123)I-metaiodobenzylguanidine imaging allows early identification of dementia with Lewy bodies during life. *Eur J Nucl Med Mol Imaging* 2008;35:1636–41.

86. Watanabe H, Ieda T, Katayama T, et al. Cardiac (123)I-meta-iodobenzylguanidine (MIBG) uptake in dementia with Lewy bodies: comparison with Alzheimer's disease. *J Neurol Neurosurg Psychiatry* 2001;70:781–3.

87. Idiaquez J, Roman GC. Autonomic dysfunction in neurodegenerative dementias. *J Neurol Sci* 2011;305:22–7.

88. Schenck CH, Mahowald MW. Rapid eye movement sleep parasomnias. *Neurol Clin* 2005;23:1107–26.

89. Postuma RB, Lang AE, Massicotte-Marquez J, Montplaisir J. Potential early markers of Parkinson disease in idiopathic REM sleep behavior disorder. *Neurology* 2006;66:845–51.

90. Montplaisir J, Gagnon JF, Fantini ML, et al. Polysomnographic diagnosis of idiopathic REM sleep behavior disorder. *Mov Disord* 2010;25:2044–51.

91. McKeith IG, Galasko D, Kosaka K, et al. Consensus guidelines for the clinical and pathologic diagnosis of dementia with Lewy bodies (DLB): report of the consortium on DLB international workshop. *Neurology* 1996;47:1113–24.

92. McKeith IG. Consensus guidelines for the clinical and pathologic diagnosis of dementia with Lewy bodies (DLB): report of the Consortium on DLB International Workshop. *J Alzheimers Dis* 2006;9:417–23.

93. Ballard CG, Aarsland D, McKeith I, et al. Fluctuations in attention: PD dementia vs DLB with parkinsonism. *Neurology* 2002;59:1714–20.

94. Aarsland D, Ballard C, McKeith I, Perry RH, Larsen JP. Comparison of extrapyramidal signs in dementia with Lewy bodies and Parkinson's disease. *J Neuropsychiatry Clin Neurosci* 2001;13:374–9.

95. Gomez-Isla T, Growdon WB, McNamara M, et al. Clinicopathologic correlates in temporal cortex in dementia with Lewy bodies. *Neurology* 1999;53:2003–9.

96. Simard M, van Reekum R, Myran D, et al. Differential memory impairment in dementia with Lewy bodies and Alzheimer's disease. *Brain Cogn* 2002; 49:244–9.

97. Aarsland D, Litvan I, Salmon D, et al. Performance on the dementia rating scale in Parkinson's disease with dementia and dementia with Lewy bodies: comparison with progressive supranuclear palsy and Alzheimer's disease. *J Neurol Neurosurg Psychiatry* 2003;74:1215–20.

98. Olichney JM, Galasko D, Salmon DP, et al. Cognitive decline is faster in Lewy body variant than in Alzheimer's disease. *Neurology* 1998;51:351–7.

99. Stavitsky K, Brickman AM, Scarmeas N, et al. The progression of cognition, psychiatric symptoms, and functional abilities in dementia with Lewy bodies and Alzheimer disease. *Arch Neurol* 2006;63:1450–6.

100. Gaig C, Valldeoriola F, Gelpi E, et al. Rapidly progressive diffuse Lewy body disease. *Mov Disord* 2011;26:1316–23.

101. Williams MM, Xiong C, Morris JC, Galvin JE. Survival and mortality differences between dementia with Lewy bodies vs Alzheimer disease. *Neurology* 2006;67:1935–41.

102. Barber R, Panikkar A, McKeith IG. Dementia with Lewy bodies: diagnosis and management. *Int J Geriatr Psychiatry* 2001;16 Suppl 1:S12–8.

103. Ahlskog JE, *Parkinson's Disease Treatment Guide for Physicians*. Oxford University Press: New York, NY, 2009.

104. Samuel W, Caligiuri M, Galasko D, et al. Better cognitive and psychopathologic response to donepezil in patients prospectively diagnosed as dementia with Lewy bodies: a preliminary study. *Int J Geriatr Psychiatry* 2000;15:794–802.

105. Kurtz AL, Kaufer DI. Dementia in Parkinson's disease. *Curr Treat Options Neurol* 2011;13:242–54.

106. Emre M, Aarsland D, Albanese A, et al. Rivastigmine for dementia associated with Parkinson's disease. *N Engl J Med* 2004;351:2509–18.

107. McLaren AT, Allen J, Murray A, Ballard CG, Kenny RA. Cardiovascular effects of donepezil in patients with dementia. *Dement Geriatr Cogn Disord* 2003;15:183–8.

108. Burke WJ, Pfeiffer RF, McComb RD. Neuroleptic sensitivity to clozapine in dementia with Lewy bodies. *J Neuropsychiatry Clin Neurosci* 1998;10:227–9.

109. Nielsen J, Graff C, Kanters JK, et al. Assessing QT interval prolongation and its associated risks with antipsychotics. *CNS Drugs* 2011;25:473–90.

110. Arnulf I. Excessive daytime sleepiness in parkinsonism. *Sleep Med Rev* 2005; 9:185–200.

CHAPTER 10
Corticobasal Degeneration

Keith A. Josephs, Jr.

Department of Neurology, Divisions of Movement Disorders and Behavioral Neurology, Mayo Clinic, Rochester, Minnesota, USA

Clinical definition and epidemiology

Corticobasal degeneration (CBD) is a rare neurodegenerative disease that is characterized histologically by the presence of abnormal tau deposition in specific regions of the brain. The deposited tau shows characteristic morphological appearances that aid with the diagnosis. Corticobasal degeneration is not a clinical syndrome but is associated with many different clinical syndromes.

The first report of cases of CBD occurred in 1968 by Rebeiz and colleagues [1] who published a series of three patients with unusual neurological signs and symptoms including abnormal posture and gait, as well as involuntary movements. All three patients had died and underwent pathological examination which revealed focal frontoparietal atrophy, the presence of achromatic swollen neurons, and neuronal loss and gliosis of the substantia nigra and cerebellar dentate nuclei. Given these specific findings the authors proposed the term corticodentatonigral degeneration with neuronal achromasia. After the original description, there were few reports of additional cases with similar presenting features until Riley and colleagues published a series of 15 patients in 1990 [2]. In that large series, additional features were reported, and it was suggested that the cardinal clinical features of CBD were cortical sensory loss, focal reflex myoclonus, alien limb phenomena, apraxia, rigidity, akinesia, postural-action tremor, limb dystonia, and postural instability. It was also recognized that CBD was associated with significant asymmetry, one side of the body and the contralateral brain hemisphere being strikingly more affected than the other. Since 1968, there have been major advances in our understanding of CBD including the fact that there is no one syndrome, sign, or symptom characteristic of, or associated with, CBD. In fact, CBD is no longer considered a distinct clinicopathological entity, but instead, the term CBD is now reserved for pathological diagnosis [3]. Prior to the usage of the term CBD however [4], this disease has also been called cortical-basal ganglionic degeneration [2]. Many clinical criteria for the diagnosis of CBD have been proposed [5]; however, clinicopathological studies have demonstrated that although there are clinical features associated with CBD, these same clinical features are also associated with many other neurodegenerative and non-neurodegenerative diseases. This clinical heterogeneity has rendered it extremely difficult to make an ante mortem diagnosis of CBD. Recently, newly proposed criteria for the diagnosis of CBD were published [6]. In this instance, two sets of criteria were developed: one to be specific for research where the term "prob-

able CBD" applies, and the other to be sensitive to capture other tau entities where the term "possible CBD" applies. Neither, however, has been validated.

Epidemiology

CBD is a relatively rare neurodegenerative disease in which incidence and prevalence estimates are crude at best. In one prevalence study looking at cases of parkinsonian disorders, of 121,628 subjects, no case of CBD was identified [7]. It has been estimated however that CBD may account for approximately 5% of parkinsonism, which would translate into an incidence of 0.62–0.92/100,000 and a prevalence of 4.9–7.3/100,000 [8]. The onset of symptoms is typically around the fifth to seventh decade of life and disease duration is approximately 7 years [9]. Cases with a rapid progression and much shorter disease duration have also been described [10].

Spectrum of clinical phenotype

Clinical signs and symptoms associated with CBD

The clinical features associated with CBD include: cogwheel and Gegenhalten rigidity, action and postural tremor (less commonly rest tremor), bradykinesia, myoclonus, limb apraxia, alien limb phenomena, limb and neck dystonia, gait and posture difficulties, dysarthria, aphasia, apraxia of speech, and dementia [11]. There have been increasing reports demonstrating that cognitive impairment [12], including aphasia [13–15], visual spatial and perceptual deficits [16, 17], and even episodic memory loss [18, 19], can be associated with CBD.

Parkinsonism

The most common motor feature associated with CBD is asymmetric parkinsonism which typically, although not always, affects the upper extremity first. Rigidity, followed by bradykinesia, postural instability, and then tremor, in order of decreasing frequency, have been reported [20]. Unlike Parkinson disease in which the tremor is typically approximately 4 Hz, the tremor in CBD is faster at 6–8 Hz, and appears more irregular and jerky [21]. In addition, very early reports have suggested that the tremor tends to be seen with posture or action, rather than at rest [2]. Postural instability may lead to falls and eventually the patient becomes wheelchair bound.

Neurodegeneration, First Edition. Edited by Anthony Schapira, Zbigniew Wszolek, Ted M. Dawson and Nicholas Wood.
© 2017 John Wiley & Sons, Ltd. Published 2017 by John Wiley & Sons, Ltd.

Dystonia

Dystonia is a common feature of CBD [22]. In the majority of cases dystonia affects the limbs, although there have been reports of patients having neck and trunk dystonia as well as blepharospasm. Dystonia can be one of the most disabling features in CBD, rendering the affected limb or limbs immobile and essentially useless. Most patients with dystonia later will develop contractures and associated pain. Pain may accompany dystonia in almost 50% of the patients [23].

Apraxia

One of the most studied features of CBD is apraxia [24–31]. Apraxia is more commonly associated with CBD than the other neurodegenerative disorders, however it is not pathognomonic for CBD. Apraxia has been a consistent feature across all the proposed diagnostic criteria for CBD [6, 21, 32–34]. In CBD both limb-kinetic apraxia and ideomotor apraxia have been well described although ideational apraxia clearly also occurs. Ideomotor limb apraxia tends to be bilateral but typically asymmetric, particularly early in the disease course. It has been reported that ideomotor apraxia in CBD consists of spatial, temporal, and sequencing errors [35]. One study demonstrated that imitative transitive and intransitive limb non-representational gestures are abnormal, but intransitive limb representational gestures are not [26]. In addition to limb apraxia, truncal apraxia [29] and orofacial apraxia [28] can occur in CBD.

Alien limb phenomenon

A subset of patients with limb apraxia will develop what is called an "alien limb phenomenon". In alien limb phenomenon, the patient observes that the limb behaves as though it has a mind of its own. Furthermore, the limb moves involuntarily and uncontrollably. Alien limb phenomenon typically is observed in the upper extremities but can also affect the lower extremities [18]. Patients with an alien limb may personify the limb and refer to it as "my little friend", or term it "this thing". Alien limb phenomenon is not specific to CBD, though; it has also been described in other neurodegenerative diseases, for example in Creutzfeldt–Jakob disease [36, 37] and Alzheimer's disease [38]. When it occurs in CBD, however, it appears to be associated with right parietal lobe pathology [39]. In addition, alien limb phenomenon can occur in non-neurodegenerative diseases, such as in strokes or in patients who have undergone surgical dissection of the corpus callosum [40, 41].

Myoclonus

Myoclonus in CBD is strongly suspected to be of cortical origin given the presence of long-latency reflex response [42]. However, most studies on myoclonus in CBD have been in patients suspected to have CBD and not in patients diagnosed with CBD.

Neuropsychiatric features

Neuropsychiatric features are present in patients with CBD [43]. The most common neuropsychiatric features in one study with 36 cases of CBD included depression and compulsive behavior, which were present in 22% of patients, while psychosis was absent.

Less common signs and symptoms

Other less common features have also been described in patients suspected to have CBD. However, it is unclear whether these are associated with CBD, since none of these cases have had autopsy confirmation. RBD, which has been reported to suggest underlying synucleinopathy [44], has been reported in patients suspected to have CBD [45–47]. Vertical supranuclear gaze palsy, on the other hand, has been identified in patients with CBD [22]. Progressive frontal gait disturbances have been described in a CBD case [48].

Clinical syndromes associated with CBD

Over the past two decades there have been many case reports and small case series that have identified clinical syndromes associated with CBD. Recently, larger case series have been published that have confirmed earlier reports. Although these syndromes are not pathognomonic for CBD, a few are worth discussing in some detail since together they account for the great majority of cases of CBD.

Corticobasal syndrome

The corticobasal syndrome is characterized by the presence of asymmetric parkinsonism and cortical dysfunction [32]. This syndrome was initially thought to be specific to CBD. However, studies have demonstrated that patients presenting with the corticobasal syndrome may not have CBD pathology [49]. In fact, in one clinicopathological series of corticobasal syndrome and CBD, of 21 patients with corticobasal syndrome, only 5 (23%) had CBD. In that same series, of 19 cases with CBD, only 5 cases (26%) had presented as corticobasal syndrome. Other series, however, have reported a higher likelihood of CBD given a corticobasal syndrome presentation [9, 50]. Therefore, although the corticobasal syndrome is most likely to be associated with CBD, its presentation can also be associated with many other non-CBD diagnoses, and CBD is not necessarily associated with a corticobasal syndrome presentation.

Progressive supranuclear palsy syndrome

Another presentation of CBD is that of progressive supranuclear palsy syndrome [50], also known as Richardson's syndrome [51]. This syndrome is characterized by symmetric parkinsonism, with postural instability and falls and vertical supranuclear gaze palsy. This presentation may in fact be as common or even be more commonly associated with CBD than the corticobasal syndrome [22]. Therefore, CBD may present as a relatively symmetric syndrome and is not always associated with asymmetry. Neuropathological studies of such cases have revealed a shifting of the tau deposition with more tau deposited in limbic and hindbrain structures in those presenting with a progressive supranuclear palsy syndrome [52, 53]. Sometimes there can be overlap between features of the corticobasal syndrome and features of the progressive supranuclear palsy syndrome, known as the hybrid syndrome [54]. In such instances the underlying pathology can be CBD, but more likely will be that of progressive supranuclear palsy.

Symmetric CBD

A recent case series described five patients with CBD who presented without asymmetric features. Some patients had features of the progressive supranuclear palsy syndrome but many either presented with, or also had, relatively severe behavioral changes and executive dysfunction [55]. These patients tended to be on average 5 years younger than those with an asymmetric presentation.

Progressive apraxia of speech with or without aphasia

There have been many reports of CBD patients presenting with a progressive speech and language disorder [9, 14, 56, 57]. Careful characterization of such cases has identified a motor speech disorder, known as apraxia of speech, in which there is difficulty with the planning and programming of speech [58]. In such instances the speech output is characterized by the production of distorted sounds and sound substitutions. In addition, patients with CBD and apraxia of speech can also have a coexisting progressive aphasia [14]. The aphasia in such instances is typically characterized by agrammatism; pure aphasia without apraxia of speech is less commonly associated with CBD [14].

Other syndromes

While the three most common syndromes associated with CBD are the corticobasal syndrome, the progressive supranuclear palsy syndrome, and progressive apraxia of speech with or without aphasia, there are other less common syndromes associated with CBD. One such syndrome is posterior cortical atrophy in which patients have visual spatial and visuoperceptual deficits [9, 17]. Another syndrome is that of behavioral variant frontotemporal dementia in which patients present with behavioral dyscontrol and executive dysfunction [9, 50, 57].

Pathology/pathophysiology of CBD

Pathology

Macroscopic and microscopic findings of CBD were first reported in 1968 by Rebeiz and colleagues [1]. Since that first report there have been many studies on neuropathology, including morphology, distribution, biochemistry, and ultrastructure of the lesions characteristic of CBD. Dickson and colleagues have published consensus neuropathological criteria for CBD [3] which currently serve as the gold standard for diagnosis.

Macroscopic features of CBD

In CBD, cortical atrophy is often focal and asymmetric, affecting parasagittal, peri-Sylvian, and peri-Rolandic regions (Figure 10.1A). The superior frontal gyrus is typically more affected than middle and inferior frontal gyri [3]. The pre-central and post-central gyri are also affected. Unless the patient had a posterior cortical atrophy presentation, the occipital lobe is usually spared. On sectioning the brain, cerebral white matter volume loss and thinning of the corpus callosum are observed [59]. The white matter may have a gelatinous consistency. The ventricular system may be enlarged. The anterior limb of the internal capsule is usually affected. The substantia nigra tends to be severely affected with depigmentation. Regions of the basal ganglia, including globus pallidus, striatum, and subthalamic nuclei, as well as thalamic nuclei and brainstem regions, are variably affected. Typically the medulla, pons, and cerebellar dentate nucleus are spared.

Microscopic features of CBD

Microscopic features of CBD include neuronal loss and gliosis affecting frontal and parietal neocortex and substantia nigra. Other neocortical regions can also be affected, as can basal ganglia, brainstem, and cerebellar regions, but to a lesser degree. Cases with spinal cord involvement have been reported [60]. The cardinal histological lesions observed in CBD are balloon neurons, neuronal inclusions, pre-tangles, coiled bodies, threads, and astrocytic plaques (Figure 10.1B–F). Balloon neurons are swollen, achromatic neurons that are observed with routine hematoxylin and eosin stain and immunohistochemistry (Figure 10.1B and C). Balloon neurons are not specific to CBD and can be seen in other neurodegenerative diseases, such as argyrophilic grain disease [61]. The other lesions are best identified with either silver stain or with tau immunohisto-

chemistry. Coiled bodies are oligodendroglial in origin (Figure 10.1D and F) but, like balloon neurons, they are not specific to CBD and can be found in other neurodegenerative diseases, such as progressive supranuclear palsy [62]. Neuronal inclusions tend to be found in small neurons in the upper lamina of the cortex, or they may be observed in brainstem nuclei, for example in the substantia nigra or locus coeruleus. In original descriptions, neuronal inclusions in the substantia nigra were referred to as corticobasal bodies [4]. Threads can be of neuronal or glial origin. They tend to be numerous in gray and white matter in CBD (Figure 10.1F) and are one of the defining features of CBD. The astrocytic plaques, however, are considered the lesion most specific to CBD. Astrocytic plaques (Figure 10.1E), as the name implies, are astrocytic in origin and characterized by tau deposition in the terminal processes of astrocytes.

CBD biochemistry

CBD is considered a tauopathy because tau is abnormally deposited in brain cells and cellular processes. Tau is a microtubule associated protein that functions to promote assembly and to stabilize microtubules. Alternative RNA splicing of exons 2, 3, and 10 produces six tau isoforms that exist with either 3 or 4 conserved repeat sequences. Tauopathies can therefore be divided into those in which exon 10 is spliced in, and there are 4 conserved repeat sequences (4R tau), and those in which exon 10 is spliced out, and there are 3 conserved repeat sequences (3R tau). The insoluble tau found in CBD is predominantly 4R tau. Hence, CBD is considered a 4R tauopathy.

Biochemical studies have also revealed a specific tau profile associated with CBD. The detergent-insoluble cleaved tau fragments in CBD migrate as a doublet of approximately 37 kDa [63].

Distinguishing CBD from other tauopathies

CBD can be difficult to differentiate from progressive supranuclear palsy. However, unlike in CBD where astrocytic plaques are observed, another lesion known as the tufted astrocyte is pathognomonic for progressive supranuclear palsy. The two lesions do not coexist in CBD or in progressive supranuclear palsy, making distinction possible [64]. Biochemically, CBD can be differentiated from progressive supranuclear palsy because detergent-insoluble cleaved fragments in progressive supranuclear palsy migrate as a single band of 33 kDa [63].

Genetics

Almost all cases of CBD have been sporadic with only rare reports of so-called "familial CBD". At present, the evidence does *not* support CBD having a genetic underpinning, although CBD is clearly linked to the microtubule associated protein tau. The chromosomal region containing the microtubule associated protein tau gene has been shown to involve two major haplotypes, H1 and H2, defined by linkage disequilibrium between several polymorphisms over the entire gene. One large study demonstrated that there is an association between CBD and the microtubule associated protein tau H1 haplotype [65]. There have been reported families with mutations in the *MAPT* gene in which autopsy has demonstrated pathological features similar to those of CBD [66–68]. It remains unclear however whether these cases are truly CBD or whether they are cases of frontotemporal dementia and parkinsonism linked to chromosome 17. There has however been a report of a single case of CBD associated with a pathological mutation in exon 13 of the tau gene [69]. There is no clear association between CBD and the apolipoprotein E epsilon 4 allele [70, 71].

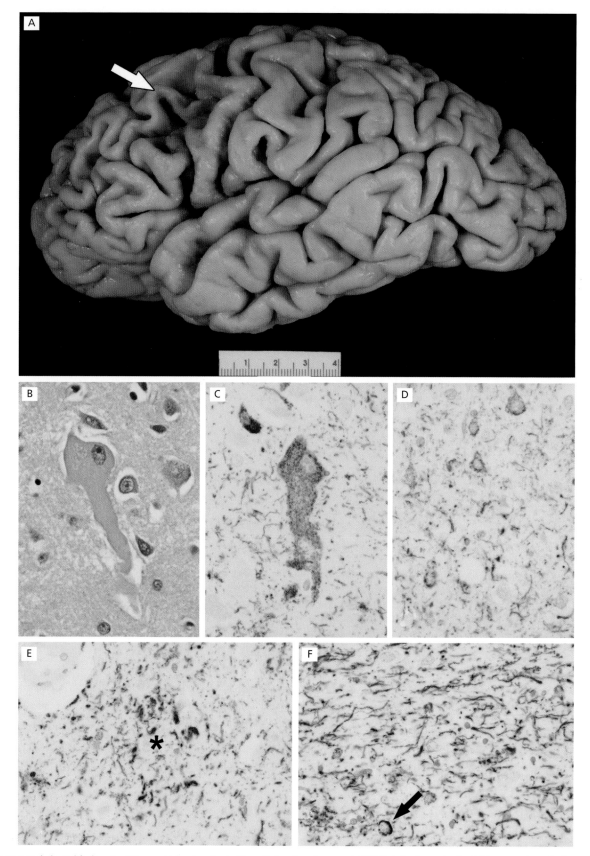

Figure 10.1 Pathological findings in a 70-year-old female patient with corticobasal syndrome and CBD. Note focal superior frontal (premotor) atrophy (arrow) (A), and microscopic findings of balloon neurons on hematoxylin and eosin (B) and tau (C), cortical pre-tangles on tau (D), astrocytic plaque (asterisk) on tau (E), and white matter threads (arrow indicates a coiled body) on tau (F) staining. All microscopic images are ×400. Courtesy of Dennis W. Dickson, MD, Mayo Clinic, Jacksonville, Florida.

Biomarkers

Neuroimaging

Voxel-based morphometry (VBM) is an unbiased technique that allows for statistical comparisons of volume loss on magnetic resonance imaging (MRI) across groups of subjects. VBM has been applied to subjects with CBD compared to controls and to patients with other neurodegenerative diseases [9, 72–74]. Patterns of frontoparietal atrophy, with predominant involvement of posterior frontal regions and relative sparing of temporal and occipital regions, are associated with CBD (Figure 10.2). One study using VBM compared autopsy confirmed subjects with CBD to those with progressive supranuclear palsy [74], and showed that atrophy in CBD was more cortical, whereas progressive supranuclear palsy showed greater involvement of the white matter, including superior cerebellar peduncle, as well as the midbrain. The authors also found that the pattern of atrophy in CBD differed depending on whether the predominant presenting symptom was dementia or an extrapyramidal syndrome [74]. One study showed that the pattern of atrophy in CBD cases presenting as corticobasal syndrome differed from cases with corticobasal syndrome with other neurodegenerative diseases, suggesting that results from previous studies assessing patients with corticobasal syndrome do not necessarily reflect CBD [73]. This finding was later confirmed [9].

Similar to VBM, there are techniques that allow assessment of white matter tract degeneration at the group level. Using diffusion tensor imaging, studies have demonstrated white matter tract degeneration in subjects with corticobasal syndrome compared to controls and to other neurodegenerative diseases [75–77], although none has been reported in CBD. One other potential imaging biomarker is the rate of whole brain volume loss. One study demonstrated that the rate of loss was higher in CBD compared to many other neurodegenerative diseases, including progressive supranuclear palsy [78].

Cerebrospinal fluid

Cerebrospinal fluid (CSF) studies, including CSF total tau and phospho-tau [79], CSF beta-amyloid [80], CSF neurofilament heavy chain [81], and CSF orexin [82], have been assessed in patients with corticobasal syndrome, but are lacking in CBD.

Examination and investigations

Laboratory testing

There is no one specific test that allows for a diagnosis of CBD. However, laboratory testing is important to exclude other conditions that may have a clinical presentation suggestive of CBD, especially those conditions that are treatable. Routine laboratory studies including a complete blood count, electrolytes, and liver, renal, and thyroid function studies should be performed, at least once. Additional testing should be considered, including vitamin B_{12} level, ceruloplasmin and copper levels, and urine analysis. If the condition is rapidly progressive, consider a serum paraneoplastic panel and other markers of autoimmune disease. CSF evaluations are important to exclude infectious, autoimmune, and inflammatory conditions that could have a presentation suggestive of CBD. CSF neuron-specific enolase, 14-3-3 protein, and S-100 protein, are useful to differentiate rapidly progressive CBD from Creutzfeldt–Jakob disease [10], because levels are typical normal or mildly abnormal in CBD. Electroencephalogram (EEG) may also be useful in such circumstances. In CBD, focal slow wave patterns may be observed [83].

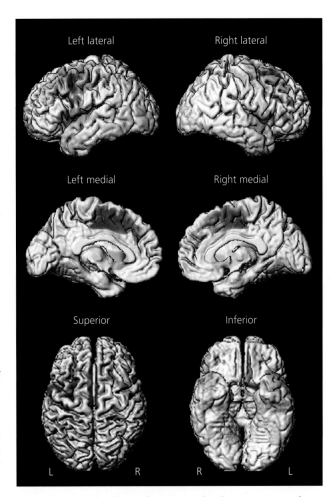

Figure 10.2 Voxel-based morphometry results showing regions of gray matter loss in patients with corticobasal syndrome and CBD compared to healthy controls. The 3D surface renders show cortical gray matter loss in the medial and lateral posterior frontal lobes, particularly premotor cortex, with relative sparing of the temporal, parietal, and occipital lobes and frontal pole. L = left, R = right. Courtesy of Jennifer L. Whitwell, PhD, Mayo Clinic, Rochester, Minnesota.

Myoclonus occurs in CBD and is thought to be cortically mediated. It has the characteristic features of absent cortical spikes preceding myoclonic jerks, absent giant evoked potentials, and enhanced long latency reflex [84, 85]. Therefore, electrophysiological studies may have some clinical utility in CBD. Somatosensory evoked potentials [86], visual event related potentials [87], and motor evoked potentials [88], measured by transcranial magnetic stimulation of the cortex, have not been assessed in CBD, only in cases of corticobasal syndrome [89, 90]. These studies may be useful in differentiating CBD from other neurodegenerative diseases [91, 92], but further work is needed.

Magnetic resonance imaging

Single-subject MRI studies in CBD are lacking and the utility of MRI to predict CBD or to differentiate CBD from other neurodegenerative diseases in individual cases is questionable. Early studies were performed in patients with corticobasal syndrome and suggested that asymmetric posterior frontal and superior parietal neocortical atrophy and atrophy of the corpus callosum are indicative of CBD [59, 93–95]. However these findings can also be seen in other neurodegenerative diseases and are not specific to CBD [96]. Furthermore, the pattern of atrophy will vary depending on the presenting clinical syndrome [9, 73]. Therefore a CBD patient presenting as posterior cortical atrophy will have a different neocortical pattern of atrophy than a CBD patient presenting as behavioral variant frontotemporal dementia.

Molecular imaging

Molecular studies using positron emission tomography (PET) or single photon emission computer tomography (SPECT) are lacking in CBD. There has been one case reported of [18F]fluorodeoxyglucose PET (FDG-PET) in CBD showing asymmetric hypometabolism of the parietal lobe [97]. Similar to MRI studies in corticobasal syndrome, however, hypometabolism is reported to be asymmetric and worse in the hemisphere contralateral to the more affected side of the body [98]. FDG-PET typically shows hypometabolism in frontal and parietal lobes (Figure 10.3), as well as in basal ganglia and thalamus in corticobasal syndrome [99–103], a pattern that can be observed in any neurodegenerative disease presenting as corticobasal syndrome. Studies using SPECT in corticobasal syndrome have found similar findings to those reported with PET, showing predominantly frontoparietal and striatal hypoperfusion [104, 105].

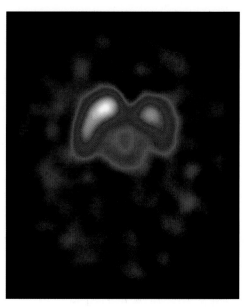

Figure 10.4 ^{123}I-fluoropropyl-CIT dopamine transporter SPECT imaging reveals asymmetric striatal dopamine transporter binding in a patient with corticobasal syndrome suspected to have CBD.

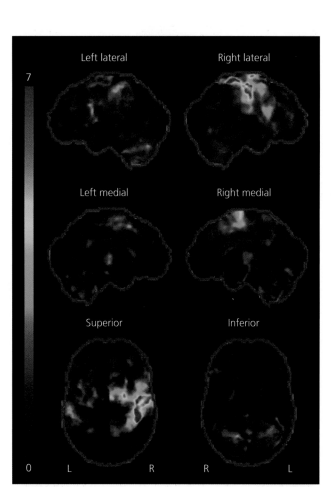

Figure 10.3 ^{18}F-FDG-PET with CT fusion demonstrates decreased metabolism of the right medial and lateral superior posterior frontal lobe almost 7 standard deviations from the norm when compared to an age-matched normal database.

Striatal dopamine transporter (DAT) imaging and assessment of striatal receptors has not been performed in CBD cases, although studies have observed abnormalities in patients with corticobasal syndrome [106–108]. Striatal DAT imaging, for example, typically shows asymmetric presynaptic dopamine transporter binding with greater reduction observed on the side contralateral to the more affected limb (Figure 10.4).

Diagnosis and prognosis

The diagnosis of CBD requires histological examination of the brain. Ante mortem diagnosis of CBD should take into account the presenting clinical signs and symptoms and syndromic diagnosis. Imaging characteristics on MRI, FDG-PET, or SPECT should be assessed and the clinician should give a differential diagnosis. A family history of dementia, parkinsonism, or ALS should exclude a diagnosis of CBD. A syndromic presentation of corticobasal syndrome, asymmetric progressive supranuclear palsy-like syndrome with limb apraxia and mixed apraxia of speech and agrammatic aphasia must have CBD in the differential diagnosis. An imaging pattern of very focal posterior frontal atrophy affecting medial and lateral superior, mid and inferior premotor cortex, whether asymmetric or not, should move CBD up the differential ladder. Whenever a diagnosis of CBD is being considered, the prognosis is poor. Disease duration is likely less than 7 years. The patient and family should be counseled that progression will occur in the order of most affected limb, then ipsilateral limb, then contralateral limbs. Speech and swallowing function and gait and posture will be affected. The patient will likely become wheelchair bound and possibly mute. The most affected limb will likely become fixed and eventually useless. The most common cause of death is aspiration pneumonia although in some patients death occurs when the patient suddenly, without known reason, stops accepting any oral intake.

Treatment

At present there is no treatment to slow or stop the progression of CBD. However, some CBD patients may get some benefit from certain types of therapies aimed at ameliorating specific signs or symptoms. Therefore, treatment approaches should be tailored towards the most bothersome symptoms.

One of the most disabling features of CBD is rigidity and bradykinesia. Therefore, it is important that there is a trial of high-dose levodopa (>1000 mg daily, on an empty stomach), as tolerated. A rare patient without any response to levodopa at lower doses may experience mild to moderate transient benefit at doses greater than 1000 mg [20]. Levodopa side effects can occur, especially at higher doses, but levodopa-induced dyskinesias are extremely rare [109]. Visual hallucinations are also rare. More common side effects are nausea and orthostatic hypotension.

Dystonia and myoclonus are also very disabling to patients suspected to have CBD. Benzodiazepines, primarily clonazepam, may provide some benefit [20]. In a retrospective study of patients suspected to have CBD, improvement in myoclonus and dystonia was observed with clonazepam therapy [20]. Anticholinergics and baclofen have not been beneficial but are still worth a trial; anticholinergic side effects may limit their usage however. Dystonia treatment with botulism toxin injections has been studied [110]. Of three patients with a dystonic clenched fist and suspected to have CBD who were treated with botulism toxin A, all had significant relief of pain and two had marked improvement of posture, however no patient experienced any functional improvement [110]. Another study reported that six out of nine patients also experienced improvement of dystonia with botulinum toxin injections [20]. Deep brain stimulation was inadvertently completed in one patient suspected to have CBD without significant improvement [111]. No studies have been completed in CBD.

Palliative therapies in patients suspected to have CBD are extremely important to obtain the best possible quality of life. Therefore, symptoms causing significant concern to patients should be addressed individually with appropriate intervention. Physical therapy is very important and should be tailored to the most disabling signs. Subjects with difficulty swallowing should undergo swallowing evaluations and be assisted with adaptive feeding techniques depending on how they perform on the swallow evaluation. Speech and language therapy are very important for patients with significant dysarthria and apraxia of speech. Patients who are mute can benefit from the use of devices that allow for communication depending on their physical state, i.e. the preserved ability to type. Depression and emotional lability may respond to serotonin specific reuptake inhibitors. However, careful evaluation is needed to differentiate apathy from depression. Patient and family support should be addressed and information regarding diagnosis, prognosis, and support groups such as www.curepsp.org should be provided.

Future developments

Identification of biomarkers

The majority of research performed to date has focused on the corticobasal syndrome. However, given current knowledge that the corticobasal syndrome is not specific to CBD, future biomarker development must focus on tau and CBD instead. Similar to Alzheimer's disease, another neurodegenerative entity in which amyloid binding ligands have been developed and CSF protein detection levels characterized, biomarkers for the detection of underlying tau pathologies are needed. Two areas that show promise are CSF biomarkers and imaging biomarkers. Imaging biomarkers that have so far been assessed include PET ligands [112], MRI patterns of atrophy [9, 73], and rates of whole brain and regional volume loss [78]. One case report showing correlation between ante mortem tau-PET with the ligand AV-1451 and histological tau burden in the brain of a corticobasal syndrome case with CBD pathology has been published [113].

Tau-directed therapies

There are many different approaches being directed at tau. These approaches include stabilizing microtubules, decreasing hyperphosphorylated tau, inhibiting protein kinases, inhibiting aggregation of tau fibril, and enhancing intracellular tau degradation. Four different agents have been tested so far in human Phase I–III trials including methylene blue, lithium chloride, the octapeptide NAP, and tideglusib. None of these compounds has shown efficacy as yet but data are scant and some agents are still currently being assessed.

References

1. Rebeiz JJ, Kolodny EH, Richardson EP, Jr. Corticodentatonigral degeneration with neuronal achromasia. *Arch Neurol.* 1968 Jan;18(1):20–33.
2. Riley DE, Lang AE, Lewis A, Resch L, Ashby P, Hornykiewicz O, et al. Cortical-basal ganglionic degeneration. *Neurology.* 1990 Aug;40(8):1203–12.
3. Dickson DW, Bergeron C, Chin SS, Duyckaerts C, Horoupian D, Ikeda K, et al. Office of Rare Diseases neuropathologic criteria for corticobasal degeneration. *J Neuropathol Exp Neurol.* 2002 Nov;61(11):935–46.
4. Gibb WR, Luthert PJ, Marsden CD. Corticobasal degeneration. *Brain.* 1989 Oct;112 (Pt 5):1171–92.
5. Litvan I, Bhatia KP, Burn DJ, Goetz CG, Lang AE, McKeith I, et al. Movement Disorders Society Scientific Issues Committee report: SIC Task Force appraisal of clinical diagnostic criteria for Parkinsonian disorders. *Mov Disord.* 2003 May;18(5):467–86.
6. Armstrong MJ, Litvan I, Lang AE, Bak TH, Bhatia KP, Borroni B, et al. Criteria for the diagnosis of corticobasal degeneration. *Neurology.* [Multicenter Study Research Support, Non-U.S. Gov't]. 2013 Jan 29;80(5):496–503.
7. Schrag A, Ben-Shlomo Y, Quinn NP. Prevalence of progressive supranuclear palsy and multiple system atrophy: a cross-sectional study. *Lancet.* 1999 Nov 20;354(9192):1771-5.
8. Togasaki DM, Tanner CM. Epidemiologic aspects. *Adv Neurol.* 2000;82:53-9.
9. Lee SE, Rabinovici GD, Mayo MC, Wilson SM, Seeley WW, DeArmond SJ, et al. Clinicopathological correlations in corticobasal degeneration. *Ann Neurol.* 2011 Aug;70(2):327–40.
10. Josephs KA, Ahlskog JE, Parisi JE, Boeve BF, Crum BA, Giannini C, et al. Rapidly progressive neurodegenerative dementias. *Arch Neurol.* 2009 Feb;66(2):201–7.
11. Wenning GK, Litvan I, Jankovic J, Granata R, Mangone CA, McKee A, et al. Natural history and survival of 14 patients with corticobasal degeneration confirmed at postmortem examination. *J Neurol Neurosurg Psychiatry.* 1998 Feb;64(2):184–9.
12. Bergeron C, Davis A, Lang AE. Corticobasal ganglionic degeneration and progressive supranuclear palsy presenting with cognitive decline. *Brain Pathol.* 1998 Apr;8(2):355–65.
13. Frattali CM, Grafman J, Patronas N, Makhlouf F, Litvan I. Language disturbances in corticobasal degeneration. *Neurology.* 2000 Feb 22;54(4):990–2.
14. Josephs KA, Duffy JR, Strand EA, Whitwell JL, Layton KF, Parisi JE, et al. Clinicopathological and imaging correlates of progressive aphasia and apraxia of speech. *Brain.* 2006 Jun;129(Pt 6):1385–98.
15. McMonagle P, Blair M, Kertesz A. Corticobasal degeneration and progressive aphasia. *Neurology.* 2006 Oct 24;67(8):1444–51.
16. Bak TH, Caine D, Hearn VC, Hodges JR. Visuospatial functions in atypical parkinsonian syndromes. *J Neurol Neurosurg Psychiatry.* 2006 Apr;77(4):454–6.
17. Tang-Wai DF, Josephs KA, Boeve BF, Dickson DW, Parisi JE, Petersen RC. Pathologically confirmed corticobasal degeneration presenting with visuospatial dysfunction. *Neurology.* 2003 Oct 28;61(8):1134–5.
18. Hu WT, Josephs KA, Ahlskog JE, Shin C, Boeve BF, Witte RJ. MRI correlates of alien leg-like phenomenon in corticobasal degeneration. *Mov Disord.* 2005 Jul;20(7):870–3.
19. Shelley BP, Hodges JR, Kipps CM, Xuereb JH, Bak TH. Is the pathology of corticobasal syndrome predictable in life? *Mov Disord.* 2009 Aug 15;24(11):1593–9.

20. Kompoliti K, Goetz CG, Boeve BF, Maraganore DM, Ahlskog JE, Marsden CD, et al. Clinical presentation and pharmacological therapy in corticobasal degeneration. *Arch Neurol.* 1998 Jul;55(7):957–61.

21. Watts RL, Mirra SS, Richardson EP, Jr. Corticobasal ganglionic degeneration. In: MarsdenCD, editor. *Movement disorders 3.* Oxford: Butterworths-Heinemann; 1994. p. 282–99.

22. Ling H, O'Sullivan SS, Holton JL, Revesz T, Massey LA, Williams DR, et al. Does corticobasal degeneration exist? A clinicopathological re-evaluation. *Brain.* 2010 Jul;133(Pt 7):2045–57.

23. Vanek Z, Jankovic J. Dystonia in corticobasal degeneration. *Mov Disord.* 2001 Mar;16(2):252–7.

24. Soliveri P, Piacentini S, Paridi D, Testa D, Carella F, Girotti F. Distal-proximal differences in limb apraxia in corticobasal degeneration but not progressive supranuclear palsy. *Neurol Sci.* 2003 Oct;24(3):213–4.

25. Soliveri P, Piacentini S, Girotti F. Limb apraxia in corticobasal degeneration and progressive supranuclear palsy. *Neurology.* 2005 Feb 8;64(3):448–53.

26. Salter JE, Roy EA, Black SE, Joshi A, Almeida Q. Gestural imitation and limb apraxia in corticobasal degeneration. *Brain Cogn.* 2004 Jul;55(2):400–2.

27. Pharr V, Uttl B, Stark M, Litvan I, Fantie B, Grafman J. Comparison of apraxia in corticobasal degeneration and progressive supranuclear palsy. *Neurology.* 2001 Apr 10;56(7):957–63.

28. Ozsancak C, Auzou P, Dujardin K, Quinn N, Destee A. Orofacial apraxia in corticobasal degeneration, progressive supranuclear palsy, multiple system atrophy and Parkinson's disease. *J Neurol.* 2004 Nov;251(11):1317–23.

29. Okuda B, Tanaka H, Kawabata K, Tachibana H, Sugita M. Truncal and limb apraxia in corticobasal degeneration. *Mov Disord.* 2001 Jul;16(4):760–2.

30. Leiguarda R, Lees AJ, Merello M, Starkstein S, Marsden CD. The nature of apraxia in corticobasal degeneration. *J Neurol Neurosurg Psychiatry.* 1994 Apr;57(4):455–9.

31. Jacobs DH, Adair JC, Macauley B, Gold M, Gonzalez Rothi LJ, Heilman KM. Apraxia in corticobasal degeneration. *Brain Cogn.* 1999 Jul;40(2):336–54.

32. Boeve BF, Lang AE, Litvan I. Corticobasal degeneration and its relationship to progressive supranuclear palsy and frontotemporal dementia. *Ann Neurol.* 2003;54 Suppl 5:S15–9.

33. Lang AE, Riley DE, Bergeron C. Cortico-basal ganglionic degeneration. In: Calne D, editor. *Neurodegenerative diseases.* Philadelphia: WB Saunders; 1994. p. 877–94.

34. Watts RL, Brewer RP, Schneider JA, Mirra SS. Corticobasal degeneration. In: Watts RL, KollerWC, editors. *Movement disorders: neurologic principles and practice.* New York: McGraw Hill; 1997. p. 611–21.

35. Leiguarda R, Merello M, Balej J. Apraxia in corticobasal degeneration. *Adv Neurol.* 2000;82:103-21.

36. Fogel B, Wu M, Kremen S, Murthy K, Jackson G, Vanek Z. Creutzfeldt-Jakob disease presenting with alien limb sign. *Mov Disord.* 2006 Jul;21(7):1040–2.

37. Rubin M, Graff-Radford J, Boeve B, Josephs KA, Aksamit AJ. The alien limb phenomenon and Creutzfeldt-Jakob disease. *Parkinsonism Related Disord.* 2012 Aug;18(7):842–6.

38. Chand P, Grafman J, Dickson D, Ishizawa K, Litvan I. Alzheimer's disease presenting as corticobasal syndrome. *Mov Disord.* 2006 Nov;21(11):2018–22.

39. Graff-Radford J, Rubin MN, Jones DT, Aksamit AJ, Ahlskog JE, Knopman DS, et al. The alien limb phenomenon. *J Neurol.* [Research Support, N.I.H., Extramural Research Support, Non-U.S. Gov't]. 2013 Jul;260(7):1880–8.

40. Goldberg G, Bloom KK. The alien hand sign. Localization, lateralization and recovery. *Am J Phys Med Rehabil.* 1990 Oct;69(5):228–38.

41. Leiguarda R, Starkstein S, Berthier M. Anterior callosal haemorrhage. A partial interhemispheric disconnection syndrome. *Brain.* 1989 Aug;112 (Pt 4):1019–37.

42. Carella F, Ciano C, Panzica F, Scaioli V. Myoclonus in corticobasal degeneration. *Mov Disord.* 1997 Jul;12(4):598–603.

43. Geda YE, Boeve BF, Negash S, Graff-Radford NR, Knopman DS, Parisi JE, et al. Neuropsychiatric features in 36 pathologically confirmed cases of corticobasal degeneration. *J Neuropsychiatry Clin Neurosci.* 2007 Winter;19(1):77–80.

44. Boeve BF, Silber MH, Parisi JE, Dickson DW, Ferman TJ, Benarroch EE, et al. Synucleinopathy pathology and REM sleep behavior disorder plus dementia or parkinsonism. *Neurology.* 2003 Jul 8;61(1):40–5.

45. Kimura K, Tachibana N, Aso T, Kimura J, Shibasaki H. Subclinical REM sleep behavior disorder in a patient with corticobasal degeneration. *Sleep.* 1997 Oct;20(10):891–4.

46. Thomas A, Bonanni L, Onofrj M. Symptomatic REM sleep behaviour disorder. *Neurol Sci.* 2007 Jan;28 Suppl 1:S21–36.

47. Gatto EM, Uribe Roca MC, Martinez O, Valiensi S, Hogl B. Rapid eye movement (REM) sleep without atonia in two patients with corticobasal degeneration (CBD). *Parkinsonism Relat Disord.* 2007 Mar;13(2):130–2.

48. Rossor MN, Tyrrell PJ, Warrington EK, Thompson PD, Marsden CD, Lantos P. Progressive frontal gait disturbance with atypical Alzheimer's disease and corticobasal degeneration. *J Neurol Neurosurg Psychiatry.* 1999 Sep;67(3):345–52.

49. Boeve BF, Maraganore DM, Parisi JE, Ahlskog JE, Graff-Radford N, Caselli RJ, et al. Pathologic heterogeneity in clinically diagnosed corticobasal degeneration. *Neurology.* 1999 Sep 11;53(4):795–800.

50. Josephs KA, Petersen RC, Knopman DS, Boeve BF, Whitwell JL, Duffy JR, et al. Clinicopathologic analysis of frontotemporal and corticobasal degenerations and PSP. *Neurology.* 2006 Jan 10;66(1):41–8.

51. Williams DR, de Silva R, Paviour DC, Pittman A, Watt HC, Kilford L, et al. Characteristics of two distinct clinical phenotypes in pathologically proven progressive supranuclear palsy: Richardson's syndrome and PSP-parkinsonism. *Brain.* 2005 Jun;128(Pt 6):1247–58.

52. Kouri N, Murray ME, Hassan A, Rademakers R, Uitti RJ, Boeve BF, et al. Neuropathological features of corticobasal degeneration presenting as corticobasal syndrome or Richardson syndrome. *Brain.* 2011 Nov;134(Pt 11):3264–75.

53. Kouri N, Whitwell JL, Josephs KA, Rademakers R, Dickson DW. Corticobasal degeneration: a pathologically distinct 4R tauopathy. *Nat Rev Neurol.* 2011 May;7(5):263–72.

54. Josephs KA, Eggers SD, Jack CR, Jr., Whitwell JL. Neuroanatomical correlates of the progressive supranuclear palsy corticobasal syndrome hybrid. *Eur J Neurol.* [Research Support, Non-U.S. Gov't]. 2012 Nov;19(11):1440–6.

55. Hassan A, Whitwell JL, Boeve BF, Jack CR, Jr., Parisi JE, Dickson DW, et al. Symmetric corticobasal degeneration (S-CBD). *Parkinsonism Relat Disord.* 2010 Mar;16(3):208–14.

56. Kertesz A, McMonagle P, Blair M, Davidson W, Munoz DG. The evolution and pathology of frontotemporal dementia. *Brain.* 2005 Sep;128(Pt 9):1996–2005.

57. Rohrer JD, Lashley T, Schott JM, Warren JE, Mead S, Isaacs AM, et al. Clinical and neuroanatomical signatures of tissue pathology in frontotemporal lobar degeneration. *Brain.* 2011 Sep;134(Pt 9):2565–81.

58. Josephs KA, Duffy JR. Apraxia of speech and nonfluent aphasia: a new clinical marker for corticobasal degeneration and progressive supranuclear palsy. *Curr Opin Neurol.* 2008 Dec;21(6):688–92.

59. Yamauchi H, Fukuyama H, Nagahama Y, Katsumi Y, Dong Y, Hayashi T, et al. Atrophy of the corpus callosum, cortical hypometabolism, and cognitive impairment in corticobasal degeneration. *Arch Neurol.* 1998 May;55(5):609–14.

60. Iwasaki Y, Yoshida M, Hattori M, Hashizume Y, Sobue G. Widespread spinal cord involvement in corticobasal degeneration. *Acta Neuropathol.* 2005 Jun;109(6):632–8.

61. Togo T, Dickson DW. Ballooned neurons in progressive supranuclear palsy are usually due to concurrent argyrophilic grain disease. *Acta Neuropathol (Berl).* 2002 Jul;104(1):53–6.

62. Hauw JJ, Daniel SE, Dickson D, Horoupian DS, Jellinger K, Lantos PL, et al. Preliminary NINDS neuropathologic criteria for Steele-Richardson-Olszewski syndrome (progressive supranuclear palsy). *Neurology.* 1994 Nov;44(11):2015–9.

63. Arai T, Ikeda K, Akiyama H, Nonaka T, Hasegawa M, Ishiguro K, et al. Identification of amino-terminally cleaved tau fragments that distinguish progressive supranuclear palsy from corticobasal degeneration. *Ann Neurol.* 2004 Jan;55(1):72–9.

64. Komori T, Arai N, Oda M, Nakayama H, Mori H, Yagishita S, et al. Astrocytic plaques and tufts of abnormal fibers do not coexist in corticobasal degeneration and progressive supranuclear palsy. *Acta Neuropathol.* 1998 Oct;96(4):401–8.

65. Houlden H, Baker M, Morris HR, MacDonald N, Pickering-Brown S, Adamson J, et al. Corticobasal degeneration and progressive supranuclear palsy share a common tau haplotype. *Neurology.* 2001 Jun 26;56(12):1702–6.

66. Mirra SS, Murrell JR, Gearing M, Spillantini MG, Goedert M, Crowther RA, et al. Tau pathology in a family with dementia and a P301L mutation in tau. *J Neuropathol Exp Neurol.* 1999 Apr;58(4):335–45.

67. Spillantini MG, Yoshida H, Rizzini C, Lantos PL, Khan N, Rossor MN, et al. A novel tau mutation (N296N) in familial dementia with swollen achromatic neurons and corticobasal inclusion bodies. *Ann Neurol.* 2000 Dec;48(6):939–43.

68. Brown J, Lantos PL, Roques P, Fidani L, Rossor MN. Familial dementia with swollen achromatic neurons and corticobasal inclusion bodies: a clinical and pathological study. *J Neurol Sci.* 1996 Jan;135(1):21–30.

69. Kouri N, Carlomagno Y, Baker M, Liesinger AM, Caselli RJ, Wszolek ZK, et al. Novel mutation in MAPT exon 13 (p.N410H) causes corticobasal degeneration. *Acta Neuropathol.* [Research Support, N.I.H., Extramural Research Support, Non-U.S. Gov't]. 2014 Feb;127(2):271–82.

70. Schneider JA, Gearing M, Robbins RS, de l'Aune W, Mirra SS. Apolipoprotein E genotype in diverse neurodegenerative disorders. *Ann Neurol.* 1995 Jul;38(1):131–5.

71. Schneider JA, Watts RL, Gearing M, Brewer RP, Mirra SS. Corticobasal degeneration: neuropathologic and clinical heterogeneity. *Neurology.* 1997 Apr;48(4):959–69.

72. Josephs KA, Whitwell JL, Boeve BF, Knopman DS, Petersen RC, Hu WT, et al. Anatomical differences between CBS-corticobasal degeneration and CBS-Alzheimer's disease. *Mov Disord.* 2010 Jul 15;25(9):1246–52.

73. Whitwell JL, Jack CR, Jr., Boeve BF, Parisi JE, Ahlskog JE, Drubach DA, et al. Imaging correlates of pathology in corticobasal syndrome. *Neurology.* 2010 Nov 23;75(21):1879–87.

74. Josephs KA, Whitwell JL, Dickson DW, Boeve BF, Knopman DS, Petersen RC, et al. Voxel-based morphometry in autopsy proven PSP and CBD. *Neurobiol Aging.* 2008 Feb;29(2):280–9.

75. Whitwell JL, Schwarz CG, Reid RI, Kantarci K, Jack CR, Jr., Josephs KA. Diffusion tensor imaging comparison of progressive supranuclear palsy and corticobasal syndromes. *Parkinsonism Relat Disord.* [Research Support, Non-U.S. Gov't]. 2014 May;20(5):493–8.

76. Tovar-Moll F, de Oliveira-Souza R, Bramati IE, Zahn R, Cavanagh A, Tierney M, et al. White matter tract damage in the behavioral variant of frontotemporal and corticobasal dementia syndromes. *PLoS One.* [Research Support, N.I.H., Intramural]. 2014;9(7):e102656.

77. Borroni B, Garibotto V, Agosti C, Brambati SM, Bellelli G, Gasparotti R, et al. White matter changes in corticobasal degeneration syndrome and correlation with limb apraxia. *Arch Neurol.* [Comparative Study Research Support, Non-U.S. Gov't]. 2008 Jun;65(6):796–801.

78. Whitwell JL, Jack CR, Jr., Parisi JE, Knopman DS, Boeve BF, Petersen RC, et al. Rates of cerebral atrophy differ in different degenerative pathologies. *Brain.* 2007 Apr;130(Pt 4):1148–58.

79. Borroni B, Gardoni F, Parnetti L, Magno L, Malinverno M, Saggese E, et al. Pattern of Tau forms in CSF is altered in progressive supranuclear palsy. *Neurobiol Aging.* 2009 Jan;30(1):34–40.

80. Noguchi M, Yoshita M, Matsumoto Y, Ono K, Iwasa K, Yamada M. Decreased beta-amyloid peptide42 in cerebrospinal fluid of patients with progressive supranuclear palsy and corticobasal degeneration. *J Neurol Sci.* 2005 Oct 15;237(1-2):61-5.

81. Brettschneider J, Petzold A, Sussmuth SD, Landwehrmeyer GB, Ludolph AC, Kassubek J, et al. Neurofilament heavy-chain NfH(SMI35) in cerebrospinal fluid supports the differential diagnosis of Parkinsonian syndromes. *Mov Disord.* 2006 Dec;21(12):2224–7.

82. Yasui K, Inoue Y, Kanbayashi T, Nomura T, Kusumi M, Nakashima K. CSF orexin levels of Parkinson's disease, dementia with Lewy bodies, progressive supranuclear palsy and corticobasal degeneration. *J Neurol Sci.* 2006 Dec 1;250(1-2):120-3.

83. Tashiro K, Ogata K, Goto Y, Taniwaki T, Okayama A, Kira J, et al. EEG findings in early-stage corticobasal degeneration and progressive supranuclear palsy: a retrospective study and literature review. *Clin Neurophysiol.* 2006 Oct;117(10):2236–42.

84. Lu CS, Ikeda A, Terada K, Mima T, Nagamine T, Fukuyama H, et al. Electrophysiological studies of early stage corticobasal degeneration. *Mov Disord.* 1998 Jan;13(1):140–6.

85. Grosse P, Kuhn A, Cordivari C, Brown P. Coherence analysis in the myoclonus of corticobasal degeneration. *Mov Disord.* 2003 Nov;18(11):1345–50.

86. Monza D, Ciano C, Scaioli V, Soliveri P, Carella F, Avanzini G, et al. Neurophysiological features in relation to clinical signs in clinically diagnosed corticobasal degeneration. *Neurol Sci.* 2003 Apr;24(1):16–23.

87. Wang L, Kuroiwa Y, Kamitani T, Li M, Takahashi T, Suzuki Y, et al. Visual event-related potentials in progressive supranuclear palsy, corticobasal degeneration, striatonigral degeneration, and Parkinson's disease. *J Neurol.* 2000 May;247(5):356–63.

88. Frasson E, Bertolasi L, Bertasi V, Fusina S, Bartolomei L, Vicentini S, et al. Paired transcranial magnetic stimulation for the early diagnosis of corticobasal degeneration. *Clin Neurophysiol.* 2003 Feb;114(2):272–8.

89. Wolters A, Classen J, Kunesch E, Grossmann A, Benecke R. Measurements of transcallosally mediated cortical inhibition for differentiating parkinsonian syndromes. *Mov Disord.* 2004 May;19(5):518–28.

90. Trompetto C, Buccolieri A, Marchese R, Marinelli L, Michelozzi G, Abbruzzese G. Impairment of transcallosal inhibition in patients with corticobasal degeneration. *Clin Neurophysiol.* 2003 Nov;114(11):2181–7.

91. Takeda M, Tachibana H, Okuda B, Kawabata K, Sugita M. Electrophysiological comparison between corticobasal degeneration and progressive supranuclear palsy. *Clin Neurol Neurosurg.* 1998 Jun;100(2):94–8.

92. Kuhn AA, Grosse P, Holtz K, Brown P, Meyer BU, Kupsch A. Patterns of abnormal motor cortex excitability in atypical parkinsonian syndromes. *Clin Neurophysiol.* 2004 Aug;115(8):1786–95.

93. Soliveri P, Monza D, Paridi D, Radice D, Grisoli M, Testa D, et al. Cognitive and magnetic resonance imaging aspects of corticobasal degeneration and progressive supranuclear palsy. *Neurology.* 1999 Aug 11;53(3):502–7.

94. Hauser RA, Murtaugh FR, Akhter K, Gold M, Olanow CW. Magnetic resonance imaging of corticobasal degeneration. *J Neuroimaging.* 1996 Oct;6(4):222–6.

95. Winkelmann J, Auer DP, Lechner C, Elbel G, Trenkwalder C. Magnetic resonance imaging findings in corticobasal degeneration. *Mov Disord.* 1999 Jul;14(4):669–73.

96. Josephs KA, Tang-Wai DF, Edland SD, Knopman DS, Dickson DW, Parisi JE, et al. Correlation between antemortem magnetic resonance imaging findings and pathologically confirmed corticobasal degeneration. *Arch Neurol.* 2004 Dec;61(12):1881–4.

97. Zalewski N, Botha H, Whitwell JL, Lowe V, Dickson DW, Josephs KA. FDG-PET in pathologically confirmed spontaneous 4R-tauopathy variants. *J Neurol.* 2014 Apr;261(4):710–6.

98. Blin J, Vidailhet MJ, Pillon B, Dubois B, Feve JR, Agid Y. Corticobasal degeneration: decreased and asymmetrical glucose consumption as studied with PET. *Mov Disord.* 1992 Oct;7(4):348–54.

99. Coulier IM, de Vries JJ, Leenders KL. Is FDG-PET a useful tool in clinical practice for diagnosing corticobasal ganglionic degeneration? *Mov Disord.* 2003 Oct;18(10):1175–8.

100. Laureys S, Salmon E, Garraux G, Peigneux P, Lemaire C, Degueldre C, et al. Fluorodopa uptake and glucose metabolism in early stages of corticobasal degeneration. *J Neurol.* 1999 Dec;246(12):1151–8.

101. Nagasawa H, Tanji H, Nomura H, Saito H, Itoyama Y, Kimura I, et al. PET study of cerebral glucose metabolism and fluorodopa uptake in patients with corticobasal degeneration. *J Neurol Sci.* 1996 Aug;139(2):210–7.

102. Hirono N, Ishii K, Sasaki M, Kitagaki H, Hashimoto M, Imamura T, et al. Features of regional cerebral glucose metabolism abnormality in corticobasal degeneration. *Dement Geriatr Cogn Disord.* 2000 May-Jun;11(3):139–46.

103. Garraux G, Salmon E, Peigneux P, Kreisler A, Degueldre C, Lemaire C, et al. Voxel-based distribution of metabolic impairment in corticobasal degeneration. *Mov Disord.* 2000 Sep;15(5):894–904.

104. Koyama M, Yagishita A, Nakata Y, Hayashi M, Bandoh M, Mizutani T. Imaging of corticobasal degeneration syndrome. *Neuroradiology.* 2007 Nov;49(11):905–12.

105. Okuda B, Tachibana H, Takeda M, Kawabata K, Sugita M, Fukuchi M. Focal cortical hypoperfusion in corticobasal degeneration demonstrated by three-dimensional surface display with 123I-IMP: a possible cause of apraxia. *Neuroradiology.* 1995 Nov;37(8):642–4.

106. Cilia R, Rossi C, Frosini D, Volterrani D, Siri C, Pagni C, et al. Dopamine transporter SPECT imaging in corticobasal syndrome. *PLoS One.* 2011;6(5):e18301.

107. Klaffke S, Kuhn AA, Plotkin M, Amthauer H, Harnack D, Felix R, et al. Dopamine transporters, D2 receptors, and glucose metabolism in corticobasal degeneration. *Mov Disord.* 2006 Oct;21(10):1724–7.

108. Plotkin M, Amthauer H, Klaffke S, Kuhn A, Ludemann L, Arnold G, et al. Combined 123I-FP-CIT and 123I-IBZM SPECT for the diagnosis of parkinsonian syndromes: study on 72 patients. *J Neural Transm.* 2005 May;112(5):677–92.

109. Frucht S, Fahn S, Chin S, Dhawan V, Eidelberg D. Levodopa-induced dyskinesias in autopsy-proven cortical-basal ganglionic degeneration. *Mov Disord.* 2000 Mar;15(2):340–3.

110. Cordivari C, Misra VP, Catania S, Lees AJ. Treatment of dystonic clenched fist with botulinum toxin. *Mov Disord.* 2001 Sep;16(5):907–13.

111. Okun MS, Tagliati M, Pourfar M, Fernandez HH, Rodriguez RL, Alterman RL, et al. Management of referred deep brain stimulation failures: a retrospective analysis from 2 movement disorders centers. *Arch Neurol.* 2005 Aug;62(8):1250–5.

112. Fodero-Tavoletti MT, Okamura N, Furumoto S, Mulligan RS, Connor AR, McLean CA, et al. 18F-THK523: a novel in vivo tau imaging ligand for Alzheimer's disease. *Brain.* 2011 Apr;134(Pt 4):1089–100.

113. Josephs KA, Whitwell JL, Tacik P, Duffy JR, Senjem ML, Tosakulwong N, et al. 18F]AV-1451 tau-PET uptake does correlate with quantitatively measured 4R-tau burden in autopsy-confirmed corticobasal degeneration. *Acta Neuropathol.* 2016 Dec;132(6):931–933

CHAPTER 11

Alzheimer's Disease

Qurat ul Ain Khan and Neill R. Graff-Radford

Mayo College of Medicine, Jacksonville, Florida, USA

Clinical definition

The classic definition of Alzheimer's disease (AD) is a clinicopathological entity with: (i) a clinical phenotype including impaired episodic memory, decline in other cognitive domains, and decreased ability to function in instrumental activities of daily living; and (ii) specific neuropathological changes including intraneuronal (neurofibrillary tangles) and extracellular parenchymal lesions (senile plaques), which are often accompanied by synaptic loss and inflammatory and oxidative processes [1].

Epidemiology

AD accounts for 70% of cases of dementia with a prevalence of 6.4% and incidence of 10.5/1000 per year in North Americans aged 60 or over [1]. The incidence and prevalence increase with age and are highest in the eighth and ninth decades. While some studies have suggested that the incidence of AD is higher in African Americans, after adjusting for education and socioeconomic status results have been inconsistent [2]. Recently epidemiology studies have shown a decline in the prevalence of dementia and it has been hypothesized this may be related to better treatment of vascular risk factors [3].

AD Criteria

Historical background

Until 1950, dementia in people 65 years of age or less was diagnosed as presenile dementia; those older than 65 were diagnosed as having senile dementia, with a vascular component thought to be a major contributing factor. From 1950 to 1980, the cutoff age of 65 for diagnosing AD was abandoned and the concept of early- and late-onset AD was embraced because the histopathological findings of early- and late-onset AD were determined to be similar and there was less emphasis on vascular burden as a cause of most dementia [1]. In 1984 the NINCDS-ADRDA (National Institute of Neurological and Communicative Disorders and Stroke and the Alzheimer's Disease and Related Disorders Association) criteria were published which defined AD as a clinicopathologic entity, and these became the gold standard [4].

As a result of advances in the field, biomarkers are now considered diagnostic tools. A series of papers defining a preclinical stage of AD [5], mild cognitive impairment (MCI) due to AD [6], and the dementia phase of AD [7] have been published; these are discussed in the following paragraphs.

Preclinical stage of AD

The key concept behind the notion of the preclinical stage is that the pathophysiological process of amyloid β (Aβ) brain deposition starts years, or maybe more than a decade, before the disease manifests itself clinically as MCI or AD. It can be detected by using Aβ biomarkers, specifically a decrease in Aβ42 levels in the cerebrospinal fluid (CSF) or Aβ deposition in the brain measured with positron emission tomography (PET). This asymptomatic period when AD pathogenesis is beginning could be a very important window for intervention to delay or even prevent the symptoms of AD. By the time clinical features appear there is a very large pathological load and damage to the brain. At present we do not know how many cognitively normal persons with brain Aβ deposition detected either using PET or CSF will go on to develop symptoms or how long it will take (see prognosis section further on). The most recent study [8] evaluating this indicates that the prognosis or conversion to dementia is dependent on other biomarkers that accompany the low Aβ42 in the CSF or high Aβ seen on the PET. If there is high tau and low hippocampal volume the majority (80%) will have AD dementia in 5 years but if there is no increase in tau or hippocampal volume loss less than 20% convert at 5 years. The stages of the new preclinical criteria are outlined in Table 11.1.

MCI due to AD

On the continuum of the AD pathophysiological process, MCI is an intermediate stage between the preclinical and dementia phases of AD. In this phase people start experiencing cognitive decline but they are mostly able to function. According to the Einstein Aging Study, the prevalence of amnestic MCI is 11.6% and the incidence

Table 11.1 Stages of preclinical criteria.

Stages	Aβ (PET or CSF)	Neuronal injury markers (tau, FDG, sMRI)	Subtle cognitive change	Description
Stage 1	Positive	Negative	Negative	Asymptomatic amyloidosis
Stage 2	Positive	Positive	Negative	Asymptomatic amyloidosis + neuronal injury
Stage 3	Positive	Positive	Positive	Amyloidosis + neuronal injury + subtle cognitive decline

Abbreviations: AD, Alzheimer's disease; Aβ, amyloid beta; CSF, cerebrospinal fluid; FDG, [18F]fluorodeoxyglucose; PET, positron emission tomography; sMRI, structural magnetic resonance imaging.
Source: Sperling 2011 [4]. Reproduced with permission of Elsevier.

Neurodegeneration, First Edition. Edited by Anthony Schapira, Zbigniew Wszolek, Ted M. Dawson and Nicholas Wood.
© 2017 John Wiley & Sons, Ltd. Published 2017 by John Wiley & Sons, Ltd.

is 3.8/100 persons per year. The prevalence and incidence of non-amnestic MCI are 9.9% and 3.9/100 persons per year, respectively [2]. The criteria for MCI are divided into two main classes: (i) the core clinical criteria, and (ii) the clinical research criteria.

The core clinical criteria

These criteria [6] were developed to help clinicians identify MCI despite not having access to specialized diagnostic tools. According to these criteria, patients and/or informants and/or clinicians become concerned about change in cognitive function. However the change may be subtle and cannot always be detected accurately on bedside screening tools such as the Mini Mental Status Examination (MMSE) [9]. The criteria require objective evidence of this change. If, on neuropsychological testing, the individual falls 1–1.5 standard deviations below scores matched for age, education, and cultural norms, this is in keeping with MCI. AD-related MCI patients often have anterograde memory loss but some patients have cognitive decline in other domains such as language, visuospatial skills, and executive function. Further, some patients may have impairments in more than one domain but still function well. The algorithm described using the Petersen criteria [10] thus includes persons with MCI fitting into four categories:

1 Amnestic single domain.
2 Amnestic multiple domain.
3 Non-amnestic single domain.
4 Non-amnestic multiple domain.

An important issue is that in most longitudinal studies some persons diagnosed with MCI may revert back to normal; this return to normal can be as high as 30% [10]. Ideally, MCI diagnosis is based on progressive cognitive decline so obtaining an informant history is very helpful.

The clinical research criteria

Because most clinical sites do not use brain amyloid imaging or CSF measures to diagnose MCI, at present these criteria are used in the research setting. According to these criteria, Aβ biomarkers and structural and functional biomarkers such as CSF tau, FDG-PET, and MRI are used to diagnose MCI due to AD with different degrees of certainty. There is a *high likelihood* that AD is the cause when biomarkers for both amyloid and structural/functional biomarkers such as tau/MRI/FDG-PET are positive. There is *intermediate likelihood* that AD is the cause of MCI when either amyloid or structural/functional biomarkers are positive but the other one is negative. The *lowest likelihood* that AD is the etiology is when biomarkers for both amyloid and structural/functional are negative. In this case other etiologies such as depression, frontotemporal dementia (FTD), vascular disease (VD), LBD, or prion disease should be considered. AD as the etiology of MCI is *undetermined* when neither amyloid nor tau biomarkers are available or test results are uninformative or conflicting (Table 11.2).

Prognosis using biomarkers and the concept of Suspected Non Alzheimer Pathology.(SNAP)

As data has accumulated in several prospective studies [8, 11–13] it became clear that some patients were Aβ -ve in the CSF and on PET scan but had either hippocampal atrophy, high CSF tau or abnormal deoxyglucose PET scans. This group was designated as having SNAP(14). Recently Dr. Jack and colleagues(15) have published the prognosis of in 5 groups based on 4 studies, MCSA, ADNI, Wash U and the Rotterdam study [8, 11-13]). Follow up ranged from 1.3 to 6 years.

1 Normal
2 Amyloid +ve and neurodegeneration -ve (Stage 1)

Table 11.2 MCI criteria incorporating biomarkers.

Diagnostic category	Aβ (PET or CSF)	Neuronal injury markers (CSF tau, FDG, sMRI)	Probability of AD
MCI – core clinical criteria	Indeterminate/ untested	Indeterminate/ untested	Uninformative
MCI due to AD – high likelihood	Positive	Positive	Highest
MCI due to AD – intermediate likelihood	Positive Untested	Untested Positive	Intermediate Intermediate
MCI – unlikely due to AD	Negative	Negative	Lowest

Abbreviations: AD, Alzheimer's disease; Aβ, amyloid beta peptide; PET, positron emission tomography; CSF, cerebrospinal fluid; FDG, [18F]fluorodeoxyglucose; sMRI, structural magnetic resonance imaging.
Source: Albert 2011 [5]. Reproduced with permission of Elsevier.

3 Amyloid +ve and neurodegeneration +ve (Stages 2 and 3)
4 Amyloid -ve and neurodegeneration +ve (SNAP)

Less than 5% in the normal converted, 10–15% of stage 1 converted, 20–-25% of stage 2 converted, 45–60% of Stage 3 converted and 5–15% of SNAP converted.

Dementia phase of AD

The NINCDS-ADRDA criteria for AD published in 1984 [4] have now been updated to include the following seven changes [7]:

1 Evidence of AD "pathophysiological process", i.e. by the presence of Aβ biomarkers (in CSF or with Aβ brain PET).
2 Takes into account the described criteria for LBD [16], FTD [17,18], and VD [19].
3 Includes presence of neuronal injury as evidenced by increased CSF tau and/or atrophy on the MRI and/or hypometabolism seen on the FDG-PET scan.
4 May not present with memory loss but with a focal onset such as the cases of visual variant AD [20], logopenic aphasia [17], and some cases of frontotemporal dementia [21].
5 Takes into account patients with known gene mutations causing AD [22].
6 Includes persons below age 40.
7 Excludes those with MCI from the category of possible AD.
The new criteria are in Table 11.3.

Table 11.3 AD dementia criteria incorporating biomarkers.

Diagnostic category	Aβ (PET or CSF)	Neuronal injury markers (CSF tau, FDG, sMRI)	Probability of AD
Probable AD			
• Based on clinical criteria	Unavailable/ indeterminate	Unavailable/indeterminate	Uninformative
• Three levels of AD-P	Positive	Positive	High
	Positive	Unavailable/indeterminate	Indeterminate
	Unavailable/ indeterminate	Positive	Indeterminate
Possible AD (atypical presentation)			
• Based on clinical criteria	Unavailable/ indeterminate	Unavailable/indeterminate	Uninformative
• Evidence of AD-P	Positive	Positive	High but does not rule out second etiology
Dementia unlikely due to AD	Negative	Negative	Lowest

Abbreviations: AD, Alzheimer's disease; Aβ, amyloid beta; AD-P, Alzheimer's disease pathophysiological process; CSF, cerebrospinal fluid; FDG, [18F]fluorodeoxyglucose; MRI, magnetic resonance imaging; PET, positron emission tomography.
Source: McKhann 2011 [4]. Reproduced with permission of Elsevier.

Atypical phenotype

AD patients may present with focal cortical symptoms but without memory loss initially.

Visual variant of AD

Patients with posterior cortical atrophy (PCA) present with signs and symptoms of cortical visual dysfunction, including some features of Balint syndrome, and may have some signs of Gerstmann syndrome, visual agnosia, alexia, agraphia, and transcortical sensory aphasia [20]. Their orientation and memory are relatively preserved at the start. Neuroimaging usually confirms posterior atrophy.

Logopenic aphasia

This is a relatively newly described entity in which word retrieval (in spontaneous speech and confrontation naming) and sentence repetition deficits are the core features. Spontaneous speech is characterized by its slow rate, with frequent pauses due to significant word-finding problems, but there is no frank agrammatism [17]. At the start patients often have good orientation and preserved anterograde memory.

Frontotemporal dementia

Some patients presenting with the clinical syndrome of FTD may actually have AD. In a study [21] using Pittsburg Compound B (PIB) to image persons with FTD, 16% were positive for brain Aβ.

Many of the patients with an atypical presentation have the pathological pattern called "hippocampal sparing AD", which made up 16% of one large autopsy series [23]. Because of this they often are oriented and initially have relatively preserved anterograde memory.

Pathophysiology of AD

When Alzheimer described the disease histologically, he noted the deposition of a substance in the form of plaques which was later identified as the beta amyloid protein by Dr Glenner and colleagues [19]. Subsequently, many lines of evidence have led to the hypothesis that brain deposition of this protein leads to AD.

Aβ is produced by the sequential proteolytic cleavage of the amyloid precursor protein (APP) (coded for on chromosome 21) by enzymes known as secretases. There are two pathways: one leading to the production of the Aβ peptides, the other not. In the amyloidogenic pathway the first step involves cleavage of APP at the amino terminus by an aspartyl protease (β-secretase, resulting in the formation of soluble APPβ (sAPPβ) and a membrane-bound APP carboxyl terminal fragment (CTF-β) [25]. Cleavage of CTF-β by γ-secretase results in the formation of Aβ peptides of varying length, including a 40 amino acid peptide (Aβ40) and a 42 amino acid peptide (Aβ42). The γ-secretase cleavage requires the presence of two membrane proteases, presenilin 1 (PSEN 1) and presenilin 2 (PSEN 2); it is thought that these presenilins may, in fact, be part of the γ-secretase complex. Other parts of this complex include nicastrin, a type I membrane protein that was originally found to include, APH-1, and PEN-2 [26]. Together with presenilin, the three components appear to comprise a minimal functional γ-secretase complex. It is also possible that these "accessory" proteins are involved in substrate presentation.

The non-amyloidogenic pathway is carried out by α-secretase, which cleaves the APP protein in the middle into sAPPα and CTF-β, which in turn is cleaved by γ-secretase into P3 and CTF-γ [27] (see Figure 11.1).

Aβ42 comprises less than 10% of the total secreted amyloid protein. It has been found to be more likely to form fibrils and is more toxic than the Aβ40 protein [28]. Aβ42 is found in the brains of all patients with AD and Aβ40 in two-thirds of patients [29]. Both accumulate as extracellular plaques consisting of β-pleated sheets, but prior to plaque formation a combination of fewer Aβ molecules form oligomers which may mediate the neurotoxic effects seen in AD [30]. Understanding of the generation of Aβ has proceeded at a faster rate than understanding of the pathways that lead to neuronal dysfunction and death. Aβ may be directly neurotoxic, initiate inflammation, cause oxidative stress, affect calcium homeostasis, or any combination of all of these. The relationship of Aβ to tau is also unknown but a clue comes from the triple transgenic mouse model JNPL3 [31]. In this model, mice have tau mutations, APP mutations, and a construct that allows the activation or inactivation of the tau pathway by the mouse taking doxycycline or not. Compared to the tau-only mouse model, mice with both tau and Aβ pathway mutations have more tau pathology, suggesting that the presence of Aβ increases tau pathology.

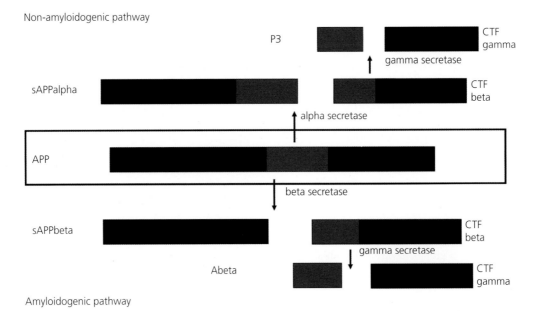

Figure 11.1 Amyloid precursor protein processing pathways. Abeta, amyloid beta; CTF, carboxyl terminal fragment; sAPP, soluble amyloid precursor protein.

Neuropathology of AD

Microcopic findings

On gross examination, the brain weighs 900–1200 g and atrophy is more pronounced in early-onset than in late-onset AD brain, when matched with controls. Cortical degeneration is evident in medial temporal and parietal lobes more often than frontal lobes (Figure 11.2A). Focal atrophy may be seen in atypical cases such as logopenic aphasia and posterior cortical atrophy. There is dilation of the third and lateral ventricles. The brainstem shows normal pigmentation of the substantia nigra and lack of pallor in the locus coeruleus in advanced cases. The olfactory bulb is consistently smaller than expected.

Histological findings

The classic histopathologic lesions of AD are senile plaques and neurofibrillary tangles [32]. *Senile plaques* are extracellular amyloid deposits that can be seen with silver (Bielschowsky) stain and thioflavin S or Congo Red stains. The β-pleated sheet structure of amyloid protein gives rise to characteristic birefringent apple green under polarized light. Amyloid plaques are of two types: diffuse, and cored or neuritic plaques. Diffuse plaques (Figure 11.2B) are not

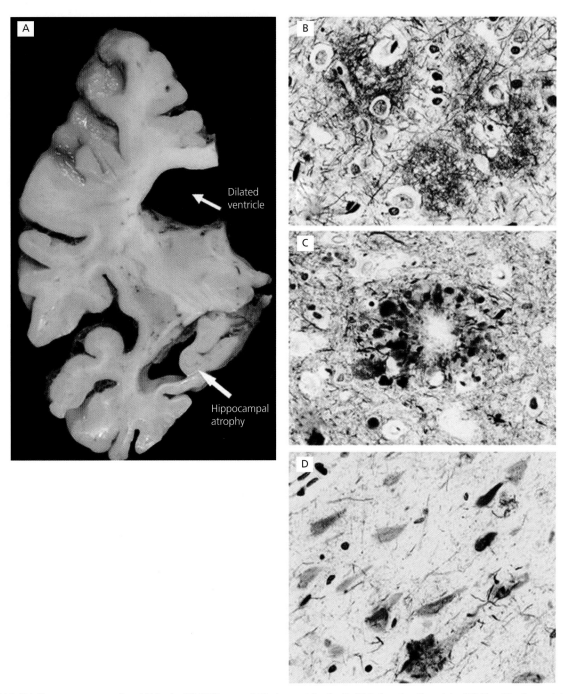

Figure 11.2 (A) Gross appearance of an AD brain. (B) Diffuse amyloid plaque stained with Bielschowsky silver stain. (C) Neuritic plaque stained with Bielschowsky silver stain. (D) Neurofibrillary tangle stained with Bielschowsky silver stain. Courtesy of Dr. Dennis Dickson, Department of Neuroscience, Mayo Clinic, Jacksonville, Florida.

specific for AD, are also seen in non-demented persons, and consist of extracellular amyloid aggregates with no neurites (nerve endings with tau); whereas neuritic plaques (Figure 11.2C) consist of extracellular cored amyloid aggregates surrounded by neurites [33]. *Neurofibrillary tangles* (Figure 11.2D) are intraneuronal aggregates of hyperphosphorylated tau, which is a microtubule associated protein (MAPT) [34]. Tau first accumulates in the nucleus and forms paired helical filaments which may then attach to the protein ubiquitin [35]. This tau aggregate disrupts the microtubular structure of the neuron, resulting in cell death. Phagocytes then surround these neurons to remove debris and ultimately the tangles become extracellular structures.

Other changes that take place in AD brains are as follows:

- *Inflammation*: This involves microglia, components of the complement cascade, pro-inflammatory cytokines, and α1-antichymotrypsin. Microglia are more evident in neuritic plaques and especially those with Aβ40 [36]. Microglia also respond to tangle formation and degeneration of synapses and neurons in the hippocampus and other parts of the brain. Discovery that variants of TREM2 are associated with AD [37] and that relative TREM2 deficiency related to the genetic variants results enhances Aβ accumulation from microglial dysfunction suggest immune dysregulation in AD pathogenesis [38].
- *Extracellular components* found in senile plaques are proteoglycans, amyloid P component, and apolipoprotein E. Amyloid P is a serum protein which is thought to accumulate due to possible damage to blood–brain barrier [39].
- Deposition of amyloid in cerebral blood vessels, called *cerebral amyloid angiopathy* (CAA) [40].
- *Granulovacuolar degeneration*, which is seen as a basophilic vesicle [41].

Atypical pathology

Recently two new atypical pathological subtypes of AD were recognized – hippocampal sparing and limbic predominant – according to the number and distribution of tangles in the brain [23] (Figure 11.3).

Hippocampal sparing AD

This pathological pattern seen in some AD cases is characterized by a lower neurofibrillary tangle burden in the hippocampus with relative sparing of the CA1 subiculum, and a higher neurofibrillary count in the cortices than in typical and limbic predominant AD. Braak staging is higher compared to the other two types. Disease duration is correlated with a high tangle count in middle frontal cortex. This pattern has early onset and rapid decline with predilection for men and frequently presents with focal cortical syndromes such as behavioral variant frontotemporal dementia, logopenic aphasia, or visual variant AD. Hippocampal sparing AD is associated with the H1H2 *MAPT* gene, rapid progression, and early disease onset [23].

Limbic predominant AD

This type of AD is characterized by a high neurofibrillary tangle count in the hippocampus as compared to association cortices than the other two forms of AD. It is more common in women and has a slower decline and prolonged course with less severe cognitive impairment than in typical AD. The number of senile plaques is lower in the visual cortex as compared to typical AD. H1H1 homozygous gene for *MAPT* and ApoE4 are more commonly seen than in limbic predominant AD. Limbic predominant AD might show some similarities with tangle-predominant dementia but differs in the extent of senile plaques, longer disease duration, and relation to ApoE4 [23].

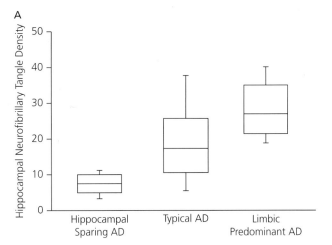

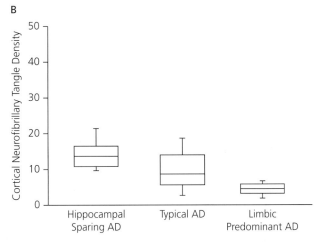

Figure 11.3 Hippocampal (A) and cortical (B) neurofibrillary tangle densities by AD subtype. Hippocampal data are the average neurofibrillary tangle count per 1.025 mm³ for the superior temporal, middle frontal, and inferior parietal regions. Source: Murray 2011 [18]. Reproduced with permission of Elsevier.

Genetics of AD

Genetic risk factors

Twin studies indicate that 60–80% of AD is related to genetic factors [42]. For an update see http://www.alzgene.org/.

From a genetic point of view, AD can be classified into two main types: early-onset, familial, autosomal dominant type AD (EOFAD); and late onset AD (LOAD).

Early-onset familial AD

Early-onset AD accounts for fewer than 2% of all cases of AD. Genes with mutations associated with this form are *APP, PSEN1* [43], and *PSEN 2* [44], which are located on chromosomes 21, 14, and 1 respectively. To date the numbers of mutations found for each of these genes are 32, 177, and 14 respectively. These can be seen on the Alzheimer Disease & Frontotemporal Dementia Mutation Database, curated by Marc Cruts (http://www.molgen.ua.ac.be/ADMutations/). The location of *APP* on chromosome 21 has been associated with early-onset AD in Down syndrome [45].

Late-onset AD

The gene most strongly associated with LOAD is apolipoprotein E (*APOE*) on chromosome 19 [46]. It is estimated by population-based studies in European subjects that a heterozygous carrier of this gene has a 2- to 4-fold greater risk of developing AD than a non-carrier. The odds ratio is 6–30 times greater in homozygous carriers of the gene [22]. The effect of this gene is strongly influenced by age and is strongest from 70 to 80 years of age. The presence of ApoE4 is not used clinically for diagnosis and is neither necessary nor sufficient to cause AD [47]. Linkage and smaller scale association studies have identified some other genes associated with AD, which are at present *BIN1* (bridging integrator 1), *CLU* (clusterin), *ABCA7* (ATP-binding cassette, sub-family A, ABC1, member 7), *CR1* (complement component 3b/4b receptor 1, Knops blood group), *PICALM* (phosphatidylinositol binding clathrin assembly protein), *MS4A6A* (membrane-spanning 4-domains, subfamily A, member 6A), *CD33* (protein CD33), *MS4A4E* (membrane-spanning 4-domains, subfamily A, member 4E) and *CD2AP* (CD2-associated protein). Results of genome-wide association studies (GWAS), whole exome sequencing and (WES) and whole genome sequencing (WGS), are updated regularly on AlzGene (http://www.alzgene.org/).

Environment

Risk factors

Risk factors associated with AD include aging, family history, head injury, female gender, and vascular risk factors such as hypertension and high cholesterol [1]. While type 2 diabetes has been associated with an increased risk of AD, some pathological studies have found diabetes to be associated more with vascular than with AD pathology [48, 49]. Depression is a common finding in people who develop AD; it is unclear at this time if it is a risk factor, prodrome, or consequence of the disease [50].

Protective factors

Protective factors for AD include diet and physical and mental activity. The Mediterranean diet may be protective. It includes a high intake of vegetables, legumes, fruits, and cereals; high intake of unsaturated fatty acids (mostly in the form of olive oil), but low intake of saturated fatty acids; a moderately high intake of fish; a low-to-moderate intake of dairy products (mostly cheese or yogurt); a low intake of meat and poultry; and a regular but moderate amount of ethanol, primarily in the form of wine and generally during meals [51]. A randomized prospective study in cognitively normal older persons found that those on a Mediterranean diet had improved cognition [52]. Some studies report that mental activities such as reading, learning, or playing games are associated with a decrease in cognitive decline and there are some prospective studies showing that certain cognitive exercises may enhance cognition [53].

Environmental enrichment has been shown to reduce Aβ deposition and increase the expression of certain protective transcripts in brains of transgenic mice [54]. Midlife systolic hypertension (≥160 mmHg) and hypercholesterolemia (≥6.5 mmol/L) may also increase the risk of AD in later life [55]. Several studies show that treating hypertension are associated with a decreased chance of dementia [56, 57]. Further in an observation from France treating vascular risk factors when person have Alzheimer disease seems to slow the rate of cognitive decline [58]. In a randomized controlled trial, there was no effect of reducing homocystine levels by taking high-dose vitamin B on slowing cognitive decline in AD [59]. Reviews summarize the evidence that physical activity is associated with protection against several types of dementia [60, 61]. Studies have shown that physical exercise and stretching improve cognition by several mechanisms including release of neutrotrophic factors, increasing hippocampal volume, and decreasing risk of vascular disease in general [62] (Figure 11.4). Exercise has also been shown to decrease Aβ and tau deposition in transgenic mice [63]. Moderate alcohol consumption (about 1 drink or <15.0 g of alcohol/day) seems to decrease the risk of cognitive decline in women [64]. A diet rich in polyunsaturated and nonhydrogenated fats may be protective whereas saturated or trans-unsaturated fats may increase the risk of AD [65]. Consumption of fish (at least once a week) and n-3 fatty acids might also be protective against incident AD by providing docosahexaenoic acid (DHA), which is an important component of membrane phospholipids in the brain [66]. In a randomized prospective study from Finland [66] the Finnish Geriatric Intervention Study to Prevent Cognitive Impairment and Disability (FINGER) patients were randomized to a multi domain intervention group (diet, exercise, cognitive training and vascular risk monitoring) compared to a control group. After two years patients in the active group had improved significantly on the neuropsychological battery compared to the control group.

Box 11.1 lists healthy brain behaviors.

Diagnosis

When completing an evaluation for dementia it is essential to keep in mind the differential diagnosis (Table 11.4).

Evaluation of dementia patients includes history taking, examination, laboratory tests, imaging, neuropsychological evaluation, and special tests.

History

In dementia cases, in addition to history provided by the patient, collateral history from an informant is also very important because patients might not be able to remember or articulate symptoms or might not be aware of them due to lack of insight, as happens in anosognosia. The history in dementia should cover the following aspects:

- *Onset* (acute vs subacute vs chronic) and *course* (slow, rapid, stepwise).
- *Evaluation of all cognitive domains,* which are:
  - *Memory*: type of memory (immediate vs-. short-term vs long-term, or anterograde vs retrograde, or declarative vs nondeclarative)
  - *Language*: difficulty naming, speaking, understanding, or repeating words/sentences
  - *Visuospatial*: ability to remember directions or faces
  - *Executive*: ability to make decisions, attention, concentration, and judgment.
- *Personality changes*: changes in behavior and social conduct, apathy, lack of empathy, disinhibition, changes in eating habits, increased jocularity, etc.
- *Level of functioning*: ability to function in occupational, personal, or social life (instrumental activities of daily living) can be assessed by asking about activities such as cooking, performing chores of the house such as laundry, using appliances such as microwave or phones, shopping, traveling in public transportation, managing finances, and medication management. Basic activities

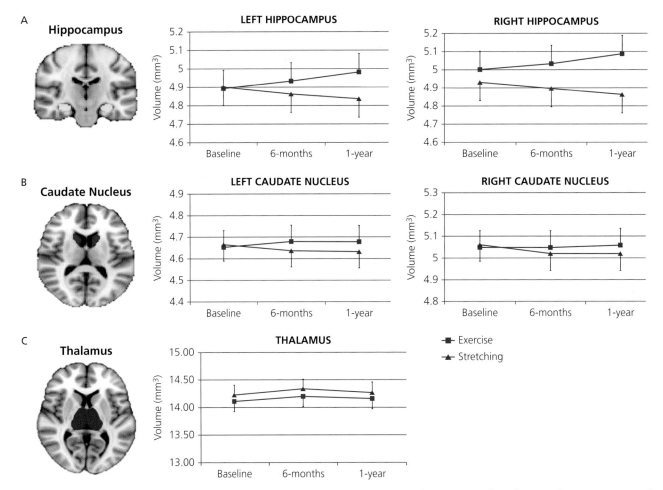

Figure 11.4 (A) Example of hippocampus segmentation and graphs demonstrating an increase in hippocampus volume for an aerobic exercise group and a decrease in volume for a stretching control group. The Time × Group interaction was significant ($P <.001$) for both left and right regions. (B) Example of caudate nucleus segmentation and graphs demonstrating the changes in volume for both groups. Although the exercise group showed an attenuation of decline, this did not reach significance (both $P >.10$). (C) Example of thalamus segmentation and graph demonstrating the change in volume for both groups. None of the changes were significant for the thalamus. Source: Erickson et al. 2011 [62]. Reproduced with permission from PNAS.

of daily living such as bathing, dressing, toileting, and feeding are usually affected late in the course of the disease.

- *Neuropsychiatric symptoms*:
  - *Depression* is often a comorbid condition with dementia and can be assessed by asking about feelings of sadness, hopelessness, worthlessness or guilt, negative thoughts, anger, anhedonia, changes in sleep, appetite or energy level, passive or active thoughts of suicide, etc. Impairment in cognition, especially attention, concentration, and short-term memory, can also be a symptom of depression.
  - *Anxiety* can be assessed by asking about feelings of restlessness, apprehension, irritability, fear or uneasiness about being alone, ruminative thoughts, and panic attacks.
  - *Agitation and aggression*: assessment should include potential for physical and verbal aggression, and danger to self or others.
  - *Psychosis*: questions should be asked about paranoia, delusions, or hallucinations. Common delusional themes may be that someone is stealing money, delusions of jealousy, and phantom boarder late in the disease. Auditory and visual hallucinations may be present in the late stages of AD; however visual hallucinations can be an early feature in Lewy body disease.

- *Sleep*: evaluation of sleep patterns, insomnia, REM sleep disorders, especially dream enactment, sleep apnea, daytime sleepiness, fluctuations in alertness and cognition, periodic limb movement disorder (PLMD), etc., is often helpful.
- *Motor symptoms*: asking about motor or extrapyramidal symptoms such as tremor, slowness of movements, falls, difficulty with balance and gait, change in handwriting, and softer voice often helps.
- *Autonomic symptoms*: symptoms of dysautonomia such as orthostatic hypotension (dizziness, light headedness), urinary incontinence, and dysphagia should be inquired about.
- *Medical and neurological conditions*: inquire about conditions such as hypertension, hypercholesterolemia, diabetes, stroke/transient ischemic attack, thyroid disease, vitamin B_{12} deficiency, cardiac arrest, multiple sclerosis, history of head injury, loss of consciousness, and seizures.
- *Social history*: knowing about the level of education, occupational history, and time of retirement gives insight into the IQ level and baseline functioning, as well as decline. Use of alcohol and other recreational drugs can have significant effects on memory and cognition.
- *Family history*: history of dementia in first degree relatives (parents, siblings, children), and other relatives (grandparents, uncles,

Box 11.1 A dozen healthy brain tips.

Human epidemiology and mouse experiments suggest that the following may be associated with a decreased chance of memory loss.

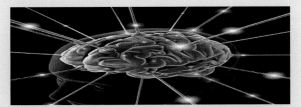

1 Mental exercise (e.g., reading, doing puzzles, learning something new).
2 Moderate aerobic exercise, 50 minutes, three times per week (e.g., walking, bicycling).
3 B-complex vitamins (one per day).
4 Vitamin C (500 mg per day).
5 A handful (1.5 oz) of nuts daily (e.g., almonds, walnuts).
6 Fish three times per week (e.g., salmon, halibut, mackerel).
7 Foods with curry spice including curcumin.
8 Foods high in antioxidants (e.g., grape juice, pomegranate juice, beans, berries, green tea).
9 The Mediterranean diet (e.g., vegetables, legumes, fruit, cereal, olive oil, fish, moderate dairy products, wine, low intake of meat and poultry).
10 Treating cardiac risk factors such as hypertension, high cholesterol, diabetes, and being overweight.
11 Socialization (e.g., frequent time with family and friends).
12 Quality sleep (e.g., tell your doctor if you have loud snoring or episodes of stopping breathing or gasping).

aunts, cousins) including age of onset, symptoms, and specific diagnosis, if known, is an important part of evaluation.

• *Medication*: all the medications and supplements that the patient takes should be thoroughly reviewed. Information about any over-the-counter and prn medications should be obtained. Table 11.5 lists medications that can contribute to cognitive impairment.

Examination

Bedside screening tests of cognition such as the MMSE [9], the Kokmen Short Test of Mental Status [67], or the Montreal Cognitive Assessment [68] are important tools in evaluation of AD patients. The screening test can be further supplemented by questions testing for anterograde memory such as name of the current president and spouse and names of past presidents and spouses. The medical exam should include examining for carotid bruits, hypertension, cardiac murmurs, and arrhythmias. A complete neurological examination should be completed. Assessment of gait including stability and balance, length of steps, steps required for turning, arm swing, and distance between the legs provides important information. Special attention should be paid to any focal findings or deficits on exam. Features of parkinsonism including tremor, rigidity, hypomimia, slowing of finger, hand, and foot rapid alternating movements, and glabellar reflex should be looked for. Cerebellar function should be assessed by the finger to nose test, alternating rapid movements of hands, and heel to shin test. The palmomental and snout reflexes are not particularly useful as they are also common in normal individuals.

Investigation

The indicated routine workup for dementia patients includes blood work and brain imaging. The blood work includes complete blood count (CBC), thyroid stimulating hormone (TSH), serum vitamin B_{12} level, and rapid plasma reagin (RPR), which helps mainly to exclude

Table 11.4 Differential diagnosis of dementia.

Degenerative
• Alzheimer's disease
• Lewy body dementia
• Frontotemporal dementia
• Semantic dementia
• Progressive non-fluent aphasia
• Frontal dementia
• Corticobasal degeneration
• Progressive supranuclear palsy
• Multiple system atrophy
• Huntington disease

Vascular
• Single strategic stroke
• Multiple strokes
• Multiple lacunes
• Small vessel disease
• Amyloid angiopathy
• Subarachnoid hemorrhage
• Superficial siderosis
• Cerebral autosomal dominant arteriopathy with subcortical infarcts and leukoencephalopathy (CADASIL)
• Subdural hematoma

Infectious
• Acute and chronic fungal and bacterial meningitis
• Sequel of herpes encephalitis
• Other viral encephalitis
• HIV dementia
• Neurosyphilis
• Transmissible prion disease
• Subacute sclerosing panencephalitis (SSPE)
• Progressive multifocal leukoencephalopathy (PML)

Toxic, metabolic, and deficiency states
• Medications (see Table 11.5)
• Glue sniffing
• Heavy metal, for example mercury
• Hypothyroidism
• Vitamin B_{12}, B_1, B_3, and B_6 deficiency
• Organ failure (heart, lung, kidney, and liver)
• Substance abuse

Psychiatric
• Mood disorder (depression, bipolar disorder)
• Psychosis

Neurological diseases
• Anoxic brain damage
• Cerebral neoplasm
• Limbic encephalitis
• Head injury
• Multiple sclerosis
• Hydrocephalus
• Leukodystrophies (for example metachromatic, and adrenoleukodystrophy)
• Hashimoto's encephalopathy
• Non-vasculitic autoimmune inflammatory meningoencephalitis

other reversible causes of cognitive impairment. CT or structural MRI changes typical of AD are atrophy of medial and lateral temporal lobes, inferior parietal lobe, and insula. With advances in the field, other modalities of imaging are now available including Aβ imaging using Pittsburg Compound B (PIB) and FDA approved florbetapir and florbetaben positron emission tomography (PET) (Figure 11.5) and fluorodeoxyglucose (FDG) PET scanning (Figure 11.6). Several companies are now evaluating tau imaging agents and they the tau deposition correlates with the clinical findings [69].

Neuropsychological testing is often helpful in looking for the typical pattern of cognitive impairment in AD (rapid forgetting, impaired semantic or letter fluency, decreased naming, and

Table 11.5 Commonly used drugs that may cause memory loss.

Over-the-counter
- Sleep aids, cold medications, and antihistamines that contain doxylamine or diphenhydramine:
  - Tylenol PM
  - Nyquil PM
  - Advil PM
  - Sominex
  - Unisom
  - Benadryl
  - Sudafed Sinus Nighttime
  - Tylenol Allergy Sinus

Stimulants (amphetamines)
- Ritalin, Concerta, Metadate, Methylin (methylphenidate)
- Adderall (dextroamphetamine)
- Provigil (modafinil)

Mood stabilizers (antipsychotics)
- Seroquel (quetiapine)
- Zyprexa (olanzapine)
- Abilify (aripiprazole)
- Risperdal (risperidone)

Blood pressure (antihypertensives)
- Cozaar (losartan)
- Lisinopril
- Hyzaar (losartan-hydrochlorothiazide)
- Catapress (clonidine)
- Beta blockers:
  - Toprolol (metoprolol)
  - Atenolol
  - Coreg (carvedilol)
  - Propranolol
  - Labetalol

Anti-anxiety (benzodiazepines)
- Xanax (alprazolam)
- Klonopin (clonazepam) Ativan (lorazepam)
- Valium (diazepam)

Antidepressants
- Celexa (citalopram)
- Wellbutrin, Budeprion, Buproban (bupropion)
- Trazodone
- Amitriptyline
- Imipramine

Transplant (immunosuppressants)
- Prograf (tacrolimus)
- Neoral (cyclosporine)

Nausea
- Transderm Scop patch (scopolamine)
- Reglan (metoclopramide)
- Meclizine

Antiparkinson (dopamine agonists)
- Parcopa, Sinemet (carbidopa/levodopa)
- Cogentin (benzatropine)

Sleep (hypnotics)
- Ambien (zolpidem)
- Lunesta (eszopiclone)
- Restoril (temazepam)

Migraine (serotonin 5-HT agonists)
- Imitrex (sumatriptan)
- Maxalt (rizatriptan)

Heart (antiarrhythmic)
- Lanoxin (digoxin)
- Sotalol

Seizure (anticonvulsants)
- Lamictal (lamotrigine)
- Phenobarbital
- Dilantin (phenytoin)
- Keppra (levetiracetam)
- Topamax (topiramate)
- Zonegran (zonisamide)

Overactive bladder (anticholinergics)
- Detrol (tolterodin)
- Ditropan (oxybutynin)

Pain
- Opiates
  - Oxycontin, Percocet, Percodan (oxycodone)
  - Atvinza, Kadian, MS Contin (morphine)
  - Lortab, Lorcet, Vicoprofen (hydrocodone)
  - Duragesic patch (fentanyl)
  - Suboxone (buprenorphine and naloxone)
  - Darvocet (propoxyphene and acetaminophen)
  - Methadone
- Salicylates
  - Aspirin
- Other
  - Baclofen

Acid blocker (H$_2$ antagonist)
- Pepcid (famotidine)
- Tagamet (cimetidine)

Antibiotics
- Flagyl (metronidazole)

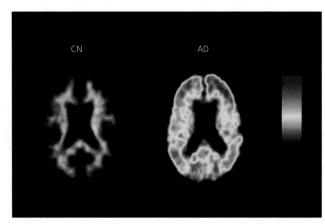

Figure 11.5 PIB-PET in a control patient (left) and an AD patient (right). The yellow and red areas indicate retention of amyloid binding tracer, reflecting amyloid deposits. The patient with normal cognition (left) has no tracer retention, whereas the patient with AD has prominent tracer retention (right). Courtesy of Dr. Val Lowe.

impaired visuospatial ability). Further, neuropsychology is excellent for following progression of the disease.

Biomarkers in CSF at present are used for research and can be used to distinguish patients with an atypical presentation from causes other than AD. The typical CSF biomarker pattern in AD is low CSF Aβ42 and high total tau (tTau) and phospho tau (pTau).

Management

Pharmacological treatment
See Table 11.6 for FDA-approved treatment for AD.

Safety issues
Driving
Patients with memory impairment are at increased risk for automobile accidents and therefore should be made aware of this [70]. The American Academy of Neurology (AAN) guidelines [70] on driving and Alzheimer's disease indicate that persons with a Clini-

Parietal lobe hypometabolism

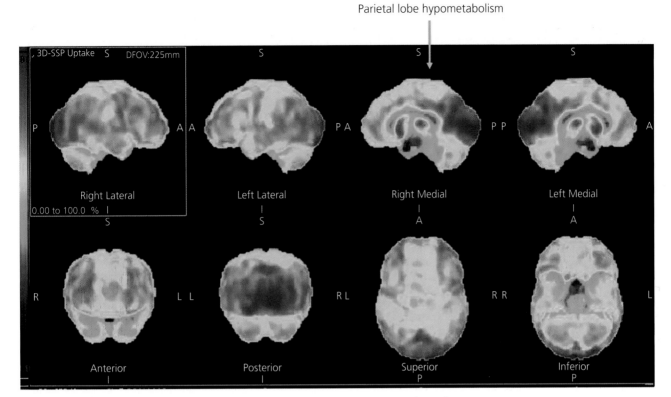

Figure 11.6 FDG-PET showing parietal lobe hypometabolism in a patient with AD. Courtesy of Dr. Val Lowe.

Table 11.6 FDA-approved medications for AD.

Class	Name	Dose	Disease stage	Comment
Cholinesterase inhibitors	Donepezil	Start 5 mg q.d. Effective: 5–10 mg q.d.	Mild to moderate, perhaps severe	Easiest compliance; mild diarrhea
	Rivastigmine	Start 1.5 mg b.i.d. Titrate up monthly to 3–6 mg b.i.d.	Mild to moderate, perhaps severe	Inhibits acetyl and butyrylcholinesterase; requires gradual titration because of GI intolerance; follow weight
	Galantamine	Start 4 mg b.i.d. Effective: 8–12 mg b.i.d.	Mild to moderate, perhaps severe	Allosteric modulator of nicotinic receptor; nausea most common adverse side effects
NMDA antagonist	Memantine	Start 5 mg q.d. Titrate weekly to 10 mg b.i.d.	Moderate to severe, perhaps mild (in those who do not tolerate cholinesterase inhibitors)	Headache, transient confusion may occur

cal Dementia Rating Scale (CDR) of 0.5 (equivalent to an MMSE score of about 25/30 or above) are at increased risk for accidents but no greater than other increased risk groups such as males 18–25 years or those with blood alcohol levels less than 0.08%. They can be offered an on-the-road test to evaluate their driving ability. Patients with a CDR of 1 or greater (equivalent to MMSE score <25) are at great risk and should be advised not to drive.

Medication supervision

Health workers should advise patients and their caregivers to have an organized system for taking medication such as a "day of the week" medication organizer. The caregiver and patient should share this responsibility.

Wandering

If the patient has a tendency to wander, an identity bracelet may be obtained from a local branch of the Alzheimer's Association.

Living situation

The health provider should assess the patient's living situation to make sure the patient is safe. Tailor advice for each situation. Factors to account for include severity of the problem, amount of family support available, patients' behaviors, finances, and community options. Weapons should be removed or disabled. At the beginning, patients often live with a spouse or independently with regular monitoring by family members. Later, options include in-home respite care, day care, and assisted living facilities. In the later stages, the family may need to place a person in a nursing home. Determining factors in making the decision to place a person in a nursing home include severity of the disease, behavioral symptoms, incontinence, caregiver stress or health, and the family's financial situation

Durable power of attorney

The healthcare provider should address the patient to designate a person with durable power of attorney for health decisions.

Finances

The family should create a situation so that the patient is less subject to financial errors, for example paying bills more than once or forgetting to pay them. Family members can oversee paying bills, or payment can be automated through the bank. Families should prevent exploitation of patients (which is all too common) and monitor investment decisions, another area of vulnerability.

Medication supervision

It is imperative that patients with memory problems have their medicines supervised by a spouse or other family member. It is helpful to have a "day of the week" container into which medicines for each day of the week can be placed. The patient's spouse is ideally suited to this role; quite often it is taken over by the spouse before the patient is seen at the tertiary clinic.

Management of agitation in dementia

Establish the cause:

- *Medical*: infection (especially urinary infection), medication (particularly anticholinergics, pain medications, sedatives, and antipsychotics; see Table 11.5), dehydration, electrolyte imbalance, constipation, pain, system dysfunction (liver, heart, pulmonary, kidney, and endocrine), neurological (stroke, seizure, subdural hemorrhage).
- *Environmental*: noisy roommate, change of environment, social isolation, interruptions from staff, change of caregiver, room lighting and temperature.
- *Sleep disorders*: establish quantity, quality (for example apneic spells, dream enactment behavior, or restless legs syndrome), and pattern of sleep.
- *Psychiatric*: evaluate for mood disorder, psychosis, and anxiety disorder.

Grade severity

Management of agitation depends on the severity, amount of disruption, and risk of physical harm to the patient or others.

- *Mild agitation*: may be disruptive but non-aggressive with little risk of danger to patient or staff; includes wandering and repetitive movements.
- *Severe agitation*: aggressive behavior with threat of physical harm to self or others, not controlled by verbal redirection (patient throws objects or food items, screams, grabs, bites, attempts to hit caregiver or injure self).

There are no good studies showing effective medication management of agitation. If the cause can be determined, non-medication intervention is ideal. Empiric trials of different medications are often instituted. We caution that there is a Federal Drug Administration (FDA) black box warning about the use of atypical antipsychotics in this situation.

The future in Alzheimer's disease

In the last two decades advances have been made towards identification of genes causing EOFAD. Until recently only ApoE4 has been consistently related to increased risk of LOAD, but excellent candidates are now summarized on AlzGene. Discovery of these and other genes will be helpful in understanding the underlying pathophysiological mechanisms of AD and would open doors for new treatment strategies.

The amyloid hypothesis has long been proposed as a major pathogenic mechanism of AD. Traditionally, insoluble amyloid plaques are associated with AD pathology; however, recent research has emphasized the possible role of soluble Aβ oligomers in AD pathogenesis. Further, mechanisms of excessive Aβ production vs impaired clearance leading to disturbance of homeostasis need to be explored. The role and mechanism of Aβ to tau accumulation are also unclear at this time and the role of the tau protein in AD pathogenesis is an area of extensive research. Better mouse models more closely resembling human expression of the disease are needed to understand the sequence of events [71].

One of the most challenging areas in the field is the treatment of AD. Several medications reached Phase II and III trails but failed, see for example Doody et al. [72]. At present there are several phase I or II or III trial either directed at early onset AD or at the presymptomatic phase of AD (called secondary prevention because the pathogenesis has started) . All of these studies can be found on www.Clinicaltrials.gov. Using Aβ PET candidates are screened and only those who are Aβ PET +ve are included. Monoclonal antibodies against Aβ fibrils (e.g. aducanumab [73]) or Aβ monomer (e.g. solanezumab [72]) are being tried. In addition there are several studies underway directed against Aβ using beta secretase inhibitors see www.Alzforum.org summarized the latest findings in a report on November 3rd 2016. Anti tau drugs are also in development and are being tried in AD.

Research in AD has come a long way in the last three decades. We have good hypotheses to test and improving biomarkers will help us follow the effects of intervention. Hopefully we shall be able to delay or even prevent this dreaded disease in the future.

References

1. Reitz C, Brayne C, Mayeux R. Epidemiology of Alzheimer disease. *Nat Rev Neurol.* [Review]. 2011 Mar;7(3):137–52.
2. Katz MJ, Lipton RB, Hall CB, Zimmerman ME, Sanders AE, Verghese J, et al. Age-specific and sex-specific prevalence and incidence of mild cognitive impairment, dementia, and Alzheimer dementia in blacks and whites: a report from the Einstein Aging Study. Alzheimer disease and associated disorders. [Research Support, N.I.H., Extramural]. 2012 Oct-Dec;26(4):335–43.
3. Matthews FE, Arthur A, Barnes LE, Bond J, Jagger C, Robinson L, et al. A two-decade comparison of prevalence of dementia in individuals aged 65 years and older from three geographical areas of England: results of the Cognitive Function and Ageing Study I and II. Lancet. [Comparative Study Research Support, Non-U.S. Gov't]. 2013 Oct 26;382(9902):1405–12.
4. McKhann G, Drachman D, Folstein M, Katzman R, Price D, Stadlan EM. Clinical diagnosis of Alzheimer's disease: report of the NINCDS-ADRDA Work Group under the auspices of Department of Health and Human Services Task Force on Alzheimer's Disease. *Neurology.* 1984 Jul;34(7):939–44.
5. Sperling RA, Aisen PS, Beckett LA, Bennett DA, Craft S, Fagan AM, et al. Toward defining the preclinical stages of Alzheimer's disease: Recommendations from the National Institute on Aging and the Alzheimer's Association workgroup. *Alzheimers Dement.* 2011 Apr 20.
6. Albert MS, DeKosky ST, Dickson D, Dubois B, Feldman HH, Fox NC, et al. The diagnosis of mild cognitive impairment due to Alzheimer's disease: recommendations from the National Institute on Aging-Alzheimer's Association workgroups on diagnostic guidelines for Alzheimer's disease. Alzheimer's & dementia : the journal of the Alzheimer's Association. [Consensus Development Conference, NIH Research Support, Non-U.S. Gov't]. 2011 May;7(3):270–9.
7. McKhann GM, Knopman DS, Chertkow H, Hyman BT, Jack CR, Jr., Kawas CH, et al. The diagnosis of dementia due to Alzheimer's disease: recommendations from the National Institute on Aging-Alzheimer's Association workgroups on diagnostic guidelines for Alzheimer's disease. Alzheimer's & dementia : the journal of the Alzheimer's Association. [Consensus Development Conference, NIH Research Support, Non-U.S. Gov't]. 2011 May;7(3):263–9.
8. Vos SJ, Gordon BA, Su Y, Visser PJ, Holtzman DM, Morris JC, et al. NIA-AA staging of preclinical Alzheimer disease: discordance and concordance of CSF and imaging biomarkers. *Neurobiology of aging.* 2016 Aug;44:1–8.

9. Folstein MF, Folstein SE, McHugh PR. "Mini-mental state". A practical method for grading the cognitive state of patients for the clinician. *J Psychiatr Res.* 1975 Nov;12(3):189–98.

10. Petersen RC. Clinical practice. Mild cognitive impairment. *The New England journal of medicine. [Review].* 2011 Jun 9;364(23):2227–34.

11. Weiner MW, Veitch DP, Aisen PS, Beckett LA, Cairns NJ, Green RC, et al. The Alzheimer's Disease Neuroimaging Initiative: a review of papers published since its inception. Alzheimer's & dementia : the journal of the Alzheimer's Association. *[Multicenter Study Review].* 2012 Feb;8(1 Suppl):S1–68.

12. Roberts RO, Geda YE, Knopman DS, Cha RH, Pankratz VS, Boeve BF, et al. The Mayo Clinic Study of Aging: design and sampling, participation, baseline measures and sample characteristics. *Neuroepidemiology.* 2008;30(1):58–69.

13. van Harten AC, Smits LL, Teunissen CE, Visser PJ, Koene T, Blankenstein MA, et al. Preclinical AD predicts decline in memory and executive functions in subjective complaints. *Neurology.* 2013 Oct 15;81(16):1409–16.

14. Jack CR, Jr., Knopman DS, Weigand SD, Wiste HJ, Vemuri P, Lowe V, et al. An operational approach to National Institute on Aging-Alzheimer's Association criteria for preclinical Alzheimer disease. *Annals of neurology. [Research Support, N.I.H., Extramural Research Support, Non-U.S. Gov't].* 2012 Jun;71(6):765–75.

15. Jack CR, Jr., Knopman DS, Chetelat G, Dickson D, Fagan AM, Frisoni GB, et al. Suspected non-Alzheimer disease pathophysiology–concept and controversy. *Nat Rev Neurol. [Research Support, N.I.H., Extramural Research Support, Non-U.S. Gov't Review].* 2016 Feb;12(2):117–24.

16. McKeith IG, Dickson DW, Lowe J, Emre M, O'Brien JT, Feldman H, et al. Diagnosis and management of dementia with Lewy bodies: third report of the DLB Consortium. *Neurology.* 2005 Dec 27;65(12):1863–72.

17. Gorno-Tempini ML, Hillis AE, Weintraub S, Kertesz A, Mendez M, Cappa SF, et al. Classification of primary progressive aphasia and its variants. Neurology. [Consensus Development Conference Research Support, N.I.H., Extramural Research Support, Non-U.S. Gov't]. 2011 Mar 15;76(11):1006–14.

18. Rascovsky K, Hodges JR, Knopman D, Mendez MF, Kramer JH, Neuhaus J, et al. Sensitivity of revised diagnostic criteria for the behavioural variant of frontotemporal dementia. Brain : a journal of neurology. *[Research Support, N.I.H., Extramural Research Support, Non-U.S. Gov't].* 2011 Sep;134(Pt 9):2456–77.

19. Roman GC, Tatemichi TK, Erkinjuntti T, Cummings JL, Masdeu JC, Garcia JH, et al. Vascular dementia: diagnostic criteria for research studies. Report of the NINDS-AIREN International Workshop. *Neurology.* 1993 Feb;43(2):250–60.

20. Tang-Wai DF, Graff-Radford NR, Boeve BF, Dickson DW, Parisi JE, Crook R, et al. Clinical, genetic, and neuropathologic characteristics of posterior cortical atrophy. *Neurology.* 2004 Oct 12;63(7):1168–74.

21. Rabinovici GD, Rosen HJ, Alkalay A, Kornak J, Furst AJ, Agarwal N, et al. Amyloid vs FDG-PET in the differential diagnosis of AD and FTLD. *Neurology.* 2011 Dec 6;77(23):2034–42.

22. Ertekin-Taner N. Genetics of Alzheimer disease in the pre- and post-GWAS era. *Alzheimers Res Ther.* 2010 Mar 05;2(1):3.

23. Murray ME, Graff-Radford NR, Ross OA, Petersen RC, Duara R, Dickson DW. Neuropathologically defined subtypes of Alzheimer's disease with distinct clinical characteristics: a retrospective study. The Lancet Neurology. *[Comparative Study Research Support, N.I.H., Extramural Research Support, Non-U.S. Gov't Research Support, U.S. Gov't, Non-P.H.S.].* 2011 Sep;10(9):785–96.

24. Glenner GG. The proteins and genes of Alzheimer's disease. *Biomed Pharmacother.* 1988;42(9):579–84.

25. Murphy MP, Hickman LJ, Eckman CB, Uljon SN, Wang R, Golde TE. gamma-Secretase, evidence for multiple proteolytic activities and influence of membrane positioning of substrate on generation of amyloid beta peptides of varying length. *The Journal of biological chemistry. [Research Support, Non-U.S. Gov't Research Support, U.S. Gov't, P.H.S.].* 1999 Apr 23;274(17):11914–23.

26. Murphy MP, Das P, Nyborg AC, Rochette MJ, Dodson MW, Loosbrock NM, et al. Overexpression of nicastrin increases Abeta production. *Faseb J.* 2003 Jun;17(9):1138–40.

27. Gotz J, Ittner LM. Animal models of Alzheimer's disease and frontotemporal dementia. *Nat Rev Neurosci. [Research Support, Non-U.S. Gov't Review].* 2008 Jul;9(7):532–44.

28. Seubert P, Vigo-Pelfrey C, Esch F, Lee M, Dovey H, Davis D, et al. Isolation and quantification of soluble Alzheimer's beta-peptide from biological fluids. *Nature.* 1992 Sep 24;359(6393):325–7.

29. Gravina SA, Ho L, Eckman CB, Long KE, Otvos L, Jr., Younkin LH, et al. Amyloid beta protein (A beta) in Alzheimer's disease brain. Biochemical and immunocytochemical analysis with antibodies specific for forms ending at A beta 40 or A beta 42(43). The Journal of biological chemistry. [Comparative Study Research Support, Non-U.S. Gov't Research Support, U.S. Gov't, P.H.S.]. 1995 Mar 31;270(13):7013–6.

30. Ngo S, Guo Z. Key residues for the oligomerization of Abeta42 protein in Alzheimer's disease. Biochemical and biophysical research communications. *[Research Support, Non-U.S. Gov't].* 2011 Oct 28;414(3):512–6.

31. Lewis J, Dickson DW, Lin WL, Chisholm L, Corral A, Jones G, et al. Enhanced neurofibrillary degeneration in transgenic mice expressing mutant tau and APP. *Science.* 2001 Aug 24;293(5534):1487–91.

32. Hyman BT. The neuropathological diagnosis of Alzheimer's disease: clinical-pathological studies. *Neurobiol Aging.* 1997 Jul-Aug;18(4 Suppl):S27–32.

33. Dickson DW. Neuropathology of Alzheimer's disease and other dementias. *Clin Geriatr Med.* 2001 May;17(2):209–28.

34. Ksiezak-Reding H, Yen SH. Two monoclonal antibodies recognize Alzheimer's neurofibrillary tangles, neurofilament, and microtubule-associated proteins. Journal of neurochemistry. *[Research Support, U.S. Gov't, P.H.S.].* 1987 Feb;48(2):455–62.

35. Manetto V, Perry G, Tabaton M, Mulvihill P, Fried VA, Smith HT, et al. Ubiquitin is associated with abnormal cytoplasmic filaments characteristic of neurodegenerative diseases. Proceedings of the National Academy of Sciences of the United States of America. *[Research Support, Non-U.S. Gov't Research Support, U.S. Gov't, P.H.S.].* 1988 Jun;85(12):4501–5.

36. Johnston H, Boutin H, Allan SM. Assessing the contribution of inflammation in models of Alzheimer's disease. *Biochemical Society transactions. [Review].* 2011 Aug;39(4):886–90.

37. Guerreiro R, Hardy J. TREM2 and neurodegenerative disease. The New England journal of medicine. *[Comment Letter Research Support, Non-U.S. Gov't].* 2013 Oct 17;369(16):1569–70.

38. Tharp WG, Sarkar IN. Origins of amyloid-beta. BMC Genomics. *[Research Support, N.I.H., Extramural].* 2013 Apr 30;14:290.

39. Perlmutter LS, Barron E, Myers M, Saperia D, Chui HC. Localization of amyloid P component in human brain: vascular staining patterns and association with Alzheimer's disease lesions. J Comp Neurol. *[Research Support, Non-U.S. Gov't Research Support, U.S. Gov't, Non-P.H.S. Research Support, U.S. Gov't, P.H.S.].* 1995 Jan 30;352(1):92–105.

40. Bergeron C, Ranalli PJ, Miceli PN. Amyloid angiopathy in Alzheimer's disease. The Canadian journal of neurological sciences Le journal canadien des sciences neurologiques. *[Research Support, Non-U.S. Gov't].* 1987 Nov;14(4):564–9.

41. Mott RT, Hulette CM. Neuropathology of Alzheimer's disease. Neuroimaging Clin N Am. *[Research Support, N.I.H., Extramural Review].* 2005 Nov;15(4):755–65, ix.

42. Gatz M, Reynolds CA, Fratiglioni L, Johansson B, Mortimer JA, Berg S, et al. Role of genes and environments for explaining Alzheimer disease. *Arch Gen Psychiatry.* 2006 Feb;63(2):168–74.

43. Sherrington R, Rogaev EI, Liang Y, Rogaeva EA, Levesque G, Ikeda M, et al. Cloning of a gene bearing missense mutations in early-onset familial Alzheimer's disease. *Nature.* 1995 Jun 29;375(6534):754–60.

44. Levy-Lahad E, Wijsman EM, Nemens E, Anderson L, Goddard KA, Weber JL, et al. A familial Alzheimer's disease locus on chromosome 1. *Science.* 1995 Aug 18;269(5226):970–3.

45. Goldgaber D, Lerman MI, McBride OW, Saffiotti U, Gajdusek DC. Characterization and chromosomal localization of a cDNA encoding brain amyloid of Alzheimer's disease. *Science.* 1987 Feb 20;235(4791):877–80.

46. Pericak-Vance M, Bebout J, Gaskell P, Yamaoka L, Hung W, Alberts M, et al. Linkage studies in familial Alzheimer's disease: evidence for chromosome 19 linkage. *Am J Hum Genet.* 1991;48(6):1034–50.

47. Ertekin-Taner N. Genetics of Alzheimer's disease: a centennial review. *Neurologic clinics. [Review].* 2007 Aug;25(3):611–67, v.

48. Peila R, Rodriguez BL, Launer LJ. Type 2 diabetes, APOE gene, and the risk for dementia and related pathologies: The Honolulu-Asia Aging Study. Diabetes. *[Research Support, U.S. Gov't, P.H.S.].* 2002 Apr;51(4):1256–62.

49. Arvanitakis Z, Schneider JA, Wilson RS, Li Y, Arnold SE, Wang Z, et al. Diabetes is related to cerebral infarction but not to AD pathology in older persons. *Neurology.* 2006 Dec 12;67(11):1960–5.

50. Sun X, Steffens DC, Au R, Folstein M, Summergrad P, Yee J, et al. Amyloid-associated depression: a prodromal depression of Alzheimer disease? *Arch Gen Psychiatry.* 2008 May;65(5):542–50.

51. Scarmeas N, Luchsinger JA, Mayeux R, Stern Y. Mediterranean diet and Alzheimer disease mortality. Neurology. *[Research Support, N.I.H., Extramural Research Support, Non-U.S. Gov't].* 2007 Sep 11;69(11):1084–93.

52. Valls-Pedret C, Sala-Vila A, Serra-Mir M, Corella D, de la Torre R, Martinez-Gonzalez MA, et al. Mediterranean Diet and Age-Related Cognitive Decline: A Randomized Clinical Trial. *JAMA Intern Med. [Randomized Controlled Trial Research Support, Non-U.S. Gov't].* 2015 Jul;175(7):1094–103.

53. Barnes DE, Yaffe K. The projected effect of risk factor reduction on Alzheimer's disease prevalence. The Lancet Neurology. *[Research Support, N.I.H., Extramural Research Support, Non-U.S. Gov't Review].* 2011 Sep;10(9):819–28.

54. Lazarov O, Robinson J, Tang YP, Hairston IS, Korade-Mirnics Z, Lee VM, et al. Environmental enrichment reduces Abeta levels and amyloid deposition in transgenic mice. *Cell.* 2005 Mar 11;120(5):701–13.

55. Kivipelto M, Helkala EL, Hanninen T, Laakso MP, Hallikainen M, Alhainen K, et al. Midlife vascular risk factors and late-life mild cognitive impairment: A population-based study. *Neurology.* 2001 Jun 26;56(12):1683–9.

56. Yasar S, Xia J, Yao W, Furberg CD, Xue QL, Mercado CI, et al. Antihypertensive drugs decrease risk of Alzheimer disease: Ginkgo Evaluation of Memory Study. Neurology. *[Randomized Controlled Trial Research Support, N.I.H., Extramural Research Support, Non-U.S. Gov't Research Support, U.S. Gov't, P.H.S.].* 2013 Sep 3; 81(10):896–903.

57. Gelber RP, Ross GW, Petrovitch H, Masaki KH, Launer LJ, White LR. Antihypertensive medication use and risk of cognitive impairment: the Honolulu-Asia Aging Study. Neurology. *[Research Support, N.I.H., Extramural Research Support, U.S. Gov't, Non-P.H.S.].* 2013 Sep 3;81(10):888–95.

58. Deschaintre Y, Richard F, Leys D, Pasquier F. Treatment of vascular risk factors is associated with slower decline in Alzheimer disease. *Neurology. [Research Support, Non-U.S. Gov't].* 2009 Sep 1;73(9):674–80.

59. Aisen PS, Schneider LS, Sano M, Diaz-Arrastia R, van Dyck CH, Weiner MF, et al. High-dose B vitamin supplementation and cognitive decline in Alzheimer disease: a randomized controlled trial. *JAMA. [Multicenter Study Randomized Controlled Trial Research Support, N.I.H., Extramural].* 2008 Oct 15;300(15):1774–83.

60. Lautenschlager NT, Cox KL, Flicker L, Foster JK, van Bockxmeer FM, Xiao J, et al. Effect of physical activity on cognitive function in older adults at risk for Alzheimer disease: a randomized trial. *Jama.* 2008 Sep 3;300(9):1027–37.

61. Graff-Radford NR. Can aerobic exercise protect against dementia? *Alzheimers Res Ther.* 2011 Feb 28;3(1):6.

62. Erickson KI, Voss MW, Prakash RS, Basak C, Szabo A, Chaddock L, et al. Exercise training increases size of hippocampus and improves memory. *Proc Natl Acad Sci U S A.* 2011 Jan 31.

63. Garcia-Mesa Y, Lopez-Ramos JC, Gimenez-Llort L, Revilla S, Guerra R, Gruart A, et al. Physical exercise protects against Alzheimer's disease in 3xTg-AD mice. *Journal of Alzheimer's disease : JAD. [Research Support, Non-U.S. Gov't].* 2011;24 (3):421–54.

64. Stampfer MJ, Kang JH, Chen J, Cherry R, Grodstein F. Effects of moderate alcohol consumption on cognitive function in women. The New England journal of medicine. *[Research Support, Non-U.S. Gov't Research Support, U.S. Gov't, P.H.S.].* 2005 Jan 20;352(3):245–53.

65. Morris MC, Evans DA, Bienias JL, Tangney CC, Bennett DA, Wilson RS, et al. Consumption of fish and n-3 fatty acids and risk of incident Alzheimer disease. *Arch Neurol.* 2003 Jul;60(7):940–6.

66. Ngandu T, Lehtisalo J, Solomon A, Levalahti E, Ahtiluoto S, Antikainen R, et al. A 2 year multidomain intervention of diet, exercise, cognitive training, and vascular risk monitoring versus control to prevent cognitive decline in at-risk elderly people (FINGER): a randomised controlled trial. Lancet. *[Multicenter Study Randomized Controlled Trial Research Support, Non-U.S. Gov't].* 2015 Jun 6;385(9984):2255–63.

67. Kokmen E, Naessens JM, Offord KP. A short test of mental status: description and preliminary results. *Mayo Clin Proc.* 1987 Apr;62(4):281–8.

68. Nasreddine ZS, Phillips NA, Bedirian V, Charbonneau S, Whitehead V, Collin I, et al. The Montreal Cognitive Assessment, MoCA: a brief screening tool for mild cognitive impairment. *Journal of the American Geriatrics Society. [Evaluation Studies Research Support, Non-U.S. Gov't Research Support, U.S. Gov't, P.H.S.].* 2005 Apr;53(4):695–9.

69. Ossenkoppele R, Schonhaut DR, Scholl M, Lockhart SN, Ayakta N, Baker SL, et al. Tau PET patterns mirror clinical and neuroanatomical variability in Alzheimer's disease. *Brain : a journal of neurology.* 2016 May;139(Pt 5):1551–67.

70. Dubinsky RM, Stein AC, Lyons K. Practice parameter: risk of driving and Alzheimer's disease (an evidence-based review): report of the quality standards subcommittee of the American Academy of Neurology. *Neurology. [Review].* 2000 Jun 27; 54(12):2205–11.

71. Selkoe DJ. Resolving controversies on the path to Alzheimer's therapeutics. *Nature medicine.* 2011 Sep 07;17(9):1060–5.

72. Doody RS, Farlow M, Aisen PS. Phase 3 trials of solanezumab and bapineuzumab for Alzheimer's disease. *The New England journal of medicine. [Comment Letter].* 2014 Apr 10;370(15):1460.

73. Sevigny J, Chiao P, Bussiere T, Weinreb PH, Williams L, Maier M, et al. The antibody aducanumab reduces Abeta plaques in Alzheimer's disease. *Nature.* 2016 Aug 31;537(7618):50–6.

CHAPTER 12

Frontotemporal Dementia

Christian W. Wider[1], Barbara Jasinska-Myga[2], Takuya Konno[3], and Zbigniew K. Wszolek[3]

[1]Formerly of Department of Clinical Neuroscience, Lausanne University Hospital (CHUV-UNIL), Lausanne, Switzerland
[2]Department of Neurology, Medical University of Silesia, Katowice, Poland
[3]Department of Neurology, Mayo Clinic, Jacksonville, Florida, USA

Introduction

In his classic monograph published in 1892 while working at the German University in Prague, Arnold Pick described a patient with dementia, language impairment, and behavioral changes, in whom autopsy revealed temporal lobe atrophy [1]. He then reported four additional patients with progressive language difficulties, developing a strong interest in comparing clinical deficits and macroscopic changes in brain tissue. However, it was Alois Alzheimer who later identified the characteristic argyrophilic inclusions and ballooned cells found in patients with the condition soon to be known as Pick disease [2].

Frontotemporal dementia (FTD) is the third most prevalent form of dementia with onset before the age of 65 years, after Alzheimer's disease (AD) and vascular dementia [3]. It also represents the third overall cause of cortical dementia. Patients with FTD present with various combinations of cognitive impairment, behavioral changes, and language difficulties, which negatively impact on quality of life [4]. The most common clinical presentation is the behavioral variant (bvFTD), followed by the aphasic syndromes: progressive non-fluent aphasia (PNFA), semantic dementia (SD), and logopenic progressive aphasia (LPA) [5–7]. Disease progression is relentless. Autopsy findings are dominated by neuronal inclusions of one of three proteins: tau, 43-kDa transactive response DNA-binding protein (TDP-43), or fused in sarcoma (FUS) [8]. When defined more broadly as a clinical–pathological spectrum of neurodegenerative conditions, FTD also encompasses closely related entities such as the motor syndromes progressive supranuclear palsy (PSP, see Chapter 8) and corticobasal degeneration (CBD, see Chapter 10) [9]. Finally, the syndrome of FTD overlaps with motor neuron disease (MND), both at the clinical and pathological levels, and some patients present with FTD and motor neuron impairment (FTD-MND).

Over the past decades, major progress has been achieved in the understanding of the molecular events involved in FTD, mainly through autopsy studies and the discovery of monogenic forms of FTD. This has led to thorough reappraisal of the FTD spectrum with significant nosologic changes. In the present overview, we discuss relevant and recent advances in the field of FTD, with particular emphasis on clinical, pathological, and genetic aspects.

Clinical definition and epidemiology

Patients with FTD present with progressive behavioral or language impairment that significantly impacts their daily activities. The disease typically affects men and women in their fifties to sixties. Prevalence figures differ widely depending on the study design; in one series from the United Kingdom prevalence was estimated at 15/100,000 among individuals 45 to 64 years old, comparable to figures for AD within the same age range [10]. Another series examining a population from The Netherlands found prevalence rates of 3.6 per 100,000 between ages 50 and 59, 9.4/100,000 between ages 60 and 69, and 3.8/100,000 between ages 70 and 79 [11]. Few studies have estimated the incidence of FTD; in Rochester, Minnesota, Knopman and colleagues found incidence (new cases per year per 100,000 inhabitants) to be 2.2 for ages 40–49, 3.3 for ages 50–59, and 8.9 for ages 60–69 [12]. Expectedly, the incidence of Alzheimer's disease in the same series was lower for ages 40–49, similar for ages 50–59, and higher for ages 60–69. No significant gender bias exists for FTD, and there is no known environmental risk factor.

Spectrum of clinical phenotype

Symptoms tend to correlate well with the regional distribution of atrophy, less so with the underlying pathology. However, while cases with bvFTD are evenly distributed between tau-positive and tau-negative pathology, there is evidence that PSP-like and CBD-like cases tend to be tau-positive, and that cases with FTD-MND are almost always tau-negative [9]. The spectrum of clinical presentation ranges from behavioral disturbances (bvFTD) to difficulties communicating with reduced language (PNFA, LPA) or fluent aphasia (SD) [4, 7, 13]. Movement disorders such as parkinsonian features may also be seen, as well as motor neuron disease (FTD-MND) or supranuclear gaze palsy. The clinical phenotype often changes over time and it has been shown in prospective studies that patients with initial aphasic presentation may evolve into a more behavioral phenotype; conversely, some patients initially present with behavioral abnormalities and later develop non-fluent aphasia [14–16]. The following subsections provide detailed descriptions of the most important phenotypic presentations in FTD.

Neurodegeneration, First Edition. Edited by Anthony Schapira, Zbigniew Wszolek, Ted M. Dawson and Nicholas Wood.
© 2017 John Wiley & Sons, Ltd. Published 2017 by John Wiley & Sons, Ltd.

Behavioral variant (bvFTD)

This is the most common clinical presentation of FTD [5]. The core features consist of progressive behavioral changes whereby patients interact differently with the outside world (Table 12.1) [13]. Early on there are modifications of interpersonal conduct, personality, and emotional modulation, however a precise beginning is often difficult to define. Patients display loss of insight together with a tendency for disinhibition, leading them to perform tactless actions they would previously have considered inappropriate, rude, or embarrassing. Those include behaviors linked to sexual or other intimate actions. Emotional blunting is also present, along with lack of empathy, mental rigidity, and reduced ability to predict and comprehend future consequences of specific actions or decisions. Apathy is very common and manifests with inertia and lack of interest in others and in activities the person previously enjoyed such as hobbies. Adherence to systems of values may change including religious beliefs or political preferences, which may be challenging for spouses and caregivers. Some degree of language difficulties is often present. Food habits are dramatically altered with binge eating a common manifestation leading to weight gain [17]. Patients often present ritualistic behavior and motor stereotypies such as humming, foot tapping, or lip licking; perseveration also manifests with a tendency to repeat sentences, stories, or jokes. There is self-neglect in many aspects of daily life including personal hygiene, as well as inability to manage grocery shopping or personal finances. Compared to AD, memory is relatively spared early in the disease, although this has been challenged by several studies that identified memory deficits in bvFTD [18]. In fact behavioral changes such as euphoria, stereotypical motor behavior, and changes in eating preferences seem to discriminate best between bvFTD and AD [19, 20]. Morphological imaging shows atrophy of the mesial frontal lobes as well as anterior insula cortices (see section Morphologic and functional imaging).

Primary non-fluent aphasia (PNFA)

In the mostly expressive language disorder PNFA, early on there is reduction of spontaneous speech, often with some degree of inertia and apathy (Table 12.1). Patients speak less and do so with effortful speech, short sentences, and numerous grammatical errors (agrammatic speech). There is disordered prosody (altered melody of speech) and speech sound errors including apraxia of speech [21,

22]. Word finding difficulties worsen sometimes to a state of muteness, whereas there is relative preservation of word comprehension. As the disease progresses patients may display motor abnormalities including parkinsonian features such as bradykinesia or rigidity, as well as dystonia, supranuclear gaze palsy, gait difficulties, muscle wasting, or fasciculations [21, 23, 24]. Imaging shows atrophy in the left posterior frontal region and in the insula (see section Morphologic and functional imaging).

Semantic dementia (SD)

In contrast with PNFA, language impairment in SD consists of altered word comprehension with relative preservation of speech fluency and syntax (fluent aphasia) (Table 12.1) [25]. Patients have difficulties finding words, with anomia an early manifestation. In addition to reduced word comprehension there is altered object knowledge (semantic representation). Speech becomes empty of content with overuse of words that have imprecise meanings [21]. There is some degree of surface dyslexia, whereby words are pronounced as spelled. With disease progression, patients lose access to all but the simplest words, which causes distress. There is often some degree of behavioral changes with loss of empathy and reduced insight [26, 27]. When the right temporal lobe is involved there are difficulties recognizing faces, along with a tendency for compulsive behavior centered on words or symbols. Patients can experience radical changes in political or religious beliefs, which they may express in offensive ways to strangers on the street. Morphological imaging often shows asymmetric atrophy of the anterior part of the temporal lobes (see section Morphologic and functional imaging).

Logopenic progressive aphasia (LPA)

Patients with LPA present with reduced speech output due to major word finding difficulties [28]. In contrast with PNFA the grammatical structure of language is preserved (Table 12.1). Repetition is also altered with reduced auditory–verbal short-term memory, but word meaning is retained. With disease progression patients may experience difficulty in word comprehension. Given the phenotype and the finding of more posterior atrophy on imaging, some authors have suggested that LPA overlaps with posterior cortical atrophy and may represent a variant of AD. Along the same lines it has been suggested that patients with LPA who turn out to have AD pathology have more pronounced episodic memory alteration compared to those LPA patients with FTD pathology [29]. However, LPA does not share the genetic factors involved in AD, in particular the *APOE* genotype does not modify the risk for LPA.

Frontotemporal dementia with parkinsonism linked to chromosome 17 (FTDP-17)

In the 1980s and 1990s, families were reported with autosomal dominant FTD and parkinsonism, which led to the discovery of two major FTD genes: microtubule-associated protein tau (*MAPT*) and granulin (*GRN*) (see subsection Genetics). The term FTDP-17 was coined at a consensus conference in 1996, based on the most consistently reported symptoms and the observed linkage to chromosome 17 [30].

In patients with mutations in *MAPT* the cardinal clinical features are behavioral and personality changes, cognitive impairment, and motor symptoms (Table 12.2) [31–34]. bvFTD combined with semantic impairment has been suggested to be typical for *MAPT*-linked FTD [35]. Parkinsonism consists of

Table 12.1 Summary of behavioral variant frontotemporal dementia and primary progressive aphasia.

Syndrome	Main characteristics
bvFTD	• Loss of insight, emotional blunting, impairment of personal and interpersonal conduct • Mental rigidity, hyperorality, dietary changes, stereotyped behavior, lack of personal hygiene • Economy of speech, stereotypy of speech, echolalia, mutism
PNFA	• Agrammatic speech, reduced speech output, errors in language production • Effortful speech, speech sound errors, preserved word comprehension • Preserved object knowledge, impaired syntax
SD	• Altered naming by confrontation • Impaired word comprehension and object knowledge • Surface dyslexia, spared motor speech
LPA	• Altered word retrieval • Impaired sentence repetition, speech sound errors • Spared motor speech and word comprehension

bvFTD, behavioral variant frontotemporal dementia; LPA, logopenic progressive aphasia; PNFA, progressive non-fluent aphasia; SD, semantic dementia.

Table 12.2 Clinical, imaging, and pathological characteristics of major forms of monogenic FTD.

	MAPT	GRN	C9ORF72
Clinical features	Mostly bvFTD parkinsonism, MND	Mostly bvFTD parkinsonism, CBS, PNFA Rarely MND	Mostly bvFTD MND/ALS, PNFA, psychosis, parkinsonism
Onset age (years)	48 (33–71)	59 (28–83)	57 (30–76)
Percentage of FTD series – familial	5–10	5–10	11–25
Percentage of FTD series – sporadic	1.5	3	3–6
Pathology	Tau positive	TDP-43 positive	TDP-43 positive

ALS, amyotrophic lateral sclerosis; bvFTD, behavioral variant frontotemporal dementia; CBS, corticobasal syndrome; MND, motor neuron disease; PNFA, progressive nonfluent aphasia; SD, semantic dementia.

bradykinesia, rigidity, postural tremor, and gait difficulties, and usually develops with bvFTD [31]. Other forms of parkinsonism include CBD-like and PSP-like manifestations, such as lateralized dystonia or supranuclear gaze palsy (Figure 12.1). Pyramidal signs exist in some patients [31]. *MAPT* mutations have been rarely identified in patients with PNFA [36]. Some patients have been reported with an episodic memory deficit [37, 38]. Patients display prominent and rapidly progressive frontal and temporal atrophy on MRI (Figure 12.2).

There is more phenotype variability in *GRN* mutation carriers than in those patients with a *MAPT* mutation. The most common phenotype in *GRN* mutation carriers is bvFTD, however a significant proportion of patients display PNFA [35, 39–41]. Additional phenotypes in *GRN* mutation carriers include corticobasal syndrome (CBS), AD, and parkinsonism, which occurs later in the disease in as many as 50% of the patients [42–44]. Associated MND is distinctly rare, although evidence indicates it may be found in up to 5% of *GRN* mutation carriers [39]. Compared to FTD in general, patients with FTDP-17 tend to display an earlier onset (late forties for *MAPT* mutations, late fifties for *GRN* mutations) and a more rapid course. Imaging shows variable severity of frontal, temporal, and basal ganglia atrophy (see section Morphologic and functional imaging).

Frontotemporal dementia with motor neuron disease (FTD-MND)

The association of FTD and MND occurs in about 10% of bvFTD cases, with variable proportions of either the cortical or the motor manifestations [24, 45]. However, some degree of motor neuron symptoms occurs in up to half of bvFTD patients [23] and may even be subclinical [46]. In fact the notion that FTD and ALS are two diseases at different ends of one spectrum has gained strong support from findings at the clinical, pathological (TDP-43-positive inclusions), and genetic levels (discovery of the *C9ORF72* expansion and others, see subsection Genetics).

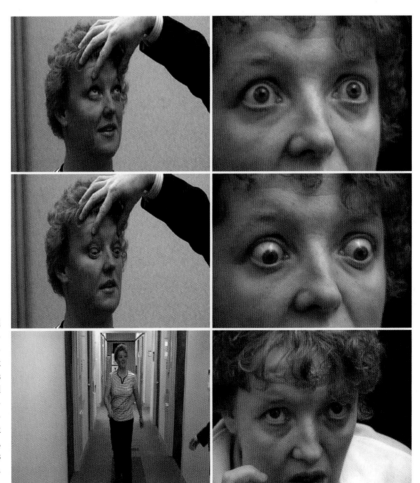

Figure 12.1 Patient from the pallido-ponto-nigral degeneration (PPND) family carrying the N279K mutation in the *MAPT* gene. Left panel: a 42-year-old patient who complained of reduced performance at work for four years, as well as a staring expression that was noticed by her family. Ocular movements were normal and she was able to walk almost unremarkably, however she had mild parkinsonian signs (mostly rigidity). Right panel: same patient at age 46, unable to walk and entirely dependent for activities of daily living, displaying supranuclear vertical gaze palsy, as well as cognitive decline, parkinsonism, and pyramidal signs. See Figure 12.2 for MRI of the patient.

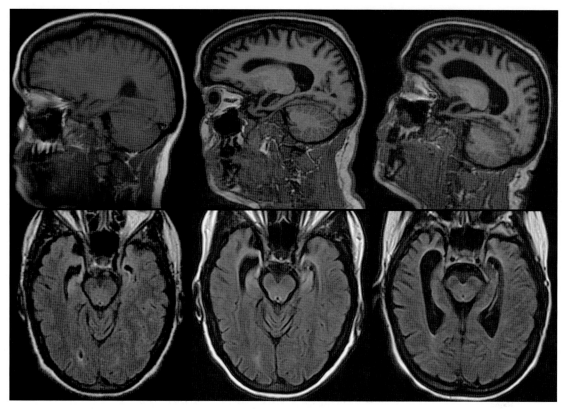

Figure 12.2 MRI of the same patient as Figure 12.1 (pallido-ponto-nigral degeneration family carrying the N279K mutation in the *MAPT* gene), showing sagittal (upper part) and transverse views (lower part) at ages 42 (left), 45 (middle), and 46 (right) years, with progressive worsening of frontal and temporal atrophy.

Pathology /pathophysiology

Genetics

The past 20 years have witnessed tremendous progress in the genetics of FTD, which has proved invaluable in understanding the molecular mechanisms involved. A positive family history is reported by 30–40% of FTD patients, yet autosomal dominant inheritance can be demonstrated only in about 10%. bvFTD is the most heritable phenotype, followed by PNFA, with SD only rarely displaying familial aggregation. Mutations in several genes have been linked to dominantly inherited FTD, with microtubule-associated protein (*MAPT*) [47], granulin (*GRN*) [48, 49], and chromosome 9 open reading frame 72 (*C9ORF72*) [50, 51] being the most important (Table 12.2), and mutations in transactive response DNA-binding protein (*TARDBP*) [52, 53], fused in sarcoma (*FUS*) [54], valosin containing protein (*VCP*) [55], charged multivesicular body protein 2B (*CHMP2B*) [56], ubiquilin-2 (*UBQLN2*) [57], p62/sequestosome 1 (*SQSTM1*) [58], and TANK-binding kinase 1 (*TBK1*) [59] being much rarer.

Microtubule-associated protein tau (*MAPT*)

Mutations in the *MAPT* gene account for 5–20% of cases with FTD [60]. Over 50 mutations have been identified in more than 100 families [61], most of them clustered in exons 9 to 12 which code for the microtubule binding repeats (see the FTD mutation database, http://www.molgen.vib-ua.be/FTDMutations). *MAPT* encodes the tau protein, which plays a major role in microtubule assembly and stabilization. Six tau isoforms are produced from a single gene in

humans, by alternatively splicing out exons 2, 3, and 10. Based on the number of microtubule binding domains, tau isoforms can be divided into those with three (3R) and those with four (4R) microtubule binding repeats. A wide range of diseases in humans display hyperphosphorylated tau-positive inclusions including Pick disease, AD, PSP, CBD, argyrophilic grain disease, and familial FTD with a mutation in *MAPT*.

Most mutations in *MAPT* influence the expression of all six tau isoforms, however mutations in exon 10 only affect the expression of 4R tau [62]. *MAPT* mutations exert their pathogenic effects through altered interaction with microtubules, fibril formation, or increased splicing out of exon 10. The majority of pathogenic mutations in exons 9, 11, 12, and 13 reduce the ability of the mutant protein to promote microtubule assembly, and some also display pro-fibrillogenic properties [63, 64]. Intronic mutations, which are located in the introns flanking the alternatively spliced exon 10, act on exon 10 splicing, thereby increasing the relative proportion of 4R tau isoforms. Several coding *MAPT* mutations also increase the 4R:3R tau isoform ratio by affecting splicing regulating elements in exon 10. It has been suggested that 4R tau is more fibrillogenic than 3R tau [65]. Interestingly, it has been observed that mutations in exons 9 and 13 are usually associated with a phenotype devoid of motor symptoms, whereas mutations altering *MAPT* splicing are more commonly found in patients with FTD and parkinsonism [66]. Similarly, mutations altering the first two microtubule binding domains seem to be associated with an earlier age of onset and shorter disease duration than other mutations [67].

Granulin (*GRN*)

Mutations in *GRN* account for up to 20% of patients with FTD [60]. Ten years after its discovery nearly 80 mutations have been reported; these include large deletions as well as missense, nonsense, frameshift, and splice site mutations [35, 41, 42, 48, 49, 68]. In most cases the mechanism appears to be haploinsufficiency, with the mutated allele being degraded by nonsense-mediated decay. Although its exact role remains to be elucidated, the encoded protein progranulin has been involved as an antagonist to tumor necrosis factor alpha signaling and shown to act on nerve cells by binding to sortilin following release from activated microglial cells [69]. At autopsy, patients with *GRN* mutations display neuronal inclusions that stain positive for the TDP-43 protein [70, 71]. In addition to clinical investigation and genetic testing, measurement of blood levels of the granulin protein has been suggested to predict mutation status in FTD patients [72, 73].

Chromosome 9 open reading frame 72 (*C9ORF72*)

A hexanucleotide (GGGGCC) expansion in the non-coding region of the *C9ORF72* gene was identified as the cause of chromosome 9p21-linked FTD-MND [50, 51]. The discovery has major implications given the number of previously reported families linked to chromosome 9p [74–77]. Moreover, the expansion was also found in a substantial proportion of patients with either FTD or MND. In the Mayo Clinic series it was identified in 11.7% of familial FTD cases and in 3% of sporadic cases, representing the most common mutation in overall FTD patients [50]. For ALS, 23.5% of familial and 4.1% of sporadic patients harbored the expansion. Most FTD patients displayed the behavioral variant, with about a third having associated MND. Another series also found bvFTD to be the most common presentation; however PNFA was also present in over 20% of the patients [51]. Subsequent series have largely confirmed *C9ORF72* expansion as a major cause of familial and sporadic FTD, FTD-MND, and ALS [78–81]. In the largest White/European population examined, the *C9ORF72* repeat expansion was found in 24.8% of patients with familial FTD and in 6% of patients with sporadic FTD [81]. This study also estimated penetrance, with non-penetrance at age 35, 50% penetrance by 58 years, and almost full penetrance by age 80. In the same study 85.5% of patients displayed bvFTD, 8.9% PNFA, and 5.6% SD. An association with psychosis was also reported [79]. In addition, one study identified a few patients with AD, although the authors acknowledge that the patients may have represented the amnestic subtype of FTD [82]. While the exact function of the encoded protein remains unknown, three potential mechanisms by which the repeat expansion induces neurodegeneration have been proposed: loss of function of C9ORF72, toxic RNA foci formation, and toxic dipeptide repeat proteins translated from the expanded repeat [83].

Valosin-containing protein (*VCP*), transactive response DNA binding protein 43 (*TARDBP*), fused in sarcoma (*FUS*), charged multivesicular body protein 2B (*CHMP2B*), ubiquilin-2 (*UBQLN2*), p62/sequestosome 1 (*SQSTM1*), and TANK-binding kinase 1 (*TBK1*)

Mutations in the *VCP* gene cause FTD with inclusion body myopathy and Paget's disease of the bone (IBMPFD), a rare cause of dominantly inherited muscle weakness and Paget's disease, with early-onset FTD in approximately 30% of the patients [55, 84, 85]. Recent findings also indicate that *VCP* mutations may cause MND [86]. While a number of families have been reported with IBMPFD

[87, 88], the molecular mechanisms involved in pathogenicity remain elusive. These may include altered ubiquitin-proteasome system activity, with accumulation of protein material such as TDP-43 [89].

Most patients with mutations in *TARDBP* develop MND; however there have been a few descriptions of *TARDBP* mutation carriers with bvFTD, SD, and even parkinsonism [52, 90–92]. Overall, more data will be required to establish the role of *TARDBP* mutations in FTD. Similarly, mutations in the *FUS* gene cause MND, yet patients have been reported who presented with FTD [54, 93]. More studies are warranted to establish the role of *FUS* in FTD.

Mutations in *CHMP2B* as a cause of FTD were first reported in a Danish family with autosomal dominant disease [56]. Subsequent studies have indicated that it is a very rare condition, with no mutation identified in a series of 141 familial cases of FTD [94]. Pathogenetic mechanisms may include altered endosomal trafficking with the finding of dysmorphic organelles in *CHMP2B* mutants [56, 95].

UBQLN2 mutations cause dominant X-linked ALS and FTD [57, 96]. The mutations have also been found in sporadic cases with ALS or FTD [97]. Mutation carriers develop not only ALS/FTD but also diverse phenotypes including involuntary movements, dystonia, and spastic paraplegia [96, 98]. The age of symptom onset ranges from 16 to 71 years. However, in three affected males with p.P497L mutation the first symptoms occurred below the age of 10 years [98]. *UBQLN2* encodes the ubiquitin-like protein, ubiquilin-2, which plays a role in the ubiquitin-proteasome system.

Although rare, mutations in *SQSTM1*, which were first reported in ALS [99], have been identified in patients with FTD with or without ALS [58, 100]. The most frequent phenotype is bvFTD. Similar to *VCP*, mutations in *SQSTM1* also cause Paget's disease. *SQSTM1* encodes p62/sequestosome 1, which is involved in autophagy.

Recently, mutations in *TBK1* were identified in patients with ALS, FTD, and ALS/FTD [59, 101, 102]. Most of them are loss-of-function mutations. It is considered that haploinsufficiency of *TBK1* causes the disease [59]. In a Belgian cohort, *TBK1* is the third most frequent causative gene of FTD, accounting for 3.4% of FTD [103]. TANK-binding kinase 1, which is encoded by *TBK1*, interacts with p62/sequestosome 1 and facilitates autophagy.

These newly discovered genes, *VCP*, *UBQLN2*, *SQSTM1*, and *TBK1*, are implicated in dysfunction of the protein degradation system, and thus may underlie the pathomechanism of ALS/FTD [101].

Pathology

Classification of FTD based on pathology differs somewhat from that used to describe clinical syndromes. Briefly, the umbrella term frontotemporal lobar degeneration (FTLD) encompasses entities with atrophy of the frontal and temporal lobes such as FTD, PNFA, SD, CBD, or PSP. Most forms of FTLD fall into one of three main categories based on the dominant protein aggregates, which are named FTLD-tau, FTLD-TDP, and FTLD-FUS [104–107]. Recent developments have prompted the publication of an updated version of consensus criteria [108], of which a simplified summary is provided in Table 12.3. Overall, cases with FTD display bilateral frontotemporal atrophy with neuronal loss, microvacuolation, and astrocytic gliosis.

FTLD-tau represents around 40% of FTLD cases; it includes classical Pick disease with Pick cells and Pick bodies, PSP, CBD, argyrophilic grain disease, familial cases of FTLD with a mutation in the *MAPT* gene, and a few other rare entities [108]. Tau pathology appears to be distinctly rare in SD [13, 109]. By contrast, about

Table 12.3 Simplified pathologic classification of frontotemporal lobar degeneration.

Category	Pattern	Gene involved
FTLD-tau	Pick disease	*MAPT**
	CDB	
	PSP	
	AGD	
	MSTD	
	NFT-dementia	
	WMT-GGI	
FTLD-TDP	Type A	*GRN***
	Type B	*C9ORF72*
	Type C	
	Type D	*VCP*
FTLD-FUS	aFTLD-U	
	NIFID	
	BIBD	
FTLS-UPS	FTD-3	*CHMP2B*

*Cases with *MAPT* mutations are associated with several pathologic patterns.
**Most cases of FTLD-TDP type A are not due to *GRN* mutations.
aFTLD-U, atypical frontotemporal lobar degeneration with ubiquitinated inclusions; AGD, argyrophilic grain disease; BIBD, basophilic inclusion body disease; *C9ORF72*, chromosome 9 open reading frame 72; CBD, corticobasal degeneration; *CHMP2B*, charged multivesicular body protein 2B; FTD-3, frontotemporal dementia linked to chromosome 3; FTLD, frontotemporal lobar degeneration; FUS, fused in sarcoma; *GRN*, granulin gene; IF, intermediate filaments; *MAPT*, microtubule associated protein tau; MSTD, multiple system tauopathy with dementia; NFT-dementia, neurofibrillary tangle predominant dementia; NIFID, neuronal intermediate filament inclusion disease; PiD, Pick disease; PSP, progressive supranuclear palsy; TARDBP, transactive response DNA binding protein; TDP, TDP-43 protein; UPS, ubiquitin-proteasome system; *VCP*, valosin containing protein; WMT-GGI, white matter tauopathy with globular glial inclusions.
Adapted from Mackenzie et al. 2010 [108].

45% of cases with bvFTD have tau pathology. In addition to neuronal loss that predominates in the frontal and temporal lobes, there is gliosis and accumulation of hyperphosphorylated tau in the cytoplasm of neurons and glial cells. There is some degree of specificity with regards to tau isoforms in that, for example, PSP and CBD display predominantly 4R tau deposits, whereas 3R tau accumulates in Pick disease [104, 110].

Approximately 50% of cases with FTLD display ubiquitin-positive immunoreactivity, with the majority having inclusions positive to TDP-43 (FTLD-TDP) and the remaining ~10% of cases to FUS. A classification of four FTLD-TDP forms (A–D) was proposed that combines previously reported classifications by Mackenzie et al. and Sampathu et al. [71]. Briefly, distinction is based on the distribution of dystrophic neurites, neuronal cytoplasmic inclusions (NCI), and neuronal intranuclear inclusions (NII) (Table 12.3). Type A is associated with bvFTD and PNFA, type B with bvFTD and FTD-MND, type C with SD, and type D with IBMPFD. FTLD-TDP includes sporadic FTD as well as monogenic forms caused by mutations in the *GRN*, *C9ORF72*, *VCP*, *SQSTM1*, *UBQLN2*, and *TBK1* genes. In the Mayo Clinic brain bank series, *TBK1* is the third most common gene in FTLD-TDP following *C9ORF72* and *GRN* [102]. The clinical correlates of FTLD-TDP include most cases of SD, about 45% of bvFTD, and some cases of LPA, FTDP-17, CBS, and PNFA [13, 109].

The most recently identified pathologic category is FTLD-FUS [106, 111, 112]. This includes atypical forms of ubiquitin-positive FTLD, neuronal intermediate filament inclusion disease, and basophilic inclusion body disease (Table 12.3). Clinically, patients have an early onset and display atrophy of frontoinsular and cingulate cortex, as well as of the head of the caudate nucleus [113].

Clinical prodrome and biomarkers

In addition to imaging (see section Morphologic and functional imaging) there is strong interest in identifying early markers/predictors that would help diagnose FTD but also correctly discriminate between different types of dementia. Clinically, early manifestations of FTD include diverse symptoms such as behavioral/social changes, character changes, or language difficulties. However, some degree of memory impairment may exist, and imaging does not always help decide which type of dementing illness is in progress.

Over the past years there has been growing interest in biomarkers that can be measured in the CSF of affected individuals. Based on knowledge of the proteins implicated in various neurodegenerative conditions, several studies have measured CSF levels of α-synuclein, amyloid-β42 (Aβ42), total tau (tau), or phosphorylated tau (p-tau). The most consistent findings in FTD patients have been reduced Aβ42, increased tau, and no change in p-tau. One study examined CSF from 512 patients with AD, 272 patients with other dementia including 144 patients with FTD, and controls [114]. Although overall observed abnormalities in FTD (moderately reduced Aβ42, moderately increased tau, normal p-tau) differed from those in controls (normal findings) and in AD cases (markedly reduced Aβ42, markedly increased tau, markedly increased p-tau), as many as 28% of FTD cases in fact had AD "CSF profiles". This overlap was seen preferentially among older patients. Other studies have also shown the importance of p-tau levels in discriminating AD from non-AD dementia [115]. In addition to Aβ42, tau, and p-tau, one study comparing 55 patients with FTD, 60 patients with AD, and 40 controls found that adding Aβ40 into the predictive model significantly improved diagnostic accuracy [116].

Based on the notion that *GRN* mutations cause disease through a mechanism of haploinsufficiency, CSF and plasma progranulin levels were reduced in FTD patients with a *GRN* mutation [117–119], which could have important diagnostic implications.

Morphologic and functional imaging

Early in the disease morphological imaging often shows few if any abnormalities, however with progression atrophy can be readily demonstrated by regular CT or MRI examination [120]. Overall, atrophy tends to predominate in the frontal and temporal lobes (particularly mesial frontal) in patients with bvFTD, whereas in PNFA it affects more the left frontal lobe (particularly the insula), and in SD the rostral temporal areas (often left) [121, 122]. One morphometric study found strong discriminative power of regional atrophy to predict the clinical syndrome [123]. However there is wide variability and overlap of atrophy patterns, presence or absence of asymmetry, and even abnormalities in other brain areas such as the parietal lobe [124]. Overall, there is some degree of correlation between volumetric MRI atrophy profile and underlying pathology [125, 126], although with some conflicting results [122]. One volumetric study in bvFTD patients found that frontal, limbic, and temporal cortices were affected early in the disease, with posterior regions and white matter involved later [127]. Normal or borderline MR scan early into the disease was found to represent a favorable prognostic factor, whereas age and clinical features were not [128]. Overall, it seems that patients with FTD display higher rates of atrophy progression over time compared to patients with AD, consistent with more rapid clinical progression [129]. Interestingly, a voxel-based morphometric MRI study examined FTD patients with or without binge eating disorder and found atrophy in the right ventral insula, striatum, and orbitofrontal areas to be associated with binge eating [130]. Another study identified abnormalities in the posterior hypothalamus in bvFTD patients, particularly pronounced in those with feeding problems, in whom pathology examination also confirmed hypothalamus atrophy [131]. FTD patients with apathy and disinhibition were shown to have more atrophy in prefrontal and temporal areas [132]. In addition to morphometry, other MRI techniques including diffusion tensor imaging (DTI) and fractional anisotropy (FA) have been used and showed significant involvement of white matter in FTD, more so than in AD [133].

Genetically determined forms of FTD have been compared in a number of MRI studies. Overall, mutations in *MAPT* have been associated with predominant involvement of the anteromedial temporal lobes, whereas *GRN* mutations showed more widespread patterns of atrophy in frontal, temporal, and parietal regions [134–136]. Using a voxel-based morphometry (VBM) approach, one study compared 9 patients with *GRN* mutations and 11 patients with *MAPT* mutations [135]. Differences included greater asymmetry and a faster rate of whole brain atrophy in *GRN* mutation carriers compared with those carrying a *MAPT* mutation. Overall, overlapping but distinct anatomical networks were affected. Another study compared bvFTD patients with no mutation and sporadic disease (20 patients) to those who had a mutation in *C9ORF72* (19 patients), *MAPT* (25 patients), or *GRN* (12 patients) [137]. *C9ORF72* associated with symmetric atrophy of the dorsolateral, medial, and orbitofrontal areas, whereas *MAPT* associated with anteromedial temporal atrophy, *GRN* with temporoparietal atrophy, and the sporadic group with frontal and anterior temporal atrophy. Taken together, these data suggest that MR-based imaging may help differentiate subtypes of genetically determined forms of FTD even at the single subject level.

Functional imaging using glucose positron emission tomography (FDG-PET) and single photon emission computed tomography (SPECT) is very useful in early diagnosis of FTD, often showing hypometabolism/hypoperfusion in frontal and temporal areas [138, 139]. Longitudinal studies have found hypometabolism in the lateral and medial prefrontal cortices, insula, and thalamus, with later involvement of temporal and parietal cortices [140, 141]. Posterior orbitofrontal cortex hypometabolism was correlated with apathy and disinhibition in one study, and ventromedial prefrontal and temporal hypoperfusion with disinhibition in another study [141, 142].

Functional imaging studies of patients with FTDP-17 have consistently shown abnormalities in temporal and frontal regions [143], and examination of presymptomatic mutation carriers showed frontal hypoperfusion [144]. In patients with parkinsonism, a mostly postsynaptic dopaminergic deficit was reported, consistent with the poor/short-lasting response to treatment with levodopa [143, 145]. Dopaminergic pathway imaging of the PPND family carrying the N279K mutation in *MAPT* showed reduced tracer uptake in a presymptomatic mutation carrier, which was of lesser magnitude than the reduction seen in symptomatic patients, illustrating the potential to identify early, presymptomatic biomarkers of the disease [145, 146].

Diagnosis and prognosis

A diagnosis of FTD should be suspected in patients with a history of progressive behavioral changes or language difficulties. However, early manifestations may be subtle, confused with psychiatric problems, or simply overlooked. Careful questioning of not only the patient but also spouses/caregivers is of paramount importance to detect early symptoms.

Clinical diagnostic criteria for FTD were established in 1998 and have been widely used since [4]. Diagnosis focuses on the main symptoms and signs defining the various FTD subtypes (Table 12.1). For bvFTD the core criteria consist of the insidious onset and gradual progression of loss of insight, emotional blunting, impairment in regulation of personal conduct, and decline in social interpersonal conduct. Supportive features include behavioral changes (e.g., mental rigidity, decline in personal hygiene) and speech and language alterations (e.g., echolalia, perseveration), along with other physical signs and findings on a range of investigations such as brain imaging. Improvements have been proposed, particularly with the development of criteria that include diagnosis of possible, probable, and definite bvFTD [147]. Diagnosis of the language syndromes PNFA, SD, and LPA focuses on their respective deficits (Table 12.1).

Overall studies have found these diagnostic criteria to be both sensitive (85%) and specific (99%) [148, 149], with the revised version for bvFTD having higher sensitivity [147]. Brain imaging is widely used and improves sensitivity of clinical criteria [150]. Several authors have argued that the Neary Consensus criteria were more appropriate for a research setting than for use in routine clinical practice [151]. Hence criteria were developed that are easier to use on a daily basis; these include early and progressive changes in language or personality; impairment in social and occupational functioning; gradual and progressive course; exclusion of other causes; absence of delirium; and exclusion of an active psychiatric condition [151]. A detailed evaluation of sensitivity and specificity has not yet been carried out, however the criteria are prone to miss cases with SD.

The overall prognosis in FTD is poorer than in AD, with a mean survival from initial symptoms of approximately 7 years [152–154]. Prognosis depends on the underlying subtype of FTD. In patients with bvFTD disease duration is usually between 7 and 9 years [152]. In contrast, patients with FTD-MND tend to have a more rapid progression with death after 3–4 years [154, 155]. Patients with genetic forms due to *MAPT* and *GRN* mutations also have a more rapid progression.

Treatment options

No known treatment has any proven influence on disease course and no specific substance is FDA approved for FTD. Therefore current therapeutic strategies rely on symptomatic measures. In contrast to the usefulness of acetylcholinesterase inhibitors or memantine for AD, several studies showed that these drugs had no beneficial effects for FTD patients and might worsen cognition and behavioral symptoms [156, 157]. Some clinicians recommend using atypical antipsychotics and antidepressants in patients displaying significant behavioral or mood alterations. Speech therapy may benefit patients with language impairment, and physical therapy may help with gait and activities of daily living. Driving ability should be carefully assessed and driving discouraged in patients with significant cognitive impairment, as is the case in other types of dementia.

Future developments

Major progress has been achieved over the past decade, mainly in the fields of genetics and pathology of FTD. Also, imaging and CSF studies have provided evidence that a reliable biomarker for diagnosis and disease progression monitoring may become available soon. The challenge for the years to come will be to further enhance our knowledge of the molecular mechanisms involved in neurodegeneration, in order to nominate pathways and potential targets for future therapeutic strategies. Such developments will only be successful if a complete set of biomarkers are developed that allow reliable and early detection of FTD, as well as monitoring of the effects of therapeutic measures. Ultimately, it is hoped that future progress will lead to the discovery of treatments that will prevent or cure the disease.

References

1. Pick A. Uber die Beziehungen der senilen Hirnatrophie zur Aphasie. *Prager Med Wochenschr.* 1892;17:165–7.
2. Alzheimer A. Uber eigenartige Krankheitsfälle des späteren Alters. *Z ges Neurol Psychiat.* 1911;4:356–85.
3. Rossor MN, Fox NC, Mummery CJ, Schott JM, Warren JD. The diagnosis of young-onset dementia. *Lancet Neurol.* 2010 Aug;9(8):793–806.
4. Neary D, Snowden JS, Gustafson L, Passant U, Stuss D, Black S, et al. Frontotemporal lobar degeneration: a consensus on clinical diagnostic criteria. *Neurology.* 1998 Dec;51(6):1546–54.
5. Neary D, Snowden J, Mann D. Frontotemporal dementia. *Lancet Neurol.* 2005 Nov;4(11):771–80.
6. Clinical and neuropathological criteria for frontotemporal dementia. The Lund and Manchester Groups. *J Neurol Neurosurg Psychiatry.* 1994 Apr;57(4):416–8.
7. Gorno-Tempini ML, Hillis AE, Weintraub S, Kertesz A, Mendez M, Cappa SF, et al. Classification of primary progressive aphasia and its variants. *Neurology.* 2011 Mar 15;76(11):1006–14.
8. Mackenzie IR, Neumann M, Bigio EH, Cairns NJ, Alafuzoff I, Kril J, et al. Nomenclature for neuropathologic subtypes of frontotemporal lobar degeneration: consensus recommendations. *Acta Neuropathol.* 2009 Jan;117(1):15–8.
9. Josephs KA, Petersen RC, Knopman DS, Boeve BF, Whitwell JL, Duffy JR, et al. Clinicopathologic analysis of frontotemporal and corticobasal degenerations and PSP. *Neurology.* 2006 Jan 10;66(1):41–8.
10. Ratnavalli E, Brayne C, Dawson K, Hodges JR. The prevalence of frontotemporal dementia. *Neurology.* 2002 Jun 11;58(11):1615–21.
11. Rosso SM, Donker Kaat L, Baks T, Joosse M, de Koning I, Pijnenburg Y, et al. Frontotemporal dementia in The Netherlands: patient characteristics and prevalence estimates from a population-based study. *Brain.* 2003 Sep;126(Pt 9):2016–22.
12. Knopman DS, Petersen RC, Edland SD, Cha RH, Rocca WA. The incidence of frontotemporal lobar degeneration in Rochester, Minnesota, 1990 through 1994. *Neurology.* 2004 Feb 10;62(3):506–8.
13. Piguet O, Hornberger M, Mioshi E, Hodges JR. Behavioural-variant frontotemporal dementia: diagnosis, clinical staging, and management. *Lancet Neurol.* 2011 Feb;10(2):162–72.
14. Kertesz A, McMonagle P, Blair M, Davidson W, Munoz DG. The evolution and pathology of frontotemporal dementia. *Brain.* 2005 Sep;128(Pt 9):1996–2005.
15. Le Rhun E, Richard F, Pasquier F. Natural history of primary progressive aphasia. *Neurology.* 2005 Sep 27;65(6):887–91.
16. Kertesz A, Blair M, McMonagle P, Munoz DG. The diagnosis and course of frontotemporal dementia. *Alzheimer Dis Assoc Disord.* 2007 Apr-Jun;21(2):155–63.
17. Piguet O. Eating disturbance in behavioural-variant frontotemporal dementia. *J Mol Neurosci.* 2011 Nov;45(3):589–93.
18. Hornberger M, Piguet O, Graham AJ, Nestor PJ, Hodges JR. How preserved is episodic memory in behavioral variant frontotemporal dementia? *Neurology.* 2010 Feb 9;74(6):472–9.
19. Bozeat S, Gregory CA, Ralph MA, Hodges JR. Which neuropsychiatric and behavioural features distinguish frontal and temporal variants of frontotemporal dementia from Alzheimer's disease? *J Neurol Neurosurg Psychiatry.* 2000 Aug;69(2):178–86.
20. Liu W, Miller BL, Kramer JH, Rankin K, Wyss-Coray C, Gearhart R, et al. Behavioral disorders in the frontal and temporal variants of frontotemporal dementia. *Neurology.* 2004 Mar 9;62(5):742–8.
21. Grossman M. Primary progressive aphasia: clinicopathological correlations. *Nat Rev Neurol.* 2010 Feb;6(2):88–97.
22. Josephs KA, Duffy JR, Strand EA, Whitwell JL, Layton KF, Parisi JE, et al. Clinicopathological and imaging correlates of progressive aphasia and apraxia of speech. *Brain.* 2006 Jun;129(Pt 6):1385–98.
23. Lomen-Hoerth C, Anderson T, Miller B. The overlap of amyotrophic lateral sclerosis and frontotemporal dementia. *Neurology.* 2002 Oct 8;59(7):1077–9.
24. Neary D, Snowden JS, Mann DM, Northen B, Goulding PJ, Macdermott N. Frontal lobe dementia and motor neuron disease. *J Neurol Neurosurg Psychiatry.* 1990 Jan;53(1):23–32.
25. Hodges JR, Patterson K. Semantic dementia: a unique clinicopathological syndrome. *Lancet Neurol.* 2007 Nov;6(11):1004–14.
26. Snowden JS, Bathgate D, Varma A, Blackshaw A, Gibbons ZC, Neary D. Distinct behavioural profiles in frontotemporal dementia and semantic dementia. *J Neurol Neurosurg Psychiatry.* 2001 Mar;70(3):323–32.
27. Czarnecki K, Duffy JR, Nehl CR, Cross SA, Molano JR, Jack CR, Jr., et al. Very early semantic dementia with progressive temporal lobe atrophy: an 8-year longitudinal study. *Arch Neurol.* 2008 Dec;65(12):1659–63.
28. Gorno-Tempini ML, Dronkers NF, Rankin KP, Ogar JM, Phengrasamy L, Rosen HJ, et al. Cognition and anatomy in three variants of primary progressive aphasia. *Ann Neurol.* 2004 Mar;55(3):335–46.
29. Forman MS, Farmer J, Johnson JK, Clark CM, Arnold SE, Coslett HB, et al. Frontotemporal dementia: clinicopathological correlations. *Ann Neurol.* 2006 Jun;59(6):952–62.
30. Foster NL, Wilhelmsen K, Sima AA, Jones MZ, D'Amato CJ, Gilman S. Frontotemporal dementia and parkinsonism linked to chromosome 17: a consensus conference. *Conference Participants. Ann Neurol.* 1997 Jun;41(6):706–15.
31. Tsuboi Y, Uitti RJ, Delisle MB, Ferreira JJ, Brefel-Courbon C, Rascol O, et al. Clinical features and disease haplotypes of individuals with the N279K tau gene mutation: a comparison of the pallidopontonigral degeneration kindred and a French family. *Arch Neurol.* 2002 Jun;59(6):943–50.
32. Wszolek ZK, Tsuboi Y, Ghetti B, Pickering-Brown S, Baba Y, Cheshire WP. Frontotemporal dementia and parkinsonism linked to chromosome 17 (FTDP-17). *Orphanet J Rare Dis.* 2006;1:30.
33. Wszolek ZK, Kardon RH, Wolters EC, Pfeiffer RF. Frontotemporal dementia and parkinsonism linked to chromosome 17 (FTDP-17): PPND family. *A longitudinal videotape demonstration. Mov Disord.* 2001 Jul;16(4):756–60.
34. Arvanitakis Z, Witte RJ, Dickson DW, Tsuboi Y, Uitti RJ, Slowinski J, et al. Clinical-pathologic study of biomarkers in FTDP-17 (PPND family with N279K tau mutation). *Parkinsonism Relat Disord.* 2007 May;13(4):230–9.
35. Pickering-Brown SM, Rollinson S, Du Plessis D, Morrison KE, Varma A, Richardson AM, et al. Frequency and clinical characteristics of progranulin mutation carriers in the Manchester frontotemporal lobar degeneration cohort: comparison with patients with MAPT and no known mutations. *Brain.* 2008 Mar;131(Pt 3):721–31.
36. Rossi G, Bastone A, Piccoli E, Morbin M, Mazzoleni G, Fugnanesi V, et al. Different mutations at V363 MAPT codon are associated with atypical clinical phenotypes and show unusual structural and functional features. *Neurobiol Aging.* 2014 Feb;35(2):408–17.
37. Tolboom N, Koedam EL, Schott JM, Yaqub M, Blankenstein MA, Barkhof F, et al. Dementia mimicking Alzheimer's disease owing to a tau mutation: CSF and PET findings. *Alzheimer Dis Assoc Disord.* 2010 Jul-Sep;24(3):303–7.
38. Rovelet-Lecrux A, Hannequin D, Guillin O, Legallic S, Jurici S, Wallon D, et al. Frontotemporal dementia phenotype associated with MAPT gene duplication. *J Alzheimers Dis.* 2010;21(3):897–902.
39. Chen-Plotkin AS, Martinez-Lage M, Sleiman PM, Hu W, Greene R, Wood EM, et al. Genetic and clinical features of progranulin-associated frontotemporal lobar degeneration. *Arch Neurol.* 2011 Apr;68(4):488–97.
40. Yu CE, Bird TD, Bekris LM, Montine TJ, Leverenz JB, Steinbart E, et al. The spectrum of mutations in progranulin: a collaborative study screening 545 cases of neurodegeneration. *Arch Neurol.* 2010 Feb;67(2):161–70.
41. Gass J, Cannon A, Mackenzie IR, Boeve B, Baker M, Adamson J, et al. Mutations in progranulin are a major cause of ubiquitin-positive frontotemporal lobar degeneration. *Hum Mol Genet.* 2006 Oct 15;15(20):2988–3001.
42. Rademakers R, Baker M, Gass J, Adamson J, Huey ED, Momeni P, et al. Phenotypic variability associated with progranulin haploinsufficiency in patients with the common 1477C-->T (Arg493X) mutation: an international initiative. *Lancet Neurol.* 2007 Oct;6(10):857–68.
43. Kelley BJ, Haidar W, Boeve BF, Baker M, Shiung M, Knopman DS, et al. Alzheimer disease-like phenotype associated with the c.154delA mutation in progranulin. *Arch Neurol.* 2010 Feb;67(2):171–7.
44. Di Fabio R, Tessa A, Simons EJ, Santorelli FM, Casali C, Serrao M, et al. Familial frontotemporal dementia with parkinsonism associated with the progranulin c.C1021T (p.Q341X) mutation. *Parkinsonism Relat Disord.* 2010 Aug;16(7):484–5.
45. Lomen-Hoerth C. Characterization of amyotrophic lateral sclerosis and frontotemporal dementia. *Dement Geriatr Cogn Disord.* 2004;17(4):337–41.
46. Josephs KA, Parisi JE, Knopman DS, Boeve BF, Petersen RC, Dickson DW. Clinically undetected motor neuron disease in pathologically proven frontotemporal lobar degeneration with motor neuron disease. *Arch Neurol.* 2006 Apr;63(4):506–12.
47. Hutton M, Lendon CL, Rizzu P, Baker M, Froelich S, Houlden H, et al. Association of missense and 5'-splice-site mutations in tau with the inherited dementia FTDP-17. *Nature.* 1998 Jun 18;393(6686):702–5.

48. Baker M, Mackenzie IR, Pickering-Brown SM, Gass J, Rademakers R, Lindholm C, et al. Mutations in progranulin cause tau-negative frontotemporal dementia linked to chromosome 17. *Nature.* 2006 Aug 24;442(7105):916–9.

49. Cruts M, Gijselinck I, van der Zee J, Engelborghs S, Wils H, Pirici D, et al. Null mutations in progranulin cause ubiquitin-positive frontotemporal dementia linked to chromosome 17q21. *Nature.* 2006 Aug 24;442(7105):920–4.

50. DeJesus-Hernandez M, Mackenzie IR, Boeve BF, Boxer AL, Baker M, Rutherford NJ, et al. Expanded GGGGCC hexanucleotide repeat in noncoding region of C9ORF72 causes chromosome 9p-linked FTD and ALS. *Neuron.* 2011 Oct 20; 72(2):245–56.

51. Renton AE, Majounie E, Waite A, Simon-Sanchez J, Rollinson S, Gibbs JR, et al. A hexanucleotide repeat expansion in C9ORF72 is the cause of chromosome 9p21-linked ALS-FTD. *Neuron.* 2011 Oct 20;72(2):257–68.

52. Benajiba L, Le Ber I, Camuzat A, Lacoste M, Thomas-Anterion C, Couratier P, et al. TARDBP mutations in motoneuron disease with frontotemporal lobar degeneration. *Ann Neurol.* 2009 Apr;65(4):470–3.

53. Borroni B, Bonvicini C, Alberici A, Buratti E, Agosti C, Archetti S, et al. Mutation within TARDBP leads to frontotemporal dementia without motor neuron disease. *Hum Mutat.* 2009 Nov;30(11):E974–83.

54. Ticozzi N, Silani V, LeClerc AL, Keagle P, Gellera C, Ratti A, et al. Analysis of FUS gene mutation in familial amyotrophic lateral sclerosis within an Italian cohort. *Neurology.* 2009 Oct 13;73(15):1180–5.

55. Watts GD, Wymer J, Kovach MJ, Mehta SG, Mumm S, Darvish D, et al. Inclusion body myopathy associated with Paget disease of bone and frontotemporal dementia is caused by mutant valosin-containing protein. *Nat Genet.* 2004 Apr;36(4):377–81.

56. Skibinski G, Parkinson NJ, Brown JM, Chakrabarti L, Lloyd SL, Hummerich H, et al. Mutations in the endosomal ESCRTIII-complex subunit CHMP2B in frontotemporal dementia. *Nat Genet.* 2005 Aug;37(8):806–8.

57. Deng HX, Chen W, Hong ST, Boycott KM, Gorrie GH, Siddique N, et al. Mutations in UBQLN2 cause dominant X-linked juvenile and adult-onset ALS and ALS/dementia. *Nature.* 2011 Aug 21;477(7363):211–5.

58. Rubino E, Rainero I, Chiò A, Rogaeva E, Galimberti D, Fenoglio P, et al. SQSTM1 mutations in frontotemporal lobar degeneration and amyotrophic lateral sclerosis. *Neurology.* 2012 Oct 9;79(15):1556–62.

59. Freischmidt A, Wieland T, Richter B, Ruf W, Schaeffer V, Müller K, et al. Haploinsufficiency of TBK1 causes familial ALS and fronto-temporal dementia. *Nat Neurosci.* 2015 May;18(5):631–6.

60. Rademakers R, Neumann M, Mackenzie IR. Advances in understanding the molecular basis of frontotemporal dementia. *Nat Rev Neurol.* 2012 Aug;8(8): 423–34.

61. Ghetti B, Oblak AL, Boeve BF, Johnson KA, Dickerson BC, Goedert M. Invited review: Frontotemporal dementia caused by microtubule-associated protein tau gene (MAPT) mutations: a chameleon for neuropathology and neuroimaging. *Neuropathol Appl Neurobiol.* 2015 Feb;41(1):24–46.

62. van Swieten J, Spillantini MG. Hereditary frontotemporal dementia caused by Tau gene mutations. *Brain Pathol.* 2007 Jan;17(1):63–73.

63. Hasegawa M, Smith MJ, Goedert M. Tau proteins with FTDP-17 mutations have a reduced ability to promote microtubule assembly. *FEBS Lett.* 1998 Oct 23;437(3):207–10.

64. Rizzini C, Goedert M, Hodges JR, Smith MJ, Jakes R, Hills R, et al. Tau gene mutation K257T causes a tauopathy similar to Pick's disease. *J Neuropathol Exp Neurol.* 2000 Nov;59(11):990–1001.

65. Lee VM, Goedert M, Trojanowski JQ. Neurodegenerative tauopathies. *Annu Rev Neurosci.* 2001;24:1121–59.

66. Ingram EM, Spillantini MG. Tau gene mutations: dissecting the pathogenesis of FTDP-17. *Trends Mol Med.* 2002 Dec;8(12):555–62.

67. Heutink P. Untangling tau-related dementia. *Hum Mol Genet.* 2000 Apr 12;9(6):979–86.

68. Le Ber I, van der Zee J, Hannequin D, Gijselinck I, Campion D, Puel M, et al. Progranulin null mutations in both sporadic and familial frontotemporal dementia. *Hum Mutat.* 2007 Sep;28(9):846–55.

69. Hu F, Padukkavidana T, Vaegter CB, Brady OA, Zheng Y, Mackenzie IR, et al. Sortilin-mediated endocytosis determines levels of the frontotemporal dementia protein, progranulin. *Neuron.* 2010 Nov 18;68(4):654–67.

70. Mackenzie IR, Baker M, Pickering-Brown S, Hsiung GY, Lindholm C, Dwosh E, et al. The neuropathology of frontotemporal lobar degeneration caused by mutations in the progranulin gene. *Brain.* 2006 Nov;129(Pt 11):3081–90.

71. Mackenzie IR, Neumann M, Baborie A, Sampathu DM, Du Plessis D, Jaros E, et al. A harmonized classification system for FTLD-TDP pathology. *Acta Neuropathol.* 2011 Jul;122(1):111–3.

72. Schofield EC, Halliday GM, Kwok J, Loy C, Double KL, Hodges JR. Low serum progranulin predicts the presence of mutations: a prospective study. *J Alzheimers Dis.* 2010;22(3):981–4.

73. Carecchio M, Fenoglio C, De Riz M, Guidi I, Comi C, Cortini F, et al. Progranulin plasma levels as potential biomarker for the identification of GRN deletion carriers. A case with atypical onset as clinical amnestic Mild Cognitive Impairment converted to Alzheimer's disease. *J Neurol Sci.* 2009 Dec 15;287(1-2):291–3.

74. Valdmanis PN, Dupre N, Bouchard JP, Camu W, Salachas F, Meininger V, et al. Three families with amyotrophic lateral sclerosis and frontotemporal dementia with evidence of linkage to chromosome 9p. *Arch Neurol.* 2007 Feb;64(2):240–5.

75. Vance C, Al-Chalabi A, Ruddy D, Smith BN, Hu X, Sreedharan J, et al. Familial amyotrophic lateral sclerosis with frontotemporal dementia is linked to a locus on chromosome 9p13.2-21.3. *Brain.* 2006 Apr;129(Pt 4):868–76.

76. Boxer AL, Mackenzie IR, Boeve BF, Baker M, Seeley WW, Crook R, et al. Clinical, neuroimaging and neuropathological features of a new chromosome 9p-linked FTD-ALS family. *J Neurol Neurosurg Psychiatry.* 2011 Feb;82(2):196–203.

77. Pearson JP, Williams NM, Majounie E, Waite A, Stott J, Newsway V, et al. Familial frontotemporal dementia with amyotrophic lateral sclerosis and a shared haplotype on chromosome 9p. *J Neurol.* 2011 Apr;258(4):647–55.

78. Gijselinck I, Van Langenhove T, van der Zee J, Sleegers K, Philtjens S, Kleinberger G, et al. A C9orf72 promoter repeat expansion in a Flanders-Belgian cohort with disorders of the frontotemporal lobar degeneration-amyotrophic lateral sclerosis spectrum: a gene identification study. *Lancet Neurol.* 2012 Jan;11(1):54–65.

79. Snowden JS, Rollinson S, Thompson JC, Harris JM, Stopford CL, Richardson AM, et al. Distinct clinical and pathological characteristics of frontotemporal dementia associated with C9ORF72 mutations. *Brain.* 2012 Mar;135(Pt 3):693–708.

80. Simon-Sanchez J, Dopper EG, Cohn-Hokke PE, Hukema RK, Nicolaou N, Seelaar H, et al. The clinical and pathological phenotype of C9ORF72 hexanucleotide repeat expansions. *Brain.* 2012 Mar;135(Pt 3):723–35.

81. Majounie E, Renton AE, Mok K, Dopper EG, Waite A, Rollinson S, et al. Frequency of the C9orf72 hexanucleotide repeat expansion in patients with amyotrophic lateral sclerosis and frontotemporal dementia: a cross-sectional study. *Lancet Neurol.* 2012 Apr;11(4):323–30.

82. Majounie E, Abramzon Y, Renton AE, Perry R, Bassett SS, Pletnikova O, et al. Repeat expansion in C9ORF72 in Alzheimer's disease. *N Engl J Med.* 2012 Jan 19;366(3):283–4.

83. Todd TW, Petrucelli L. Insights into the pathogenic mechanisms of Chromosome 9 open reading frame 72 (C9orf72) repeat expansions. *J Neurochem.* 2016 Aug;138 Suppl 1:145–62.

84. Kovach MJ, Waggoner B, Leal SM, Gelber D, Khardori R, Levenstien MA, et al. Clinical delineation and localization to chromosome 9p13.3-p12 of a unique dominant disorder in four families: hereditary inclusion body myopathy, Paget disease of bone, and frontotemporal dementia. *Mol Genet Metab.* 2001 Dec;74(4):458–75.

85. Kim EJ, Park YE, Kim DS, Ahn BY, Kim HS, Chang YH, et al. Inclusion body myopathy with Paget disease of bone and frontotemporal dementia linked to VCP p.Arg155Cys in a Korean family. *Arch Neurol.* 2011 Jun;68(6):787–96.

86. Johnson JO, Mandrioli J, Benatar M, Abramzon Y, Van Deerlin VM, Trojanowski JQ, et al. Exome sequencing reveals VCP mutations as a cause of familial ALS. *Neuron.* 2010 Dec 9;68(5):857–64.

87. Watts GD, Thomasova D, Ramdeen SK, Fulchiero EC, Mehta SG, Drachman DA, et al. Novel VCP mutations in inclusion body myopathy associated with Paget disease of bone and frontotemporal dementia. *Clin Genet.* 2007 Nov;72(5):420–6.

88. Bersano A, Del Bo R, Lamperti C, Ghezzi S, Fagiolari G, Fortunato F, et al. Inclusion body myopathy and frontotemporal dementia caused by a novel VCP mutation. *Neurobiol Aging.* 2009 May;30(5):752–8.

89. Weihl CC, Temiz P, Miller SE, Watts G, Smith C, Forman M, et al. TDP-43 accumulation in inclusion body myopathy muscle suggests a common pathogenic mechanism with frontotemporal dementia. *J Neurol Neurosurg Psychiatry.* 2008 Oct;79(10):1186–9.

90. Kovacs GG, Murrell JR, Horvath S, Haraszti L, Majtenyi K, Molnar MJ, et al. TARDBP variation associated with frontotemporal dementia, supranuclear gaze palsy, and chorea. *Mov Disord.* 2009 Sep 15;24(12):1843–7.

91. Quadri M, Cossu G, Saddi V, Simons EJ, Murgia D, Melis M, et al. Broadening the phenotype of TARDBP mutations: the TARDBP Ala382Thr mutation and Parkinson's disease in Sardinia. *Neurogenetics.* 2011 Aug;12(3):203–9.

92. Chio A, Calvo A, Moglia C, Restagno G, Ossola I, Brunetti M, et al. Amyotrophic lateral sclerosis-frontotemporal lobar dementia in 3 families with p.Ala382Thr TARDBP mutations. *Arch Neurol.* 2010 Aug;67(8):1002–9.

93. Broustal O, Camuzat A, Guillot-Noel L, Guy N, Millecamps S, Deffond D, et al. FUS mutations in frontotemporal lobar degeneration with amyotrophic lateral sclerosis. *J Alzheimers Dis.* 2010;22(3):765–9.

94. Cannon A, Baker M, Boeve B, Josephs K, Knopman D, Petersen R, et al. CHMP2B mutations are not a common cause of frontotemporal lobar degeneration. *Neurosci Lett.* 2006 May 1;398(1-2):83–4.

95. van der Zee J, Urwin H, Engelborghs S, Bruyland M, Vandenberghe R, Dermaut B, et al. CHMP2B C-truncating mutations in frontotemporal lobar degeneration

are associated with an aberrant endosomal phenotype in vitro. *Hum Mol Genet.* 2008 Jan 15;17(2):313–22.

96. Vengoechea J, David MP, Yaghi SR, Carpenter L, Rudnicki SA. Clinical variability and female penetrance in X-linked familial FTD/ALS caused by a P506S mutation in UBQLN2. *Amyotroph Lateral Scler Frontotemporal Degener.* 2013 Dec;14(7-8):615–9.

97. Synofzik M, Maetzler W, Grehl T, Prudlo J, Vom Hagen JM, Haack T, et al. Screening in ALS and FTD patients reveals 3 novel UBQLN2 mutations outside the PXX domain and a pure FTD phenotype. *Neurobiol Aging.* 2012 Dec;33(12):2949.e13–7.

98. Fahed AC, McDonough B, Gouvion CM, Newell KL, Dure LS, Bebin M, et al. UBQLN2 mutation causing heterogeneous X-linked dominant neurodegeneration. *Ann Neurol.* 2014 May;75(5):793–8.

99. Fecto F, Yan J, Vemula SP, Liu E, Yang Y, Chen W, et al. SQSTM1 mutations in familial and sporadic amyotrophic lateral sclerosis. *Arch Neurol.* 2011 Nov;68(11):1440–6.

100. Le Ber I, Camuzat A, Guerreiro R, Bouya-Ahmed K, Bras J, Nicolas G, et al. SQSTM1 mutations in French patients with frontotemporal dementia or frontotemporal dementia with amyotrophic lateral sclerosis. *JAMA Neurol.* 2013 Nov;70(11):1403–10.

101. Cirulli ET, Lasseigne BN, Petrovski S, Sapp PC, Dion PA, Leblond CS, et al. Exome sequencing in amyotrophic lateral sclerosis identifies risk genes and pathways. *Science.* 2015 Mar 27;347(6229):1436–41.

102. Pottier C, Bieniek KF, Finch N, van de Vorst M, Baker M, Perkersen R, et al. Whole-genome sequencing reveals important role for TBK1 and OPTN mutations in frontotemporal lobar degeneration without motor neuron disease. *Acta Neuropathol.* 2015 Jul;130(1):77–92.

103. Gijselinck I, Van Mossevelde S, van der Zee J, Sieben A, Philtjens S, Heeman B, et al. Loss of TBK1 is a frequent cause of frontotemporal dementia in a Belgian cohort. *Neurology.* 2015 Dec 15;85(24):2116–25.

104. Cairns NJ, Bigio EH, Mackenzie IR, Neumann M, Lee VM, Hatanpaa KJ, et al. Neuropathologic diagnostic and nosologic criteria for frontotemporal lobar degeneration: consensus of the Consortium for Frontotemporal Lobar Degeneration. *Acta Neuropathol.* 2007 Jul;114(1):5–22.

105. Neumann M, Sampathu DM, Kwong LK, Truax AC, Micsenyi MC, Chou TT, et al. Ubiquitinated TDP-43 in frontotemporal lobar degeneration and amyotrophic lateral sclerosis. *Science.* 2006 Oct 6;314(5796):130–3.

106. Neumann M, Rademakers R, Roeber S, Baker M, Kretzschmar HA, Mackenzie IR. A new subtype of frontotemporal lobar degeneration with FUS pathology. *Brain.* 2009 Nov;132(Pt 11):2922–31.

107. Goedert M, Ghetti B, Spillantini MG. Frontotemporal dementia: implications for understanding Alzheimer disease. *Cold Spring Harb Perspect Med.* 2012 Feb;2(2):a006254.

108. Mackenzie IR, Neumann M, Bigio EH, Cairns NJ, Alafuzoff I, Kril J, et al. Nomenclature and nosology for neuropathologic subtypes of frontotemporal lobar degeneration: an update. *Acta Neuropathol.* 2010 Jan;119(1):1–4.

109. Piguet O, Halliday GM, Reid WG, Casey B, Carman R, Huang Y, et al. Clinical phenotypes in autopsy-confirmed Pick disease. *Neurology.* 2011 Jan 18;76(3):253–9.

110. Trojanowski JQ, Dickson D. Update on the neuropathological diagnosis of frontotemporal dementias. *J Neuropathol Exp Neurol.* 2001 Dec;60(12):1123–6.

111. Neumann M, Roeber S, Kretzschmar HA, Rademakers R, Baker M, Mackenzie IR. Abundant FUS-immunoreactive pathology in neuronal intermediate filament inclusion disease. *Acta Neuropathol.* 2009 Nov;118(5):605–16.

112. Urwin H, Josephs KA, Rohrer JD, Mackenzie IR, Neumann M, Authier A, et al. FUS pathology defines the majority of tau- and TDP-43-negative frontotemporal lobar degeneration. *Acta Neuropathol.* 2010 Jul;120(1):33–41.

113. Josephs KA, Whitwell JL, Parisi JE, Petersen RC, Boeve BF, Jack CR, Jr., et al. Caudate atrophy on MRI is a characteristic feature of FTLD-FUS. *Eur J Neurol.* 2010 Jul;17(7):969–75.

114. Schoonenboom NS, Reesink FE, Verwey NA, Kester MI, Teunissen CE, van de Ven PM, et al. Cerebrospinal fluid markers for differential dementia diagnosis in a large memory clinic cohort. *Neurology.* 2012 Jan 3;78(1):47–54.

115. Le Bastard N, Martin JJ, Vanmechelen E, Vanderstichele H, De Deyn PP, Engelborghs S. Added diagnostic value of CSF biomarkers in differential dementia diagnosis. *Neurobiol Aging.* 2010 Nov;31(11):1867–76.

116. Verwey NA, Kester MI, van der Flier WM, Veerhuis R, Berkhof H, Twaalfhoven H, et al. Additional value of CSF amyloid-beta 40 levels in the differentiation between FTLD and control subjects. *J Alzheimers Dis.* 2010;20(2):445–52.

117. Finch N, Baker M, Crook R, Swanson K, Kuntz K, Surtees R, et al. Plasma progranulin levels predict progranulin mutation status in frontotemporal dementia patients and asymptomatic family members. *Brain.* 2009 Mar;132(Pt 3):583–91.

118. Ghidoni R, Benussi L, Glionna M, Franzoni M, Binetti G. Low plasma progranulin levels predict progranulin mutations in frontotemporal lobar degeneration. *Neurology.* 2008 Oct 14;71(16):1235–9.

119. Van Damme P, Van Hoecke A, Lambrechts D, Vanacker P, Bogaert E, van Swieten J, et al. Progranulin functions as a neurotrophic factor to regulate neurite outgrowth and enhance neuronal survival. *J Cell Biol.* 2008 Apr 7;181(1):37–41.

120. Koedam EL, Van der Flier WM, Barkhof F, Koene T, Scheltens P, Pijnenburg YA. Clinical characteristics of patients with frontotemporal dementia with and without lobar atrophy on MRI. *Alzheimer Dis Assoc Disord.* 2010 Jul-Sep;24(3):242–7.

121. Williams GB, Nestor PJ, Hodges JR. Neural correlates of semantic and behavioural deficits in frontotemporal dementia. *Neuroimage.* 2005 Feb 15;24(4):1042–51.

122. Pereira JM, Williams GB, Acosta-Cabronero J, Pengas G, Spillantini MG, Xuereb JH, et al. Atrophy patterns in histologic vs clinical groupings of frontotemporal lobar degeneration. *Neurology.* 2009 May 12;72(19):1653–60.

123. Lindberg O, Ostberg P, Zandbelt BB, Oberg J, Zhang Y, Andersen C, et al. Cortical morphometric subclassification of frontotemporal lobar degeneration. *AJNR Am J Neuroradiol.* 2009 Jun;30(6):1233–9.

124. Chow TW, Binns MA, Freedman M, Stuss DT, Ramirez J, Scott CJ, et al. Overlap in frontotemporal atrophy between normal aging and patients with frontotemporal dementias. *Alzheimer Dis Assoc Disord.* 2008 Oct-Dec;22(4):327–35.

125. Rohrer JD, Geser F, Zhou J, Gennatas ED, Sidhu M, Trojanowski JQ, et al. TDP-43 subtypes are associated with distinct atrophy patterns in frontotemporal dementia. *Neurology.* 2010 Dec 14;75(24):2204–11.

126. Rohrer JD, Lashley T, Schott JM, Warren JE, Mead S, Isaacs AM, et al. Clinical and neuroanatomical signatures of tissue pathology in frontotemporal lobar degeneration. *Brain.* 2011 Sep;134(Pt 9):2565–81.

127. Kril JJ, Macdonald V, Patel S, Png F, Halliday GM. Distribution of brain atrophy in behavioral variant frontotemporal dementia. *J Neurol Sci.* 2005 May 15;232(1-2):83–90.

128. Davies RR, Kipps CM, Mitchell J, Kril JJ, Halliday GM, Hodges JR. Progression in frontotemporal dementia: identifying a benign behavioral variant by magnetic resonance imaging. *Arch Neurol.* 2006 Nov;63(11):1627–31.

129. Krueger CE, Dean DL, Rosen HJ, Halabi C, Weiner M, Miller BL, et al. Longitudinal rates of lobar atrophy in frontotemporal dementia, semantic dementia, and Alzheimer's disease. *Alzheimer Dis Assoc Disord.* 2010 Jan-Mar;24(1):43–8.

130. Woolley JD, Gorno-Tempini ML, Seeley WW, Rankin K, Lee SS, Matthews BR, et al. Binge eating is associated with right orbitofrontal-insular-striatal atrophy in frontotemporal dementia. *Neurology.* 2007 Oct 2;69(14):1424–33.

131. Piguet O, Petersen A, Yin Ka Lam B, Gabery S, Murphy K, Hodges JR, et al. Eating and hypothalamus changes in behavioral-variant frontotemporal dementia. *Ann Neurol.* 2011 Feb;69(2):312–9.

132. Zamboni G, Huey ED, Krueger F, Nichelli PF, Grafman J. Apathy and disinhibition in frontotemporal dementia: Insights into their neural correlates. *Neurology.* 2008 Sep 2;71(10):736–42.

133. Zhang Y, Schuff N, Du AT, Rosen HJ, Kramer JH, Gorno-Tempini ML, et al. White matter damage in frontotemporal dementia and Alzheimer's disease measured by diffusion MRI. *Brain.* 2009 Sep;132(Pt 9):2579–92.

134. Whitwell JL, Josephs KA, Rossor MN, Stevens JM, Revesz T, Holton JL, et al. Magnetic resonance imaging signatures of tissue pathology in frontotemporal dementia. *Arch Neurol.* 2005 Sep;62(9):1402–8.

135. Rohrer JD, Ridgway GR, Modat M, Ourselin S, Mead S, Fox NC, et al. Distinct profiles of brain atrophy in frontotemporal lobar degeneration caused by progranulin and tau mutations. *Neuroimage.* Nov 15;53(3):1070–6.

136. Whitwell JL, Jack CR, Jr., Baker M, Rademakers R, Adamson J, Boeve BF, et al. Voxel-based morphometry in frontotemporal lobar degeneration with ubiquitin-positive inclusions with and without progranulin mutations. *Arch Neurol.* 2007 Mar;64(3):371–6.

137. Whitwell JL, Weigand SD, Boeve BF, Senjem ML, Gunter JL, Dejesus-Hernandez M, et al. Neuroimaging signatures of frontotemporal dementia genetics: C9ORF72, tau, progranulin and sporadics. *Brain.* 2012 Mar;135(Pt 3):794–806.

138. Pasquier F, Fukui T, Sarazin M, Pijnenburg Y, Diehl J, Grundman M, et al. Laboratory investigations and treatment in frontotemporal dementia. *Ann Neurol.* 2003;54 Suppl 5:S32–5.

139. Salmon E, Kerrouche N, Herholz K, Perani D, Holthoff V, Beuthien-Baumann B, et al. Decomposition of metabolic brain clusters in the frontal variant of frontotemporal dementia. *Neuroimage.* 2006 Apr 15;30(3):871–8.

140. Diehl-Schmid J, Grimmer T, Drzezga A, Bornschein S, Riemenschneider M, Forstl H, et al. Decline of cerebral glucose metabolism in frontotemporal dementia: a longitudinal 18F-FDG-PET-study. *Neurobiol Aging.* 2007 Jan;28(1):42–50.

141. Peters F, Perani D, Herholz K, Holthoff V, Beuthien-Baumann B, Sorbi S, et al. Orbitofrontal dysfunction related to both apathy and disinhibition in frontotemporal dementia. *Dement Geriatr Cogn Disord.* 2006;21(5-6):373–9.

142. Le Ber I, Guedj E, Gabelle A, Verpillat P, Volteau M, Thomas-Anterion C, et al. Demographic, neurological and behavioural characteristics and brain perfusion SPECT in frontal variant of frontotemporal dementia. *Brain.* 2006 Nov;129(Pt 11):3051–65.

143. Sperfeld AD, Collatz MB, Baier H, Palmbach M, Storch A, Schwarz J, et al. FTDP-17: an early-onset phenotype with parkinsonism and epileptic seizures caused by a novel mutation. *Ann Neurol.* 1999 Nov;46(5):708–15.

144. Alberici A, Gobbo C, Panzacchi A, Nicosia F, Ghidoni R, Benussi L, et al. Frontotemporal dementia: impact of P301L tau mutation on a healthy carrier. *J Neurol Neurosurg Psychiatry.* 2004 Nov;75(11):1607–10.

145. Pal PK, Wszolek ZK, Kishore A, de la Fuente-Fernandez R, Sossi V, Uitti RJ, et al. Positron emission tomography in pallido-ponto-nigral degeneration (PPND) family (frontotemporal dementia with parkinsonism linked to chromosome 17 and point mutation in tau gene). *Parkinsonism Relat Disord.* 2001 Apr;7(2):81–8.

146. Kishore A, Wszolek ZK, Snow BJ, de la Fuente-Fernandez R, Arwert F, Wijker M, et al. Presynaptic nigrostriatal function in genetically tested asymptomatic relatives from the pallido-ponto-nigral degeneration family. *Neurology.* 1996 Dec;47(6):1588–90.

147. Rascovsky K, Hodges JR, Knopman D, Mendez MF, Kramer JH, Neuhaus J, et al. Sensitivity of revised diagnostic criteria for the behavioural variant of frontotemporal dementia. *Brain.* 2011 Sep;134(Pt 9):2456–77.

148. Knopman DS, Boeve BF, Parisi JE, Dickson DW, Smith GE, Ivnik RJ, et al. Antemortem diagnosis of frontotemporal lobar degeneration. *Ann Neurol.* 2005 Apr;57(4):480–8.

149. Pijnenburg YA, Mulder JL, van Swieten JC, Uitdehaag BM, Stevens M, Scheltens P, et al. Diagnostic accuracy of consensus diagnostic criteria for frontotemporal dementia in a memory clinic population. *Dement Geriatr Cogn Disord.* 2008;25(2):157–64.

150. Mendez MF, Shapira JS, McMurtray A, Licht E, Miller BL. Accuracy of the clinical evaluation for frontotemporal dementia. *Arch Neurol.* 2007 Jun;64(6):830–5.

151. McKhann GM, Albert MS, Grossman M, Miller B, Dickson D, Trojanowski JQ. Clinical and pathological diagnosis of frontotemporal dementia: report of the Work Group on Frontotemporal Dementia and Pick's Disease. *Arch Neurol.* 2001 Nov;58(11):1803–9.

152. Roberson ED, Hesse JH, Rose KD, Slama H, Johnson JK, Yaffe K, et al. Frontotemporal dementia progresses to death faster than Alzheimer disease. *Neurology.* 2005 Sep 13;65(5):719–25.

153. Rascovsky K, Salmon DP, Lipton AM, Leverenz JB, DeCarli C, Jagust WJ, et al. Rate of progression differs in frontotemporal dementia and Alzheimer disease. *Neurology.* 2005 Aug 9;65(3):397–403.

154. Hodges JR, Davies R, Xuereb J, Kril J, Halliday G. Survival in frontotemporal dementia. *Neurology.* 2003 Aug 12;61(3):349–54.

155. Josephs KA, Knopman DS, Whitwell JL, Boeve BF, Parisi JE, Petersen RC, et al. Survival in two variants of tau-negative frontotemporal lobar degeneration: FTLD-U vs FTLD-MND. *Neurology.* 2005 Aug 23;65(4):645–7.

156. Boxer AL, Knopman DS, Kaufer DI, Grossman M, Onyike C, Graf-Radford N, et al. Memantine in patients with frontotemporal lobar degeneration: a multicentre, randomised, double-blind, placebo-controlled trial. *Lancet Neurol.* 2013 Feb;12(2):149–56.

157. Tsai RM, Boxer AL. Therapy and clinical trials in frontotemporal dementia: past, present, and future. *J Neurochem.* 2016 Aug;138 Suppl 1:211–21.

CHAPTER 13

Prion Diseases and Other Rapidly Progressive Dementias

Eric Eggenberger[1] and Daniel L. Murman[2]

[1]Michigan State University, East Lansing, Michigan, USA
[2]Department of Neurological Sciences, University of Nebraska Medical Center, Omaha, Nebraska, USA

Prion diseases

Clinical definition and epidemiology

Transmissible spongiform encephalopathies are a unique category of neurologic diseases related to toxic conformational abnormalities in the prion protein. These diseases affect both animal and human hosts (with suspected cross-species transmission capabilities under select circumstances), produce symptoms related to progressive neurologic dysfunction in various regions of the central nervous system (CNS), and appear to be uniformly fatal. Symptoms depend upon the specific strain or type of prion protein, the brain regions affected, and the route of transmission. Although generally rare, these diseases have assumed an increased public health importance since the emergence of "mad cow disease" in 1986 with subsequent human consequences in the form of "new" or "variant" Creutzfeldt–Jakob disease (vCJD) in 1996. In addition, these diseases have general neurology relevance as the well-described protein misfolding pathophysiology of these diseases serves as a model for other neurodegenerative diseases.

Spectrum of clinical phenotype

Animal prion diseases

Prion disease has been known in the animal world for hundreds of years, with scrapie in sheep serving as the best example. Scrapie was first recognized in the 1700s and occurs in most regions throughout the world. It is endemic in France and the United Kingdom. Scrapie features include incoordination, twitching, irritability, often intense pruritus prompting the animal to literally scrape their skin off (hence, the name "scrapie"), and ultimately paralysis and death. Scrapie was first shown to be transmissible in 1936; however, the majority of cases result from genetic defects.

Bovine spongiform encephalopathy (BSE), also known as "mad cow disease", appears to be a more recent animal prion disease with important human disease implications. BSE was first described in 1986 in the UK, and is characterized by insidious onset of incoordination and apprehension. The source of the outbreak was traced to a bovine food supplement derived from meat and bone meal prepared from dead sheep and cattle. The rendering process generating this food supplement was changed in the late 1970s with elimination of the prior high-temperature solvent and superheated steam extraction, which likely resulted in failure to attenuate the prion agent; this process was banned in 1988, but not before more than 150,000 cattle were affected by BSE in an epidemic peaking in 1992. Subsequently, several lines of evidence have linked BSE with the emergence of "variant" CJD (vCJD).

Human prion diseases

Human prion disease appears in sporadic, genetic (15%), and iatrogenic (<2%) forms.

Kuru

Kuru is a human prion disease that has been described among the Fore highlanders of Papua New Guinea. Kuru affects persons primarily between the ages of 5 and 60 years, with an equal sex ratio among pre-adolescents, but a marked excess in female adults. In fact, Kuru was once the most common cause of death among Fore women; however, the number of Kuru-related deaths per year has steadily declined since the 1950s, and there have been fewer than 15 deaths from kuru per year since 1985. This epidemiologic change is attributable to the cessation of ritual cannibalism: the consumption of dead kinsmen was practiced as a mourning rite, primarily by women and small children. No-one born since cannibalism ceased in a given village has died of kuru [1]. The disease can be transmitted to experimental animals orally as well as by peripheral inoculation, but not through casual contact. The incubation period in humans can be more than 30 years.

Kuru is characterized clinically by insidious onset of both cortical and brainstem dysfunction followed by rapidly progressive cerebellar dysfunction. The resultant ataxia is associated with a shivering tremor of the head, trunk, and legs (leading to the name Kuru, from the Fore word for "shiver"). Extrapyramidal and cerebellar dysfunction progresses until the patient is unable to walk or move without ataxic tremors, with the addition of cognitive decline leading to severe dementia. Dysphagia and dysarthria ensue, and patients die of inanition or respiratory failure 3–24 months after onset of symptoms.

Neurodegeneration, First Edition. Edited by Anthony Schapira, Zbigniew Wszolek, Ted M. Dawson and Nicholas Wood.
© 2017 John Wiley & Sons, Ltd. Published 2017 by John Wiley & Sons, Ltd.

Creutzfeldt–Jakob disease (CJD)

In 1920, Creutzfeldt published the case of a 22-year-old woman with dementia, tremor, spasticity, and startle myoclonus [2], and in 1921 Jakob published "About Peculiar Diseases of the Central Nervous System with Remarkable Anatomical Findings" [3]. Modern review of the pathology from these cases suggests that Creutzfeldt's case was atypical, whereas two of Jakob's cases clearly satisfied current CJD criteria [4]. Nonetheless, this disorder takes its name from these early reports.

In the 1960s, Gibbs et al. successfully transmitted CJD to a chimpanzee via intracerebral inoculation of a human brain homogenate, and subsequent investigators were able to demonstrate transmissibility to other animals including rodents [5, 6].

CJD epidemiology Sporadic CJD occurs worldwide with a prevalence and incidence of approximately 0.5–1 per million. Most cases of sporadic CJD occur between 55 and 75 years of age (mean 61 years) without gender predilection [7]. CJD pathogenesis remains enigmatic; the disease does not appear contagious through casual contact as patients who develop sporadic CJD typically have not had contact with other affected patients.

In 1995, a novel form of CJD, variant CJD (vCJD), was described in the UK. vCJD affected younger patients, presenting with atypical CJD features including prominent psychiatric symptoms followed within 6 months by more typical CJD features such as ataxia, dementia, and abnormal involuntary movements (dystonia, myoclonus, or chorea). The average age at onset of vCJD is 29 years compared to sporadic CJD average age 65 years, and death occurs after a median duration of approximately 13 months (compared to ~4 months in sporadic CJD). In contrast to sporadic CJD, vCJD may be blood transmissible. As of October 2016, 228 cases of vCJD have been recorded worldwide (178 in the UK) [8] (http://www.cjd.ed.ac.uk/data.html); although data suggest the disease may have peaked in the late 1990s, models vary on this point, and the possibility of later onset in genetically less susceptible subjects remains. vCJD was subsequently linked to BSE, although the exact mechanism of transmission remains enigmatic.

Pathology/pathophysiology specific to the disease

The main pathophysiologic theory related to prion diseases is the protein-only theory, which hypothesizes that the only (or primary) agent in prion diseases such as CJD is the abnormal conformational form of the prion protein; this abnormal conformational prion protein then acts in an enzymatic fashion to convert normal host prion into the abnormal isoform. Although PrP^C (prion protein cellular, or normal native form) and PrP^{Sc} (prion protein scrapie, or abnormal pathogenic form) have identical amino acid sequences, PrP^{Sc} is distinguished from PrP^C by the 3D conformational structure, stability, greater hydrophobic character, protease resistance, insolubility after detergent extraction, deposition in lysosomes, post-translational synthesis, and polymerization into rod-like structures similar to amyloid. Pathogenic prion proteins are resistant to normal sterilization methods, organic solvents, formalin fixation, irradiation, and heat; however, they may be inactivated through exposure to hypochlorite solutions or by prolonged high-temperature sterilization, an important procedure following surgical instrumentation of potentially infected tissues. Procedures that normally denature protein appear to diminish but may not eliminate infectivity.

Species barrier and strains

Different strains of CJD can be distinguished by varying incubation times, clinical manifestations, transmissibility, prion characteristics

Table 13.1 Codon 129 status in CJD and controls.

Codon 129 status	Caucasian	CJD	Relative risk
Val homo	11%	92–95%	4
Met homo	38%		11
Val/met hetero	51%		1

(glycoform ratios and degree of protease resistance), and experimental pathology (pattern of vacuolation and PrP accumulation). Different strains of PrP vary in their degrees of "infectivity"; these strain differences account for a degree of the species barrier, whereby pathologic forms of PrP from one species less readily induce disease after inoculation into a different species. Greater homology between the abnormal prion and the native host prion increases the chances of successful transmission and disease development.

Genetics

Genetic polymorphisms

The *PRNP* gene is highly conserved across mammalian species. In humans, there are two common polymorphisms at codon 129 and 219. Codon 129 is the site of an important polymorphism with either methionine (Met) or valine (Val), which appears to be a primary determinant of prion susceptibility [9]. Windl et al. (1996) [10] calculated the relative risk for sporadic CJD among the Met/Met:Val/Val:Met/Val genotypes as 11:4:1 (Table 13.1). In Japan, patients with sporadic CJD exhibit a significant tendency toward codon 129 M/M homogeneity, with one series reporting 92% frequency of Met/Met. Similarly, most cases of human growth hormone (HGH) related CJD occur in codon 129 homozygotes, primarily Val/Val [11].

Genetic CJD

In addition to the more common sporadic CJD, there are genetic forms of prion diseases including Gerstmann–Sträussler–Scheinker disease and fatal familial insomnia (FFI). About 15% of CJD cases are familial with an autosomal dominant hereditary pattern. Familial CJD is associated with several different mutations of chromosome 20. The *PRNP* gene codes for the precursor of the constituent amyloid protein that accumulates in the brain of such patients. Both point mutations and insertion repeats between codons 51 and 91 (the open reading frame) of the *PRNP* gene have been described; each mutation causes a 1 million-fold increase in the probability of a spontaneous configurational change to the pathologic polypeptide PrP^{Sc}.

Environmental

Iatrogenic Creutzfeldt–Jakob disease

Iatrogenic CJD was first reported in 1974 following a corneal transplant; the recipient developed ataxia 18 months postoperatively and died of CJD 8 months later. In addition to corneal tissue, the disease has been transmitted through pituitary tissue used in extraction of HGH or gonadotropins prior to recombinant technology, insertion of processed human cadaveric dural or other grafts, and use of inadequately sterilized neurosurgical equipment.

HGH-related CJD is somewhat unique among iatrogenic prion disease and typically presents with ataxia progressing over 6–18 months; some patients develop dementia later in the course. In contrast, CJD acquired through contaminated neurosurgical instruments or electroencephalographic (EEG) depth electrodes usually presents with cognitive decline. The majority of HGH-related CJD cases occurred in France due to slower transition to recombinant drug technology. In 34 patients with HGH-derived CJD, ataxia was a component of the presentation in 94%, while visual disorders including diplopia (53%) and nystagmus (47%) were reported in 88% [12]. Internuclear ophthalmoplegia occurred in 68% of patients after a mean duration of 5 months. Electroretinograms (ERG) were abnormal in the first 3 months of illness in 9 of 11 (82%) patients so tested. Myoclonic jerks were present in 82% of patients. EEG testing was not generally useful diagnostically; pseudoperiodic bursts were present in 9 patients after duration of 5–13 months, but classic triphasic waves were noted in only 2 patients after 6 and 20 months of illness.

Clinical prodrome and biomarkers

Clinical prodrome of sporadic Creutzfeldt–Jakob disease
The onset of sporadic CJD is usually insidious, with a nonspecific prodrome characterized by asthenia, anxiety, altered sleep pattern, anorexia, weight loss, fatigue, dizziness, vague memory difficulty, mood or behavior change, weakness, or slight problems with locomotion in approximately one-third of patients. During this prodrome, patients often develop increasing difficulties with higher-order mental functioning including calculations, abstract thought, memory, reasoning, and judgment. Patients subsequently develop progressive aphasia, apraxia, pyramidal signs, myoclonus, and choreiform-athetoid movements. Biomarkers useful in the diagnosis include EEG, magnetic resonance imaging (MRI), and cerebrospinal fluid (CSF) (see Examination and investigations including imaging).

The classic clinical triad of dementia, typical EEG changes, and myoclonus has been incorporated into diagnostic criteria. Visual disturbances occur often during the course of sporadic CJD. The *Heidenhain variant of CJD* is characterized by relatively sudden onset of homonymous visual field defects, usually a complete hemianopia or cerebral blindness early in the course of the disease. MRI typically shows hyperintensity on diffusion weighted imaging (DWI) within the parietal-occipital cortex, and positron emission tomography (PET) may demonstrate regional hypometabolism in these areas. EEG is often initially normal in patients with the Heidenhain variant of CJD; however, it becomes abnormal in almost all patients with this form of CJD. Visual hallucinations and palinopsia are also not uncommon in this population. Regardless of the prodromal or presenting symptoms, most patients become severely demented within 6 months, leading to death within 12 months of symptom onset, usually related to intercurrent infection (pneumonia or urosepsis) combined with cachexia.

Examination and investigations including imaging
EEG, MRI, and CSF analysis are the most helpful ancillary tests to complement clinical history and exam. Classic EEG changes of pseudoperiodic triphasic waves occur in approximately 60–70% of sporadic CJD patients, requiring at least 3 months to develop in the majority.

MRI has proven very helpful in the diagnosis of CJD and elimination of other diseases. MRI findings in CJD often take the form of bilateral hyperintensity within the basal ganglia, corpus striatum, or thalamus, best visualized on **fluid attenuated inversion recovery** (FLAIR) or diffusion-weighted imaging [13]. In one study, 63% of CJD patients exhibited basal ganglia MRI abnormalities [14].

Table 13.2 CSF 14-3-3 abnormality by prion disease state.

Disease	n positive/n total	Percent
CJD (path confirmed)	311/329	95%
Iatrogenic	6/10	60%
Genetic	35/57	61%
vCJD	5/11	45%

Data from Zerr and Poser 2002 [14].

In the appropriate clinical setting, MRI basal ganglia hyperintensity is relatively specific for CJD; similar MRI changes from ischemia typically have a patchy character (and distinct history), while other diseases that may produce such basal ganglia high signal such as Wilson disease, Leigh disease, and certain infections (e.g., mycoplasma) are distinguishable on clinical grounds. vCJD exhibits a distinct and specific MRI pattern with most patients exhibiting prominent hyperintensity within the posterior thalamus ("pulvinar sign"), a part of the vCJD diagnostic criteria [15].

CSF is perhaps the most sensitive diagnostic test. Mild pleocytosis (<10 cells/mm^3) may be present, but otherwise the routine CSF formula is normal. The CSF 14-3-3 protein is a useful marker of acute and relatively extensive neuronal damage. Elevation of CSF 14-3-3 protein may occur in several conditions such as large cerebral infarction, neoplasm, inflammation, paraneoplastic disorders, or prolonged seizure in addition to prion disease; however, these are often easily distinguished on clinical and imaging grounds. The diagnostic usefulness of CSF 14-3-3 varies by specific prion condition (Table 13.2), and CSF analysis for 14-3-3 has been consistently negative in patients with fatal familial insomnia (FFI). Occasionally, repeat CSF analysis at least 2 weeks after the initial lumbar puncture is useful in demonstrating increasing 14-3-3 in CJD compared to decreasing levels found in other acute events with an elevated 14-3-3 level [14].

Diagnosis and prognosis
The diagnosis of sporadic CJD is often difficult to make in the early stages of the disease, and the differential diagnosis may include such varied disorders as Alzheimer's disease, Pick's disease, paraneoplastic disease, Whipple's disease, stroke, viral encephalitis, or subacute sclerosing panencephalitis (SSPE) depending upon demographic and clinical evidence.

The clinical criteria for sporadic CJD include:
1 progressive dementia and
2 at least two of the following four:
  (a) myoclonus
  (b) visual/cerebellar symptoms
  (c) pyramidal/extrapyramidal symptoms
  (d) akinetic mutism.

Probable CJD is defined by the above *and* periodic slow wave complexes in EEG *or* 14-3-3 CSF protein in patients with a disease duration of less than 2 years. Possible CJD is defined by the above and the absence of EEG or CSF changes.

vCJD is distinct in its presentation and diagnostic criteria compared to sporadic CJD. The pathologic prion protein appears in lymph tissue, and tonsillar biopsy is a very useful tool for histological diagnosis. The diagnostic criteria for vCJD include:
  I A. Progressive psychiatric disorder
     B. Duration >6 months
     C. Routine investigations do not suggest alternative diagnosis
     D. No history iatrogenic exposure
     E. No evidence familial prion disease

II A. Early psychiatric symptoms
   B. Persistent painful sensory symptoms
   C. Ataxia
   D. Myoclonus, chorea, or dystonia
   E. Dementia
III A. EEG without typical periodic slow wave changes
    B. Bilateral pulvinar high signal on MRI
IV A. Positive tonsillar biopsy.

Definite diagnosis of vCJD requires IA and neuropathologic confirmation; probable diagnosis requires I and 4/5 of II and IIIA and IIIB, or I and IVA; and possible vCJD diagnosis consists of I and 4/5 of II and IIIA [15].

The genetic forms of prion disease often have a strong family history and may be confirmed through appropriate genetic testing.

All known prion diseases end fatally, regardless of current treatment.

Treatment options

At present, there are no effective therapies for prion disease and multiple challenges remain in the development of potential prion therapies. An effective agent would have to be successful against prion accumulation or pathophysiology, be deliverable to the required sites in a timely manner, and be tolerable. There is evidence that significant CNS damage and PrP accumulation occur long before clinical symptoms appear, and our current diagnostic capabilities do not easily allow for early diagnosis even if a suitable treatment was discovered. Our lack of understanding about differing prion diseases and strains and the exact pathophysiology of the pathologic form of prion protein is an additional treatment hurdle. Prophylactic therapy in high-risk patients (e.g., prion genetic aberrations or recipients of contaminated medical products) may be the easiest treatment scenario, but this represents a very small fraction of cases. Genetically based therapy is promising, and genetically engineered PrP-free animal models exist [16].

The PRION I trial recruited patients with CJD in the UK from 2004 to 2006 to investigate the therapeutic usefulness of quinacrine (mepacrine hydrochloride). Recruitment ended in 2006 with 81 subjects (approximately 50% of target accrual). Quinacrine at a dose of 300 mg q.d. appeared tolerable but did not affect the clinical course in this observational study [17]. The University of California San Francisco's randomized trial found that quinacrine 300 mg per day did not improve 2-month survival of patients with sCJD compared with placebo [18]. There are a number of additional agents (e.g., chlorpromazine, phosphorothioate oligonucleotides, plasminogen) and strategies in development including vaccines, gene therapy approaches, and other treatments targeting various presumptive facets of the prion replication, accumulation, and clearance pathways under consideration. Although these have yet to reach Phase III human trial status, there is optimism for effective prion disease therapy in the future.

Social, family, or third-party care

The burden of prion disease from a social and family perspective is enormous. Family and caregivers shoulder the tremendous burden of caring for the rapidly deteriorating sufferers, which extracts a heavy emotional and physical toll. While aspects of this burden are similar to other dementing illnesses, prion diseases progress with a rapidity rarely seen in other neurodegenerative illnesses.

Future developments

Although relatively rare, prion diseases are an important and uniformly fatal group of neurologic animal and human diseases. The protein-only toxin-like pathophysiologic theory of prions may find parallels in other conditions. BSE, vCJD, and iatrogenic CJD have taught important lessons about the food chain and contamination of medical supplies. Although our knowledge of prions has grown tremendously in the last two decades, we still lack an effective prevention or treatment strategy for prion diseases, and much basic prion biology remains enigmatic.

Non-prion, rapidly progressive dementias

Clinical definition and epidemiology

There is no standard definition of rapidly progressive dementias, although in clinical practice they are loosely defined as those cases of progressive cognitive impairment that have a rate of decline similar to that of patients with prion dementias, such as CJD. This time course implies progression from normal cognitive and functional abilities to moderate or severe dementia over a period of 6–12 months, but potentially extending up to 2 years. Just as the spectrum of clinical presentations of prion dementias is very broad, so too patients being evaluated for rapidly progressing dementias may present with many atypical clinical features including atypical or focal cognitive impairment, myoclonus, seizures, parkinsonism, and ataxia. Median survival for patients with sporadic CJD is 8 months, with 85% of patients dying from the condition within 1 year. Thus, this rapid progression of dementia over 1–2 years is the type of time course implied by the term "rapidly progressive dementia (RPD)".

The epidemiology of human prion diseases has been more thoroughly studied than that of non-prion RPD. Incidence rates for CJD are estimated at 1–1.5 cases per one million people, per year. Referral centers for prion diseases and other RPDs estimate that 30–40% of referred patients do not have a prion disease [19–22]. Thus, in a referral center setting, the incidence of non-prion RPDs would be approximately 0.5 cases per one million people, per year. Population-based estimates of non-prion RPDs are not available due to lack of consensus on the definition of RPD and absence of uniform reporting of this type of patient. However, based upon population-based prion surveillance information, both prion dementias and RPDs that mimic prion diseases are rare.

Spectrum of clinical phenotype

Prion disease referral centers provide an opportunity to understand the relative frequency of prion diseases and non-prion RPDs mimicking prion diseases. A cohort of patients seen at the University of California, San Francisco (UCSF) Memory and Aging Center that were referred for RPD between 2001 and 2007 have been described [20]. This description of 178 patients referred and evaluated at the UCSF Memory and Aging Center provides information about the relative frequency of subtypes of prion disease and non-prion RPDs in a referral population (see Table 13.3). Of the evaluated patients, 62% were found to have a prion disease, of whom 75% had confirmed sporadic CJD, 22% a genetic prion disease, and 3% an acquired prion disease. Of the evaluated patients, 38% had symptoms that were initially suggestive of prion disease but they were found to have a non-prion RPD. The most common cause of non-prion RPDs was neurodegenerative diseases, including corticobasal degeneration (CBD), frontotemporal dementia (FTD), Alzheimer's disease (AD), dementia with Lewy bodies (DLB), and progressive supranuclear palsy (PSP). The second most common cause of non-prion RPDs was autoimmune disorders including Hashimoto's encephalopathy and autoantibody-associated, paraneoplastic

Table 13.3 Causes of rapidly progressive dementia (RPD) in a cohort of patients referred for evaluation of possible prion disease.*

Cause of RPD	Percent of prion cases	Percent of non-prion cases	Percent of all cases
Sporadic CJD	75%		
Genetic CJD	22%		
Acquired CJD	3%		
All prion RPDs	100%		**62%**
Neurodegenerative		39%	
Autoimmune		22%	
Unknown		12%	
Infectious		6%	
Malignancy		6%	
Psychiatric		6%	
Toxic–metabolic		5%	
Vascular		4%	
All non-prion RPDs		100%	**38%**

*Data from Geschwind et al. 2008 [20].
A summary of the final diagnoses of 178 patients who were referred for possible prion disease and evaluated at the UCSF Memory and Aging Center between 2001 and 2007.

and non-paraneoplastic, limbic encephalopathies (LE). Other less common causes of RPDs included primary CNS lymphoma, encephalitis, toxic or metabolic encephalopathy, psychiatric and cerebrovascular disease. Other prion referral centers have reported similar types of non-prion RPDs [19, 21].

The US National Prion Disease Pathology Surveillance Center reviewed 1106 brain autopsies that had been referred to the Center for suspected CJD between 2006 and 2009 [22]. Of these referred cases, 32% (352) did not have a prion disease. Of the 352 cases, there were 71 patients who were felt to have potentially treatable conditions (20% of the non-prion RPD cases and 6% of all RPD cases referred). Of the 71 potentially treatable non-prion cases of RPD, 37% were immune-mediated conditions including limbic encephalopathy, primary CNS vasculitis, and acute demyelinating encephalomyelitis (ADEM). Thirty-five percent of the potentially treatable, non-prion RPDs were neoplastic conditions including primary CNS lymphoma, intravascular lymphoma, meningeal carcinomatosis, and diffuse glioma. Twenty percent of the potentially treatable cases were infectious including viral, fungal, and parasitic CNS infections, and 8% were metabolic encephalopathies including Wernicke's encephalopathy. Of note, 40% of these non-prion RPD cases had a positive CSF 14-3-3 protein test. This highlights the nonspecific nature of the 14-3-3 protein test as a marker for prion diseases, but more appropriately it can be interpreted as a marker of neuronal injury in RPDs. Thus, in patients with signs and symptoms of an RPD, approximately one-third will not have prion pathology and of these patients up to 20% may have a potentially treatable condition.

Pathophysiology of specific causes of RPD

Neurodegenerative disorders

RPDs can be caused by a more rapid progression of the more common neurodegenerative dementias. These include CBD, PSP, FTD, AD, and DLB [23–28]. In addition to the rapid rate of progression, these neurodegenerative causes of RPD frequently have other atypical features including early loss of language, disinhibited or apathetic behavior, rigidity, amyotrophy, early gait disorder, frequent falls, and myoclonus. Patients with CBD and PSP present with akinetic, rigid parkinsonism without resting tremor and typically have disorders of eye movements, gait impairment, poor postural balance, and focal or frontal cognitive impairment. Patients with FTD

have prominent behavioral symptoms or language impairment with or without features of motor neuron disease or parkinsonism. Most commonly, patients with AD present with poor short-term memory and gradual and progressive cognitive decline. However, rapidly progressive forms of AD have been described [25, 26]. In one series of rapidly progressive AD, 75% of the patients had myoclonus, 66% had disorders of gait, and 31% had elevated CSF 14-3-3 protein levels; the median survival was 26 months [26]. In rapidly progressive AD, CSF biomarkers for AD show high levels of total tau and phosphorylated tau and very low levels of Aβ1-42 [27]. Rapidly progressive presentations of DLB have been described [25, 28]. In one series, visual hallucinations and parkinsonism were seen in a majority of patients and myoclonus and delirium in 50% of these patients [28]. However, there was no evidence of a prion disease on MRI, EEG, or CSF studies (i.e., 14-3-3 protein). The average duration of disease in one series of rapidly progressive DLB patients was 9 months.

Each of the neurodegenerative diseases described above is associated with dysfunctional regulation of specific proteins as described in other chapters. These dysfunctional proteins include Aβ in AD; microtubule associated tau protein (MAP-tau) in CBD, PSP, and some forms of FTD; α-synuclein in DLB; and TAR-DNA binding protein (TDP-43) in some forms of FTD and FTD with motor neuron disease. Genetic mutations can cause dysregulation of these proteins in rare families including mutations in the genes for presenilin 1 (*PSEN1*), presenilin 2 (*PSEN2*), amyloid precursor protein (*APP*), MAP-tau, glucosidase beta acid, progranulin, colony stimulating factor 1 receptor (*CSF1R*), and chromosome 9 open reading frame 72 (*C9ORF72*). The abnormal accumulation of these proteins leads to neuronal dysfunction and death in selective neuronal networks leading to characteristic clinical symptoms and pathologic features in each of these diseases. The pathogenesis of rapid progression in neurodegenerative diseases is unknown.

Autoimmune encephalopathies

Autoimmune encephalopathies represent an important and potentially treatable cause of non-prion RPDs. These include autoantibody-associated, autoimmune encephalopathies such as paraneoplastic limbic encephalopathy (PLE), non-paraneoplastic limbic encephalopathy (LE), steroid-responsive encephalopathy associated with autoimmune thyroiditis (SREAT), which is also termed Hashimoto's encephalopathy (HE), and autoimmune cerebellar ataxias [29–43]. Specific autoantibodies are associated with each of these syndromes and specific cancers are more commonly associated with specific autoantibodies in PLE. In addition, autoimmune inflammatory vasculopathies can present as RPDs, including primary CNS vasculitis, Susac's syndrome (also termed retinocochleocerebral syndrome), and secondary CNS involvement in systemic vasculitis [44, 45].

PLE presents typically with short-term memory loss, partial complex seizures, and behavioral changes (e.g., depression, psychosis) [37]. Neuropathy, dysautonomia, gastrointestinal dysfunction, weight loss, and hyponatremia can be clues to autoimmunity or an underlying cancer. Commonly, the neurologic symptoms precede the diagnosis of cancer. A series of autoantibodies have been associated with PLE including ANNA-1 (anti-Hu), CRMP-5 (anti-CV2), anti-Ma2, anti-voltage-gated potassium channel antibodies (anti-VGKC), anti-NMDA receptor, anti-AMPA receptor, and anti-GABA-B receptor [37]. Individual autoantibodies are often associated with specific types of cancer. For example, ANNA-1 antibodies are highly predictive of small cell lung cancer; CRMP-5 and anti-VGKC antibodies can be associated with lung cancer or thymoma; anti-Ma2 antibodies are highly predictive of testicular cancer; anti-NMDA receptor antibodies are strongly associated with teratoma, especially in young women; and anti-AMPA receptor and anti-GABA-B receptor antibodies are commonly associated with lung and breast cancer. Despite the presence of autoantibodies, the main pathologic process is thought to be mediated by cytotoxic T cell mechanisms. Most commonly, brain MRI will demonstrate increased signal in the hippocampus and adjacent structures on FLAIR images. Medial temporal lobe structures, including the hippocampus, are selectively vulnerable in PLE and permanent neuronal loss and persistent symptoms of amnesia and seizures are common.

Even among those patients without an underlying cancer, a majority have autoantibodies to neuronal, voltage-gated potassium channels (VGKC) [41]. The most common clinical presentation in patients with VGKC autoantibodies is that of limbic encephalopathy with rapid onset of memory loss and associated seizures, often associated with hyponatremia. As in PLE, brain MRI often demonstrates abnormal signal in medial temporal lobe structures. Patients with LE have an excellent response to immunotherapy (e.g., high-dose steroids, intravenous immunoglobulin, plasma exchange, and oral immunosuppressant drugs), with near complete recovery often achieved and sustained with immunotherapy [30, 31]. Patients with autoantibodies to VGKC can also present clinically with Morvan's syndrome with symptoms of neuromyotonia, dysautonomia (e.g., hyperhidrosis, sialorrhea, blood pressure fluctuations), and insomnia in addition to encephalopathy [46]. Recent evidence suggests that VGKC autoantibodies can bind more specifically to other VGKC-associated proteins, specifically leucine-rich glioma-inactivated protein 1 (LGI1) and contactin-associated protein 2 (CASPR2) [47, 48]. Typically, patients with LGI1 autoantibodies present with LE, and patients with CASPR2 autoantibodies present with features of Morvan's syndrome.

Steroid-responsive encephalopathy associated with autoimmune thyroiditis (SREAT) or Hashimoto's encephalopathy (HE) is seen in patients with thyroid autoimmunity, with or without thyroid dysfunction, who present with subacute cognitive dysfunction with a fluctuating course, myoclonus, tremor, neuropsychiatric symptoms, and occasionally seizures [34]. Serum antibodies against thyroperoxidase (TPO) or thyroglobulin (formerly termed thyroid microsomal antibodies) are found, but the titers do not correlate with clinical symptom severity. Evidence of thyroid autoimmunity is common in the general population without neurologic symptoms (i.e., approximately 10% of an adult population would have evidence of thyroid autoimmunity), making it difficult to know in an individual patient whether their clinical symptoms are due to HE or not. MRI is often normal or shows nonspecific signal changes, and the CSF may show nonspecific elevation of protein levels and anti-thyroid antibodies, but their presence and their levels are not specific to HE and do not correlate with neurologic symptom severity. Immunotherapy with high-dose steroids (intravenous methylprednisolone 1 g daily for 5 days) can provide dramatic improvement in neurologic symptoms in some patients. Other forms of immunotherapy have been reported to be effective in some patients including intravenous immunoglobulin, plasma exchange, and azathioprine. The natural history of HE is not well understood, but relapsing or chronic neurologic symptoms have been described in some patients.

Other autoimmune encephalopathies that can cause RPD or mimic prion diseases include paraneoplastic cerebellar degeneration syndromes and inflammatory vasculopathies. Paraneoplastic cerebellar degeneration can be associated with neuronal autoantibodies such as anti-GAD65 antibodies and anti-Purkinje cell antibodies (also termed anti-Yo antibodies) [36]. Patients with paraneoplastic cerebellar degeneration present with subacute and progressive ataxia, with or without mild cognitive impairment, and often have an underlying malignancy. These paraneoplastic syndromes can mimic cerebellar presentations of prion diseases. Inflammatory vasculopathies can cause RPD and can be isolated to the CNS (e.g., isolated CNS vasculitis) or be a part of systemic vasculitic syndromes (e.g., lupus cerebritis, Sjögren's syndrome) [45]. In addition, Susac's syndrome can present as an RPD due to inflammatory lesions in the corpus callosum, in addition to lesions in the cochlea, causing hearing loss, and retina causing vision loss [44]. In each of these inflammatory vasculopathies, brain MRI typically would be suggestive of a vasculopathy and in Susac's syndrome the MRI changes can be quite characteristic (see Figure 13.1).

Other causes of RPD

The list of other causes of RPD is long and includes toxic, metabolic, infectious, and malignant causes. Toxic and metabolic causes include hepatic encephalopathy, Wernicke's encephalopathy, extrapontine myelinolysis, organic solvent ingestion, carbon monoxide poisoning, bismuth encephalopathy due to excessive consumption of bismuth subsalicylate (e.g., Pepto-Bismol), vitamin deficiency (e.g., niacin, vitamin B$_{12}$), polypharmacy, and heavy metal intoxication [49–52]. Historical information, laboratory test results, and MRI can all provide clues to the diagnosis in these conditions. Infectious causes that can produce RPD and mimic a prion disease include viral infections (e.g., HIV-associated dementia, progressive multifocal leukoencephalopathy – PML, viral encephalitis), atypical bacterial infections (e.g., syphilis, Lyme disease, Whipple's disease), and parasitic and fungal infections (e.g., *Coccidioides immitis*, *Aspergillus fumigatus*, and *Cryptococcus neoformans*) [22, 53–57]. Serum and CSF titers, polymerase chain reaction (PCR) measurement of infectious agent associated proteins, and cultures can be used diagnostically in the majority of these infections. Malignant causes of RPD include lymphoma (e.g., primary CNS, intravascular, and leptomeningeal), leptomeningeal carcinomatosis, and atypical presentations of malignant gliomas [22, 58]. Brain imaging and brain biopsy are required to diagnosis malignant causes of RPD. A case of fragile X tremor/ataxia syndrome (FXTAS) has been described that presented as an RPD [59]. Similarly, cerebral amyloid angiopathy has been described as a cause of RPD [60, 61].

Examinations and investigations

The evaluation of RPDs seeks to find supportive evidence of a prion disease; if this is not found, further investigations are initiated to look for the wide variety of other conditions that could mimic a prion disease [62]. Evaluating a patient with a potential RPD requires a detailed history and neurologic examination, obtaining basic laboratory tests, and then proceeding with additional diagnostic tests including brain imaging (ideally MRI), EEG, and CSF analysis. From the history it is important to determine the exact time course of changes in cognition and function from a knowledgeable informant since patients with memory loss may not remember the exact onset of their symptoms. Determining the time course is key to confirming that the patient is suffering from a rapidly progressive condition. The history should determine whether there have been stroke-like events, seizures, head injury, alcohol abuse, or other toxic exposure. It should focus also on whether the patient has a family history of similar neurologic symptoms.

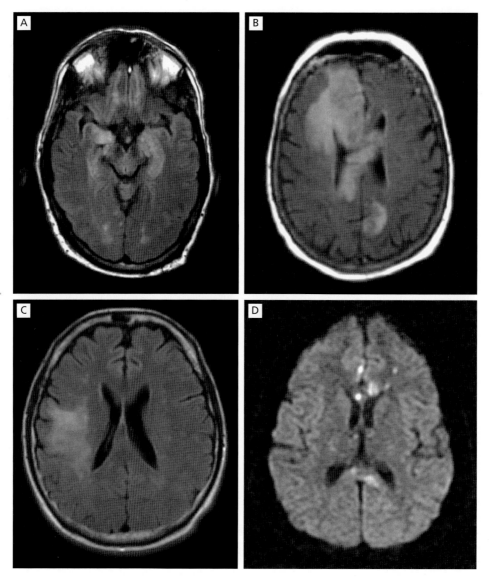

Figure 13.1 MRI findings in selected non-prion RPDs. (A) MRI FLAIR image of a patient with LE due to anti-VGKC autoantibodies. (B) MRI FLAIR image of a patient with primary CNS lymphoma. (C) MRI FLAIR image of a patient with AIDS and progressive multifocal leukoencephalopathy (PML). (D) MRI diffusion image of a patient with Susac's syndrome, showing restricted diffusion in and around the corpus callosum.

Genetic forms of prion diseases and a majority of neurodegenerative dementias have an autosomal dominant pattern of inheritance. In the setting of autosomal dominant inheritance, one of the patient's parents would have had similar symptoms and roughly half of each generation of the affected side of the family would have similar symptoms. Other forms of inheritance can be associated with rapidly progressive dementias but these would be much less common. The neurologic examination should document the pattern and severity of cognitive deficits in multiple domains including attention, orientation, language, memory, visuospatial abilities, and executive cognitive function. The presence or absence of movement disorders including myoclonus, chorea, tremor, and parkinsonism should be documented as should any signs of dysfunction in motor and sensory systems, coordination, or reflexes. A detailed description of the patient's gait and postural balance should be included as part of the neurologic examination. Neurologic exam findings can help narrow the list of possible causes of a patient's RPD.

Basic laboratory evaluations are appropriate in all patients with RPD and should include a comprehensive metabolic panel (CMP), complete blood count with differential (CBC), tests of thyroid function (e.g., thyroid stimulating hormone – TSH), vitamin B_{12} levels, and sedimentation rate. After the initial laboratory test results are available, the next step in the evaluation of an RPD would be a brain MRI scan. If the MRI results do not suggest a prion disease, then there are many additional laboratory tests that can be completed to diagnose a non-prion RPD. If the history suggests the possibility of LE or PLE, then blood should be tested for autoantibodies that have been associated with PLE or LE. Commercial autoantibody panels are available that screen for the known autoantibodies associated with LE or PLE. Similarly, if HE is in the differential then anti-thyroid antibodies, both anti-thyroperoxidase and anti-thyroglobulin autoantibodies, should be screened for. If an infectious cause of an RPD is being considered, blood should be tested for syphilis serology, HIV titer, and Lyme titer. Additional tests of possible rheumatologic causes (e.g., CNS involvement with systemic vasculitis) include C-reactive protein, antinuclear antibody screen including extractable nuclear antibody testing, anti-neutrophil cytoplasmic antibodies, and complement levels. Common additional laboratory tests of metabolic and toxic causes of RPD to consider include tests of magnesium, calcium, ammonia, vitamin B_1 and B_6 levels in blood and urine, and screening for heavy metal toxicity and drugs of abuse. If a genetic form of AD, CBD, FTD, or PSP is suspected as the cause of a patient's RPD, serum can be tested for mutations in several genes that can cause genetic forms of these neurodegenerative diseases. A commercial laboratory can test for most of these genes, but in some cases testing must be done in a research laboratory. Currently, testing for mutations in the following genes is available: PS1, PS2, APP, MAP-tau, progranulin, CSF1R, and C9ORF72.

Besides a history, neurologic exam, and basic laboratory tests, MR imaging of the brain with and without contrast is a critical diagnostic test in the evaluation of a patient with an RPD. If the patient cannot have a brain MRI scan, then head CT with and without contrast should be performed, but CT imaging is unable to identify specific findings in prion diseases and is much less sensitive in diagnosing many causes of RPD. Brain MRI can demonstrate specific findings in prion disease using DWI and FLAIR imaging [63, 64]. Gray matter hyperintensities (DWI greater than FLAIR) are seen in cortical and subcortical structures including a cortical ribbon pattern or involvement of subcortical gray structures including the basal ganglia and thalamus [65]. UCSF proposed MRI criteria for the diagnosis of prion diseases in 2005 and revised them in 2011. Using these criteria, blinded raters were able to differentiate a prion disease from a non-prion RPD with a sensitivity of 96% and specificity of 93% [63]. In the clinical evaluation of an RPD all MR images should be reviewed by a specialist who is knowledgeable of the MRI changes seen in prion diseases and non-prion RPDs; the DWI and subtle FLAIR changes in patients with prion disease are frequently not reported because they are attributed to artifact. In addition to specific findings in prion diseases, brain MR imaging is able to identify: signal changes in the medial temporal lobes and hippocampus in LE, PLE, and viral encephalitis; features of cerebrovascular disease including vasculitis, amyloid angiopathy, and CNS hemorrhage; mass lesions in CNS tumors and meningeal thickening and enhancement in meningeal carcinomatosis; demyelinating lesions in ADEM and extrapontine myelinolysis; and confluent white matter lesions in progressive multifocal leukoencephalopathy (PML) (see Figure 13.1). Nonspecific brain MRI findings may suggest a neurodegenerative cause of an RPD based upon the pattern of brain atrophy (e.g., FTD, PSP, CBD) or identify the possibility of hydrocephalus as a cause of an RPD.

Other important tests in the evaluation of patients with RPD include EEG and lumbar puncture for CSF analysis (Table 13.4). An EEG can provide important diagnostic information in the evaluation of RPD. It can show sharp waves or spikes in patients with seizures, can identify periodic sharp wave discharges in a majority of patients with prion diseases, especially those with prominent involvement of the cortex, and can identify either focal or generalized slowing in neurodegenerative or toxic–metabolic causes of RPD. The presence of triphasic waves on an EEG recording should prompt the search for a metabolic cause of encephalopathy such as that seen in patients with renal or hepatic dysfunction. CSF analysis is necessary in the diagnostic evaluation of RPD. CSF cell count with differential, protein, and glucose should be tested in all cases. The most important CSF tests are biomarkers that have been associated with prion dementias or other conditions that produce extensive neuronal damage. These biomarkers include increased levels of the 14-3-3 protein, total tau, neuron-specific enolase, and S-100B protein. Caution should be used in interpreting the 14-3-3 protein and related CSF biomarker test results, since many causes of RPD have an elevated 14-3-3 protein or positive related CSF biomarker test result, demonstrating that these tests are not specific to prion diseases but should be viewed as markers of neuronal damage or destruction [66, 67]. Combinations of these CSF biomarkers are used to improve the accuracy of diagnosing a prion disease, including use of the 14-3-3 protein and total tau in combination or combining total tau and S-100B protein levels for a diagnosis of a prion disease [68]. CSF tests can be used to look for evidence of non-prion causes of RPD. For example, the CSF IgG index and the presence of oligoclonal bands in CSF that are not present in serum are markers of an inflammatory or potentially autoimmune cause of an RPD. Cytology and in some cases tests for lymphoma cell surface markers can provide a diagnosis of a malignant cause of RPD. Tests for infectious conditions should include bacterial and fungal cultures and surface antigen tests, and tests for treatable viral infections including the herpes family of viruses by PCR and enteroviruses in the right setting. In selected cases, tests for Whipple's disease, tuberculosis, PML, syphilis, and neurosarcoidosis can be performed on spinal fluid. CSF biomarkers for AD can be tested, including measurement of CSF Aβ1-42 and phosphorylated and total tau levels, if a rapidly progressive form of AD is suspected [27]. Opening pressures should be obtained to make sure there is not evidence of symptomatic hydrocephalus. If history suggests the possibility of normal pressure hydrocephalus, then a large-volume spinal tap can be performed with evaluations of gait and cognition before and after the spinal tap.

In addition to the tests described above, some patients with an RPD will require a tissue biopsy to make a correct diagnosis and guide treatment. In patients suspected of having an underlying cancer, CT imaging of the chest, abdomen, and pelvis, with and without contrast, is indicated and may identify a mass that can be

Table 13.4 Typical results of diagnostic tests in common conditions that cause RPD.

Diagnostic test	Prion disease	Neuro degenerative	Autoimmune	Malignant	Metabolic
Chemistries	Normal	Normal	Normal or abnormal	Normal	Abnormal
EEG	Periodic sharp wave discharges	Focal or generalized slowing	Focal sharp waves or spikes	Focal slowing	Generalized slowing
Brain MRI	High signal DWI >FLAIR gray matter	Atrophy	High signal hippocampus, temporal lobe	Enhancing lesion	Normal or low signal
LP protein	Normal or high	Normal	Normal or high	Normal or high	Normal
LP 14-3-3	Increased	Normal or increased	Normal or increased	Normal or increased	Normal
LP Aβ1-42	Normal	Low in AD	Normal	Normal	Normal
LP tau	Very high	Normal or high	Normal or high	Normal or high	Normal

biopsied. Some patients may require additional focused diagnostic tests or whole body PET imaging to identify an underlying malignancy. In cases where other testing is not diagnostic and there are structural lesions on brain imaging, especially if a malignancy (e.g., primary CNS lymphoma) or primary CNS vasculitis is suspected, then a diagnostic brain biopsy should be considered. A brain biopsy provides the most yield if it targets an abnormal area on the MRI and if enough tissue can be obtained for the neuropathologist. The diagnostic sensitivity of brain biopsy in patients with RPDs ranges from 20 to 83% depending on the center, type of biopsy, and situation. In one case series of 171 patients with RPD, a brain biopsy was able to establish a diagnosis in 65% of the cases. The most commonly diagnosed conditions after brain biopsy included primary CNS lymphoma (20%), CJD (16%), viral encephalitis (14%), and CNS vasculitis (9%) [69]. Risks associated with brain biopsy include hemorrhage, seizures, postoperative delirium, and death due to cardiopulmonary causes. In the setting of a possible prion disease, special precautions are required for all involved in the biopsy and the handling of brain tissue. It must be made clear to the pathologist and staff involved that a prion disease is a possibility. If a prion disease is identified, then neurosurgical equipment needs to be destroyed or decontaminated with specific measures that have been shown to inactivate prions.

Diagnosis and prognosis

The diagnosis of a prion disease as a cause of RPD is based upon clinical history, physical examination, and findings from ancillary tests including serology, MRI of the brain, EEG, and spinal fluid biomarkers. As described earlier in the chapter, there are clinical criteria to make a diagnosis of probable CJD based upon clinical features, EEG, and CSF findings. Also, new brain MRI criteria have been established for the diagnosis of a prion disease and have been found to be very sensitive and specific. Genetic forms of a prion disease can be diagnosed by identifying a mutation in the prion protein gene. LE and PLE can be diagnosed by identifying neuronal autoantibodies and evidence of medial temporal lobe abnormalities clinically, by EEG or brain MRI, and by ruling out a viral cause of limbic encephalitis (e.g., herpes simplex encephalitis). In PLE, a search for an underlying malignancy should be undertaken. A diagnosis of HE is supported by elevated titers of anti-thyroid antibodies and a positive clinical response to a trial of high-dose steroids. Diagnostic criteria are available for the clinical diagnosis of neurodegenerative disorders, and genetic testing is available in cases with an autosomal dominant family history. CSF biomarkers and PET can be used to support a diagnosis of AD, especially in rapidly progressive and atypical presentations. Specific biomarkers for other neurodegenerative dementias are currently not available. Ancillary tests can help establish a diagnosis of a toxic, metabolic, infectious, vascular, or neoplastic cause of RPD. Brain biopsy may be required to establish a diagnosis of a vasculitic or neoplastic cause of an RPD.

There are examples of diagnostic dilemmas in the evaluation of RPDs including patients with neuronal or thyroid autoimmunity that did not respond to immunotherapy and subsequently were found to have a prion disease or neurodegenerative dementia [24, 34]. Additionally, there is a case series of patients with RPD that had a clear response to immunotherapy but were later found to have AD pathology at autopsy [70]. Thus, in patients with an RPD and neuronal or thyroid autoimmunity a trial of immunotherapy is indicated to determine if they are immunoresponsive, although response to immunotherapy does not guarantee that the patient does not have a second cause of their RPD. Clinical syndromes alone are not sufficient to diagnose an RPD. There is a case report of a patient who presented with the corticobasal syndrome, often associated with CBD, but was later found to have CJD [71]. In this case, MRI did suggest the diagnosis of CJD with bilateral gyral involvement on DWI in parietal and occipital cortices. Thus, clinical syndromes alone are not sufficient to diagnose RPD, but ancillary tests, especially brain MRI, can significantly improve diagnostic accuracy.

The prognosis for patients diagnosed with prion diseases is poor, as described previously. Rapidly progressive decline in cognition and function is expected, with survival of only 12 months in typical cases of sporadic CJD. No treatment has been shown to slow the progression of prion diseases. The prognosis for neurodegenerative causes of RPD is also poor, with continued cognitive and functional decline expected and no specific treatment to slow this progression. LE that is not associated with an underlying malignancy, such as LE associated with anti-VGKC antibodies, has the best prognosis of non-prion RPDs. Patients with this type of LE are very responsive to immunotherapy acutely and can have excellent long-term outcomes with chronic immunosuppression. Patients with PLE require the identification and treatment of their underlying malignancy to achieve better long-term outcomes. Patients with PLE often stabilize with treatment of their underlying malignancy and with immunotherapy, but residual neurologic problems (e.g., amnesia and seizures) are common. Patients with HE often have an excellent response to immunotherapy but may have a relapsing course requiring repeat acute therapy followed by chronic immunotherapy. The prognosis for the other rare causes of RPD depends on identifying the underlying cause and treating the condition where treatments are available.

Treatment options

Currently there are no treatment options that have been shown to delay the onset or slow the progression of prion diseases or neurodegenerative conditions causing RPDs such as AD, FTD, DLB, CBD, or PSP. There are specific treatments for metabolic, infectious, neoplastic, and autoimmune causes of RPD. The mainstay of treatment for autoimmune causes would be acute immunotherapy, most commonly high-dose steroids (1 g of IV methylprednisolone daily for 5 days), intravenous immunoglobulin (0.4 g/kg per day for 5 consecutive days), or plasma exchange (every other day exchange for 5–6 exchanges) [32, 34]. Many autoimmune encephalopathies require more persistent treatment that can include chronic use of steroids or steroid-sparing agents. All patients with RPDs and their families need substantial education and support. Ensuring that the patient has adequate supervision and care is essential whether that care is received at home or in a more formal long-term care setting. Involvement of palliative care specialists early in the process is appropriate because of the irreversible terminal nature of most causes of RPDs other than those caused by autoimmune encephalopathies. Early in the course of RPD patients should identify a surrogate decision maker through the process of assigning power of attorney, if they are capable of making decisions, or through the assignment of a guardian if they are already incompetent to make decisions. Patients should be asked about their end of life care wishes so that they can help determine their end of life care. Families caring for patients with prion diseases should be reassured that they are not at increased risk of developing a prion disease if they are in contact with saliva, urine, and sweat. Healthcare providers handling blood and CSF of patients with a prion disease should use universal precautions.

Future developments

The hope for the future is the development of disease-modifying therapies for prion diseases as well as other neurodegenerative disorders. Further development of biomarkers for neurodegenerative disorders and other causes of RPD such as HE is expected in the future. The identification of new neuronal autoantibodies is also expected. Both the diagnostic tools and the effectiveness of therapies are expected to improve significantly in the future.

References

1. Liberski, P.P. and D.C. Gajdusek, Kuru: forty years later, a historical note. *Brain Pathol*, 1997. 7(1): p. 555–60.
2. Creutzfeldt, H., Über eine eigenartige herdförmige Erkrankung des Zentrainervensystems. *Z Ges Neurol Psychiatr*, 1920. 57: p. 1–18.
3. Jakob, A., Über eigenartige Erkrankungen des Zentralnervensystems mit bemerkenswerten anatomischen Befunde (spastische Pseudosklerose Encephalomyelopathie mit disseminierten Degenerationsherden). *Z Ges Neurol Psychiatr*, 1921. 64: p. 147–228.
4. Richardson, E.P., Jr. and C.L. Masters, The nosology of Creutzfeldt-Jakob disease and conditions related to the accumulation of PrPCJD in the nervous system. *Brain Pathol*, 1995. 5(1): p. 33–41.
5. Gajdusek, D.C. and C.J. Gibbs, Jr., Transmission of two subacute spongiform encephalopathies of man (Kuru and Creutzfeldt-Jakob disease) to new world monkeys. *Nature*, 1971. 230(5296): p. 588–91.
6. Gajdusek, D.C., C.J. Gibbs, and M. Alpers, Experimental transmission of a Kuru-like syndrome to chimpanzees. *Nature*, 1966. 209(5025): p. 794–6.
7. Ironside, J.W., Review: Creutzfeldt-Jakob disease. *Brain Pathol*, 1996. 6(4): p. 379–88.
8. Updated Case Surveillance from UK and Europe regarding CJD and vCJD. http://www.cjd.ed.ac.uk/data.html
9. Prusiner, S.B. and K.K. Hsiao, Human prion diseases. *Ann Neurol*, 1994. 35(4): p. 385–95.
10. Windl, O., et al., Genetic basis of Creutzfeldt-Jakob disease in the United Kingdom: a systematic analysis of predisposing mutations and allelic variation in the PRNP gene. *Hum Genet*, 1996. 98(3): p. 259–64.
11. Collinge, J., et al., Presymptomatic detection or exclusion of prion protein gene defects in families with inherited prion diseases. *Am J Hum Genet*, 1991. 49(6): p. 1351–4.
12. Billette de Villemeur, T., et al., Creutzfeldt-Jakob disease from contaminated growth hormone extracts in France. *Neurology*, 1996. 47(3): p. 690–5.
13. Collie, D.A., et al., Diagnosing variant Creutzfeldt-Jakob disease with the pulvinar sign: MR imaging findings in 86 neuropathologically confirmed cases. *AJNR Am J Neuroradiol*, 2003. 24(8): p. 1560–9.
14. Zerr, I. and S. Poser, Clinical diagnosis and differential diagnosis of CJD and vCJD. With special emphasis on laboratory tests. *APMIS*, 2002. 110(1): p. 88–98.
15. Will, R.G., et al., Diagnosis of new variant Creutzfeldt-Jakob disease. *Ann Neurol*, 2000. 47(5): p. 575–82.
16. Richt, J.A., et al., Production of cattle lacking prion protein. *Nat Biotechnol*, 2007. 25(1): p. 132–8.
17. Collinge, J., et al., Safety and efficacy of quinacrine in human prion disease (PRION-1 study): a patient-preference trial. *Lancet Neurol*, 2009. 8(4): p. 334–44.
18. Geschwind, M.D., et al., Quinacrine treatment trial for sporadic Creutzfeldt-Jakob disease. *Neurology*, 2013. 81(23): p. 2015–23.
19. Poser, S., B. Mollenhauer, A. Kraub, I. Zerr, B.J. Steinhoff, A. Schroeter, M. Finkenstaedt, W.J. Schulz-Schaeffer, H.A. Kretzschmar, K. Felgenhauer, How to improve the clinical diagnosis of Creutzfeldt-Jakob disease. *Brain*, 1999. 122: p. 2345–51.
20. Geschwind, M.D., et al., Rapidly progressive dementia. *Ann Neurol*, 2008. 64(1): p. 97–108.
21. Sala, I., et al., Rapidly progressive dementia: experience in a tertiary care medical center. *Alzheimer Dis Assoc Disord*, 2012. 26(3): p. 267–71.
22. Chitravas, N., et al., Treatable neurological disorders misdiagnosed as Creutzfeldt-Jakob disease. *Ann Neurol*, 2011. 70(3): p. 437–44.
23. Roberson, E.D., et al., Frontotemporal dementia progresses to death faster than Alzheimer disease. *Neurology*, 2005. 65(5): p. 719–25.
24. Ramos, V.F., D.L. Murman, and R.D. McComb, Progressive personality and language changes in a 62-year-old woman. *Rev Neurol Dis*, 2011. 8(3-4): p. 121–2.
25. Tschampa, H.J., et al., Patients with Alzheimer's disease and dementia with Lewy bodies mistaken for Creutzfeldt-Jakob disease. *J Neurol Neurosurg Psychiatry*, 2001. 71(1): p. 33–9.
26. Schmidt, C., et al., Clinical features of rapidly progressive Alzheimer's disease. *Dement Geriatr Cogn Disord*, 2010. 29(4): p. 371–8.
27. Schmidt, C., et al., Rapidly progressive Alzheimer disease. *Arch Neurol*, 2011. 68(9): p. 1124–30.
28. Gaig, C., et al., Rapidly progressive diffuse Lewy body disease. *Mov Disord*, 2011. 26(7): p. 1316–23.
29. Gultekin, S.H., et al., Paraneoplastic limbic encephalitis: neurological symptoms, immunological findings and tumour association in 50 patients. *Brain*, 2000. 123 (Pt 7): p. 1481–94.
30. Thieben, M.J., et al., Potentially reversible autoimmune limbic encephalitis with neuronal potassium channel antibody. *Neurology*, 2004. 62(7): p. 1177–82.
31. Vincent, A., et al., Potassium channel antibody-associated encephalopathy: a potentially immunotherapy-responsive form of limbic encephalitis. *Brain*, 2004. 127 (Pt 3): p. 701–12.
32. Ances, B.M., et al., Treatment-responsive limbic encephalitis identified by neuropil antibodies: MRI and PET correlates. *Brain*, 2005. 128(Pt 8): p. 1764–77.
33. Chong, J.Y. and L.P. Rowland, What's in a NAIM? Hashimoto encephalopathy, steroid-responsive encephalopathy associated with autoimmune thyroiditis, or nonvasculitic autoimmune meningoencephalitis? *Arch Neurol*, 2006. 63(2): p. 175–6.
34. Castillo, P., et al., Steroid-responsive encephalopathy associated with autoimmune thyroiditis. *Arch Neurol*, 2006. 63(2): p. 197–202.
35. Dalmau, J., et al., Paraneoplastic anti-N-methyl-D-aspartate receptor encephalitis associated with ovarian teratoma. *Ann Neurol*, 2007. 61(1): p. 25–36.
36. Chang, C.C., et al., Anti-GAD antibody cerebellar ataxia mimicking Creutzfeldt-Jakob disease. *Clin Neurol Neurosurg*, 2007. 109(1): p. 54–7.
37. Vernino, S., M. Geschwind, and B. Boeve, Autoimmune encephalopathies. *The neurologist*, 2007. 13(3): p. 140–7.
38. Tuzun, E. and J. Dalmau, Limbic encephalitis and variants: classification, diagnosis and treatment. *Neurologist*, 2007. 13(5): p. 261–71.
39. Geschwind, M.D., et al., Voltage-gated potassium channel autoimmunity mimicking creutzfeldt-jakob disease. *Arch Neurol*, 2008. 65(10): p. 1341–6.
40. Graus, F., et al., Neuronal surface antigen antibodies in limbic encephalitis: clinical-immunologic associations. *Neurology*, 2008. 71(12): p. 930–6.
41. Tan, K.M., et al., Clinical spectrum of voltage-gated potassium channel autoimmunity. *Neurology*, 2008. 70(20): p. 1883–90.
42. McKeon, A., et al., Reversible extralimbic paraneoplastic encephalopathies with large abnormalities on magnetic resonance images. *Arch Neurol*, 2009. 66(2): p. 268–71.
43. Irani, S.R., et al., N-methyl-D-aspartate antibody encephalitis: temporal progression of clinical and paraclinical observations in a predominantly non-paraneoplastic disorder of both sexes. *Brain*, 2010. 133(Pt 6): p. 1655–67.
44. Susac, J.O., et al., Susac's Syndrome: 1975-2005 microangiopathy/autoimmune endotheliopathy. *J Neurol Sci* 2007. 257: p. 270–272.
45. Salvarani, C., R.D. Brown, and G.G. Hunder, Adult primary central nervous system vasculitis. *Lancet*, 2012. 380(9843): p. 767–77.
46. Liguori, R., A. Vincent, and L. Clover, Morvan's syndrome: peripheral, central nervous system and cardiac involvement with antibodies to voltage-gated potassium channels. *Brain*, 2001. 124: p. 2417–2426.
47. Lai, M., et al., Investigation of LGI1 as the antigen in limbic encephalitis previously attributed to potassium channels: a case series. *Lancet Neurol*, 2010. 9(8): p. 776–85.
48. Irani, S.R., et al., Antibodies to Kv1 potassium channel-complex proteins leucine-rich, glioma inactivated 1 protein and contactin-associated protein-2 in limbic encephalitis, Morvan's syndrome and acquired neuromyotonia. *Brain*, 2010. 133(9): p. 2734–48.
49. Von Bose, M.J. and M. Zaudig, Encephalopathy resembling Creutzfeldt-Jakob disease following oral, prescribed doses of bismuth nitrate. *Br J Psychiatry*, 1991. 158: p. 278–80.
50. Teepker, M., et al., Myoclonic encephalopathy caused by chronic bismuth abuse. *Epileptic Disord*, 2002. 4(4): p. 229–33.
51. Halavaara, J., et al., Wernicke's encephalopathy: is diffusion-weighted MRI useful? *Neuroradiology*, 2003. 45(8): p. 519–23.
52. Salazar, J.A., I. Poon, and M. Nair, Clinical consequences of polypharmacy in elderly: expect the unexpected, think the unthinkable. *Expert Opin Drug Saf*, 2007. 6(6): p. 695–704.
53. Waniek, C., et al., Rapidly progressive frontal-type dementia associated with Lyme disease. *J Neuropsychiatry Clin Neurosci*, 1995. 7(3): p. 345–7.
54. Bouwman, F.H., et al., Variable progression of HIV-associated dementia. *Neurology*, 1998. 50(6): p. 1814–20.
55. Weil, A.A., et al., Patients with suspected herpes simplex encephalitis: rethinking an initial negative polymerase chain reaction result. *Clin Infect Dis*, 2002. 34(8): p. 1154–7.

56. Panegyres, P.K., Diagnosis and management of Whipple's disease of the brain. *Pract Neurol*, 2008. 8(5): p. 311–7.

57. Valcour, V., et al., A case of enteroviral meningoencephalitis presenting as rapidly progressive dementia. *Nat Clin Pract Neurol*, 2008. 4(7): p. 399–403.

58. Bakshi, R., et al., Lymphomatosis cerebri presenting as a rapidly progressive dementia: clinical, neuroimaging and pathologic findings. *Dement Geriatr Cogn Disord*, 1999. 10(2): p. 152–7.

59. Goncalves, M.R., et al., Atypical clinical course of FXTAS: rapidly progressive dementia as the major symptom. *Neurology*, 2007. 68(21): p. 1864–6.

60. Sarazin, M., et al., Reversible leukoencephalopathy in cerebral amyloid angiopathy presenting as subacute dementia. *Eur J Neurol*, 2002. 9(4): p. 353–8.

61. Harkness, K.A., et al., Rapidly reversible dementia in cerebral amyloid inflammatory vasculopathy. *Eur J Neurol*, 2004. 11(1): p. 59–62.

62. Rosenbloom, M.H. and A. Atri, The evaluation of rapidly progressive dementia. *Neurologist*, 2011. 17(2): p. 67–74.

63. Vitali, P., et al., Diffusion-weighted MRI hyperintensity patterns differentiate CJD from other rapid dementias. *Neurology*, 2011. 76(20): p. 1711–9.

64. Shiga, Y., et al., Diffusion-weighted MRI abnormalities as an early diagnostic marker for Creutzfeldt-Jakob disease. *Neurology*, 2004. 63(3): p. 443–9.

65. Meissner, B., et al., MRI lesion profiles in sporadic Creutzfeldt-Jakob disease. *Neurology*, 2009. 72(23): p. 1994–2001.

66. Chapman, T., D.W. McKeel, Jr., and J.C. Morris, Misleading results with the 14-3-3 assay for the diagnosis of Creutzfeldt-Jakob disease. *Neurology*, 2000. 55(9): p. 1396–7.

67. Geschwind, M.D., et al., Challenging the clinical utility of the 14-3-3 protein for the diagnosis of sporadic Creutzfeldt-Jakob disease. *Arch Neurol*, 2003. 60(6): p. 813–6.

68. Coulthart, M.B., et al., Diagnostic accuracy of cerebrospinal fluid protein markers for sporadic Creutzfeldt-Jakob disease in Canada: a 6-year prospective study. *BMC Neurol*, 2011. 11(133): p. 1–13.

69. Josephson, S.A., et al., The diagnostic utility of brain biopsy procedures in patients with rapidly deteriorating neurological conditions or dementia. *J Neurosurg*, 2007. 106(1): p. 72–5.

70. Mateen, F.J., et al., Steroid-responsive encephalopathy subsequently associated with Alzheimer's disease pathology: a case series. *Neurocase*, 2012. 18(1): p. 1–12.

71. Valverde, A.H., et al., Rapidly progressive corticobasal degeneration syndrome. *Case Rep Neurol*, 2011. 3(2): p. 185–90.

CHAPTER 14

Amyotrophic Lateral Sclerosis and Primary Lateral Sclerosis

Kevin B. Boylan[1], Mark A. Ross[2], and Eric J. Sorenson[3]

[1]Department of Neurology, Mayo Clinic, Jacksonville, Florida, USA
[2]Department of Neurology, Mayo Clinic, Scottsdale, Arizona, USA
[3]Department of Neurology, Mayo Clinic, Rochester, Minnesota, USA

Clinical definition and epidemiology

Clinical definition

Amyotrophic lateral sclerosis (ALS) and primary lateral sclerosis (PLS) are neurodegenerative motor neuron disorders of unknown cause, each resulting in stereotypic motor impairment with some overlapping features [1, 2]. ALS and PLS are marked by variability among patients in age of onset, rate of progression, survival, degree of associated cognitive impairment, and, in ALS, the relative extent of upper motor neuron (UMN) and lower motor neuron (LMN) features [3]. The pathogenesis is unknown, although 5–10% of patients have a familial form of the disorder [3]. ALS and PLS are considered together here in light of the clinical similarities between them and the possibility, based on current knowledge, that ALS and PLS may represent disorders on a clinical spectrum rather than distinct entities [1].

ALS is commonly known in the United States (USA) as Lou Gehrig's disease, after the famous baseball player who was stricken with the disease in the 1930s. Motor neuron disease is synonymous with ALS in the United Kingdom, while the label Charcot's disease may be applied in other regions [2, 4]. In 1874, Charcot described the clinical and pathological features of UMN and LMN involvement in ALS, which remain largely accepted today [5]. The concept that PLS may represent an entity distinct from ALS also was considered by Charcot [1].

Classical ALS is defined as a mixed UMN and LMN disorder, but the relative extent of UMN and LMN involvement may differ among patients. The term "ALS" may also be applied to incomplete presentations with only LMN or UMN signs, or solely bulbar features. In pure form, however, these partial presentations may be recognized as disorders separate from ALS (Figure 14.1) [2, 3, 6]. One approach to this issue is to view this range of presentations as a spectrum of adult motor neuron diseases including variants of ALS (Table 14.1) [2]. Motor neuron disease (MND) with exclusively LMN features is classified as progressive muscular atrophy (PMA) [7]. Generalized, purely UMN disease is termed primary lateral sclerosis (PLS), although LMN signs, to a limited degree, have been accepted by some authors in defining PLS, and the diagnostic criteria for PLS are less well established than those of ALS [1, 8, 9]. Progressive bulbar palsy (PBP) is a UMN and/or LMN disorder

restricted to the bulbar region. Most patients presenting with these syndromes eventually develop the full clinical picture of ALS, but approximately 10% of adult MND patients retain the diagnosis of PMA, PLS, or PBP [6]. In life, these diagnoses are established on clinical grounds, as no confirmatory supportive test is available other than post mortem examination [10]. The diagnostic challenge is exemplified by patients clinically diagnosed with PMA who at autopsy demonstrate UMN pathology, which then establishes the correct diagnosis of ALS [11]. Diagnostic distinction is more than academic, as prognosis differs for the various syndromes [2, 12].

The World Federation of Neurology Subcommittee on ALS developed diagnostic criteria that were first published in 1994 and intended to standardize the assessment of patients with ALS for research trials. Referred to as the El Escorial criteria, the guidelines divide the central nervous system into four anatomic regions – bulbar, cervical, thoracic, and lumbosacral – and rank the level of diagnostic certainty for ALS based on signs found in each region [13] (Table 14.2). Requirements for the diagnosis of ALS include the presence of UMN and LMN signs, evidence of progression, and absence of conditions that could otherwise account for the presentation. Revised El Escorial criteria published in 2000 allowed supportive evidence for the diagnosis of ALS to be obtained from electromyography and created special guidelines for the diagnosis of familial ALS where confirmation by DNA testing is available (Table 14.2) [14]. Further revised guidelines incorporating new recommendations for use of electromyographic findings in establishing the presence of LMN involvement, referred to as the Awaji criteria, have been proposed but are not yet widely applied [15]. Although these criteria provide a diagnostic framework that is potentially useful in clinical practice, they remain arbitrary guidelines rather than staging criteria, and patients do not necessarily follow a stepwise progression from the lower levels of diagnostic certainty to clinically definite ALS [16, 17].

Epidemiology

ALS occurs throughout the world but does not appear to be uniformly distributed. The epidemiology of PLS is less well studied and may be encompassed by the definition of ALS in some reports. The following discussion represents studies investigating incidence,

Neurodegeneration, First Edition. Edited by Anthony Schapira, Zbigniew Wszolek, Ted M. Dawson and Nicholas Wood.
© 2017 John Wiley & Sons, Ltd. Published 2017 by John Wiley & Sons, Ltd.

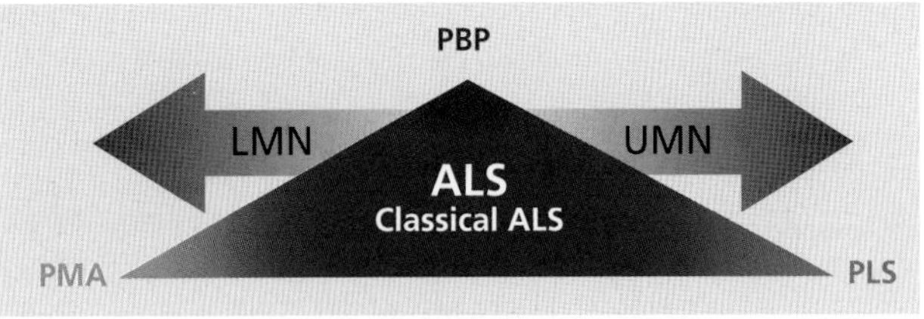

Figure 14.1 Theoretical relationships between ALS and other forms of adult motor neuron disease – progressive bulbar palsy (PBP), progressive muscular atrophy (PMA), and primary lateral sclerosis (PLS). Indistinct boundaries between these entities reflect the possibility that these disorders may represent varied expression of the same underlying disease process. Most, but not all, patients presenting with features of PBP, PMA, or PLS progress to classical ALS. LMN denotes predominance of lower motor neuron signs at one end of the spectrum and UMN denotes predominance of upper motor neuron signs at the other. Frontotemporal cognitive impairment or frontotemporal dementia may be present across the range of motor neuron disease phenotypes. Source: Boylan 2007 [327]. Reproduced with permission of Elsevier.

Table 14.1 Nomenclature of idiopathic adult motor neuron disease [6, 126, 329].

Amyotrophic lateral sclerosis	ALS	Upper and lower motor neuron signs in limbs, trunk, and bulbar regions
Progressive bulbar palsy	PBA	Upper and/or lower motor neuron signs in bulbar region only
Progressive muscular atrophy	PMA	Lower motor neuron signs of limb and trunk musculature; bulbar involvement late if at all; no upper motor neuron signs
Primary lateral sclerosis	PLS	Upper motor neuron signs in bulbar, limb, and trunk regions; no lower motor neuron signs

Table 14.2 El Escorial criteria for the diagnosis of ALS, original and revised criteria [13, 14].

The guidelines divide the central nervous system into four regions: bulbar, cervical, thoracic, and lumbosacral.

Level of certainty	Original criteria 1994	Revised criteria 2000
Definite ALS	LMN and UMN signs in 3 regions	LMN and UMN signs in 3 regions
Definite familial ALS	Not used	LMN and UMN signs in ≥1 region plus laboratory identification of DNA mutation associated with ALS
Probable ALS	LMN and UMN signs in at least 2 regions; regions may be different but some UMN signs must in part be rostral to LMN signs	LMN and UMN signs in at least 2 regions; regions may be different but some UMN signs must in part be rostral to LMN signs
Probable ALS, laboratory supported	Not used	LMN and UMN signs in only 1 region or UMN signs alone are found, plus signs of active and chronic denervation on EMG in at least 2 limbs
Possible ALS Permits diagnosis of possible ALS in monomelic ALS, PLS, and PBP	LMN and UMN signs in 1 region; or UMN signs alone in >2 regions; or LMN signs are rostral to UMN signs	LMN and UMN signs in 1 region or UMN signs alone in >2 regions or LMN signs are rostral to UMN signs and the diagnosis of Probable ALS, laboratory supported can not be made
Suspected ALS	LMN signs alone in ≥2 regions	Deleted

EMG, electromyography; LMN, lower motor neuron; UMN, upper motor neuron.

Table 14.3 Epidemiology of ALS [18–20, 28, 330].

Worldwide prevalence ~4 per 100,000
Annual incidence 1–2 per 100,000
Male to female ratio ~1.1–2.3:1.0
Peak age of onset 45–74 years

prevalence, and mortality of ALS. Epidemiological aspects of ALS are summarized in Table 14.3. Epidemiological studies suggest a higher incidence in Northern European populations and a somewhat lower incidence in non-White populations, generally with a crude incidence of 1–2/100,000 in White people and less than 1/100,000 in non-White people [18–20]. The highest reported crude incidence of ALS is 2.4/100,000 in Finland, and among the lowest is 0.31/100,000 in Hong Kong [21, 22]. In the USA, ALS incidence is reported to be higher in non-Hispanic White people than in non-White people including Black Americans or American Hispanics [23–26]. In a study conducted in Cuba covering the interval 2001–2006, ALS White mortality was 0.93/100,000, Black mortality was 0.87/100,000, and mortality in those of mixed race ethnicity was 0.55/100,000 [27]. Investigation of potential geographic effects on ALS susceptibility have not identified significant effects of geographic region on risk of ALS, but methodological limitations make it difficult to interpret these findings [18]. Overall, ALS incidence, prevalence, and mortality data suggest that ancestral origin influences ALS susceptibility, while the possibility that geographic factors impact ALS risk requires further study.

Gender effects of ALS risk are consistently reported in epidemiological studies throughout the world with a slightly higher incidence in males than females, and gender effects are seen in site of onset and age of onset. The male to female ratio in studies in which sporadic and familial ALS were considered together ranges from 1.11 to 2.32 [28]. Limited data suggest that the gender ratio in familial ALS generally is closer to 1:1 [29–31]. Bulbar onset is reported in several studies to occur more frequently in females [28]. In addition, onset of ALS at a young age (<40 years) is reported to be more likely in males [32, 33].

Spectrum of the clinical phenotype

ALS

The typical phenotype of ALS is that of gradually progressive muscle weakness with focal onset and combined UMN and LMN signs, without pain or sensory symptoms. Initial manifestations are varied owing to differences among patients in the region of onset (bulbar, cervical, thoracic, lumbosacral), degree of UMN and LMN involvement, rate of progression (rapid, average, slow), and features such as cognitive dysfunction. Physical signs indicating LMN involvement include muscle weakness, muscle atrophy, and fasciculations. The signs indicating UMN involvement are weakness, hyperreflexia, spasticity, and pathologic reflexes. The brainstem is involved, producing bulbar signs including dysarthria, dysphagia, sialorrhea, and laryngospasm.

Weakness associated with LMN pathology is generally more severe than that seen with UMN disease and is associated with muscle atrophy and fasciculations. Muscle atrophy may not be prominent early in the disorder because muscle fiber reinnervation may keep up with muscle fiber denervation, and a relatively small number of LMNs may be affected. With progressive loss of LMNs, muscle atrophy is expected. Fasciculations are common in ALS and provide supportive evidence for the diagnosis. The fasciculations in ALS are often prominent, widespread, and accompanied by muscle weakness, muscle atrophy, and UMN signs.

Signs of UMN pathology include weakness, spasticity, hyperreflexia, pathologic reflexes, and pseudobulbar emotional lability. Patients with UMN involvement experience loss of fine motor control and reduced speed of movements. They may recognize that their affected limbs are not weak but rather fail to cooperate with the expected speed and precision required for the intended movement. The weakness related to UMN disease is often accompanied by spasticity. Patients may perceive spasticity as stiffness that is aggravated by physical activity such as walking. Hyperreflexia is the most common UMN finding in ALS.

Motor neuron pathology involving brainstem motor nuclei and/or descending corticobulbar fibers produces bulbar signs with LMN, UMN, or mixed LMN/UMN features. LMN involvement includes flaccid-type dysarthria and tongue weakness with tongue atrophy and fasciculations. UMN involvement includes spastic-type dysarthria, hyperactive gag and jaw reflexes, snout reflex, and pseudobulbar palsy. Flaccid, spastic, and combined forms of dysarthria each have impaired articulation. Flaccid dysarthria may involve hypernasality, nasal air emission, and breathiness. Spastic dysarthria is characterized by a slow rate and a strained or strangulated quality. Often ALS patients have a mixed flaccid and spastic dysarthria pattern. Pseudobulbar palsy, presenting as reduced control of emotional expression, results in reduced ability to suppress laughing, crying, or both, in response to normal emotional stimuli.

Dysphagia usually presents as choking on liquids before difficulty with swallowing solid foods is evident. Patients may report difficulty chewing food or manipulating food in the mouth. Complaints about oral secretions may include sialorrhea or thick secretions that are difficult to clear from the throat, especially if the cough is reduced. Laryngospasm, a temporary inability to breathe or speak due to spasm of the laryngeal muscles, may occur in ALS and can include inspiratory stridor. The cause of laryngospasm is not known, but irritation of the larynx from oral secretions or reflux of gastric secretions may contribute.

Patients with ALS eventually develop weakness of their respiratory muscles and dyspnea, typically later in the course of the disease after limb and/or bulbar muscle weakness is apparent. Dyspnea often first manifests with physical exertion or as orthopnea, and later as dyspnea when speaking, and, ultimately, dyspnea at rest. Other respiratory symptoms include weak cough and difficulty clearing secretions. Some patients complain of morning headache related to nocturnal hypoventilation. With advanced respiratory muscle weakness, breathing requires activation of accessory respiratory muscles, and breathing appears labored. As respiratory muscles begin to fail, carbon dioxide retention develops; hypercarbia may be associated with altered mental status, usually somnolence, and in some patients hallucinations may occur.

Although typically regarded as a painless illness, pain actually occurs frequently in ALS patients but usually as a later feature of musculoskeletal origin. Causes include muscle stiffness, overuse of weak muscles, and lack of mobility. Occasionally, ALS patients may have pain that is not clearly explained.

Other relatively late features of ALS are constipation and edema. Constipation is usually related to decreased mobility and decreased oral intake of fluids. Lower extremity edema occurs frequently in patients with leg weakness and muscle atrophy due to reduced venous return. This is a natural consequence of losing muscle tissue that normally promotes venous and lymphatic return. Likewise, the leg usually becomes cool due to loss of the muscle with its rich vascular supply.

Cognitive dysfunction is a relatively common feature of ALS and may also occur in PLS [2, 34]. Cognitive and behavioral deficits include impaired executive function, disinhibition, impulsivity, apathy, affective symptoms, compulsivity, irritability, and aggressive behavior [35–38]. Up to 15% of patients with ALS may have frontotemporal dementia, and up to 50% of patients with ALS may meet criteria for frontotemporal dementia or frontotemporal cognitive impairment [2, 37, 39–42].

PLS

PLS is a form of progressive MND with purely UMN features [1]. Motor impairments in PLS typically take the form of lower limb weakness and spasticity and spastic bulbar palsy, with associated but usually less prominent upper limb involvement [1]. The clinical distinction between PLS and hereditary spastic paraparesis (HSP) may be difficult to draw, but can be made based on the general observation that bulbar features eventually develop in most patients with PLS but are only seen in HSP in rare exceptions [43, 44]. Proposed classification systems for PLS differ with regard to allowances made for the presence of LMN signs and the duration of time over which a patient may be observed with purely UMN features before the diagnosis of PLS can be made with confidence [9, 45]. A central issue in establishing a diagnosis of PLS is that patients presenting with predominantly UMN signs may progress to develop the full picture of ALS, and that any LMN features on physical examination or electromyography (EMG) may point toward eventual development of ALS [1, 9].

PLS is less common than ALS, representing 2–4% of patients reported in large MND series [45–47]. Age of onset is similar to ALS [1]. Spasticity and weakness may begin in the bulbar region or lower limbs, usually the latter. Physical findings may initially be asymmetrical (i.e., hemiparesis) [48]. Gradual progression to initially uninvolved regions is typical. The concept of PLS as a specific disease entity is supported by autopsy data demonstrating solely UMN pathology in patients given this diagnosis in life [45, 49]. However, natural history data include reports of patients initially diagnosed with PLS who after years of follow-up evolved LMN signs compatible with ALS [50]. Further, mild creatine kinase elevation is reported in some patients otherwise meeting criteria for diagnosis of PLS, needle EMG may reveal signs of active and chronic motor denervation, and muscle biopsy may show neurogenic changes [46, 51]. Also, patients diagnosed in life with PLS may at post mortem demonstrate anterior horn cell disease [52].

Cognitive dysfunction also may occur in PLS [34]. Cognitive features of PLS are less well studied compared to ALS, but basic features of cognitive dysfunction in PLS seem generally similar to those found in ALS [34].

Pathophysiology

ALS appears to be caused by an interaction of genetic and acquired mechanisms including environmental factors leading to neuronal death, although the causes remain unknown [53, 54]. Causative genes identified in several inherited forms of ALS have provided insights on the molecular pathogenesis of ALS, but how these mutations lead to the disease is not understood [55]. ALS may involve multiple CNS systems, with selective vulnerability of UMNs and LMNs as well as non-motor regions supporting cognitive function [42].

Environmental factors

It has long been suspected that environmental factors play a major role in the etiology of ALS. For over 100 years many environmental hypotheses have been suggested with little experimental evidence of support. There have been considerable advances in the monogenetic inheritance of ALS. With the recent concepts of complex genetic inheritance in neurodegenerative diseases, it is unclear at present how much ALS risk is derived from environment and how much from genetics.

In support of an environmental cause, there have been a number of case reports of ALS following certain environmental exposures, a number of geographic clusters, and additional reports of conjugal ALS. The environmental factors in question have included a diverse collection of hypotheses. These have included trace metal toxicity, agrochemical exposure, head trauma, infectious and other biological agents, smoking, and more recently, military service. Despite study of the case reports, ALS clusters, and conjugal cases, there ultimately has been little supportive evidence for a unifying environmental cause forthcoming from epidemiological studies. It appears likely that there are multiple environmental exposures, each with a weak association individually, but in aggregate, these exposures may account for a significant risk.

The hypothesis that ALS is due to trace metal toxicity dates back nearly 100 years. Possible risk factors have included lead, aluminum, and selenium, among others. A number of reports have suggested lead exposure as a risk for ALS. As recently as 2010, a case-control study demonstrated higher blood lead levels in cases of ALS but with a relatively weak odds ratio of 1.9 [56]. One report from Italy suggested that selenium exposure in drinking water may be associated when an excess of selenium was discovered in the well water of a town with a larger than expected number of ALS cases [57]. There have been additional isolated case reports suggesting an association; however, these have either not been reproducible or have been subject to methodological flaws. To date there have been no confirmatory studies linking trace metals to ALS [58, 59].

As with trace metals, agrochemical exposure has long been proposed as an environmental risk for ALS. The foundation for this hypothesis rests in case reports and case-control studies [60]. Some studies have demonstrated an association with living in rural areas, while others have not [61]. A recent systematic review of the literature on agrochemical risk in ALS was indeterminate. From a number of papers identified addressing this hypothesis, there were two independent studies finding a weak link between ALS and exposure to pesticides [62]. However, large prospective studies have failed to demonstrate any association [63].

Recent epidemiological studies have demonstrated a small but significant risk associated with cigarette smoking [64]. A pooled analysis of these studies indicates that the relative risks are small and fail to demonstrate a convincing dose-dependent effect [65]. This suggests that cigarette smoking may serve as a confounding variable for an as yet unidentified environmental agent.

Biological agents have also long been suspected as an etiology for ALS. The possibility of a viral cause has been postulated for nearly a century. Initially this was suspected because of the similarities between the acute form of poliomyelitis and the chronic motor nerve degeneration in ALS. There have been additional studies suggesting that viral DNA may be identified in a disproportionate number of ALS subjects. A number of studies initially suggested that enteroviral DNA and RNA were identified in a very large proportion of ALS cases but a very small number of controls [66, 67],

while follow-up studies could not confirm these findings [68, 69]. As with studies on other environmental risk factors, these studies have not been reproducible or have not withstood scientific scrutiny. To date there is no convincing evidence that ALS is associated with any infectious agent.

Another biological agent has come into question. Although cyanobacteria (blue-green algae) are not infectious, exposure to them has been attributed to an increased risk of developing ALS. It has been postulated that this risk is due to cyanobacterial production of cyanotoxins. Recent reports of high levels of cyanobacteria in the Persian Gulf have been suggested as an explanation for the purported increased risk among those military servicemen who served in the Gulf War [70]. In that report, it was suggested that inhalation of dust containing cyanotoxins may be responsible for the association. Much of the focus has been on the neurotoxin, β-methylamino-L-alanine (BMAA). Cyanobacteria and BMAA have also been found in high concentrations within the root system of the cycad trees of Guam. This has led to speculation that perhaps cyanobacteria are responsible for the notable geographic cluster of ALS on that island [71].

Epidemiological studies have also suggested that military service may be associated with an increased risk of ALS. This was first proposed when a study among military personnel demonstrated a nearly two-fold increase in the risk of ALS in subjects deployed to the Persian Gulf [72, 73]. Another, independent study confirmed an increased risk among all military personnel, not just those deployed to the Persian Gulf, although the odds ratios were less at 1.5 [74]. While service alone seems an unlikely cause, many environmental exposures have been postulated. These hypotheses have included exposure to chemical warfare agents and exposure to cyanotoxins [70, 75]. To date, further studies on military exposures have not identified a common risk.

Finally, trauma, and in particular head trauma, has long been suspected to have an association with ALS. Case-control studies have suggested a weak association of ALS with head trauma earlier in life. A number of studies have addressed concussions and sports-related injuries with some evidence of an association [76]. These studies have been questioned because of the potential of recall bias in those affected with ALS [77]. However, recent reports from a tissue bank of head trauma victims identified cases of MND in trauma victims demonstrating pathology of both ALS and chronic trauma, referred to as chronic traumatic encephalopathy (CTE) [78]. While these reports have been controversial, they have provided evidence in support of the association between head trauma and the development of ALS later in life.

Genetics

ALS

Genetic factors in ALS include disease-causing mutations in familial ALS (fALS) and genes that may modify disease risk in sporadic ALS. Phenotypes associated with these genes include classical ALS, ALS/FTD, PLS, and PMA, and may include non-ALS phenotypes, such as FTD without MND and extrapyramidal features [55]. fALS is estimated to represent 5–10% of people with ALS, although data suggest that a larger proportion of patients may have fALS than is generally recognized, owing to incomplete family history and reduced penetrance of disease mutations [54, 55, 79]. Inheritance of most forms of fALS is autosomal dominant, although autosomal recessive and X-linked fALS also occur; different modes of inheritance may be associated with the same gene, depending on the mutation involved [55].

Table 14.4 Genetic forms of ALS.

Type	Gene*	Locus	Inheritance	Clinical phenotype
ALS1 [97]	SOD1	21q22.1	AD AR Sporadic	ALS, PMA, PBP
ALS2 [110]	Alsin	2q33.2	AR	Juvenile onset PLS and ALS; infantile HSP
ALS3 [331]	Unknown	18q21	AD	ALS
ALS4 [332]	SETX	9q34	AD	Early adult onset ALS
ALS5 [333]	SPG11	15q21.1	AR	Juvenile or adult onset ALS
ALS6 [88, 91]	FUS	16q11.2	AD Sporadic	ALS, ALS/ FTD
ALS7 [334]	Unknown	20p13	AD	ALS
ALS8 [200]	VAPB	20q13.3	AD	ALS, PMA, PBP
ALS9 [335]	ANG	14q11.2	AD	ALS, ALS/FTD, PBP
ALS10 [84, 87, 336]	TARDBP	1p36.2	AD AR	ALS, ALS/FTD
ALS11 [108]	FIG4	6q21	AD	ALS, PLS
ALS12 [123]	OPTN	10p13	AD AR Sporadic	ALS
ALS13 [337]	ATXN2	12q24	AD	ALS
ALS14 [338]	VCP	9p13.3	AD	ALS, ALS/FTD
ALS15 [121]	UBQLN2	Xp11.21	XLD Sporadic	ALS, ALS/FTD
ALS16 [339]	SIGMAR1	9p13	AR	Juvenile ALS
FTDALS [81, 82]	C9ORF72	9q21.2	AD	ALS, ALS/FTD, PMA, FTD

*ANG, angiogenin; ATXN2, ataxin 2; C9ORF72, chromosome 9 open reading frame 72; FIG4, a phosphoinositide phosphatase; FUS, fused in sarcoma/translated in liposarcoma; OPTN, optineurin; SETX, senataxin; SIGMAR1, sigma non-opioid receptor, Type I; SOD1, Cu/Zn superoxide dismutase; SPG11, spatacsin; TARDPB, TAR DNA binding protein; UBQLN2, ubiquilin 2; VAPB, vesicle associated membrane protein/synaptobrevin-associated membrane protein B; VCP, valosin containing protein. For updated information visit Online Mendelian Inheritance in Man; http://www.ncbi.nlm.nih.gov/omim [55, 80, 95].

Genetic linkage is established for a growing number of fALS types (Table 14.4). Reports of families not linked to known loci indicate further heterogeneity. In outbred populations, approximately 50% or more of familial ALS is accounted for by known ALS-linked genes. C9ORF72 hexanucleotide expansion mutations appear to account for at least 30% of fALS in North America and Europe, while SOD1 mutations are found in about 20%, mutations of TARDBP and FUS account for a few percent each, and other, relatively rare, gene mutations are found in the remainder [80–82].

Incomplete penetrance is reported for some SOD1, TARDBP, and FUS mutations [83–88]. De novo mutation has been documented in rare cases for SOD1 and FUS mutations [81, 89, 90].

Present concepts of the pathogenesis of ALS have been strongly influenced by recent discoveries of four genes linked to fALS, fALS/FTD, and FTD. These include the recognition that mutations in the RNA binding proteins TAR DNA-binding protein 43 (TDP-43, encoded by the gene TARDBP) and fused in sarcoma/translated in liposarcoma (FUS, encoded by the gene FUS) may cause autosomal dominant ALS [84, 87, 88, 91]. The product of the TARDBP gene encodes the 43-kDa TAR DNA-binding protein, which functions in regulation of gene expression and RNA splicing [92]. FUS protein is involved in DNA and RNA metabolism, including the regulation of transcription and RNA splicing [88, 91].

A third recent ALS gene discovery that has had significant impact on concepts of ALS pathogenesis is that mutations in the ubiquilin-2 gene (UBQLN2) may cause X-linked dominant ALS

and ALS/FTD with reduced penetrance in females [93]. Ubiquilin-2 appears to be involved with protein degradation pathways, and functional analysis suggests that UBQLN2 mutations resulting in ALS and ALS/FTD are pathogenic owing to disruption of this process [94].

The most recent gene discovery with significant impact on present understanding of ALS pathogenesis is the identification of expansions of a GGGGCC hexanucleotide repeat in the first intron of a gene that encodes a protein of unknown function on chromosome 9, C9ORF72, in people with ALS, ALS/FTD, and FTD [81, 82]. Hexanucleotide repeat expansions in C9ORF72 appear to be the most common cause of familial ALS, ALS/FTD, and FTD, involving a genetic mechanism that is not found in other known genes linked to ALS or FTD pathogenesis [81, 82]. The phenotype associated with C9ORF72 hexanucleotide expansions may include familial ALS, ALS/FTD, or FTD, potentially with combinations of these in the same kindred, as well as sporadic ALS [80, 95, 96]. The possibility that onset of ALS caused by C9ORF72 hexanucleotide expansions may be earlier in affected offspring of affected parents requires confirmation [80, 95].

Approximately 20% of patients with fALS have ALS1, a mutation in the Cu/Zn superoxide dismutase gene (SOD1) linked to chromosome 21q12.1, the first causative gene identified in ALS [97, 98]. Over 100 pathogenic SOD1 mutations are known [55]. Inheritance with all but one of these is autosomal dominant. The phenotype is compatible with classical ALS or, with some mutations, PMA, but age of onset and severity may vary within families, and penetrance may be less than 100% [99–101]. Frontotemporal cognitive impairment is rare in ALS linked to SOD1 [55].

A growing list of other genes associated with ALS and related phenotypes is reported, each contributing to a relatively small proportion of fALS (Table 14.4) [55]. The protein products of several of these genes appear to share functional characteristics with proteins encoded by other genes associated with ALS, offering potential clues regarding key cellular pathways in the molecular pathogenesis of ALS [94]. Among these, VCP and OPTN are involved in autophagic protein degradation, consistent with the notion that ALS pathogenesis is associated with disruption of this process. Further, SQSTM1/p62, VCP, and OPTN have been linked to Paget's disease of bone, and ALS has been reported in association with that disorder [102, 103].

Several studies suggest the presence of a genetic component in sporadic ALS, supporting the concept that sporadic ALS may be multifactorial, contributed to in part by multiple genetic variants, each contributing to a person's overall susceptibility to the disease [55].

PLS

PLS is rarely hereditary, although there are reports of familial PLS and reports of PLS occurring in families with other members affected by ALS [104–106]. The potential clinical overlap between patients with PLS and those classified as having HSP is an additional challenge in the characterization of familial UMN conditions resembling PLS [107].

Heterozygous mutations in the gene FIG4, which encodes a phosphoinositide phosphatase, are reported to produce a PLS phenotype in some patients, but most mutation carriers appear to have an ALS phenotype [108].

A large French Canadian family with PLS inherited in an autosomal dominant pattern has been reported. Genome-wide scanning identified a candidate region on chromosome 4ptel-4p16.1; the condition is designated PLS1, but the gene has not yet been reported [109].

A juvenile onset form of PLS or a juvenile onset form of ALS with autosomal recessive inheritance may be associated with mutations in the *ALSIN* gene, which encodes alsin, a guanine nucleotide exchange factor for the small GTPase RAB5 [110, 111]. Mutations in *ALSIN* may also lead to infantile-onset spastic paralysis [112].

Pathology

ALS

The neuropathology of ALS is characterized by loss of LMNs in bulbar motor nuclei and spinal anterior horn [113, 114]. Pathological changes include myelin pallor, degeneration of the lateral and anterior corticospinal tracts, and variable pathological changes in motor cortex, such as loss of pyramidal neurons, including Betz cells and pyramidal cells, and reactive gliosis in the motor cortex. Degeneration and loss of motor neurons and accompanying reactive gliosis are also seen in affected brainstem motor nuclei and anterior horn (Figure 14.2) [114]. LMN nuclei characteristically spared are those innervating external ocular muscles (cranial nerves III, IV, and VI) and pelvic floor/sphincter muscles (Onuf's nucleus).

The pathological hallmark of sporadic and most familial forms of ALS is the presence of ubiquitin-immunoreactive inclusions in motor neurons of the anterior horns; these are also found in pyramidal neurons, Betz cells, and associated glial cells in the motor cortex [114–116]. Bunina bodies, cystatin C-containing inclusions occurring in the cell bodies of motor neurons, were considered a pathological sine qua non of ALS prior to the discovery of ubiquitinated inclusions in affected brain tissue in ALS (Figure 14.3) [117].

The occurrence of TDP-43-positive neuronal and glial inclusions in people with ALS, in those with ALS and dementia, and in approximately half of patients with frontotemporal dementia without MND, suggests that these neurodegenerative conditions represent a spectrum of diseases with overlapping features [113, 118].

The neuropathology of ALS associated with the *C9ORF74* hexanucleotide repeat expansion gene on chromosome 9 includes ubiquitin and TDP-43 pathology that is generally similar to that found in most cases of sporadic ALS [81, 82]. However, neuronal and glial inclusions immunoreactive for p62 in non-motor brain regions, including cerebellar granular neurons, and neuronal inclusions in

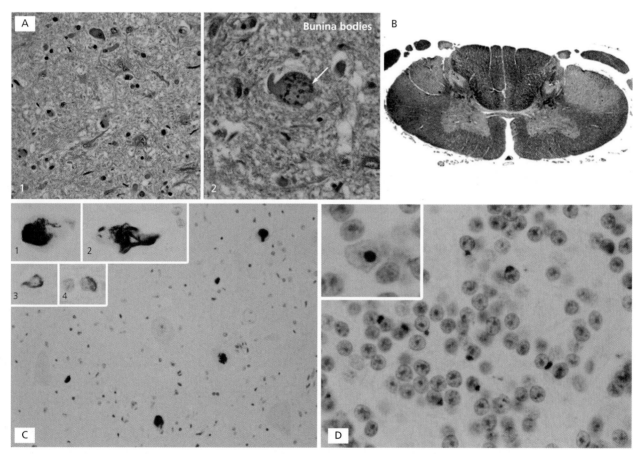

Figure 14.2 Examples of neuropathological findings in ALS. (A) (1) Neuronal loss and dense fibrillary astrocytosis in the hypoglossal nucleus. A few residual neurons have eosinophilic cytoplasmic inclusions typical of ALS; (2) enlargement showing motor neuron containing Bunina bodies (arrow). (B) Spinal cord showing loss of myelinated fibers (lack of stain) in corticospinal tracts as well as degeneration of anterior roots. (C) Motor neurons and glia containing intracytoplasmic inclusions immunoreactive for TDP-43; inset enlargement shows variable morphology of TDP-43 neuronal intracytoplasmic inclusions with dense (1) and skein-like (2) morphology, and oligodendroglia with "coiled body-like" intracytoplasmic inclusions (3, 4). (D) Neurons in the granular layer of the cerebellum in a patient with ALS associated with an expansion in the gene *C9ORF72*, demonstrating neuronal cytoplasmic inclusions immunoreactive for antibody to p62; inset enlargement shows a single neuron containing a cytoplasmic inclusion. (A, C, and D) Courtesy of Dr. Dennis Dickson, Department of Neuroscience, Mayo Clinic, Jacksonville, Florida. (B) Kumar 2010. Reproduced with permission of Elsevier.).

the hippocampal CA4 subfield appear to be specific for the mutation (Figure 14.2) [96].

Although the distribution of neuropathological changes in familial forms of ALS caused by *SOD1* mutations is generally similar to that in sporadic ALS, neuronal inclusions immunoreactive for ubiquitin and for SOD1 and not immunoreactive for TDP-43 or FUS are a distinctive feature of fALS associated with mutations in *SOD1* [119–121].

The neuropathology of ALS associated with mutations in the *FUS* gene is marked by the presence of basophilic neuronal cytoplasmic inclusions immunoreactive for FUS protein and ubiquitin, but negative for TDP-43 [122, 123].

PLS

The pathology of PLS is less well characterized than that of ALS. Few post mortem examinations have been reported in PLS, and most antedate recognition of TDP-43 pathology in MND and FTD. Pathology series reported in the early 20th century described degeneration of the corticospinal tracts and less prominent degeneration of cerebellar tracts and the fasciculus gracilis, although interpretation of earlier literature is difficult owing to the possibility that diagnoses other than neurodegenerative MND may not have been recognized, given that these studies occurred prior to the identification of Bunina bodies and ubiquitinated neuronal inclusions as diagnostic markers in the brain and spinal cord in ALS [1].

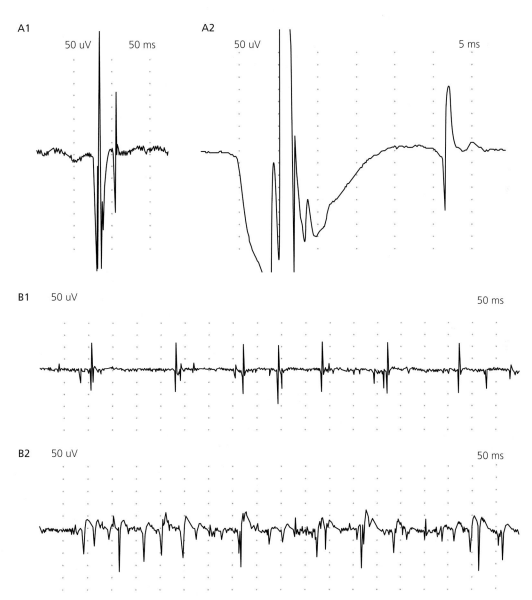

Figure 14.3 Examples of EMG findings in ALS. (A) (1) Two fasciculation potentials recorded at 50 ms/division sweep speed; (2) same fasciculation potentials shown in A. (1), at 5 ms/division sweep speed, demonstrating prolonged duration of the first potential and normal duration of the second. The configuration of fasciculation potentials in ALS reflects the state of the motor unit generating the potential, and may be that of a normal motor unit potential or show evidence of chronic motor denervation. (B) Fibrillation potentials: (1) predominantly spike configuration; (2) mixed positive wave and spike configuration. (C) Abnormal voluntary motor unit potentials seen with chronic partial motor denervation and reinnervation: (1) complex motor unit potentials; (2) neurogenic reduced recruitment; high amplitude motor unit potential firing at ~30 Hz; (3) unstable, complex motor unit potential firing at ~25 Hz; (4) motor unit potential in (3), superimposed tracings demonstrate instability of firing, including variable presence of satellite potentials (asterisk). Source: Boylan 2007 [327]. Reproduced with permission of Elsevier.

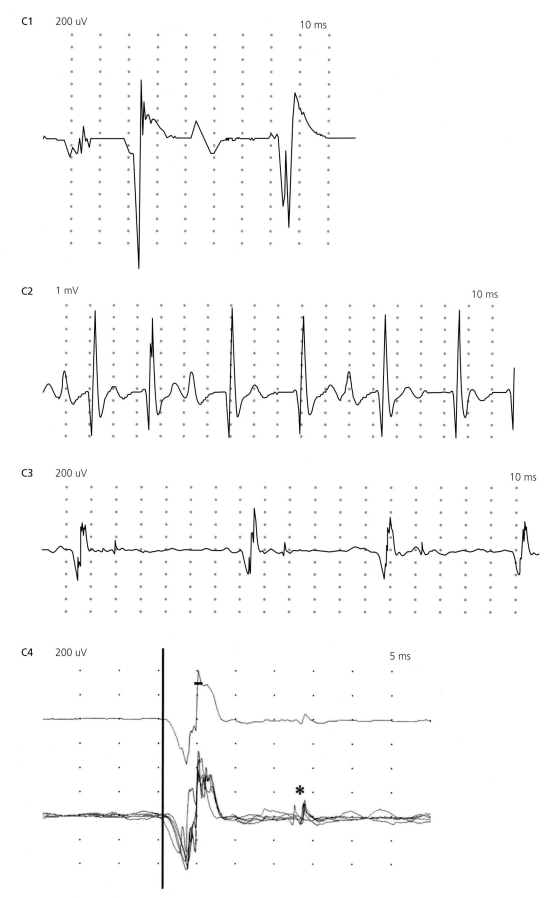

Figure 14.3 *(continued)*

Microscopic examination of brain and spinal cord tissue in less recent PLS autopsy cases reported prior to the introduction of TDP-43 immunohistochemistry, but in which ubiquitin immunohistochemistry was performed, showed corticospinal tract degeneration and Betz cell depletion in the motor cortex as common features, with sparing of anterior horn cells. The presence of Bunina bodies has been variable in reported cases, from few to none. In a more recent report of neuropathological findings, two patients with an adult onset PLS in conjunction with later onset FTD were found to have pathological findings compatible with UMN-predominant ALS with FTD-TDP, based on TDP-43 immunohistochemistry [124].

Clinical prodrome and biomarkers

Prodromal features of ALS and PLS

Initial motor deficits in ALS tend to arise focally, involving a single limb or bulbar muscles, and gradually extend to adjacent body regions [125, 126]. The ratio of limb onset to bulbar onset is around 3:1 [12, 127, 128]. Diffuse onset of weakness is uncommon [129]. Deficits tend to progress to the corresponding opposite side of the body, and ipsilaterally in a rostral or caudal direction [125, 130]. Rostral–caudal extension appears to occur more rapidly than caudal–rostral [125]. Uncommon presentations of ALS include hemiparesis with mainly UMN signs, known as Mills' variant, and cervical muscle weakness presenting as head drop and onset in the thoracic region [131–133]. Onset features distinguishing PLS from ALS include greater tendency to bilateral onset of motor signs in the upper and lower limbs and stiffness as a presenting complaint in PLS [134].

Fasciculations are not found in PLS but may be an early sign of ALS [9, 135, 136]. Muscle cramps are a common and potentially early symptom in ALS but are nonspecific and lack diagnostic importance [135, 137]. Dysphagia is an early or presenting symptom in 10–30% of ALS patients, and weight loss can occur as an early sign in ALS owing to oropharyngeal weakness and dysphagia [138–140].

Clinically significant respiratory muscle weakness may occur as an early feature of ALS and, as a presenting symptom, can be overlooked or misattributed to cardiac or pulmonary disease resulting in delayed diagnosis [141–145]. Respiratory symptoms are not typically a presenting feature of PLS [146].

Frontotemporal cognitive dysfunction may present before onset of motor features [2]. Pseudobulbar affect, involuntary outbursts of laughter or crying triggered by circumstances that normally would not provoke an overtly emotional response, also may be a presenting symptom [3, 147–149].

Biomarkers of ALS and PLS

Standard measures of disease activity and progression in ALS and PLS include neurophysiological tests, pulmonary function tests, manual muscle testing, and functional rating scales. New surrogate biomarkers are at various stages of development and validation in the areas of neurophysiology and neuroimaging, but these remain experimental. Well-validated surrogate biomarkers of LMN pathology in MND are available, but markers of UMN and extra motor involvement are not [77].

The discussion of surrogate biomarkers in this section surveys well-established tests as well as those not traditionally considered within the purview of neurology, such as the assessment of pulmonary function and the evaluation of cognitive function. Investigational biomarkers are briefly discussed. Neurophysiological and neuroimaging biomarkers and the types of pathology for which they may be useful for characterization are listed in Table 14.5.

Table 14.5 Biomarkers for the evaluation of upper and lower motor neuron involvement and cognitive dysfunction in ALS and PLS.

Biomarker	UMN*	LMN*	Cognitive*	Status in evaluation of MND
Neurophysiological biomarkers				
Electromyography (EMG)		+		Standard; may be difficult to quantitate
Motor unit estimation (MUNE)		+		Investigational
Neurophysiological index		+		Investigational
Electrical impedance myography		+		Investigational
Magnetic stimulation				
Central motor conduction time	+			Investigational
Motor evoked potentials	+			Investigational
Cortical silent period	+			Investigational
Magnetic resonance imaging				
Structural MRI	+		+	Standard; may be difficult to quantitate; limited sensitivity and specificity
Diffusion tensor imaging	+		+	Investigational
Voxel-based morphology	+		+	Investigational
Functional MRI	+		+	Investigational
Magnetization transfer	+			Investigational
Magnetic resonance spectroscopy	+		+	Investigational
Nuclear medicine imaging				
PET scanning	?		+	Investigational; standard in evaluation of dementias

*+ Denotes sensitivity and specificity in detecting the type of deficits or pathology indicated; see text for further discussion.

Neurophysiological testing

Electromyography Electromyography aids in demonstrating LMN involvement in ALS and is central to published diagnostic guidelines used in establishing the diagnosis (Table 14.2 and Table 14.6) [13, 14, 150, 151]. The revised El Escorial criteria advise electrophysiological studies to confirm signs of LMN dysfunction, identify electrophysiological evidence of LMN dysfunction in clinically uninvolved regions, and exclude other pathophysiological processes. Evidence of LMN dysfunction supports the diagnosis of ALS but is not itself diagnostic of the disorder, as similar abnormalities can be found in a wide range of conditions involving LMNs [152]. EMG in ALS typically demonstrates fasciculation potentials, fibrillation potentials, and long-duration, high-amplitude, and complex voluntary motor unit potentials (MUP) with reduced recruitment (Figure 14.3) [150–152]. Fibrillation and fasciculation potentials in particular are expected in ALS. In ALS patients, fasciculation potentials generally show some combination of features of the enlarged and complex motor unit. Thus, they might be large-amplitude, long-duration, and polyphasic, in contrast to the fasciculation potentials of the normal individual which have normal MUP morphology [153]. Large and/or complex MUP reflect chronic motor denervation and reinnervation in affected motor units. Recruitment changes signal loss of motor units. In the investigation of possible ALS, examination of muscles that do not appear to be involved may reveal subclinical LMN involvement.

As an established means to identify LMN pathology in ALS, EMG can provide a basis for documenting progression of LMN

Table 14.6 El Escorial guidelines for electrophysiological testing in the diagnosis of ALS.

Nerve conduction studies		
	Expected in ALS	**Features suggesting other diagnoses**
Motor	CV normal unless CMAP is small	• Evidence of motor conduction block • CV <70% of LLN • DL >30% above ULN • F-wave or H-wave latency >30% above ULN • Decrement >20% on repetitive stimulation
Sensory	Normal, but may be abnormal with peripheral nerve disease/entrapment coexisting with ALS; lower limb sensory responses may be difficult to elicit in the elderly	Abnormal sensory nerve conduction studies, i.e., owing to peripheral neuropathy, entrapment
Needle EMG		
Signs of active and chronic denervation* on needle EMG examination in at least 2 of the 4 CNS regions:	• Brainstem • Cervical • Thoracic • Lumbosacral	≥1 muscle; i.e., tongue, face, jaw ≥2 limb muscles innervated by different roots/peripheral nerves paraspinal region below T6 or abdominal muscles ≥2 limb muscles innervated by different roots/peripheral nerves
Other electrophysiological testing		
Somatosensory evoked potentials	Normal	Evoked response latencies greater than 20% above ULN
Autonomic testing	Normal	Significant abnormality
Electronystagmography	Normal	Significant abnormality

CMAP, compound muscle action potential; CV, conduction velocity; LLN, lower limit of normal; ULN, upper limit of normal.
*Signs of active denervation: fibrillation potentials; positive sharp waves; signs of chronic denervation: large MUP; reduced recruitment (firing rates of individual potentials >10 Hz), unstable MUP (Figure 14.3C); fasciculation potentials not required, but absence raises doubts regarding diagnosis [340].

involvement in ALS as a measure of disease progression. In patients with clinical evidence of UMN pathology, EMG can aid in confirming whether the patient has associated LMN involvement in order to distinguish ALS, in which signs of motor denervation are characteristic, from PLS, in which EMG is expected to show no evidence of motor denervation [9, 134].

Nerve conduction studies are an essential companion to EMG in establishing the diagnosis of ALS or PLS and investigating other possible diagnoses. General guidelines for interpretation of nerve conduction abnormalities in ALS have been published [150–152, 154]. Phrenic nerve conduction studies have been suggested as a prognostic indicator in ALS, but have not been fully validated for routine clinical application [155].

Central nervous system magnetic stimulation techniques Central motor conduction time (CMCT) and motor evoked potentials (MEP) have been studied as a potential means to identify UMN pathology in ALS and PLS. These techniques may provide evidence of UMN pathology in PLS and ALS, but may be more sensitive to the primary pathology in PLS than ALS [156–159]. Longitudinal data on CMCT or MEP as a measure of disease progression in these disorders are few and conflicting [160, 161]. Neither method is clearly established as a potential biomarker for disease progression.

Cortical hyperexcitability is a recognized feature of UMN involvement in ALS, and transcranial magnetic stimulation has been applied to evaluate the cortical silent period, the interval between repeated stimulation during which the cortex remains inexcitable [77, 162]. Reduced cortical silent period in ALS may represent a biomarker of UMN pathology in ALS but requires further validation [156, 163].

Motor unit estimates Motor unit estimates (MUNE) refers to neurophysiological techniques developed for quantification of the number of motor units in skeletal muscles [164, 165]. MUNE

is reported to have acceptable repeatability and correlate with disease progression in line with other standardized outcome measures of ALS, but has not been established as a standard outcome measure and remains primarily investigational [166, 167]. MUNE is not considered a useful surrogate biomarker in PLS given that it is fundamentally a measure of LMN pathology [166].

Neurophysiological index The neurophysiological index (NI) is a derivation of three neurophysiological measurements routinely performed during motor nerve conduction studies [168]. The NI has been held to represent effects of motor axonal degeneration and resulting denervation and reinnervation, as well as the electrical excitability of anterior horn cells, serving as an LMN biomarker, but the measure has yet to be fully validated [160, 168, 169].

Electrical impedance myography Electrical impedance myography (EIM) measures electrical impedance of skeletal muscle using surface electrodes and application of high-frequency direct current [170]. The procedure appears to be reproducible in experienced hands in longitudinal studies and is essentially painless. Recent studies suggest that impedance measurements may provide a surrogate measure of LMN pathology in ALS, but EIM is not yet established as a longitudinal biomarker in ALS, and there are no published data available on its role in PLS [171, 172].

Neuroimaging

Central nervous system imaging MRI of the brain and spine has a central role in initial evaluation and diagnosis of ALS and PLS, primarily to rule out disease mimics [173]. Advanced magnetic resonance-based techniques have demonstrated promise in the development of surrogate biomarkers of UMN and extra motor pathology in ALS and PLS but remain largely investigational [174–177].

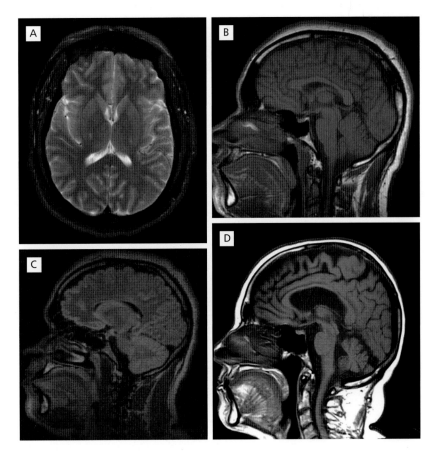

Figure 14.4 Examples of MRI findings in the brain in patients with ALS. (A) Symmetrically increased signal in the corticospinal tract in a fluid attenuated inversion recovery (FLAIR) image in a 40-year-old man with clinically definite ALS of 10 months' duration (axial view at the level of the posterior limb of the internal capsule). Clinical findings included prominent UMN signs in the upper and lower limbs. (B) Atrophy of the posterior corpus callosum with relative sparing of the splenium in a T1-weighted sagittal image of the same patient depicted in (A). (C) Hyperintensity in the corpus callosum corresponding to the region of atrophy shown in (B) demonstrated in a T2-weighted sagittal image. (D) Frontotemporal atrophy in a T1-weighted image in a 61-year-old woman with ALS and FTD of 2 years' duration (sagittal view).

Structural imaging with proton density brain MRI in ALS and PLS may reveal increased signal in the corticospinal tract with T2-weighted and fluid attenuated inversion recovery (FLAIR) sequence imaging, although this phenomenon also may be seen in normal individuals (Figure 14.4) [178]. Callosal atrophy attributed to loss of motor crossing fibers in the cerebral hemispheres may also be observed (Figure 14.4) [174]. T2-weighted and FLAIR imaging may demonstrate hypointensity (motor dark line) in the motor cortex which has been associated with UMN involvement and is attributed to iron accumulation, although this too may be seen in normal subjects [178]. Atrophy of the precentral gyrus may be detected in PLS and ALS with significant UMN involvement, but generally requires quantitative morphometric analysis and is of limited clinical utility [178]. Frontotemporal atrophy may be seen on proton density MRI in patients with ALS or PLS and FTD, especially in advanced disease (Figure 14.4) [179–183].

Advanced MRI techniques involving computer-based analysis of imaging data are emerging as potential means to noninvasively examine cerebral spinal motor and extra motor regions and pathways in ALS and PLS [174–177]. Diffusion tensor imaging, voxel-based morphometry, resting functional MRI, magnetization transfer imaging, and magnetic resonance spectroscopy hold promise in ALS biomarker development, but more work is needed to advance sensitivity and specificity beyond group level analysis to the level of individual patients [174, 176, 177]. Limitations of these techniques include physical barriers to patients who are unable to remain supine for completion of imaging protocols and relatively high cost [184].

Diffusion tensor imaging (DTI) provides information on the structural integrity of white matter by assessing the directional

movement of water in neural circuits [178]. Water in normal nerve tissue demonstrates highly confined directional movement, or anisotropy; it is more diffusible, or isotropic, in damaged axonal tracts [178]. Quantitation of diffusion anisotropy by DTI is typically by a measure referred to as fractional anisotropy (FA) [174, 176, 184]. Reviews of DTI and its application in ALS are available [174, 175, 178, 185, 186]. An association between rate of disease progression and decreased FA in the corticospinal tract is reported in ALS and in PLS [187–191]. Whole brain DTI in ALS and PLS demonstrated differences in the distribution of white matter pathology in the two conditions (Figure 14.5) [192]. DTI in conjunction with voxel-based morphometry provides support for the concept of ALS as a multisystem disorder with callosal pathology as a consistent feature of ALS [193–195].

Computer-based analysis of three-dimensional changes in brain volume obtained by MRI, referred to as voxel-based morphometry, or VBM, has allowed identification of even minor degrees of regional atrophy and changes in motor and non-motor gray and white matter regions in ALS and PLS (Figure 14.6) [196–199]. VBM studies in ALS and PLS have demonstrated decreased brain volume in primary motor cortex and the cortical spinal tract, as well as in frontotemporal regions in patients with FTD [196–198, 200]. Early data suggest that VBM, performed in combination with other advanced MRI methods such as resting functional MRI or DTI, in ALS and PLS may enhance information collected with either technique alone [201, 202].

Functional MRI (fMRI), based on blood oxygen level-dependent T2-weighted MRI, allows noninvasive investigation of brain cortical activity in patients with ALS and PLS by means of stimulation

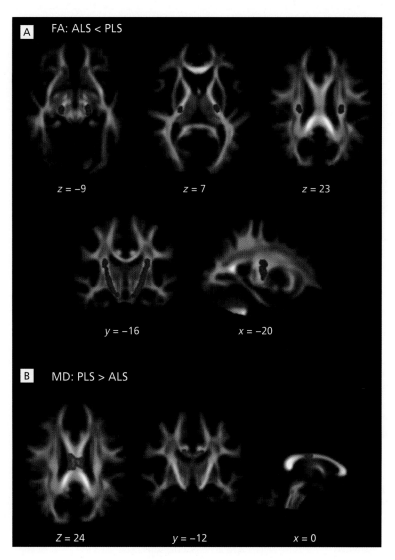

Figure 14.5 Example of tract based spatial analysis (TBSS) of images obtained with DTI, comparing findings in patients with ALS with those with PLS. TBSS analysis of clusters of voxels with significantly lower fractional anisotropy (FA) (red) in (A) patients with ALS compared with patients with primary lateral sclerosis (PLS), and significantly greater mean diffusivity (MD) (blue) in (B) patients with primary lateral sclerosis compared with patients with ALS in selected axial, coronal, and sagittal sections (P50.05), corrected for multiple comparisons across space (FWE) using threshold-free cluster enhancement. MNI coordinates are shown. Images are displayed in radiological convention (right brain on left side). Imaging data in this study suggest that white matter pathology involves the distal intracranial portion of the corticospinal tract in ALS (red), while abnormalities in PLS involve mainly the subcortical white matter underlying the motor cortex (blue). Source: Iwata et al. 2011 [192]. Reproduced with permission of Oxford University Press.

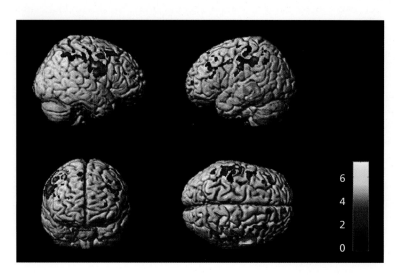

Figure 14.6 Brain cortical atrophy demonstrated by VBM imaging in patients with ALS compared to control subjects. Regional gray matter atrophy in ALS patients compared to controls. Group comparison of 17 ALS patients versus 17 healthy controls showed regional gray matter atrophy in the precentral and postcentral gyrus bilaterally, extending from the primary motor cortex to premotor, parietal, and frontal regions bilaterally (displayed at P = .001, uncorrected, extended threshold 100 voxels). The color bar represents the T-score indicating statistical significance; white–yellow is highest significance. The differences between the groups are superimposed on a standard normalized T1-weighted image. Images are shown in neurological convention. Views displayed are right hemisphere (upper left), left hemisphere (upper right), anterior (lower left), and superior (lower left). Source: Grosskreutz [328], http://bmcneurol.biomedcentral.com/articles/10.1186/1471-2377-6-17. Used under CC BY 2.0 http://creativecommons.org/licenses/by/2.0/.

paradigms intended to activate specific brain regions [176]. Resulting shifts in blood flow in response to neuronal activation produce a signal change, referred to as the blood oxygenated level-dependent effect, which is detectable on MRI and indicates activation of the involved brain region (Figure 14.7) [176]. fMRI has provided evidence of frontotemporal involvement in ALS with FTD and lesser degrees of cognitive impairment [203]. Resting state fMRI, a modification of fMRI performed with the patient at rest, identified reduced activation in multiple premotor frontal brain regions linked to executive dysfunction and changes in premotor cortical activation in ALS [184, 204]. Further developments include combined collection data using fMRI and VBM, DTI, or VBM plus DTI, to investigate structural changes and functional alterations in neuronal circuits [202, 205, 206].

MRI incorporating a spin-echo sequence with a magnetization transfer (MT) pulse on T1-weighted images may show in MND patients with UMN involvement a hyperintensity of the corticospinal tract that appears to attenuate in advanced disease [178, 207, 208]. Recent data on MT and DTI suggest that the two imaging methods may offer enhanced sensitivity in the quantitative assessment of white matter pathology in ALS and PLS [208, 209].

Proton (¹H) magnetic resonance spectroscopy (MRS) allows quantitative assessment of the levels of brain metabolites in a defined region of interest (ROI) [176]. Commonly studied metabolites include *N*-acetyl aspartate (NAA), a marker for neuronal damage, choline (Cho), a marker of cell proliferation and membrane turnover, and creatine (CR), which reflects tissue energy state [176]. Proton MRS in ALS has been reported to show reduced NAA concentration or a reduced NAA/Cho, NAA/Cr, or NAA/Cho+Cr ratio in motor cortex, interpreted as representing loss of motor neurons [176, 210, 211]. Studies with proton MRS in ALS patients have found associations between NAA concentration in motor cortex and

disease severity, as well as UMN signs and survival [176]. High field strength proton MRS at 3 Tesla is reported to allow quantitation of metabolites such as γ-aminobutyric acid (GABA) that are not readily detected at lower field strengths [212, 213]. Although promising, proton MRS is limited by lack of standardization in data acquisition and variations in analytic methodology among users [174, 178, 184].

Muscle ultrasonography Muscle ultrasonography may be useful in the evaluation of skeletal muscle signs corresponding to motor denervation in ALS and appears to be a sensitive indicator of fasciculations in ALS [214–216]. No published data are available on the utility of muscle ultrasonography in monitoring for signs of disease progression.

Evaluation of respiratory function

Several measures of pulmonary function have been evaluated as potential indicators of respiratory function for therapeutic decision-making and assessment of prognosis.

Forced vital capacity (FVC) and slow vital capacity (SVC) have been used as outcome measures in ALS therapeutic trials [16, 217]. Maximal inspiratory pressure (MIP), also called maximal respiratory force (MIF), may be decreased at baseline, and may predict survival [217]. Inability to form an adequate seal on the mouthpiece, impaired voluntary control of inspiration owing to muscle weakness or apraxia, and cognitive deficit may produce inconsistent test results [217].

Nasal sniff inspiratory pressure (SNIP) is predictive of survival and published data are available on normal values in ALS [217–219]. SNIP is more readily performed by patients with bulbar weakness, but reliability may be compromised by apraxia or cognitive impairment [217].

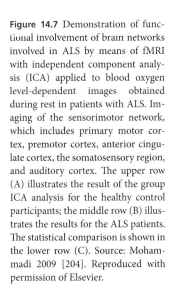

Figure 14.7 Demonstration of functional involvement of brain networks involved in ALS by means of fMRI with independent component analysis (ICA) applied to blood oxygen level-dependent images obtained during rest in patients with ALS. Imaging of the sensorimotor network, which includes primary motor cortex, premotor cortex, anterior cingulate cortex, the somatosensory region, and auditory cortex. The upper row (A) illustrates the result of the group ICA analysis for the healthy control participants; the middle row (B) illustrates the results for the ALS patients. The statistical comparison is shown in the lower row (C). Source: Mohammadi 2009 [204]. Reproduced with permission of Elsevier.

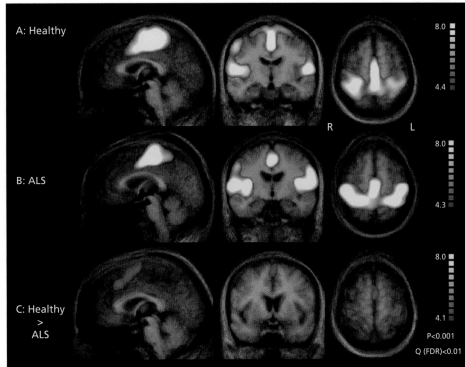

Global functional assessment

Quantitative functional assessment allows systematic evaluation of the patient's ability to perform activities of daily living. Rating scales developed and validated in ALS include the Norris Scale, the Appel Scale, and the ALS Functional Rating Scale [220, 221]. The ALS functional rating scale (ALSFRS) is the most widely used in ALS clinical trials, presently in a revised form (Table 14.7) [222, 223]. Decline in the ALSFRS-R score is generally linear, and consensus data on the clinical significance of change of decline in the ALSFRS-R have been published [224–226].

Assessment of cognitive function

Frontotemporal cognitive impairment is a manifestation of the neurodegenerative process in a subset of patients with ALS and PLS [37, 42]. Formal neuropsychological evaluation is reviewed elsewhere in this volume. Cognitive screening instruments practical for routine use in the ALS and PLS population have been proposed, but validation data are limited for most of these; controlling for motor deficits that impact test performance is a challenge [42].

Examination and investigations

Once the diagnosis of ALS is suspected, the evaluation begins with the clinical examination. The two primary objectives of the clinical examination are documentation of neurological signs supportive of the diagnosis and investigation for atypical features that may raise suspicion for a mimic syndrome. While there are no pathognomonic features on the clinical examination, in the proper clinical setting, the identification of the typical UMN and LMN features diffusely and in the absence of atypical features is strongly suggestive of ALS.

While examining for the supportive features of ALS, one has to remember that the pathology of ALS represents a mixture of degeneration within the upper and lower motor neurons. Degeneration of the LMNs is associated with the hallmark features of muscle weakness, atrophy, and fasciculations. Degeneration of the UMNs is associated with the hallmark features of spasticity, slowness of fine motor movements, and hyperreflexia. With the current El Escorial diagnostic criteria (Table 14.2), each region (bulbar, cervical, thoracic, and lumbar) should be examined carefully for each of these features [13].

Table 14.7 ALS Functional Rating Scale – revised version (ALSFRS-R).

1. SPEECH
4 normal speech processes
3 detectable speech disturbance
2 intelligible with repeating
1 speech combined with non-vocal communication
0 loss of useful speech

2. SALIVATION
4 normal
3 slight but definite excess of saliva in mouth, may have nighttime drooling
2 moderately excessive saliva, may have minimal drooling
1 marked excess of saliva with some drooling
0 marked drooling, requires constant tissue

3. SWALLOWING
4 normal eating habits
3 early eating problems, occasional choking
2 dietary consistency changes
1 needs supplemental tube feedings
0 NPO (exclusively parenteral or enteral feedings)

4. HANDWRITING
4 normal
3 slow or sloppy, all words legible
2 not all words legible
1 able to grip pen, unable to write
0 unable to grip pen

5a. CUTTING FOOD AND HANDLING UTENSILS
(patients without gastrostomy)
4 normal
3 somewhat slow and clumsy, needs no help
2 can cut most foods, slow or clumsy, some help needed
1 foods cut by someone else, can still feed slowly
0 needs to be fed

5b. CUTTING FOOD AND HANDLING UTENSILS
(patients with gastrostomy)
4 normal
3 clumsy, able to perform all manipulations
2 some help needed with closures and fasteners
1 provides minimal assistance to caregiver
0 unable to perform any aspect of task

6. DRESSING AND HYGIENE
4 normal
3 independent self-care with effort or decreased efficiency
2 intermittent assistance or substitute methods
1 needs attendant for self-care
0 total dependence

7. TURNING IN BED AND ADJUSTING BEDCLOTHES
4 normal
3 somewhat slow or clumsy, needs no help
2 can turn alone or adjust sheets with great difficulty
1 can initiate, cannot turn or adjust sheets
0 helpless

8. WALKING
4 normal
3 early ambulation difficulties
2 walks with assistance
1 non-ambulatory functional movement only
0 no purposeful leg movement

9. CLIMBING STAIRS
4 normal
3 slow
2 mild unsteadiness or fatigue
1 needs assistance
0 cannot do

10. DYSPNEA
4 none
3 occurs when walking
2 occurs with one or more: eating, bathing, dressing
1 occurs at rest, either sitting or lying
0 significant difficulty, considering mechanical support

11. ORTHOPNEA
4 none
3 some difficulty sleeping, due to shortness of breath, does not routinely use more than two pillows
2 needs extra pillows to sleep (>2)
1 can only sleep sitting up
0 unable to sleep

12. RESPIRATORY INSUFFICIENCY
4 none
3 intermittent use of NIV
2 continuous use of NIV at night
1 continuous use of NIV day and night
0 invasive mechanical ventilation by intubation/trach

Total Score: /48

NIV, noninvasive ventilation.
Source: Cedarbaum 1999 [222]. Reproduced with permission of Elsevier.

While clinical involvement of the genioglossus is commonly known to occur in ALS, the UMN and LMN degeneration is clinically manifest in a number of bulbar muscles. The genioglossus should be inspected for weakness, atrophy, fasciculations, and slowed movements. Inspection for fasciculations should be attempted with the muscle relaxed, which may be difficult in some circumstances. The jaw jerk reflex should be examined looking for supportive evidence of UMN involvement. Likewise, the patient may exhibit a pseudobulbar affect which should be noted and considered a UMN sign.

Each of the limbs should be inspected for muscle atrophy and fasciculations in addition to examination of strength and reflexes. In the upper extremity, the hands should be examined for the presence of Hoffman's reflex, which represents an exaggerated finger flexor reflex. In the lower extremity, the ankle should be tested for clonus and the foot for the Babinski sign, both pathological reflexes supportive of a UMN process. Muscle tone and the rate of fine motor movements should also be evaluated in the upper and lower extremities. Because LMN degeneration may mask or diminish the upper motor signs, these must be examined carefully, as the UMN features may be more subtle. For example, the reflexes may be diminished in amplitude but still demonstrate pathological spread to other regional reflexes.

Finally the gait should be inspected for signs of a spastic gait (limb circumduction and scissoring of the steps). Also evident may be a foot drop or gastrocnemius weakness with difficulty on heel walking.

Beyond identifying supportive motor signs, it is important to look for associated cognitive features that may occur in ALS. At a minimum, the subject should undergo a brief cognitive screen looking for evidence of executive or language dysfunction, which may be suggestive of the overlap syndrome of ALS with frontotemporal dementia.

The presence of a pure UMN syndrome (PLS) or pure LMN syndrome deserves further attention with a more comprehensive investigation to exclude central and neuromuscular mimic syndromes. In some cases, the distribution of the weakness may suggest an alternative diagnosis. For example, an LMN syndrome that preferentially affects the distribution of the radial nerve, or other individual peripheral nerve, should raise suspicion for multifocal motor neuropathy, a rare but treatable disorder that may be mistaken for ALS. Weakness preferentially affecting the flexor digitorum profundus, flexor pollicis profundus, and quadriceps muscles in the absence of fasciculations or UMN features would be suggestive of inclusion body myositis. In some cases, an LMN-only syndrome is identified that otherwise fulfills the diagnostic criteria for MND without an apparent alternative diagnosis. These cases have been referred to as progressive muscular atrophy (PMA). Presently, most neuromuscular physicians consider PMA to be a phenotypic variant of ALS associated with a more benign prognosis.

UMN-only syndromes should raise suspicion for a central nervous system disorder, and central inflammatory, structural, vascular malformation, and genetic spastic disorders should be considered. A progressive UMN-only syndrome for which no alternative cause exists supports a diagnosis of PLS. PLS may be considered a phenotypic variant of ALS, and typically carries a more benign prognosis. The EMG is important in distinguishing PLS from UMN-predominant ALS. In cases of PLS, the EMG will not demonstrate any LMN findings, in contrast to UMN- predominant ALS, where LMN features may only be identified on EMG.

The sensory system should be interrogated carefully. While a minority of ALS cases may complain of sensory symptoms, few demonstrate objective sensory loss. In the presence of sensory loss, an alternative diagnosis should be carefully sought.

Further investigation beyond the clinical examination is directed by the findings on the examination. The most important ancillary tests in suspected cases of ALS are nerve conduction studies and needle EMG. Sensory and motor nerve conduction studies should be performed in an area of clinical involvement and if abnormal should be extended to other limbs to determine the distribution of the abnormalities. Sensory involvement on EMG should raise suspicion for alternative etiologies. Signs of motor conduction block would raise suspicion for multifocal motor neuropathy. If there is a high clinical suspicion for multifocal motor neuropathy and standard motor nerve conduction studies are unrevealing, examination of proximal segments at the plexus or nerve root may be considered. Nerve conduction evidence of a peripheral demyelinating neuropathy also would raise suspicion for a diagnosis other than ALS.

Needle EMG should be initiated within a region of clinical involvement. Each muscle should be examined for evidence of abnormal spontaneous activity (fibrillation and fasciculation potentials). When examining for fasciculation potentials, it is helpful to place the needle within the muscle, have the subject relax the muscle, and listen for an extended period of time, such as 20 seconds, before moving on with the examination. Each muscle should also be evaluated during light activation. With activation the muscle should be inspected for signs of denervation: long-duration, high-amplitude, and complex motor unit potentials that are firing at excessively high frequencies. Motor unit potentials in ALS commonly demonstrate marked variation, indicative of the ongoing denervation with unstable reinnervation. The El Escorial diagnostic criteria call for examination of these features in muscles within the cervical, thoracic, and lumbar regions, and examination of bulbar muscles if there are bulbar signs and/or symptoms and the subject does not fully meet the El Escorial criteria after needle examination of other regions.

Beyond EMG, imaging studies are the next most informative ancillary tests. While not all patients require imaging of the central nervous system, given the gravity of the diagnosis one should have a low threshold to image clinically affected regions and rostrally if UMN features are apparent. MRI aids in excluding central inflammatory, structural, and vascular lesions.

Although there are no specific guidelines for additional diagnostic testing, blood, CSF, and urine testing should be guided by the clinical presentation. There have been considerable attempts in recent years to identify a sensitive and specific biomarker for ALS [227–233]. Thus far, these attempts have not yielded a reliable clinical test for the diagnosis of ALS. As a result, there is no confirmatory laboratory test at this time. Ancillary testing is indicated to exclude the mimic syndromes.

The evaluation of predominantly UMN motor syndromes should be directed at excluding other myelopathic and pseudobulbar syndromes. This should include examination of the CSF for inflammatory markers such as total nucleated cell counts, total protein, IgG index and synthesis rates, and oligoclonal banding. While these are not specific, in their presence the diagnosis of primary progressive multiple sclerosis would need to be considered as an alternative. Infectious agents associated with chronic myelopathy, such as HTLV I or II, should be sought. If a family history is present, genetic testing for hereditary spastic paraparesis and very long chain fatty acids for adrenomyeloneuropathy should be considered if there is lower limb onset.

In predominantly LMN syndromes, CSF should also be considered with similar inflammatory markers, mainly to exclude an inflammatory polyradiculopathy as can be seen in autoimmune syndromes such as Sjögren's syndrome or sarcoidosis. Consideration should be given to examining the serum for ganglioside antibodies; while a minority of ALS cases will have modest titers to ganglioside antibodies, markedly elevated titers are suggestive of multifocal motor neuropathy [234]. Serum should also be examined for evidence of a monoclonal protein, as lymphoproliferative disorders such as POEMS syndrome may present with an axonal polyradiculopathy, and this may be suggested by the presence of a monoclonal protein in the blood or urine [235]. If a monoclonal protein is detected, additional studies with X-rays of the long bones (searching for osteosclerotic lesions), abdominal fat aspirate (searching for amyloid deposition), and a bone marrow biopsy (searching for evidence of a lymphoproliferative disorder) should be considered.

In classical presentations of ALS with mixed UMN and LMN features, it is debatable how much additional work-up is necessary. Case reports of ALS phenotypes in hyperparathyroidism have suggested that elevated serum calcium warrants examination of serum parathyroid levels, and isolated reports of hexosaminidase deficiency with an ALS phenotype have suggested that hexosaminidase level may be appropriate as well, but no recent reviews have been completed to examine the true yield of such investigations.

Approximately 5–10% of all ALS cases are familial [236]. In recent years, the number of genes known to be responsible for Mendelian inherited ALS has grown, so that now a genetic mutation can be identified in over 50% of familial cases [81]. Clinical testing for several of these genes is available. It is strongly suggested that genetic testing be performed only at the request of the individual and only after that person has undergone appropriate genetic counseling to fully understand the implications of both a positive and negative test.

Diagnosis and prognosis

Diagnosis
ALS and PLS are clinical diagnoses, and presently no single diagnostic test can establish whether a person has or does not have ALS or PLS. Three basic criteria must be met to make a diagnosis of ALS: (i) progressive weakness, (ii) combined UMN and LMN signs, and (iii) no alternative disorder or combination of disorders that might possibly account for the clinical presentation. For PLS, the criteria differ only in that there should be UMN signs and no LMN signs. Clinical history and neurologic examination provide the information necessary to determine if the patient meets the first two criteria. History and physical findings aid in evaluating support for the third criterion, but differential diagnosis generally calls for further confirmation through diagnostic tests, as discussed in the section Examination and diagnostic evaluation.

ALS is a devastating diagnosis that should be given in person, under proper circumstances [237]. If the patient has a spouse or significant other, it is best to offer the patient the opportunity to have that person attend the visit, with adequate time allowed to explain the diagnosis of ALS and answer questions free of interruptions, in terms the patient can understand, avoiding information overload. The patient should be offered literature concerning ALS and contact information for organizations that provide support services for ALS patients. It is important to convey a sense of hope, with reassurance that ALS clinics are available to provide specialized care in conjunction with continuing care with the primary neurologist, and that ALS research is ongoing and that new medications for treating ALS are being evaluated.

It is also necessary to plan for what to tell the patient suspected of having MND who does not have enough clinical signs to make

the diagnosis of ALS, as may occur if the patient is evaluated soon after onset of symptoms. Such presentations include solely LMN, UMN, or bulbar abnormalities, in which case the diagnosis must be left as uncertain with plans to follow the patient and reassess. Such patients may have early ALS or another form of MND, including PMA, PBP, or PLS. These other forms of MND are usually diagnosed when the patient has been followed for several years and the typical signs of ALS have not developed.

Prognosis
Progressive degeneration of UMNs and LMNs in ALS leads to progressive, severe disability owing to diffuse skeletal muscle paresis, typically culminating in life-threatening complications of respiratory muscle weakness. More than 50% of patients die within 3 years of onset, but close to 10% may survive beyond 8 years [2]. The time course for patients with PMA, a purely LMN disorder, and PBP, which may have UMN and/or LMN features, appears to be similar to that of ALS [7, 238]. The clinical course of PLS, characterized by purely UMN features, usually results in diffuse skeletal muscle weakness and spasticity that generally evolves over a longer time course than ALS, and it is reported that patients with classical ALS in whom UMN signs predominate also appear to have a longer disease course [1, 8].

Survival is improved if the patient opts for mechanical ventilatory support and/or a gastrostomy feeding tube [239–241]. Better prognosis is reported with age less than 55 years, limb onset, presentation with purely LMN or purely UMN signs, as in PLS, absence of pulmonary symptoms at onset, minimal fasciculations, and relatively mild motor impairment and/or extended time from symptom onset to diagnosis [242, 243]. Poor prognosis is associated with shortened time from symptom onset to diagnosis, rapid progression of early ALS symptoms, rapid decline of pulmonary function, and presence of frontotemporal dementia [244–247]. About 10% of patients with ALS survive 10 years or more [248]. Survival in excess of three decades is reported, but prolonged survival does not necessarily equate with milder disability, as patients with severe impairment may experience extended survival [243]. Spontaneous improvement of ALS is reported but is rare [249]. LMN features predominated in these cases, and none had bulbar involvement; whether these patients in fact had ALS or a clinically similar disorder remains unresolved [243].

Treatment

Medical management

Medications
The search for safe and effective treatments in ALS has been disappointing. Despite the numerous clinical trials conducted in the past 15 years, only one agent, riluzole, has demonstrated any efficacy in prolonging survival in ALS subjects. The results of the first riluzole trial were first published in 1994 [250]. This study demonstrated a modest prolongation of survival. Independent clinical trials confirmed a modest mean survival benefit of about 4 months [251]. In these studies, there was a dose-dependent response with the optimal dose being 50 mg twice daily. On the strength of these studies, the US Federal Drug Administration (FDA) approved the use of riluzole in ALS in 1996. This ushered in a new era of interest in drug development for ALS. The mechanism of action of riluzole is not fully understood but is believed to inhibit the release of glutamate

and theoretically slow excitotoxicity [250]. However, clinical trials with other agents believed to reduce the effects of glutamate excitation have failed to demonstrate benefit [252, 253]. Other studies with drugs directed at alternative pathways have been equally disappointing. These have included neurotrophic factors, vitamin and nutritional supplements, anti-inflammatory agents, and, more recently, lithium [254–258]. A prime contributor to the failure of these clinical trials is the fundamental lack of understanding of the pathophysiology of the disease.

Treatment of ALS is otherwise directed at symptomatic relief. Guidelines to therapy appear in the published ALS practice parameter [219, 237]. While no Class I evidence exists in support of these symptomatic therapies in ALS, the use of these medications is supported by clinical practice. Options for treatment of spasticity include diazepam, baclofen, and tizanidine [259–261]. These medications should be used cautiously because at higher doses they may actually weaken the muscles. Intrathecal baclofen administered via an implantable pump is a consideration in patients with an extended clinical course dominated by spasticity in whom oral agents are ineffective or poorly tolerated [261, 262]. Options for sialorrhea include anticholinergics such as amitriptyline or glycopyrrolate. Subjects having difficulty clearing tracheal secretions may benefit from transdermal scopolamine. If these are not sufficient, reports have suggested benefit from botulinum toxin to the salivary glands or irradiation of the salivary glands [263–266]. These latter two treatments can be complicated by deterioration in swallowing and should only be considered as a last option in subjects where sialorrhea is a major quality of life issue and subjects who already possess a percutaneous endoscopic gastrostomy (PEG) tube, in case the subject's dysphasia is worsened.

Pseudobulbar affect is a troubling symptom in some cases of ALS. The symptom of emotional lability can most easily be treated with amitriptyline, though no Class 1 evidence exists for this indication, and it is an off-label use. A study with the combination drug dextromethorphan/quinidine has demonstrated its efficacy with pseudobulbar palsy in trials [149, 267, 268]. The FDA has approved the use of this combination drug for this indication in ALS. Use of this drug is expensive, and it is not clear that its efficacy is superior to the traditional treatments. It also carries some risk of cardiac arrhythmia [268]. It is this author's opinion that its use be limited to those who have not responded to the traditional options.

Pulmonary management

Respiratory care for ALS patients includes ventilatory support and management of secretions, and the patient's decision regarding mechanical ventilation is central to the approach taken [237]. As the respiratory muscles weaken, the options for maintaining ventilation include noninvasive ventilation (NIV) and tracheostomy with mechanical ventilation (TMV). Survival time is improved with use of NIV [269–271] or TMV [272]. Acceptance by patients and caregivers of noninvasive ventilation tends to be greater than ventilation by tracheostomy [237]. The optimal time for starting NIV is not established; the majority of ALS patients on TMV begin this because of an emergency need precipitated by ventilatory failure [273]. American Academy of Neurology practice parameters for the care of people with ALS recommend that NIV be offered if forced vital capacity (FVC) falls to <50% of the predicted value or maximal inspiratory pressure (MIP) to <−60 cmH$_2$O, nocturnal oxygen desaturation is <88% for 5 consecutive minutes on overnight oximetry, or development of orthopnea [219]. Medicare guidelines for

medical necessity of NIV also include hypercarbia with PaCO$_2$ ≥ 45 mmHg [274]. TMV is indicated if the patient on NIV is unable to maintain pO$_2$ >90%, pCO$_2$ <50 or inability to control oral secretions establishes an ongoing aspiration risk [219].

Devices used for NIV may be pressure limited or volume limited, with some equipment capable of operating in either mode [275]. Bi-level positive airway pressure (PAP) machines with pressure levels set for inspiration and expiration are the most widely used. Volume-limited machines deliver a specified tidal volume by automatically titrating the pressure needed to deliver the required air volume. The interface worn by the patient to receive air from the NIV machine, typically held in place by elastic straps, must be tight enough to ensure adequate air delivery; many styles of facemasks and nasal interfaces are available. A period of adjustment may be required, from initial brief utilization to full application as prescribed based on respiratory status. Most patients begin using NIV at night to improve orthopnea; daytime use generally becomes routine as respiratory muscles become weaker.

Weakness of the oropharyngeal and respiratory muscles leads to difficulty clearing secretions from the airway and reduced cough strength. Management includes medications and physical measures to aid clearance of secretions. Medications for management of increased oral secretions, or sialorrhea, are discussed in the section Medications. Alternatively, patients may complain of thick secretions that are difficult to clear, which, if not resolved by attention to hydration, may respond to mucolytic agents such as guaifenesin or acetylcysteine [219]. A handheld suction device can also help to clear unwanted oropharyngeal secretions. Additional methods for physical clearance of excess secretions include chest percussions and postural drainage, but the technique is labor intensive for the caregiver, and the patient may have difficulty with proper positioning owing to weakness. Mechanical insufflation/exsufflation (MIE) generates a positive–negative air flow cycle via a facemask to assist a natural cough and promote clearance of airway secretions, and may improve peak cough flow rate [276]. High-frequency chest wall oscillations administered via a vest may facilitate clearance of airway secretions but effectiveness is not fully established in ALS or PLS [277, 278]. Air-stacking, an exercise in which the patient takes in a breath, holds it, and then sequentially adds additional breaths to inflate the lungs as much as possible may facilitate generation of a more effective cough, and is reported to increase inspired volume by up to 20% [279].

Nutrition

Nutrition is an independent predictor of survival in ALS, and multiple factors contribute to nutritional compromise in ALS, including effects of the disease on metabolism and motor deficits [280, 281]. Weight loss can occur as an early sign in MND owing to oropharyngeal weakness; 25–30% of patients have bulbar weakness as a presenting sign, and nearly all patients eventually experience dysphagia [138, 280, 282–284]. A videofluoroscopic swallowing study may help to determine food textures that can be consumed safely but is not essential to establish the presence of dysphagia [219].

Management strategies for nutrition in ALS and PLS include dietary modification to ensure that nutritional needs are met, physical maneuvers to reduce aspiration risk during swallowing (i.e., chin tuck), and PEG feeding [2]. Consideration of percutaneous gastrostomy (i.e., PEG or percutaneous radiologic gastrostomy [PRG]), is warranted for loss of body weight exceeding 10% from premorbid body weight or BMI less than 18 kg/m^2[240, 280, 285]. Early patient education regarding the rationale for PEG/PRG tube placement may help to establish acceptance of the procedure, and it is appropriate to make the patient aware that a feeding tube does not necessarily eliminate oral feeding [219]. Risks of PEG/PRG placement include laryngeal spasm, infection at the site of tube placement, bleeding, failure of tube insertion because of technical difficulties, and death owing to respiratory complications [219]. Patients with significant respiratory muscle weakness (i.e., FVC less than 50% predicted) may be at increased risk for procedure-associated morbidity from gastrostomy tube placement [219]. Uncontrolled case series data suggest that patients with more advanced respiratory muscle weakness (i.e., FVC <40% predicted) may tolerate gastrostomy placement when supported with noninvasive positive pressure ventilation [286–290]. Enteric tube feeding may stabilize weight and body mass and improve survival; impact on quality of life is unclear [219, 280, 285, 291].

There is evidence that patients with ALS are hypermetabolic and that caloric needs may not be accurately predicted based on standard nutritional algorithms [292–299]. Although data on optimal dietary balance in ALS are limited, a recent general guideline advises a high-energy, high-fat diet [300]. Best practices include regular monitoring of body weight and consultations with a dietitian and speech pathologist to individualize the patient's diet to his or her activity level and physical status [280].

Rehabilitation

Rehabilitation is a central component of multidisciplinary care, incorporating occupational, physical, and speech therapy [261, 301, 302]. Dysarthria is a common feature of ALS and PLS, ranging from mildly reduced speech intelligibility to mutism [303]. A speech pathologist can assist the patient and family in adaptive approaches [301, 303, 304]. Electronic communication devices (augmentative, alternative communication [AAC]) are available with speech synthesizer and text display capabilities, with eye tracking and other control systems for patients unable to use a keyboard [303, 304].

An occupational therapist can facilitate management of upper limb and cervical muscle weakness by introducing assistive devices and instruction in adaptive maneuvers to facilitate independence [301, 305]. For gait-impaired patients, evaluation by a physical therapist is indicated for guidance in the selection and use of gait aids, ranging from a cane to a power wheelchair, and for instruction in transfer techniques [301, 305].

Flexibility and strengthening, and aerobic exercises are applicable to the care of people with ALS and PLS, but data in support of exercise therapy are largely anecdotal [301, 305, 306]. Flexibility training may transiently improve spasticity and help limit development of painful joint contractures [301, 307]. The effectiveness of strengthening exercise is not established, but a review concluded that individualizing strengthening exercises may have some therapeutic benefit in early-stage ALS [307]. Individualized aerobic exercise does not appear to be harmful in ALS and PLS, but objective data regarding benefit are not available [301, 307].

Management of spasticity in ALS and PLS includes pharmacological and non-pharmacological approaches, although efficacy data from randomized, controlled clinical trials are limited [260]. Gait stability may be improved with ankle–foot orthoses [301]. Medications are discussed in the section Medication. Data from a randomized trial suggest that a stretching exercise program may improve functional status in ALS [260].

Surgical treatment of ALS and PLS

Surgical interventions directed at the management of complications of ALS and PLS are relatively few. Gastrostomy tube placement is covered in the section Nutrition. Tracheostomy and laryngectomy, baclofen pump implantation, and implantation of an electronic diaphragm pacing device are discussed in this section.

Tracheostomy to facilitate mechanical ventilatory support is an established treatment for ventilatory failure in ALS and potentially for airway protection in patients with severe dysphagia, but is chosen by a minority of patients [217, 283, 308]. Survival with tracheostomy ventilation is indefinite, but median survival in a population-based study in Italy was less than 1 year [309–312]. Total laryngectomy in order to establish a tracheal airway for mechanical ventilation and airway protection in advanced dysphagia may be an alternative to tracheostomy in patients with MND, with potential advantages over tracheostomy owing to surgical closure of the upper airway [313].

Baclofen pump implantation for management of spasticity is an established surgical indication in people with ALS and PLS with disabling spasticity who are unable to tolerate adequate doses of oral antispasticity medications [262, 314]. The risk–benefit profile is favorable [315].

Surgical implantation of an electronic diaphragm pacing device or phrenic nerve stimulation device has been studied in ALS as a means to condition the diaphragm and delay the need for tracheostomy ventilation. However, diaphragm pacing in particular remains controversial owing to conflicting results of clinical trials that have raised questions regarding efficacy, and research to resolve these issues is ongoing [217, 316–321].

Family-based and third-party care of ALS and PLS patients

Patients with ALS and PLS face overwhelming challenges in dealing with progressive loss of motor function, and a number of organizations have been established to provide assistance. The International Alliance of ALS/MND Associations (http://www.alsmndalliance.org/) provides a directory of these organizations, listed by country, that support or facilitate multidisciplinary care and research. Multidisciplinary clinics are an established ALS care model, associated with improved quality of life, reduced hospitalizations, and possibly with improved survival [266, 322–325]. The multidisciplinary care team typically includes a neurologist; nurse; dietitian; speech, respiratory, physical, and occupational therapists; and a social worker, and may include a pulmonologist, psychologist, and chaplain.

Palliative, or end-of-life care, is a component of multidisciplinary care in advanced disease [237, 261]. Palliative care includes management of symptoms stemming from respiratory failure and severe limb and trunk muscle weakness [219, 237, 261, 326]. A role for palliative care in the terminal phase of ALS is recognized in the American Academy of Neurology Practice Parameter for the care of the patient with ALS [219]. Some have proposed that care is enhanced by involvement of palliative care specialists as early as the time of diagnosis, by providing primary continuing care and symptomatic treatment prior to development of terminal complications [326].

Hospice referral, where available, should be offered to patients with advanced disease, whether at home or in hospital, and can significantly improve quality of life during terminal care of ALS [237]. Hospice services in the USA are available to ALS patients when their survival time is estimated to be less than 6 months, typically at the stage of severe weakness and marked functional impairment. In addition to care directed to the patient, including home visits by hospice nurses to deliver and manage medications, assess pain control, and assist with skin and bowel care, hospice support may include psychosocial services that can benefit caregivers as well as the patient [323]. Hospice care is associated with improved quality of life in ALS [237].

References

1. Singer MA, Statland JM, Wolfe GI, et al. Primary lateral sclerosis. *Muscle Nerve.* 2007 Mar;35:291–302.

2. Hardiman O, van den Berg LH, Kiernan MC. Clinical diagnosis and management of amyotrophic lateral sclerosis. *Nat Rev Neurol.* 2011 Nov;7:639–49.

3. Kiernan MC, Vucic S, Cheah BC, et al. Amyotrophic lateral sclerosis. *Lancet.* 2011 Mar 12;377:942–55.

4. Cleveland DW, Rothstein JD. From Charcot to Lou Gehrig: deciphering selective motor neuron death in ALS. *Nat Rev Neurosci.* 2001 Nov;2:806–19.

5. Goldblatt D. Historical introduction. *Motor Neuron Diseases; Research on Amyotrophic Lateral Sclerosis and Related Disorders.* New York: Grune & Stratton, 1969. p. 3–11.

6. Rowland LP, Shneider NA. Amyotrophic lateral sclerosis. *N Engl J Med.* 2001 May 31;344:1688–700.

7. Visser J, van den Berg-Vos RM, Franssen H, et al. Disease course and prognostic factors of progressive muscular atrophy. *Arch Neurol.* 2007 Apr;64:522–8.

8. Strong MJ, Gordon PH. Primary lateral sclerosis, hereditary spastic paraplegia and amyotrophic lateral sclerosis: discrete entities or spectrum? *Amyotroph Lateral Scler Other Motor Neuron Disord.* 2005 Mar;6:8–16.

9. Gordon PH, Cheng B, Katz IB, et al. Clinical features that distinguish PLS, upper motor neuron-dominant ALS, and typical ALS. *Neurology.* 2009 Jun 2;72: 1948–52.

10. Ince PG. Neuropathology. In: Brown RH, Meininger V, Swash M, editors. *Amyotrophic Lateral Sclerosis.* London: Martin Dunitz; 2000. p. 83–112.

11. Ince PG, Evans J, Knopp M, et al. Corticospinal tract degeneration in the progressive muscular atrophy variant of ALS. *Neurology.* 2003 Apr 22;60:1252–8.

12. Norris F, Shepherd R, Denys E, et al. Onset, natural history and outcome in idiopathic adult motor neuron disease. *J Neurol Sci.* 1993 Aug;118:48–55.

13. Brooks BR. El Escorial World Federation of Neurology criteria for the diagnosis of amyotrophic lateral sclerosis. Subcommittee on Motor Neuron Diseases/Amyotrophic Lateral Sclerosis of the World Federation of Neurology Research Group on Neuromuscular Diseases and the El Escorial "Clinical limits of amyotrophic lateral sclerosis" workshop contributors. *J Neurol Sci.* 1994 Jul;124 Suppl:96–107.

14. Brooks BR, Miller RG, Swash M, et al. El Escorial revisited: revised criteria for the diagnosis of amyotrophic lateral sclerosis. *Amyotroph Lateral Scler Other Motor Neuron Disord.* 2000 Dec;1:293–9.

15. Douglass CP, Kandler RH, Shaw PJ, et al. An evaluation of neurophysiological criteria used in the diagnosis of motor neuron disease. *J Neurol Neurosurg Psychiatry.* 2010 Jun;81:646–9.

16. Traynor BJ, Zhang H, Shefner JM, et al. Functional outcome measures as clinical trial endpoints in ALS. *Neurology.* 2004 Nov 23;63:1933–5.

17. Traynor BJ, Codd MB, Corr B, et al. Clinical features of amyotrophic lateral sclerosis according to the El Escorial and Airlie House diagnostic criteria: A population-based study. *Arch Neurol.* 2000 Aug;57:1171–6.

18. Cronin S, Hardiman O, Traynor BJ. Ethnic variation in the incidence of ALS: a systematic review. *Neurology.* 2007 Mar 27;68:1002–7.

19. Hirtz D, Thurman DJ, Gwinn-Hardy K, et al. How common are the "common" neurologic disorders? *Neurology.* 2007 Jan 30;68:326–37.

20. Logroscino G, Traynor BJ, Hardiman O, et al. Incidence of amyotrophic lateral sclerosis in Europe. *J Neurol Neurosurg Psychiatry.* 2010 Apr;81:385–90.

21. Murros K, Fogelholm R. Amyotrophic lateral sclerosis in Middle-Finland: an epidemiological study. *Acta Neurol Scand.* 1983 Jan;67:41–7.

22. Fong KY, Yu YL, Chan YW, et al. Motor neuron disease in Hong Kong Chinese: epidemiology and clinical picture. *Neuroepidemiology.* 1996;15:239–45.

23. Annegers JF, Appel S, Lee JR, et al. Incidence and prevalence of amyotrophic lateral sclerosis in Harris County, Texas, 1985–1988. *Arch Neurol.* 1991 Jun;48: 589–93.

24. Matsumoto N, Worth RM, Kurland LT, et al. Epidemiologic study of amyotrophic lateral sclerosis in Hawaii. Identification of high incidence among Filipino men. *Neurology.* 1972 Sep;22:934–40.

25. McGuire V, Longstreth WT, Jr., Koepsell TD, et al. Incidence of amyotrophic lateral sclerosis in three counties in western Washington state. *Neurology.* 1996 Aug;47:571–3.

26. Noonan CW, White MC, Thurman D, et al. Temporal and geographic variation in United States motor neuron disease mortality, 1969–1998. *Neurology.* 2005 Apr 12;64:1215–21.

27. Zaldivar T, Gutierrez J, Lara G, et al. Reduced frequency of ALS in an ethnically mixed population: a population-based mortality study. *Neurology.* 2009 May 12;72:1640–5.

28. McCombe PA, Henderson RD. Effects of gender in amyotrophic lateral sclerosis. *Gend Med.* 2010 Dec;7:557–70.

29. Kurland LT, Mulder DW. Epidemiologic investigations of amyotrophic lateral sclerosis. 2. Familial aggregations indicative of dominant inheritance. II. *Neurology.* 1955 Apr;5:249–68.

30. Li TM, Alberman E, Swash M. Comparison of sporadic and familial disease amongst 580 cases of motor neuron disease. *J Neurol Neurosurg Psychiatry.* 1988 Jun;51:778–84.

31. Orrell RW, Habgood JJ, Malaspina A, et al. Clinical characteristics of SOD1 gene mutations in UK families with ALS. *J Neurol Sci.* 1999 Oct 31;169:56–60.

32. Beghi E, Millul A, Micheli A, et al. Incidence of ALS in Lombardy, Italy. *Neurology.* 2007 Jan 9;68:141–5.

33. Sabatelli M, Madia F, Conte A, et al. Natural history of young-adult amyotrophic lateral sclerosis. *Neurology.* 2008 Sep 16;71:876–81.

34. Grace GM, Orange JB, Rowe A, et al. Neuropsychological functioning in PLS: a comparison with ALS. *Can J Neurol Sci.* 2011 Jan;38:88–97.

35. Elamin M, Phukan J, Bede P, et al. Executive dysfunction is a negative prognostic indicator in patients with ALS without dementia. *Neurology.* 2011 Apr 5;76: 1263–9.

36. Terada T, Obi T, Yoshizumi M, et al. Frontal lobe-mediated behavioral changes in amyotrophic lateral sclerosis: are they independent of physical disabilities? *J Neurol Sci.* 2011 Oct 15;309:136–40.

37. Phukan J, Elamin M, Bede P, et al. The syndrome of cognitive impairment in amyotrophic lateral sclerosis: a population-based study. *J Neurol Neurosurg Psychiatry.* 2012 Jan;83:102–8.

38. Kiernan MC. Amyotrophic lateral sclerosis and frontotemporal dementia. *J Neurol Neurosurg Psychiatry.* 2012 Apr;83:355.

39. Lomen-Hoerth C, Murphy J, Langmore S, et al. Are amyotrophic lateral sclerosis patients cognitively normal? *Neurology.* 2003 Apr 8;60:1094–7.

40. Giordana MT, Ferrero P, Grifoni S, et al. Dementia and cognitive impairment in amyotrophic lateral sclerosis: a review. *Neurol Sci.* 2011 Feb;32:9–16.

41. Murphy JM, Henry RG, Langmore S, et al. Continuum of frontal lobe impairment in amyotrophic lateral sclerosis. *Arch Neurol.* 2007 Apr;64:530–4.

42. Strong MJ, Grace GM, Freedman M, et al. Consensus criteria for the diagnosis of frontotemporal cognitive and behavioural syndromes in amyotrophic lateral sclerosis. *Amyotroph Lateral Scler.* 2009 Jun;10:131–46.

43. Brugman F, Eymard-Pierre E, van den Berg LH, et al. Adult-onset primary lateral sclerosis is not associated with mutations in the ALS2 gene. *Neurology.* 2007 Aug 14;69:702–4.

44. Casari G, Marconi R. Spastic Paraplegia 7. 1993. GeneReviews®. University of Washington, Seattle.

45. Pringle CE, Hudson AJ, Munoz DG, et al. Primary lateral sclerosis. Clinical features, neuropathology and diagnostic criteria. *Brain.* 1992 Apr;115 (Pt 2):495–520.

46. Le Forestier N, Maisonobe T, Spelle L, et al. Primary lateral sclerosis: further clarification. *J Neurol Sci.* 2001 Apr 1;185:95–100.

47. Singer MA, Kojan S, Barohn RJ, et al. Primary lateral sclerosis: clinical and laboratory features in 25 patients. *J Clin Neuromuscul Dis.* 2005 Sep;7:1–9.

48. Gastaut JL, Bartolomei F. Mills' syndrome: ascending (or descending) progressive hemiplegia: a hemiplegic form of primary lateral sclerosis? *J Neurol Neurosurg Psychiatry.* 1994 Oct;57:1280–1.

49. Hudson AJ, Kiernan JA, Munoz DG, et al. Clinicopathological features of primary lateral sclerosis are different from amyotrophic lateral sclerosis. *Brain Res Bull..* 1993;30:359–64.

50. Younger DS, Chou S, Hays AP, et al. Primary lateral sclerosis. A clinical diagnosis reemerges. *Arch Neurol.* 1988 Dec;45:1304–7.

51. Kojan S, Goodwin W, Bryan W, et al. Clinical and laboratory features of primary lateral sclerosis. *J Child Neurol.* 2000;15:200.

52. Brownell B, Oppenheimer DR, Hughes JT. The central nervous system in motor neurone disease. *J Neurol Neurosurg Psychiatry.* 1970 Jun;33:338–57.

53. Mitchell JD, Borasio GD. Amyotrophic lateral sclerosis. *Lancet.* 2007 Jun 16;369:2031–41.

54. Rothstein JD. Current hypotheses for the underlying biology of amyotrophic lateral sclerosis. *Ann Neurol.* 2009 Jan;65 Suppl 1:S3–9.

55. Andersen PM, Al-Chalabi A. Clinical genetics of amyotrophic lateral sclerosis: what do we really know? *Nat Rev Neurol.* 2011 Nov;7:603–15.

56. Fang F, Kwee LC, Allen KD, et al. Association between blood lead and the risk of amyotrophic lateral sclerosis. *Am J Epidemiol.* 2010 May 15;171:1126–33.

57. Vinceti M, Bonvicini F, Rothman KJ, et al. The relation between amyotrophic lateral sclerosis and inorganic selenium in drinking water: a population-based case-control study. *Environ Health.* 2010;9:77.

58. Callaghan B, Feldman D, Gruis K, et al. The association of exposure to lead, mercury, and selenium and the development of amyotrophic lateral sclerosis and the epigenetic implications. *Neurodegener Dis.* 2011;8:1–8.

59. Royce-Nagel G, Cudkowicz M, Myers D, et al. Vanadium, aluminum, magnesium and manganese are not elevated in hair samples in amyotrophic lateral sclerosis. *Amyotroph Lateral Scler.* 2010 Oct;11:492–3.

60. Morahan JM, Pamphlett R. Amyotrophic lateral sclerosis and exposure to environmental toxins: an Australian case-control study. *Neuroepidemiology.* 2006;27:130–5.

61. Furby A, Beauvais K, Kolev I, et al. Rural environment and risk factors of amyotrophic lateral sclerosis: a case-control study. *J Neurol.* 2010 May;257:792–8.

62. Sutedja NA, Veldink JH, Fischer K, et al. Exposure to chemicals and metals and risk of amyotrophic lateral sclerosis: a systematic review. *Amyotroph Lateral Scler.* 2009 Oct-Dec;10:302–9.

63. Weisskopf MG, Morozova N, O'Reilly EJ, et al. Prospective study of chemical exposures and amyotrophic lateral sclerosis. *J Neurol Neurosurg Psychiatry.* 2009 May;80:558–61.

64. Armon C. Smoking may be considered an established risk factor for sporadic ALS. *Neurology.* 2009 Nov 17;73:1693–8.

65. Wang H, O'Reilly EJ, Weisskopf MG, et al. Smoking and risk of amyotrophic lateral sclerosis: a pooled analysis of 5 prospective cohorts. *Arch Neurol.* 2011 Feb;68:207–13.

66. Berger MM, Kopp N, Vital C, et al. Detection and cellular localization of enterovirus RNA sequences in spinal cord of patients with ALS. *Neurology.* 2000 Jan 11;54:20–5.

67. Giraud P, Beaulieux F, Ono S, et al. Detection of enteroviral sequences from frozen spinal cord samples of Japanese ALS patients. *Neurology.* 2001 Jun 26;56:1777–8.

68. Nix WA, Berger MM, Oberste MS, et al. Failure to detect enterovirus in the spinal cord of ALS patients using a sensitive RT-PCR method. *Neurology.* 2004 Apr 27;62:1372–7.

69. Vandenberghe N, Leveque N, Corcia P, et al. Cerebrospinal fluid detection of enterovirus genome in ALS: a study of 242 patients and 354 controls. *Amyotroph Lateral Scler.* 2010 May 3;11:277–82.

70. Cox PA, Richer R, Metcalf JS, et al. Cyanobacteria and BMAA exposure from desert dust: a possible link to sporadic ALS among Gulf War veterans. *Amyotroph Lateral Scler.* 2009;10 Suppl 2:109–17.

71. Bradley WG, Mash DC. Beyond Guam: the cyanobacteria/BMAA hypothesis of the cause of ALS and other neurodegenerative diseases. *Amyotroph Lateral Scler.* 2009;10 Suppl 2:7–20.

72. Haley RW. Excess incidence of ALS in young Gulf War veterans. *Neurology.* 2003 Sep 23;61:750–6.

73. Horner RD, Kamins KG, Feussner JR, et al. Occurrence of amyotrophic lateral sclerosis among Gulf War veterans. *Neurology.* 2003 Sep 23;61:742–9.

74. Weisskopf MG, O'Reilly EJ, McCullough ML, et al. Prospective study of military service and mortality from ALS. *Neurology.* 2005 Jan 11;64:32–7.

75. Miranda ML, Alicia Overstreet Galeano M, Tassone E, et al. Spatial analysis of the etiology of amyotrophic lateral sclerosis among 1991 Gulf War veterans. *Neurotoxicology.* 2008 Nov;29:964–70.

76. Piazza O, Siren AL, Ehrenreich H. Soccer, neurotrauma and amyotrophic lateral sclerosis: is there a connection? *Curr Med Res Opin.* 2004 Apr;20:505–8.

77. Turner MR, Abisgold J, Yeates DG, et al. Head and other physical trauma requiring hospitalisation is not a significant risk factor in the development of ALS. *J Neurol Sci.* 2010 Jan 15;288:45–8.

78. McKee AC, Gavett BE, Stern RA, et al. TDP-43 proteinopathy and motor neuron disease in chronic traumatic encephalopathy. *J Neuropathol Exp Neurol.* 2010 Sep;69:918–29.

79. Van Damme P, Robberecht W. Recent advances in motor neuron disease. *Curr Opin Neurol.* 2009 Oct;22:486–92.

80. Chio A, Borghero G, Restagno G, et al. Clinical characteristics of patients with familial amyotrophic lateral sclerosis carrying the pathogenic GGGGCC hexanucleotide repeat expansion of C9ORF72. *Brain.* 2012 Mar;135:784–93.

81. DeJesus-Hernandez M, Mackenzie IR, Boeve BF, et al. Expanded GGGGCC hexanucleotide repeat in noncoding region of C9ORF72 causes chromosome 9p-linked FTD and ALS. *Neuron.* 2011 Oct 20;72:245–56.

82. Renton AE, Majounie E, Waite A, et al. A hexanucleotide repeat expansion in C9ORF72 is the cause of chromosome 9p21-linked ALS-FTD. *Neuron.* 2011 Oct 20;72:257–68.

83. Gamez J, Caponnetto C, Ferrera L, et al. I112M SOD1 mutation causes ALS with rapid progression and reduced penetrance in four Mediterranean families. *Amyotroph Lateral Scler.* 2011 Jan;12:70–5.

84. Kabashi E, Valdmanis PN, Dion P, et al. TARDBP mutations in individuals with sporadic and familial amyotrophic lateral sclerosis. *Nat Genet.* 2008 May;40:572–4.

85. Lopate G, Baloh RH, Al-Lozi MT, et al. Familial ALS with extreme phenotypic variability due to the I113T SOD1 mutation. *Amyotroph Lateral Scler.* 2010;11:232–6.

86. Robberecht W, Aguirre T, Van den Bosch L, et al. D90A heterozygosity in the SOD1 gene is associated with familial and apparently sporadic amyotrophic lateral sclerosis. *Neurology.* 1996 Nov;47:1336–9.

87. Sreedharan J, Blair IP, Tripathi VB, et al. TDP-43 mutations in familial and sporadic amyotrophic lateral sclerosis. *Science (New York, NY).* 2008 Mar 21;319:1668–72.

88. Vance C, Rogelj B, Hortobagyi T, et al. Mutations in FUS, an RNA processing protein, cause familial amyotrophic lateral sclerosis type 6. *Science (New York, NY).* 2009 Feb 27;323:1208–11.

89. Alexander MD, Traynor BJ, Miller N, et al. "True" sporadic ALS associated with a novel SOD-1 mutation. *Ann Neurol.* 2002 Nov;52:680–3.

90. Chio A, Calvo A, Moglia C, et al. A de novo missense mutation of the FUS gene in a "true" sporadic ALS case. *Neurobiol Aging.* 2011 Mar;32:553.

91. Kwiatkowski TJ, Jr., Bosco DA, Leclerc AL, et al. Mutations in the FUS/TLS gene on chromosome 16 cause familial amyotrophic lateral sclerosis. *Science (New York, NY).* 2009 Feb 27;323:1205–8.

92. Banks GT, Kuta A, Isaacs AM, et al. TDP-43 is a culprit in human neurodegeneration, and not just an innocent bystander. *Mamm Genome.* 2008 May;19:299–305.

93. Deng HX, Chen W, Hong ST, et al. Mutations in UBQLN2 cause dominant X-linked juvenile and adult-onset ALS and ALS/dementia. *Nature.* 2011 Sep 8;477:211–5.

94. Fecto F, Siddique T. UBQLN2/P62 cellular recycling pathways in amyotrophic lateral sclerosis and frontotemporal dementia. *Muscle Nerve.* 2012 Feb;45:157–62.

95. Boeve BF, Boylan KB, Graff-Radford NR, et al. Characterization of frontotemporal dementia and/or amyotrophic lateral sclerosis associated with the GGGGCC repeat expansion in C9ORF72. *Brain.* 2012 Mar;135:765–83.

96. Cooper-Knock J, Hewitt C, Highley JR, et al. Clinico-pathological features in amyotrophic lateral sclerosis with expansions in C9ORF72. *Brain.* 2012 Mar;135:751–64.

97. Rosen DR, Siddique T, Patterson D, et al. Mutations in Cu/Zn superoxide dismutase gene are associated with familial amyotrophic lateral sclerosis. *Nature.* 1993 Mar 4;362:59–62.

98. Gros-Louis F, Gaspar C, Rouleau GA. Genetics of familial and sporadic amyotrophic lateral sclerosis. *Biochim Biophys Acta.* 2006 Nov-Dec;1762:956–72.

99. Cudkowicz ME, McKenna-Yasek D, Chen C, et al. Limited corticospinal tract involvement in amyotrophic lateral sclerosis subjects with the A4V mutation in the copper/zinc superoxide dismutase gene. *Ann Neurol.* 1998 Jun;43:703–10.

100. Cudkowicz ME, McKenna-Yasek D, Sapp PE, et al. Epidemiology of mutations in superoxide dismutase in amyotrophic lateral sclerosis. *Ann Neurol.* 1997 Feb;41:210–21.

101. Felbecker A, Camu W, Valdmanis PN, et al. Four familial ALS pedigrees discordant for two SOD1 mutations: are all SOD1 mutations pathogenic? *J Neurol Neurosurg Psychiatry.* 2010 May;81:572–7.

102. Varelas PN, Bertorini TE, Kapaki E, et al. Paget's disease of bone and motor neuron disease. *Muscle Nerve.* 1997 May;20:630.

103. Fecto F, Yan J, Vemula SP, et al. SQSTM1 mutations in familial and sporadic amyotrophic lateral sclerosis. *Arch Neurol.* 2011 Nov;68:1440–6.

104. Rowland LP. Primary lateral sclerosis, hereditary spastic paraplegia, and mutations in the alsin gene: historical background for the first International Conference. *Amyotroph Lateral Scler Other Motor Neuron Disord.* 2005 Jun;6:67–76.

105. Dupre N, Valdmanis PN, Bouchard JP, et al. Autosomal dominant primary lateral sclerosis. *Neurology.* 2007 Apr 3;68:1156–7.

106. Praline J, Guennoc AM, Vourc'h P, et al. Primary lateral sclerosis may occur within familial amyotrophic lateral sclerosis pedigrees. *Amyotroph Lateral Scler.* 2010;11:154–6.

107. Brugman F, Veldink JH, Franssen H, et al. Differentiation of hereditary spastic paraparesis from primary lateral sclerosis in sporadic adult-onset upper motor neuron syndromes. *Arch Neurol.* 2009 Apr;66:509–14.

108. Chow CY, Landers JE, Bergren SK, et al. Deleterious variants of FIG4, a phosphoinositide phosphatase, in patients with ALS. *Am J Hum Genet.* 2009 Jan;84:85–8.

109. Valdmanis PN, Dupre N, Rouleau GA. A locus for primary lateral sclerosis on chromosome 4ptel-4p16.1. *Arch Neurol.* 2008 Mar;65:383–6.

110. Hadano S, Hand CK, Osuga H, et al. A gene encoding a putative GTPase regulator is mutated in familial amyotrophic lateral sclerosis 2. *Nat Genet.* 2001 Oct;29:166–73.

111. Yang Y, Hentati A, Deng HX, et al. The gene encoding alsin, a protein with three guanine-nucleotide exchange factor domains, is mutated in a form of recessive amyotrophic lateral sclerosis. *Nat Genet.* 2001 Oct;29:160–5.

112. Eymard-Pierre E, Yamanaka K, Haeussler M, et al. Novel missense mutation in ALS2 gene results in infantile ascending hereditary spastic paralysis. *Ann Neurol.* 2006 Jun;59:976–80.

113. Ince PG, Highley JR, Kirby J, et al. Molecular pathology and genetic advances in amyotrophic lateral sclerosis: an emerging molecular pathway and the significance of glial pathology. *Acta Neuropathol.* 2011 Dec;122:657–71.

114. Hays AP. Pathology of amyotrophic lateral sclerosis. In: Mitsumoto H, Przedborski S, Gordon P, editors. Amyotrophic Lateral Sclerosis. New York: Taylor and Francis; 2006. p. 43–80.

115. Matsumoto S, Goto S, Kusaka H, et al. Ubiquitin-positive inclusion in anterior horn cells in subgroups of motor neuron diseases: a comparative study of adult-

onset amyotrophic lateral sclerosis, juvenile amyotrophic lateral sclerosis and Werdnig-Hoffmann disease. *J Neurol Sci.* 1993 Apr;115:208–13.

116. Sasaki S, Maruyama S. Immunocytochemical and ultrastructural studies of the motor cortex in amyotrophic lateral sclerosis. *Acta Neuropathol.* 1994;87:578–85.

117. Okamoto K, Hirai S, Amari M, et al. Bunina bodies in amyotrophic lateral sclerosis immunostained with rabbit anti-cystatin C serum. *Neurosci Lett.* 1993 Nov 12;162:125–8.

118. Geser F, Lee VM, Trojanowski JQ. Amyotrophic lateral sclerosis and frontotemporal lobar degeneration: a spectrum of TDP-43 proteinopathies. *Neuropathology.* 2010 Apr;30:103–12.

119. Mackenzie IR, Bigio EH, Ince PG, et al. Pathological TDP-43 distinguishes sporadic amyotrophic lateral sclerosis from amyotrophic lateral sclerosis with SOD1 mutations. *Ann Neurol.* 2007 May;61:427–34.

120. Dickson DW, Josephs KA, Amador-Ortiz C. TDP-43 in differential diagnosis of motor neuron disorders. *Acta Neuropathol.* 2007 Jul;114:71–9.

121. Deng HX, Zhai H, Bigio EH, et al. FUS-immunoreactive inclusions are a common feature in sporadic and non-SOD1 familial amyotrophic lateral sclerosis. *Ann Neurol.* 2010 Jun;67:739–48.

122. Mackenzie IR, Ansorge O, Strong M, et al. Pathological heterogeneity in amyotrophic lateral sclerosis with FUS mutations: two distinct patterns correlating with disease severity and mutation. *Acta Neuropathol.* 2011 Jul;122:87–98.

123. Maruyama H, Morino H, Ito H, et al. Mutations of optineurin in amyotrophic lateral sclerosis. *Nature.* 2010 May 13;465:223–6.

124. Kosaka T, Fu YJ, Shiga A, et al. Primary lateral sclerosis: upper-motor-predominant amyotrophic lateral sclerosis with frontotemporal lobar degeneration – immunohistochemical and biochemical analyses of TDP-43. *Neuropathology.* 2012 Aug; 32:373–84.

125. Ravits J, Paul P, Jorg C. Focality of upper and lower motor neuron degeneration at the clinical onset of ALS. *Neurology.* 2007 May 8;68:1571–5.

126. Desai J, Swash M. Essentials of diagnosis. In: KunclRW, editor. *Motor Neuron Disease.* New York: Saunders; 2002. p. 1–20.

127. Gubbay SS, Kahana E, Zilber N, et al. Amyotrophic lateral sclerosis. A study of its presentation and prognosis. *J Neurol.* 1985;232:295–300.

128. Jokelainen M. Amyotrophic lateral sclerosis in Finland. II: Clinical characteristics. *Acta Neurol Scand.* 1977 Sep;56:194–204.

129. Ferguson TA, Elman LB. Clinical presentation and diagnosis of amyotrophic lateral sclerosis. *NeuroRehabilitation.* 2007;22:409–16.

130. Brooks B. Design of clinical therapeutic trials in amyotrophic lateral sclerosis. In: Rowland LP, editor. *Amyotrophic Lateral Sclerosis and Other Motor Neuron Diseases.* New York: Raven Press; 1991. p. 521–46.

131. O'Reilly DF, Brazis PW, Rubino FA. The misdiagnosis of unilateral presentations of amyotrophic lateral sclerosis. *Muscle Nerve.* 1982;5:724–6.

132. Kuncl RW, Cornblath DR, Griffin JW. Assessment of thoracic paraspinal muscles in the diagnosis of ALS. *Muscle Nerve.* 1988 May;11:484–92.

133. Gourie-Devi M, Nalini A, Sandhya S. Early or late appearance of "dropped head syndrome" in amyotrophic lateral sclerosis. *J Neurol Neurosurg Psychiatry.* 2003 May;74:683–6.

134. Tartaglia MC, Rowe A, Findlater K, et al. Differentiation between primary lateral sclerosis and amyotrophic lateral sclerosis: examination of symptoms and signs at disease onset and during follow-up. *Arch Neurol.* 2007 Feb;64:232–6.

135. de Carvalho M, Swash M. Cramps, muscle pain, and fasciculations: not always benign? *Neurology.* 2004 Aug 24;63:721–3.

136. Singh V, Gibson J, McLean B, et al. Fasciculations and cramps: how benign? Report of four cases progressing to ALS. *J Neurol.* 2011 Apr;258:573–8.

137. Layzer RB. Diagnostic implications of clinical fasciculation and cramps. *Adv Neurol.* 1982;36:23–9.

138. Moirangthem V, Ouseph MM. Atypical presentations of amyotrophic lateral sclerosis: a case report. *J Neuropsychiatry Clin Neurosci.* 2011 Summer;23:362–4.

139. Robbins J. Swallowing in ALS and motor neuron disorders. *Neurol Clin.* 1987 May;5:213–29.

140. Rubin AD, Griffin GR, Hogikyan ND, et al. A new member of the multidisciplinary ALS team: the otolaryngologist. *Amyotroph Lateral Scler.* 2012 Feb;13: 229–32.

141. Chen R, Grand'Maison F, Brown JD, et al. Motor neuron disease presenting as acute respiratory failure: electrophysiological studies. *Muscle Nerve.* 1997 Apr;20:517–9.

142. Fromm GB, Wisdom PJ, Block AJ. Amyotrophic lateral sclerosis presenting with respiratory failure. Diaphragmatic paralysis and dependence on mechanical ventilation in two patients. *Chest.* 1977 May;71:612–4.

143. Hill R, Martin J, Hakim A. Acute respiratory failure in motor neuron disease. *Arch Neurol.* 1983 Jan;40:30–2.

144. Krvickas L. Pulmonary function and respiratory failure. In: MitsumotoH, ChadD, Pioro E, editors. *Amyotrophic Lateral Sclerosis.* Philadelphia: F.A. Davis; 1998. p. 382–404.

145. Nightingale S, Bates D, Bateman DE, et al. Enigmatic dyspnoea: an unusual presentation of motor-neurone disease. *Lancet.* 1982 Apr 24;1:933–5.

146. Gordon PH, Cheng B, Katz IB, et al. The natural history of primary lateral sclerosis. *Neurology.* 2006 Mar 14;66:647–53.

147. Gallagher JP. Pathologic laughter and crying in ALS: a search for their origin. *Acta Neurol Scand.* 1989 Aug;80:114–7.

148. Parvizi J, Anderson SW, Martin CO, et al. Pathological laughter and crying: a link to the cerebellum. *Brain.* 2001 Sep;124:1708–19.

149. Pioro EP, Brooks BR, Cummings J, et al. Dextromethorphan plus ultra low-dose quinidine reduces pseudobulbar affect. *Ann Neurol.* 2010 Nov;68:693–702.

150. de Carvalho M, Dengler R, Eisen A, et al. Electrodiagnostic criteria for diagnosis of ALS. *Clin Neurophysiol.* 2008 Mar;119:497–503.

151. Lambert EH, Mulder DW. *Electromyography in amyotrophic lateral sclerosis.* New York: Grune & Stratton; 1968. p. 135–53.

152. Daube JR. Electrodiagnostic studies in amyotrophic lateral sclerosis and other motor neuron disorders. *Muscle Nerve.* 2000 Oct;23:1488–502.

153. Eisen A, Stewart H. Not-so-benign fasciculation. *Ann Neurol.* 1994 Mar;35:375–6.

154. Cornblath DR, Kuncl RW, Mellits ED, et al. Nerve conduction studies in amyotrophic lateral sclerosis. *Muscle Nerve.* 1992 Oct;15:1111–5.

155. Singh D, Verma R, Garg RK, et al. Assessment of respiratory functions by spirometry and phrenic nerve studies in patients of amyotrophic lateral sclerosis. *J Neurol Sci.* 2011 Jul 15;306:76–81.

156. Attarian S, Verschueren A, Pouget J. Magnetic stimulation including the triple-stimulation technique in amyotrophic lateral sclerosis. *Muscle Nerve.* 2007 Jul;36:55–61.

157. Kaufmann P, Pullman SL, Shungu DC, et al. Objective tests for upper motor neuron involvement in amyotrophic lateral sclerosis (ALS). *Neurology.* 2004 May 25;62:1753–7.

158. Osei-Lah AD, Mills KR. Optimising the detection of upper motor neuron function dysfunction in amyotrophic lateral sclerosis – a transcranial magnetic stimulation study. *J Neurol.* 2004 Nov;251:1364–9.

159. Kuipers-Upmeijer J, de Jager AE, Hew JM, et al. Primary lateral sclerosis: clinical, neurophysiological, and magnetic resonance findings. *J Neurol Neurosurg Psychiatry.* 2001 Nov;71:615–20.

160. de Carvalho M, Chio A, Dengler R, et al. Neurophysiological measures in amyotrophic lateral sclerosis: markers of progression in clinical trials. *Amyotroph Lateral Scler Other Motor Neuron Disord.* 2005 Mar;6:17–28.

161. Mills KR. The natural history of central motor abnormalities in amyotrophic lateral sclerosis. *Brain.* 2003 Nov;126:2558–66.

162. Vucic S, Cheah BC, Kiernan MC. Defining the mechanisms that underlie cortical hyperexcitability in amyotrophic lateral sclerosis. *Exp Neurol.* 2009 Nov;220:177–82.

163. Vucic S, Cheah BC, Yiannikas C, et al. Cortical excitability distinguishes ALS from mimic disorders. *Clin Neurophysiol.* 2011 Sep;122:1860–6.

164. Boe SG, Stashuk DW, Doherty TJ. Motor unit number estimates, quantitative motor unit analysis and clinical outcome measures in amyotrophic lateral sclerosis. *Suppl Clin Neurophysiol.* 2009;60:181–8.

165. Olney RK, Lomen-Hoerth C. Motor unit number estimation (MUNE): how may it contribute to the diagnosis of ALS? *Amyotroph Lateral Scler Other Motor Neuron Disord.* 2000 Jun;1 Suppl 2:S41–4.

166. Gooch CL, Pullman SL, Shungu DC, et al. Motor unit number estimation (MUNE) in diseases of the motor neuron: utility and comparative analysis in a multimodal biomarker study. *Suppl Clin Neurophysiol.* 2009;60:153–62.

167. Shefner JM, Watson ML, Simionescu L, et al. Multipoint incremental motor unit number estimation as an outcome measure in ALS. *Neurology.* 2011 Jul 19;77:235–41.

168. Swash M, de Carvalho M. The neurophysiological index in ALS. *Amyotroph Lateral Scler Other Motor Neuron Disord.* 2004 Sep;5 Suppl 1:108–10.

169. Cheah BC, Vucic S, Krishnan AV, et al. Neurophysiological index as a biomarker for ALS progression: validity of mixed effects models. *Amyotroph Lateral Scler.* 2011 Jan;12:33–8.

170. Tarulli AW, Garmirian LP, Fogerson PM, et al. Localized muscle impedance abnormalities in amyotrophic lateral sclerosis. *J Clin Neuromuscul Dis.* 2009 Mar;10:90–6.

171. Rutkove SB, Zhang H, Schoenfeld DA, et al. Electrical impedance myography to assess outcome in amyotrophic lateral sclerosis clinical trials. *Clin Neurophysiol.* 2007 Nov;118:2413–8.

172. Wang LL, Spieker AJ, Li J, et al. Electrical impedance myography for monitoring motor neuron loss in the SOD1 G93A amyotrophic lateral sclerosis rat. *Clin Neurophysiol.* 2011 Dec;122:2505–11.

173. Grosskreutz J, Peschel T, Unrath A, et al. Whole brain-based computerized neuroimaging in ALS and other motor neuron disorders. *Amyotroph Lateral Scler.* 2008 Aug;9:238–48.

174. Kassubek J, Ludolph AC, Muller HP. Neuroimaging of motor neuron diseases. *Ther Adv Neurol Disord.* 2012 Mar;5:119–27.

175. Turner MR, Kiernan MC, Leigh PN, et al. Biomarkers in amyotrophic lateral sclerosis. *Lancet Neurol.* 2009 Jan;8:94–109.

176. Wang S, Melhem ER, Poptani H, et al. Neuroimaging in amyotrophic lateral sclerosis. *Neurotherapeutics.* 2011 Jan;8:63–71.

177. Turner MR, Grosskreutz J, Kassubek J, et al. Towards a neuroimaging biomarker for amyotrophic lateral sclerosis. *Lancet Neurol.* 2011 May;10:400–3.

178. Wang S, Melhem ER. Amyotrophic lateral sclerosis and primary lateral sclerosis: The role of diffusion tensor imaging and other advanced MR-based techniques as objective upper motor neuron markers. *Ann N Y Acad Sci.* 2005 Dec;1064:61–77.

179. de Brito-Marques PR, de Mello RV. Amyotrophic lateral sclerosis with dementia. Case report. *Arq Neuropsiquiatr.* 1999 Jun;57:277–83.

180. Kato S, Hayashi H, Yagishita A. Involvement of the frontotemporal lobe and limbic system in amyotrophic lateral sclerosis: as assessed by serial computed tomography and magnetic resonance imaging. *J Neurol Sci.* 1993 May;116:52–8.

181. Tan CF, Kakita A, Piao YS, et al. Primary lateral sclerosis: a rare upper-motor-predominant form of amyotrophic lateral sclerosis often accompanied by frontotemporal lobar degeneration with ubiquitinated neuronal inclusions? Report of an autopsy case and a review of the literature. *Acta Neuropathol.* 2003 Jun;105:615–20.

182. Tsuchiya K, Ozawa E, Fukushima J, et al. Rapidly progressive aphasia and motor neuron disease: a clinical, radiological, and pathological study of an autopsy case with circumscribed lobar atrophy. *Acta Neuropathol.* 2000 Jan;99:81–7.

183. Tartaglia MC, Rosen HJ, Miller BL. Neuroimaging in dementia. *Neurotherapeutics.* 2011 Jan;8:82–92.

184. Turner MR. MRI as a frontrunner in the search for amyotrophic lateral sclerosis biomarkers? *Biomark Med.* 2011 Feb;5:79–81.

185. Bosma R, Stroman PW. Diffusion tensor imaging in the human spinal cord: development, limitations, and clinical applications. *Crit Rev Biomed Eng.* 2012;40:1–20.

186. Li J, Pan P, Song W, et al. A meta-analysis of diffusion tensor imaging studies in amyotrophic lateral sclerosis. *Neurobiol Aging.* 2012 Aug;33:1833–8.

187. Ciccarelli O, Behrens TE, Altmann DR, et al. Probabilistic diffusion tractography: a potential tool to assess the rate of disease progression in amyotrophic lateral sclerosis. *Brain.* 2006 Jul;129:1859–71.

188. Ciccarelli O, Behrens TE, Johansen-Berg H, et al. Investigation of white matter pathology in ALS and PLS using tract-based spatial statistics. *Hum Brain Mapp.* 2009 Feb;30:615–24.

189. Agosta F, Rocca MA, Valsasina P, et al. A longitudinal diffusion tensor MRI study of the cervical cord and brain in amyotrophic lateral sclerosis patients. *J Neurol Neurosurg Psychiatry.* 2009 Jan;80:53–5.

190. Nickerson JP, Koski CJ, Boyer AC, et al. Linear longitudinal decline in fractional anisotropy in patients with amyotrophic lateral sclerosis: preliminary results. *Klin Neuroradiol.* 2009 Jun;19:129–34.

191. Zhang Y, Schuff N, Woolley SC, et al. Progression of white matter degeneration in amyotrophic lateral sclerosis: A diffusion tensor imaging study. *Amyotroph Lateral Scler.* 2011 Nov;12:421–9.

192. Iwata NK, Kwan JY, Danielian LE, et al. White matter alterations differ in primary lateral sclerosis and amyotrophic lateral sclerosis. *Brain.* 2011 Sep;134:2642–55.

193. Sage CA, Van Hecke W, Peeters R, et al. Quantitative diffusion tensor imaging in amyotrophic lateral sclerosis: revisited. *Hum Brain Mapp.* 2009 Nov;30:3657–75.

194. Senda J, Kato S, Kaga T, et al. Progressive and widespread brain damage in ALS: MRI voxel-based morphometry and diffusion tensor imaging study. *Amyotroph Lateral Scler.* 2011 Jan;12:59–69.

195. Filippini N, Douaud G, Mackay CE, et al. Corpus callosum involvement is a consistent feature of amyotrophic lateral sclerosis. *Neurology.* 2010 Nov 2;75:1645–52.

196. Chang JL, Lomen-Hoerth C, Murphy J, et al. A voxel-based morphometry study of patterns of brain atrophy in ALS and ALS/FTLD. *Neurology.* 2005 Jul 12;65:75–80.

197. Whitwell JL, Jack CR, Jr., Senjem ML, et al. Patterns of atrophy in pathologically confirmed FTLD with and without motor neuron degeneration. *Neurology.* 2006 Jan 10;66:102–4.

198. Kassubek J, Unrath A, Huppertz HJ, et al. Global brain atrophy and corticospinal tract alterations in ALS, as investigated by voxel-based morphometry of 3-D MRI. *Amyotroph Lateral Scler Other Motor Neuron Disord.* 2005 Dec;6:213–20.

199. Chen Z, Ma L. Grey matter volume changes over the whole brain in amyotrophic lateral sclerosis: A voxel-wise meta-analysis of voxel based morphometry studies. *Amyotroph Lateral Scler.* 2010 Dec;11:549–54.

200. Chen HJ, Anagnostou G, Chai A, et al. Characterization of the properties of a novel mutation in VAPB in familial amyotrophic lateral sclerosis. *J Biol Chem.* 2010 Dec 17;285:40266–81.

201. Douaud G, Filippini N, Knight S, et al. Integration of structural and functional magnetic resonance imaging in amyotrophic lateral sclerosis. *Brain.* 2011 Dec;134:3470–9.

202. Cosottini M, Pesaresi I, Piazza S, et al. Structural and functional evaluation of cortical motor areas in amyotrophic lateral sclerosis. *Exp Neurol.* 2012 Mar;234:169–80.

203. Lule D, Ludolph AC, Kassubek J. MRI-based functional neuroimaging in ALS: an update. *Amyotroph Lateral Scler.* 2009 Oct-Dec;10:258–68.

204. Mohammadi B, Kollewe K, Samii A, et al. Changes of resting state brain networks in amyotrophic lateral sclerosis. *Exp Neurol.* 2009 May;217:147–53.

205. Verstraete E, van den Heuvel MP, Veldink JH, et al. Motor network degeneration in amyotrophic lateral sclerosis: a structural and functional connectivity study. *PLoS ONE.* 2010;5:e13664.

206. Poujois A, Schneider FC, Faillenot I, et al. Brain plasticity in the motor network is correlated with disease progression in amyotrophic lateral sclerosis. *Hum Brain Mapp.* 2013 Oct;34:2391–401.

207. da Rocha AJ, Oliveira AS, Fonseca RB, et al. Detection of corticospinal tract compromise in amyotrophic lateral sclerosis with brain MR imaging: relevance of the T1-weighted spin-echo magnetization transfer contrast sequence. *AJNR Am J Neuroradiol.* 2004 Oct;25:1509–15.

208. da Rocha AJ, Maia AC, Jr., Valerio BC. Corticospinal tract MR signal-intensity pseudonormalization on magnetization transfer contrast imaging: a potential pitfall in the interpretation of the advanced compromise of upper motor neurons in amyotrophic lateral sclerosis. *AJNR Am J Neuroradiol.* 2012 May;33:E79–80.

209. Carrara G, Carapelli C, Venturi F, et al. A distinct MR imaging phenotype in amyotrophic lateral sclerosis: correlation between T1 magnetization transfer contrast hyperintensity along the corticospinal tract and diffusion tensor imaging analysis. *AJNR Am J Neuroradiol.* 2012 Apr;33:733–9.

210. Pioro EP, Antel JP, Cashman NR, et al. Detection of cortical neuron loss in motor neuron disease by proton magnetic resonance spectroscopic imaging in vivo. *Neurology.* 1994 Oct;44:1933–8.

211. Gredal O, Rosenbaum S, Topp S, et al. Quantification of brain metabolites in amyotrophic lateral sclerosis by localized proton magnetic resonance spectroscopy. *Neurology.* 1997 Apr;48:878–81.

212. Kalra S, Hanstock CC, Martin WR, et al. Detection of cerebral degeneration in amyotrophic lateral sclerosis using high-field magnetic resonance spectroscopy. *Arch Neurol.* 2006 Aug;63:1144–8.

213. Foerster BR, Callaghan BC, Petrou M, et al. Decreased motor cortex gamma-aminobutyric acid in amyotrophic lateral sclerosis. *Neurology.* 2012 May 15;78:1596–600.

214. Arts IM, Overeem S, Pillen S, et al. Muscle ultrasonography: A diagnostic tool for amyotrophic lateral sclerosis. *Clin Neurophysiol.* 2012 Aug;123:1662–7.

215. Boekestein WA, Schelhaas HJ, van Dijk JP, et al. Ultrasonographic detection of fasciculations markedly increases diagnostic sensitivity of ALS. *Neurology.* 2012 Jan 31;78:370; author reply -1.

216. Swash M, Carvalho M. Muscle ultrasound detects fasciculations and facilitates diagnosis in ALS. *Neurology.* 2011 Oct 18;77:1508–9.

217. Hardiman O. Management of respiratory symptoms in ALS. *J Neurol.* 2011 Mar;258:359–65.

218. Uldry C, Fitting JW. Maximal values of sniff nasal inspiratory pressure in healthy subjects. *Thorax.* 1995 Apr;50:371–5.

219. Miller RG, Jackson CE, Kasarskis EJ, et al. Practice parameter update: The care of the patient with amyotrophic lateral sclerosis: multidisciplinary care, symptom management, and cognitive/behavioral impairment (an evidence-based review): report of the Quality Standards Subcommittee of the American Academy of Neurology. *Neurology.* 2009 Oct 13;73:1227–33.

220. Appel V, Stewart SS, Smith G, et al. A rating scale for amyotrophic lateral sclerosis: description and preliminary experience. *Ann Neurol.* 1987 Sep;22:328–33.

221. Hillel AD, Miller RM, Yorkston K, et al. Amyotrophic lateral sclerosis severity scale. *Neuroepidemiology.* 1989;8:142–50.

222. Cedarbaum JM, Stambler N, Malta E, et al. The ALSFRS-R: a revised ALS functional rating scale that incorporates assessments of respiratory function. BDNF ALS Study Group (Phase III). *J Neurol Sci.* 1999 Oct 31;169:13–21.

223. The Amyotrophic Lateral Sclerosis Functional Rating Scale. Assessment of activities of daily living in patients with amyotrophic lateral sclerosis. The ALS CNTF treatment study (ACTS) phase I-II Study Group. *Arch Neurol.* 1996 Feb 1;53:141–7.

224. Gordon PH, Miller RG, Moore DH. ALSFRS-R. *Amyotroph Lateral Scler Other Motor Neuron Disord.* 2004 Sep;5 Suppl 1:90–3.

225. Gordon PH, Moore DH, Miller RG, et al. Efficacy of minocycline in patients with amyotrophic lateral sclerosis: a phase III randomised trial. *Lancet Neurol.* 2007 Dec;6:1045–53.

226. Castrillo-Viguera C, Grasso DL, Simpson E, et al. Clinical significance in the change of decline in ALSFRS-R. *Amyotroph Lateral Scler.* 2010;11:178–80.

227. Cudkowicz ME, Swash M. CSF markers in amyotrophic lateral sclerosis: has the time come? *Neurology.* 2010 Mar 23;74:949–50.

228. Ganesalingam J, An J, Shaw CE, et al. Combination of neurofilament heavy chain and complement C3 as CSF biomarkers for ALS. *J Neurochem.* 2011 May;117:528–37.

229. Noto Y, Shibuya K, Sato Y, et al. Elevated CSF TDP-43 levels in amyotrophic lateral sclerosis: specificity, sensitivity, and a possible prognostic value. *Amyotroph Lateral Scler.* 2011 Mar;12:140–3.

230. Sussmuth SD, Sperfeld AD, Hinz A, et al. CSF glial markers correlate with survival in amyotrophic lateral sclerosis. *Neurology.* 2010 Mar 23;74:982–7.

231. Tateishi T, Yamasaki R, Tanaka M, et al. CSF chemokine alterations related to the clinical course of amyotrophic lateral sclerosis. *J Neuroimmunol.* 2010 May;222:76–81.

232. Valentino F, Bivona G, Butera D, et al. Elevated cerebrospinal fluid and plasma homocysteine levels in ALS. *Eur J Neurol.* 2010 Jan;17:84–9.

233. Yamamoto-Watanabe Y, Watanabe M, Jackson M, et al. Quantification of cystatin C in cerebrospinal fluid from various neurological disorders and correlation with G73A polymorphism in CST3. *Brain Res.* 2010 Nov 18;1361:140–5.

234. Taylor BV, Gross L, Windebank AJ. The sensitivity and specificity of anti-GM1 antibody testing. *Neurology.* 1996 Oct;47:951–5.

235. Rowland LP. Amyotrophic lateral sclerosis with paraproteins and autoantibodies. *Adv Neurol.* 1995;68:93–105; discussion 7–11.

236. Sorenson EJ, Stalker AP, Kurland LT, et al. Amyotrophic lateral sclerosis in Olmsted County, Minnesota, 1925 to 1998. *Neurology.* 2002 Jul 23;59:280–2.

237. Miller RG, Rosenberg JA, Gelinas DF, et al. Practice parameter: the care of the patient with amyotrophic lateral sclerosis (an evidence-based review): report of the Quality Standards Subcommittee of the American Academy of Neurology: ALS Practice Parameters Task Force. *Neurology.* 1999 Apr 22;52:1311–23.

238. Karam C. IBP is a form of PLS and should be distinguished from PBP. *Amyotroph Lateral Scler.* 2012 Jan;13:158.

239. Mazzini L, Corra T, Zaccala M, et al. Percutaneous endoscopic gastrostomy and enteral nutrition in amyotrophic lateral sclerosis. *J Neurol.* 1995 Oct;242:695–8.

240. Chio A, Galletti R, Finocchiaro C, et al. Percutaneous radiological gastrostomy: a safe and effective method of nutritional tube placement in advanced ALS. *J Neurol Neurosurg Psychiatry.* 2004 Apr;75:645–7.

241. Aboussouan LS, Khan SU, Banerjee M, et al. Objective measures of the efficacy of noninvasive positive-pressure ventilation in amyotrophic lateral sclerosis. *Muscle Nerve.* 2001 Mar;24:403–9.

242. Magnus T, Beck M, Giess R, et al. Disease progression in amyotrophic lateral sclerosis: predictors of survival. *Muscle Nerve.* 2002 May;25:709–14.

243. Mitsumoto H, Chad D, Pioro E. Course and prognosis. In: MitsumotoH, ChadDA, PioroEP, editors. *Amyotrophic Lateral Sclerosis: Contemporary Neurology Series; 49.* Philadelphia: F.A. Davis; 1998. p. 151–63.

244. del Aguila MA, Longstreth WT, Jr., McGuire V, et al. Prognosis in amyotrophic lateral sclerosis: a population-based study. *Neurology.* 2003 Mar 11;60:813–9.

245. Chio A, Mora G, Leone M, et al. Early symptom progression rate is related to ALS outcome: a prospective population-based study. *Neurology.* 2002 Jul 9;59:99–103.

246. Turner M, Al-Chalabi A. Early symptom progression rate is related to ALS outcome: a prospective population-based study. *Neurology.* 2002 Dec 24;59:2012-3; author reply 3.

247. Chio A, Logroscino G, Hardiman O, et al. Prognostic factors in ALS: A critical review. *Amyotroph Lateral Scler* 2009 Oct-Dec;10:310–23.

248. Mulder DW, Howard FM, Jr. Patient resistance and prognosis in amyotrophic lateral sclerosis. *Mayo Clin Proc.* 1976 Sep;51:537–41.

249. Tucker T, Layzer RB, Miller RG, et al. Subacute, reversible motor neuron disease. *Neurology.* 1991 Oct;41:1541–4.

250. Bensimon G, Lacomblez L, Meininger V. A controlled trial of riluzole in amyotrophic lateral sclerosis. ALS/Riluzole Study Group. *N Engl J Med.* 1994 Mar 3;330:585–91.

251. Miller RG, Bouchard JP, Duquette P, et al. Clinical trials of riluzole in patients with ALS. ALS/Riluzole Study Group-II. *Neurology.* 1996 Oct;47:S86–90; discussion S-2.

252. Cudkowicz ME, Shefner JM, Schoenfeld DA, et al. A randomized, placebo-controlled trial of topiramate in amyotrophic lateral sclerosis. *Neurology.* 2003 Aug 26;61:456–64.

253. Miller RG, Moore DH, 2nd, Gelinas DF, et al. Phase III randomized trial of gabapentin in patients with amyotrophic lateral sclerosis. *Neurology.* 2001 Apr 10;56:843–8.

254. Cudkowicz ME, Shefner JM, Schoenfeld DA, et al. Trial of celecoxib in amyotrophic lateral sclerosis. *Ann Neurol.* 2006 Jul;60:22–31.

255. Graf M, Ecker D, Horowski R, et al. High dose vitamin E therapy in amyotrophic lateral sclerosis as add-on therapy to riluzole: results of a placebo-controlled double-blind study. *J Neural Transm.* 2005 May;112:649–60.

256. Pasquali L, Longone P, Isidoro C, et al. Autophagy, lithium, and amyotrophic lateral sclerosis. *Muscle Nerve.* 2009 Aug;40:173–94.

257. Sorenson EJ, Windbank AJ, Mandrekar JN, et al. Subcutaneous IGF-1 is not beneficial in 2-year ALS trial. *Neurology.* 2008 Nov 25;71:1770–5.

258. Testa D, Caraceni T, Fetoni V, et al. Chronic treatment with L-threonine in amyotrophic lateral sclerosis: a pilot study. *Clin Neurol Neurosurg.* 1992;94:7–9.

259. Forshew DA, Bromberg MB. A survey of clinicians' practice in the symptomatic treatment of ALS. *Amyotroph Lateral Scler Other Motor Neuron Disord.* 2003 Dec;4:258–63.

260. Ashworth NL, Satkunam LE, Deforge D. Treatment for spasticity in amyotrophic lateral sclerosis/motor neuron disease. *Cochrane Database Syst Rev.* 2012;2:CD004156.

261. Andersen PM, Abrahams S, Borasio GD, et al. EFNS guidelines on the clinical management of amyotrophic lateral sclerosis (MALS) – revised report of an EFNS task force. *Eur J Neurol.* 2012 Mar;19:360–75.

262. Marquardt G, Lorenz R. Intrathecal baclofen for intractable spasticity in amyotrophic lateral sclerosis. *J Neurol.* 1999 Jul;246:619–20.

263. Guidubaldi A, Fasano A, Ialongo T, et al. Botulinum toxin A versus B in sialorrhea: a prospective, randomized, double-blind, crossover pilot study in patients with amyotrophic lateral sclerosis or Parkinson's disease. *Mov Disord.* 2011 Feb 1;26:313–9.

264. Jackson CE, Gronseth G, Rosenfeld J, et al. Randomized double-blind study of botulinum toxin type B for sialorrhea in ALS patients. *Muscle Nerve.* 2009 Feb;39:137–43.

265. Neppelberg E, Haugen DF, Thorsen L, et al. Radiotherapy reduces sialorrhea in amyotrophic lateral sclerosis. *Eur J Neurol.* 2007 Dec;14:1373–7.

266. Rodriguez de Rivera FJ, Oreja Guevara C, Sanz Gallego I, et al. Outcome of patients with amyotrophic lateral sclerosis attending in a multidisciplinary care unit. *Neurologia.* 2011 Oct;26:455–60.

267. Brooks BR, Thisted RA, Appel SH, et al. Treatment of pseudobulbar affect in ALS with dextromethorphan/quinidine: a randomized trial. *Neurology.* 2004 Oct 26;63:1364–70.

268. Garnock-Jones KP. Dextromethorphan/quinidine: in pseudobulbar affect. *CNS Drugs.* 2011 May;25:435–45.

269. Pinto AC, Evangelista T, Carvalho M, et al. Respiratory assistance with a non-invasive ventilator (Bipap) in MND/ALS patients: survival rates in a controlled trial. *J Neurol Sci.* 1995 May;129 Suppl:19–26.

270. Aboussouan LS, Khan SU, Meeker DP, et al. Effect of noninvasive positive-pressure ventilation on survival in amyotrophic lateral sclerosis. *Ann Intern Med.* 1997 Sep 15;127:450–3.

271. Bourke SC, Tomlinson M, Williams TL, et al. Effects of non-invasive ventilation on survival and quality of life in patients with amyotrophic lateral sclerosis: a randomised controlled trial. *Lancet Neurol.* 2006 Feb;5:140–7.

272. Hayashi H, Oppenheimer EA. ALS patients on TPPV: totally locked-in state, neurologic findings and ethical implications. *Neurology.* 2003 Jul 8;61:135–7.

273. Moss AH, Oppenheimer EA, Casey P, et al. Patients with amyotrophic lateral sclerosis receiving long-term mechanical ventilation. Advance care planning and outcomes. *Chest.* 1996 Jul;110:249–55.

274. Gruis KL, Lechtzin N. Respiratory therapies for amyotrophic lateral sclerosis: a primer. *Muscle Nerve.* 2012 Sep;46:313–31.

275. Lechtzin N. Respiratory effects of amyotrophic lateral sclerosis: problems and solutions. *Respir Care.* 2006 Aug;51:871–81; discussion 81–4.

276. Mustfa N, Aiello M, Lyall RA, et al. Cough augmentation in amyotrophic lateral sclerosis. *Neurology.* 2003 Nov 11;61:1285–7.

277. Lange DJ, Lechtzin N, Davey C, et al. High-frequency chest wall oscillation in ALS: an exploratory randomized, controlled trial. *Neurology.* 2006 Sep 26;67:991–7.

278. Chaisson KM, Walsh S, Simmons Z, et al. A clinical pilot study: high frequency chest wall oscillation airway clearance in patients with amyotrophic lateral sclerosis. *Amyotroph Lateral Scler.* 2006 Jun;7:107–11.

279. Baker WL, Lamb VJ, Marini JJ. Breath-stacking increases the depth and duration of chest expansion by incentive spirometry. *Am Rev Respir Dis.* 1990 Feb;141:343–6.

280. Heffernan C, Jenkinson C, Holmes T, et al. Nutritional management in MND/ALS patients: an evidence based review. *Amyotroph Lateral Scler Other Motor Neuron Disord.* 2004 Jun;5:72–83.

281. Kasarskis EJ, Mendiondo MS, Wells S, et al. The ALS Nutrition/NIPPV Study: design, feasibility, and initial results. *Amyotroph Lateral Scler.* 2011 Jan;12:17–25.

282. Beghi E, Millul A, Logroscino G, et al. Outcome measures and prognostic indicators in patients with amyotrophic lateral sclerosis. *Amyotroph Lateral Scler.* 2008 Jun;9:163–7.

283. Kuhnlein P, Gdynia HJ, Sperfeld AD, et al. Diagnosis and treatment of bulbar symptoms in amyotrophic lateral sclerosis. *Nat Clin Pract Neurol.* 2008 Jul;4:366–74.

284. Noh EJ, Park MI, Park SJ, et al. A case of amyotrophic lateral sclerosis presented as oropharyngeal Dysphagia. *J Neurogastroenterol Motil.* 2010 Jul;16:319–22.

285. Spataro R, Ficano L, Piccoli F, et al. Percutaneous endoscopic gastrostomy in amyotrophic lateral sclerosis: effect on survival. *J Neurol Sci.* 2011 May 15;304:44–8.

286. Bach JR, Gonzalez M, Sharma A, et al. Open gastrostomy for noninvasive ventilation users with neuromuscular disease. *Am J Phys Med Rehabil.* 2010 Jan;89:1–6.

287. Park JH, Kang SW. Percutaneous radiologic gastrostomy in patients with amyotrophic lateral sclerosis on noninvasive ventilation. *Arch Phys Med Rehabil.* 2009 Jun;90:1026–9.

288. Rowin J, Meriggioli MN. Noninvasive ventilation allows gastrostomy tube placement in patients with advanced ALS. *Neurology*. 2001 Oct 9;57:1351; author reply -2.

289. Rio A, Leigh N. Noninvasive ventilation allows gastrostomy tube placement in patients with advanced ALS. *Neurology*. 2001 Oct 9;57:1351; discussion -2.

290. Boitano LJ, Jordan T, Benditt JO. Noninvasive ventilation allows gastrostomy tube placement in patients with advanced ALS. *Neurology*. 2001 Feb 13;56:413–4.

291. Katzberg HD, Benatar M. Enteral tube feeding for amyotrophic lateral sclerosis/motor neuron disease. *Cochrane Database Syst Rev*. 2011:CD004030.

292. Desport JC, Preux PM, Magy L, et al. Factors correlated with hypermetabolism in patients with amyotrophic lateral sclerosis. *Am J Clin Nutr*. 2001 Sep;74:328–34.

293. Desport JC, Torny F, Lacoste M, et al. Hypermetabolism in ALS: correlations with clinical and paraclinical parameters. *Neurodegener Dis*. 2005;2:202–7.

294. Kasarskis EJ, Berryman S, Vanderleest JG, et al. Nutritional status of patients with amyotrophic lateral sclerosis: relation to the proximity of death. *Am J Clin Nutr*. 1996 Jan;63:130–7.

295. Sherman MS, Pillai A, Jackson A, et al. Standard equations are not accurate in assessing resting energy expenditure in patients with amyotrophic lateral sclerosis. *JPEN J Parenter Enteral Nutr*. 2004 Nov-Dec;28:442–6.

296. Vaisman N, Lusaus M, Nefussy B, et al. Do patients with amyotrophic lateral sclerosis (ALS) have increased energy needs? *J Neurol Sci*. 2009 Apr 15;279:26–9.

297. Weijs PJ. Hypermetabolism, is it real? The example of amyotrophic lateral sclerosis. *J Am Diet Assoc*. 2011 Nov;111:1670–3.

298. Dupuis L, Pradat PF, Ludolph AC, et al. Energy metabolism in amyotrophic lateral sclerosis. *Lancet Neurol*. 2011 Jan;10:75–82.

299. Ellis AC, Rosenfeld J. Which equation best predicts energy expenditure in amyotrophic lateral sclerosis? *J Am Diet Assoc*. 2011 Nov;111:1680–7.

300. Rio A, Cawadias E. Nutritional advice and treatment by dietitians to patients with amyotrophic lateral sclerosis/motor neurone disease: a survey of current practice in England, Wales, Northern Ireland and Canada. *J Hum Nutr Diet*. 2007 Feb;20:3–13.

301. Krvickas L, Dal Bello-Haas V, Danforth SE, et al. Rehabilitation. In: Mitsumoto H, PrzedborskiS, GordonP, editors. *Amyotrophic Lateral Sclerosis*. New York: Taylor and Francis; 2006. p. 691–720.

302. Mitsumoto H, Borasio GD, Genge A, et al. The multidisciplinary care clinic: the principles and an international perspective. In: Mitsumoto H, Przedborski S, GordonP, editors. *Amyotrophic Lateral Sclerosis*. New York: Taylor and Francis; 2006. p. 605–31.

303. Tomik B, Guiloff RJ. Dysarthria in amyotrophic lateral sclerosis: A review. *Amyotroph Lateral Scler*. 2010;11:4–15.

304. Brownlee A, Palovcak M. The role of augmentative communication devices in the medical management of ALS. *NeuroRehabilitation*. 2007;22:445–50.

305. Lewis M, Rushanan S. The role of physical therapy and occupational therapy in the treatment of amyotrophic lateral sclerosis. *NeuroRehabilitation*. 2007;22:451–61.

306. Dalbello-Haas V, Florence JM, Krivickas LS. Therapeutic exercise for people with amyotrophic lateral sclerosis or motor neuron disease. *Cochrane Database Syst Rev*. 2008:CD005229.

307. Chen A, Montes J, Mitsumoto H. The role of exercise in amyotrophic lateral sclerosis. *Phys Med Rehabil Clin N Am*. 2008 Aug;19:545–57, ix–x.

308. Benditt JO, Boitano L. Respiratory treatment of amyotrophic lateral sclerosis. *Phys Med Rehabil Clin N Am*. 2008 Aug;19:559–72, x.

309. Cazzolli PA, Oppenheimer EA. Home mechanical ventilation for amyotrophic lateral sclerosis: nasal compared to tracheostomy-intermittent positive pressure ventilation. *J Neurol Sci*. 1996 Aug;139 Suppl:123–8.

310. Marchese S, Lo Coco D, Lo Coco A. Outcome and attitudes toward home tracheostomy ventilation of consecutive patients: a 10-year experience. *Respir Med*. 2008 Mar;102:430–6.

311. Sancho J, Servera E, Banuls P, et al. Prolonging survival in amyotrophic lateral sclerosis: efficacy of noninvasive ventilation and uncuffed tracheostomy tubes. *Am J Phys Med Rehabil*. 2010 May;89:407–11.

312. Chio A, Calvo A, Ghiglione P, et al. Tracheostomy in amyotrophic lateral sclerosis: a 10-year population-based study in Italy. *J Neurol Neurosurg Psychiatry*. 2010 Oct;81:1141–3.

313. Garvey CM, Boylan KB, Salassa JR, et al. Total laryngectomy in patients with advanced bulbar symptoms of amyotrophic lateral sclerosis. *Amyotroph Lateral Scler*. 2009 Oct-Dec;10:470–5.

314. Panourias IG, Themistocleous M, Sakas DE. Intrathecal baclofen in current neuromodulatory practice: established indications and emerging applications. *Acta Neurochir Suppl*. 2007;97:145–54.

315. Dario A, Tomei G. A benefit-risk assessment of baclofen in severe spinal spasticity. *Drug Saf*. 2004;27:799–818.

316. Onders RP, Carlin AM, Elmo M, et al. Amyotrophic lateral sclerosis: the Midwestern surgical experience with the diaphragm pacing stimulation system shows that general anesthesia can be safely performed. *Am J Surg*. 2009 Mar;197:386–90.

317. Onders RP, Elmo M, Khansarinia S, et al. Complete worldwide operative experience in laparoscopic diaphragm pacing: results and differences in spinal cord injured patients and amyotrophic lateral sclerosis patients. *Surg Endosc*. 2009 Jul;23:1433–40.

318. Gonzalez-Bermejo J, Morelot-Panzini C, Salachas F, et al. Diaphragm pacing improves sleep in patients with amyotrophic lateral sclerosis. *Amyotroph Lateral Scler*. 2012 Jan;13:44–54.

319. Gonzalez-Bermejo J, Morélot-Panzini C, Tanguy ML, et al. Early diaphragm pacing in patients with amyotrophic lateral sclerosis (RespiStimALS): a randomised controlled triple-blind trial. *Lancet Neurol*. 2016 Nov;15:1217–27.

320. Miller RG, Lewis RA. Diaphragm pacing in patients with amyotrophic lateral sclerosis. *Lancet Neurol*. 2016 May;15:542.

321. DiPALS Writing Committee; DiPALS Study Group Collaborators, McDermott CJ, Bradburn MJ, Maguire C, et al. Safety and efficacy of diaphragm pacing in patients with respiratory insufficiency due to amyotrophic lateral sclerosis (DiPALS): a multicentre, open-label, randomised controlled trial. *Lancet Neurol*. 2015 Sep;14:883–92.

322. Ng L, Khan F, Mathers S. Multidisciplinary care for adults with amyotrophic lateral sclerosis or motor neuron disease. *Cochrane Database Syst Rev*. 2009:CD007425.

323. Mayadev AS, Weiss MD, Distad BJ, et al. The amyotrophic lateral sclerosis center: a model of multidisciplinary management. *Phys Med Rehabil Clin N Am*. 2008 Aug;19:619–31, xi.

324. Van den Berg JP, Kalmijn S, Lindeman E, et al. Multidisciplinary ALS care improves quality of life in patients with ALS. *Neurology*. 2005 Oct 25;65:1264–7.

325. Traynor BJ, Alexander M, Corr B, et al. Effect of a multidisciplinary amyotrophic lateral sclerosis (ALS) clinic on ALS survival: a population based study, 1996–2000. *J Neurol Neurosurg Psychiatry*. 2003 Sep;74:1258–61.

326. Blackhall LJ. Amyotrophic lateral sclerosis and palliative care: where we are, and the road ahead. *Muscle Nerve*. 2012 Mar;45:311–8.

327. Boylan K. Amyotrophic lateral sclerosis. In: Shapira AHV, Byrne E, DiMauro S, Frackowiak RSJ, Johnson RT, Mizuno Y, et al., editors. *Neurology and Clinical Neuroscience*. Philadelphia: Mosby Elsevier; 2007. p. 859–78.

328. Grosskreutz J, Kaufmann J, Fradrich J, et al. Widespread sensorimotor and frontal cortical atrophy in amyotrophic lateral sclerosis. *BMC Neurol*. 2006;6:17.

329. Swash M, Desai J. Motor neuron disease: classification and nomenclature. *Amyotroph Lateral Scler Other Motor Neuron Disord*. 2000 Mar;1:105–12.

330. Chancellor AM, Warlow CP. Adult onset motor neuron disease: worldwide mortality, incidence and distribution since 1950. *J Neurol Neurosurg Psychiatry*. 1992 Dec;55:1106–15.

331. Hand CK, Khoris J, Salachas F, et al. A novel locus for familial amyotrophic lateral sclerosis, on chromosome 18q. *Am J Hum Genet*. 2002 Jan;70:251–6.

332. Chen YZ, Bennett CL, Huynh HM, et al. DNA/RNA helicase gene mutations in a form of juvenile amyotrophic lateral sclerosis (ALS4). *Am J Hum Genet*. 2004 Jun;74:1128–35.

333. Orlacchio A, Babalini C, Borreca A, et al. SPATACSIN mutations cause autosomal recessive juvenile amyotrophic lateral sclerosis. *Brain*. 2010 Feb;133:591–8.

334. Sapp PC, Hosler BA, McKenna-Yasek D, et al. Identification of two novel loci for dominantly inherited familial amyotrophic lateral sclerosis. *Am J Hum Genet*. 2003 Aug;73:397–403.

335. van Es MA, Diekstra FP, Veldink JH, et al. A case of ALS-FTD in a large FALS pedigree with a K17I ANG mutation. *Neurology*. 2009 Jan 20;72:287–8.

336. Gitcho MA, Baloh RH, Chakraverty S, et al. TDP-43 A315T mutation in familial motor neuron disease. *Ann Neurol*. 2008 Apr;63:535–8.

337. Elden AC, Kim HJ, Hart MP, et al. Ataxin-2 intermediate-length polyglutamine expansions are associated with increased risk for ALS. *Nature*. 2010 Aug 26;466:1069–75.

338. Johnson JO, Mandrioli J, Benatar M, et al. Exome sequencing reveals VCP mutations as a cause of familial ALS. *Neuron*. 2010 Dec 9;68:857–64.

339. Al-Saif A, Al-Mohanna F, Bohlega S. A mutation in sigma-1 receptor causes juvenile amyotrophic lateral sclerosis. *Ann Neurol*. 2011 Dec;70:913–9.

340. Mitsumoto H, Chad D, Pioro E. Electrodiagnosis. In: Mitsumoto H, Chad DA, Pioro EP, editors. *Amyotrophic Lateral Sclerosis: Contemporary Neurology Series; 49*. Philadelphia: F.A. Davis; 1998. p. 80–2.

CHAPTER 15

Hereditary Spastic Paraplegia

Pawel P. Liberski[1] and Craig Blackstone[2]

[1]Departments of Molecular Pathology and Neuropathology, Medical University of Lodz, Lodz, Poland
[2]Cell Biology Section, Neurogenetics Branch, National Institutes of Neurological Disorders and Stroke, National Institutes of Health, Bethesda, Maryland, USA

Introduction

Hereditary spastic paraplegia (HSP or SPG), or Strümpell disease, was described by Seeligmüller in 1876 and Adolf Strümpell in 1880, 1886, and 1904 [1–6]. It has since become an umbrella term that encompasses a diverse group of inherited neurological diseases characterized by the defining feature of prominent spastic paraparesis. Currently, well over 70 distinct genetic loci (SPG1–73, plus others) and more than 60 gene products have been identified for this group of disorders. The prevalence of HSP is 1.27–9.6/100,000, depending upon geography and ethnicity [7–9]. HSPs are divided further on the basis of the mode of inheritance (autosomal dominant, autosomal recessive, X-linked, and maternal, with some sporadic cases as well) or by the presence of signs and symptoms different from those of "pure" forms of HSP. If additional signs and symptoms are present, the disease is often referred to as "complicated" or "complex" HSP.

Neuropathology

The cardinal feature of HSPs is lower extremity spasticity and typically more mild weakness due to a length-dependent axonopathy of corticospinal motor neurons (Figures 15.1 and 15.2). Even so, there are limited data on the neuropathology of genetically confirmed HSPs, as most of these studies pre-date the identification of the vast majority of SPG gene loci. Also, apart from degeneration of pyramidal tracts in the spinal cord, significant heterogeneity is present.

Appel and Van Bogaert [10] described degeneration of large pyramidal (Betz) neurons in Brodmann's area 4, plus severe astrocytic gliosis in pyramids, pons and medulla, substantia nigra, and cerebellum. Degeneration of both anterior and lateral (crossed and uncrossed) pyramidal tracts was observed. Schwarz and collaborators [11, 12] reported severe demyelination in axons in pyramidal tracts, with lateral pyramidal tracts more severely affected than anterior pyramidal tracts. Additionally, depopulation of Betz neurons in motor cortex, or central chromatolysis of those cells, was noted along with degeneration of cells in spinal cord anterior horn and Clarke's nucleus, accompanied by astrocytic gliosis. A detailed pathologic description for one patient was reported by Schwarz [11]. At the second sacral level of the spinal cord, a few swollen fibers and demyelination were observed using Weil's myelin stain. Lateral columns demonstrated loss of fibers. At the third lumbar level,

anterior columns were relatively spared while lateral columns were demyelinated. At the eighth cervical level, the fasciculus cuneatus (Burdach) of dorsal columns was intact, while the fasciculus gracilis (tract of Goll) showed demyelination. At the second cervical level, in the lateral pyramidal tract, loss of myelin was less than that described above, while the dorsal columns remained demyelinated. At the decussation of pyramids in the medulla, the pyramids were pale, and demyelination was observed along the medial and lateral surfaces of the gracile nuclei.

More recently, a case of hereditary spastic paraplegia (crystalloid oligodendrogliopathy) was reported (Figure 15.3) [13]. This was a 64-year-old woman with onset at age 40 of progressive spastic paraparesis. Some cognitive impairment was also noted. Neurologic examination showed bilateral ptosis, reduced bulbar motility and anisocoria, perioral dyskinesis, spastic tetraparesis, and bilateral Babinski signs. The most prominent findings at autopsy were crystalloid deposits (cubic or trapezoid shapes) accompanied by astrocytic gliosis and microglial proliferation. The crystalloids were PAS positive, accumulated cathepsin D, ubiquitin, and p62, and were α-tubulin immunoreactive. On electron microscopy, they appeared as lattice- or ladder-like structures. Unfortunately, the molecular genetic basis for this condition remains unknown.

Ferrer et al. [14] described a case of a 49-year-old woman from a family whose parents were first cousins. The case was characterized by spastic paraparesis of the lower limbs. Furthermore, generalized muscle atrophy, contractures, dysphasia, and alternating, rapid horizontal eye movements were observed. The brain was highly atrophic (1100 g), and atrophy of the corpus callosum was readily noticed. Lateral and anterior pyramidal tracts were atrophic, and loss of nerve fibers was seen in dorsal spinocerebellar and posterior columns, in particular in fasciculus gracilis. Mild spongiosis was seen in the hippocampal formation. Parvalbumin immunostaining of neurons was reduced, and calbindin D28K immunoreactivity was markedly reduced. Many neurons demonstrated varicose and fragmented neuronal processes. Axonal enlargements were also visualized.

Autosomal recessive hereditary spastic paraplegia with atrophy of corpus callosum is particularly common in Japan [15–17]. This variant of HSP is labeled "spastic paraplegia with thin corpus callosum" (TCC). A case of HSP with dementia and TCC was published by Wakabayashi et al. [15]. On pathologic examination, practically complete loss of Betz cells in the precentral gyrus was seen. Grumose degeneration [18], comprising degenerating axons, was

Neurodegeneration, First Edition. Edited by Anthony Schapira, Zbigniew Wszolek, Ted M. Dawson and Nicholas Wood.
© 2017 John Wiley & Sons, Ltd. Published 2017 by John Wiley & Sons, Ltd.

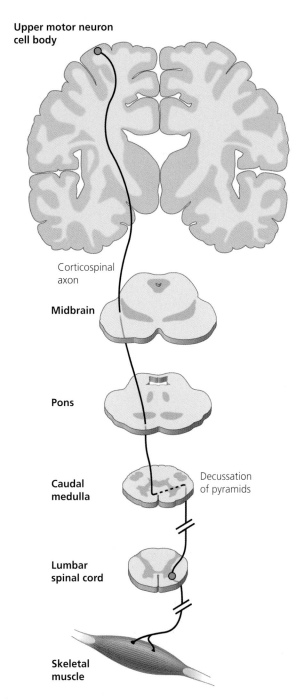

Figure 15.1 Schematic diagram of the corticospinal tract's path through the central nervous system. Although most fibers decussate in the caudal medulla, a minority of fibers descend uncrossed as the ventral corticospinal tract (not shown). Adapted from Blackstone 2012 [117].

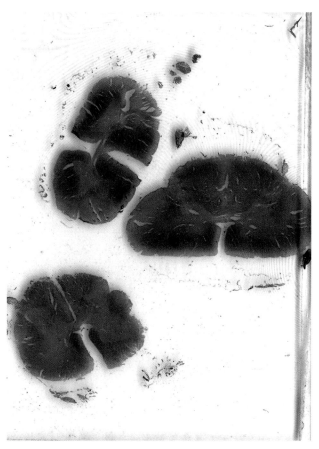

Figure 15.2 Cross-sections through the spinal cord in a case with HSP. Courtesy of Dr. Romana Hoftberger, Clinical Institute of Neurology, Medical University Vienna, Vienna, Austria.

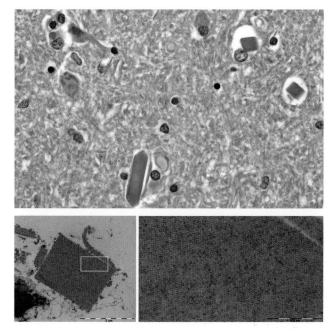

Figure 15.3 Crystalloids from a case of HSP (crystalloid oligodendrogliopathy) [13]. Source: Woehrer et al. 2012 [13]. Reproduced with permission of Springer.

seen. In the neuronal cytoplasm, coarse eosinophilic granules were found; they were ubiquitin positive and MAP/tau negative. Nomura et al. [17] described a case of HSP with onset in the mid teens. Upper extremities were also involved, and dementia was present. There was severe atrophy of skeletal muscle and brain atrophy with white matter changes and TCC. Depigmentation of substantia nigra was severe, and spinal cord and ventral roots were atrophic. Neurons throughout the brain accumulated large amounts of lipofuscin, and they were markedly reduced in number. Hippocampus and substantia nigra were depleted of neurons. Pyramidal tracts were atrophic, and loss of neurons was detected readily in the spinal cord anterior horn. Additionally, the dorsal spinocerebellar tract and fasciculus gracilis were atrophic. Increased ubiquitin immunoreactivity was also observed.

Many of these pathologic cases pre-dated the genetic identification of the HSPs, but spastic gait (SPG) loci are increasingly the predominant way that HSPs are classified, and over time better genetic and pathologic correlations will be possible. Currently there are 73 SPG loci (named in order of discovery and discussed in the section Hereditary spastic paraplegia syndromes) as well as a number of other syndromes in which spastic paraplegia can be prominent, but which are not formally classified as HSPs [19].

Hereditary spastic paraplegia syndromes

Spastic paraplegia 1, MASA or CRASH syndrome, X-linked, SPG1

SPG1 is commonly referred to as MASA syndrome (derived from: Mental retardation, Aphasia, Shuffling gait, and Adducted thumbs) [20]. Additional signs include microcephaly, lumbar lordosis, and hyperreflexia in the lower extremities; corpus callosum agenesis and enlargement of lateral and third ventricles can be seen on brain imaging. Kenwrick et al. [21] used the term "SPG1" and noticed the absence of the extensor pollicis longus muscle. Rosenthal et al. [22] found mutations in the *L1CAM* (L1 cell adhesion molecule; neural cell adhesion molecule L1) gene. An alternative name has been suggested – CRASH (derivative of Corpus callosum hypoplasia, Retardation, Adducted thumbs, Spastic paraplegia, and Hydrocephalus) – which emphasizes the presence of spastic paraplegia.

Spastic paraplegia 2, X-linked, SPG2

This HSP was discovered by Johnston and McKusick [23] in a family with spastic paraplegia, nystagmus, dysarthria, sensory impairment, joint contractures, and cognitive impairment. Magnetic resonance imaging (MRI) can reveal a "patchy leukodystrophy," and polyneuropathy is sometimes present. Saugier-Veber et al. [24] later identified mutations in the *PLP1* gene encoding proteolipid protein. Alterations in this gene also cause Pelizaeus–Merzbacher disease.

Spastic paraplegia 3A, autosomal dominant, SPG3

This is the most common early-onset form of HSP, and second most common overall. Mutations in the *ATL1* gene were first described by Zhao et al. [25]. It is known for very slow or no progression in many patients. Most mutations are missense changes giving rise to pure HSP, but complex forms have also been described, and a single dominant missense change also underlies hereditary and sensory neuropathy type 1D [26].

Spastic paraplegia 4, autosomal dominant, SPG4

Mutations in the *SPAST* gene for this, the most common form of HSP, were described by Hazan et al. [27] in a large Dutch family. Age at onset of symptoms can vary widely, and although many cases are pure, a number of complex cases are known. Additional features include cognitive impairment (in particular visuospatial dysfunction), TCC, low back pain (a late symptom), severe amyotrophy of the thenar eminence, peroneal muscle wasting, and peripheral neuropathy [28, 29]. Neuropathologic evaluation in a small number of cases has revealed atrophy of the spinal cord due to degeneration of the pyramidal tract, accompanied by spongiosis with ubiquitin-immunopositive granules.

Spastic paraplegia 5, autosomal recessive, SPG5

SPG5A was reported by Rothschild et al. [30]. Onset is typically in the twenties or later. In addition to spastic paraplegia, dysarthria, significantly impaired vibratory sensation in the lower extremities, dysfunction of cranial nerves IX, X, and XII, and disrupted visual pathways have been observed. Brain MRI can show white matter abnormalities [31]. In a large English consanguineous family, Tsaousidou et al. [32] found a mutation in the *CYP7B1* gene. More cases have subsequently been identified.

Spastic paraplegia 6, autosomal dominant, SPG6

This HSP was described by Fink and colleagues [33, 34]. Age of onset has ranged from 8 to 37 years. The clinical picture consists of spastic paraplegia and impaired vibratory sensation. Rarely, patients may have neuropathy or cognitive impairment. Mutations in the *NIPA1* gene were identified by Rainier et al. [35] and have also been reported de novo [36].

Spastic paraplegia 7, autosomal recessive, SPG7

SPG7 was initially reported in a large consanguineous family by De Michele et al. [37], and age of onset can range from childhood to the forties. Additional symptomatology can include optic atrophy, cerebellar ataxia, impairment of vibratory sensation, scoliosis, axonal neuropathy, and pes cavus. Mutations are found in the *SPG7* gene encoding the mitochondrial protein paraplegin.

Spastic paraplegia 8, autosomal dominant, SPG8

This HSP was first reported by de Bot et al. [38] in a Dutch family. Symptom onset ranges widely from about 10 to 60 years. The clinical picture consists of severe lower limb spasticity, upper extremity spasticity, and ataxia (not observed in all patients). Mild dysphagia has also been observed, and rarely neuropathy. Valdmanis et al. [39] reported mutations in the *KIAA0196* gene encoding strumpellin. It is allelic with autosomal recessive Ritscher–Schnitzel syndrome.

Spastic paraplegia 9, autosomal dominant, SPG9

SPG9 was reported by Slavotinek et al. [40] in a family with motor neuropathy, spasticity, developmental delay, and skeletal deformities. Bilateral lamellar cataracts, delayed age of bone, shallow acetabulum, small carpal bones, dysplastic cranial base, and decreased muscle mass are other features. Age of onset was the first year of life in a proband but 22 years in his mother and 37 years in an earlier generation. Ocular abnormalities, myopia, and chorioretinal dystrophy were reported along with persistent vomiting and gastroesophageal reflux. The gene was mapped to 10q23.3–q14.2 [41].

Spastic paraplegia 10, autosomal dominant, SPG10

This HSP was reported by Reid et al. [42] and is due to mutations in the *KIF5A* gene that encodes a kinesin heavy chain protein. Age of onset varies from 8 to 40 years. The clinical picture consists of pure spastic paraplegia plus distal impairment of vibratory sensation. Crimella et al. [43] also found a case of axonal sensorimotor peripheral neuropathy consistent with type 2 Charcot–Marie–Tooth disease. The age of onset was 16 years and the clinical picture consisted of lower limb atrophy, weakness of small muscles of the hands, impairment of vibration sensation and joint position sense, pes cavus, and impairment of gait, but without spasticity. Peripheral axonal neuropathy is frequent, and cerebellar ataxia has been reported.

Spastic paraplegia 11, autosomal recessive, SPG11

First reported by Nakamura et al. [44] in two Japanese families, this is the most common autosomal recessive HSP. Onset in the first family was in the second decade, and the clinical picture consisted of lower limb spastic paraplegia, ataxia, mild sensory impairment, and mental dysfunction (IQ <60). Neuroimaging studies revealed TCC, mild frontal and temporal atrophy, and enlarged ventricles. Additional signs can include parkinsonism, retinopathy, pseudobulbar signs, urinary dysfunction, peripheral motor or sensorimotor polyneuropathy, and distal amyotrophy. Stevanin et al. [45] identified mutations in the *KIAA1840* gene that encodes the spatacsin protein.

Spastic paraplegia 12, autosomal dominant, SPG12

SPG12 was reported by Reid et al. [46] in a Welsh family. Age of onset varies between 5 and 24 years and the clinical picture is mostly pure. Montenegro et al. [47] identified a mutation in the *RTN2* gene encoding the endoplasmic reticulum (ER) protein reticulon 2.

Spastic paraplegia 13, autosomal dominant, SPG13

This was reported by Fontaine et al. [48] in a French family. The majority of patients with SPG13 did not have the Babinski sign. The gene for SPG13 was mapped to 2q24-q25. Hansen et al. [49] found a mutation in the gene encoding the chaperonin HSP60 (*HSPD1*).

Spastic paraplegia 14, autosomal recessive, SPG14

The original report of a family with SPG14 was by Vazza et al. [50]; the average age of onset was 30 years. The clinical picture consisted of spastic paraplegia with distal motor neuropathy, mild cognitive dysfunction, and pes cavus.

Spastic paraplegia 15, autosomal recessive, SPG15

This SPG reported by Goizet al. [51] is also known as spastic paraplegia with retinal degeneration or Kjellin syndrome. In addition to spastic paraplegia, patients suffer from mental retardation, parkinsonism, retinopathy, and cerebellar ataxia. Kjellin [52] in 1959 reported two pairs of siblings with spastic paraplegia, wasting of distal muscles, mental retardation, and central degeneration of the retina [53]. This is the second most common autosomal recessive HSP, and clinically it is virtually identical to SPG11. Imaging of both forms often shows prominent TCC as well as "ears of the lynx" white matter changes (Figure 15.4).

Spastic paraplegia 16, X-linked, SPG16

This HSP was reported by Steinmuller et al. [54]. Onset occurred in the first 3 years. Features are quadriplegia, aphasia, and impairment of vision and sphincter function. The gene has been mapped to Xq11.2-q23.

Spastic paraplegia 17, autosomal dominant, SPG 17 (Silver syndrome)

SPG17 was described in two families with spastic paraplegia and amyotrophy of the hands by Silver [55]. Onset of gait impairment varied from 8 to 40 years, and hand amyotrophy was noted at 14–60 years. Other presentations can be consistent with distal spinal muscular atrophy, pure spastic paraplegia, and peroneal muscular atrophy; the latter has been accompanied by pyramidal signs and symptoms [56]. Windpassinger et al. [57] reported missense mutations in the *BSCL2* gene encoding seipin. It is allelic with autosomal recessive congenital lipodystrophy type 2.

Spastic paraplegia 18, autosomal recessive, SPG18

This form of spastic paraplegia was reported by Al-Yahyaee et al. [58] in Omani families. The age of onset varied between 4 and 6 years. Epilepsy and TCC were observed, as well as joint contractures, febrile seizures, and severe mental retardation. Electron microscopic examination of leukocytes revealed electron-dense membrane-bound vacuoles. Yildirim et al. [59] found truncation mutations in the *ERLIN2* (endoplasmic reticulum lipid raft-associated

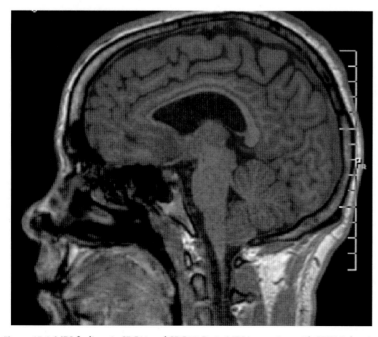
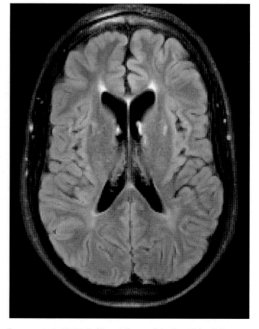

Figure 15.4 MRI findings in SPG11 and SPG15. Brain MRI in a patient with SPG15 showing characteristic TCC (left) and "ears of the lynx" (right). Source: Renvoisé et al. 2014 [193]. Reproduced with permission of John Wiley and Sons.

protein 2) gene on 8p11.2, encoding a protein involved in ERAD (ER-associated degradation).

Spastic paraplegia 19, autosomal dominant, SPG19

This HSP was described in an Italian family by Valente et al. [60]. Age of onset varied from 36 to 55 years. The clinical picture consists of spastic paraplegia, pes cavus, and slowing of motor and sensory conduction in the lower extremities. The gene was mapped to 9q33-q34.

Spastic paraplegia 20, autosomal recessive, SPG20 (Troyer syndrome)

This complex spastic paraplegia was reported in the Old Order Amish by Cross and McKusick [61]. Onset occurred in early childhood. Drooling, pseudobulbar affect, short stature, distal amyotrophy, and cerebellar signs were also observed. Patel et al. [62] identified a loss-of-function mutation in the SPG20 gene encoding spartin [63, 64].

Spastic paraplegia 21, autosomal recessive, SPG21 (Mast syndrome)

This HSP was also reported in the Old Order Amish by Cross and McKusick [65]. Onset was in adulthood, with speech decline, personality changes, psychosis, and cerebellar dysfunction in addition to spastic paraplegia. Mutations in the SPG21/ACP33 gene were identified by Cross and colleagues [66].

Spastic paraplegia 22, X-linked, SPG22

This HSP is in the Allan–Herndon–Dudley syndrome (AHDS) disease spectrum. It was reported in 1944 [67] in a family with hypotonia at birth, inability to raise the head, reduced motor milestones, generalized muscle atrophy, and hyperreflexia. Ataxia, dysarthria, athetoid movements, and spastic paraplegia were also observed. Vaurs-Barrière et al. [68] detected mutations in the MCT8 (monocarboxylic acid transporter-8, member 2; SLC16A2) gene. The protein encoded by the MCT8 gene is involved in the transport of triiodothyronine (T_3) to neurons.

Spastic paraplegia 23, autosomal recessive, SPG23 (Lison syndrome)

Although originally described in a consanguineous Arab Israeli family in 1985, the locus was refined by Blumen et al. [69]. Onset is in infancy, with abnormal skin and hair pigmentation, skeletal deformities, and sensorimotor neuropathy. On brain MRI, ventricles may be enlarged or microcephaly may be noted. The locus has been mapped to 1q24-32.

Spastic paraplegia 24, autosomal recessive, SPG24

SPG24 was reported by Hodgkinson et al. [70] in a Saudi family. The disease starts in childhood, and associated features can include spastic dysarthria and pseudobulbar signs. The locus has been mapped to 13q14.

Spastic paraplegia 25, autosomal recessive, SPG25

SPG25 was reported by Zortea et al. [71] in a consanguineous Italian family. Disease onset ranged between 30 and 46 years. The paraparesis was preceded by back pain due to disc herniations. Peripheral neuropathy can also be present. Linkage to chromosome 6q23.3-q24.1 has been reported.

Spastic paraplegia 26, autosomal recessive, SPG26

SPG26 was reported in a Kuwaiti family by Farag et al. [72]. Age at disease onset has ranged from 2 to 19, with difficulties in walking and dysarthria. Associated signs include pes cavus, atrophy of small hand muscles, and ataxia. MRI has demonstrated cortical atrophy and white matter hyperintensities. Mutations were found in the B4GALNT1 (β-1,4-N-acetylgalactosaminyltransferase) gene encoding an enzyme that catalyzes the synthesis of complex gangliosides.

Spastic paraplegia 27, autosomal recessive, SPG27

This was reported by Meijer et al. [73] in a large French-Canadian family. Onset of disease for the more pure forms is 25–45 years; complex forms originate in childhood. Additional signs and symptoms have included skeletal abnormalities, cerebellar signs, and polyneuropathy. The gene has been mapped to 10q22.1-q24.1.

Spastic paraplegia 28, autosomal recessive, SPG28

SPG28 was reported in a consanguineous Moroccan family by Bouslam et al. [74]. Disease onset ranged from 6 to 15 years. In addition to spastic paraplegia, axonal neuropathy and cerebellar oculomotor dysfunction have been observed. Mutations were identified in DDHD1 (DDHD domain-containing protein 1; phosphatidic acid-preferring phospholipase A1), which encodes a lipase that catalyzes degradation of phosphatidic acid.

Spastic paraplegia 29, autosomal dominant, SPG29

This was first described in a large Scottish family by Orlacchio et al. [75]. Onset is in infancy, and associated signs included sensorineural hearing deficits and persistent vomiting due to hiatal hernia. The gene was mapped to 1p31.1-p21.1. In the neonatal period, hyperbilirubinemia (without kernicterus) was detected.

Spastic paraplegia 30, autosomal recessive, SPG30

This was reported in an Algerian consanguineous family by Klebe et al. [76]. Onset of disease varied between 12 and 21 years with distal sensory loss, mild cerebellar signs, and saccadic ocular pursuits. MRI revealed cerebellar atrophy. Another family was reported by Erlich et al. [77], who described mutations in the KIF1A (kinesin family member) gene which encodes for a motor protein. This gene is also mutated in hereditary sensory neuropathy, type IIC.

Spastic paraplegia 31, autosomal dominant, SPG31

This HSP was originally described in two Caucasian families [78, 79]. Mild weakness of small muscles of the hands was observed. Züchner et al. [79] detected mutations in the REEP1 gene, with haploinsufficiency as a proposed mechanism. Numerous mutations have been identified subsequently, and this is the third most common form of autosomal dominant HSP.

Spastic paraplegia 32, autosomal recessive, SPG32

SPG32 was reported by Stevanin et al. [80] in a Portuguese family. Disease onset was 6–7 years. In addition to spastic paraplegia, mild cognitive impairment was reported. MRI revealed TCC and cortical and cerebellar atrophy as well as pontine dysraphia. The gene was mapped to 14q12-q21.

Spastic paraplegia 33, autosomal dominant, SPG33

A large German family with spastic paraplegia was described by Mannan et al. [81]. SPG33 is a pure form of HSP with spastic paraplegia, Babinski signs, ankle clonus, and pes cavus. A missense mutation was identified in the *ZFYVE27* gene which encodes for the protrudin protein, which is an interactor of the SPG4 protein spastin and SPG3A protein atlastin-1 [81, 82]. This identification remains questionable, and Rugarli and colleagues have reported that this mutation is a benign polymorphism [83].

Spastic paraplegia 34, X-linked, SPG34

This X-linked spastic paraplegia was reported by Zatz et al. [84] in a Brazilian family. The clinical picture consists of pure spastic paraplegia. Onset of disease was in late teens or twenties. A candidate locus is on Xq24-q25.

Spastic paraplegia 35, autosomal recessive, SPG35

This form was described in a large Omani family by Dick et al. [85]. Age of onset varied from 2 to 17 years. There is a rapidly progressive spasticity of lower and upper extremities. Additional signs and symptoms are clonus, dystonia, seizures, cognitive decline, and cerebellar signs. MRI revealed periventricular white matter hyperintensities in parietal and occipital lobes, TCC, and hypointensities in the globus pallidus. Dick et al. [86] found mutations in the *FA2H* gene encoding fatty acid-2 hydroxylase. It is allelic with neurodegeneration with brain iron accumulation (NBIA) and leukodystrophy.

Spastic paraplegia 36, autosomal dominant, SPG36

SPG36 was described in a German family by Schüle et al. [87]. Age of onset varied from 14 to 33 years. The clinical picture consists of spastic paraplegia and peripheral sensorimotor neuropathy. Linkage to 12q23-q24 was reported.

Spastic paraplegia 37, autosomal dominant, SPG37

This HSP was described in a French family by Hanein et al. [88]. Age of onset varied from 8 to 60 years. The clinical picture consisted mostly of a pure spastic paraplegia. A candidate locus on 8p21.1.-q13.3 was identified.

Spastic paraplegia 38, autosomal dominant, SPG38

This HSP was described by Orlacchio et al. [89] in a four-generation family. Age of onset was in the late teens. The clinical picture is one of predominantly pure spastic paraplegia. The locus was identified as 4p16-p15.

Spastic paraplegia 39, autosomal recessive, SPG39

This HSP was detected in an Ashkenazi Jewish family by Rainier et al. [90]. Electrophysiology revealed motor axonopathy. MRI revealed spinal cord atrophy. Rainier et al. [90] and Synofzik et al. [91] reported mutations in the *PNPLA6/NTE* gene (patatin-like phospholipase domain-containing protein 6; neuropathy-target esterase) on 19p32.

Spastic paraplegia 40, autosomal dominant, SPG40

This locus is reserved. This is provisionally considered an autosomal dominant, pure HSP with possible memory deficits and genetic anticipation.

Spastic paraplegia 41, autosomal dominant, SPG41

This HSP was identified in a Chinese family by Zhao et al. [92]. It is a mostly pure spastic paraplegia with age of onset in the mid teens. The clinical picture consists of spastic paraplegia, hyperreflexia, and mild weakness in the upper extremities.

Spastic paraplegia 42, autosomal dominant, SPG42

Lin et al. [93] described this HSP in a Chinese family. Age of onset has varied from 4 to 42 years. The clinical picture consisted of spastic paraplegia, hyperreflexia, pes cavus, and atrophy of the lower limb muscles. It is reportedly caused by mutations in the *SLC33A1* gene encoding the acetyl-CoA transporter.

Spastic paraplegia 43, autosomal recessive, SPG43

Meilleur et al. [94] reported two siblings with HSP beginning in childhood. Other signs included Babinski sign, involvement of upper extremities, and impairment of vibration sense. Landouré et al. [95] found a missense mutation in the *C19ORF12* gene in those two siblings; the same mutation was detected in a Brazilian family with NBIA4, and genetic analysis revealed a founder effect between those families.

Spastic paraplegia 44, autosomal recessive, SPG44

This form of spastic paraplegia was reported in an Italian family by Orthmann-Murphy et al. [96]. Symptoms started in the first or second decade. The clinical picture consisted of spastic paraparesis, pes cavus, dysarthria, loss of subtle movements of fingers, and cerebellar signs. One patient demonstrated lumbar hyperlordosis and scoliosis. Tonic-clonic seizures were also seen. MRI revealed hypomyelinating leukodystrophy and TCC. A mutation in the *GJC2* (GAP-junction protein gamma 2) gene was identified, and the same gene is mutated in hypomyelinating leukodystrophy 2.

Spastic paraplegia 45, autosomal recessive, SPG45

This was reported by Dursun et al. [97] in a consanguineous Turkish family. The onset of disease varied from 5 to 8 years. It is a complicated HSP with joint contractures, myopia, pendular nystagmus, and optic atrophy. Patients could neither write nor read. Novarino et al. [98] reported additional families with SPG45 but labeled them SPG65. They also demonstrated a thin or dysplastic corpus callosum. Mutations were found in the *NT5C2* gene which encodes for purine 5′-nucleotidase that hydrolyzes inosine 5′-monophosphate.

Spastic paraplegia 46, autosomal recessive, SPG46

This form of spastic paraplegia was reported by Boukhris et al. [99] in a consanguineous Tunisian family. Age of onset was in the first and second decades. Spastic bladder, upper limb cerebellar dysmetria, congenital cataracts, and pes cavus were also observed. Martin et al. [100] reported an additional three families. All patients developed cataracts, cerebellar ataxia, dementia, hearing loss, and axonal neuropathy. Brain MRI showed atrophy of corpus callosum and cerebellum. Of interest, spermatozoid heads were malformed. Martin et al. [100] found mutations in the *GBA2* (glucosidase, β, acid 2) gene which encodes for an enzyme initially identified as a microsomal β-glucosidase that catalyzes the hydrolysis of endogenous bile acid 3-O-glucosides.

Spastic paraplegia 47, autosomal recessive, SPG47

SPG47 was reported by Abou Jamra et al. [101] in an Israeli-Arab family with dementia and paraplegia. Symptoms noticed at birth included microcephaly and hypotonia which eventually evolved to hypertonia. Other signs include high palate, wide nasal bridge, short stature, hypermobility of joints, and genu recurvatum (a knee joint deformity, such that the knee bends backwards). A truncation mutation was found in AP4B1 (adaptor-related protein complex 4, β-1 subunit).

Spastic paraplegia 48, autosomal recessive, SPG48
This HSP was identified by Slabicki et al. [102]. The clinical picture consists of spastic paraplegia and bladder impairment. A homozygous indel (the term implies insertion or deletion) truncation mutation and another mutation in the *KIAA0415* gene were found. This gene encodes an adaptor protein complex 5 subunit that co-precipitates with two other proteins involved in SPG: spatacsin (SPG 11) and spastizin (SPG15). Recently identified cases have parkinsonism and retinal abnormalities as additional features [103].

Spastic paraplegia 49, autosomal recessive, SPG49 (by OMIM, no HUGO designation)
Oz-Levi et al. [104] reported this HSP in a family of Jewish Bukharian (Binai Israel; Jews from the emirate of Bukhara) descent. Onset of symptoms was at about 2 years. The clinical picture consists of dysmorphic features, developmental delay, brachycephaly, microcephaly, dental crowding, dysarthria, and dysmetria. Episodes of central dyspnea and seizures were recorded. Truncating mutations were identified in the *TECPR2* (tectonin β-propeller repeat-containing protein 2) gene, causing defects in autophagy.

Spastic paraplegia 50, autosomal recessive, SPG50
SPG50 was reported in a Moroccan family by Verkerk et al. [105]. The five affected siblings demonstrated signs and symptoms of infantile hypotonia, severe mental retardation, quadriplegia, and strabismus. Speech never developed or was very poor. They also demonstrated signs of pseudobulbar palsy, compulsive laughter, and sphincter impairment. MRI revealed enlarged ventricles, white matter changes, and cerebellar degeneration. A loss-of-function mutation was identified in the *AP4M1* (adaptor-related protein complex 4) gene on chromosome 7q22.1.

Spastic paraplegia 51, autosomal recessive, SPG51
This form of spastic paraplegia was described by Moreno-De-Luca et al. [106] in a consanguineous Palestinian-Jordanian family. The affected children showed signs and symptoms at birth. The clinical picture consisted of quadriplegia, microcephaly, psychomotor retardation, seizures, and dysmorphic features. MRI revealed cortical and cerebellar atrophy, ventriculomegaly, and diffuse white matter loss. A 192-kb deletion was detected on chromosome 15q21.2 within the *AP4E1* (adaptor-related protein complex 4, ε-1 subunit) gene.

Spastic paraplegia 52, autosomal recessive, SPG52
This form of spastic paraplegia was reported by Abou Jamra et al. [101] in a consanguineous Syrian family. The disease started in infancy, and the clinical picture comprises mental retardation, contractures, pes equinovarus (club foot), microcephaly, dysmorphic features, inappropriate laughter, and short stature. A truncating mutation in the *AP4S1* (adaptor-related protein complex 4, σ-1 subunit) gene was identified.

Spastic paraplegia 53, autosomal recessive, SPG53
This form of spastic paraplegia was reported by Zivony-Elboum et al. [107] in two Arab families. Symptom onset was about the second year of life. The clinical picture consists of quadriplegia, developmental delay, marked kyphosis, and pectus carinatum. A mutation in the *VPS37A* (vacuolar protein sorting 37A) gene was identified.

Spastic paraplegia 54, autosomal recessive, SPG54
This HSP was identified in two unrelated families, and subsequently in Omani and Iranian families by Schuurs-Hoeijmakers et al. [108]. Clinically, there is spastic paraplegia, mental retardation, foot contractures, dysarthria, dysphagia, strabismus, and optic hypoplasia. MRI demonstrated TCC, white matter hyperintensities, and spinal syrinx. Mutations were identified in the *DDHD2* (DDHD domain-containing protein 2) gene.

Spastic paraplegia 55, autosomal recessive, SPG55
This form of spastic paraplegia was described by Yoshita et al. [109]. The disease started at age 7 with impairment of vision, with walking difficulties several years later. Optic atrophy and decreased motor and sensory velocities were detected. Nerve biopsy revealed decreased numbers of large-diameter nerve fibers as well as onion bulbs. Shimazaki et al. [110] identified a truncating mutation of the *C12ORF56* gene encoding a protein involved in releasing proteins from mitochondrial ribosomes. Defects of the same gene cause combined oxidative phosphorylation deficiency 7 (OMIM 613559).

Spastic paraplegia 56, autosomal recessive, SPG56 (denoted SPG49 by HUGO)
SPG56 was reported by Tesson et al. [111] in two Saudi Arabian consanguineous families. Age of onset varied from birth to 8 years. The clinical picture consists of spastic paraplegia or quadriparesis, dystonic postures, dementia, and axonal neuropathy. Brain MRI revealed TCC or basal ganglia calcifications. Mutations in *CYP2U1* were identified.

Spastic paraplegia 57, autosomal recessive, SPG57
This form of spastic paraplegia was identified by Beetz et al. [112] in two siblings of Indian descent. In addition to spastic paraplegia, axonal demyelinating motor neuropathy and optic atrophy are present. A mutation in *TFG (TRK-fused* gene) was identified.

Spastic paraplegia 58, autosomal recessive, SPG58
SPG58 was reported by Caballero Oteyza et al. [113] in a family with spastic paraplegia, cervical dystonia, chorea, and cerebellar ataxia. Mutations were found in the *KIF1C* (kinesin family member 1C) gene. This is allelic with spastic ataxia SPAX2 (OMIM 611302).

Spastic paraplegia 59, autosomal recessive, SPG59
This HSP was identified by Novarino et al. [98]. Age of onset was 20 months. Pes equinovarus and nystagmus were reported. Mutations were found in the *USP8* gene encoding ubiquitin-specific protease 8.

Spastic paraplegia 61, autosomal recessive, SPG61
Discovered by Novarino et al. [98] through exome sequencing, SPG61 is a complex spastic paraplegia with associated sensory and motor polyneuropathy and acropathy mutilation. A mutation in the *ARL61P1* (ADP-ribosylation-like factor 6-interacting protein 1) gene was found.

Spastic paraplegia 62, autosomal recessive, SPG62
This HSP was identified by Novarino et al. [98] and is caused by mutation in the *ERLIN1* gene. It is a pure HSP with onset in infancy.

Spastic paraplegia 63, autosomal recessive, SPG63
This form of spastic paraplegia was reported by Novarino et al. [98]. Disease onset was in early life. The clinical picture includes short

stature, and brain MRI has shown TCC and white matter hyperintensities. Mutations were identified in the *AMPD2* gene.

Spastic paraplegia 64, autosomal recessive, SPG64
This HSP has onset at 1–4 years of age. Additional symptoms include dysarthria, borderline IQ, aggressiveness, and microcephaly. Missense and nonsense mutations in the *ENTPD1* gene encoding ectonucleoside triphosphate diphosphohydrolase 1 were found [98].

Spastic paraplegia 65, autosomal recessive, SPG65
This spastic paraplegia is the same as SPG45 [98].

Spastic paraplegia 66, autosomal recessive, SPG66
SPG66 was reported by Novarino et al. [98] in a consanguineous family. Age of onset was in infancy, and the clinical picture in addition to spastic paraplegia consisted of pes equinovarus, amyotrophy, and a severe sensorimotor polyneuropathy. MRI revealed corpus callosal and cerebellar hypoplasia. An insertion mutation in the *ARSI* (arylsulfatase I) gene at 5q32 was reported.

Spastic paraplegia 67, autosomal recessive, SPG67
This HSP was identified by Novarino et al. [98] in another consanguineous family. Age of onset was early childhood, and the clinical picture includes amyotrophy. MRI revealed agenesis of corpus callosum and cortical as well as cerebellar atrophy, plus defective myelination. A splice site mutation in the *PGAP1* (post-GPI attachment to proteins 1) gene was responsible.

Spastic paraplegia 68, autosomal recessive, SPG68
The gene involved is fibronectin-like domain-containing leucine-rich transmembrane protein 1 (*FLRT1*) [98]. Age of onset is early childhood, and associated symptoms include optic atrophy, nystagmus, and mild neuropathy.

Spastic paraplegia 69, autosomal recessive, SPG69
This form of HSP is caused by mutations in the *RAB3GAP2* gene encoding a RAB3 GTPase-activating protein, non-catalytic subunit [98]. The clinical picture consists of dementia, cataract, and deafness. This gene is also mutated in Martsolf syndrome and Warburg micro syndrome 2.

Spastic paraplegia 70, autosomal recessive, SPG70
This form of spastic paraplegia was identified by Novarino et al. [98] in a consanguineous family. Disease onset was before the age of 1, and the clinical picture includes Achilles tendon contractures and amyotrophy. Mutations were found in the *MARS* gene encoding methionyl-tRNA synthetase.

Spastic paraplegia 71, autosomal recessive, SPG71
SPG71 is another gene found by Novarino et al. [98] through exome sequencing in a child in whom signs and symptoms appeared at 1 year of age. MRI revealed TCC. Mutations in *ZFR* (zinc finger RNA-binding protein) were detected.

Spastic paraplegia 72, autosomal recessive/dominant, SPG72
This pure form of HSP was reported in 2014 in a large French family. Age of onset varied from infancy to 8 years, and the clinical picture is notable for slowly progressive lower extremity spasticity.

Upper limb spasticity was also noticed as well as pes cavus, urinary problems, slight postural tremor, and impaired vibratory sensation. Mutations in the *REEP2* gene were identified [114].

Spastic paraplegia 73, autosomal dominant, SPG73
This predominantly pure form of adult-onset HSP was reported in 2015 in a multigenerational Italian family by Rinaldi et al. [115]. It resulted from a missense mutation in the *CPT1C* gene that encodes a carnitine palmitoyltransferase. Patients also have loss of vibratory sensation at the ankles, and a couple of those affected have a mild foot deformity.

Common cellular pathogenic themes
The overlapping clinical and pathologic features of different HSPs prefigure a relatively small number of common abnormalities at the cellular level, and the remarkable genetic heterogeneity of the HSPs provides a significant advantage in identifying such convergent pathogenic themes. Indeed, most proteins encoded by HSP genes fall into a small number of functional groups, and these groupings have been fundamental to understanding the cell biology and pathogenesis underpinning various HSP subtypes (Figure 15.5 and Table 15.1). Importantly, many HSP proteins function in a number of different pathways, and thus pathogenic groupings may evolve over time [116, 117].

Membrane modeling and organelle morphogenesis
The largest group of HSP proteins are either known or suspected to be involved in intracellular trafficking, distribution, biogenesis, and/or shaping of membrane compartments [116, 117]. This is not surprising, given the great length and extreme polarity of corticospinal axons, which can extend to 1 meter in length. Indeed, this is a particularly important and relevant subgroup, since mutations in the genes responsible for autosomal dominant SPG4, SPG3A, and SPG31 represent about half of HSP cases in North America and Northern Europe. Furthermore, loss-of-function mutations in the two most common autosomal recessive HSPs, SPG11 and SPG15, affect proteins that also settle within this category [19].

Spastin: coupling membrane modeling to microtubule severing
The *SPAST* gene mutated in the most common form of HSP, SPG4, encodes four main cellular isoforms of the spastin protein, a multimeric AAA ATPase. These isoforms include a 616 amino acid full-length protein (M1 spastin] and a shorter isoform lacking the first 86 residues of the full-length protein (M87 spastin), generated via alternative initiation of protein translation from different AUG start codons. Splice variants exist for both which lack a 32 amino acid stretch encoded by exon 4 [118].

Spastin is a hexameric, microtubule-severing ATPase that causes internal breaks in microtubules, thus regulating microtubule-dependent cellular functions [119]. The C-terminal half of the spastin protomer contains domains required for binding and severing microtubules, including the AAA ATPase domain. The N-terminal half mediates interaction with proteins that recruit spastin to various cellular compartments. In addition to microtubules, these include the ER, endosomes, and midbodies [120]. Spastin localization patterns are isoform specific, with the membrane-bound M1 isoform predominantly found in ER and to a much lesser extent on endosomes, while the smaller, soluble M87 isoform is present in a cytoplasmic pool that can be recruited to structures such as endosomes and midbodies [120, 121].

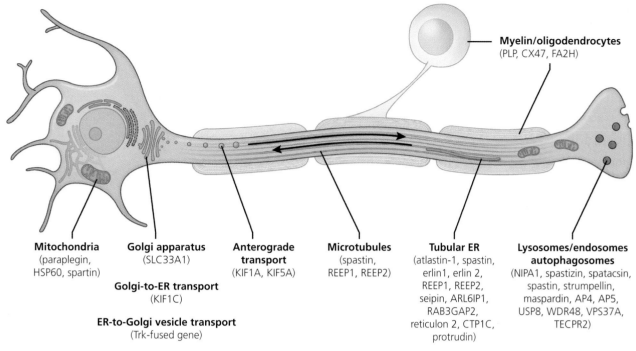

Figure 15.5 Common pathogenic themes in the HSPs. This schematic representation of a corticospinal motor neuron emphasizes where HSP gene products are proposed to function. A number of gene products are not shown, pending more detailed studies of their sites of action. Adapted from Blackstone 2012 [117].

Table 15.1 Identified SPG gene products, grouped functionally.

Disease/gene[a](OMIM)	Protein name	Inheritance	Cellular functions
Membrane traffic, organelle shaping, and biogenesis			
SPG3A/*ATL1*	Atlastin-1	AD	ER morphogenesis, BMP signaling, lipid droplet biogenesis
SPG4/*SPAST*	Spastin (M1 and M87 isoforms)	AD	Microtubule severing, ER morphogenesis, endosomal dynamics, BMP signaling, lipid droplet biogenesis, cytokinesis
SPG6/*NIPA1*	NIPA1	AD	Endosomal traffic, Mg^{2+} transport, BMP signaling
SPG8/*KIAA0196*	Strumpellin	AD	Endosomal dynamics, cytoskeletal (actin) regulation
SPG10/*KIF5A*	Kinesin heavy chain isoform 5A	AD	Microtubule-based motor protein, axon transport
SPG11	Spatacsin	AR	Endosomal traffic, lysosomal biogenesis, autophagy
SPG12/*RTN2*	Reticulon 2	AD	ER morphogenesis
SPG15/*ZFYVE26*	Spastizin/ZFYVE26/FYVE-CENT	AR	Endosomal traffic, lysosomal biogenesis, autophagy
SPG17/*BSCL2*	Seipin/BSCL2	AD	Lipid droplet biogenesis
SPG18/*ERLIN2*	Erlin2	AR	ER-associated degradation, lipid raft-associated
SPG20	Spartin	AR	Endosomal traffic, BMP signaling, cytokinesis, lipid droplet turnover, mitochondrial regulation
SPG21	Maspardin	AR	Endosomal traffic
SPG30/*KIF1A*	Kinesin family member 1A	AR	Microtubule-based motor protein
SPG31/*REEP1*	REEP1	AD	ER morphogenesis, microtubule interactions
SPG33/*ZFYVE27*	Protrudin	AD	ER morphogenesis, endosome interactions
SPG47/*AP4B1*	AP-4 β1 subunit	AR	Endocytic adaptor protein complex
SPG48/*KIAA0415*	KIAA0415 (AP-5 ζ1 subunit)	AR	Endocytic adaptor protein complex
SPG49/*TECPR2*	TECPR2	AR	Autophagy
SPG50/*AP4M1*	AP-4 μ1 subunit	AR	Endocytic adaptor protein complex
SPG51/*AP4E1*	AP-4 ε1 subunit	AR	Endocytic adaptor protein complex
SPG52/*AP4S1*	AP-4 σ1 subunit	AR	Endocytic adaptor protein complex
SPG53/*VPS37A*	VPS37A	AR	Retromer component
SPG57/*TFG*	Trk-fused gene	AR	ER morphogenesis and vesicle biogenesis
SPG58/*KIF1C*	Kinesin family member 1C	AR, ?AD	Motor protein, retrograde Golgi-to-ER transport
SPG61/*ARL6IP1*	ADP-ribosylation factor-like interacting protein 1	AR	ER morphogenesis
SPG62/*ERLIN1*	Erlin1	AR	ER-associated degradation, lipid raft-associated
SPG67/*PGAP1*	GPI inositol-deacylase	AR	Transport of GPI-anchored proteins from ER to Golgi apparatus
SPG69/*RAB3GAP2*	RAB3 GTPase-activating protein 2	AR	ER morphogenesis
SPG72/*REEP2*	REEP2	AR/AD	ER morphogenesis, microtubule interactions
Mitochondrial regulation			
SPG7	Paraplegin	AR	Mitochondrial *m*-AAA ATPase
SPG13/*HSPD1*	HSP60	AD	Mitochondrial chaperonin
SPG55/*C12orf65*	C12orf65	AR	Mitochondrial protein translation

Continued

Table 15.1 *Continued*

Myelination and lipid/sterol modification			
SPG2/*PLP1*	Proteolipid protein	X-linked	Major myelin protein
SPG5/*CYP7B1*	CYP7B1/OAH1	AR	Cholesterol metabolism
SPG26/*B4GALNT1*	β-1,4-*N*-acetyl-galactosaminyl transferase	AR	Ganglioside biosynthesis
SPG28/*DDHD1*	Phospholipase A1	AR	Phosphatidic acid metabolism, membrane traffic
SPG35/*FA2H*	Fatty acid 2-hydroxylase	AR	Myelin lipid hydroxylation
SPG39/*PNPLA2*	Neuropathy target esterase	AR	Phospholipid homeostasis
SPG42/*SLC33A1*	Solute carrier family 33, acetyl-CoA transporter, member 1	AD	Acetyl-CoA transporter
SPG44/*GJC2*	Connexin-47	AR	Intercellular gap junction channel
SPG46/*GBA2*	Glucocerebrosidase 2	AR	Lipid metabolism
SPG54/*DDHD2*	Phospholipase A1	AR	Phosphatidic acid metabolism, membrane traffic
SPG56/*CYP2U1*	CYP2U1	AR	Long-chain fatty acid metabolism
SPG73/*CPT1C*	Carnitine palmitoyltransfer-ase 1C	AD	Lipid metabolism
Axon pathfinding			
SPG1/*L1CAM*	L1CAM	X-linked	Cell adhesion and signaling
Other/unknown			
SPG22/*SLC16A2*	Solute carrier family 16 (monocarboxylic acid transporter) member 2	X-linked	Thyroid hormone (T_3) transporter
SPG43/*C19orf12*	C19orf12	AR	Unknown
SPG59/*USP8*	Ubiquitin-specific peptidase 8	AR	Deubiquitination enzyme
SPG60/*WDR48*	WD repeat domain 48	AR	Regulation of deubiquitination
SPG63/*AMPD2*	Adenosine monophosphate deaminase 2	AR	Deaminates AMP to IMP (purine metabolism)
SPG64/*ENTPD1*	Ectonucleoside triphosphate diphosphohydrolase 1	AR	Hydrolyzes ATP and other nucleotides (purinergic transmission)
SPG65/*NT5C2*	Cytosolic 5′-nucleotidase	AR	IMP hydrolysis, purine/pyrimidine nucleotide metabolism
SPG66/*ARSI*	Arylsulfatase I	AR	Sulfate ester hydrolysis, hormone biosynthesis
SPG68/*FLRT1*	Fibronectin leucine-rich transmembrane protein 1	AR	Fibroblast growth factor pathway
SPG70/*MARS*	Methionyl-tRNA synthetase	AR	Cytosolic methionyl-tRNA synthesis
SPG71/*ZFR*	Zinc finger RNA binding protein	AR	Unknown

AD, autosomal dominant; AR, autosomal recessive; BMP, bone morphogenetic protein; ER, endoplasmic reticulum.
^aWhen different from disease name.

The N-terminal half of spastin contains two distinct domains that can explain this isoform specificity. A hydrophobic hairpin, which mediates membrane localization and interactions with multiple classes of ER proteins – including atlastins, REEPs, and reticulons – lies within a portion of spastin's N-terminal region that is absent in the smaller M87 isoform [121–124]. By contrast, all known spastin isoforms possess a Microtubule Interacting and Trafficking (MIT) domain (residues 116–194 of the full-length M1 protein) that binds a family of proteins termed CHarged Multivesicular body Proteins (CHMP1–7 as well as IST1). These proteins form a protein complex termed Endosomal Sorting Complex Required for Transport (ESCRT)-III. ESCRT comprises a series of cytosolic protein complexes, ESCRT-0, ESCRT-I, ESCRT-II, and ESCRT-III, and sequential activities of these complexes are required for the recognition and sorting of ubiquitin-conjugated proteins into internal vesicles of multivesicular bodies [125]. Cellular roles for the ESCRT complex have been described for a variety of other membrane modeling processes, including viral budding and the abscission phase of cell division [126].

The MIT domain is necessary for recruitment of spastin to endosomes and midbodies, and spastin interacts selectively with the C-terminal helix of two specific ESCRT-III proteins, CHMP1B and IST1 [127–129]. Interestingly this C-terminal helix typically exists in an autoinhibited, unexposed state, but it is revealed upon ESCRT-III oligomerization, providing an oligomerization-dependent switch for interaction with MIT-domain proteins that permits selective, temporally-regulated recruitment.

Spastin's cellular functions are increasingly well understood. M87 spastin is required for completion of abscission at the terminal stage of cytokinesis, when the midbody is densely packed with an anti-parallel array of microtubules. In cells lacking spastin, the microtubule disruption that normally accompanies abscission does not occur, suggesting that it requires spastin-mediated microtubule severing [120]. ESCRT proteins are also required for abscission by participating in the resolution of the midbody membrane [130]. Thus, this exemplifies how microtubule regulation can be linked to membrane modeling events through spastin. Another example is provided by spastin's function at endosomes. Cells lacking spastin have increased tubulation of endosomal tubular recycling compartments, with resulting defects in receptor sorting. Cells lacking IST1 also have increased endosomal tubulation. Thus, inclusion of the ESCRT-III subunit IST1 into the ESCRT complex triggers recruitment of spastin to facilitate fission of recycling tubules from endosomes. These functions may be of particular relevance for the CNS, as loss of spastin decreases axon branching in cultured neurons, and axon branching also involves coordinated microtubule regulation and membrane modeling [131, 132].

Atlastin: a large GTPase that fuses ER tubules
The ER is a continuous membrane system comprising the nuclear envelope, ribosome-studded sheets, and a polygonal network of smooth tubules extending throughout the cell. M1 spastin binds numerous proteins that localize selectively to the tubular ER [133].

This tubular ER extends well into axons, including the long axons impaired in the HSPs. Spastin interacts with the atlastin-1 protein that is mutated in SPG3A, the second most common cause of HSP. Atlastin-1 is a member of a superfamily of membrane-bound, multimeric, ER-localized dynamin-related GTPases. In humans, atlastin-1 is one of three mammalian atlastin proteins that likely represent functional paralogs to mediate fusion of ER tubules to generate the reticular network, and it is the form most highly enriched in the CNS [134, 135]. Atlastin orthologs are present in all eukaryotic cells and include RHD3 in *Arabidopsis* and Sey1p in *S. cerevisiae*. Species such as *Drosophila* and *C. elegans* have only one atlastin ortholog, facilitating functional studies [124]. Atlastins across all species harbor an N-terminal GTP-binding domain and two very closely-spaced hydrophobic segments near the C-terminus that likely form a transmembrane hairpin domain. Atlastin GTPases participate in homotypic fusion of ER tubules, generating the three-way junctions in ER tubules that give the ER its characteristic polygonal appearance in the cell periphery [124, 134, 135].

Depletion of atlastin-1 in rat cortical neurons in primary culture inhibits axon elongation [136] and similar findings are found in human forebrain neurons derived from induced pluripotent stem cells (iPSCs) prepared from SPG3A patient fibroblasts [137]. The importance of ER morphology in the formation and maintenance of long processes is further supported by studies of the atlastin ortholog in *Arabidopsis*, RHD3. Mutant *rhd3* plants have short, wavy root hairs and abnormal-appearing, tubular ER bundles. Also, the morphology of the ER changes significantly during the elongation phase of root hair growth [138]. Thus, long cellular protrusions appear highly reliant on the dynamic morphology of the tubular ER.

Numerous HSP proteins shape the ER network

Remarkably, numerous HSP proteins localize to the tubular ER and interact with one another in various combinations to shape the distinctive features of the tubular ER network. These include the proteins just discussed, M1 spastin and atlastin-1, as well as REEP1 (SPG31, the third most common HSP), reticulon 2 (SPG12), ARL6IP1 (SPG61), RAB3GAP2 (SPG69), protrudin (SPG33, although there is controversy regarding this locus), and REEP2 (SPG72). These proteins participate in several cellular mechanisms governing the formation and maintenance of the heterogeneous architecture of the ER [133]. For instance, several classes of proteins are important for the generating the high curvature of tubular ER membranes, most notably the proteins of the DP1/REEP/Yop1p and reticulon families as well as ARL6IP1. Although there is little overall sequence homology across these families, they exhibit a common structural feature – elongated, hydrophobic segments that form paired hairpin domains that insert into the membrane, generating high curvature through hydrophobic wedging and scaffolding [133, 139] and also serve as interaction motifs. Lastly, in the absence of RAB3GAP2, which is a GDP/GTP exchange factor for the ER-localized Rab18 GTPase, ER tubular networks are disrupted [140].

In highly polarized cells such as neurons, distribution of the ER is tightly coordinated with cytoskeletal dynamics, mostly involving microtubules in mammalian cells [133]. Expression of ATPase-defective M1 spastin causes dramatic tubulation of the ER and redistribution of ER markers, including atlastin-1, into abnormally thickened microtubule bundles [123]. In addition to interactions with tubule-shaping reticulons, both atlastins and M1 spastin appear to interact directly with DP1/REEPs in the tubular ER [121]. REEPs comprise six members in humans – REEP1–6 (REEP5 is

also known as DP1) – with structural and phylogenetic distinctions between REEP1–4 and REEP5–6 [121]. REEP1–4 proteins harbor hydrophobic hairpins but also interact with microtubules [121, 141]. These proteins may help mediate the formation or stabilization of the tubular ER network, since deletion of a microtubule-interacting domain of REEP1 decreases the number of three-way junctions in the peripheral ER [121]. These interactions among REEPs, atlastins, and M1 spastin via hydrophobic hairpins provide a compelling mechanism for coupling ER membrane remodeling to cytoskeletal dynamics.

How does the common link to ER shaping and network formation potentially explain the pathogenesis of HSPs linked to mutations in these proteins? In a zebrafish model, spastin was required for axon outgrowth during embryonic development [142], reminiscent of effects of atlastin-1 depletion in rat cortical neurons [136]. Also, SPG4 mouse models expressing mutant spastin proteins exhibit axonal transport defects [143, 144]. Finally, microtubule-binding agents can rescue axonal phenotypes in neurons derived from both SPG3A and SPG4 forebrain neurons derived from iPSCs [137, 145]. Thus, although how ER morphology is linked to the formation or maintenance of long protrusions, particularly axons, remains unknown, spastin- and microtubule-dependent transport and distribution of ER tubules in axons is an attractive possibility.

Lipid droplet defects in HSP models

The ER has many roles in cells, and whether impairment in any one is particularly important for HSP pathogenesis remains unclear. One key function of the tubular ER is the synthesis, metabolism, and distribution of lipids and sterols, employing both vesicular and non-vesicular mechanisms. Lipid droplets (LDs) are prominent organelles formed from ER, and they are the major fat storage organelles in eukaryotic cells [146]. In a variety of organisms including *C. elegans* and *Drosophila*, loss-of-function mutations in atlastin cause not only changes in ER morphology, but also a reduction in LD size. Similar results are obtained after depletion of atlastin, whereas over-expression of atlastin has the opposite effect. In mammalian cells, co-overexpression of atlastin-1 and REEP1 generates large LDs. The effect of atlastin-1 on LD size correlates with its activity to promote membrane fusion *in vitro* [147]. Similarly, increasing M1 spastin levels affects LDs, decreasing the number but increasing size. Over-expression of *Drosophila* spastin (Dspastin) leads to larger and less numerous LDs in fat bodies, plus increased triacylglycerol levels. By contrast, Dspastin overexpression increases LD number when expressed specifically in skeletal muscles or nerves. Down-regulation of Dspastin or expression of a dominant-negative variant decreases LD number in skeletal muscle, nerves, and fat bodies, and reduces triacylglycerol levels in larvae [148]. Taken together, these studies demonstrate an evolutionarily conserved role for these ER network proteins in LD formation and size and support the notion that dysfunction of LDs in axons may contribute to HSP pathogenesis.

Further support for pathogenic significance of LD changes in HSP pathogenesis is provided by other known HSP gene products. The complex, autosomal recessive Troyer syndrome (SPG20) is caused by mutations that result in loss of spartin protein [149]. Spartin has been implicated in a number of processes including cytokinesis and epidermal growth factor (EGF) receptor trafficking [150–153]. Spartin also regulates LD biogenesis by promoting atrophin-1 interacting protein 4 (AIP4)-mediated ubiquitination of a number of LD proteins [154–156] and by recruiting PKC-ζ to LDs via the PKC-ζ-interacting proteins ZIP1 (p62/sequestosome) and ZIP3 [157]. The SPG17 protein seipin and its yeast ortholog Fld1p also regulate LD formation, further indicating that alterations in LD biogenesis or turnover could conceivably affect lipid distribution, organelle shaping, or signaling pathways important for axonal health [117].

Although not directly implicated in LD biogenesis, other HSP proteins are enzymes involved in related lipid and sterol biosynthetic pathways. SPG42 results from mutations in *SLC33A1* that encodes the acetyl-CoA transporter. In animals, acetyl-CoA is essential for maintaining a proper balance between carbohydrate and fat metabolism. Under normal circumstances, acetyl-CoA from fatty acid metabolism enters the citric acid cycle, contributing to the energy supply of the cell. SLC33A1 transports acetyl-CoA into the lumen of the Golgi apparatus and has been directly linked to the growth of axons, since knockdown of *slc33a1* in zebrafish causes defective outgrowth from spinal cord [93].

Neuropathy target esterase (NTE)/patatin-like phospholipase domain-containing protein 6 is an integral membrane protein of the ER in neurons that is mutated in autosomal recessive SPG39, a complicated HSP with prominent amyotrophy. NTE deacylates the major membrane phospholipid, phosphatidylcholine. Mutation of the NTE gene *PNPLA2* or chemical inhibition of NTE with organophosphates changes membrane composition and results in distal degeneration of long spinal axons in mice and man [90, 158]. Another HSP protein, cytochrome P450-7B1 (CYP7B1), is mutated in autosomal recessive SPG5 [32] and functions in cholesterol metabolism; in patients with SPG5 there is a dramatic increase in oxysterol substrates in plasma and cerebrospinal fluid [159]. Finally, recently discovered HSP genes within this broad category include *B4GALNT1* (SPG26), *DDHD1* (SPG28), *DDHD2* (SPG54), *CYP2U1* (SPG56), and *CPT1C* (SPG73) [98, 115], plus several others that will be discussed later in this chapter as myelination is described. Given the fundamental roles played by lipids and sterols in neuronal functions, it seems very likely that more genes will be identified within this category.

Spatacsin and spastizin: regenerating lysosomes
The most common forms of autosomal recessive HSPs are SPG11 and SPG15, virtually identical clinical disorders with prominent additional features including early-onset parkinsonism, retinal abnormalities, ataxia, thin corpus callosum, and white matter changes. The SPG11 protein spatacsin and SPG15 protein spastizin bind one another and function together in a process called autophagic lysosome reformation (ALR), a pathway that generates new lysosomes [160]. Autophagy allows cells to adapt to changes in their environment by coordinating the degradation and recycling of cellular components to maintain homeostasis. Lysosomes are organelles critical for terminating autophagy through their fusion with mature autophagosomes to generate autolysosomes that degrade autophagic materials; thus, maintenance of the lysosomal population is essential for autophagy-dependent cellular clearance. Loss of spatacsin and spastizin, as occurs in SPG11 and SPG15, results in depletion of free lysosomes, which are competent to fuse with autophagosomes, and an accumulation of autolysosomes, reflecting a failure in ALR. Moreover, spastizin and spatacsin are essential components for the initiation of lysosomal tubulation [160]. Together, these results link dysfunction of the autophagy/lysosomal biogenesis machinery to neurodegeneration.

Adaptor proteins in HSPs
Spastizin and spatacsin were identified as proteins that co-precipitate with one another and also with the SPG48 protein KIAA0415/

AP5Z1 [102, 161], a subunit of a hetero-tetrameric adaptor protein complex, AP-5, involved in endosomal dynamics [162]. To date, only a handful of SPG48 patients have been described, and further studies will clarify both the clinical presentation and functional role of these interactions. Along these lines, mutations in multiple proteins of the AP-4 adaptor protein complex, which is involved in trafficking of amyloid precursor protein from the *trans*-Golgi to endosomes [163], cause autosomal recessive syndromes (SPG47, SPG50–SPG52), with clinical features ranging from intellectual disability to progressive spastic paraplegia [101]. Thus, these adaptor protein complexes appear highly relevant for pathogenesis of HSPs, and represent areas for future emphasis.

Strumpellin and endosomal tubulation
The membrane shaping and trafficking theme in the endolysosomal pathway continues with SPG8, an HSP with mutations in the *KIAA1096* gene coding for the strumpellin protein. Strumpellin is part of a large protein complex, the WASH complex, which associates with endosomes via interaction with VPS35, a component of retromer, itself an endosomal complex responsible for sorting certain cargoes from endosomes to the *trans*-Golgi network. Depletion of members of the WASH complex increases tubulation at early endosomes, resulting in impaired trafficking via early endosomal compartments. The WASH complex helps generate an actin network on early endosomes by activating the Arp2/3 complex to nucleate new actin filaments that branch off of existing filaments. Increased tubulation associated with WASH complex depletion may reflect a lack of actin-mediated forces that are required for fission of tubular transport intermediates from the endosome [164]. Thus, the WASH complex (containing strumpellin) exemplifies another HSP protein functioning in coordinating membrane modeling and cytoskeletal organization [116].

Interestingly, strumpellin interacts with valosin-containing protein (VCP/p97), an AAA ATPase mutated in frontotemporal dementia with Paget's disease of bone and inclusion body myopathy [165], and *VPS35* is mutated in a number of families with autosomal dominant, late-onset Parkinson disease [166, 167]. A mutation in the WASH subunit SWIP has been described for autosomal recessive intellectual disability [168]. Thus, roles of the WASH-retromer axis in neurodegenerative disease pathogenesis extend beyond the HSPs and represent a very important area for investigation.

As noted earlier, the SPG20 protein spartin functions in LD turnover, but it is also required for efficient EGF receptor degradation [151]. Spartin also may regulate a variety of signaling pathways through ubiquitin modification through its interactions with E3 ubiquitin ligases such as AIP4 and AIP5. Spartin harbors an MIT domain as well and interacts selectively with the ESCRT-III subunit IST1 [152].

Organelle shaping defects and axonopathy
The shared functions of several common HSP proteins in membrane shaping, for example M1 spastin, atlastin, and REEP1 at the ER and strumpellin, spatacsin, and spastizin at endosomes and lysosomes, suggests that membrane modeling is mechanistically important for disease pathogenesis, but the nature of this link is not yet clear. One possibility is that defects in membrane modeling events within the axon, perhaps required for axonal functions such as synaptic plasticity or efficient axonal transport, are the primary cause of the disease. Another possibility is that these membrane defects affect the traffic of receptors controlling specific signaling pathways that are important for axonal function.

Bone morphogenetic protein (BMP) signaling

Several proteins that have been associated with HSP regulate signaling pathways that are known to be important for axonal function. One compelling candidate that cuts across HSP categories and is widely implicated in neurodegenerative diseases is BMP signaling [169]. BMPs are ligands of the transforming growth factor β (TGF-β) superfamily, and BMP signaling has crucial roles in many developmental processes, including organogenesis, dorso-ventral patterning, cellular differentiation, and tissue remodeling. HSP-associated mutations are found in at least four proteins – atlastin-1, NIPA1 (SPG6), spastin and spartin – that function as inhibitors of BMP signaling [116]. In *Drosophila* and mammalian nerve cells, BMP signaling functions in regulating axonal growth and synaptic function, and impairment of BMP signaling in *Drosophila* results in axon transport defects [170]. In rodents, BMP signaling is up-regulated following lesioning of the corticospinal tract, and suppressing this up-regulation can promote regrowth of axons [171].

Of the HSP proteins known to function in inhibition of BMP signaling, the best characterized mechanistically is NIPA1, a protein with nine predicted transmembrane domains that localizes to endosomes and the plasma membrane and functions in Mg^{2+} transport [172]. *Drosophila* larvae lacking spichthyin (a NIPA1 ortholog) have increased synaptic boutons at neuromuscular junctions and increased phosphorylated MAD, a downstream messenger of BMP signaling. These changes can be suppressed by genetic changes that inhibit BMP signaling [170]. NIPA1/spichthyin is thought to inhibit BMP signaling by promoting internalization of BMP type II receptors and their subsequent degradation. NIPA1 missense changes found in SPG6 patients interfere with this process, up-regulating signaling. Similarly, depletion of spartin or spastin, both of which localize partially to endosomes, up-regulates BMP signaling [173]. Dysregulated BMP signaling linked to axonal abnormalities has also been demonstrated for atlastin. Depletion of atlastin-1 in zebrafish results in abnormal spinal motor axon morphology, with increased branching and decreased larval mobility. BMP signaling is up-regulated in these larvae, and inhibition of BMP signaling rescues the *atl1* knockdown phenotype [174].

In summary, these results suggest that abnormal BMP signaling, in many cases probably caused by abnormal BMP receptor trafficking, could be a unifying mechanism for some classes of HSP, including the two most common – SPG4 and SPG3A – that comprise almost 50% of patients [116]. Studies in HSP animal models will be critical to determine whether inhibition of BMP signaling using small-molecule inhibitors, several of which are already available, can rescue disease phenotypes.

Motor-based transport

Correct shaping and positioning of organelles, signaling complexes, and other molecules within highly-polarized corticospinal neurons depends on motor proteins. Thus, it is not surprising that several kinesins are mutated in HSPs. The identification of mutations in the *KIF5A* gene encoding kinesin **heavy chain 5A** in families with SPG10, a pure or complicated HSP, has provided direct evidence for motor-based transport impairments underlying HSPs [175, 176]. KIF5 proteins are ATP-dependent motors that move cargoes in the anterograde direction along axons, and most mutations are missense changes in the motor domain. *Drosophila* harboring mutations in the *KIF5* ortholog *Khc* have posterior paralysis, with axon swellings jammed with cargoes and organelles [177]. In mammals, the KIF5A motor protein shuttles neurofilament subunits, and possibly other anterograde cargoes such as vesicles, along axons.

KIF5 also regulates transport of cargoes in dendrites and has roles in a number of membrane traffic pathways. The efficiency of cargo transport to the distal axon is thought to be affected either because the mutated KIF5A are slower motors or because they have reduced microtubule binding affinity and act in a dominant-negative manner by competing with wild-type motors for cargo binding [178]. More recently, mutations have been described in the *KIF1A* gene encoding kinesin family member 1A (also involved in anterograde axon transport) in SPG30 and in the *KIF1C* gene encoding the kinesin family member 1C (involved in vesicle transport between ER and Golgi apparatus) in SPG58 [19].

Mitochondrial function

Mitochondrial dysfunction has been implicated in a host of developmental and degenerative neurological disorders, manifesting clinically broadly as peripheral neuropathies, movement disorders, myopathies, visual disturbances, and cognitive disability [179]. Given this fundamental link to neurological disease, it is perhaps surprising that so few HSP genes encode proteins directly associated with mitochondrial functions. Two mitochondrial proteins mutated in HSPs are paraplegin (SPG7) and HSP60 (SPG13). Paraplegin is an *m*-AAA metalloprotease of the inner mitochondrial membrane, where it functions in ribosomal assembly and protein quality control. Muscle tissue from SPG7 patients exhibits defects in oxidative phosphorylation, and *Spg7* null mice have axonal swellings with accumulated mitochondria and neurofilaments, indicating that both mitochondrial function and axonal transport are impaired [180]. SPG13 is a typically later-onset, pure HSP, and a causative missense mutation (p.V98I) impairs HSP60 chaperonin activity, impairing mitochondrial quality control [181]. The SPG20 protein spartin has been localized to mitochondria as well, and of course it remains possible that mitochondrial function could be impaired downstream in other HSPs.

Axon pathfinding

Among the first HSP mutations described were in the *L1CAM* gene, encoding a cell surface glycoprotein of the immunoglobulin (Ig) superfamily. Loss-of-function mutations in *L1CAM* are implicated in X-linked, early-onset, complicated HSP (SPG1) as well as other X-linked syndromes including MASA (mental retardation, aphasia, shuffling gait, and adducted thumbs), hydrocephalus, and agenesis of the corpus callosum [182, 183]. In each of these disorders there is corticospinal tract impairment, and they are often lumped together along a disease spectrum known as L1 disease or CRASH syndrome [117].

The L1CAM protein has a large extracellular segment harboring six Ig-like domains and five fibronectin type III domains, a single transmembrane domain, and a short cytoplasmic tail. L1CAM participates in a complex set of extracellular and intracellular interactions, binding to other L1CAM molecules as well as a host of extracellular ligands – including other cell adhesion molecules, integrins, and proteoglycans – plus intracellular proteins such as ankyrins. Disease mutations are found broadly throughout the protein, and partial or complete loss of L1CAM function seems critical for the disease phenotype. In *L1CAM* null mice, corticospinal tracts are abnormal, with a conspicuous failure to decussate within the medulla [184, 185].

How does this pathfinding defect occur? In the developing central nervous system (CNS), L1CAM associates with neuropilin-1 (Nrp1), which itself interacts with plexin-A proteins to form the Semphorin3A (Sema3A) receptor complex. Upon Sema3A binding to Nrp1, L1CAM and Nrp1 become co-internalized in an

L1CAM-dependent manner. Sema3A is a repulsive guidance cue released from cells in the ventral spinal cord to help steer corticospinal neurons away from the midline spinal cord/medullary junction. L1CAM mutations may affect Sema3A signaling when axons are crossing the midline by interfering with receptor internalization and signaling at growth cones [186]. In fact, the association of Nrp1 with L1CAM mediates the activation of a focal adhesion kinase-mitogen-activated protein kinase pathway controlling a critical aspect of the repulsive behavior, the disassembly of adherent zones in growth cones and their subsequent collapse [187]. This compelling role of L1CAM in axon pathfinding during development is consistent with the early onset of SPG1 [117].

Myelination

A distinguishing feature of axons in the central and peripheral nervous systems is an insulating myelin sheath, a specialization important for increasing the speed of electrical impulse propagation. Schwann cells supply myelin for peripheral neurons, whereas oligodendrocytes myelinate axons of CNS neurons. Spastic paraplegia as a manifestation of abnormal myelination in the CNS is fairly common; for example, this occurs in multiple sclerosis and a variety of acquired and inherited leukodystrophies. Thus, it is not surprising that genetic mutations that impair CNS myelination would have prominent spastic paraplegia as a manifestation [117]. Indeed, mutations in the *PLP1* gene encoding the tetraspan integral membrane proteolipid protein (PLP) and its smaller DM20 isoform give rise to two major diseases along a clinical spectrum: a pure or complicated HSP (SPG2), and the typically much more severe Pelizaeus–Merzbacher disease (PMD) [188].

Although PLP and DM20 are major protein constituents of CNS myelin (~50% of total protein), *PLP1* duplications paradoxically cause more severe disease than deletions, while complete absence of PLP/DM20 is usually associated with SPG2 or mild PMD presentations. *Plp1* null mice have been widely studied as a model for SPG2. Unexpectedly, the myelin sheath attains its normal thickness in these mice, though with subtle anomalies at the intraperiod lines. In the underlying axons, anterograde transport is impaired, and cargoes undergoing retrograde transport apparently become stuck at distal juxtaparanodal regions [189, 190]. Thus, oligodendrocytes may modulate the activities of motor proteins involved in intracellular cargo transport via signaling cascades in the underlying axon, with this modulation sensitive to PLP/DM20 [190].

Mutations in another HSP gene similarly define a disease spectrum comprising HSP and PMD-like disease where cell–cell communication is impaired. SPG44 is caused by homozygous mutations in the *GJC2* gene encoding connexin 47 (CX47). Connexins are oligomeric proteins forming gap junction channels, which establish connections between apposed cell membranes to permit the intercellular diffusion of ions and small molecules (typically <1000 Da). CX47 forms connections between astrocytes and oligodendrocytes in concert with CX43. Because CX47/CX43 heterotypic channels appear essential for the maintenance of CNS myelin, alterations in CX47 that result in CX47/CX43 channel dysfunction likely underlie SPG44 [96].

Another HSP with a compelling link to myelination is autosomal recessive SPG35. This disorder is part of a disease spectrum spanning NBIA, leukodystrophy, and HSP, and results from loss-of-function mutations in the fatty acid-2 hydroxylase gene *FA2H* [86, 191]. The fatty acid-2 hydroxylase protein is an NADPH-dependent mono-oxygenase that catalyzes the conversion of free fatty acids to 2-hydroxy fatty acids. These are incorporated into myelin galac-tolipids containing hydroxy fatty acid as the *N*-acyl chain, which maintain the myelin sheath. *Fa2h* null mice have been developed as a model for SPG35, and these animals exhibit significant demyelination, axon loss/enlargement, cerebellar anomalies, and spatial learning and memory deficits. Interestingly, animals lacking *Fa2h* only in oligodendrocytes and Schwann cells do not exhibit memory deficits, indicating that some neurological manifestations may derive from lack of fatty acid-2 hydroxylase in other cell types [192].

Considered together, this subgroup of HSPs most convincingly exemplifies a non-cell autonomous disease pathogenesis [117]. In this regard, oligodendrocytes from *Plp1* null mice are able to induce a focal axonopathy when transplanted into the dorsal columns of the *shiverer* mouse that is myelin deficient [189]. Thus, HSP-associated alterations in oligodendrocyte-mediated myelination can directly cause changes in the underlying axon, impairing corticospinal tract function [117].

Conclusions

With the falling cost and increasing throughput of next generation exome and whole genome sequencing technologies, many additional genes for HSPs and related disorders will likely be uncovered over the next few years. With compelling cellular pathogenic mechanisms already identified, pharmacologic manipulation of these pathways and evaluations in cellular and animal preclinical models will be increasingly possible. Currently, pathways such as BMP signaling, microtubule stability, and lipid metabolism seem to be particularly attractive targets, since they could be relevant for a significant percentage of HSP patients and appear particularly amenable to modulation by small molecules.

The past several years have yielded remarkable advancements in our understanding of the pathogenesis underlying the HSPs, and with increasing interest in the fascinating biology of HSP proteins and technological advances in genetics and imaging, prospects for effective therapies are improving.

Acknowledgments

PPL is supported in part by the Healthy Ageing Research Centre project (REGPOT-2012-2013-1, 7FP) and CB is supported by the Intramural Research Program of the National Institute of Neurological Disorders and Stroke, NIH. Ewa Skarzynska is kindly acknowledged for excellent secretarial assistance.

References

1. Seeligmüller A. Sklerose der seitenstränge des rückenmarks bei vier kindern derselben familie. *Dtsch Med Wschr* 1876;2:185–186.
2. Strümpell A. Beiträge zur pathologie des rückenmarks. *Arch Psychiat Nervenkr* 1880;10:676–717.
3. Strümpell A. Ueber eine bestimmte form der primären combinierten systemerkrankung des rückenmarks. *Arch Psychiat Nervenkr* 1886;17:217–238.
4. Strümpell A. Die primäre seitenstrang-sklerose. *Dtsch Z Nervenheilk* 1904;27: 291–339.
5. Sutherland JM. Familial spastic parapalegia. In: Vinken PJ, Bruyn GW, eds. *Handbook of Clinical Neurology. System Disorders and Atrophies, part II.* Amsterdam: North-Holland Publishing Company, 1975:421–431.
6. Fink JK. Hereditary spastic paraplegia. In: Rosenberg RN, Pascual JM, eds. *Rosenberg's Molecular and Genetic Basis of Neurological and Psychiatric Disease.* Fifth edition. San Diego: Elsevier, 2015:891–906.
7. Polo AE, Calleja J, Combarros O, Bericiano J. Hereditary ataxias and paraplegias in Cantabria, Spain: An epidemiological and clinical study. *Brain* 1991; 114:855–856.

8. Filla A, DeMichele G, Marconi R, et al. Prevalence of hereditary ataxias and spastic paraplegias in Molise, a region of Italy. *J Neurol* 1992;239:351–353.

9. Ruano L1, Melo C, Silva MC, Coutinho P. The global epidemiology of hereditary ataxia and spastic paraplegia: a systematic review of prevalence studies. *Neuroepidemiology* 2014;42:174–183.

10. Appel L, Bogaert L. [Studies on familial spastic paraplegia. III. The Tib family . . . ; very early forms of familial spastic paraplegia with idiocy and oligophrenia in collateral branches of the family]. *Acta Neurol Psychiatr Belg* 1951;51:716–730.

11. Schwarz GA. Hereditary (familial) spastic paraplegia. *AMA Arch Neurol Psychiatry* 1952;68:655–662.

12. Schwarz GA, Liu CN. Hereditary (familial) spastic paraplegia; further clinical and pathologic observations. *AMA Arch Neurol Psychiatry* 1956;75:144–162.

13. Woehrer A, Laszlo L, Finsterer J, et al. Novel crystalloid oligodendrogliopathy in hereditary spastic paraplegia. *Acta Neuropathol* 2012;124:583–591.

14. Ferrer I, Olivé M, Rivera R, et al. Hereditary spastic paraparesis with dementia, amyotrophy and peripheral neuropathy. A neuropathological study. *Neuropathol Appl Neurobiol* 1995;21:255–261.

15. Wakabayashi K, Kobayashi H, Kawasaki S, et al. Autosomal recessive spastic paraplegia with hypoplastic corpus callosum, multisystem degeneration and ubiquitinated eosinophilic granules. *Acta Neuropathol* 2001;101:69–73.

16. Kuru S, Sakai M, Konagaya M, et al. Autopsy case of hereditary spastic paraplegia with thin corpus callosum showing severe gliosis in the cerebral white matter. *Neuropathology* 2005;25:346–352.

17. Nomura H, Koike F, Tsuruta Y, et al. Autopsy case of autosomal recessive hereditary spastic paraplegia with reference to the muscular pathology. *Neuropathology* 2001;21:212–217.

18. Ishizawa K, Lin WL, Tiseo P, et al. A qualitative and quantitative study of grumose degeneration in progressive supranuclear palsy. *J Neuropathol Exp Neurol* 2000;59:513–524.

19. Tesson C, Koht J, Stevanin G. Delving into the complexity of hereditary spastic paraplegias: how unexpected phenotypes and inheritance modes are revolutionizing their nosology. *Hum Genet* 2015;134:511–538.

20. Bianchine JW, Lewis RC Jr. The MASA syndrome: a new heritable mental retardation syndrome. *Clin Genet* 1974;5:298–306.

21. Kenwrick S, Ionasescu G, Searby C, et al. Linkage studies of X-linked recessive spastic paraplegia using DNA probes. *Hum Genet* 1986;73:264–266.

22. Rosenthal A, Joulet M, Kenwrick S. Aberrant splicing of neural cell adhesion molecule L1 mERNA in a family with X-linked hydrocephalus. *Nat Genet* 1992;2:107–112.

23. Johnston AW, McKusick VA. A sex-linked recessive form of spastic paraplegia. *Am J Hum Genet* 1962;14:83–94.

24. Saugier-Veber P, Munnich A, Bonneau D, et al. X-linked spastic paraplegia and Pelizaeus-Merzbacher disease are allelic disorders at the proteolipid protein locus. *Nat Genet* 1994;6:257–262.

25. Zhao X, Alvarado D, Rainier S, et al. Mutations in a newly identified GTPase gene cause autosomal dominant hereditary spastic paraplegia. *Nat Genet* 2001;29:326–331.

26. Guelly C, Zhu P-P, Leonardis L, et al. Targeted high-throughput sequencing identifies mutations in atlastin-1 as a cause of hereditary sensory neuropathy type I. *Am J Hum Genet* 2011;88:99–105.

27. Hazan J, Fontaine B, Bruyn RPM, et al. Linkage of a new locus for autosomal dominant familial spastic paraplegia to chromosome 2p. *Hum Mol Genet* 1994;3:1569–1573.

28. Racis L, Storti E, Pugliatti M, et al. Novel SPAST deletion and reduced DPY30 expression in a Spastic Paraplegia type 4 kindred. *BMC Med Genet* 2014;15:39.

29. Murphy S, Gorman G, Beetz C, et al. Dementia in SPG4 hereditary spastic paraplegia: clinical, genetic, and neuropathologic evidence. *Neurology* 2009;73:378–84.

30. Rothschild H, Happel L, Rampp D, Hackett E. Autosomal recessive spastic paraplegia: evidence for demyelination. *Clin Genet* 1979;15:356–360.

31. Arnoldi A, Crimella C, Tenderini E, et al. Clinical phenotype variability in patients with hereditary spastic paraplegia type 5 associated with CYP7B1 mutations. *Clin Genet* 2012;81:150–157.

32. Tsaousidou MK, Ouahchi K, Warner TT, et al. Sequence alterations within CYP7B1 implicate defective cholesterol homeostasis in motor-neuron degeneration. *Am J Hum Genet* 2008;82:510–515.

33. Fink JK, Sharp GB, Lange BM, et al. Autosomal dominant, familial spastic paraplegia, type I: clinical and genetic analysis of a large North American family. *Neurology* 1995;45:325–331.

34. Fink JK, Wu CB, Jones SM, et al. Autosomal dominant familial spastic paraplegia: tight linkage to chromosome 15q. *Am J Hum Genet* 1995;56:188–192.

35. Rainier S, Chai J-H, Tokarz D, et al. NIPA1 gene mutations cause autosomal dominant hereditary spastic paraplegia (SPG6). *Am J Hum Genet* 2003;73:967–971.

36. Arkadir D, Noreau A, Goldman JS, et al. Pure hereditary spastic paraplegia due to a de novo mutation in the NIPA1 gene. *Eur J Neurol* 2014;21:e2.

37. De Michele G, De Fusco M, Cavalcanti F, et al. A new locus for autosomal recessive hereditary spastic paraplegia maps to chromosome 16q24.3. *Am J Hum Genet* 1998;63:135–139.

38. de Bot ST, Vermeer S, Buijsman W, et al. Pure adult-onset spastic paraplegia caused by a novel mutation in the KIAA0196 (SPG8) gene. *J Neurol* 2013;260:1765–1769.

39. Valdmanis PN, Meijer IA, Reynolds A, et al. Mutations in the KIAA0196 gene at the SPG8 locus cause hereditary spastic paraplegia. *Am J Hum Genet* 2007;80:152–161.

40. Slavotinek AM, Pike M, Mills K, Hurst JA. Cataracts, motor system disorder, short stature, learning difficulties, and skeletal abnormalities: a new syndrome? *Am J Med Genet* 1996;62:42–47.

41. Panza E, Pippucci T, Cusano R, et al. Refinement of the SPG9 locus on chromosome 10q23.3-24.2 and exclusion of candidate genes. *Eur J Neurol* 2008;15:520–524.

42. Reid E, Dearlove AM, Rhodes M, Rubinsztein DC. A new locus for autosomal dominant 'pure' hereditary spastic paraplegia mapping to chromosome 12q13, and evidence for further genetic heterogeneity. *Am J Hum Genet* 1999;65:757–763.

43. Crimella C, Baschirotto C, Arnoldi A, et al. Mutations in the motor and stalk domains of KIF5A in spastic paraplegia type 10 and in axonal Charcot-Marie-Tooth type 2. *Clin Genet* 2012;82:157–164.

44. Nakamura A, Izumi K, Umehara F, et al. Familial spastic paraplegia with mental impairment and thin corpus callosum. *J Neurol Sci* 1995;131:35–42.

45. Stevanin G, Santorelli FM, Azzedine H, et al. Mutations in SPG11, encoding spatacsin, are a major cause of spastic paraplegia with thin corpus callosum. *Nature Genet* 2007;39:366–372.

46. Reid E, Dearlove AM, Osborn O, et al. A locus for autosomal dominant 'pure' hereditary spastic paraplegia maps to chromosome 19q13. *Am J Hum Genet* 2000;66:728–732.

47. Montenegro G, Rebelo AP, Connell J, et al. Mutations in the ER-shaping protein reticulon 2 cause the axon-degenerative disorder hereditary spastic paraplegia type 12. *J Clin Invest* 2012;122:538–544.

48. Fontaine B, Davoine C-S, Dürr A, et al. A new locus for autosomal dominant pure spastic paraplegia, on chromosome 2q24-q34. *Am J Hum Genet* 2000;66:702–707.

49. Hansen J, Corydon TJ, Palmfeldt J, et al. Decreased expression of the mitochondrial matrix proteases Lon and ClpP in cells from a patient with hereditary spastic paraplegia (SPG13). *Neuroscience* 2008;153:474–482.

50. Vazza G, Zortea M, Boaretto F, et al. A new locus for autosomal recessive spastic paraplegia associated with mental retardation and distal motor neuropathy, SPG14, maps to chromosome 3q27-q28. *Am J Hum Genet* 2000;67:504–509.

51. Goizet C, Boukhris A, Maltete D, et al. SPG15 is the second most common cause of hereditary spastic paraplegia with thin corpus callosum. *Neurology* 2009;73:1111–1119.

52. Kjellin K. Familial spastic paraplegia with amyotrophy, oligophrenia, and central retinal degeneration. *Arch Neurol* 1959;1:133–140.

53. Hanein S, Martin E, Boukhris A, et al. Identification of the SPG15 gene, encoding spastizin, as a frequent cause of complicated autosomal-recessive spastic paraplegia, including Kjellin syndrome. *Am J Hum Genet* 2008;82:992–1002.

54. Steinmuller R, Lantigua-Cruz A, Garcia-Garcia R, et al. Evidence of a third locus in X-linked recessive spastic paraplegia. *Hum Genet* 1997;100:287–289.

55. Silver JR. Familial spastic paraplegia with amyotrophy of the hands. *J Neurol Neurosurg Psychiatry* 1966;29:135–144.

56. van Gent EM, Hoogland RA, Jennekens FGI. Distal amyotrophy of predominantly the upper limbs with pyramidal features in a large kinship. *J Neurol Neurosurg Psychiatry* 1985;48:266–269.

57. Windpassinger C, Auer-Grumbach M, Irobi J, et al. Heterozygous missense mutations in BSCL2 are associated with distal hereditary motor neuropathy and Silver syndrome. *Nat Genet* 2004;36:271–276.

58. Al-Yahyaee S, Al-Gazali LI, De Jonghe P, et al. A novel locus for hereditary spastic paraplegia with thin corpus callosum and epilepsy. *Neurology* 2006;66:1230–1234.

59. Yildirim Y, Orhan EK, Iseri SAU, et al. A frameshift mutation of ERLIN2 in recessive intellectual disability, motor dysfunction and multiple joint contractures. *Hum Mol Genet* 2011;20:1886–1892.

60. Valente EM, Brancati F, Caputo V, et al. Novel locus for autosomal dominant pure hereditary spastic paraplegia (SPG19) maps to chromosome 9q33-q34. *Ann Neurol* 2002;51:681–685.

61. Cross HE, McKusick VA. The Troyer syndrome: a recessive form of spastic paraplegia with distal muscle wasting. *Arch Neurol* 1967;16:473–485.

62. Patel H, Cross H, Proukakis C, et al. SPG20 is mutated in Troyer syndrome, an hereditary spastic paraplegia. *Nat Genet* 2002;31:347–348.

63. Tawamie H, Wohlleber E, Uebe S, et al. Recurrent null mutation in SPG20 leads to Troyer syndrome. *Mol Cell Probes* 2015;29:315–318.

64. Bakowska JC, Wang H, Xin B, et al. Lack of spartin protein in Troyer syndrome: a loss-of-function disease mechanism? *Arch Neurol* 2008;65:520–524.

65. Cross HE, McKusick VA. The Mast syndrome: a recessively inherited form of presenile dementia with motor disturbances. *Arch Neurol* 1967;16:1–13.

66. Simpson MA, Cross H, Proukakis C, et al. Maspardin is mutated in Mast syndrome, a complicated form of hereditary spastic paraplegia associated with dementia. *Am J Hum Genet* 2003;73:1147–1156.

67. Allan W, Herndon CN, Dudley FC. Some examples of the inheritance of mental deficiency: apparently sex-linked idiocy and microcephaly. *Am J Ment Defic* 1944;48:325–334.

68. Vaurs-Barrière C, Deville M, Sarret C, et al. Pelizaeus-Merzbacher-like disease presentation of MCT8 mutated male subjects. *Ann Neurol* 2009;65:114–118.

69. Blumen SC, Bevan S, Abu-Mouch S, et al. A locus for complicated hereditary spastic paraplegia maps to chromosome 1q24-32. *Ann Neurol* 2003;54:796–803.

70. Hodgkinson CA, Bohlega S, Abu-Amero SN, et al. A novel form of autosomal recessive pure hereditary spastic paraplegia maps to chromosome 13q14. *Neurology* 2002;59:1905–1909.

71. Zortea M, Vettori A, Trevisan CP, et al. Genetic mapping of a susceptibility locus for disc herniation and spastic paraplegia on 6q23.3-q24.1. *J Med Genet* 2002;39:387–390.

72. Farag TI, El-Badramany MH, Al-Sharkawy S. Troyer syndrome: report of the first 'non-Amish' sibship and review. *Am J Med Genet* 1994;53:383–385.

73. Meijer IA, Cossette P, Roussel J, et al. A novel locus for pure recessive hereditary spastic paraplegia maps to 10q22.1-10q24.1. *Ann Neurol* 2004;56:579–582.

74. Bouslam N, Benomar A, Azzedine H, et al. Mapping of a new form of pure autosomal recessive spastic paraplegia (SPG28). *Ann Neurol* 2005;57:567–571.

75. Orlacchio A, Kawarai T, Gaudiello F, et al. New locus for hereditary spastic paraplegia maps to chromosome 1p31.1-1p21.1. *Ann Neurol* 2005;58:423–429.

76. Klebe S, Azzedine H, Dürr A, et al. Autosomal recessive spastic paraplegia (SPG30) with mild ataxia and sensory neuropathy maps to chromosome 2q37.3. *Brain* 2006;129:1456–1462.

77. Erlich Y, Edvardson S, Hodges E, et al. Exome sequencing and disease-network analysis of a single family implicate a mutation in KIF1A in hereditary spastic paraparesis. *Genome Res* 2011;21:658–664.

78. Züchner S, Kail ME, Nance MA, et al. A new locus for dominant hereditary spastic paraplegia maps to chromosome 2p12. *Neurogenetics* 2006;7:127–129.

79. Züchner S, Wang G, Tran-Viet K-N, et al. Mutations in the novel mitochondrial protein REEP1 cause hereditary spastic paraplegia type 31. *Am J Hum Genet* 2006;79:365–369.

80. Stevanin G, Paternotte C, Coutinho P, et al. A new locus for autosomal recessive spastic paraplegia (SPG32) on chromosome 14q12-q21. *Neurology* 2007; 68:1837–1840.

81. Mannan AU, Krawen P, Sauter SM, et al. ZFYVE27 (SPG33), a novel spastin-binding protein, is mutated in hereditary spastic paraplegia. *Am J Hum Genet* 2006;79:351–357.

82. Chang J, Lee S, Blackstone C. Protrudin binds atlastins and endoplasmic reticulum-shaping proteins and regulates network formation. *Proc Natl Acad Sci USA* 2013;110:14954–14959.

83. Martignoni M, Riano E, Rugarli EI. The role of ZFYVE27/protrudin in hereditary spastic paraplegia. *Am J Hum Genet* 2008;83:127–128.

84. Zatz M, Penha-Serrano C, Otto PA. X-linked recessive type of pure spastic paraplegia in a large pedigree: absence of detectable linkage with Xg. *J Med Genet* 1976;13:217–222.

85. Dick KJ, Al-Mjeni R, Baskir W, et al. A novel locus for an autosomal recessive hereditary spastic paraplegia (SPG35) maps to 16q21-q23. *Neurology* 2008;71:248–252.

86. Dick KJ, Eckhardt M, Paisán-Ruiz C, et al. Mutation of FA2H underlies a complicated form of hereditary spastic paraplegia (SPG35). *Hum Mutat* 2010;31:E1251–E1260.

87. Schüle R, Bonin M, Dürr A, et al. Autosomal dominant spastic paraplegia with peripheral neuropathy maps to chr12q23-24. *Neurology* 2009;72:1893–1898.

88. Hanein S, Dürr A, Ribai P, et al. A novel locus for autosomal dominant 'uncomplicated' hereditary spastic paraplegia maps to chromosome 8p21.1-q13.3. *Hum Genet* 2007;122:261–273.

89. Orlacchio A, Patrono C, Gaudiello F, et al. Silver syndrome variant of hereditary spastic paraplegia: a locus to 4p and allelism with SPG4. *Neurology* 2008; 70:1959–1966.

90. Rainier S, Bui M, Mark E, et al. Neuropathy target esterase gene mutations cause motor neuron disease. *Am J Hum Genet* 2008;82:780–785.

91. Synofzik M, Gonzalez MA, Lourenco CM, et al. PNPLA6 mutations cause Boucher-Neuhauser and Gordon Holmes syndromes as part of a broad neurodegenerative spectrum. *Brain* 2014;137:69–77.

92. Zhao G, Hu Z, Shen L, et al. A novel candidate locus on chromosome 11p14.1-p11.2 for autosomal dominant hereditary spastic paraplegia. *Chin Med J* 2008;121:430–434.

93. Lin P, Li J, Liu Q, et al. A missense mutation in SLC33A1, which encodes the acetyl-CoA transporter, causes autosomal-dominant spastic paraplegia (SPG42). *Am J Hum Genet* 2008;83:752–759.

94. Meilleur KG, Traore M, Sangare M, et al. Hereditary spastic paraplegia and amyotrophy associated with a novel locus on chromosome 19. *Neurogenetics* 2010;11:313–318.

95. Landouré G, Zhu P-P, Lourenco CM, et al. Hereditary spastic paraplegia type 43 (SPG43) is caused by mutation in C19orf12. *Hum Mutat* 2013;34:1357–1360.

96. Orthmann-Murphy JL, Salsano E, Abrams CK, et al. Hereditary spastic paraplegia is a novel phenotype for GJA12/GJC2 mutations. *Brain* 2009;132:426–438.

97. Dursun U, Koroglu C, Orhan EK, et al. Autosomal recessive spastic paraplegia (SPG45) with mental retardation maps to 10q24.3-q25.1. *Neurogenetics* 2009;10:325–331.

98. Novarino G, Fenstermaker AG, Zaki MS, et al. Exome sequencing links corticospinal motor neuron disease to common neurodegenerative disorders. *Science* 2014;343:506–511.

99. Boukhris A, Stevanin G, Feki I, et al. Hereditary spastic paraplegia with mental impairment and thin corpus callosum in Tunisia: SPG11, SPG15, and further genetic heterogeneity. *Arch Neurol* 2008;65:393–402.

100. Martin E, Schule R, Smets K, et al. Loss of function of glucocerebrosidase GBA2 is responsible for motor neuron defects in hereditary spastic paraplegia. *Am J Hum Genet* 2013;92:238–244.

101. Abou Jamra R, Philippe O, Raas-Rothschild A, et al. Adaptor protein complex 4 deficiency causes severe autosomal-recessive intellectual disability, progressive spastic paraplegia, shy character, and short stature. *Am J Hum Genet* 2011;88:788–795.

102. Slabicki M, Theis M, Krastev DB, et al. A genome-scale DNA repair RNAi screen identifies SPG48 as a novel gene associated with hereditary spastic paraplegia. *PLoS Biol* 2010;8:e1000408.

103. Hirst J, Edgar JR, Esteves T, et al. Loss of AP-5 results in accumulation of aberrant endolysosomes, defining a new type of lysosomal storage disease. *Hum Mol Genet* 2015;24:4984–4996.

104. Oz-Levi D, Ben-Zeev B, Ruzzo EK, et al. Mutation in TECPR2 reveals a role for autophagy in hereditary spastic paraparesis. *Am J Hum Genet* 2012;91:1065–1072.

105. Verkerk AJMH, Schot R, Dumee B, et al. Mutation in the AP4M1 gene provides a model for neuroaxonal injury in cerebral palsy. *Am J Hum Genet* 2009;85:40–52.

106. Moreno-De-Luca A, Helmers SL, Mao H, et al. Adaptor protein complex-4 (AP-4) deficiency causes a novel autosomal recessive cerebral palsy syndrome with microcephaly and intellectual disability. *J Med Genet* 2011;48:141–144.

107. Zivony-Elboum Y, Westbroek W, Kfir N, et al. A founder mutation in Vps37A causes autosomal recessive complex hereditary spastic paraplegia. *J Med Genet* 2012;49:462–472.

108. Schuurs-Hoeijmakers JHM, Geraghty MT, Kamsteeg E-J, et al. Mutations in DDHD2, encoding an intracellular phospholipase A91), cause a recessive form of complex hereditary spastic paraplegia. *Am J Hum Genet* 2012;91:1073–1081.

109. Yoshita Y, Atsumi T, Miyatake T. Two siblings with spastic paraplegia, optic atrophy and peripheral neuropathy. *Rinsho Shinkeigaku* 1982;22:901–908.

110. Shimazaki H, Takiyama Y, Ishiura H, et al. A homozygous mutation of C12orf65 causes spastic paraplegia with optic atrophy and neuropathy (SPG55). *J Med Genet* 2012;49:777–784.

111. Tesson C, Nawara M, Salih MAM, et al. Alteration of fatty-acid-metabolizing enzymes affects mitochondrial form and function in hereditary spastic paraplegia. *Am J Hum Genet* 2012;91:1051–1064.

112. Beetz C, Johnson A, Schuh AL, et al. Inhibition of TFG function causes hereditary axon degeneration by impairing endoplasmic reticulum structure. *Proc Nat Acad Sci USA* 2013;110:5091–5096.

113. Caballero Oteyza A, Battaloğlu E, Ocek L, et al. Motor protein mutations cause a new form of hereditary spastic paraplegia. *Neurology*. 2014;82:2007–2016.

114. Esteves T, Dürr A, Mundwiller E, et al. Loss of association of REEP2 with membranes leads to hereditary spastic paraplegia. *Am J Hum Genet* 2014;94:268–277.

115. Rinaldi C, Schmidt T, Situ AJ, et al. Mutation in CPT1C associated with pure autosomal dominant spastic paraplegia. *JAMA Neurol* 2015;72:561–570.

116. Blackstone C, O'Kane CJ, Reid E. Hereditary spastic paraplegias: membrane traffic and the motor pathway. *Nat Rev Neurosci* 2011;12:31–42.

117. Blackstone C. Cellular pathways of hereditary spastic paraplegia. *Annu Rev Neurosci* 2012;35:25–47.

118. Claudiani P, Riano E, Errico A, et al. Spastin subcellular localization is regulated through usage of different translation start sites and active export from the nucleus. *Exp Cell Res* 2005;309:358–369.

119. Roll-Mecak A, McNally FJ. Microtubule-severing enzymes. *Curr Opin Cell Biol* 2010;22:96–103.

120. Connell JW, Lindon C, Luzio JP, Reid E. Spastin couples microtubule severing to membrane traffic in completion of cytokinesis and secretion. *Traffic* 2009;10:42–56.

121. Park SH, Zhu P-P, Parker RL, Blackstone C. Hereditary spastic paraplegia proteins REEP1, spastin, and atlastin-1 coordinate microtubule interactions with the tubular ER network. *J Clin Invest* 2010;120:1097–1110.

122. Voeltz GK, Prinz WA, Shibata Y, et al. A class of membrane proteins shaping the tubular endoplasmic reticulum. *Cell* 2006;124:573–586.

123. Sanderson CM, Connell JW, Edwards TL, et al. Spastin and atlastin, two proteins mutated in autosomal-dominant hereditary spastic paraplegia, are binding partners. *Hum Mol Genet* 2006;15:307–318.

124. Hu J, Shibata Y, Zhu P-P, et al. A class of dynamin-like GTPases involved in the generation of the tubular ER network. *Cell* 2009;138:549–561.

125. Hurley JH, Hanson PI. Membrane budding and scission by the ESCRT machinery: it's all in the neck. *Nat Rev Mol Cell Biol* 2010;11:556–566.

126. Schuh AL, Audhya A. The ESCRT machinery: from the plasma membrane to endosomes and back again. *Crit Rev Biochem Mol Biol* 2014;49:242–261.

127. Reid, E. Connell J, Edwards TL, et al. The hereditary spastic paraplegia protein spastin interacts with the ESCRT-III complex-associated endosomal protein CHMP1B. *Hum Mol Genet* 2005;14:19–38.

128. Agromayor M, Carlton JG, Phelan JP, et al. Essential role of hIST1 in cytokinesis. *Mol Biol Cell* 2009;20:1374–1387.

129. Renvoisé B, Stadler J, Singh R, et al. Spg20-/- mice reveal multimodal functions for Troyer syndrome protein spartin in lipid droplet maintenance, cytokinesis and BMP signaling. *Hum Mol Genet* 2012;21:3604–3618.

130. Carlton JG, Martin-Serrano J. Parallels between cytokinesis and retroviral budding: a role for the ESCRT machinery. *Science* 2007;316:1908–1912.

131. Riano E, Martignoni M, Mancuso G, et al. Pleiotropic effects of spastin on neurite growth depending on expression levels. *J Neurochem* 2009;108:1277–1288.

132. Yu PB, Hong CC, Sachidanandan C, et al. Dorsomorphin inhibits BMP signals required for embryogenesis and iron metabolism. *Nat Chem Biol* 2008;4:33–41.

133. Goyal U, Blackstone C. Untangling the web: mechanisms underlying ER network formation. *Biochim Biophys Acta* 2013;1833:2492–2498.

134. Rismanchi N, Soderblom C, Stadler J, et al. Atlastin GTPases are required for Golgi apparatus and ER morphogenesis. *Hum Mol Genet* 2008;17:1591–1604.

135. Orso G, Pendin D, Liu S, et al. Homotypic fusion of ER membranes requires the dynamin-like GTPase atlastin. *Nature* 2009;460:978–983.

136. Zhu P-P, Soderblom C, Tao-Cheng J-H, et al. SPG3A protein atlastin-1 is enriched in growth cones and promotes axon elongation during neuronal development. *Hum Mol Genet* 2006;15:1343–1353.

137. Zhu P-P, Denton KR, Pierson TM, et al. Pharmacologic rescue of axon growth defects in a human iPSC model of hereditary spastic paraplegia SPG3A. *Hum Mol Genet* 2014;23:5638–5648.

138. Ridge RW, Uozumi Y, Plazinski J, et al. Developmental transitions and dynamics of the cortical ER of Arabidopsis cells seen with green fluorescent protein. *Plant Cell Physiol* 1999;40:1253–1261.

139. Brady JP, Claridge JK, Smith PG, Schnell JR. A conserved amphipathic helix is required for membrane tubule formation by Yop1p. *Proc Natl Acad Sci USA* 2015;112:E639–E648.

140. Gerondopoulos A, Bastos RN, Yoshimura S, et al. Rab18 and a Rab18 GEF complex are required for normal ER structure. *J Cell Biol* 2014;205:707–720.

141. Schlaitz AL, Thompson J, Wong CC, et al. REEP3/4 ensure endoplasmic reticulum clearance from metaphase chromatin and proper nuclear envelope architecture. *Dev Cell* 2013;26:315–323.

142. Wood JD, Landers JA, Bingley M, et al. The microtubule-severing protein spastin is essential for axon outgrowth in the zebrafish embryo. *Hum Mol Genet* 2006;15:2763–2771.

143. Tarrade A, Fassier C, Courageot S, et al. A mutation of spastin is responsible for swellings and impairment of transport in a region of axon characterized by changes in microtubule composition. *Hum Mol Genet* 2006;15:3544–3558.

144. Kasher PR, De Vos KJ, Wharton SB, et al. Direct evidence for axonal transport defects in a novel mouse model of mutant spastin-induced hereditary spastic paraplegia (HSP) and human HSP patients. *J Neurochem* 2009;110:34–44.

145. Denton KR, Lei L, Grenier J, et al. Loss of spastin function results in disease-specific axonal defects in human pluripotent stem cell-based models of hereditary spastic paraplegia. *Stem Cells* 2014;32:414–423.

146. Welte MA. Expanding roles for lipid droplets. *Curr Biol* 2015;25:R470–R481.

147. Klemm RW, Norton JP, Cole RA, et al. A conserved role for atlastin GTPases in regulating lipid droplet size. *Cell Rep* 2013;3:1465–1475.

148. Papadopoulos C, Orso G, Mancuso G, et al. 2015. Spastin binds to lipid droplets and affects lipid metabolism. *PLoS Genet* 2015;11:e1005149.

149. Bakowska JC, Wang H, Xin B, et al. Lack of spartin protein in Troyer syndrome: a loss-of-function disease mechanism? *Arch Neurol* 2008;65:520–524.

150. Robay D, Patel H, Simpson MA, et al. Endogenous spartin, mutated in hereditary spastic paraplegia, has a complex subcellular localization suggesting diverse roles in neurons. *Exp Cell Res* 2006;312:2764–2777.

151. Bakowska JC, Jupille H, Fatheddin P, et al. Troyer syndrome protein spartin is mono-ubiquitinated and functions in EGF receptor trafficking. *Mol Biol Cell* 2007;18:1683–1692.

152. Renvoisé B, Parker RL, Yang D, et al. SPG20 protein spartin is recruited to midbodies by ESCRT-III protein Ist1 and participates in cytokinesis. *Mol Biol Cell* 2010;21:3293–3303.

153. Lind GE, Raiborg C, Danielsen SA, et al. SPG20, a novel biomarker for early detection of colorectal cancer, encodes a regulator of cytokinesis. *Oncogene* 2011;30:3967–3978.

154. Eastman SW, Yassaee M, Bieniasz PD. A role for ubiquitin ligases and Spartin/SPG20 in lipid droplet turnover. *J Cell Biol* 2009;184:881–894.

155. Edwards TL, Clowes VE, Tsang HTH, et al. Endogenous spartin (SPG20) is recruited to endosomes and lipid droplets and interacts with the ubiquitin E3 ligases AIP4 and AIP5. *Biochem J* 2009;423:31–39.

156. Hooper C, Puttamadappa SS, Loring Z, et al. Spartin activates atrophin-1-interacting protein 4 (AIP4) E3 ubiquitin ligase and promotes ubiquitination of adipophilin on lipid droplets. *BMC Biol* 2010;8:72.

157. Urbanczyk A, Enz R. Spartin recruits PKC-ζ via the PKC-ζ-interacting proteins ZIP1 and ZIP3 to lipid droplets. *J Neurochem* 2011;118(5):737–748.

158. Read DJ, Li Y, Chao MV, et al. Neuropathy target esterase is required for adult vertebrate axon maintenance. *J Neurosci* 2009;29:11594–11600.

159. Schüle R, Siddique T, Deng HX, et al. Marked accumulation of 27-hydroxycholesterol in SPG5 patients with hereditary spastic paresis. *J Lipid Res* 2010;51:819–823.

160. Chang J, Lee S, Blackstone C. Spastic paraplegia proteins spastizin and spatacsin mediate autophagic lysosome reformation. *J Clin Invest* 2014;124:5249–5262.

161. Murmu RP, Martin E, Rastetter A, et al. Cellular distribution and subcellular localization of spatacsin and spastizin, two proteins involved in hereditary spastic paraplegia. *Mol Cell Neurosci* 2011;47:191–202.

162. Hirst J, Barlow L, Francisco GC, et al. The fifth adaptor protein complex. *PLoS Biol* 2011;9:e1001170.

163. Burgos PV, Mardones GA, Rojas AL, et al. Sorting of the Alzheimer's disease amyloid precursor protein mediated by the AP-4 complex. *Dev Cell* 2010;18:425–436.

164. Campellone KG, Welch MD. A nucleator arms race: cellular control of actin assembly. *Nat Rev Mol Cell Biol* 2010;11:237–251.

165. Clemen CS, Tangavelou K, Strucksberg K-H, et al. Strumpellin is a novel valosin-containing protein binding partner linking hereditary spastic paraplegia to protein aggregation diseases. *Brain* 2010;133:2920–2941.

166. Vilariño-Güell C, Wider C, Ross OA, et al. VPS35 mutations in Parkinson disease. *Am J Hum Genet* 2011;89:162–167.

167. Zimprich A, Benet-Pagès A, Struhal W, et al. A mutation in VPS35, encoding a subunit of the retromer complex, causes late-onset Parkinson disease. *Am J Hum Genet* 2011;89:168–175.

168. Ropers F, Derivery E, Hu H, et al. Identification of a novel candidate gene for non-syndromic autosomal recessive intellectual disability: the WASH complex member SWIP. *Hum Mol Genet* 2011;20:2585–2590.

169. Bayat V, Jaiswal M, Bellen HJ. The BMP signaling pathway at the Drosophila neuromuscular junction and its links to neurodegenerative diseases. *Curr Opin Neurobiol* 2011;21:182–188.

170. Wang X, Shaw WR, Tsang HTH, et al. Drosophila spichthyin inhibits BMP signaling and regulates synaptic growth and axonal microtubules. *Nat Neurosci* 2007;10:177–185.

171. Matsuura I, Taniguchi J, Hata K, et al. BMP inhibition enhances axonal growth and functional recovery after spinal cord injury. *J Neurochem* 2008;105:1471–1479.

172. Goytain A, Hines RM, El-Husseini A, Quamme GA. NIPA1(SPG6), the basis for autosomal dominant form of hereditary spastic paraplegia, encodes a functional Mg2+ transporter. *J Biol Chem* 2007;282:8060–8068.

173. Tsang HTH, Edwards TL, Wang X, et al. The hereditary spastic paraplegia proteins NIPA1, spastin and spartin are inhibitors of mammalian BMP signalling. *Hum Mol Genet* 2009;18:3805–3821.

174. Fassier C, Hutt JA, Scholpp S, et al. Zebrafish atlastin controls motility and spinal motor axon architecture via inhibition of the BMP pathway. *Nat Neurosci* 2010;13:1380–1387.

175. Reid E, Kloos M, Ashley-Koch A, et al. A kinesin heavy chain (KIF5A) mutation in hereditary spastic paraplegia (SPG10). *Am J Hum Genet* 2002;71:1189–1194.

176. Goizet C, Boukhris A, Mundwiller E, et al. Complicated forms of autosomal dominant hereditary spastic paraplegia are frequent in SPG10. *Hum Mutat* 2009;30:E376–E385.

177. Hurd DD, Saxton WM. Kinesin mutations cause motor neuron disease phenotypes by disrupting fast axonal transport in Drosophila. *Genetics* 1996;144:1075–1085.

178. Ebbing B, Mann K, Starosta A, et al. Effect of spastic paraplegia mutations in KIF5A kinesin on transport activity. *Hum Mol Genet* 2008;17:1245–1252.

179. DiMauro S, Schon EA. Mitochondrial disorders in the nervous system. *Annu Rev Neurosci* 2008;31:91–123.

180. Ferreirinha F, Quattrini A, Pirozzi M, et al. Axonal degeneration in paraplegin-deficient mice is associated with abnormal mitochondria and impairment of axonal transport. *J Clin Invest* 2004;113:231–242.

181. Bross P, Naundrup S, Hansen J, et al. The Hsp60-(p.V98I) mutation associated with hereditary spastic paraplegia SPG13 compromises chaperonin function both in vitro and in vivo. *J Biol Chem* 2008;283:15694–15700.

182. Jouet M, Rosenthal A, Armstrong G, et al. X-linked spastic paraplegia (SPG1), MASA syndrome and X-linked hydrocephalus result from mutations in the L1 gene. *Nat Genet* 1994;7:402–407.

183. Weller S, Gärtner J. Genetic and clinical aspects of X-linked hydrocephalus (L1 disease): mutations in the L1CAM gene. *Hum Mutat* 2001;18:1–12.

184. Dahme M, Bartsch U, Martini R, et al. Disruption of the mouse L1 gene leads to malformations of the nervous system. *Nat Genet* 1997;17:346–349.

185. Cohen NR, Taylor JS, Scott LB, et al. Errors in corticospinal axon guidance in mice lacking the neural cell adhesion molecule L1. *Curr Biol* 1998;8:26–33.

186. Castellani V, Falk J, Rougon G. Semaphorin3A-induced receptor endocytosis during axon guidance responses is mediated by L1 CAM. *Mol Cell Neurosci* 2004;26:89–100.

187. Bechara A, Nawabi H, Moret F, et al. FAK-MAPK-dependent adhesion disassembly downstream of L1 contributes to semaphorin3A-induced collapse. *EMBO J* 2008;27:1549–1562.

188. Inoue K. PLP1-related inherited dysmyelinating disorders: Pelizaeus-Merzbacher disease and spastic paraplegia type 2. *Neurogenetics* 2005;6:1–16.

189. Edgar JM, McLaughlin M, Yool D, et al. Oligodendroglial modulation of fast axonal transport in a mouse model of hereditary spastic paraplegia. *J Cell Biol* 2004;166:121–131.

190. Gruenenfelder FI, Thomson G, Penderis J, Edgar JM. Axon-glial interaction in the CNS: what we have learned from mouse models of Pelizaeus-Merzbacher disease. *J Anat* 2011;219:33–43.

191. Schneider SA, Bhatia KP. Three faces of the same gene: FA2H links neurodegeneration with brain iron accumulation, leukodystrophies, and hereditary spastic paraplegias. *Ann Neurol* 2010;68:575–577.

192. Potter KA, Kern MJ, Fullbright G, et al. Central nervous system dysfunction in a mouse model of FA2H deficiency. *Glia* 2011;59:1009–1021.

193. Renvoisé B, Chang J, Singh R, et al. Lysosomal abnormalities in hereditary spastic paraplegia types SPG15 and SPG11. *Ann Clin Transl Neurol* 2014;1:379–389.

CHAPTER 16

Spinal Muscular Atrophy

Joseph R. Wooley[1], Melissa E. Crowder[1], Noah J. Pyles[1], and Charlotte J. Sumner[1,2]

Departments of Neurology[1] and Neuroscience[2], Johns Hopkins University School of Medicine, Baltimore, Maryland, USA

Introduction

Spinal muscular atrophy (SMA) is an autosomal recessively inherited neurodegenerative disease characterized by motor neuron cell loss and muscle weakness and atrophy. One in 40–50 adults are genetic carriers and 1 in 6000–10,000 live births are affected, making SMA the leading inherited cause of infant mortality [1, 2]. SMA is caused by homozygous mutations in the survival motor neuron 1 (*SMN1*) gene and retention of the *SMN2* gene, which together lead to reduced expression levels of the SMN protein. Since the genetic basis of the disease was elucidated in 1995, research efforts have focused on characterizing the SMN protein, understanding the molecular mechanisms of disease, generating SMA animal models, and identifying targets for therapeutic intervention [3]. Although no disease-modifying treatment is currently available, advances in medical technology and supportive care have improved clinical disease management and patient quality of life. Ongoing clinical trials are showing efficacy and thus we are on the brink of new treatments for SMA patients.

In addition to SMA caused by SMN protein deficiency, also known as "proximal" or "5q" SMA, there are multiple other inherited lower motor neuron disorders. These are known collectively as the "non-5q" spinal muscular atrophies [4]. They are defined by their inheritance pattern and distribution of muscle weakness [5]. For example, SMA caused by SMN deficiency presents with a stereotypical pattern of proximal predominant weakness, but another infantile onset SMA, SMA with respiratory distress (SMARD), primarily affects distal muscles [6]. Distal SMA variants can clinically overlap with axonal forms of Charcot–Marie–Tooth disease. In many of these alternate forms of SMA, causative genes have been identified and research into disease mechanisms is ongoing [7]. In the future, it is likely that the ease of genetic testing will facilitate the early diagnosis of such patients and continued improvements in sequencing technology will continue to define the genetic causes of these disorders. Although this is an area of active research, the remainder of this chapter will focus on proximal SMA caused by SMN deficiency.

Genetic basis of disease

Approximately 95% of all SMA patients carry homozygous deletions that affect exon 7 of *SMN1*, while 5% are compound heterozygotes for a deletion and an alternate mutation, such as a small deletion, insertion, or point mutation, which can disrupt SMN protein function [3]. Crucially, all SMA patients retain at least one copy of the centromeric copy of SMN (*SMN2*), despite the fact that perhaps 5–10% of the unaffected population has no *SMN2* [2]. The genes differ by only five nucleotides, one of which lies within an exonic splicing region of exon 7 and affects splicing such that exon 7 is frequently excluded from *SMN2*-derived transcripts [8, 9]. Protein lacking exon 7 is unable to oligomerize, and is rapidly degraded [10, 11]. Thus, the loss of *SMN1* and retention of *SMN2* cause SMA by leading to reduced expression levels of functional SMN protein (see Figure 16.1).

Due to the instability of the genomic region and gene conversion events, the number of copies of *SMN1* and *SMN2* can vary. Examinations of copy number variation among patients demonstrate a significant inverse correlation between the number of *SMN2* copies and disease severity [12]. Thus, among Type 1 cases, 87.5% possess one (25%) or two (62.5%) *SMN2* copies, while 85.6% of Type 2 cases possess two or more copies, and 86.7% of Type 3 cases have three or more copies [13]. Similar results have been seen in multiple studies and the correlation extends to patient-derived cell lines, in which increased *SMN2* copy number correlates with higher protein levels and milder disease [14–17]. About 10% of *SMN2*-derived transcripts do encode for the full-length SMN protein, thus a greater number of copies of *SMN2* would be expected to produce more functional SMN protein and a milder disease [18]. Indeed, rare asymptomatic individuals with no *SMN1*, but 5 copies of *SMN2*, have been reported [15].

Epidemiology

SMA is the most frequent monogenic cause of infant mortality. The incidence ranges from 1 in 6000 to 1 in 10,000 live births in all ethnic populations that have been investigated. Type I SMA cases account for 50–60% of all cases [2, 19]. The carrier frequency within the general population has been estimated at 1 in 50 [20]. This carrier frequency would predict a higher incidence of SMA, but the discordance is likely accounted for by some *in utero* mortality. Fetuses with no functional *SMN1* or *SMN2* gene and no SMN protein expression would not be expected to be born because complete SMN knockout in other species is known to be uniformly embryonic lethal [21]. Studies have examined carrier frequencies in

Neurodegeneration, First Edition. Edited by Anthony Schapira, Zbigniew Wszolek, Ted M. Dawson and Nicholas Wood.
© 2017 John Wiley & Sons, Ltd. Published 2017 by John Wiley & Sons, Ltd.

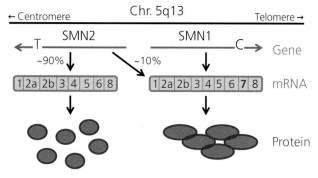

Figure 16.1 SMN genomic locus. The human *SMN1* and *SMN2* genes are located on chromosome 5 in inverse orientation. They are highly similar in their nucleotide sequence. One key difference between them is the presence of a C in *SMN1* and a T in *SMN2* within a splicing motif located in exon 7. The presence of the T alters the splicing of *SMN2*-derived transcripts such that exon 7 is frequently excluded. These transcripts lacking exon 7 code for a truncated SMN protein that is unstable and rapidly degraded. A minority of the time, exon 7 is retained in *SMN2*-derived transcripts and these transcripts encode a normal SMN protein identical to that arising from *SMN1*-derived transcripts. SMA is thus caused by insufficient expression levels of SMN protein.

different ethnic populations and found some variation. In southern China the frequency was estimated to be 1 in 42 [22], while a study from Cuba estimated the incidence at 1 in 84 [23]. A large analysis of different populations in North America documented an overall frequency of 1 in 54 with slight variation among groups (Caucasians 1:47, Ashkenazi Jews 1:67, African Americans 1:72, Asians 1:59, Asian Indians 1:52, Hispanics 1:68) [24]. It has also been estimated that approximately 2% of SMA cases arise from de novo *SMN1* mutations, which helps to explain why such a severe disease can maintain a high carrier frequency within the population [25].

Clinical characteristics

SMA was first described in a series of articles published in the 1890s by Guido Werdnig of the University of Vienna and Johann Hoffmann of the University of Heidelberg [26–28]. They each independently described a hereditary form of infantile-onset neuromuscular disease characterized by progressive weakness, muscle atrophy, and death due to respiratory failure. They documented degeneration of motor neurons in the anterior horn of the spinal cord. Patients with SMA have muscle weakness that is symmetrical and affects proximal muscles of the limbs more than distal muscles. The legs are more affected than the arms, and the face and diaphragm muscles are relatively spared. Disease severity is extremely heterogeneous and prior to the identification of the causative gene was believed to represent multiple disorders. This monogenic disorder is now known as "proximal" or "5q" SMA.

The range of clinical symptoms seen in proximal SMA patients has driven clinicians to develop a classification system that groups patients based on the "maximum functional status" approach, which defines SMA type by the highest motor milestones achieved [29]: Type 1 refers to patients who can never sit independently; Type 2 patients can sit, but never stand or walk independently; and Type 3 patients are able to stand and walk at some point during their disease course (see Table 16.1). More recently, the terms Type 0 and Type 4 have been introduced to refer to the extreme ends of the spectrum and define the most severely and most mildly

Table 16.1 SMA disease classification.

Type	Name	Onset	Lifespan	Milestones
0	Congenital	Prenatal	<6 months	None
1	Werdnig–Hoffmann	<6 months	<2 years	Never sit
2	Intermediate	6–18 months	~½ normal	Never stand
3	Kugelberg–Welander	>18 months	Slightly reduced	Walk
4	Adult	>18 years	Normal	Normal

affected cases, respectively [30]. Although these classifications are extremely useful, it is important to remember that they are arbitrary and define a spectrum of disease rather than distinct entities.

Type 0 SMA

The most severe cases are Type 0 SMA patients. They typically present with profound and generalized weakness and hypotonia at birth. Most are unable to achieve any motor milestones. Due to respiratory failure, they will require ventilation support and endotracheal intubation early in life. These complications greatly reduce lifespan and few are able to survive past 6 months of age. Maternal reports often note decreased fetal movements in the third trimester, which likely contributes to congenital arthrogryposis in some patients. These decreased movements, combined with the gravity of symptoms at birth, suggest a prenatal onset of disease [30].

Type 1 SMA

Patients with Type 1 SMA (Werdnig–Hoffmann disease) constitute 50–60% of all cases [2]. By definition, these infants are never able to sit up independently. Disease onset is typically before 6 months and often proceeds rapidly with patients regressing from normal to markedly weak in just days. They present with severe and generalized hypotonia. Often, muscle weakness causes infants to adopt a stereotypical posture with open hips ("frog-legged") and internally or externally rotated shoulders (see Figure 16.2A) [31]. Wrist and ankle contractures may also occur. Patients demonstrate progressive proximal weakness evidenced by minimal movements of the hip and shoulder with frequent hand and foot control and rare fasciculations and hand tremor. Facial and extraocular movements are also usually preserved although facial diplegia can be seen in severe cases. Areflexia is typically observed, while sensory and sphincter functions are normal. Babies have an alert state and auditory and visual responses are normal. Sucking and swallowing are often affected and can cause aspiration. Impairment of intercostal muscles combined with relatively spared diaphragm function can lead to the appearance of an anteriorly collapsed and "bell-shaped" chest and contribute to hypoventilation (see Figure 16.2A). Although these respiratory complications often lead to death by age 2, recent increases in lifespan have been achieved with the use of assisted ventilation technologies [32].

SMA symptoms were previously thought to be confined to the neuromuscular system; however, recent evidence suggests that some severe cases can present with clinical symptoms involving multiple other organ systems. (Autopsy data also suggest involvement of other organs and systems, but this is largely thought to be subclinical and is discussed in the Pathology section.) Reports of four unrelated patients with severe SMA found digital tissue necrosis, thought to be secondary to vascular perfusion abnormalities caused by autonomic dysfunction [33, 34]. Studies in small groups of patients have found evidence for autonomic dysfunction, although it remains unclear if it results from a primary defect of

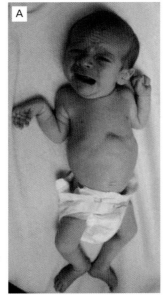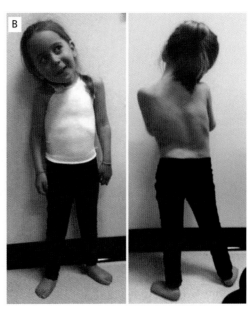

Figure 16.2 SMA patients. (A) A severely affected Type 1 infant has severe proximal limb and truncal muscle weakness. Intercostal muscle weakness results in a depressed sternum and compromised respiratory function. Source: Wee, Kong, & Sumner 2010 [4]. Reproduced with permission of Wolters Kluwer Health, Inc. (B) A child with Type 3 SMA can stand and walk, but has diffuse muscle weakness and atrophy, scoliosis, pes planovalgus, and small stature. Courtesy of Thomas Crawford. [290] Reproduced with permission of Elsevier.

SMN reduction [35]. The occurrence of congenital heart defects in Type 1 SMA has also been proposed to be related to disease pathogenesis; however, as both are relatively common disorders, coincidence has not been excluded. A retrospective study of 20 patients reported that left ventricular outflow abnormalities were overrepresented in the Type 1 SMA population [36]. Another study found that three of four SMA patients with only one copy of *SMN2* had significant atrial or ventricular septal defects [37]. A similar phenomenon has been observed regarding fatty acid metabolism, with severe SMA patients showing abnormalities that are absent in mild cases and controls [38]. These observations raise the possibility that different organ systems may be differentially susceptible to reduced SMN protein levels, and in severe cases SMN deficiency may cause multisystem dysfunction. Interestingly, models of severe SMA mice also show cardiac and vascular perfusion abnormalities, and may provide insight to primary defects of SMN reduction in these systems [39, 40].

Type 2 SMA

Patients with Type 2 (intermediate) SMA are able to sit unsupported at some point during their disease course, but are never able to stand or walk independently. Signs are typically identified between 7 and 18 months of age, because children fail to reach developmental milestones. Similar to Type 1 patients, initial symptoms consist of proximal weakness and hypotonia. Although all children can sit unsupported at some point, motor function can still vary significantly within this group. Some patients can struggle to sit and roll over, while others can do so easily and may even crawl unaided. Hand tremors and joint contractures may occur. Progressive scoliosis usually develops. This can contribute to restrictive lung disease and frequently requires surgical intervention. Weak swallowing is common and may affect weight gain, while weak bulbar musculature and intercostals strength may impair clearing of tracheal secretions and contribute to respiratory complications. Indeed, outcomes in this group are generally dependent on the degree of respiratory involvement. Aggressive management can extend lifespan. One large study found survival rates of 98.5% at 5 years and 68.5% at 25 years in this group [41].

Type 3 SMA

Type 3 SMA (Kugelberg–Welander) patients reach all major motor milestones, including the ability to walk unaided. They typically experience their first symptoms of disease between 18 months of age and early childhood. Disease severity is remarkably heterogeneous in this group: some require wheelchair assistance in childhood while others may remain ambulatory into adulthood with only minor weakness. This is correlated with age of onset, such that patients who experience their first symptoms later in life tend to have a longer ambulant period. However, onset itself is not predictive for individual patients, as many with early onset can walk for decades. Patients may develop scoliosis (see Figure 16.2B) or symptoms of joint overuse, but rarely suffer from serious respiratory complications. As a result, life expectancy is nearly normal. Intelligence and cognition are within the normal range, and verbal IQ scores (an indication of environmentally mediated knowledge) tend to be higher in adolescent SMA patients, perhaps because these children focus on developing cognitive skills to deal with restrictions associated with their physical handicaps [42].

Type 4 SMA

This designation is used to refer to individuals with adult disease onset sometimes as late as the fifth or sixth decade. Motor impairment is generally mild and there is little to no respiratory involvement [29]. These individuals represent an extremely small proportion of all SMA cases. Their mild disease course is often related to high *SMN2* copy number and in some cases to the presence of other genetic modifiers.

Disease course

In proximal SMA, the course of disease and outcome are dependent on the age of symptom onset, with those affected earlier likely to experience a rapid disease course and poor outcome. Among severe cases, those with clear prenatal involvement are unlikely to live past 3 months of age, those affected between 0 and 2 months will typically die before 1 year, and patients whose symptoms present between 2 and 6 months will likely die before age 2 without aggressive respiratory intervention [43, 44]. The most frequent causes of death are associated with intercurrent respiratory complications caused by weak bulbar and respiratory muscle function. In recent years, the use of mechanical ventilation devices and nutritional support have been associated with increases in life expectancy among Type 1 patients [32].

SMA progression is unique among neurodegenerative disorders. Typically, insidious onset is followed by inexorable progression in these disorders. In SMA, the greatest loss of muscle power is seen at disease onset and is often followed by a period of symptom stabilization. In some children there may be a clear loss of strength; in others it may manifest only as the inability to gain strength or to achieve developmental milestones. A prospective study of over 70 Type 2 and 3 patients over a 4-year period found no evidence for quantitative loss of muscle strength, seemingly indicating a lack of disease progression [45]. Many patients, however, were seen to lose functional abilities during this period. This seeming contradiction raises the question of whether disease is progressive at the level of clinical function, but not in the primary pathology. In these patients, complications associated with weakness, including progressive contractures, place increasing demands on their limited muscle strength and, in turn, cause progressive loss of function perhaps without any further decrease in motor neuron number. The timing of disease onset (during the development of the neuromuscular system) combined with the unusual progression and pathological observations have suggested that failed initial maturation of the motor system may play an important role in disease pathogenesis in addition to neurodegeneration.

Pathology

A majority of the pathological studies of SMA tissues have been carried out in Type 1 infants, as most fatalities are concentrated within this group. The primary pathological change observed is a paucity of motor neurons in the anterior horn of the spinal cord (see Figure 16.3) [46], (reviewed in [47]). A group of five Type 1 patients ranging from 5 to 22 months old showed a 73% reduction in motor neuron number compared to controls [48]. In SMA cases, 0.2–6.4% of remaining motor neurons were TUNEL positive indicating active degeneration. Motor neuron loss can also be seen in cranial motor nerve nuclei in the lower brainstem [49]. Motor neurons that remain are characterized by perikaryon swelling and chromatolysis, signs of degeneration. Immunocytochemistry studies have revealed phosphorylated neurofilaments concentrated near the perikaryon periphery, while granular ubiquitin-positive deposits occupy the central region. Studies of these tissues at the ultrastructural level also showed evidence of peripheral neurofilament accumulation and found mitochondria, lysosomes, and other vesicular bodies concentrated at the center [50]. Abnormally migrated motor neurons are also observed within ventral horn white matter, but it remains unclear if these contribute to disease pathogenesis [51]. Microglial and astrocytic invasion of the anterior horn is common, and thought to be secondary to motor neuron death.

Since these autopsy findings represent the end-stage of disease and are limited in their ability to reveal primary pathologic mechanisms, fetal tissues have recently been used to study presymptomatic stages of disease. Motor neurons establish contact with their target muscles by around 7–8 weeks post conception, and their continued survival depends on trophic signals from muscle. Large numbers of motor neurons lacking those signals then die as part of a normal developmental culling process, and motor neuron numbers stabilize at a

much lower number by 25 weeks [52]. SMA fetuses have fewer neurons at 12 weeks (the earliest time point examined), and further loss progresses at a similar pace as in control fetuses [53]. By 25 weeks, SMA fetuses have 50% fewer neurons, indicating that SMN deficiency can manifest as defects in fetal life.

On examination, spinal cord ventral roots have demonstrated axonal atrophy, a selective loss of large myelinated fibers, and an increased amount of connective tissue. Furthermore, they are frequently invaded by fibrous glial processes enclosed by a basal lamina [54, 55]. These "glial bundles" were initially proposed as a pathogenic mechanism but were subsequently found with lower frequency in other motor neuron disorders and are now thought to be secondary to substantial motor neuron loss early in development [56]. Intramuscular nerves are notable for the selective loss of large, myelinated fibers, evidence of Wallerian degeneration, and some distal axonal sprouting.

Other changes can be seen throughout the central nervous system. Although they may be largely subclinical, these findings suggest that SMN deficiency may affect other neuronal cell types [57]. Chromatolytic neurons were found within Clarke's column in the spinal cord, in subsets of neurons in the lateral geniculate nucleus and ventrolateral thalamus, and within the dorsal root ganglia in some Type 1 patients. A study of sural nerves in patients with Types 1–3 found evidence for sensory nerve degeneration in Type 1, but not Type 2 or 3, patients [58]. These data suggest differential vulnerability to SMN depletion among different cell types.

Biopsies of SMA muscle show myofiber atrophy that varies in appearance depending on disease severity. In Type 1 patients, muscles often show significant atrophy of both myofiber types, often involving entire fascicles. This panfascicular atrophy combined with clusters of hypertrophic type I fibers likely indicates advanced denervation followed by at least some reinnervation. Electron microscopy analysis demonstrated that many of these small fibers appear immature, contain central nuclei, and tend to cluster near larger, isolated myotubes [59]. Some fibers resemble developing myotubes and are undergoing apoptosis [60]. Whether this appearance is due to denervation very early in development or a primary failure of muscle development remains unclear. Cases with later onset typically show a milder pathology consistent with normal muscle development, followed by chronic neurogenic atrophy, as indicated by grouped, angulated atrophic fibers and fiber type grouping [61]. Overall, the pathological changes observed in SMA patients suggest that motor neurons, muscle fibers, and the connections between them are all involved in disease pathogenesis.

Diagnosis

A diagnosis of SMA was formerly made based on findings obtained from the clinical examination, electromyography, and muscle biopsy. The discovery of the disease-causing gene in 1995 now allows noninvasive genetic testing that has largely eliminated the need for invasive muscle biopsies.

Clinical investigation and findings

Initial investigations in a patient with suspected SMA generally focus on differentiating between a myopathic versus a neurogenic condition. Mildly elevated serum creatine kinase levels have been reported in SMA patients of all types, however they are often normal. Levels in Type 1 and 2 patients range from normal to a fourfold increase, while a slight elevation that is not correlated with disease progression may

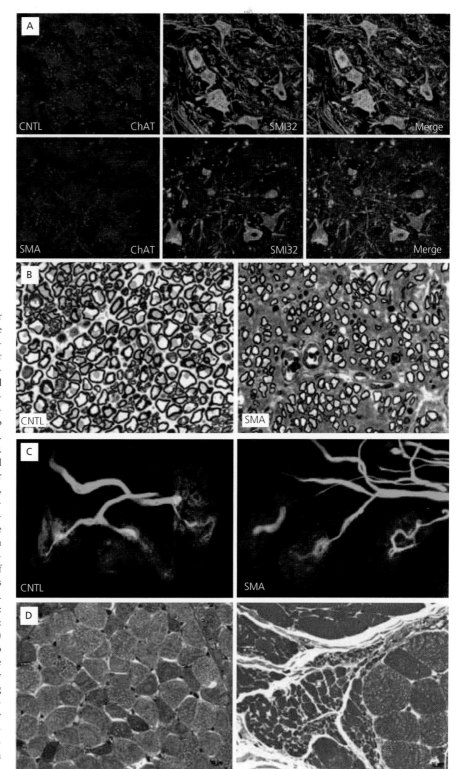

Figure 16.3 The pathology of SMA. (A) Motor neuron cell loss from the anterior horn of the spinal cord is a characteristic feature of human Type 1 SMA pathology at autopsy. Motor neurons are identified immunohistochemically by co-localization of choline acetyl transferase (ChAT) and a non-phosphorylated neurofilament (SMI32). They are markedly reduced in number in SMA patients (top panel) compared to controls (bottom panel). Reproduced with permission from Elsevier. (B) Control (left) and SMA (right) ventral roots at the lumbar level. Total axon number is reduced in ventral roots of SMA patients, with occasional myelin ovoids demonstrating active axonal degeneration. (C) Neuromuscular junctions of the diaphragm muscle are innervated, but structurally abnormal in SMA. Analysis at the light level reveals neurofilament accumulation and a paucity of synaptic vesicles in presynaptic terminals as well as thin axons in SMA patients (right). (Green: SMI312, pan-axonal marker; blue: synaptophysin, synaptic vesicle marker; red: mAB35, acetylcholine receptor marker.) (D) Muscles are differentially susceptible to denervation in human SMA patients. The diaphragm muscle (left) shows little atrophy compared to the iliopsoas (right) indicating relative sparing of phrenic nerve motor neurons in SMA. In the iliopsoas muscle, many small myofibers coexist with scattered hypertrophic ones. Source: (A, C & D) Perez-Garcia et al. [291] Reproduced with permission from Elsevier.

be observed in Type 3. Levels above 10 times the normal limit should raise concern about an alternative diagnosis [62, 63].

Nerve conduction studies show a reduction in compound muscle action potential (CMAP) amplitudes in motor, but not sensory nerves [64]. Slight abnormalities in sensory studies have been noted in a small number of SMA cases, but substantial abnormalities exclude a SMA diagnosis. One study reported a correlation between

the magnitude of CMAP reduction and disease severity as measured by earlier onset age with shortened life expectancy [65].

Needle electromyography reveals evidence of denervation and reinnervation [64, 66]. A neurogenic pattern is observed in all cases. Denervation, but rarely reinnervation, is reported in EMGs of Type 1 patients, possibly because the disease process occurs too quickly for reinnervation to take place [30]. High-amplitude, increased-duration motor unit potentials suggesting robust reinnervation are evident in Types 2 and 3. Fibrillation potentials tend to occur to the greatest extent in Type 2, followed by Type 3, and are rare in Type 1 [67]. In contrast, fasciculations are most commonly observed in Type 1 [68]. Before the era of widespread genetic testing, muscle biopsy – usually from the quadriceps muscle – was a diagnostic test in SMA. An SMA diagnosis is suspected if small, normal-sized, and hypertrophic fibers coexist (see Pathology section). In some cases, especially in Type 1 SMA, small, round myofibers are present in large groups. Muscle samples from less severely affected patients may exhibit fiber type grouping indicative of reinnervation, a finding that is less common in Type 1 SMA children. Although muscle biopsy was previously a useful diagnostic tool, the pathology has not been shown to predict severity or disease course [69, 70].

Genetic testing

Homozygous deletion of *SMN1* exon 7 is present in approximately 95% of all SMA cases. The *SMN1* deletion test is therefore the first test that should be pursued in an individual with suspected SMA (see Figure 16.4). A polymerase chain reaction using a restriction fragment length polymorphism (PCR-RFLP) technique uses restriction enzymes that recognize and digest the proper exon 7 base pairs resulting in the appearance of bands. A homozygous deletion in exon 7 corresponds to undigested DNA for which a band does not appear, and SMA diagnosis is confirmed. Although this test is highly accurate and produces results quickly, it cannot detect carrier status or *SMN2* copy number [71]. Nonetheless, many laboratories now report *SMN2* copy number together with *SMN1* deletion analysis. Copy number analysis is performed using quantitative PCR or multiplex ligation-dependent probe amplification techniques and is used by some as prognostic information regarding disease severity. We urge caution because although *SMN2* copy number does correlate inversely overall with SMA type, there are many individual exceptions to this rule.

Importantly, a negative result for the PCR-RFLP does not necessarily exclude SMA. Approximately 5% of SMA cases are compound heterozygotes and have one *SMN1* deletion combined with a second SMN mutation, usually a missense or small deletion on the other allele. If an SMA diagnosis is still suspected after further clinical examination, *SMN1* copy number analysis is necessary. If *SMN1*

copy number analysis detects a single *SMN1* copy, DNA sequencing should be performed to evaluate for the possibility of a second *SMN1* mutation [71].

The 5q genomic region is in an area with numerous repeated sequences and is therefore vulnerable to recombination and unequal crossover events that may result in *de novo* mutation [72]. In addition, evidence for gene conversion of *SMN1* to *SMN2*, and more recently *SMN2* to *SMN1*, has been reported [73]. A 2% incidence of *de novo* mutation is believed to account for the high carrier frequency in the general population in spite of the lethality associated with Type 1 SMA [25]. Although carrier screening via determination of *SMN1* copy number will detect most SMA carriers, carrier status cannot be definitively ruled out because this testing detects neither rare point mutations nor the presence of two *SMN1* alleles in *cis* on a single chromosome. Although carrier frequency is high among all ethnicities, carrier screening is currently only recommended for individuals with a family history of the disease or upon request, but not as a standard test for all individuals receiving genetic counseling [72]. This is rapidly evolving, however, as many obstetricians are now offering SMA carrier screening at the same time as cystic fibrosis screening.

There has been great interest in including SMA as part of the panel of diseases tested during population-wide neonatal screening. As it has been shown that loss of over 95% of motor units and severe denervation take place within the first 6 months after birth in Type 1 SMA patients, early detection would allow affected infants to be enrolled in clinical trials during this critical window for successful intervention [74, 75]. The criteria for a genetic condition to become part of population-based screening include disease severity, the possibility of prenatal diagnosis, high carrier frequency, and highly sensitive genetic testing, all of which apply to SMA [76]. The American College of Medical Genetics advocates its addition to population-based screening, while the American College of Obstetricians and Gynecologists' Committee on Genetics does not, citing a lack of pilot screening programs and cost effectiveness concerns [77]. The advantages and challenges of newborn screening are currently being investigated in pilot studies [78]. As newborn screening practices currently do not include DNA testing, and SMA lacks a biochemical marker, liquid microbead array would be used to detect homozygous *SMN1* deletion if SMA testing were to be implemented soon [72, 79].

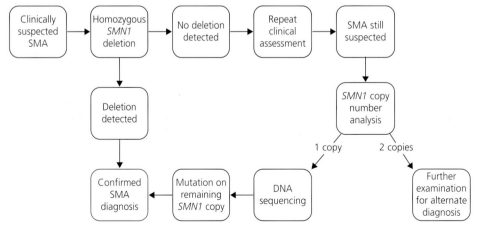

Figure 16.4 SMA genetic diagnosis. Homozygous *SMN1* deletion accounts for approximately 95% of SMA cases and is detected by the *SMN1* gene deletion test. Approximately 5% of individuals with SMA receive a negative result for the gene deletion test and may be compound heterozygotes. If the suspicion for a SMA diagnosis remains high after further clinical examination, *SMN1* copy number analysis should be performed. If this testing reveals only one *SMN 1* copy, DNA sequencing should be performed to identify a second mutation on the other allele.

Medical care and treatment

The phenotypic variation in SMA calls for an individualized approach to treatment that evolves based on disease course within a given patient. Medical caregivers and families must be aware of quality of life considerations when implementing procedures intended to prolong life. Variability between clinical presentation, intervention strategies, and situational factors contributes to the lack of standardized care for SMA, thereby making clinical studies difficult to interpret. In an effort to minimize such discrepancies, the International Standard of Care Committee for Spinal Muscular Atrophy was established in 2005 and has set forth guidelines for care in each of the areas listed below [29].

Respiratory

Pulmonary disease with ultimate respiratory failure is the leading cause of mortality in Type 1 and 2 patients [80]. Weakness of the inspiratory, expiratory, and bulbar-innervated muscle groups limits chest expansion during respiration and secretion release, and contributes to swallowing dysfunction. Without clinical intervention to ameliorate these symptoms, chest infections may ensue and, in some cases, result in death [81].

In Type 1 patients, depression of the sternum is caused by the compensatory action of diaphragm muscle in the face of severe intercostal muscle weakness. This phenotype is associated with inadequate lung development, and breathing exercises with mechanical insufflators-exsufflators should be performed to strengthen these muscles, thereby allowing a greater degree of lung inflation [1, 82]. Type 2 patients who are able to sit breathe with greater ease, but may require additional support as a result of scoliosis, disease progression, or illness.

Weak cough, a secondary effect of chest muscle weakness, is especially problematic during a cold, flu, or viral infection because secretions may remain in the lungs for long enough to block airways, further complicating inspiration. Several noninvasive therapies are recommended for loosening secretions, including chest physiotherapy, manually assisted cough, and postural drainage [29].

Individuals with SMA may need additional ventilatory support as a result of disease progression, sleep hypoventilation, or during an infection. A range of treatments are available, from noninvasive ventilation (NIV) to more aggressive options such as intubation and tracheostomy [81]. The degree of intervention is largely based on family preference. NIV can relieve symptoms, stabilize breathing patterns and gas exchange, improve sleep patterns, improve quality of life, and prolong survival [81, 83]. In addition, it has been shown to improve pectus excavatum and lung development in Type 1 SMA patients [84]. NIV is believed to provide these improvements by resting chronically fatigued muscles, reversing microatelectasis, and shifting the carbon dioxide set point [83]. Reduced disruption of breathing patterns facilitates more restful sleep, with improved appetite and concentration, and fewer headaches during the daytime are reported [29, 85]. Providing a sufficiently small interface is an important consideration in successfully implementing NIV in young SMA patients [81].

Bi-level positive airway pressure (BiPAP), mechanical ventilators, and negative pressure ventilators (NPV) are examples of NIV devices that can be used during both sleep and wakeful periods. A study with Type 2 SMA males reported that sleep-administered BiPAP did not negatively affect hemodynamics when pressures were well controlled and the mask was appropriately positioned [86]. A more complex alternative to BiPAP is the mechanical ventilator, which offers greater lifestyle flexibility via numerous setting options and wheelchair models [80, 87]. Due to the improved technology in BiPAP and mechanical ventilators, physicians rarely prescribe NPV to treat respiratory problems in SMA [80].

Invasive respiratory care in the form of intubation or tracheotomy is available for severely affected patients or during illness for stronger patients. The question of whether tracheotomy is appropriate for a particular individual with SMA is a controversial subject that should be carefully considered [29]. Following tracheotomy, Type 1 children often lose their ability to speak and are unable to breathe independently at any time [88]. For Type 2 children, tracheotomy is rarely needed [81]. Regardless of the chosen course of care, respiratory status must be monitored closely in order to adjust treatment as necessary.

Gastrointestinal and nutritional

Difficulties in nutrient intake and gastrointestinal function are universal in SMA and vary depending on disease severity and course. Weakness in facial and masticatory muscles hinders the ability to chew and swallow food. These muscles fatigue quickly in severely affected patients, prolonging feeding time [29, 89]. Additional limiting factors include dental malocclusion and poor head control [90]. Involvement of the bulbar muscles in Type 1 and occasionally Type 2 and 3 contributes to these symptoms and can lead to aspiration pneumonia [91]. Signals of aspiration include coughing and choking, but silent aspiration should be considered especially if pneumonia infections are recurrent [29]. In studies with Type 2 and 3 patients, the most prevalent difficulties reported were in chewing, adequately opening the mouth to take in food, and choking, particularly in those over 20 years old [92, 93]. To verify the existence and nature of swallowing deficiencies, a videofluoroscopic swallowing study should be obtained [29].

Because SMA individuals have unique nutritional considerations and are at risk for being under- or over-weight, close monitoring is imperative. Type 1 and 2 children generally need 20–50% fewer calories than their unaffected counterparts, but should avoid long periods of fasting that can cause muscle catabolism [38, 94]. Undernourishment increases the risk of illness, pressure sores, and loss of strength, while overnutrition increases the risk of diabetes, hypertension, pain, and loss of ambulation (Type 3) [17]. Furthermore, abnormal fatty acid metabolism has been reported in severely affected infants and is thought to be directly related to the loss of SMN function rather than the disease process [38]. In a study that compared fat mass index in patients grouped by functional status, nearly 75% of high-functioning, non-ambulatory individuals were above the 85th percentile for their age and gender compared to nearly 50% in both the ambulatory and the non-ambulatory low-functioning groups [95]. Nutritional status monitoring may include skinfold thickness tests and dual-energy X-ray absorptiometry scans to measure levels of body fat and blood work to monitor amino acids, blood glucose, and prealbumin [94].

Enteral feeding may be necessary if a patient struggles with oral feeding, acquiring adequate nutrition, digestion, illness, or is undergoing surgery. Short-term options include nasogastric or nasojejunal tubes while gastrostomy tubes (G-tube) and percutaneous gastrostomies are recommended for periods longer than 1 month.

A number of gastrointestinal and digestive problems are associated with SMA, including delayed gastric emptying, constipation, diarrhea, yeast infection, and vomiting after meals. The most severe of these comorbid conditions is gastroesophageal reflux disease (GERD), with greatest severity in Type 1 followed by 2 and 3.

Laparoscopic Nissen fundoplication is recommended for serious GERD, and has been noted to improve nutritional status, reduce aspiration-related events, and decrease average number of pneumonias and hospitalizations, especially when coupled with enteral feeding [96, 97]. Some physicians believe this procedure should be performed in all severely affected patients even if reflux is not present [96]. Whether severe or minor, gastrointestinal and nutrition complications that arise in SMA contribute to pulmonary function, and should be monitored closely by caregivers and physicians.

Orthopedic

Muscle weakness in SMA limits motor ability and can result in contracture formation, scoliosis, pelvic obliquity, osteopenia, pain, and bone fracture [29]. Truncal muscle weakness predisposes patients to scoliosis, one of the most prevalent symptoms in the disease affecting nearly 100% of Type 2 and most Type 3 patients [98, 99]. Orthotic devices are useful in controlling posture but cannot override the need for eventual surgical intervention [100, 101]. Spinal fusion surgery effectively corrects scoliosis and is typically recommended for wheelchair-bound patients [101]. The main goals of this surgery are to improve balance, comfort, and respiratory function. Abilities reported to decline after surgery include gross motor activities—rolling, bathing, toileting—and fine motor activities—eating, self-hygiene [102, 103]. Treatment immediately following surgery includes physical therapy, respiratory support, and pain control [100, 104].

Since their introduction in the 1960s, growing rods have been used to maintain spinal correction performed during the initial fusion surgery. Single rod techniques were widely used before the advent of dual rods, which demonstrated more effective long-term results [105–107]. Growing rods are also capable of improving pelvic obliquity, a prevalent symptom in SMA that is associated with scoliosis [108, 109]. Pelvic obliquity often leads to lead to hip dislocation in most non-ambulant Type 2 and some Type 3 individuals, but is not associated with significant pain and therefore does not require surgical intervention [110, 111]. Non-ambulatory Type 2 and 3 patients also experience contractures that cause discomfort and contribute to a decreased range of motion [112, 113]. Physical therapy that incorporates stretching and exercise is recommended to prevent contractures [29].

Osteopenia is commonly observed in several pediatric neuromuscular diseases, and very low bone mineral densities (BMD) have been reported in SMA patients [114]. Fractures can occur at birth and in neonatal SMA patients, possibly a result of *in utero* spinal motor neuron death [115]. BMD levels are reportedly normal in young SMA patients yet significantly reduced in ambulatory patients over 10 years old, indicating that a greater degree of movement does not prevent osteopenia in SMA [114, 116]. Interestingly, a study in yeast cells revealed protein–protein interactions between exon 7 of SMN splice variants and osteoclast-stimulating-factor that may cause increased osteoclast activity, thereby promoting bone resorption [117]. This may indicate supplemental intake of vitamin D and calcium for patients with lowered BMD, and caregivers should be aware that there is an increased risk of fracture even with minimal trauma [29].

Palliative care

The universal aim of palliative care is to improve quality of life by minimizing pain and suffering associated with terminal illness. The disease process in SMA is active and ongoing, and disease-modifying treatments are currently not available. Invasive therapies that extend life are controversial, leading physicians to question the extent to which they are appropriate when considering relative quality of life. The optimal course of therapy varies depending on each unique case and on the family's wishes as guided by trained specialists. Some families of Type 1 children choose a palliative approach from the point of diagnosis and take advantage of non-invasive ventilation and cough assistance to increase comfort while the disease follows its natural course [81].

Disease pathophysiology

The SMN gene

Approximately a century after SMA was first described, it was linked to a 10 centimorgan region of chromosome 5q13 [118, 119]. Further examinations of the region revealed that it was extremely unstable and frequently subject to large deletions, intrachromosomal rearrangements, and de novo alterations. Due to a 500-kb inverted duplication that occurred sometime during primate evolution, four genes are present in both telomeric and centromeric copies within 5q13 (see Figure 16.1). Refinement of the disease interval progressed until 1995, when a group in France showed that the telomeric copy of SMN (*SMN1*) was absent or mutated in 229 of 229 patients [3]. Both the telomeric (*SMN1*) and centromeric (*SMN2*) copies contain nine exons and eight introns and cover approximately 20 kb of genomic DNA. The two genes differ by only five nucleotides and predict identical, 294 amino acid proteins. Although these proteins are identical, only deletions of *SMN1* are associated with SMA.

The critical difference between the two genes results from alternative splicing of their pre-RNAs. In addition to the full-length messenger RNA, four splice variants have been detected that involve the exclusion of various exons (Δ5, Δ7, Δ5+7, and Δ4–7). The last isoform, consisting of only exons 1–3, is unlikely to have any role in disease, as previously identified point mutations lie in downstream exons and would not affect this protein [120]. Experiments examining each gene's mRNA products revealed that *SMN1* produces full-length mRNA, while 90% of *SMN2*-derived transcripts are missing exon 7 (Δ7) [8, 9]. The Δ7 transcript encodes a truncated protein that is unstable and rapidly degraded via the ubiquitin-proteasome system [10]. As a result, individuals lacking *SMN1* produce only a small amount of functional SMN protein, while those that lack *SMN2*, but retain *SMN1*, express functional protein and have no symptoms. Furthermore, disease severity is inversely correlated with SMN protein and *SMN2* expression levels [17, 121].

SMN splicing

The difference in the mRNA products produced by each of the two genes arises from a translationally silent sequence variant that affects mRNA splicing. *SMN1* contains a cytosine at the sixth position of exon 7 (ex7+6), while *SMN2* contains a thymidine (uridine in the mRNA). Multiple hypotheses have been proposed to explain the difference in splice products. The first posits that the C in *SMN1* is part of an exonic splice enhancer motif that recruits splicing factor 2 (SF2/ASF) to the mRNA [122]. SF2/ASF then can bind to the U2 small nuclear ribonucleoprotein (snRNP), which induces the removal of intron 6, and promotes inclusion of exon 7 in the resulting transcript. The second hypothesis suggests that the U at position ex7+6 in *SMN2* acts as part of an exonic splice suppression motif and recruits hnRNPA1, a negative splicing factor [123, 124]. This prevents SF2/ASF and U2 snRNP from binding and prevents inclusion of exon 7 into the transcript. An intronic sequence variant has also been shown to create an alternative hnRNPA1 binding site in *SMN2*-derived transcripts, which is absent in *SMN1* and essential for exon 7 exclusion, suggesting that both intronic and exonic sequence variations are involved in splicing differences [125]. An exonic splice enhancer found further downstream in exon 7 can bind Htra2-β1, a positive regulator, and promote inclusion of exon 7 in both *SMN1* and *SMN2* derived transcripts [126]. This is further enhanced by an interaction with hnRNP-G and demonstrates that recombinant trans-acting factors may be used to correct exon 7 skipping [127]. It is important to note that none of these mechanisms is mutually exclusive and all might contribute to SMN splicing *in vivo*. Estimates have suggested as many as 90% of *SMN2*-derived transcripts lack exon 7; however whether there are specific splicing patterns in different tissues, especially motor neurons, remains unclear.

SMN expression

The promoter sequences for *SMN1* and *SMN2* are nearly identical in sequence and activity [128, 129]. Both use two transcription start sites; one, −246 from the translations start site, is used primarily during fetal development, and the second, −163, is used later in development and throughout adult life. The minimal sequences required for activity are contained within a region −107 and +150 from the transcription start site, although it is likely that regulatory sequences lie further up- and down-stream [130]. SMN expression occurs in all somatic tissue, but is subject to both cell-type-specific and temporal regulation. Activity is high during fetal and early postnatal development, but decreases coincidental with, and perhaps in response to, cellular differentiation [131]. Transcription factors known to bind near and regulate expression include the cyclic AMP-response element binding protein (CREB), members of the Specificity protein (Sp) and E Twenty-six (Ets) families, nuclear factor interleukin6 (NF-IL6), and the interferon regulatory factor (IRF-1) [130, 132, 133]. Attempts to define other regulatory mechanisms have identified many putative factors whose relevance still needs to be determined [131]. In addition to transcription factor control, SMN expression is also regulated by epigenetic modifications, specifically histone acetylation [134]. Acetylated histones promote transcription by relaxing chromatin structure and the removal of the acetyl group can repress transcription by condensing chromatin. Studies have shown that the histones' acetylation within the SMN promoter decreases during development, consistent with

reduced expression. Chromatin immunoprecipitation revealed that the individual histone deacetylases HDAC1 and 2 both bound to the SMN promoter *in vivo*, and further work has suggested that HDACs may regulate acetylation in a class-specific manner [134, 135]. Further work to understand the *trans*- and *cis*-elements that can regulate SMN expression may have significant therapeutic benefit as increasing *SMN2* expression may ameliorate disease symptoms [121].

Genetic modifiers

Despite the established correlation between *SMN2* copy number and disease severity, individuals with identical *SMN1/SMN2* genotypes can present with variable disease severities. For example, individuals with three *SMN2* copies can present with Type 1, 2, or 3 disease, indicating that other genes can modulate the SMA phenotype [136, 137]. One way to identify these genetic modifiers is to identify SMA-discordant families in which individuals with identical *SMN2* copy number manifest variable severities of disease. A transcriptome-wide study of six such SMA families found that plastin 3 (an actin-binding protein) was expressed at higher levels in patients with less severe symptoms [138]. Increased plastin 3 levels were shown to result in increased F-actin levels, suggesting that modification of the actin cytoskeleton may be protective against SMA. Interestingly, the effects of plastin 3 were shown to be confined to females [139]. A sequence variant within *SMN2* itself was also shown to modify disease severity in individuals with low *SMN2* copy number. The nucleotide change (G859C) in exon 7 creates a splice enhancer site that promotes exon 7 inclusion [140]. These studies demonstrate the importance of considering genetic context when considering *SMN1/SMN2* genotyping and prognosis. In addition, they highlight the potential of genetic studies to uncover novel SMA genetic modifiers.

The SMN protein

Both *SMN1* and *SMN2* encode a 294 amino acid, 38-kDa protein with no homology to any other human protein (see Figure 16.5). The sequence contains a lysine-rich domain, a tudor domain, a proline-rich domain, and a tyrosine–glycine box, and is highly conserved from yeast to human. In mammals, it is expressed in all somatic tissues, with higher expression in the brain, spinal cord, and muscle, and relatively less in lymphocytes and fibroblasts [141, 142]. The protein can be seen throughout the cells, including nuclear, cytoplasmic, and axonal/ dendritic subcellular compartments. Within

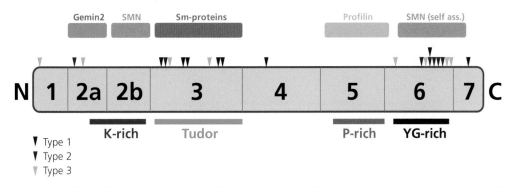

Figure 16.5 The SMN protein. The SMN protein contains several functional domains. The protein contains a lysine-rich domain, which is involved in Gemin2 binding and SMN self-association; a tudor domain, which interacts with Sm proteins; a proline-rich domain, which is important for profilin binding; and a tyrosine and glycine-rich domain, which is also involved in SMN self-association. Over 25 missense mutations have been identified and tend to cluster in known functional regions, suggesting that disruptions of these functions are associated with disease pathogenesis (for a complete list of mutations, see reference [145]).

nuclei, SMN localizes to dot-like structures that frequently overlap with coiled (Cajal) bodies, which are rich in snRNPs and are known to be sites of RNA metabolism [143]. These SMN-containing structures were named gems (gemini of coiled bodies), and their numbers have since been shown to correlate with disease severity [144]. Cells derived from SMA patients possess fewer gems per nucleus than control cells, indicating that gem function may be involved in disease pathogenesis.

As SMA is caused by a reduction in SMN protein levels, understanding the molecular functions of the SMN protein can provide insights into SMA pathogenic mechanisms and potential therapeutic targets (see Figure 16.6). Although many proteins have been proposed to bind to or interact with SMN, the validation of functional complexes remains challenging. Recently, four criteria were suggested to be required to define functional interactions [145]. They include reciprocal immunoprecipitation of the endogenous proteins, isolation of the complex from cells or tissues, co-localization, and a functional dependency on SMN levels.

To date, the role of SMN in a large, multimeric complex involved in snRNPs assembly is the best characterized function of the protein (see Figure 16.6, reviewed in [146]). In the cytoplasm, the protein forms a complex with Gemin 2–8 and Unrip (upstream of Nras-interacting protein) [147]. SMN likely exists as an oligomer within this complex as SMN oligomerizes rapidly *in vitro* and incorporation shifts its stability from hours to days [10]. This complex then functions as an "assemblysome" that allows for specific RNAs and RNA-binding proteins to interact. snRNPs are large RNA–protein complexes that catalyze the removal of introns from pre-mRNA transcripts in the nucleus. Each snRNP consists of one small nuclear RNA (snRNA), which allows it to recognize splicing signals, a core of 7 Sm proteins (B/B′, D1, D2, D3, E, F, and G), and other snRNA-specific proteins. The snRNAs are transcribed in the nucleus and exported to the cytoplasm, where Gemin 5 recognizes a large 50–60

nucleotide sequence called the "snRNP code" and brings them to the SMN complex [148]. Simultaneously, Gemin 2 binds to a heptameric ring of Sm proteins and structural features of this interaction prevent this promiscuous Sm core from binding non-snRNAs [149]. SMN can also bind directly to SmB/D3 via its tudor domain, which recognizes the protein's arginine (R) and glycine (G) rich domains. Interestingly, this interaction is enhanced by the symmetrical dimethylation of specific R residues within the Sm proteins by a protein arginine *N*-methyltransferase (PRMT5)/methylosome complex [150]. Once the proper components are assembled, the SMN complex mediates the adenosine triphosphate (ATP)-dependent assembly of the Sm proteins onto the correct snRNA. Further RNA maturation including 5′ cap hypermethylation and 3′ processing occurs and then the complex is imported to the nucleus, where the snRNPs begin to participate in pre-mRNA splicing.

Although the role of SMN in snRNP assembly has been the most extensively studied, SMN has been shown to interact with a variety of other proteins, and may function in multiple cellular pathways. Previously reported SMN interactors include Sm-like proteins (LSm), heterogeneous nuclear ribonucleoproteins (hnRNP-U/Q/R), fibrillarin, group A rotavirus protein 1 (GAR1), coilin, RNA helicase A, zinc finger protein 1 (ZPR1), plastin 3, profilin, the fragile X mental retardation protein, human antigen D (HuD), and a variety of others (reviewed in [151]). Analyses of this group reveal that a large portion of these proteins function within known RNP complexes and are involved in various aspects of RNA metabolism including transcription, pre-mRNA splicing, transfer and ribosomal RNA processing, and mRNA stabilization and decay.

The specific role of SMN in many of these processes remains to be characterized and may provide important insights into which, if any, are sensitive to reductions in SMN levels and may be involved in disease pathogenesis. Mutations in the RNA-binding proteins TAR-DNA binding protein 43 (TDP-43) and fused in sarcoma

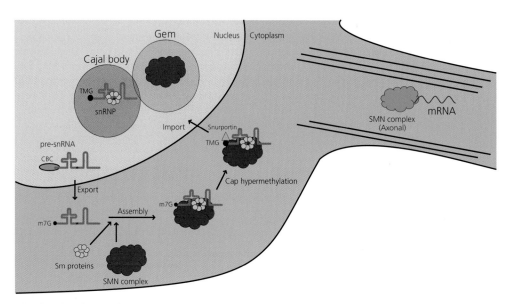

Figure 16.6 The molecular roles of SMN. The SMN protein is involved in the assembly of spliceosomal snRNP particles. Sm-site containing snRNAs are transcribed in the nucleus and are bound by cap binding complex (CBC) proteins and exported to the cytoplasm. In the cytoplasm, SMN oligomerizes and forms a large, multimeric complex with the Gemin proteins (2–8) and Unrip. Sm proteins assemble into a ring and interact with the SMN complex via Gemin 2 and SMN. Gemin 5 then recognizes Sm-site containing snRNAs and the SMN complex facilitates the assembly of the Sm proteins onto the snRNA. 5′-cap hypermethylation and further maturation steps allow the assembled snRNPs to be imported back into the nucleus. Once inside, snRNPs are targeted to Cajal bodies, and SMN complexes can be found throughout the nucleus but are especially concentrated in gems. SMN has also been shown to exist in distinct axonal RNP complexes, and may be involved in mRNA metabolism and transport.

(Fus) have been shown to cause amyotrophic lateral sclerosis (ALS). Studies utilizing TDP-43 transgenic mice have demonstrated that TDP-43 protein levels can affect gem number and subcellular distribution [152]. Researchers elucidated a potential TDP-43, Fus, and SMN pathway by which Fus associates upstream with TDP-43 and downstream with SMN regulating gem formation [153]. Further studies are needed to examine potential functional interactions between SMN and these other RNA processing proteins; however, these recent developments suggest that abnormalities of RNA metabolism may play a key role in the pathogenesis of multiple motor neuron diseases.

The set of SMN-interacting proteins also includes multiple proteins involved in regulating the actin cytoskeleton or in β-actin mRNA transport and processing. As motor neurons are particularly susceptible to reductions in SMN, and axonal transport over long distances is essential to motor neuron survival, this raises the possibility that SMN may have specific functions in axons of motor neurons. In cultured neurons, SMN can be visualized in β-actin mRNA-containing RNP granules that are actively transported down axons. Further work demonstrated that SMN bound to and co-localized with hnRNPR, which is known to bind to the 3′ untranslated region of β-actin mRNA [154]. At growth cones in developing neurons, actin polymerization drives axonogenesis by pushing the leading edge forward. In motor neurons grown from SMN-deficient mice, axons appear shorter than controls and have reduced levels of β-actin mRNA and protein in growth cones [154]. Profilin, a small actin-binding protein, can bind to the proline-rich domain of SMN and is known to be involved in actin polymerization and growth [155]. Furthermore, plastin 3 can bind to SMN and was able to rescue axon-length defects in SMN-deficient motor neurons [138]. SMN-containing complexes have also been shown to contain HuD, a neuron-specific RNA-binding protein known to transport mRNAs into growth cones during neuron growth and differentiation [156]. In this context, SMN interacts with the mRNA of candidate plasticity related gene 15 (cpg15), which is highly expressed in ventral spinal cord, transported into growth cones, and capable of promoting axon branching and neuromuscular junction (NMJ) synaptogenesis [157]. Importantly, cpg15 levels were reduced in SMN-knockdown motor neurons, and cpg15 overexpression partially rescued motor neuron defects in a zebrafish model. These data suggest that SMN is important for the transport of multiple mRNAs involved in motor neuron growth and that functional SMN reduction may affect distinct aspects of axon outgrowth and maturation.

An additional source of insight about the SMN protein function can come directly from patients. In approximately 5% of patients, small mutations, including missense mutations, cause disease [3]. Examining where these mutations are and the changes they induce in the protein sequence can provide insights into the functions of SMN that are disrupted in disease. In these patients, slightly different forms of SMN from *SMN1* and varying amount of full-length SMN from *SMN2* can produce different severities of disease. Mutations identified from patients can be expressed *in vitro* and can be screened for their ability to oligomerize, bind Sm proteins, perform snRNP assembly, or rescue animal models of disease [11, 158]. A pattern has emerged whereby mutations known to cause milder (Type 2 or 3) disease have been able to form heteromers with full-length SMN protein and to increase survival in SMN-deficient mice [159, 160]. This indicates that *in vivo* large amounts of SMN protein with missense mutations can oligomerize with full-length protein from the *SMN2* locus, which results in more functional SMN complexes and mild disease. However, missense mutations alone cannot

rescue the lethality of SMN null animals, indicating that at least some full-length protein is absolutely required [161]. Mutations that cause Type 1 disease often are found to abolish SMN's ability to oligomerize or bind Sm proteins [159].

Animal models

Because the SMN protein is present in all metazoan cells and because it has been functionally conserved in all species, model organisms are well suited for explorations of disease pathogenesis. All other organisms have only one copy of the SMN gene in their genomes, and its absence is uniformly embryonic lethal. However, in an effort to mimic the human disease various genetic models have been constructed to model disease. Each species has unique strengths as a model organism and some are thus more suited to particular experiments. Using multiple organisms also allows hypotheses to be easily validated; results that can be replicated in multiple organisms may be more likely to be relevant to human disease. A proper animal model should mirror the disease condition in humans: SMN protein levels sufficient to maintain essential cellular functions, but reduced enough to induce motor neuron-specific symptoms.

Drosophila

Many known disease-causing genes have *Drosophila* orthologs and the wide range of genetic tools available in these invertebrates provides a powerful means of investigation. Screening of known lethal mutations within the SMN genetic region identified a missense mutation that abolished oligomerization activity and was lethal during development [162]. Larval flies showed abnormal motor behavior, reduced postsynaptic currents at the NMJ, and impaired postsynaptic neurotransmitter receptor clustering. These defects could be rescued by expressing SMN under neuronal-specific and mesodermal-specific drivers together, but not by either alone. This evidence suggests that both neural and muscle tissue can contribute to SMA and that primary defects may manifest at the NMJ. Another group reported a *Drosophila* line in which SMN levels were reduced specifically in the adult thorax. This resulted in flies that were unable to fly and showed evidence of muscular atrophy [163]. The investigators showed that SMN was localized to Z lines of the sarcomere and interacted with α-actinin, which suggested a cytoskeletal role for SMN in muscle. Large databases of mutations are extremely valuable tools within the *Drosophila* field and genetic screens have tremendous potential to identify novel pathway components. A genetic modifier screen of a transposon-induced mutation collection sought to identify genes that could modify the NMJ phenotype caused by a lethal SMN mutation [164]. Interestingly, wishful thinking (*wit*), a BMP receptor, was shown to alter the *Drosophila* SMA phenotype by rescuing NMJ defects. These results implicate muscle–nerve trophic interactions in SMA disease pathogenesis and suggest that modification of BMP signaling may provide therapeutic value.

Work in the *Drosophila* SMA model suggests that SMN deficiency in additional neuronal cell populations causes CNS circuit abnormalities. SMN knockdown specific to the *Drosophila* motor neuron population was not sufficient to recapitulate the SMA disease phenotype. Rather, knockdown in cholinergic subpopulations, was necessary. SMN rescue only in motor neurons failed to ameliorate the disease, but genetic or pharmacological rescue of SMN in cholinergic sensory or spinal interneurons was sufficient to rescue the disease phenotype. Emphasizing SMN-derived abnormalities in additional cell populations, this study highlighted a novel paradigm that suggests that SMA might be a disease of the motor circuit [165].

Zebrafish

Zebrafish are prized as model organisms because of their rapid embryonic development and the ease of morpholino-mediated genetic manipulation. The use of antisense oligonucleotides targeted to SMN and injected at the 1–4 cell stage achieved a 60% decrease in SMN protein levels [166]. The embryos died in late gastrulation, consistent with essential SMN functions. Analysis of motor neuron development revealed significant numbers of motor neuron axon truncations and ectopic branchpoints, while other neurons and muscle developed normally. Significantly, single motor neuron-specific knockdown also produced defects, independent of motor neuron death. These data suggest a cell-autonomous role for SMN in motor axon development and implicate impaired motor axon outgrowth as an early consequence of SMN deficiency. A large screen later identified specific zebrafish *Smn* mutations including a point mutation found in Type 1 patients [167]. Homozygous mutants revealed a defect in the presynaptic accumulation of the synaptic vesicle protein 2 (SV2), which was rescued by introducing human SMN into motor neurons. The same group also introduced the human *SMN2* gene into SMN null zebrafish and rescued the presynaptic defect and increased survival [168]. This model, which mirrors the human condition (loss of *SMN1* and retention of splicing-defective *SMN2*), can potentially be used as an *in vivo* model for therapeutics testing or genetic screens.

Mouse

Although fish and fly models can provide important insights about SMA, the basic biology of these organisms limits their usefulness as human disease models. Mice, which share the same essential elements and organizational principles of the neuromuscular system as humans, are one of the best suited models for addressing questions about SMA biology or testing potential therapeutics (see Figure 16.7) [169]. The mouse *Smn* ortholog shares 82% amino acid identity with the human protein and its homozygous deletion is embryonically lethal with massive cell death at very early stages. *Smn* +/− heterozygous mice develop normally and live a full lifespan with no motor symptoms or weakness, mirroring unaffected heterozygous human carriers [21]. These mice do show a significant reduction (40%) in spinal motor neuron number by 6 months of age without subsequent loss, suggesting subclinical motor neuron degeneration followed by stabilization.

In order to generate more useful SMA mouse models, two separate approaches were undertaken: Cre-loxP mediated deletion of exon 7, and introduction of human *SMN2* into the *Smn* −/−background. The creation of a floxed SMN allele with loxP sites flanking of exon 7 allowed for exon 7 excision and the exclusive production of SMNΔ7 transcripts in the presence of Cre recombinase [170]. As expected, ubiquitous Cre expression in mice homozygous for the floxed *Smn* allele resulted in early embryonic lethality. Restriction of Cre to neuronal cells produced an SMA-like phenotype including

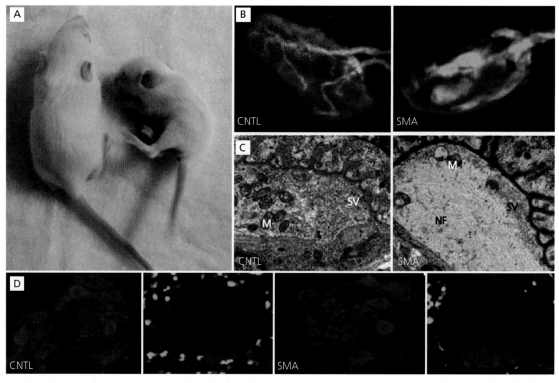

Figure 16.7 SMA pathology in mouse models of SMA. (A) The SMNΔ7 mouse model recapitulates aspects of severe SMA in humans. SMA mice (right) show reduced weight gain, impaired motor function with inability to right, and reduced survival with death at 2 weeks compared to control littermates (left). (B) Neuromuscular junctions visualized at the light level show accumulation of neurofilament and a paucity of synaptic vesicle staining in the presynaptic terminals of SMA (right) compared to wild-type (left) mice. (Green: SMI312, neurofilament, an axonal marker; blue: synaptophysin, synaptic vesicle marker; red: bungarotoxin, acetylcholine receptor marker.) (C) Electron microscope images of a control (left) and an SMA (right) neuromuscular junction. Pathological features in the SMA mouse include neurofilament accumulation and a paucity of synaptic vesicles in presynaptic terminals. (M, mitochondria; NF, neurofilament; SV, synaptic vesicles.) (D) Spinal motor neurons at the first lumbar spinal segment labeled with ChAT (red) and VGLUT (green). Motor neuron number (left panels) is reduced in the SMA mouse compared to the control. A reduction in VGLUT+ proprioceptive inputs onto individual spinal motor neurons (right panels) is also observed in the SMA mouse.

severe motor defects and death around postnatal day 25. Neurogenic muscle atrophy without motor neuron loss suggested distal axonal degeneration. Further analysis of NMJs in these mice revealed massive neurofilament accumulation at terminal axons [171]. Similar experiments designed to remove SMN from muscle led to muscle necrosis and severe muscle dystrophy resulting in paralysis and death [172]. It is important to note that conclusions from these experiments must be considered in light of the fact that the complete removal of full-length SMN, as occurs with this allele, is never seen in human patients. Cre-mediated excision of SMN has also been performed in motor neuron progenitors in mice that also express human *SMN2* as a transgene [173]. This produced a mild phenotype likely owing to the normal expression of SMN in all non-motor neuron cells. Inducible alleles have also been developed in which Cre-activity can swap exon 7 sequences, effectively converting splicing-defective *SMN2*-like alleles into properly spliced alleles [174]. Work with these mice has demonstrated that post-symptomatic SMN restoration can rescue disease symptoms and has also defined a temporal "window of opportunity" outside of which restoration does not improve symptoms. Interestingly, this window suggests that the primary consequences of disease manifest at NMJs, and that the extent of damage there determines the responsiveness of symptoms to SMN induction.

An alternate approach to modeling SMA was sought by transgenically introducing the human *SMN2* gene into mice that are homozygous mouse *Smn* null [175, 176]. The presence of one or two copies of *SMN2* was able to rescue the embryonic lethality, although a majority of the pups were either stillborn or died within 6 hours of birth. Some appeared normal at birth, but showed decreased movement and breathing within 48 hours and died within 6 days of birth. Spinal motor neuron counts revealed normal numbers at birth, but a significant decrease by postnatal day 5 (P5). A separate transgenic line, which expressed eight copies of *SMN2*, did not develop the SMA phenotype, thus confirming *SMN2* expression as a disease modifier and therapeutic target. The two copy mouse (Smn −/−, SMN2 +/+) model has also been used as a backbone upon which several other models have been created. The introduction of a transgene containing SMN cDNA lacking exon 7 (SMNΔ7) was found to increase the lifespan of this severe model from 5 to 13 days [160]. SMN Δ7 protein was shown to form heterologous complexes with full-length SMN, an interaction predicted to increase the amount of oligomeric (functional) SMN. The "SMAΔ7 mouse" as it is now known has become the most widely used model in SMA research. It shows pathology similar to the human disease (see Figure 16.7), displays symptoms severe enough that subtle improvements can be easily observed, and lives long enough for therapeutic interventions to yield results. Multiple other transgenes encoding for SMN with known human mutations (A2G, A111G) have been shown to increase survival in the severe model [177]. Interestingly, the Δ7, A2G, and A111G transgenes all fail to rescue the lethality of *Smn*−/− embryos, which suggests that some full-length SMN is an absolute requirement and that the transgenes exert their positive effects by interacting with it.

Efforts have been underway to develop mice with milder disease phenotypes and longer lifespan (for a review, see reference [169]). One strategy has been to modify the mouse *Smn* gene to alter splicing patterns and reduce SMN protein [178, 179]. Mice carrying these mutations have later disease onset, an extended lifespan, and can be useful for examinations of therapeutics delivered over longer time periods. These models, combined with continued detailed phenotypic and pathological analysis, will be useful in resolving unanswered questions regarding SMA biology and in characterizing therapeutic effectiveness.

Pig

Recently, a large animal model has been developed by the Burghes lab at Ohio State University (OSU). Researchers found that a single intrathecal dose of an scAAV9 vector expressing a short-hairpin RNA (shRNA) that targets pig SMN demonstrates effective SMN knockdown in motor neurons as well as in other neuronal tissues. When the vector is administered on P5, SMN knockdown pigs begin to effectively recapitulate key features of SMA pathology 3–4 weeks following the injection. Key disease manifestations in the pig model are the development of severe hindlimb weakness, decreased compound muscle action potential amplitudes on nerve conduction studies (CMAP), and decreased estimated number of motor neurons (MUNE). The pig model may offer significant advantages for therapeutic development efforts due to the close anatomical similarities to humans, particularly of the CNS [180].

Disease mechanisms

The disease course of SMA is unusual among the neurodegenerative diseases because a rapid disease onset is often followed by symptom stabilization. As the timing of onset can vary from *in utero* until the fifth decade of life in humans, it is also unclear whether the primary mechanisms of disease relate to developmental defects, degenerative processes, or both. Furthermore, the causative gene encodes a ubiquitously expressed protein with essential functions for all cells, yet reduced SMN protein levels appear to selectively affect motor neurons with only minor involvement of other systems. Why motor neurons seem to be uniquely susceptible to reductions in SMN protein levels remains to be established.

Multiple lines of evidence suggest that there may be a developmental aspect to SMA. Severe forms of disease (Types 0 and 1) are the most common with onset in either prenatal or early postnatal life. Pathological examinations in SMA fetuses and patients have found abnormalities in myotube development and exacerbated motor neuron cell death consistent with prenatal onset and arrested motor unit development [53, 59]. Studies of primary motor neurons isolated from SMA mice show defects in axon elongation, reductions in distal β-actin mRNA and protein levels, and defective spontaneous excitability caused by poor calcium channel clustering [154, 181]. These studies might suggest particular abnormalities of motor neuron terminals in SMA. Indeed, multiple studies have highlighted abnormalities of NMJ synapses in SMA mice that include presynaptic terminal neurofilament accumulation and immature endplates [171, 182, 183]. These pathological abnormalities are accompanied by impaired NMJ function including reduced quantal content (i.e. the number of synaptic vesicles released in response to an evoked stimulus) and altered presynaptic calcium homeostasis [184, 185]. Synaptic defects also extend to synaptic inputs to motor neuron soma [186]. Normally, sensory afferent–motor neuron synapses increase in the early postnatal period. In SMA mice, no increase in connectivity is observed, suggesting a failure of maturation, and monosynaptic responses are drastically reduced early in disease (P4). These studies have highlighted that early consequences of SMN deficiency are structural and functional abnormalities of both peripheral and central synapses that precede synaptic retraction or motor neuron loss. It appears that these synaptic abnormalities not only contribute to a failure of normal neuromuscular development, but may also subsequently cause motor neuron degeneration. In addition to the morphological abnormalities that suggest impaired development there also appears to be a temporal dependence to disease pathogenesis. Genetic rescue experiments in mice suggest that SMN induction must occur in the early neonatal period to be effective. Similarly, genetic reduction of

SMN expression must occur in the neonatal period in order to fully recapitulate SMA disease features [187].

Although the cellular consequences of SMN protein deficiency are being increasingly defined in SMA models, how they are caused by SMN protein deficiency remains unclear. The most well established molecular function of SMN is in snRNP assembly. The proper assembly and function of snRNPs is essential to proper alternative splicing and cellular viability. As such, reductions in SMN levels have been proposed to cause disease symptoms by reducing either the amount or the profile of snRNPs within affected tissues. Examinations of snRNP assembly in spinal cords from mouse models revealed a direct correlation between disease severity and assembly ability [188]. Furthermore, the injection of pre-assembled snRNPs into SMN-deficient zebrafish was able to rescue motor axon development defects, suggesting that snRNP assembly alterations manifest as axonal development defects [123]. However, an examination of Gemin 2-deficient motor neurons indicated that their pathfinding was unaffected [189]. As Gemin 2 is also required for snRNP assembly, these data suggest that snRNP assembly deficiency may not be the basis of abnormal motor axon development [189, 190]. Because snRNPs are thought to be relatively long-lived within cells, discordance exists between the rate of snRNP assembly levels and the amount of functional snRNPs. Patient cells show normal snRNP levels with severely reduced SMN levels; furthermore, specific point mutations are fully capable of assembling snRNPs [188, 191]. In SMA mice, overall snRNA levels are only mildly affected, despite huge changes in snRNP assembly. However, analysis of different tissue types in SMA mutant mice showed specific decreases of both U11 and U12 snRNAs in brain and spinal cord tissue, indicating both tissue- and target-specific differences [188, 192]. U11 and U12 are specific components of the minor spliceosome and regulate the splicing of approximately 700 genes. Longitudinal studies of exon-level changes have been undertaken and show a small number of splicing changes early in disease and extensive splicing alterations in late stages [193]. Some of these late changes likely represent non-SMN specific responses to near-death disease and cellular injury. In a recent study, defects of specific U12-dependent splicing events affected gene expression levels in an SMA *Drosophila* model. Strikingly, restoration of one of these genes,

Stasimon, restored motor circuit function in these flies, suggesting that defects of U12 splicing could play a direct role in SMA pathogenesis [194]. Further studies will be needed to define the functional consequences of impaired snRNP assembly and defects of splicing in other model systems.

An alternate explanation for why the ubiquitously expressed SMN gene causes a motor neuron-specific disease posits that the protein has a motor neuron-specific function that is essential to their survival. In cultured motor neurons, SMN appears within axons and axon terminals where it is known to interact with cytoskeletal regulators and mRNA-containing RNP granules, including axonal complexes containing the Sm-like proteins (LSm) [154, 195]. One unique aspect of motor neurons is their extraordinary length. In order to maintain proper synaptic function, mRNAs must be transported long distances to the presynaptic terminals. SMN may be involved in the assembly of RNP complexes that are crucial for this process, including ones containing hnRNPs Q and R, which bind mRNAs and may prevent decay during transport [196]. Cultures of primary motor neurons show multiple defects, including reduced outgrowth, shrunken growth cones, low levels of β-actin mRNA, and impaired calcium channel activity, while ex vivo electrophysiology reported reduced synaptic vesicle release [154, 181, 184]. SMN also interacts with many actin-binding proteins, including plastin 3 and profilin, and may be involved in regulating cytoskeletal dynamics at the distal axon, but this has not been directly demonstrated.

In summary, two main hypotheses have been proposed to link SMN deficiency to SMA disease pathogenesis. The first suggests that defects in snRNP assembly cause motor neurons to die, while the second posits that SMN has an alternate function specific to motor neurons that determines the specific vulnerability of these cells.

Therapeutics development

The development of SMA animal models has not only increased understanding of the cellular consequences of SMN protein deficiency, but has also allowed investigations of possible treatment strategies for SMA (see Figure 16.8). Given the inverse correlation

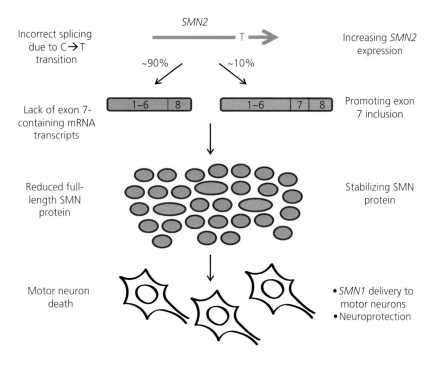

Figure 16.8 Therapeutic targets. Therapeutic strategies that could ameliorate SMA include increasing *SMN2* gene expression, promoting exon 7 inclusion into *SMN2*-derived transcripts, stabilizing the SMN protein, or replacing the *SMN1* gene.

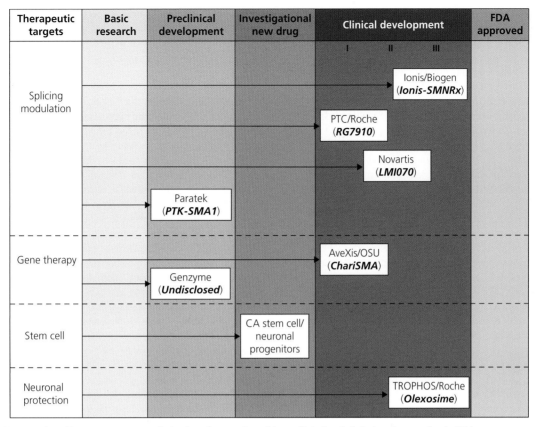

Figure 16.9 Drug pipeline. Therapeutic compounds that have been evaluated in preclinical and clinical settings as of early 2014.

between *SMN2* gene copy number and disease severity in human patients and animal models, increasing SMN expression has become a primary goal of SMA therapeutics development. Importantly, widespread genetic restoration of SMN expression in SMA mouse models can markedly ameliorate disease features if achieved early in the disease course [174, 176]. This provides extremely promising proof of principle that increased SMN expression will be effective in SMA patients. In recent years, the growing SMA therapeutics field has examined both repurposed drugs and newly developed compounds for their potential to increase SMN protein levels through a variety of mechanisms (see Figure 16.9). Some of these therapies have shown remarkable efficacy in preclinical animal models and have moved forward to clinical trials in SMA patients.

SMN2 gene activation

As all patients retain at least one copy of the *SMN2* gene, one pursued SMA treatment strategy has been to identify compounds that increase *SMN2* expression. Histone deacetylase (HDAC) inhibitors are known to modify gene expression by inhibiting the activity of HDAC enzymes. HDACs remove acetyl groups from histone proteins resulting in more compact chromatin structure and decreased transcription. HDAC inhibitors (HDACis) promote a more transcriptionally active form of chromatin. *SMN2* activation by HDAC inhibitors was first demonstrated with sodium butyrate, which improved survival in SMA-like mice when administered prenatally. It did not, however, advance to clinical trials due to its short half-life [197]. Subsequent HCDACis tested for *SMN2* activation include trichostatin A (TSA), suberoylanilide hydroxamic acid (SAHA), valproic acid (VPA), and phenylbutyrate [40, 198–202]. Median

survival in SMA mice that received TSA and SAHA was increased by 40% and 30%, respectively [40, 202]. Furthermore, postsymptomatic TSA delivery in mice resulted in phenotypic improvement with extended survival [40, 201]. VPA is an HDACi that is already in clinical use. It was shown to increase SMN levels in SMA mice and patient fibroblasts and this prompted several clinical trials of VPA in SMA patients [200, 203]. These studies noted improved muscle strength in some young patients, while others experienced no effect or further decline [204, 205]. Depleted carnitine levels were also reported in a significant number of patients, making carnitine supplementation a standard in future VPA trials [205]. A double-blind, placebo-controlled study in which non-ambulatory children received VPA with carnitine (CARNI-VAL) resulted in no significant difference between treated and untreated groups [206]. A follow-up study in ambulatory Type 3 children yielded similar results, suggesting that VPA treatment cannot improve muscle strength or function in SMA children [207]. Yet another study indicated improvements in motor abilities in Type 2, but not Type 3 patients, indicating that the viability of VPA as treatment still remains in question [208].

Phenylbutyrate (PB) is another HDACi in clinical use for other indications that has been investigated in clinical trials with SMA patients. Pilot trials that delivered PB orally reported increased SMN expression in leukocytes and improved strength and Hammersmith Functional Motor Scale (HFMS) scores [209, 210]. A randomized, placebo-controlled study, however, noted no improvement in HFMS scores [211].

Another *SMN2* activator is hydroxyurea, which is FDA approved for treating sickle cell disease. It was shown to increase full-length

SMN mRNA in a dose-dependent manner in SMA patient-derived cell lines [212, 213], possibly through a nitric oxide activator [214]. When tested in patients, one study reported a slight improvement in manual muscle testing scores, a finding that was contradicted by a placebo-controlled, double-blind study that reported no motor improvement in Type 2 and 3 patients [213, 215].

Initially discovered to up-regulate *SMN* promoter activity in a screening assay and later found to modestly increase SMN protein levels in patient-derived fibroblasts, quinazoline RG3039 advanced to Phase I clinical trials in 2012, but development of this compound is currently halted [216, 217]. Although mechanistic details are still being investigated, quinazolines are known to strongly inhibit DcpS, an enzyme that degrades the 5′ cap during mRNA decay [218, 219]. A recent study that tested one such compound in SMA mice showed an increase in survival and an improvement in motor behavior when delivered prior to motor neuron loss [220–222]. The signal transducer and activator of transcription 5 (STAT5) pathway has been implicated as a downstream target of several compounds that promote *SMN2* activity, with STAT5 knockdown corresponding to decreased SMN expression [223]. Prolactin activates the STAT5 pathway and a recombinant form of prolactin is FDA approved to stimulate lactation. Severe SMA mice injected with prolactin exhibited a 60% increase in median survival, suggesting possible therapeutic use [224].

Promoting exon 7 inclusion in SMN2-derived transcripts

The majority of SMN2 mRNA transcripts lack exon 7 as a result of alternative splicing and are translated into a truncated form of SMN protein that is rapidly degraded. Small molecules that target exon 7 inclusion through a variety of mechanisms are therefore being investigated for therapeutic potential. The first compound discovered to increase exon 7 inclusion was sodium vanadate [225]. Subsequently, albuterol (salbutamol), a β2 adrenoceptor agonist, was documented to increase SMN transcript levels in patient-derived cell lines [226]. Albuterol was also well tolerated in patients, indicating modest motor function improvement in Types 2 and 3 when administered orally for at least 6 months [227–229]. Aclarubicin also increased SMN protein levels *in vitro* via exon 7 inclusion, but cannot be tolerated for long-term use due to toxicity [230]. Other tetracycline derivatives that lack aclarubicin's prohibitive toxicity are therefore being investigated, including PTK-SMA1 (Figure 16.9). This synthetic small molecule was tested in a cell-free splicing assay and found to specifically stimulate exon 7 inclusion without altering the splicing patterns of other genes tested. Subsequent testing showed that SMN protein levels increased by approximately 40% in patient-derived fibroblasts and significantly in SMA mice after PTK-SMA1 treatment [231].

PTC Therapeutics together with Roche identified small molecules that promote exon 7 inclusion and have shown impressive efficacy in SMA mice [232]. Orally available and highly specific, these small molecules represent a major breakthrough in therapeutic development. These compounds have dose-dependently increased full-length SMN mRNA and protein in patient-derived cell lines with limited off-target effects. In addition, they have been shown to increase motor function and lifespan in two separate SMA mouse models, with similar efficacy observed for oral and intraperitoneal administration. A separate small molecule developed by Novartis has demonstrated similar efficacy as a highly specific splicing modifier of exon 7 and similarly promotes increased levels of full-length SMN mRNA and protein [233]. Both small molecules are in Phase II clinical trials [233].

Antisense oligonucleotides (ASOs) are chemically modified nucleic acids that bind to complementary sequences of mRNA. Specific ASOs have been shown to promote exon 7 inclusion through binding to, and inhibiting, exonic or intronic silencers. Of the SMN mRNA sequences targeted by ASOs, the most successful inhibition was achieved by targeting an intronic splicing silencer (ISS-N1) within the 5′ end of intron 7 [234–236]. Ionis Pharmaceuticals, partnering with Biogen Idec and in collaboration with the Krainer lab at CSHL, observed increased exon 7 inclusion in transfected cell lines, patient-derived fibroblasts, and a severe SMA mouse model treated with an ISS-N1 targeting ASO (recently denoted Ionis-SMNRx) [234, 236–239]. Subsequent research with Ionis-SMNRx demonstrated the importance of SMN restoration in peripheral tissues, with systemic injections resulting in a 25-fold increase in median survival and intracerebroventricular (ICV) injections resulting in only a twofold increase as compared to untreated SMA mice [239]. At a histological level, researchers observed marked improvements in motor neuron count, myofiber size, and NMJ integrity relative to heterozygous littermates [239]. Researchers hypothesize that elevated levels of liver-secreted, circulating Igf1 are a contributing factor to the greater efficacy observed in systemically treated SMA mice [239]. Further research is needed to determine whether the profound systemic rescue is specific to the particular SMA mouse model used or whether similar effects might be relevant to patients. Following a successful tolerability testing in cynomolgus monkeys, Ionis Pharmaceuticals/Biogen Idec reported that Ionis-SMNRx is well tolerated when administered intrathecally in Phase I (2013) and Phase II (2013) clinical trials (Figure 16.9) [240]. Phase III clinical trials to determine drug efficacy are nearly complete.

Several other ASOs of various chemistries have been studied in patient-derived cells and animal models. Studies in a mild mouse model demonstrated a 10-day median increase in survival with a reversal of tail and ear necrosis following ICV injection [237, 238]. In addition, trans-splicing and bifunctional RNAs processed into viral vectors have been investigated in animal models [241, 242].

SMN protein stabilization

Preventing SMN protein degradation is another strategy that has been pursued to increase SMN levels. Several compounds used to treat other human disorders were discovered to have SMN protein-stabilizing ability. Indoprofen is an anti-inflammatory drug that was shown to increase SMN protein levels, to modestly enhance gem numbers in SMA patient fibroblasts, and to extend survival in SMA mouse embryos [243]. Aminoglycosides, a class of antibiotics known to extend protein length by reading through stop codons, were also tested for the potential to stabilize the truncated SMN protein by extending its C-terminus. Indeed, patient-derived fibroblast cells treated with several different aminoglycosides displayed increased SMN protein levels and gem numbers [244, 245]. A novel aminoglycoside, TC007, was subsequently developed and noted to increase gem numbers in induced pluripotent stem cells (iPSCs) derived from SMA patients. When injected subcutaneously and intracerebroventricularly in mice, survival was more markedly increased with the latter method (approximately 30% vs 16%) [246]. Another study noted increased protein levels in patient fibroblasts and phenotypic improvements in mice following delivery of Geneticin [247]. Both indoprofen and aminoglycosides poorly penetrate the blood–brain barrier and therefore have limited use for treatment of humans with SMA.

Recent efforts have investigated the therapeutic potential behind SMN complex stabilization. The half-life of the SMNΔ7 protein is nearly twice as short as that of its full-length counterpart, perhaps due to a disruption in proper complex formation. Cyclic AMP-mediated activation of protein kinase A (PKA) appears to inhibit SMN degradation by promoting its uptake into the complex [10]. This degradation is mediated by the ubiquitin proteasome system, another cellular target for drug development. Patient fibroblast cells treated with the proteasome inhibitor MG132 exhibited a marked increase in SMN protein levels in two separate studies [10, 248]. SMN levels as well as motor function were also increased in mice injected intraperitoneally with bortezomib, an FDA-approved ubiquitin proteasome inhibitor. Delivering bortezomib intraperitoneally with the CNS-penetrant TSA resulted in a greater increase in median survival than TSA alone and bortezomib alone [249]. In spite of their promising effects on mice and in patient cells, aminoglycosides and proteasome inhibitors are not promising candidates for the treatment of human SMA patients because of their toxicity profiles.

Gene therapy

Gene therapy aims to treat SMA by delivery of a normal *SMN1* gene. An early study delivered *SMN1* packaged in a lentiviral vector (EAIV-SMN) intramuscularly at the second postnatal day, and mice showed a 20% increase in median survival [250]. Subsequently, self-complementary adeno-associated viral vector 9 (scAAV9) was shown to have particular tropism for motor neurons when injected intravascularly during the neonatal period [251]. SMA mice injected intravenously (IV) with a single dose of SMN-scAAV9 showed a remarkable increase in survival beyond 250 days when injected on day 1 or 2 after birth. Later injections corresponded to shorter increases in survival suggesting a short therapeutic window for treatment [252]. In a separate study, another group showed a 157-day median survival in SMA mice injected intracerebroventricularly with SMN-scAAV8 [253]. Other studies have also reported significantly extended survival, including an increase from 14 to 69 days and 27 to 199 days in mice that received IV scAAV9 injections [254, 255].

In subsequent research, cynomolgus macaques that received scAAV9-GFP intravenously shortly after birth showed robust reporter gene expression in dorsal root ganglia and motor neurons when sacrificed 25 days post injection [252]. Successful CNS penetrance and effective transduction in the SMA mouse model and non-human primates have motivated AveXis to start Phase I clinical trials at OSU to assess safety and tolerability in Type 1 SMA patients (Figure 16.9). Having had similar success with scAAV9, Genzyme is independently developing a gene therapy (Figure 16.9).

Stem cell therapy

Cell replacement in SMA became a possible route of treatment when embryonic stem (ES) cells were first successfully converted to motor neurons via neural stem cell intermediates. Motor neurons developed from ES cells after receiving appropriate inductive signals during differentiation and were able to innervate target muscles [256, 257]. When neural stem cells derived from pluripotent ES cells were injected intrathecally into SMA mice on the first postnatal day, they migrated to the spinal cord and expressed neuronal antigens. Increased survival, motor neuron numbers, and improved motor abilities were reported in treated mice [258]. The obstacle of producing highly pure human neuronal progenitor cells has recently been surmounted by using unique physical parameters, and injection into ALS and SMA animal models results in phenotypic improvement [259, 260].

Neuroprotection

One important target for effective neuroprotection may be glutamate reuptake, as prolonged presence of glutamate at the synapse can contribute to eventual motor neuron death. First discovered to increase glutamate reuptake and ameliorate the phenotype of ALS mice in a dose-dependent manner, the β-lactam antibiotic ceftriaxone was also found to modestly increase survival in SMA mice [261, 262]. Riluzole, another drug that mediates glutamate dynamics, is FDA approved for ALS treatment and is being investigated for similar use in SMA. Although the drug is toxic in neonatal SMA mice, older mice treated with riluzole from 21 days until death exhibited improved motor abilities [263]. A Phase I clinical trial indicated riluzole's safety in Type 1 patients [264]. Subsequent research revealed the drug's similar pharmacokinetics in both ALS and SMA patients [265, 266]. Clinical trials with gabapentin, another compound that inhibits glutamate action, resulted in no significant drug efficacy [267, 268].

Olesoxime, a cholesterol-like molecule, was discovered in a screen for compounds that rescued cultured rat motor neurons deprived of neurotrophic factors from death. Although its mechanism is not fully understood, olesoxime may inhibit the mitochondrial permeability transition pore's ability to activate the apoptotic pathway [269]. A double-blind, placebo-controlled, 2-year clinical trial finished enrolling non-ambulatory patients between 3 and 25 years of age [270, 271]. The study reported that olesoxime prevented motor function loss in Type 2 and Type 3 SMA patients when compared to a placebo-treated group [270, 271]. This drug is now being further developed by Roche.

Neurotrophic compounds are also being investigated for promoting motor neuron survival. One such compound, cardiotrophin-1 (CT-1), is a cytokine that is active during the embryonic period to promote the growth of selected motor neuron groups. In the context of therapeutics, the median survival of SMA mice was increased after even low doses of intramuscular adenoviral CT-1 injection [272].

Clinical trial development

As the field of SMA therapeutics development builds momentum, the question of how to assess drug efficacy most effectively in patients has become an increasingly urgent concern. Because the greatest degree of deterioration occurs shortly after symptom onset, many patients may be enrolled in clinical trials once the critical window for most successful intervention has passed. A future goal is to identify SMA presymptomatically through population-based genetic screening, and thereby test compounds before disease onset. In the meantime, however, efforts focus on identifying the most instructive outcome measures for current treatment methods.

Outcome measures

Eliminating bias is a key concern in clinical trials, requiring as tightly controlled a trial design as possible. Investigators can exert such control by choosing appropriate outcome measures that are consistent, easy to understand, and relatively comfortable for patients [273]. As previously discussed, Type 1 patients are especially weak, which poses a unique challenge in choosing valid and age-appropriate outcome measures. The Test of Strength in SMA, renamed as the Children Hospital of Pennsylvania Infant Test for Neuromuscular Disease, is a measure of observed and induced movement [273]. In addition, two tests for motor performance in infants and one specifically developed for infants with SMA have been deemed suitable for Type 1 children. The Alberta Infant Motor

Scale and Test of Motor Performance are recommended for children 0–18 months and under 4 months, respectively [274, 275]. The latter test has been used in a screening version specifically in the context of SMA, but has not been used in any published clinical trials [276].

Outcome measures of motor ability in Type 2 and 3 patients must account for the phenotypic variability seen among these patients. The Gross Motor Function Measure distinguishes between patients who are able to walk and those who sit and was previously used as a primary outcome measure in a hydroxyurea trial [210, 273]. The SMA-specific Hammersmith Functional Motor Scale, designed for non-ambulatory patients, accounts for changes due to surgery or illness and correlates with *SMN2* copy number [277–279]. Trials that tested phenylbutyrate and albuterol used an earlier version of this test, which was later modified and has been used in the 2010 L-carnitine and valproic acid study [206, 210, 211, 229]. The Spinal Muscular Atrophy Functional Rating Scale has been used in trials with adult patients testing gabapentin, and more recently valproic acid [279, 280]. Additional tests that have not yet been applied to trials include the Motor Function Measure, Quantitative Muscle Testing, Wee Functional Independence Measure, and Egen Klassification Scale [274]. Quantitative muscle ultrasound is an emerging technique that is minimally invasive and promising for future trials [281].

Gait assessments measured by observation have been used in other neuromuscular diseases and, although not yet widely implemented, may be appropriate for SMA studies. Both a 10-minute walk test and a time to ascend/descend stair test correlate with leg strength in SMA patients [282]. In addition, forced vital capacity has been commonly used as a secondary measurement for respiratory function in clinical trials, but is limited by its tendency to remain static over time [274].

In an effort to characterize disease burden on individuals and families, the Pediatric Quality of Life Inventory (PedsQL) has been tested and demonstrated validity and reliability in SMA [283–285]. Furthermore, several multisite groups, including the American Spinal Muscular Atrophy Randomized Trial (AmSMART), have been formed to further assess the effectiveness of outcome measures for strength, respiration, and motor function [284].

Biomarkers

SMA clinical trials have also been challenged by a lack of informative disease biomarkers that could provide further information about disease progression. Although circulating blood cell SMN mRNA and protein levels seem like obvious biomarkers, SMN expression in blood samples may not adequately characterize SMN expression in the CNS [285, 286]. In addition, targeting levels of SMN alone may fail to characterize disease features downstream of SMN expression [287]. Finally, measuring SMN mRNA and protein levels in patients' peripheral blood may be useful for characterizing changes within, but perhaps not between, individuals with SMA [223, 284–287]. This restriction highlights the need to identify a more easily measured biomarker whose levels correlate with those of restored SMN protein [287]. Researchers throughout the SMA community have collaborated in an effort to screen thousands of different blood plasma proteins to identify a reliable biomarker for SMA pathogenesis in a study denoted BforSMA [288]. In early 2013, the committee reported the identification of 13 different blood plasma proteins that paralleled SMA progression with regards to motor performance. Researchers noted that many of the potential markers were pleiotropic connective tissue, extracellular matrix, and growth factor pathway proteins [289]. Although this research is still very early in development, continued statistical analysis may elucidate an ideal protein for tracking disease progression and thus provide greater insight into the efficacy of various therapeutic efforts.

Concluding remarks

Although significant progress has been made in understanding SMA since the molecular basis was determined over 15 years ago, many important questions about disease pathophysiology and clinical care remain to be addressed. It remains unclear which molecular functions of the SMN protein are disrupted in disease. In addition, when and where these functions are required remain to be definitively established. These answers are crucial, as they will help to define a window of opportunity within which therapeutic compounds should be delivered to patients. In the next 5–10 years many promising treatments are likely to enter clinical trials, and may produce effective disease treatment.

Resources for physicians, researchers, patients, and families are readily available online at a number of websites. The SMA Foundation (http://www.smafoundation.org) provides funding for basic, translational, and clinical research and also includes useful information about these aspects of the field. Cure SMA (http://curesma.org/) is a non-profit organization that provides support to both research efforts and families, with an extensive website that gives an overview on all aspects of the disease. FightSMA (http://www.fightsma.org) is another non-profit organization that provides funding for research and useful information to families. The Muscular Dystrophy Association (http://www.mdausa.org/) is a health agency dedicated to curing all forms of neuromuscular disease by funding research efforts and also providing comprehensive healthcare and advocacy services.

References

1. Pearn, J., Incidence, prevalence, and gene frequency studies of chronic childhood spinal muscular atrophy. *J Med Genet*, 1978. 15(6): p. 409–13.
2. Ogino, S., R.B. Wilson, and B. Gold, New insights on the evolution of the SMN1 and SMN2 region: simulation and meta-analysis for allele and haplotype frequency calculations. *Eur J Hum Genet*, 2004. 12(12): p. 1015–23.
3. Lefebvre, S., et al., Identification and characterization of a spinal muscular atrophy-determining gene. *Cell*, 1995. 80(1): p. 155–65.
4. Wee, C.D., L. Kong, and C.J. Sumner, The genetics of spinal muscular atrophies. *Curr Opin Neurol*, 2010. 23(5): p. 450–8.
5. Darras, B.T., Non-5q spinal muscular atrophies: the alphanumeric soup thickens. *Neurology*, 2011. 77(4): p. 312–4.
6. Kaindl, A.M., et al., Spinal muscular atrophy with respiratory distress type 1 (SMARD1). *J Child Neurol*, 2008. 23(2): p. 199–204.
7. Grohmann, K., et al., Mutations in the gene encoding immunoglobulin mu-binding protein 2 cause spinal muscular atrophy with respiratory distress type 1. *Nat Genet*, 2001. 29(1): p. 75–7.
8. Monani, U.R., et al., A single nucleotide difference that alters splicing patterns distinguishes the SMA gene SMN1 from the copy gene SMN2. *Hum Mol Genet*, 1999. 8(7): p. 1177–83.
9. Lorson, C.L., et al., A single nucleotide in the SMN gene regulates splicing and is responsible for spinal muscular atrophy. *Proc Natl Acad Sci U S A*, 1999. 96(11): p. 6307–11.
10. Burnett, B.G., et al., Regulation of SMN protein stability. *Mol Cell Biol*, 2009. 29(5): p. 1107–15.
11. Lorson, C.L., et al., SMN oligomerization defect correlates with spinal muscular atrophy severity. *Nat Genet*, 1998. 19(1): p. 63–6.
12. Taylor, J.E., et al., Correlation of SMNt and SMNc gene copy number with age of onset and survival in spinal muscular atrophy. *Eur J Hum Genet*, 1998. 6(5): p. 467–74.

13. Cusco, I., et al., SMN2 copy number predicts acute or chronic spinal muscular atrophy but does not account for intrafamilial variability in siblings. *J Neurol*, 2006. 253(1): p. 21–5.

14. Feldkotter, M., et al., Quantitative analyses of SMN1 and SMN2 based on real-time lightCycler PCR: fast and highly reliable carrier testing and prediction of severity of spinal muscular atrophy. *Am J Hum Genet*, 2002. 70(2): p. 358–68.

15. Mailman, M.D., et al., Molecular analysis of spinal muscular atrophy and modification of the phenotype by SMN2. *Genet Med*, 2002. 4(1): p. 20–6.

16. Arkblad, E., et al., A population-based study of genotypic and phenotypic variability in children with spinal muscular atrophy. *Acta Paediatr*, 2009. 98(5): p. 865–72.

17. Lefebvre, S., et al., Correlation between severity and SMN protein level in spinal muscular atrophy. *Nat Genet*, 1997. 16(3): p. 265–9.

18. Lorson, C.L. and E.J. Androphy, An exonic enhancer is required for inclusion of an essential exon in the SMA-determining gene SMN. *Hum Mol Genet*, 2000. 9(2): p. 259–65.

19. Mostacciuolo, M.L., et al., Epidemiology of spinal muscular atrophies in a sample of the Italian population. *Neuroepidemiology*, 1992. 11(1): p. 34–8.

20. Ogino, S., et al., Genetic risk assessment in carrier testing for spinal muscular atrophy. *Am J Med Genet*, 2002. 110(4): p. 301–7.

21. Schrank, B., et al., Inactivation of the survival motor neuron gene, a candidate gene for human spinal muscular atrophy, leads to massive cell death in early mouse embryos. *Proc Natl Acad Sci U S A*, 1997. 94(18): p. 9920–5.

22. Ge, X., et al., The natural history of infant spinal muscular atrophy in China: a study of 237 patients. *J Child Neurol*, 2012. 27(4): p. 471–7.

23. Zaldivar, T., et al., Evidence of reduced frequency of spinal muscular atrophy type I in the Cuban population. *Neurology*, 2005. 65(4): p. 636–8.

24. Sugarman, E.A., et al., Pan-ethnic carrier screening and prenatal diagnosis for spinal muscular atrophy: clinical laboratory analysis of >72,400 specimens. *Eur J Hum Genet*, 2012. 20(1): p. 27–32.

25. Wirth, B., et al., De novo rearrangements found in 2% of index patients with spinal muscular atrophy: mutational mechanisms, parental origin, mutation rate, and implications for genetic counseling. *Am J Hum Genet*, 1997. 61(5): p. 1102–11.

26. Werdnig, G., Zwei fruhinfantile hereditare falle von progressive Muskelatrophie unter dem Bilde der Dystrophy, aber auch neurotischer Grundlage. *Arch Psychiatr Nervenkr Z Gesamte Neurol Psychiatr*, 1891. 22: p. 437.

27. Werdnig, G., Die fruhinfantile progressive spinale Amyotrophie. *Arch Psychiatr Nervenkr Z Gesamte Neurol Psychiatr*, 1894. 26: p. 706.

28. Hoffmann, J., Ueber chronische spinale Muskelatrophie im Kindesalter auf familiarer Basis. *Dtsch Z Nervenheilkd*, 1893. 3: p. 427.

29. Wang, C.H., et al., Consensus statement for standard of care in spinal muscular atrophy. *J Child Neurol*, 2007. 22(8): p. 1027–49.

30. Markowitz, J.A., P. Singh, and B.T. Darras, Spinal muscular atrophy: a clinical and research update. *Pediatr Neurol*, 2012. 46(1): p. 1–12.

31. Volpe, J.J. *Neurology of the Newborn*. Philadelphia: Saunders/Elsevier, 2008.

32. Oskoui, M., et al., The changing natural history of spinal muscular atrophy type 1. *Neurology*, 2007. 69(20): p. 1931–6.

33. Araujo Ade, Q., M. Araujo, and K.J. Swoboda, Vascular perfusion abnormalities in infants with spinal muscular atrophy. *J Pediatr*, 2009. 155(2): p. 292–4.

34. Rudnik-Schoneborn, S., et al., Digital necroses and vascular thrombosis in severe spinal muscular atrophy. *Muscle Nerve*, 2010. 42(1): p. 144–7.

35. Arai, H., et al., Finger cold-induced vasodilatation, sympathetic skin response, and R-R interval variation in patients with progressive spinal muscular atrophy. *J Child Neurol*, 2005. 20(11): p. 871–5.

36. Menke, L.A., et al., Congenital heart defects in spinal muscular atrophy type I: a clinical report of two siblings and a review of the literature. *Am J Med Genet A*, 2008. 146A(6): p. 740–4.

37. Rudnik-Schoneborn, S., et al., Congenital heart disease is a feature of severe infantile spinal muscular atrophy. *J Med Genet*, 2008. 45(10): p. 635–8.

38. Crawford, T.O., et al., Abnormal fatty acid metabolism in childhood spinal muscular atrophy. *Ann Neurol*, 1999. 45(3): p. 337–43.

39. Shababi, M., et al., Cardiac defects contribute to the pathology of spinal muscular atrophy models. *Hum Mol Genet*, 2010. 19(20): p. 4059–71.

40. Narver, H.L., et al., Sustained improvement of spinal muscular atrophy mice treated with trichostatin A plus nutrition. *Ann Neurol*, 2008. 64(4): p. 465–70.

41. Zerres, K., et al., A collaborative study on the natural history of childhood and juvenile onset proximal spinal muscular atrophy (type II and III SMA): 569 patients. *J Neurol Sci*, 1997. 146(1): p. 67–72.

42. von Gontard, A., et al., Intelligence and cognitive function in children and adolescents with spinal muscular atrophy. *Neuromuscul Disord*, 2002. 12(2): p. 130–6.

43. Thomas, N.H. and V. Dubowitz, The natural history of type I (severe) spinal muscular atrophy. *Neuromuscul Disord*, 1994. 4(5-6): p. 497–502.

44. Ignatius, J., The natural history of severe spinal muscular atrophy—further evidence for clinical subtypes. *Neuromuscul Disord*, 1994. 4(5-6): p. 527–8.

45. Iannaccone, S.T., et al., Prospective analysis of strength in spinal muscular atrophy. DCN/Spinal Muscular Atrophy Group. *J Child Neurol*, 2000. 15(2): p. 97–101.

46. Volpe, J.J., Neurology of the newborn. *Major Probl Clin Pediatr*, 1981. 22: p. 1–648.

47. Crawford, T.O. and C.A. Pardo, The neurobiology of childhood spinal muscular atrophy. *Neurobiol Dis*, 1996. 3(2): p. 97–110.

48. Simic, G., et al., Ultrastructural analysis and TUNEL demonstrate motor neuron apoptosis in Werdnig-Hoffmann disease. *J Neuropathol Exp Neurol*, 2000. 59(5): p. 398–407.

49. Lippa, C.F. and T.W. Smith, Chromatolytic neurons in Werdnig-Hoffmann disease contain phosphorylated neurofilaments. *Acta Neuropathol*, 1988. 77(1): p. 91–4.

50. Murayama, S., T.W. Bouldin, and K. Suzuki, Immunocytochemical and ultrastructural studies of Werdnig-Hoffmann disease. *Acta Neuropathol*, 1991. 81(4): p. 408–17.

51. Simic, G., et al., Abnormal motoneuron migration, differentiation, and axon outgrowth in spinal muscular atrophy. *Acta Neuropathol*, 2008. 115(3): p. 313–26.

52. Forger, N.G. and S.M. Breedlove, Motoneuronal death during human fetal development. *J Comp Neurol*, 1987. 264(1): p. 118–22.

53. Soler-Botija, C., et al., Neuronal death is enhanced and begins during foetal development in type I spinal muscular atrophy spinal cord. *Brain*, 2002. 125(Pt 7): p. 1624–34.

54. Ghatak, N.R., Spinal roots in Werdnig-Hoffmann disease. *Acta Neuropathol*, 1978. 41(1): p. 1–7.

55. Chou, S.M. and A.V. Fakadej, Ultrastructure of chromatolytic motoneurons and anterior spinal roots in a case of Werdnig-Hoffmann disease. *J Neuropathol Exp Neurol*, 1971. 30(3): p. 368–79.

56. Iwata, M. and A. Hirano, "Glial bundles" in the spinal cord late after paralytic anterior poliomyelitis. *Ann Neurol*, 1978. 4(6): p. 562–3.

57. Towfighi, J., R.S. Young, and R.M. Ward, Is Werdnig-Hoffmann disease a pure lower motor neuron disorder? *Acta Neuropathol*, 1985. 65(3-4): p. 270–80.

58. Rudnik-Schoneborn, S., et al., Classical infantile spinal muscular atrophy with SMN deficiency causes sensory neuronopathy. *Neurology*, 2003. 60(6): p. 983–7.

59. Martinez-Hernandez, R., et al., The developmental pattern of myotubes in spinal muscular atrophy indicates prenatal delay of muscle maturation. *J Neuropathol Exp Neurol*, 2009. 68(5): p. 474–81.

60. Fitzsimons, R.B. and J.F. Hoh, Embryonic and foetal myosins in human skeletal muscle. The presence of foetal myosins in duchenne muscular dystrophy and infantile spinal muscular atrophy. *J Neurol Sci*, 1981. 52(2-3): p. 367–84.

61. Mastaglia, F.L. and J.N. Walton, An electron microscopic study of skeletal muscle from cases of the Kugelberg-Welander syndrome. *Acta Neuropathol*, 1971. 17(3): p. 201–19.

62. Eng, G.D., H. Binder, and B. Koch, Spinal muscular atrophy: experience in diagnosis and rehabilitation management of 60 patients. *Arch Phys Med Rehabil*, 1984. 65(9): p. 549–53.

63. Dorsher, P.T., et al., Wohlfart-Kugelberg-Welander syndrome: serum creatine kinase and functional outcome. *Arch Phys Med Rehabil*, 1991. 72(8): p. 587–91.

64. Russell, J.W., A.K. Afifi, and M.A. Ross, Predictive value of electromyography in diagnosis and prognosis of the hypotonic infant. *J Child Neurol*, 1992. 7(4): p. 387–91.

65. Hausmanowa-Petrusewicz, I., et al., Is Kugelberg-Welander spinal muscular atrophy a fetal defect? *Muscle Nerve*, 1980. 3(5): p. 389–402.

66. Packer, R.J., M.J. Brown, and P.H. Berman, The diagnostic value of electromyography in infantile hypotonia. *Am J Dis Child*, 1982. 136(12): p. 1057–9.

67. Hausmanowa-Petrusewicz, I. and A. Karwanska, Electromyographic findings in different forms of infantile and juvenile proximal spinal muscular atrophy. *Muscle Nerve*, 1986. 9(1): p. 37–46.

68. Buchthal, F. and P.Z. Olsen, Electromyography and muscle biopsy in infantile spinal muscular atrophy. *Brain*, 1970. 93(1): p. 15–30.

69. Zalneraitis, E.L., et al., Muscle biopsy and the clinical course of infantile spinal muscular atrophy. *J Child Neurol*, 1991. 6(4): p. 324–8.

70. Han, J.J. and C.M. McDonald, Diagnosis and clinical management of spinal muscular atrophy. *Phys Med Rehabil Clin N Am*, 2008. 19(3): p. 661–80, xii.

71. Prior, T.W., et al., Technical standards and guidelines for spinal muscular atrophy testing. *Genet Med*, 2011. 13(7): p. 686–94.

72. Prior, T.W., et al., Newborn and carrier screening for spinal muscular atrophy. *Am J Med Genet A*, 2010. 152A(7): p. 1608–16.

73. Ogino, S., et al., Inverse correlation between SMN1 and SMN2 copy numbers: evidence for gene conversion from SMN2 to SMN1. *Eur J Hum Genet*, 2003. 11(9): p. 723.

74. Swoboda, K.J., Seize the day: Newborn screening for SMA. *Am J Med Genet A*, 2010. 152A(7): p. 1605–7.

75. Swoboda, K.J., et al., Natural history of denervation in SMA: relation to age, SMN2 copy number, and function. *Ann Neurol*, 2005. 57(5): p. 704–12.

76. Prior, T.W., for the Professional Practice and Guidelines Committee, Carrier screening for spinal muscular atrophy. *Genet Med*, 2008. 10(11): p. 840–2.

77. Prior, T. W. Spinal muscular atrophy: newborn and carrier screening. *Obstet Gynecol Clin North Am*, 2010. 37(1): p. 23–36.

78. Su, Y.N., et al., Carrier screening for spinal muscular atrophy (SMA) in 107,611 pregnant women during the period 2005-2009: a prospective population-based cohort study. *PLoS One*, 2011. 6(2): p. e17067.

79. Pyatt, R.E., D.C. Mihal, and T.W. Prior, Assessment of liquid microbead arrays for the screening of newborns for spinal muscular atrophy. *Clin Chem*, 2007. 53(11): p. 1879–85.

80. Families of Spinal Muscular Atrophy. Breathing Basics: Respiratory Care for Children with Spinal Muscular Atrophy. http://www.fsma.org.hk/popup/fsma_caring_brochure.pdf (accessed 04 October 2016).

81. Schroth, M.K., Special considerations in the respiratory management of spinal muscular atrophy. *Pediatrics*, 2009. 123 Suppl 4: p. S245–9.

82. Bach, J.R., The use of mechanical ventilation is appropriate in children with genetically proven spinal muscular atrophy type 1: the motion for. *Paediatr Respir Rev*, 2008. 9(1): p. 45–50; quiz 50; discussion 55-6.

83. Mehta, S. and N.S. Hill, Noninvasive ventilation. *Am J Respir Crit Care Med*, 2001. 163(2): p. 540–77.

84. Bach, J.R. and C. Bianchi, Prevention of pectus excavatum for children with spinal muscular atrophy type 1. *Am J Phys Med Rehabil*, 2003. 82(10): p. 815–9.

85. Mellies, U., et al., Sleep disordered breathing in spinal muscular atrophy. *Neuromuscul Disord*, 2004. 14(12): p. 797–803.

86. Markstrom, A., G. Cohen, and M. Katz-Salamon, The effect of long term ventilatory support on hemodynamics in children with spinal muscle atrophy (SMA) type II. *Sleep Med*, 2010. 11(2): p. 201–4.

87. Schroth, M. Respiratory Care of SMA and Choices. http://www.fsma.org.hk/popup/fsma_caring_brochure.pdf (accessed 04 October 2016).

88. Bach, J.R., et al., Spinal muscular atrophy type 1: management and outcomes. *Pediatr Pulmonol*, 2002. 34(1): p. 16–22.

89. Granger, M.W., et al., Masticatory muscle function in patients with spinal muscular atrophy. *Am J Orthod Dentofacial Orthop*, 1999. 115(6): p. 697–702.

90. Houston, K., et al., Craniofacial morphology of spinal muscular atrophy. *Pediatr Res*, 1994. 36(2): p. 265–9.

91. Willig, T.N., et al., Swallowing problems in neuromuscular disorders. *Arch Phys Med Rehabil*, 1994. 75(11): p. 1175–81.

92. Chang, Y.C., et al., A 2-year follow-up of swallowing function after radiation therapy in patients with nasopharyngeal carcinoma. *Arch Phys Med Rehabil*, 2011. 92(11): p. 1814–9.

93. Messina, S., et al., Feeding problems and malnutrition in spinal muscular atrophy type II. *Neuromuscul Disord*, 2008. 18(5): p. 389–93.

94. Families of Spinal Muscular Atrophy. Nutrition basics: fostering health and growth for spinal muscular atrophy. http://www.curesma.org/documents/support//care-documents/nutrition-basics.pdf (accessed 04 October 2016).

95. Sproule, D.M., et al., Adiposity is increased among high-functioning, non-ambulatory patients with spinal muscular atrophy. *Neuromuscul Disord*, 2010. 20(7): p. 448–52.

96. Yuan, N., et al., Laparoscopic Nissen fundoplication during gastrostomy tube placement and noninvasive ventilation may improve survival in type I and severe type II spinal muscular atrophy. *J Child Neurol*, 2007. 22(6): p. 727–31.

97. Durkin, E.T., et al., Early laparoscopic fundoplication and gastrostomy in infants with spinal muscular atrophy type I. *J Pediatr Surg*, 2008. 43(11): p. 2031–7.

98. Granata, C., et al., Spinal muscular atrophy: natural history and orthopaedic treatment of scoliosis. *Spine (Phila Pa 1976)*, 1989. 14(7): p. 760–2.

99. Evans, G.A., J.C. Drennan, and B.S. Russman, Functional classification and orthopaedic management of spinal muscular atrophy. *J Bone Joint Surg Br*, 1981. 63B(4): p. 516–22.

100. Schwentker, E.P. and D.A. Gibson, The orthopaedic aspects of spinal muscular atrophy. *J Bone Joint Surg Am*, 1976. 58(1): p. 32–8.

101. Merlini, L., et al., Scoliosis in spinal muscular atrophy: natural history and management. *Dev Med Child Neurol*, 1989. 31(4): p. 501–8.

102. Brown, J.C., et al., Surgical and functional results of spine fusion in spinal muscular atrophy. *Spine (Phila Pa 1976)*, 1989. 14(7): p. 763–70.

103. Furumasu, J., et al., Functional activities in spinal muscular atrophy patients after spinal fusion. *Spine (Phila Pa 1976)*, 1989. 14(7): p. 771–5.

104. Aprin, H., et al., Spine fusion in patients with spinal muscular atrophy. *J Bone Joint Surg Am*, 1982. 64(8): p. 1179–87.

105. Akbarnia, B.A., et al., Dual growing rod technique for the treatment of progressive early-onset scoliosis: a multicenter study. *Spine (Phila Pa 1976)*, 2005. 30(17 Suppl): p. S46–57.

106. Thompson, G.H., et al., Comparison of single and dual growing rod techniques followed through definitive surgery: a preliminary study. *Spine (Phila Pa 1976)*, 2005. 30(18): p. 2039–44.

107. Akbarnia, B.A., et al., Dual growing rod technique followed for three to eleven years until final fusion: the effect of frequency of lengthening. *Spine (Phila Pa 1976)*, 2008. 33(9): p. 984–90.

108. McElroy, M.J., et al., Growing rods for scoliosis in spinal muscular atrophy: structural effects, complications, and hospital stays. *Spine (Phila Pa 1976)*, 2011. 36(16): p. 1305–11.

109. Granata, C., et al., Spine surgery in spinal muscular atrophy: long-term results. *Neuromuscul Disord*, 1993. 3(3): p. 207–15.

110. Granata, C., et al., Hip dislocation in spinal muscular atrophy. *Chir Organi Mov*, 1990. 75(2): p. 177–84.

111. Sporer, S.M. and B.G. Smith, Hip dislocation in patients with spinal muscular atrophy. *J Pediatr Orthop*, 2003. 23(1): p. 10–4.

112. Carter, G.T., et al., Profiles of neuromuscular diseases. Hereditary motor and sensory neuropathy, types I and II. *Am J Phys Med Rehabil*, 1995. 74(5 Suppl): p. S140–9.

113. Willig, T.N., et al., Correlation of flexion contractures with upper extremity function and pain for spinal muscular atrophy and congenital myopathy patients. *Am J Phys Med Rehabil*, 1995. 74(1): p. 33–8.

114. Khatri, I.A., et al., Low bone mineral density in spinal muscular atrophy. *J Clin Neuromuscul Dis*, 2008. 10(1): p. 11–7.

115. Garcia-Cabezas, M.A., et al., Neonatal spinal muscular atrophy with multiple contractures, bone fractures, respiratory insufficiency and 5q13 deletion. *Acta Neuropathol*, 2004. 107(5): p. 475–8.

116. Kinali, M., et al., Bone mineral density in a paediatric spinal muscular atrophy population. *Neuropediatrics*, 2004. 35(6): p. 325–8.

117. Kurihara, N., et al., Osteoclast-stimulating factor interacts with the spinal muscular atrophy gene product to stimulate osteoclast formation. *J Biol Chem*, 2001. 276(44): p. 41035–9.

118. Brzustowicz, L.M., et al., Genetic mapping of chronic childhood-onset spinal muscular atrophy to chromosome 5q11.2-13.3. *Nature*, 1990. 344(6266): p. 540–1.

119. Melki, J., et al., Mapping of acute (type I) spinal muscular atrophy to chromosome 5q12-q14. The French Spinal Muscular Atrophy Investigators. *Lancet*, 1990. 336(8710): p. 271–3.

120. Setola, V., et al., Axonal-SMN (a-SMN), a protein isoform of the survival motor neuron gene, is specifically involved in axonogenesis. *Proc Natl Acad Sci U S A*, 2007. 104(6): p. 1959–64.

121. Gavrilov, D.K., et al., Differential SMN2 expression associated with SMA severity. *Nat Genet*, 1998. 20(3): p. 230–1.

122. Cartegni, L. and A.R. Krainer, Disruption of an SF2/ASF-dependent exonic splicing enhancer in SMN2 causes spinal muscular atrophy in the absence of SMN1. *Nat Genet*, 2002. 30(4): p. 377–84.

123. Kashima, T., et al., hnRNP A1 functions with specificity in repression of SMN2 exon 7 splicing. *Hum Mol Genet*, 2007. 16(24): p. 3149–59.

124. Kashima, T. and J.L. Manley, A negative element in SMN2 exon 7 inhibits splicing in spinal muscular atrophy. *Nat Genet*, 2003. 34(4): p. 460–3.

125. Kashima, T., N. Rao, and J.L. Manley, An intronic element contributes to splicing repression in spinal muscular atrophy. *Proc Natl Acad Sci U S A*, 2007. 104(9): p. 3426–31.

126. Hofmann, Y., et al., Htra2-beta 1 stimulates an exonic splicing enhancer and can restore full-length SMN expression to survival motor neuron 2 (SMN2). *Proc Natl Acad Sci U S A*, 2000. 97(17): p. 9618–23.

127. Hofmann, Y. and B. Wirth, hnRNP-G promotes exon 7 inclusion of survival motor neuron (SMN) via direct interaction with Htra2-beta1. *Hum Mol Genet*, 2002. 11(17): p. 2037–49.

128. Echaniz-Laguna, A., et al., The promoters of the survival motor neuron gene (SMN) and its copy (SMNc) share common regulatory elements. *Am J Hum Genet*, 1999. 64(5): p. 1365–70.

129. Monani, U.R., J.D. McPherson, and A.H. Burghes, Promoter analysis of the human centromeric and telomeric survival motor neuron genes (SMNC and SMNT). *Biochim Biophys Acta*, 1999. 1445(3): p. 330–6.

130. Rouget, R., et al., Characterization of the survival motor neuron (SMN) promoter provides evidence for complex combinatorial regulation in undifferentiated and differentiated P19 cells. *Biochem J*, 2005. 385(Pt 2): p. 433–43.

131. Germain-Desprez, D., et al., The SMN genes are subject to transcriptional regulation during cellular differentiation. *Gene*, 2001. 279(2): p. 109–17.

132. Majumder, S., et al., Identification of a novel cyclic AMP-response element (CRE-II) and the role of CREB-1 in the cAMP-induced expression of the survival motor neuron (SMN) gene. *J Biol Chem*, 2004. 279(15): p. 14803–11.

133. Baron-Delage, S., et al., Interferons and IRF-1 induce expression of the survival motor neuron (SMN) genes. *Mol Med*, 2000. 6(11): p. 957–68.

134. Kernochan, L.E., et al., The role of histone acetylation in SMN gene expression. *Hum Mol Genet*, 2005. 14(9): p. 1171–82.

135. Evans, M.C., J.J. Cherry, and E.J. Androphy, Differential regulation of the SMN2 gene by individual HDAC proteins. *Biochem Biophys Res Commun*, 2011. 414(1): p. 25–30.

136. Petit, F., et al., Insights into genotype-phenotype correlations in spinal muscular atrophy: a retrospective study of 103 patients. *Muscle Nerve*, 2011. 43(1): p. 26–30.

137. Rudnik-Schoneborn, S., et al., Genotype-phenotype studies in infantile spinal muscular atrophy (SMA) type I in Germany: implications for clinical trials and genetic counselling. *Clin Genet*, 2009. 76(2): p. 168–78.

138. Oprea, G.E., et al., Plastin 3 is a protective modifier of autosomal recessive spinal muscular atrophy. *Science*, 2008. 320(5875): p. 524–7.

139. Stratigopoulos, G., et al., Association of plastin 3 expression with disease severity in spinal muscular atrophy only in postpubertal females. *Arch Neurol*, 2010. 67(10): p. 1252–6.

140. Prior, T.W., et al., A positive modifier of spinal muscular atrophy in the SMN2 gene. *Am J Hum Genet*, 2009. 85(3): p. 408–13.

141. Battaglia, G., et al., Expression of the SMN gene, the spinal muscular atrophy determining gene, in the mammalian central nervous system. *Hum Mol Genet*, 1997. 6(11): p. 1961–71.

142. Coovert, D.D., et al., The survival motor neuron protein in spinal muscular atrophy. *Hum Mol Genet*, 1997. 6(8): p. 1205–14.

143. Liu, Q. and G. Dreyfuss, A novel nuclear structure containing the survival of motor neurons protein. *EMBO J*, 1996. 15(14): p. 3555–65.

144. Patrizi, A.L., et al., SMN protein analysis in fibroblast, amniocyte and CVS cultures from spinal muscular atrophy patients and its relevance for diagnosis. *Eur J Hum Genet*, 1999. 7(3): p. 301–9.

145. Burghes, A.H. and C.E. Beattie, Spinal muscular atrophy: why do low levels of survival motor neuron protein make motor neurons sick? *Nat Rev Neurosci*, 2009. 10(8): p. 597–609.

146. Yong, J., L. Wan, and G. Dreyfuss, Why do cells need an assembly machine for RNA-protein complexes? *Trends Cell Biol*, 2004. 14(5): p. 226–32.

147. Grimmler, M., et al., Unrip, a factor implicated in cap-independent translation, associates with the cytosolic SMN complex and influences its intracellular localization. *Hum Mol Genet*, 2005. 14(20): p. 3099–111.

148. Yong, J., et al., Gemin5 delivers snRNA precursors to the SMN complex for snRNP biogenesis. *Mol Cell*, 2010. 38(4): p. 551–62.

149. Zhang, R., et al., Structure of a key intermediate of the SMN complex reveals Gemin2's crucial function in snRNP assembly. *Cell*, 2011. 146(3): p. 384–95.

150. Chari, A., et al., An assembly chaperone collaborates with the SMN complex to generate spliceosomal SnRNPs. *Cell*, 2008. 135(3): p. 497–509.

151. Rossoll, W. and G.J. Bassell, Spinal muscular atrophy and a model for survival of motor neuron protein function in axonal ribonucleoprotein complexes. *Results Probl Cell Differ*, 2009. 48: p. 289–326.

152. Shan, X., et al., Altered distributions of Gemini of coiled bodies and mitochondria in motor neurons of TDP-43 transgenic mice. *Proc Natl Acad Sci U S A*, 2010. 107(37): p. 16325–30.

153. Yamazaki, T., et al., FUS-SMN protein interactions link the motor neuron diseases ALS and SMA. *Cell Rep* 2012. 2(4): p. 799–806.

154. Rossoll, W., et al., Smn, the spinal muscular atrophy-determining gene product, modulates axon growth and localization of beta-actin mRNA in growth cones of motoneurons. *J Cell Biol*, 2003. 163(4): p. 801–12.

155. Giesemann, T., et al., A role for polyproline motifs in the spinal muscular atrophy protein SMN. Profilins bind to and colocalize with smn in nuclear gems. *J Biol Chem*, 1999. 274(53): p. 37908–14.

156. Fallini, C., et al., The survival of motor neuron (SMN) protein interacts with the mRNA-binding protein HuD and regulates localization of poly(A) mRNA in primary motor neuron axons. *J Neurosci*, 2011. 31(10): p. 3914–25.

157. Akten, B., et al., Interaction of survival of motor neuron (SMN) and HuD proteins with mRNA cpg15 rescues motor neuron axonal deficits. *Proc Natl Acad Sci U S A*, 2011. 108(25): p. 10337–42.

158. Sun, Y., et al., Molecular and functional analysis of intragenic SMN1 mutations in patients with spinal muscular atrophy. *Hum Mutat*, 2005. 25(1): p. 64–71.

159. Shpargel, K.B. and A.G. Matera, Gemin proteins are required for efficient assembly of Sm-class ribonucleoproteins. *Proc Natl Acad Sci U S A*, 2005. 102(48): p. 17372–7.

160. Le, T.T., et al., SMNDelta7, the major product of the centromeric survival motor neuron (SMN2) gene, extends survival in mice with spinal muscular atrophy and associates with full-length SMN. *Hum Mol Genet*, 2005. 14(6): p. 845–57.

161. Monani, U.R., et al., A transgene carrying an A2G missense mutation in the SMN gene modulates phenotypic severity in mice with severe (type I) spinal muscular atrophy. *J Cell Biol*, 2003. 160(1): p. 41–52.

162. Chan, Y.B., et al., Neuromuscular defects in a Drosophila survival motor neuron gene mutant. *Hum Mol Genet*, 2003. 12(12): p. 1367–76.

163. Rajendra, T.K., et al., A Drosophila melanogaster model of spinal muscular atrophy reveals a function for SMN in striated muscle. *J Cell Biol*, 2007. 176(6): p. 831–41.

164. Chang, H.C., et al., Modeling spinal muscular atrophy in Drosophila. *PLoS One*, 2008. 3(9): p. e3209.

165. Roselli, F., and P. Caroni. A circuit mechanism for neurodegeneration. *Cell* 2012. 151(2): 250–52.

166. McWhorter, M.L., et al., Knockdown of the survival motor neuron (Smn) protein in zebrafish causes defects in motor axon outgrowth and pathfinding. *J Cell Biol*, 2003. 162(5): p. 919–31.

167. Boon, K.L., et al., Zebrafish survival motor neuron mutants exhibit presynaptic neuromuscular junction defects. *Hum Mol Genet*, 2009. 18(19): p. 3615–25.

168. Hao le, T., A.H. Burghes, and C.E. Beattie, Generation and characterization of a genetic zebrafish model of SMA carrying the human SMN2 gene. *Mol Neurodegener*, 2011. 6(1): p. 24.

169. Sleigh, J.N., T.H. Gillingwater, and K. Talbot, The contribution of mouse models to understanding the pathogenesis of spinal muscular atrophy. *Dis Model Mech*, 2011. 4(4): p. 457–67.

170. Frugier, T., et al., Nuclear targeting defect of SMN lacking the C-terminus in a mouse model of spinal muscular atrophy. *Hum Mol Genet*, 2000. 9(5): p. 849–58.

171. Cifuentes-Diaz, C., et al., Neurofilament accumulation at the motor endplate and lack of axonal sprouting in a spinal muscular atrophy mouse model. *Hum Mol Genet*, 2002. 11(12): p. 1439–47.

172. Cifuentes-Diaz, C., et al., Deletion of murine SMN exon 7 directed to skeletal muscle leads to severe muscular dystrophy. *J Cell Biol*, 2001. 152(5): p. 1107–14.

173. Park, G.H., et al., Reduced survival of motor neuron (SMN) protein in motor neuronal progenitors functions cell autonomously to cause spinal muscular atrophy in model mice expressing the human centromeric (SMN2) gene. *J Neurosci*, 2010. 30(36): p. 12005–19.

174. Lutz, C.M., et al., Postsymptomatic restoration of SMN rescues the disease phenotype in a mouse model of severe spinal muscular atrophy. *J Clin Invest*, 2011. 121(8): p. 3029–41.

175. Hsieh-Li, H.M., et al., A mouse model for spinal muscular atrophy. *Nat Genet*, 2000. 24(1): p. 66–70.

176. Monani, U.R., et al., The human centromeric survival motor neuron gene (SMN2) rescues embryonic lethality in Smn(-/-) mice and results in a mouse with spinal muscular atrophy. *Hum Mol Genet*, 2000. 9(3): p. 333–9.

177. Monani, U.R., et al., A transgene carrying an A2G missense mutation in the SMN gene modulates phenotypic severity in mice with severe (type I) spinal muscular atrophy. *J Cell Biol*, 2003. 160(1): p. 41–52.

178. Bowerman, M., et al., A critical Smn threshold in mice dictates onset of an intermediate spinal muscular atrophy phenotype associated with a distinct neuromuscular junction pathology. *Neuromuscul Disord*, 2012. 22(3): p. 263–76.

179. Gladman, J.T., et al., A humanized Smn gene containing the SMN2 nucleotide alteration in exon 7 mimics SMN2 splicing and the SMA disease phenotype. *Hum Mol Genet*, 2010. 19(21): p. 4239–52.

180. Duque, S., et al., A large animal model of spinal muscular atrophy and correction of phenotype. *Ann Neurol*, 2015. 77(3): p. 399–414.

181. Jablonka, S., et al., Defective Ca2+ channel clustering in axon terminals disturbs excitability in motoneurons in spinal muscular atrophy. *J Cell Biol*, 2007. 179(1): p. 139–49.

182. Murray, L.M., et al., Selective vulnerability of motor neurons and dissociation of pre- and post-synaptic pathology at the neuromuscular junction in mouse models of spinal muscular atrophy. *Hum Mol Genet*, 2008. 17(7): p. 949–62.

183. Kariya, S., et al., Reduced SMN protein impairs maturation of the neuromuscular junctions in mouse models of spinal muscular atrophy. *Hum Mol Genet*, 2008. 17(16): p. 2552–69.

184. Kong, L., et al., Impaired synaptic vesicle release and immaturity of neuromuscular junctions in spinal muscular atrophy mice. *J Neurosci*, 2009. 29(3): p. 842–51.

185. Ruiz, R., et al., Altered intracellular Ca2+ homeostasis in nerve terminals of severe spinal muscular atrophy mice. *J Neurosci*, 2010. 30(3): p. 849–57.

186. Mentis, G.Z., et al., Early functional impairment of sensory-motor connectivity in a mouse model of spinal muscular atrophy. *Neuron*, 2011. 69(3): p. 453–67.

187. Kariya, S., et al. Requirement of enhanced survival motoneuron protein imposed during neuromuscular junction maturation. *J Clin Invest*, 2014. 124(2): p. 785–800.

188. Gabanella, F., et al., Ribonucleoprotein assembly defects correlate with spinal muscular atrophy severity and preferentially affect a subset of spliceosomal snRNPs. *PLoS One*, 2007. 2(9): p. e921.

189. McWhorter, M.L., et al., The SMN binding protein Gemin2 is not involved in motor axon outgrowth. *Dev Neurobiol*, 2008. 68(2): p. 182–94.

190. Winkler, C., et al., Reduced U snRNP assembly causes motor axon degeneration in an animal model for spinal muscular atrophy. *Genes Dev*, 2005. 19(19): p. 2320–30.

191. Wan, L., et al., The survival of motor neurons protein determines the capacity for snRNP assembly: biochemical deficiency in spinal muscular atrophy. *Mol Cell Biol*, 2005. 25(13): p. 5543–51.

192. Zhang, Z., et al., SMN deficiency causes tissue-specific perturbations in the repertoire of snRNAs and widespread defects in splicing. *Cell*, 2008. 133(4): p. 585–600.

193. Baumer, D., et al., Alternative splicing events are a late feature of pathology in a mouse model of spinal muscular atrophy. *PLoS Genet*, 2009. 5(12): p. e1000773.

194. Lotti, F., et al., An SMN-dependent U12 splicing event essential for motor circuit function. *Cell*, 2012. 151(2): p. 440–54.

195. di Penta, A., et al., Dendritic LSm1/CBP80-mRNPs mark the early steps of transport commitment and translational control. *J Cell Biol*, 2009. 184(3): p. 423–35.

196. Mourelatos, Z., et al., SMN interacts with a novel family of hnRNP and spliceosomal proteins. *EMBO J*, 2001. 20(19): p. 5443–52.

197. Miller, A.A., et al., Clinical pharmacology of sodium butyrate in patients with acute leukemia. *Eur J Cancer Clin Oncol*, 1987. 23(9): p. 1283–7.

198. Andreassi, C., et al., Phenylbutyrate increases SMN expression in vitro: relevance for treatment of spinal muscular atrophy. *Eur J Hum Genet*, 2004. 12(1): p. 59–65.

199. Brichta, L., et al., Valproic acid increases the SMN2 protein level: a well-known drug as a potential therapy for spinal muscular atrophy. *Hum Mol Genet*, 2003. 12(19): p. 2481–9.

200. Sumner, C.J., et al., Valproic acid increases SMN levels in spinal muscular atrophy patient cells. *Ann Neurol*, 2003. 54(5): p. 647–54.

201. Avila, A.M., et al., Trichostatin A increases SMN expression and survival in a mouse model of spinal muscular atrophy. *J Clin Invest*, 2007. 117(3): p. 659–71.

202. Riessland, M., et al., SAHA ameliorates the SMA phenotype in two mouse models for spinal muscular atrophy. *Hum Mol Genet*, 2010. 19(8): p. 1492–506.

203. Tsai, L.K., et al., Multiple therapeutic effects of valproic acid in spinal muscular atrophy model mice. *J Mol Med (Berl)*, 2008. 86(11): p. 1243–54.

204. Weihl, C.C., A.M. Connolly, and A. Pestronk, Valproate may improve strength and function in patients with type III/IV spinal muscle atrophy. *Neurology*, 2006. 67(3): p. 500–1.

205. Swoboda, K.J., et al., Phase II open label study of valproic acid in spinal muscular atrophy. *PLoS One*, 2009. 4(5): p. e5268.

206. Swoboda, K.J., et al., SMA CARNI-VAL trial part I: double-blind, randomized, placebo-controlled trial of L-carnitine and valproic acid in spinal muscular atrophy. *PLoS One*, 2010. 5(8): p. e12140.

207. Kissel, J.T., et al., SMA CARNIVAL TRIAL PART II: a prospective, single-armed trial of L-carnitine and valproic acid in ambulatory children with spinal muscular atrophy. *PLoS One*, 2011. 6(7): p. e21296.

208. Darbar, I.A., et al., Evaluation of muscle strength and motor abilities in children with type II and III spinal muscle atrophy treated with valproic acid. *BMC Neurol*, 2011. 11: p. 36.

209. Brahe, C., et al., Phenylbutyrate increases SMN gene expression in spinal muscular atrophy patients. *Eur J Hum Genet*, 2005. 13(2): p. 256–9.

210. Mercuri, E., et al., Pilot trial of phenylbutyrate in spinal muscular atrophy. *Neuromuscul Disord*, 2004. 14(2): p. 130–5.

211. Mercuri, E., et al., Randomized, double-blind, placebo-controlled trial of phenylbutyrate in spinal muscular atrophy. *Neurology*, 2007. 68(1): p. 51–5.

212. Grzeschik, S.M., et al., Hydroxyurea enhances SMN2 gene expression in spinal muscular atrophy cells. *Ann Neurol*, 2005. 58(2): p. 194–202.

213. Liang, W.C., et al., The effect of hydroxyurea in spinal muscular atrophy cells and patients. *J Neurol Sci*, 2008. 268(1-2): p. 87–94.

214. Xu, C., et al., Hydroxyurea enhances SMN2 gene expression through nitric oxide release. *Neurogenetics*, 2011. 12(1): p. 19–24.

215. Chen, T.H., et al., Randomized, double-blind, placebo-controlled trial of hydroxyurea in spinal muscular atrophy. *Neurology*, 2010. 75(24): p. 2190–7.

216. Jarecki, J., et al., Diverse small-molecule modulators of SMN expression found by high-throughput compound screening: early leads towards a therapeutic for spinal muscular atrophy. *Hum Mol Genet*, 2005. 14(14): p. 2003–18.

217. Repligen Corporation. RG3039: An Innovative Approach to Treating Spinal Muscular Atrophy. [Online]. Available from: http://www.repligen.com/products/pipeline/rgsma [Accessed 15 January 2012].

218. Wang, Z. and M. Kiledjian, Functional link between the mammalian exosome and mRNA decapping. *Cell*, 2001. 107(6): p. 751–62.

219. Singh, J., et al., DcpS as a therapeutic target for spinal muscular atrophy. *ACS Chem Biol*, 2008. 3(11): p. 711–22.

220. Butchbach, M.E., et al., Effects of 2,4-diaminoquinazoline derivatives on SMN expression and phenotype in a mouse model for spinal muscular atrophy. *Hum Mol Genet*, 2010. 19(3): p. 454–67.

221. Gogliotti, R.G., et al. The DcpS inhibitor RG3039 improves survival, function and motor unit pathologies in two SMA mouse models. *Hum Mol Genet*, 2013. 22(20): p. 4084–101.

222. Van Meerbeke, J.P., et al. The DcpS inhibitor RG3039 improves motor function in SMA mice. *Hum Mol Genet*, 2013. 22(20): p. 4074–83.

223. Ting, C.H., et al., Stat5 constitutive activation rescues defects in spinal muscular atrophy. *Hum Mol Genet*, 2007. 16(5): p. 499–514.

224. Farooq, F., et al., Prolactin increases SMN expression and survival in a mouse model of severe spinal muscular atrophy via the STAT5 pathway. *J Clin Invest*, 2011. 121(8): p. 3042–50.

225. Zhang, M.L., et al., An in vivo reporter system for measuring increased inclusion of exon 7 in SMN2 mRNA: potential therapy of SMA. *Gene Ther*, 2001. 8(20): p. 1532–8.

226. Angelozzi, C., et al., Salbutamol increases SMN mRNA and protein levels in spinal muscular atrophy cells. *J Med Genet*, 2008. 45(1): p. 29–31.

227. Tiziano, F.D., et al., SMN transcript levels in leukocytes of SMA patients determined by absolute real-time PCR. *Eur J Hum Genet*, 2010. 18(1): p. 52–8.

228. Kinali, M., et al., Pilot trial of albuterol in spinal muscular atrophy. *Neurology*, 2002. 59(4): p. 609–10.

229. Pane, M., et al., Daily salbutamol in young patients with SMA type II. *Neuromuscul Disord*, 2008. 18(7): p. 536–40.

230. Andreassi, C., et al., Aclarubicin treatment restores SMN levels to cells derived from type I spinal muscular atrophy patients. *Hum Mol Genet*, 2001. 10(24): p. 2841–9.

231. Hastings, M.L., et al., Tetracyclines that promote SMN2 exon 7 splicing as therapeutics for spinal muscular atrophy. *Sci Transl Med*, 2009. 1(5): p. 5ra12.

232. Naryshkin, N.A., et al. SMN2 splicing modifiers improve motor function and longevity in mice with spinal muscular atrophy. *Science*, 2014. 345: p. 688–93.

233. Palacino, J., et al. SMN2 splice modulators enhance U1-pre-mRNA association and rescue SMA mice. *Nat Chem Biol* 2015. 11(7): p. 511–17.

234. Hua, Y., et al., Antisense masking of an hnRNP A1/A2 intronic splicing silencer corrects SMN2 splicing in transgenic mice. *Am J Hum Genet*, 2008. 82(4): p. 834–48.

235. Singh, N.K., et al., Splicing of a critical exon of human survival motor neuron is regulated by a unique silencer element located in the last intron. *Mol Cell Biol*, 2006. 26(4): p. 1333–46.

236. Hua, Y., et al., Enhancement of SMN2 exon 7 inclusion by antisense oligonucleotides targeting the exon. *PLoS Biol*, 2007. 5(4): p. e73.

237. Hua, Y., et al., Antisense correction of SMN2 splicing in the CNS rescues necrosis in a type III SMA mouse model. *Genes Dev*, 2010. 24(15): p. 1634–44.

238. Passini, M.A., et al., Antisense oligonucleotides delivered to the mouse CNS ameliorate symptoms of severe spinal muscular atrophy. *Sci Transl Med*, 2011. 3(72): p. 72ra18.

239. Hua, Y., et al., Peripheral SMN restoration is essential for long-term rescue of a severe spinal muscular atrophy mouse model. *Nature*, 2011. 478(7367): p. 123–6.

240. IONIS Pharmaceuticals. An open-label for patients with Spinal Muscular Atrophy (SMA) who participated in studies with IONIS-SMNRx. In: clinicaltrials.gov [Internet]. Bethesda (MD): National Library of Medicine (US). 2015-[cited 2016 Oct 13]. Available from https://clinicaltrials.gov/ct2/show/NCT02594124?term=ionis+sma&rank=1

241. Coady, T.H. and C.L. Lorson, Trans-splicing-mediated improvement in a severe mouse model of spinal muscular atrophy. *J Neurosci*, 2010. 30(1): p. 126–30.

242. Baughan, T., et al., Stimulating full-length SMN2 expression by delivering bifunctional RNAs via a viral vector. *Mol Ther*, 2006. 14(1): p. 54–62.

243. Lunn, M.R., et al., Indoprofen upregulates the survival motor neuron protein through a cyclooxygenase-independent mechanism. *Chem Biol*, 2004. 11(11): p. 1489–93.

244. Wolstencroft, E.C., et al., A non-sequence-specific requirement for SMN protein activity: the role of aminoglycosides in inducing elevated SMN protein levels. *Hum Mol Genet*, 2005. 14(9): p. 1199–210.

245. Mattis, V.B., et al., Novel aminoglycosides increase SMN levels in spinal muscular atrophy fibroblasts. *Hum Genet*, 2006. 120(4): p. 589–601.

246. Mattis, V.B., et al., Delivery of a read-through inducing compound, TC007, lessens the severity of a spinal muscular atrophy animal model. *Hum Mol Genet*, 2009. 18(20): p. 3906–13.

247. Heier, C.R. and C.J. DiDonato, Translational readthrough by the aminoglycoside geneticin (G418) modulates SMN stability in vitro and improves motor function in SMA mice in vivo. *Hum Mol Genet*, 2009. 18(7): p. 1310–22.

248. Chang, H.C., et al., Degradation of survival motor neuron (SMN) protein is mediated via the ubiquitin/proteasome pathway. *Neurochem Int*, 2004. 45(7): p. 1107–12.

249. Kwon, D.Y., et al., Increasing expression and decreasing degradation of SMN ameliorate the spinal muscular atrophy phenotype in mice. *Hum Mol Genet*, 2011. 20(18): p. 3667–77.

250. Azzouz, M., et al., Lentivector-mediated SMN replacement in a mouse model of spinal muscular atrophy. *J Clin Invest*, 2004. 114(12): p. 1726–31.

251. Foust, K.D., et al., Intravascular AAV9 preferentially targets neonatal neurons and adult astrocytes. *Nat Biotechnol*, 2009. 27(1): p. 59–65.

252. Foust, K.D., et al., Rescue of the spinal muscular atrophy phenotype in a mouse model by early postnatal delivery of SMN. *Nat Biotechnol*, 2010. 28(3): p. 271–4.

253. Passini, M.A., et al., CNS-targeted gene therapy improves survival and motor function in a mouse model of spinal muscular atrophy. *J Clin Invest*, 2010. 120(4): p. 1253–64.

254. Valori, C.F., et al., Systemic delivery of scAAV9 expressing SMN prolongs survival in a model of spinal muscular atrophy. *Sci Transl Med*, 2010. 2(35): p. 35ra42.

255. Dominguez, E., et al., Intravenous scAAV9 delivery of a codon-optimized SMN1 sequence rescues SMA mice. *Hum Mol Genet*, 2011. 20(4): p. 681–93.

256. Bevan, A.K., et al. Systemic gene delivery in large species for targeting spinal cord, brain, and perihperal tissues for pediatric disorders. *Mol Ther,* 2009. 19: p. 1971–80.

257. Wichterle, H., et al., Directed differentiation of embryonic stem cells into motor neurons. *Cell,* 2002. 110(3): p. 385–97.

258. Shin, S., S. Dalton, and S.L. Stice, Human motor neuron differentiation from human embryonic stem cells. *Stem Cells Dev,* 2005. 14(3): p. 266–9.

259. Corti, S., et al., Embryonic stem cell-derived neural stem cells improve spinal muscular atrophy phenotype in mice. *Brain,* 2010. 133(Pt 2): p. 465–81.

260. Nistor, G., et al., Derivation of high purity neuronal progenitors from human embryonic stem cells. *PLoS One,* 2011. 6(6): p. e20692.

261. Wyatt, T.J., et al., Human motor neuron progenitor transplantation leads to endogenous neuronal sparing in 3 models of motor neuron loss. *Stem Cells Int,* 2011. 2011: p. 207230.

262. Rothstein, J.D., et al., Beta-lactam antibiotics offer neuroprotection by increasing glutamate transporter expression. *Nature,* 2005. 433(7021): p. 73–7.

263. Nizzardo, M., et al., Beta-lactam antibiotic offers neuroprotection in a spinal muscular atrophy model by multiple mechanisms. *Exp Neurol,* 2011. 229(2): p. 214–25.

264. Haddad, H., et al., Riluzole attenuates spinal muscular atrophy disease progression in a mouse model. *Muscle Nerve,* 2003. 28(4): p. 432–7.

265. Russman, B.S., S.T. Iannaccone, and F.J. Samaha, A phase 1 trial of riluzole in spinal muscular atrophy. *Arch Neurol,* 2003. 60(11): p. 1601–3.

266. Abbara, C., et al., Riluzole pharmacokinetics in young patients with spinal muscular atrophy. *Br J Clin Pharmacol,* 2011. 71(3): p. 403–10.

267. Merlini, L., et al., Role of gabapentin in spinal muscular atrophy: results of a multicenter, randomized Italian study. *J Child Neurol,* 2003. 18(8): p. 537–41.

268. Miller, R.G., et al., A placebo-controlled trial of gabapentin in spinal muscular atrophy. *J Neurol Sci,* 2001. 191(1–2): p. 127–31.

269. Bordet, T., et al., Identification and characterization of cholest-4-en-3-one, oxime (TRO19622), a novel drug candidate for amyotrophic lateral sclerosis. *J Pharmacol Exp Ther,* 2007. 322(2): p.709–20.

270. Trophos. Safety and efficacy of olesoxime (TRO19622) in 3-25 years SMA patients. In: clinicaltrials.gov [Internet]. Bethesda (MD): National Library of Medicine (US). 2011- [cited 2012 Feb 27]. Available from: http://www.clinicaltrials.gov/ct2/show/NCT01302600 NLM Identifier: NCT01302600.

271. Dessaud, E., et al. Results of a Phase II study to assess safety and efficacy of olesoxime (TRO19622) in 3-25 year old spinal muscular atrophy patients. 2014 In: 18th Annual International Spinal Muscular Atrophy Research Group Meeting abstract book.

272. Lesbordes, J.C., et al., Therapeutic benefits of cardiotrophin-1 gene transfer in a mouse model of spinal muscular atrophy. *Hum Mol Genet,* 2003. 12(11): p. 1233–9.

273. Montes, J., et al., Clinical outcome measures in spinal muscular atrophy. *J Child Neurol,* 2009. 24(8): p. 968–78.

274. Piper, M.C., et al., Construction and validation of the Alberta Infant Motor Scale (AIMS). *Can J Public Health,* 1992. 83 **Suppl 2**: p. S46–50.

275. Campbell, S.K., et al., Construct validity of the test of infant motor performance. *Phys Ther,* 1995. 75(7): p. 585–96.

276. Finkel, R.S., et al., The test of infant motor performance: reliability in spinal muscular atrophy type I. *Pediatr Phys Ther,* 2008. 20(3): p. 242–6.

277. Mercuri, E., et al., Reliability of the Hammersmith functional motor scale for spinal muscular atrophy in a multicentric study. *Neuromuscul Disord,* 2006. 16(2): p. 93–8.

278. Tiziano, F.D., et al., The Hammersmith functional score correlates with the SMN2 copy number: a multicentric study. *Neuromuscul Disord,* 2007. 17(5): p. 400–3.

279. Kissel JT, E.B., Kolb SJ, King W, Chelnick S, Scott CB, LaSalle B, Krosschell KJ, Reyna SP, Swoboda KJ. A prospective, randomized controlled trial of valproic acid in ambulant adults with SMA: theVALIANT trial. Presented at the 15th Annual International Spinal Muscular Atrophy Research Group Meeting. Lake Buena Vista, Florida, USA, 2011.

280. Wu, J.S., B.T. Darras, and S.B. Rutkove, Assessing spinal muscular atrophy with quantitative ultrasound. *Neurology,* 2010. 75(6): p. 526–31.

281. Merlini, L., et al., Motor function-muscle strength relationship in spinal muscular atrophy. *Muscle Nerve,* 2004. 29(4): p. 548–52.

282. Iannaccone, S.T., et al., The PedsQL in pediatric patients with Spinal Muscular Atrophy: feasibility, reliability, and validity of the Pediatric Quality of Life Inventory Generic Core Scales and Neuromuscular Module. *Neuromuscul Disord,* 2009. 19(12): p. 805–12.

283. Iannaccone, S.T. and American Spinal Muscular Atrophy Randomized Trials Group, Outcome measures for pediatric spinal muscular atrophy. *Arch Neurol,* 2002. 59(9): p. 1445–50.

284. Iannaccone, S.T., L.S. Hynan, and American Spinal Muscular Atrophy Randomized Trials Group, Reliability of 4 outcome measures in pediatric spinal muscular atrophy. *Arch Neurol,* 2003. 60(8): p. 1130–6.

285. Sumner, C.J., et al., SMN mRNA and protein levels in peripheral blood: biomarkers for SMA clinical trials. *Neurology,* 2006. 66(7): p. 1067–73.

286. Tsai, L.K., et al., Correlation of survival motor neuron expression in leukocytes and spinal cord in spinal muscular atrophy. *J Pediatr,* 2009. 154(2): p. 303–5.

287. Crawford, T.O., Concerns about the design of clinical trials for spinal muscular atrophy. *Neuromuscul Disord,* 2004. 14(8-9): p. 456–60.

288. Finkel, R.S., et al., Candidate proteins, metabolites and transcripts in the Biomarkers for Spinal Muscular Atrophy (BforSMA) Clinical Study. *PLoS One,* 2012. 7(4): e35462.

289. Kobayashi, D.T., et al., SMA-MAP: a plasma protein panel for spinal muscular atrophy. *PLoS One,* 2013. 8(4): e60113.

290. Crawford, T.O. Standard of care for spinal muscular atrophy. In: Sumner, C.J., Paushkin, S., and Ko, C-P., (eds). *Spinal Muscular Atrophy Disease and Therapy.* Elsevier, San Diego, 2016.

291. Perez-Garcia, K., Sumner, C.J., and Tizzano, E. Developmental aspects of pathological findings in spinal muscular atrophy. In: Sumner, C.J., Paushkin, S., and Ko, C-P., (eds). *Spinal Muscular Atrophy Disease and Therapy.* Elsevier, San Diego, 2016.

CHAPTER 17

Spinal and Bulbar Muscular Atrophy (Kennedy Disease)

Erich Peter Bosch

Department of Neurology, Mayo Clinic Arizona, Scottsdale, Arizona, and Mayo College of Medicine, Rochester, Minnesota, USA

Clinical definition and epidemiology

Spinal and bulbar muscular atrophy (SBMA) is a rare, adult-onset, X-linked motor neuron disease characterized by slowly progressive muscular atrophy and weakness, bulbar lower motor neuron involvement with fasciculations of the tongue and perioral region, and postural tremor. SBMA affects only adult men, who often have gynecomastia, testicular atrophy, and reduced fertility as a result of androgen insensitivity. In 1968, Kennedy and co-workers [1] described the cardinal clinical features in 11 males from two large families. Owing to this initial description the disorder was later named Kennedy disease. Earlier reports from Japan have failed to attract attention in the English literature [2]. Subclinical sensory involvement discovered by abnormal sensory conduction studies led Harding and co-workers [3] to suggest the descriptive term X-linked bulbospinal neuronopathy, thereby emphasizing the involvement of both motor and sensory neurons.

SBMA has been mapped to Xq11-12 on the proximal long arm of the X chromosome [4]. The androgen receptor gene has been localized to the same region on the X chromosome, and therefore became a candidate gene for SBMA. SBMA is caused by an unstable CAG trinucleotide repeat which encodes a polyglutamine tract in the first exon of the androgen receptor (AR) gene [5, 6]. SBMA was the first of nine neurodegenerative disorders found to be caused by CAG repeats encoding elongated polyglutamine tracts in their respective proteins including Huntington's disease, dentato-rubral-pallido-luysian atrophy, and six forms of spinocerebellar ataxia [7].

SBMA is a rare motor neuron disorder that occurs primarily in individuals of European or Asian racial background. An epidemiological survey in Northern Italy reported a mean annual incidence of 0.2/100,000 and a prevalence rate of 3.3/100,000 for the male population [8]. In this population the average age at disease onset was 45 and the average period of survival was 27 years. Whereas the annual incidence rate of SBMA is more than 10 times lower than that of amyotrophic lateral sclerosis (ALS), its prevalence is only slightly lower than that of ALS. The disease is more common in certain regions of Japan, western Finland, and northern Sweden because of a founder effect [9, 10].

Clinical phenotype

Phenotypic expression may vary between and within affected families [6]. The typical age of onset is 30–60 years [11]. In two large clinical series of 280 patients the average age of onset of muscle weakness fell between 41 and 44 years [12, 13]. Before the onset of weakness patients may present with muscle cramps, postural and action tremor, fasciculations, and even asymptomatic hyper-CK-emia (CK, creatine kinase) [14]. Fasciculations are prominent in the lower face and the tongue, and often pre-date any functional impairment in speech and swallowing. Some patients may experience laryngospasm, which is an abrupt closure of the vocal cords that results in sudden gasping for air. Dysphagia develops in advanced stages resulting in choking, aspiration, and impaired nutrition. Early manifestations of cramps and fasciculations are followed by slowly progressive weakness and atrophy of limb and bulbar muscles. Lower extremities are initially twice as often affected than the upper extremities; proximal muscles are weaker than distal muscle groups. This results in progressive gait impairment and may lead to wheelchair dependence 20–30 years after onset [13]. Deep tendon reflexes are decreased or absent. Upper motor neuron signs are consistently absent. Patients rarely complain of sensory symptoms. Reduced vibration sense in the feet can be detected in half of the patients [1, 3, 15]. Although involvement of sensory ganglia is often subclinical, sensory nerve conduction studies show reduced or absent sensory nerve action potentials in almost all patients [3, 16, 17].

Clinical signs of partial androgen insensitivity usually appear later in life in up to 80% of SBMA patients, including gynecomastia, testicular atrophy, oligo/azoospermia, and infertility [18, 19]. Gynecomastia, however, frequently appears before the onset of muscular weakness. Hormonal changes of androgen insensitivity are more frequent than clinical signs and consist of elevated serum testosterone associated with high gonadotropin levels [20]. Adult-onset diabetes is seen in some patients but this association may be coincidental and is not known to influence the course of disease [21].

Heterozygous women who are carriers of extended CAG repeats are largely asymptomatic although minor symptoms such as muscle cramps, isolated fasciculations, and mild tremor have been described [22]. Two unique sisters homozygous for the CAG repeat expansion were reported to have occasional muscle cramps and fasciculations without muscular weakness [23].

Genotype–phenotype correlations

SBMA is caused by an increased number (>38) of CAG repeats in the first exon of the AR gene. Several studies have addressed a potential relationship of CAG repeats and clinical phenotypic

Neurodegeneration, First Edition. Edited by Anthony Schapira, Zbigniew Wszolek, Ted M. Dawson and Nicholas Wood.
© 2017 John Wiley & Sons, Ltd. Published 2017 by John Wiley & Sons, Ltd.

expression. The number of CAG repeats correlates inversely with the age of disease onset, with longer repeats associated with earlier onset [12, 24, 25]. The occurrence of gynecomastia is likewise inversely correlated with CAG expansion [20]. Disease progression was found not to be influenced by the repeat length whereas the age of developing certain activities of daily living milestones such as difficulty climbing stairs or wheelchair dependence was inversely correlated with the length of CAG repeats [12].

Pathology and pathogenesis

SBMA is caused by a trinucleotide CAG repeat (cytosine-adenine-guanine) expansion in the first exon of the androgen receptor (AR) gene on the X chromosome encoding a polyglutamine tract in its amino-terminal transactivation domain. The polymorphic repeat length ranges from a normal length of 11–35 CAG repeats to a disease-causing length of 38–62 [5]. Intergenerational CAG repeat expansion is observed via paternal transmission suggesting that the instability of the CAG repeat occurs during spermatogenesis. SBMA belongs to at least nine inherited neurodegenerative disorders caused by expanded CAG/polyglutamine tracts in the coding regions of unrelated disease-causing genes, which affect different populations of CNS neurons [26, 27]. In addition to SBMA, this group of polyglutamine extension diseases includes Huntington's disease, dentato-rubral-pallido-luysian atrophy, and six forms of spinocerebellar ataxia. The polyglutamine diseases have in common neuronal intranuclear inclusions consisting of misfolded polyglutamine-expanded proteins in affected neuronal populations. The exact mechanism by which polyglutamine expansion causes neurodegeneration is still unknown but there is increasing evidence that a toxic gain of function caused by the aggregated abnormal protein leads to neuronal dysfunction and neuronal cell loss [7, 26]. In contrast to all other polyglutamine diseases, which are inherited in an autosomal dominant fashion, SBMA is an X-linked disease. Carrier females may be protected from the CAG repeat expansion in the AR gene by random X chromosome inactivation and by lower circulating levels of testosterone.

The main pathological finding in SBMA is the loss of motor neurons in the spinal cord and in brainstem motor nuclei except for those of the sixth, fourth, and third cranial nerves [28] (Figure 17.1). Primary sensory neurons and their axons are less severely affected. A morphometric autopsy study of central and peripheral sensory pathways documented a mild loss of dorsal root ganglia together with a loss of large myelinated sensory fibers in dorsal roots and fasciculus gracilis, and distally accentuated loss of myelinated fibers in sural nerves [29]. Muscle histopathology includes both neurogenic atrophy and myopathic changes (see section Laboratory investigations).

A hallmark of polyglutamine diseases is the presence of neuronal nuclear inclusions [2, 27]. In SBMA, nuclear inclusions containing the amino-terminal epitopes of the AR protein are found in spinal cord and brainstem motor neurons as well as non-neuronal tissues

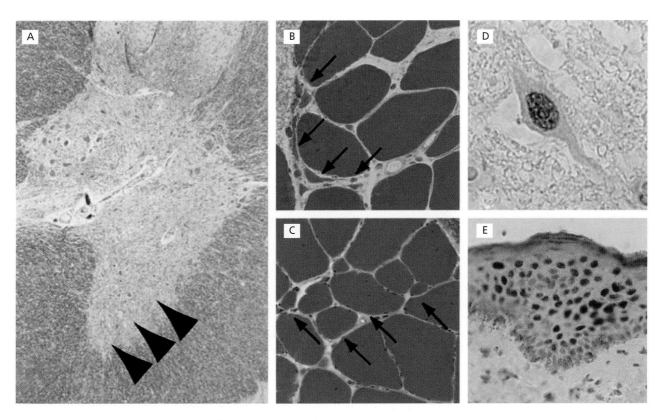

Figure 17.1 Pathology of spinal and bulbar muscular atrophy (SBMA). (A) Transverse section of spinal cord demonstrates the loss of motor neurons in the anterior horn (arrowheads). (B) Skeletal muscle shows neurogenic atrophy (arrows point to angular atrophic fibers) and myopathic changes; (C) arrows indicate fiber splitting and increased central nuclei. (D) A residual motor neuron demonstrates nuclear accumulation of mutant androgen receptor (AR). (E) Nuclear accumulation of pathogenic AR is also seen in scrotal skin cells. (B, C) Hematoxylin and eosin; (D, E) anti-polyglutamine antibody. Source: Katsuno 2006 [2]. Reproduced with permission of Elsevier.

such as testis, prostate, skeletal and heart muscle, and scrotal skin [30]. Recent observations from a unique transgenic mouse model suggest that the mutant AR gene in skeletal muscle plays an important role in the disease mechanism [31]. Knockin mice in which a human mutant AR transgene is expressed exclusively in muscle develop an androgen-dependent SBMA phenotype including myopathic changes before motor neuron pathology is detected in the spinal cord. Conversely, muscle-specific knockout of the mutant AR gene in a transgenic SBMA mouse model ameliorated the disease phenotype despite continued expression of the mutant AR in motor neurons. The AR nuclear inclusions also contain ubiquitin, which marks aggregated, misfolded proteins for degradation. An autopsy study using an anti-polyglutamine antibody which recognizes expanded polyglutamine tracts found diffuse nuclear and cytoplasmic accumulation of polyglutamine-expanded AR protein in spinal motor neurons and non-neuronal tissues far more frequently than dense ubiquinated nuclear inclusions [32]. Furthermore, the extent of diffuse nuclear accumulation of mutant AR in spinal motor neurons correlated with CAG repeat length of the AR gene. The nuclear localization of the abnormal AR containing an elongated polyglutamine tract in motor neurons and muscle is considered essential to the pathogenesis of SBMA [2, 31, 33]. Because human AR is widely expressed in various organs, nuclear accumulation of mutant AR is also detected in non-neuronal tissues such as scrotal skin. A clinical–pathological study of SBMA patients found that the degree of polyglutamine-expanded AR accumulation in scrotal skin cells correlated with that in spinal motor neurons in autopsy specimens and with the CAG repeat length of the AR gene. The nuclear accumulation of polyglutamine-expanded AR protein in scrotal skin inversely correlated with clinical deficits as measured by the Norris ALS functional scale [34]. These results indicate that scrotal skin biopsy with polyglutamine immunostaining is a reliable biomarker of SBMA, and this test has been used as a surrogate endpoint in clinical trials.

The AR is a 110-kDa nuclear receptor belonging to the steroid receptor superfamily that binds to testosterone and dihydrotestosterone. It contains an amino-terminal domain in which the CAG repeat is located, a DNA-binding domain and a ligand-binding domain. In the absence of androgen, AR is sequestered in the cytoplasm in an inactive complex with heat shock protein 90 and other chaperones. When androgens bind to the AR, the AR–ligand complex translocates to the nucleus where it functions as a transcription factor regulating the expression of a large variety of genes. Transgenic mouse models expressing the full-length mutant human AR with an expanded polyglutamine tract have shed light on the testosterone-dependent nuclear translocation of the AR [2]. That the phenotypic expression of SBMA is androgen dependent is based on several observations:

1 Only male transgenic mice, having higher androgen levels than females, develop full disease manifestations.

2 Surgical castration of male transgenic mice improved motor function and lifespan, and these animals showed fewer histopathologic findings and fewer neuronal nuclear inclusions compared to sham operated animals.

3 Androgen administration produced the full disease phenotype in female transgenic mice.

4 Androgen-reducing treatment with leuprorelin, a luteinizing hormone-releasing hormone agonist that suppresses the release of gonadotropins and reduces testosterone levels, ameliorates motor dysfunction and inhibits nuclear accumulation of mutant AR in motor neurons of male transgenic mice [2].

5 The report that two sisters homozygous for the CAG repeat expansion had only minimal clinical manifestations further confirms that the toxicity of the expanded polyglutamine AR is ligand dependent [23].

Such observations suggest that anti-androgen treatment may mitigate the disease process in SBMA [35]. Human clinical trials with leuprorelin and dutasteride, a 5α-reductase inhibitor, have been completed but have not resulted in clinically meaningful effects.

The critical cause of neurodegeneration in SBMA is thought to be a toxic gain of function of the polyglutamine-expanded AR. This hypothesis is supported by the observation that motor neuron like disorders are never seen in testicular feminization patients totally lacking AR function or AR knockout mice [2]. Nuclear localization of the polyglutamine-expanded AR is essential for inducing several molecular events such as transcriptional dysregulation, mitochondrial dysfunction, JNK pathway activation, and impaired axonal transport that are thought to result in neuronal dysfunction and cell death [2, 35, 36].

Heat shock proteins (HSP) are essential for the function and stability of AR and act as chaperones in regulating protein folding and targeting misfolded proteins for degradation. The carboxy-terminus of the AR has a high affinity for HSP90, which is important for its nuclear translocation after ligand binding [33, 36]. Inhibitors of HSP90 reduce ligand binding and promote proteasomal degradation of AR. Treatment with geldanamycin analogs, which are potent HSP90 inhibitors, reduced the diffuse nuclear accumulation of mutant AR in transgenic mice and led to improved motor performance [33]. The ability to promote degradation of disease-causing proteins by modulation of HSP90 function holds promise for the treatment of SBMA and other polyglutamine diseases.

Examination and laboratory investigations

When SBMA patients are referred to a neurologist, most will have signs of bulbar involvement. Some have surprisingly few bulbar symptoms such as mild dysarthria characterized by imprecise articulation and mild dysphagia not interfering with nutrition despite prominent tongue atrophy and fasciculations. This striking mismatch between obvious bulbar signs on examination and only minor functional deficits is a clinical hallmark of SBMA. Prominent fasciculations in the lower face and to a lesser degree in arms and legs are frequently present. Some patients develop quivering of the chin when pursing the lips. Occasional patients may present with a drooping jaw caused by severe jaw closure weakness [37]. The extraocular muscles are spared. Symmetrical atrophy and weakness initially affects proximal limb muscles more than distal muscles and legs more often than arms. Some degree of asymmetrical weakness is not unusual [13]. Tendon reflexes are reduced or absent. Upper motor neuron signs are never elicited. A postural and action tremor of the distal upper limbs may precede the onset of weakness by years [12]. Although sensory loss is often undetectable, impaired vibratory sensation in distal limbs can be found in half of the patients by careful examination [15]. Gynecomastia, a physical sign of partial androgen insensitivity, is reported to occur in up to 70% of patients and may develop before the onset of muscular weakness [20].

The case presentation in Box 17.1 highlights the clinical manifestations of SBMA.

Box 17.1 Case presentation: SBMA

A 64-year-old Filipino male presented with hand tremor, longstanding swallowing difficulties, and "prickling sensations" in his feet. Ten years earlier he had developed a postural tremor. He was aware of muscle twitches of his face, easy fatigability, and mild dysphagia resulting in occasional choking episodes. His libido had been impaired for years. Previous evaluations were inconclusive. Family history suggested that one of his six brothers had a similar undiagnosed "nervous condition". The examination revealed prominent fasciculations of the lower face producing quivering of the chin, and tongue atrophy with fasciculations. The mismatch between obvious bulbar involvement on examination and the barely detectable dysarthria was striking. He had atrophy of shoulder girdle muscles with occasional fasciculations, and mild symmetrical, proximal weakness of upper and lower limbs. Deep tendon reflexes were absent; plantar responses were flexor. Vibration sense was absent at the toes. His gait was normal. A postural tremor of his hands and gynecomastia were noted (Figure 17.2).

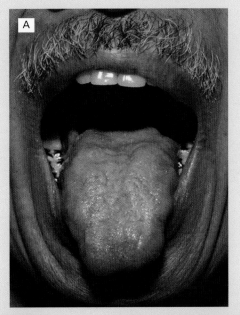

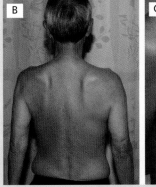

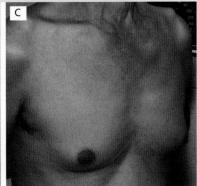

Figure 17.2 Patient with spinal and bulbar muscular atrophy: (A) tongue atrophy; (B, C) atrophy of shoulder girdle and gynecomastia.

Motor nerve conduction studies were normal. Sensory nerve action potentials were absent in the ulnar nerve and reduced in the median and sural nerves. Needle EMG showed high-amplitude, long-duration, polyphasic motor unit action potentials with decreased recruitment without fibrillation potentials in multiple muscles of upper and lower limbs. The study indicated a chronic generalized disorder of motor neurons or their axons combined with a mild sensory neuronopathy. The serum CK level was elevated to 572 u/L. Gene testing revealed an expanded number of CAG repeats (45) in the AR gene confirming the diagnosis of SBMA or Kennedy disease.

The clinical and laboratory features of eight genetically confirmed cases personally seen at Mayo Clinic are summarized in Tables 17.1A and 17.1B. In none of the patients was the diagnosis suspected by the referring physician. The interval from disease onset to diagnosis ranged from 4 to 30 years. The presenting symptoms ranged from tremor, muscle cramps, dysphagia, to upper and lower extremity weakness. Only two patients had a positive family history. The majority had elevated serum CK and reduced creatinine levels. The electrophysiologic studies confirmed chronic denervation and reinnervation and reduced to absent sensory nerve action potentials, predominantly in upper limbs. These electrophysiologic abnormalities together with a chronic lower motor neuron disorder in men should trigger gene testing for SBMA.

Table 17.1A Clinical features of SBMA cases observed personally.

Case	Age at exam (yrs)	Initial symptoms at onset (yrs)	Family history	Weakness		Bulbar signs	Ambulation	Sensory signs	Tremor	Gynecomastia
				UE	LE					
1	63	LE weakness (43)	N	+ p+d	+ p+d	+	Y	–	+	+
2ˣ	64	Tremor (54)	Y	+ p+d	+ p	+	Y	+(V)	+	+
3	37	UE weakness (33)	N	+ p+d	+ p	+	Y	–	+	–
4	48	Dysphagia (46)	N	–	–	+	Y	–	–	–
5	59	Cramps, tremor, CK↑ (39)	N	+ p+d	–	+	Y	–	+	+
6	39	UE weakness (29)	N	+ p+d	+ p+d	+	Y	–	–	–
7	81	Tremor, tingling (51)	N	+ p+d	+ p+d	++	Y with assist.	+(V)	+	–
8	50	LE weakness (48), dysphagia	Y	+ p	+ p	+	Y	+(V)	–	+

d, distal, LE, lower extremities; p, proximal; UE, upper extremities; V, vibration sense reduced to absent; Y, yes.

Table 17.1B Laboratory features of SBMA cases observed personally.

Case	CK u/L (<336)	Creatinine mg/dL (>0.8)	SNAPs	EMG chronic denervation	AR (CAG)ⁿ
1	486	0.6	Median, ulnar NR; sural nl	UE + LE	44
2	572	0.8	Ulnar NR; sural ↓	MUPs ↑, UE + LE	45
3	564	0.6	Median, sural nl	UE, LE, thoracic paraspinal	49
4	70	–	Median, ulnar ↓; sural nl	MUPs ↑, UE	40
5	609	0.7	Median ↓; ulnar NR; sural nl	UE	44
6	891	0.5	Median, sural nl	UE, LE, thoracic paraspinal	39
7	288	0.7	Median ↓; sural NR	UE + LE	41
8	2,649	0.4	Median, ulnar NR; Sural nl	UE + LE, thoracic paraspinals	47

AR(CAG)$_n$, androgen receptor gene, number of expanded CAG repeats; CK, creatine kinase; EMG, electromyography; MUPs, enlarged motor unit potentials; nl, normal; NR, no response; SNAPs, sensory nerve action potentials.

Laboratory investigations

Serum CK levels are consistently elevated up to 10 times the upper limit of normal, which is higher than the more modest elevations typically seen in other anterior horn cell or chronic denervating disorders. Below normal serum creatinine levels are frequently seen in patients with SBMA. Because serum creatinine represents a simple estimate of whole muscle mass it may be a useful biomarker of disease progression [38]. Electrodiagnostic studies indicate a chronic anterior horn cell disorder combined with a sensory neuronopathy [3, 16]. Motor nerve conduction studies show preserved distal latencies and conduction velocities but low-amplitude compound muscle action potentials (CMAP) when recorded from atrophic muscles. The reported frequency of reduced CMAP amplitudes ranges from 37 to 52% [13, 17]. Most patients have low-amplitude or absent sensory nerve action potentials [13, 17]. In a study of 57 patients, sensory nerve action potential amplitudes were reduced in 94–100% of patients, depending on the nerve examined [13]. These abnormalities are more pronounced in the nerves of the upper limbs than those of the lower limbs. In a study of 106 patients with confirmed SBMA, correlations were found between the frequency of either motor or sensory abnormalities and the size of the CAG expansion [39]. Longer CAG repeats were more closely linked to reduced CMAP amplitudes while shorter CAG repeats were more frequently associated with abnormal sensory nerve action potentials. Motor unit number estimates (MUNE), using the statistical MUNE program, were significantly reduced in the abductor pollicis brevis compared to healthy controls [13].

The needle EMG documents widespread, long-duration, high-amplitude, polyphasic motor unit action potentials associated with scant fibrillation and fasciculation potentials and reduced recruitment at maximal contraction [17]. The relative paucity of fibrillation potentials together with large neurogenic motor unit action potentials indicates chronic motor axonal loss with reinnervation. Jaw quivering is the result of grouped repetitive discharges of motor unit action potentials of lower facial muscles during mild voluntary activation [16].

Muscle biopsies confirm neurogenic atrophy and ongoing reinnervation by the presence of angular atrophic fibers arranged in groups, clumping of sarcolemmal nuclei, and fiber type grouping (Figure 17.3). In addition, many biopsies have typical myopathic changes such as increased central nuclei, hypertrophic fibers, fiber splitting, and occasional necrotic fibers. The myopathic changes are the result of impaired satellite cell activation caused by the mutant AR as both skeletal muscle and satellite cells express androgen receptors [40] and point to muscle as an important site of mutant AR toxicity.

MR imaging of skeletal muscle may show atrophy and hyperintense signals on T1-weighted images due to denervation [41].

Although a cardiomyopathy has not been associated with SBMA, it is best to obtain a baseline ECG in order to detect the Brugada-type ECG changes. Brugada-type ECG abnormalities consist of coved or saddleback-type ST segment elevations among right precordial leads, and may cause sudden death by ventricular fibrillation. Brugada-type ECG abnormalities were detected in 12% of

Figure 17.3 Quadriceps muscle biopsy. (A) Hypertrophic fibers with increased central nuclei indicate myopathic changes. Pyknotic nuclear clumps and an entire fascicle of severely atrophic fibers point to chronic neurogenic atrophy. (B) Fiber type grouping is confirmed by a large group of type 1 fibers indicating reinnervation. Angular atrophic fibers of both fiber types demonstrate ongoing denervation. (A) Hematoxylin and eosin; (B) ATPase reaction pH 9.

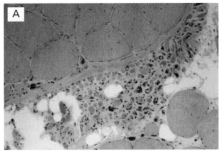
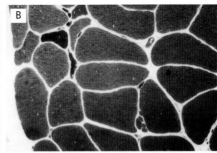

144 consecutive Japanese patients with SBMA, which is 10 times higher than in community-based populations [42].

The diagnosis of SBMA is confirmed by molecular genetic testing for the CAG trinucleotide expansion in the AR gene. The CAG repeat number is determined by polymerase chain reaction amplification of the CAG repeat region within the AR gene. Molecular gene testing is 100% sensitive and specific, and readily available in clinical reference laboratories. All patients with SBMA have expanded trinucleotide repeats of 38 or more, compared to 34 or fewer repeats in normal individuals [43]. The clinical significance of 35–37 CAG repeats needs to be interpreted in the context of the clinical phenotype and the repeat length of affected family members. Genetic testing is indicated whenever a positive family history, clinical manifestations, and electrodiagnostic findings suggest the diagnosis of SBMA. Early genetic testing can avoid more invasive testing such as nerve or muscle biopsies.

Pulmonary function studies with maximal respiratory pressures or sniff nasal inspiratory pressures are helpful in detecting early restrictive pulmonary deficits due to respiratory muscle weakness. A swallowing evaluation by videofluoroscopy will uncover silent aspiration. Both studies are needed at baseline and should be repeated periodically to assess the need for noninvasive ventilation or gastrostomy placement.

Diagnosis and prognosis

Clinical features in support of SBMA include X-linked inheritance affecting only men, prominent bulbar signs producing only mild bulbar symptoms, slowly progressive weakness over decades, mild distal large fiber sensory involvement, signs of androgen insensitivity such as gynecomastia, and the lack of upper motor neuron signs. These features, together with electrodiagnostic studies indicating a chronic anterior horn cell disorder combined with a sensory neuronopathy, warrant gene testing for CAG repeat expansion in the AR gene. The absence of a family history should not dissuade the clinician from the diagnosis of SBMA. In my own experience only two of eight genetically confirmed patients had a positive family history (Table 17.1, B). About one-third of patients in a large series of patients with SBMA had no known family history [13]. The existence of small families with few male offspring, late age of onset, premature death of at-risk male relatives, and the possibility of new mutations may explain apparently sporadic cases. Despite the increased knowledge about the clinical manifestations and readily available genetic testing, SBMA is still confused with other neuromuscular disorders including acquired or inherited anterior horn cell disorders, polyradiculoneuropathies, and myopathies including polymyositis.

The most frequent misdiagnosis is "atypical" amyotrophic lateral sclerosis (ALS). Approximately 1–2% of patients attending ALS

clinics had their diagnosis revised to SBMA after genetic testing was obtained [44]. Differentiation from ALS can be made by the presence of both lower and upper motor neuron signs including hyperreflexia, extensor plantar responses, and spasticity. Individuals with bulbar onset ALS or progressive bulbar palsy typically present with more prominent bulbar symptoms and have a more rapid disease progression. In progressive muscular atrophy distal lower motor neuron weakness prevails over bulbar symptoms, which occur late in the course of disease, whereas gynecomastia and sensory involvement are absent [45]. Facial-onset sensory and motor neuronopathy (FOSMN) syndrome, a recently described sporadic degenerative sensory and motor neuronopathy, may mimic SBMA although these patients typically present with early-onset facial numbness followed by progressive facial, bulbar, and upper extremity lower motor neuron weakness in a cranial to caudal distribution [46]. Among the autosomal recessive spinal muscular atrophies only SMA type 4 presents in adulthood with proximal lower motor neuron weakness. A missense mutation in the vesicle trafficking protein VAPB may cause an adult-onset, autosomal dominant motor neuron disease with variable clinical manifestations ranging from slowly progressive SMA with proximal weakness to classic amyotrophic lateral sclerosis [47]. An autosomal dominant inherited distal spinal and bulbar muscular atrophy caused by a mutation in the p150 subunit of dynactin, which is a microtubule protein important in retrograde axonal transport, has a distinct clinical phenotype. Affected individuals present with stridor resulting from vocal fold paresis followed later by weakness and atrophy in the face, hands, and distal legs [48]. The most common referral diagnoses of patients with unrecognized SBMA include atypical motor neuron disease, multifocal motor neuropathy, polyradiculoneuropathy, and myopathy. Accurate diagnosis is important to avoid unnecessary treatment, to provide genetic counseling for the patient and his family, and to give information about prognosis.

Prognosis

SBMA is characterized by slowly progressive weakness of bulbar and proximal extremity muscles. Progressive leg weakness results in gait impairment and may lead to wheelchair dependence 20–30 years after onset [1, 13]. The natural course of SBMA was assessed in a study of 223 genetically confirmed Japanese patients [12]. Individuals developed muscular weakness at the median age of 44 years, required handrail assistance when climbing stairs at 49 years, started to use a cane at 59 years, and required a wheelchair at 61 years. Despite the early presence of tongue atrophy and fasciculations, symptomatic dysarthria and dysphagia developed late in the sixth decade of life [12]. Life expectancy may be shortened by recurrent aspiration pneumonia and respiratory failure in about 10% of elderly individuals [1, 3, 12]. Fifteen of 223 patients died at the mean age of 65 years in the Japanese natural history study

[12]. A retrospective review of 39 patients referred to Mayo Clinic with confirmed SBMA indicated that their long-term survival was nearly as good as the normal unaffected population [49]. The study found 10-year survival to be 82% in the SBMA patients compared to 95% among age-matched controls. After a mean follow-up of 13 years patients remained independent in most activities of daily living. Climbing stairs and ambulation were impaired as 50% required some gait aids, but only 8% used wheelchairs. Although all patients had bulbar symptoms, none required gastrostomy placement or speech augmentation devices. A prospective observational study of a small cohort of confirmed SBMA patients over 3 years found that disease progression was more likely to be detected by objective motor functional tests such as the 6-minute walk, grip power, and decline in serum creatinine than by questionnaire-based functional rating scales [38].

Treatment

Currently there is no effective disease-modifying treatment available for patients with SBMA but there are symptomatic treatment options. Most patients will be relieved when they can be reassured about the slow disease progression and the normal or only minimally reduced life expectancy [12, 49].

Genetic counseling should be offered to the genetically confirmed affected individual and his family. The affected patient's daughters are obligate carriers and therefore have a 50% chance of having an affected son and a 50% chance of having a daughter who will be a carrier. None of his sons will be affected. All mothers of affected men who have been tested have been found to carry the CAG expansion. Due to the late onset of disease mothers may not be available for gene testing. The incidence of de novo mutations in men with SBMA is not known [43]. Male siblings who inherit the CAG expansion will be affected. Gene testing of at-risk asymptomatic adult males is not useful in predicting age of onset, disease severity, and progression.

Muscle cramps may be alleviated by adequate hydration, avoiding over-exertion of weakened muscles, and gentle stretching exercises. Quinine derivatives previously used for treating muscle cramps have been withdrawn by the US Food and Drug Administration due to safety concerns. Vitamin B complex, magnesium sulfate, and diltiazem are potentially helpful medications [50]. Baclofen, carbamazepine, gabapentin, and levetiracetam have been used in clinical practice but without the support of evidence-based studies. A randomized clinical trial of mexiletine reduced the frequency and intensity of muscle cramps in ALS patients and may warrant use for cramps in SBMA [51]. Patients should be seen annually for assessment of muscle strength, gait safety, aspiration risk, and pulmonary function tests. Evaluations by physical and occupational therapists are helpful to assist in activities of daily living and to delay the onset of disability. Braces, canes, and walkers are used to reduce the risk of falls and prolong the ability to ambulate. A minority of patients will require wheelchairs late in the disease. Patients with symptomatic dysphagia should be evaluated by swallowing videofluoroscopy supervised by a speech pathologist. Dietary modifications such as a mechanical soft diet, thickening of liquids to nectar consistency, and taking oral medications in yogurt or apple sauce may lessen swallowing difficulties. Indications for a percutaneous endoscopic gastrostomy (PEG) include progressive weight loss, frequent choking while eating, and aspiration on videofluoroscopy. According to the experience of patients with ALS, a PEG should be recommended when vital capacity is still greater than 50% predicted to avoid an increased risk of the procedure in patients with declining respiratory function [52]. Although rarely needed, speech-generating devices or computer tablets with speech applications are available in case the dysarthria is severe enough to interfere with communication. Orthopnea, morning headaches, and daytime drowsiness are symptoms suggestive of nocturnal hypoventilation. Nocturnal noninvasive positive pressure ventilation should be initiated when the vital capacity falls to or below 50% of predicted [52]. Administration of testosterone and its analogs is not effective in overcoming androgen insensitivity and is potentially harmful [53]. Gynecomastia can be corrected by breast reduction surgery.

There are no well-designed, large-scale studies in support of aerobic exercise programs in patients with SBMA. A study of eight patients participating in daily cycle exercises for 4 months showed little beneficial effect [54]. In a small open-label clinical trial, clenbuterol, a β2 agonist with anabolic effects on muscle, when given for 12 months improved the 6-minute walking distance and forced vital capacity between baseline and 12-month assessments [55],

Anti-androgen treatment

Anti-androgen therapy is very effective at blocking the disease onset and reducing progression of motor deficits in male transgenic mice harboring the human AR gene with expanded CAG repeats [2, 33, 36]. These findings have led to three randomized, placebo-controlled clinical trials of androgen reduction therapy in patients with SBMA. A randomized controlled trial with the testosterone-reducing agent leuprorelin in 50 patients with SBMA given for 48 weeks showed no clinically meaningful results [56]. At 48 weeks there was no significant difference in the primary outcome, the revised ALS functional rating scale, between treated and placebo groups. However, several positive biological effects were observed in the leuprorelin-treated group: swallowing function was improved by prolonging the cricopharyngeal opening duration; serum CK levels decreased; and the number of polyglutamine-positive scrotal skin cells was reduced. The promising results of this Phase 2 trial led to a large, multicenter, randomized, placebo-controlled trial of leuprorelin [57]. Two hundred patients were randomized to receive leuprorelin or placebo for 48 weeks. The study failed to show a beneficial effect of leuprorelin on swallowing function or secondary outcome measures such as the revised ALS functional rating scale although improved swallowing function was reported in a subgroup of patients whose disease duration was less than 10 years. At week 48, serum testosterone, CK levels, and the number of polyglutamine-positive scrotal skin cells were significantly reduced in the treated patients compared to those on placebo. The third anti-androgen clinical trial was undertaken at the National Institute of Neurological Disorders and Stroke with dutasteride, a 5α-reductase inhibitor that blocks the conversion of testosterone to dihydrotestosterone [58]. Based on differential levels of expression of the 5α-reductase in skeletal muscle and motor neurons, the suppression of dihydrotestosterone production was expected to reduce the toxicity of the mutant AR in motor neurons without losing the anabolic benefits of testosterone in muscle. This 2-year randomized, placebo-controlled trial failed to show a beneficial effect on the progression of muscle weakness measured by quantitative muscle strength assessment [58].

Why did anti-androgen treatments fail in human clinical trials despite showing benefits in animal models and having definite biological effects in humans? First, the chosen primary endpoints may not have been sensitive enough to detect any changes during the observation periods. The observation periods of 48 weeks or even 2 years may have been too short to show a beneficial effect in this slowly progressive disorder. Long-term androgen reduction with leuprorelin for 3.5 years also failed to prevent progression of leg weakness in a small open-label study [59]. Finally, the disease duration may be a crucial factor for treatment success as the loss of motor neurons, which increases over time, could only be prevented by early treatment [60]. Due to the slow rate of disease progression more sensitive outcome measures need to be explored in future clinical trials.

Future developments

New targets for therapeutic intervention are currently pursued in cell culture and transgenic animal models [61, 62]. The ubiquitin-proteasome system constitutes an important cellular defense mechanism against the accumulation of misfolded proteins. Heat shock protein 90 inhibition and increased expression of heat shock protein 70 facilitate proteasomal degradation of pathogenic AR, and ameliorate motor deficits in transgenic mice. Geldanamycin analogs that are potent HSP90 inhibitors have shown benefit in transgenic mice but are too toxic for long-term use. Arimoclomol, a co-inducer of the heat shock stress response, was reported to delay disease progression and to enhance motor neuron survival in transgenic mice [63]. A synthetic curcumin-related drug, ASC-JM17, has been reported to ameliorate motor weakness in transgenic SBMA mice by inducing anti-oxidant and heat shock responses and by promoting degradation of the mutant AR aggregation [64]. SBMA transgenic mice overexpressing muscle-restricted insulin-like growth factor 1 (IGF-1) showed increased clearance of the toxic AR aggregates through the ubiquitin-proteasome system. Systemic administration of IGF-1 complexed with IGF-1 binding protein also mitigated the muscle pathology and reduced both soluble and aggregated AR protein [62]. Tirasemtiv, a fast skeletal troponin activator that sensitizes the sarcomere to calcium and thereby increases the force of muscle contraction in denervated muscle, is currently in clinical trials for ALS and may warrant investigation in SBMA [65]. Gene silencing using micro-RNA or antisense oligonucleotides to reduce expression of the mutant AR gene in motor neurons or skeletal muscle has already had success in transgenic animal models and holds promise as an effective treatment strategy [66, 67].

Since the discovery of the expanded AR gene more than 25 years ago, basic and clinical research has deepened our understanding of the clinical phenotype and pathophysiology of SBMA. Hopefully, this better understanding will translate into effective disease-modifying treatments in the near future.

References

1. Kennedy WR, Alter M, Sung JH. Progressive proximal spinal and bulbar muscular atrophy of late onset. *Neurology* 1968; 18: 671–680.
2. Katsuno M, Adachi H, Waza M *et al.* Pathogenesis, animal models and therapeutics in spinal and bulbar muscular atrophy (SBMA). *Experimental Neurology* 2006; 200: 8–18.
3. Harding AE, Thomas PK, Baraitser M *et al.* X-linked recessive bulbospinal neuronopathy: a report of ten cases. *Journal of Neurology, Neurosurgery, and Psychiatry* 1982; 45: 1012–1019.
4. Fischbeck KH, Ionasescu V, Ritter AW *et al.* Localization of the gene for X-linked spinal muscular atrophy. *Neurology* 1986; 36: 1595–1598.
5. La Spada AR, Wilson EM, Lubahn DB *et al.* Androgen receptor gene mutations in X-linked spinal and bulbar muscular atrophy. *Nature* 1991; 352: 77–79.
6. Amato AA, Prior TW, Barohn RJ *et al.* Kennedy's disease: a clinicopathologic correlation with mutations in the androgen receptor gene. *Neurology* 1993; 43: 791–794.
7. Fischbeck KH. Polyglutamine expansion neurodegenerative disease. *Brain Research Bulletin* 2001; 56: 161–163.
8. Guidetti D, Sabadini R, Ferlini A *et al.* Epidemiological survey of X-linked bulbar and spinal muscular atrophy, or Kennedy disease, in the province of Reggio Emilia, Italy. *European Journal of Epidemiology* 2001; 17: 587–591.
9. Tanaka F, Manabu D, Yasuhiro I *et al.* Founder effect in spinal and bulbar muscular atrophy (SBMA). *Human Molecular Genetics* 1996; 5: 1253–1257.
10. Lund A, Udd B, Juvonen V *et al.* Founder effect in spinal and bulbar muscular atrophy (SBMA) in Scandinavia. *European Journal of Human Genetics* 2000; 8: 631–636.
11. Finsterer J. Perspectives of Kennedy's disease. *Journal of Neurological Sciences* 2010; 298: 1–10.
12. Atsuta N, Watanabe H, Ito M *et al.* Natural history of spinal and bulbar muscular atrophy (SBMA): a study of 223 Japanese patients. *Brain* 2006; 129: 1446–1455.
13. Rhodes LE, Freeman BK, Auh S *et al.* Clinical features of spinal and bulbar muscular atrophy. *Brain* 2009; 132: 3242–3251.
14. Sorenson EJ, Klein CJ. Elevated creatine kinase and transaminases in asymptomatic SMBA. *Amyotrophic Lateral Sclerosis* 2007; 8: 62–64.
15. Sperfeld AD, Karitzky J, Brummer D *et al.* X-linked bulbospinal neuronopathy. *Archives of Neurology* 2002; 59: 1921–1926.
16. Olney RK, Aminoff MJ, So YT. Clinical and electrodiagnostic features of X-linked recessive bulbospinal neuronopathy. *Neurology* 1991; 41: 823–828.
17. Ferrante MA, Wilbourn AJ. The characteristic electrodiagnostic features of Kennedy's disease. *Muscle & Nerve* 1997; 20: 323–329.
18. Arbizu T, Santamaría J, Gomez JM *et al.* A family with adult spinal and bulbar muscular atrophy, X-linked inheritance and associated testicular failure. *Journal of the Neurological Sciences* 1983; 59: 371–382.
19. Warner CL, Griffin JE, Wilson JD *et al.* X-linked spinomuscular atrophy: a kindred with associated abnormal androgen receptor binding. *Neurology* 1992; 42: 2181–2184.
20. Dejager S, Bry-Gauillard H, Bruckert E *et al.* A comprehensive endocrine description of Kennedy's disease revealing androgen insensitivity linked to CAG repeat length. *The Journal of Clinical Endocrinology & Metabolism* 2002; 87: 3893–3901.
21. Sinnreich M, Sorenson EJ, Klein CJ. Neurologic course, endocrine dysfunction and triplet repeat size in spinal bulbar muscular atrophy. *The Canadian Journal of Neurological Sciences* 2004; 31: 378–382.
22. Mariotti C, Castellotti B, Pareyson D *et al.* Phenotype manifestations associated with CAG-repeat expansion in the androgen receptor gene in male patients and heterozygous females: a clinical and molecular study of 30 families. *Neuromuscular Disorders* 2000; 10: 391–397.
23. Schmidt BJ, Greenberg CR, Allingham-Hawkins DJ *et al.* Expression of X-linked bulbospinal muscular atrophy (Kennedy's disease) in two homozygous women. *Neurology* 2002; 59: 770–772.
24. Doyu M, Sobue G, Mukai E *et al.* Severity of X-linked recessive bulbospinal neuronopathy correlates with size of the tandem CAG repeat in androgen receptor gene. *Annals of Neurology* 1992; 32: 707–710.
25. Shimada N, Sobue G, Doyu M *et al.* X-linked recessive bulbospinal neuronopathy: clinical phenotypes and CAG repeat size in androgen receptor gene. *Muscle & Nerve* 1995; 18: 1378–1384.
26. Liebermann AP, Fischbeck KH. Triplet repeat expansion in neuromuscular disease. *Muscle & Nerve* 2000; 23: 843–850.
27. Yamada M, Sato T, Tsuji S *et al.* CAG repeat disorder models and human neuropathology: similarities and differences. *Acta Neuropathologica* 2008; 115:71–86.
28. Sobue G, Hashizume Y, Mukai E *et al.* X-linked recessive bulbospinal neuronopathy: a clinicopathological study. *Brain* 1989; 112(1): 209–232.
29. Li M, Sobue G, Doyu M *et al.* Primary sensory neurons in X-linked recessive bulbospinal neuronopathy: histopathology and androgen receptor gene expression. *Muscle & Nerve* 1995; 18: 301–308.
30. Li M, Miwa S, Kobayashi Y *et al.* Nuclear inclusions of the androgen receptor protein in spinal and bulbar muscular atrophy. *Ann Neurol* 1998; 44: 249–254.
31. Cortes JC, Ling S-C, Guo LT *et al.* Muscle expression of mutant androgen receptor accounts for systemic and motor neuron disease phenotypes in spinal and bulbar muscular atrophy. *Neuron* 2014; 82: 295–307.
32. Adachi H, Katsuno M, Minamiyama M *et al.* Widespread nuclear and cytoplasmic accumulation of mutant androgen receptor in SBMA patients. *Brain* 2005; 128: 659–670.
33. Adachi H, Waza M, Katsuno M *et al.* Pathogenesis and molecular targeted therapy of spinal and bulbar muscular atrophy. *Neuropathology and Applied Neurobiology* 2007; 33: 135–151.
34. Banno H, Adachi H, Katsuno M *et al.* Mutant androgen receptor accumulation in spinal and bulbar muscular atrophy scrotal skin: a pathogenic marker. *Annals of Neurology* 2006; 59:520–526.

35. Katsuno M, Tanaka F, Adachi H et al. Pathogenesis and therapy of spinal and bulbar muscular atrophy (SBMA). *Progress in Neurobiology* 2012; 99:246–256.

36. Ranganathan S, Fischbeck KH. Therapeutic approaches to spinal and bulbar muscular atrophy. *Trends in Pharmacological Sciences* 2010; 31: 523–527.

37. Sumner CJ, Fischbeck KH. Jaw drop in Kennedy's disease. *Neurology* 2002; 59: 1471–1472.

38. Hashizume A, Katsuno M, Banno H et al. Longitudinal changes of outcome measures in spinal and bulbar muscular atrophy. *Brain* 2012; 135: 2838–2848.

39. Suzuki K, Katsuno M, Banno H et al. CAG repeat correlates to electrophysiological motor and sensory phenotypes in SBMA. *Brain* 2008; 131: 229–239.

40. Sorarù G, D'Ascenzo C, Polo A et al. Spinal and bulbar muscular atrophy: skeletal muscle pathology in male patients and heterozygous females. *Journal of the Neurological Sciences* 2008; 264: 100–105.

41. Hamano T, Mutoh T, Hirayama M et al. Muscle MRI findings of X-linked spinal and bulbar muscular atrophy. *Journal of the Neurological Sciences* 2004; 222: 93–97.

42. Araki A, Katsuno M, Suzuki K et al. Brugada syndrome in spinal and bulbar muscular atrophy. *Neurology* 2014; 82:1813–1821.

43. La Spada A. *Spinal and Bulbar Muscular Atrophy.* GeneReviews – NCBI Bookshelf. http://www.ncbi.nlm.nih.gov/books/NBK1333 (accessed 16 October 2011).

44. Parboosingh JS, Figlewicz DA, Krizus A et al. Spinobulbar muscular atrophy can mimic ALS: The importance of genetic testing in male patients with atypical ALS. *Neurology* 1997; 49: 568–572.

45. Kim W-K, Liu X, Sandner J et al. Study of 962 patients indicates progressive muscular atrophy is a form of ALS. *Neurology* 2009; 73: 1686–1692.

46. Vucic S, Tian D, Siao Tick Chong P et al. Facial onset sensory and motor neuronopathy (FOSMN syndrome): a novel syndrome in neurology. *Brain* 2006; 129: 3384–3390.

47. Nishimura AL, Mitne-Neto M, Silva HC et al. A mutation in the vesicle-trafficking protein VAPB causes late-onset spinal muscular atrophy and amyotrophic lateral sclerosis. *American Journal of Human Genetics* 2004; 75: 822–831.

48. Puls I, Oh SJ, Sumner CJ et al. Distal spinal and bulbar muscular atrophy caused by dynactin mutation. *Annals of Neurology* 2005; 57: 687–694.

49. Chahin N, Klein C, Mandrekar J et al. Natural history of spinal-bulbar muscular atrophy. *Neurology* 2008; 70: 1967–1971.

50. Katzberg HD, Khan AH, So YT. Assessment: Symptomatic treatment for muscle cramps (an evidence-based review). *Neurology* 2010; 74: 691–696.

51. Weiss MD, Macklin EA, Simmons Z et al. A randomized trial of mexiletine in ALS: Safety and effects on muscle cramps and progression. *Neurology* 2016; 86: 1474–1481.

52. Miller RG, Jackson CE, Kasarskis EJ et al. Practice Parameter update: The care of the patient with amyotrophic lateral sclerosis: Drug, nutritional, and respiratory therapies (an evidence-based review). *Neurology* 2009; 73: 1218–1226.

53. Kinirons P, Rouleau GA. Administration of testosterone results in reversible deterioration in Kennedy's disease. *Journal of Neurology, Neurosurgery, and Psychiatry* 2008; 79: 106–107.

54. Preisler N, Andersen G, Thøgersen F et al. Effect of aerobic training with spinal and bulbar muscular atrophy (Kennedy disease). *Neurology* 2009; 72: 317–323.

55. Querin G, D'Ascenzo C, Peterle E et al. Pilot trial of clenbuterol in spinal and bulbar muscular atrophy. *Neurology* 2013; 80: 2095–2098.

56. Banno H, Katsuno M, Suzuki K et al. Phase 2 trial of leuprorelin in patients with spinal and bulbar muscular atrophy. *Annals of Neurology* 2009; 65: 140–150.

57. Katsuno M, Banno H, Suzuki K et al. Efficacy and safety of leuprorelin in patients with spinal and bulbar muscular atrophy (JASMITT study): a multicentre, randomised, double-blind, placebo-controlled trial. *Lancet Neurology* 2010; 9:875–884.

58. Fernández-Rhodes LE, Kokkinis AD, White MJ et al. Efficacy and safety of dutasteride in patients with spinal and bulbar muscular atrophy: a randomised placebo-controlled trial. *Lancet Neurology* 2011; 10: 140–147.

59. Yamamoto T, Yokota K, Amao R, et al. An open trial of long-term testosterone suppression in spinal and bulbar muscular atrophy. *Muscle & Nerve* 2013; 47: 816–822.

60. Dengler R. Renewed hope for treatment of spinal and bulbar muscular atrophy? *Lancet Neurology* 2010; 9: 845–846.

61. Katsuno M, Banno H, Suzuki K et al. Molecular pathophysiology and disease-modifying therapies for spinal and bulbar muscular atrophy. *Archives of Neurology* 2012; 69: 436–440.

62. Fischbeck KH. Developing treatment for spinal and bulbar muscular atrophy. *Progress in Neurobiology* 2012; 99: 257–261.

63. Malik B, Nirmalananthan N, Gray AL et al. Co-induction of the heat shock response ameliorates disease progression in a mouse model of human spinal and bulbar muscular atrophy: implications for therapy. *Brain* 2013; 136; 926–943.

64. Bott LC, Badders NM, Chen K-L et al. A small molecule Nsf1 and Nrf2 activator mitigates polyglutamine toxicity in spinal and bulbar muscular atrophy. *Human Molecular Genetics* 2016; 25: 1979–1989.

65. Shefner JM, Watson ML, Meng L et al. A study to evaluate the safety and tolerability of repeated doses of tirasemtiv in patients with amyotrophic lateral sclerosis. *Amyotrophic Lateral Sclerosis and Frontotemporal Degeneration* 2013; 14: 574–581.

66. Pourshafie N, Lee PR, Chen KL et al. MiR counteracts mutant androgen receptor toxicity in spinal and bulbar muscular atrophy. *Molecular Therapy* 2016; 24: 937–945.

67. Sahashi K, Katsuno M, Hung G et al. Silencing neuronal mutant receptor in a mouse model of spinal and bulbar muscular atrophy. *Human Molecular Genetics* 2015; 24: 5985–5994.

CHAPTER 18
Optic Neuropathies

Desmond Kidd

Department of Clinical Neurosciences and Department of Neuro-ophthalmology, Royal Free Hospital, London, and University College London, UK

Introduction

There are 1.2 million retinal ganglion cells within each retina: 80% are midget cells, which form the parvocellular pathway, 10% are parasol cells, which constitute the magnocellular pathway, and the remainder form the melanopsin-containing koniocellular pathway. The parvocellular network has a very high cellular density at the fovea, leading to high spatial acuity, color vision, contrast sensitivity, and stereopsis, since each cell receives input from a single cone. Parasol and midget cells have the same density in the peripheral retina. Midget cells receive input from many photoreceptor cells, and so the spatial resolution is lower. These cells contribute more to motion detection and coarse stereopsis than to spatial acuity. Melanopsin-containing cells in the koniocellular pathway are thought to contribute to the integrity and function of the pupillary light reflex, as well as circadian rhythm [1].

The axons that arise from the foveal retinal ganglion cells form the papillomacular bundle. These unmyelinated axons pass through the retinal nerve fiber layer and enter the disc on the temporal side. The axons acquire myelin within the optic nerve. Unmyelinated fibers are more energy dependent since they conduct continuously rather than with the saltatory mechanism. This energy requirement must be appeased by provision of a higher density of mitochondria in the unmyelinated region, and the spread of mitochondria is much less dense in the myelinated axons within the optic nerve, being found predominantly at the nodes of Ranvier. Mitochondria are delivered to the axons via an axoplasmic transport mechanism which itself requires energy. Thus the unmyelinated retinal nerve fibers are vulnerable to oxidative stress and dysfunction of the respiratory chain mechanism of energy production.

Optic neuropathies that arise in the context of an inherited or degenerative neurological disease tend to have the same clinical characteristics: virtually without exception a disturbance of the function of the central visual field, color vision, and central acuity. This is due to a preferential involvement of the axons that form the papillomacular bundle [2]. It stands to reason, therefore, that provision of energy to these high-functioning, high-energy-requiring cells requires efficient mitochondrial function, and that these cells are vulnerable to damage if mitochondrial function is suboptimal or fails.

This chapter will describe the primary inherited optic neuropathies in detail, since these are the most common, then those in which optic neuropathy often arises within the clinical syndrome of a more widespread neurodegenerative disease, and finally uncommon conditions in which optic neuropathy may be seen, but not always. It will be seen that the majority of disorders shown share as a common etiological pathway a deficiency of mitochondrial function.

Leber's hereditary optic neuropathy (LHON)

Leber described the optic neuropathy that bears his name in 1871 [3]. It was appreciated early on that the disorder passed through maternal lines, and in 1988 gene mutations within the mitochondrial genome were first identified [4].

The prevalence in English, Dutch, and Finnish populations has been shown to be 1/30,000 to 1/50,000 [5–8] but it is seen in all ethnic groups. It is likely to be more common than has been documented, however, owing to a low clinical penetrance and underdiagnosis [8].

Clinical features

Men become affected five times more commonly than women, most often in the second and third decades, although the disorder has been seen in children and also in late age. In 95% of those affected the disorder will have become clinically manifest by the sixth decade [9]. The majority present with a subacute painless unilateral optic neuropathy. In 25% the visual loss is bilateral and synchronous [10, 11]. The acuity drop varies; some still see 6/6 (20/20) while others lose all sight in the eye. The majority reduce to 6/60 (20/200) or counting fingers. Color vision is lost in the affected eye, but in contrast to inflammatory optic neuropathies the pupillary response is not delayed (because the melanopsin ganglion cells in the photoreceptor layer are not involved) [12, 13]. The field defect varies, but the common defect is a central or centrocecal scotoma (Figure 18.1), which was seen in 87% of one series [11]. This increases in size and density over days after onset of symptoms and often becomes absolute, that is, there is no light perception within the defect. The chambers of the eye are quiet, but the disc often shows characteristic appearances: a circumpapillary telangiectatic microangiopathy, in which there is capillary dilatation within the disc, and sometimes vascular engorgement in the retinal vessels. There is swelling not of the disc but of the retina immediately around the disc, and (for the same reason) an absence of leakage of fluorescein from the disc at angiography (Figure 18.2). These signs may arise during acute visual loss, but also later in the other presymptomatic eye, and in unaffected carrier relatives. Other abnormalities may also be seen, for example

Neurodegeneration, First Edition. Edited by Anthony Schapira, Zbigniew Wszolek, Ted M. Dawson and Nicholas Wood.
© 2017 John Wiley & Sons, Ltd. Published 2017 by John Wiley & Sons, Ltd.

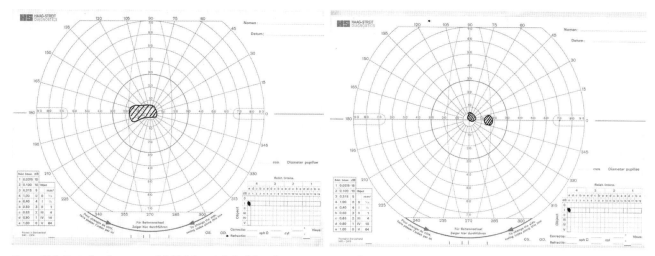

Figure 18.1 Central and centrocecal field defects in Leber's hereditary optic neuropathy.

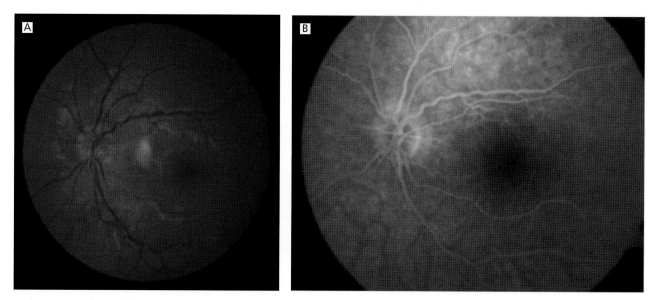

Figure 18.2 Disc photograph (A) and fluorescein angiogram (B) in Leber's hereditary optic neuropathy showing swelling around the disc and an absence of leakage from the disc itself.

a general disc swelling, macular edema, and retinal hemorrhage. In 20% of cases the disc is normal [10].

Visual loss deteriorates over 4–6 weeks and in the majority of cases does not improve (but see section Clinical course and prognosis). Over time the retinal swelling settles and the disc becomes pale, and often, since it is the retinal ganglion cells of the papillomacular bundle that are predominantly affected, cupped in the temporal quadrants [14].

In the vast majority of cases the other eye becomes affected within a year, normally within 8 weeks; persisting unilateral involvement is exceedingly rare [15].

Investigations

All blood investigation results are normal. MRI scans of the orbits may be normal initially, and high signal develops in the affected nerve over time; in others enhancement may be seen in the early stages [16]. In some cases enhancement and enlargement may be seen within the chiasm [17].

The CSF shows no abnormalities and an absence of oligoclonal bands [10, 11].

The visual evoked potential (VEP) in the early phase shows delay in the p100 and a diminished amplitude on the affected sides and the electroretinogram (ERG) is normal. Later the VEP becomes markedly attenuated or absent [18].

Clinical course and prognosis

Over time visual improvement may arise; this may be modest, for example islands of vision appearing within the central scotoma, but may be appreciable. Those with the 14484 mutation are most likely to improve and those with the 11778 the least likely. This improvement often begins slowly a year after symptom onset but has been seen to occur many years after a constant severe visual impairment [10, 11, 19].

Box 18.1 Mitochondrial structure and function

Mitochondria are organelles present in all cells. Their primary function is to produce energy in the form of ATP through the oxidative phosphorylation pathway. They also mediate cell death through apoptosis. Mitochondrial DNA is a 16.6 kb, circular, double-stranded molecule that encodes 37 genes, including 13 proteins that make up the OXPHOS system (see Figure X.X from mitochondrial chapter). This consists of a series of five enzymatic complexes situated on the inner mitochondrial membrane where, along with ubiquinone and cytochrome c, an electrochemical gradient develops that drives ATP production from ADP [65].

Mitochondria are bound by an inner and an outer membrane. The outer membrane is permeable, the inner not, leading to the establishment of an electrochemical gradient. The inner membrane contains the proteins that form an essential role in tissue and organ function and homeostasis, particularly in oxidative phosphorylation and in protein and fatty acid metabolism. Mitochondria also regulate energy production and metabolism. They undergo constant change undergoing fission and fusion, which is important in the regulation of mitochondrial function. Mutations within the complex I region of the mitochondrial genome lead to defective oxidative phosphorylation. Mitofusin 1 and 2 are important signaling proteins

that regulate fusion of the outer mitochondrial membrane, and OPA-1 performs the same function in the inner membrane. Abnormalities of these proteins can reduce energy synthesis leading to an increase in free radical production; together these reduce membrane potential and so increase the chance of apoptosis of the cell.

Mitochondrial function is also dependent on nuclear genes such as polymerase gamma (*POLG*), twinkle, and MtDNA transcription factor A, which deal with mitochondrial maintenance and repair, so that genetic abnormalities outside of the mitochondrion also affect mitochondrial function and trigger apoptosis.

Mutations, duplications, and deletions within the genome and within nuclear genes that interact with the respiratory chain lead to a variety of neurological and systemic disorders, for example mitochondrial encephalomyopathy, lactic acidosis, and stroke-like episodes (MELAS), myoclonic epilepsy with ragged red fibers (MERRF), and neuropathy, ataxia, and retinitis pigmentosa (NARP). Mitochondrial dysfunction is also implicated in many other neurodegenerative diseases, for example Parkinson and Huntington's diseases, Friedreich's ataxia, and hereditary spastic paraparesis [65].

Other neurological features

In most families the disorder is manifest only as a visual impairment. Some families also have cardiac conduction defects, myoclonus, neuropathy, and myopathy. In others, more widespread neurological problems may be associated, for example dystonia, chorea, brainstem disorders such as ataxia and tremor, and episodes of encephalopathy with lactic acidosis [10, 20–22]. These have been shown to be associated with additional mutations elsewhere within the mitochondrial genome [23].

Anita Harding observed in 1992 that some female patients with Leber mutations may develop a relapsing inflammatory neurological disease indistinguishable from multiple sclerosis (MS); women are affected twice as often as men and oftentimes have a greater than average visual loss. MRI shows characteristic abnormalities and the CSF contains oligoclonal bands [24]. The disorder arises in those with each of the three mutations known [25]. It is not yet known if the two disorders arise because of the stress of the inflammatory illness inducing phenotypic presentation of the inherited disorder or if the mitochondrial disorder itself induces an immune cascade leading to demyelination.

Genetics and pathogenesis

For an explanation of mitochondrial structure and the deleterious effects of genetic mutation on mitochondrial function see Box 18.1.

Three point mutations in the mitochondrial genome account for 90% of cases of LHON [8, 9, 11]. That located at position 11778 accounts for 70% of cases, and those at positions 14484 and 3460 account for around 14% each, although these proportions vary in different populations [9]. These mutations are found only in families with LHON. Secondary mutations are found with higher frequency in LHON families although their significance is not yet understood [9]. The 10% without any of the above mutations have been shown to have nucleotide mutations when the genome has been sequenced.

The genetic defect has a low rate of penetrance; around 50% of men with the mutation will present with optic neuropathy and only 10% of females. The risk is greatest in the third decade (the median age of onset is 20 years in men and older in females), so the risk reduces with age. A family history of diagnosed optic neuropathy is absent in around 40% of cases. The risk of visual loss in asymptomatic carriers of any of the three pathogenic mutations is 46% in men and 11% in women [9, 26–28]. Genetic heteroplasmy may

also influence the risk; it is thought that the mutational load must exceed 60% before the clinical features can develop [29]. The haplotype background is also important [30].

The mutation leads to an impairment of oxidative phosphorylation with underproduction of ATP. If this arises suddenly and in circumstances of oxidative stress, ATP production fails, free radicals and reactive oxygen species are produced, and increased glutamate production leads to cell death [31]. The retinal ganglion cell becomes swollen then degenerates through apoptosis. Atrophy ensues. The cells of the retinal pigment epithelium and the photoreceptor layer are not involved.

Why males are affected so much more than females is not understood; it is thought that nuclear modifier genes on the X chromosome may be involved [30]. Hormonal factors may also be important. In certain families the prevalence of disease manifestation reduces very substantially over time; the reasons are not known.

Environmental triggers remain important in addition; the fact that there exist several pairs of monozygotic twins, only one of whom has expressed the disease, proves this point. Cigarette smoking seems to have an important link [32], with 93% of affected men being smokers in a retrospective study. Drugs, in particular antibiotics such as ethambutol and erythromycin and antiretroviral drugs, have shown a close link to the development of visual loss in those with mutations.

Treatment

Vitamins and antioxidants such as coenzyme Q-10 have not been shown to provoke benefits [33]. Idebenone, a derivative of coenzyme Q-10, has shown an effect; a double-blind, placebo-controlled study showed a mean change in acuity over 24 months of therapy of −0.135 vs −0 071 logMAR units, which did not reach statistical significance; however with subgroup analysis a greater improvement was seen in patients with discordant visual acuities, suggesting that earlier treatment may proffer greater benefits [34]. Affected carriers receive genetic counselling and are strongly encouraged not to smoke.

Future therapies under investigation include gene insertion and shifting, and nuclear transfer (reviewed in [35]).

Dominant optic atrophy

This autosomal dominant disorder is as common as LHON, with a prevalence of 1/35,000. It is particularly common in Denmark, where it was first described in 1956 by Kjer.

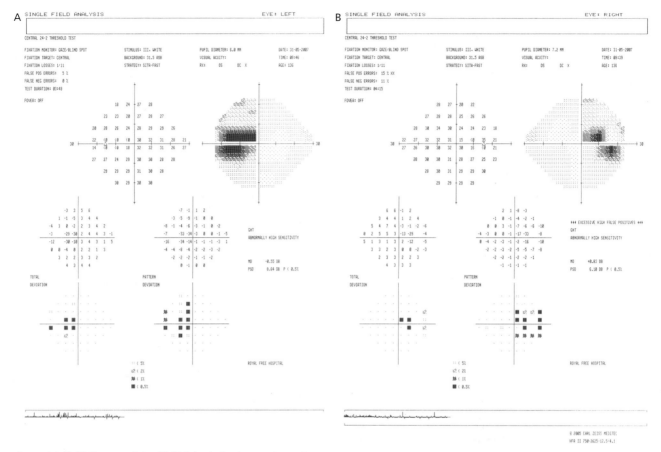

Figure 18.3 (A, B) Centrocecal visual field defect in dominant optic atrophy.

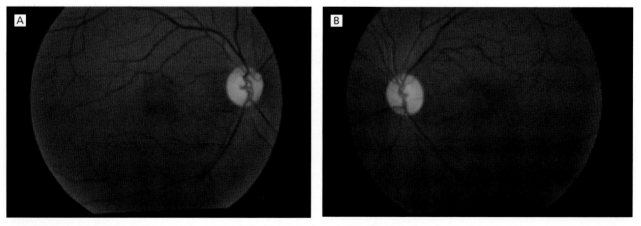

Figure 18.4 (A, B) Disc photographs in dominant optic atrophy showing disc pallor.

Clinical features

There is a progressive synchronous bilateral visual loss which usually begins late in the first decade of life [36–39]. Visual loss may be unnoticed, and may only deteriorate very slowly indeed. There is much variation in the phenotype within families and between families. In general it is uncommon for the acuity to drop below 6/60 (20/200). Some families find that the visual loss continues into late years whilst in the majority a plateau develops in middle age [39]. Color vision for both red–green and blue–yellow is lost, although only some 10% are tritanopic [40].

The fields show central or centrocecal defects for the most part (Figure 18.3), although bitemporal defects have also been seen. The discs are pale throughout or only in the temporal regions (Figure 18.4), and sometimes excavated. Retinal nerve fiber layer thickness measured using optical coherence tomography is reduced in most cases, even those discs that appear normal at slit lamp biomicroscopy [41]. This is most pronounced within the papillomacular bundle [42]. As in LHON, the retinal ganglion cells that subserve the light reflex are not affected so that the pupillary responses tend to be normal.

Investigations

Imaging is normal, and electrophysiological testing reveals a reduced amplitude rather than prolonged VEP (which is not as prolonged as that seen in inflammatory optic neuropathies), with reduced amplitude of the N95 component of the ERG, in keeping with retinal ganglion cell dysfunction.

Genetics and pathogenesis

The genetic abnormalities are widespread, with many different single base pair substitution mutations within the OPA-1 gene, and also missense mutations, deletions, and insertions. The result is that the OPA-1 protein is reduced and abnormal, leading to oxidative stress and retinal ganglion cell death. The majority of families have OPA-1 mutations, mutations in OPA-3 being much less common [43].

X-linked and recessive forms

An X-linked disorder has been described (OPA-2) [44] as have two recessive disorders related to OPA-6 and -7 [45]. OPA-7 is associated with other neurological abnormalities.

Other neurological features

Some families show additional neurological abnormalities, for example deafness, ocular motor abnormalities simulating chronic progressive external ophthalmoplegia, ataxia, myopathy, and neuropathy. These were formerly considered to be uncommon, but a series from England showed a prevalence of neuropathy and myopathy of 30–40% and of deafness of 62% [46]. Histochemical analysis of muscle has revealed a higher prevalence of cytochrome c oxidase deficiency associated with secondary mitochondrial DNA deletions in patients with additional clinical features [46]. OPA-3, -4, and -8 are associated with additional neurological abnormalities (reviewed in [39]).

Treatment

No treatment is available. Like carriers of LHON, patients are advised not to smoke.

Optic neuropathy and hereditary neuropathy

The association between optic neuropathy and inherited neuropathy has been known for some time, and has been designated hereditary motor and sensory neuropathy (HMSN) type VI. There are dominant and recessive forms [47, 48], and sporadic forms also exist. In general these are axonal-type sensorimotor neuropathies that are slowly progressive, and the optic neuropathy follows a similar course. The clinical features and relative severity vary between families; in some cases either of the systems involved can be entirely asymptomatic.

The disorder has been studied in more detail with the discovery of mutations within the mitofusin 2 (MFN2) gene; MSN2 functions as a signalling protein in the maintenance of the integrity of the outer mitochondrial membrane [49].

The optic neuropathy is most often progressive and becomes severe over many years, precluding useful vision. However in a few cases the visual disorder may be subacute and may in time recover. In a Korean series [50], 3 of 26 patients studied had optic neuropathy and in all cases it was progressive. Those affected had central scotomata and pale optic discs. The acuities were around 20/200.

In an American series of 10 patients with MFN2 mutations and optic neuropathy [51], the neuropathy began in early childhood and became progressively severe; only one patient was not wheelchair bound. The optic neuropathy was progressive in four patients, with a subacute onset with "partial recuperation" in the remainder. Each showed clear signs of optic neuropathy with pale discs, normal retinae, central visual field defects, and a low-amplitude, slightly delayed VEP. The onset of the visual impairment varied and in some cases it arose years after the neuropathy had been diagnosed. Many of these patients had white matter abnormalities on MRI which appear to have been asymptomatic.

The author has seen a family of seven members in which a subacute optic neuropathy arose in childhood and remained stable for around 10 years before improving spontaneously and not recurring. The optic neuropathy at presentation was typical of that seen in LHON, with swelling around the disc and capillary telangiectasia formation followed by pallor due to atrophy. The majority of cases have regained normal vision in their thirties. The sensorimotor neuropathy is progressive, very mild (in three cases entirely asymptomatic) until late middle age, and the penetrance of the disorder within the family is high. There is a new mutation in the MFN2 gene.

Optic neuropathy and other central nervous system degenerative disorders

Friedreich's ataxia

This autosomal recessive disorder is caused by a trinucleotide repeat within the FXN gene on chromosome 9q13. The gene lies within the mitochondria, but its exact function has not yet been determined [52]. Deficient frataxin protein is associated with reductions in mitochondrial respiration and impairments of proteins and enzymes containing iron and sulfur. There is cell loss in the dorsal root ganglia and dentate nucleus of the cerebellum, and degeneration of the axons within the dorsal columns and corticospinal and spinocerebellar tracts of the cord. There is an axonal neuropathy.

Involvement of the visual system is very common, with most patients showing evidence of optic neuropathy on examination. Some are seemingly asymptomatic; others show more striking abnormalities. There is no relationship between the number of GAA repeats and severity or incidence of visual loss. The disorder is progressive in most cases, and there is evidence for a reduction in color appreciation. A series of visual field defects is seen, including a general constriction, central scotoma, or arcuate defect [53]. The disc is pale and optical coherence tomography (OCT) examination shows atrophy in most cases. The VEP is abnormal with evidence of axonal loss leading to reduction in VEP amplitude, without slowing. In one series an abrupt visual loss resembling LHON was seen in two patients and was associated with a particularly large number of triplet repeats [53].

The spinocerebellar ataxias

One study has shown involvement of the retinal nerve fiber layer in spinocerebellar ataxia (SCA) 1 [54]. Another study of small groups of patients with SCA1, SCA2, SCA3, and SCA6 has also shown thinning of the retinal nerve fiber layer in all groups [55], although no data on the visual function of any of the patients studied were supplied. Only those patients with SCA3 are considered to be affected frequently with signs of optic neuropathy [56]. Patients with SCA7 do not have neuropathy but often have significant involvement of the retinae.

Hereditary spastic paraplegia (HSP)

Optic neuropathy may be seen in many of the "HSP plus" syndromes, particularly that associated with mutations in *SPG7*, which causes a recessive form associated with prominent bilateral optic neuropathy, HSP7 [57]. These cases had ragged red fibers and defective oxidative phosphorylation.

DIDMOAD (Wolfram) syndrome

Insulin-dependent diabetes develops early in childhood and is characterized by earlier than usual microvascular complications. Optic atrophy is noted first towards the end of the first decade and is progressive, leading to complete blindness over years. In their teens patients develop diabetes insipidus and deafness [58]. In the second and third decades, progressive ataxia and dementia with cortical atrophy develop; death occurs with respiratory complications due to brainstem atrophy in the fourth or fifth decade.

The disorder relates to a number of frameshift and splice site mutations in the gene *WFS1* on 4p16.1 [59], which encodes an endoplasmic reticulum membrane-embedded protein, wolframin. Nonsense *WFS1* transcripts are unstable and are degraded, so that membrane transport proteins are not created and the cell dies.

In the eye wolframin is located in the retinal ganglion cells and photoreceptors, and in glial cells in the proximal portion of the optic nerve [59].

Other neurodegenerative disorders

Other disorders have been described in which optic neuropathy coexists with deafness, ophthalmoparesis, ataxia, paraparesis, neuropathy, and cognitive decline to varying degrees, including progressive encephalopathy with edema, hypsarrhythmia, and optic atrophy (PEHO) syndrome, Behr's syndrome, and Costeff syndrome. It would be anticipated that with time these disorders will be shown to be associated with defects in mitochondrial function, for example *POLG* [60] and *OPA3* mutations [61].

Deafness, dystonia, optic neuropathy (Mohr–Tranebjaerg) syndrome

This is an uncommon X-linked disorder of childhood onset in which progressive deafness and dystonia develop in childhood. The disorder evolves and the patient develops blindness due to optic neuropathy and cortical degeneration in early adulthood, then a progressive dementia ensues in the fourth and fifth decades [62]. Imaging in the late stages shows a striking atrophy of the occipital and parietal cortices, and the discs are atrophic. The disorder is linked to mutations in the DDP1/*TIMM8A* gene which is involved in the transport and organization of nuclear-encoded precursor proteins to the inner membrane of the mitochondrion [63, 64].

References

1. Prasad S, Galetta SL. Anatomy and physiology of the afferent visual system. In: Kennard C, Leigh RJ (eds), *Handbook of Clinical Neurology*, vol 102 (3rd series), Neuro-ophthalmology. Elsevier, Oxford; 2011: 3–12.
2. Carelli V, Ross-Cisneros FN, Sadun AA. Mitochondrial dysfunction as a cause of optic neuropathies. *Progr Retin Eye Res* 2004; 23: 53–89.
3. Leber T. Uber hereditare und congenitalangelegte schnervenleiden. *Von Graefes Archiv fur Ophthalmol* 1871; 17: 249–91.
4. Wallace DC, Singh G, Lott MT, Hodge JA, Schurr TG, Lezza AM, Elsas LJ, Nikoskelainen EK. Mitochondrial DNA mutation associated with Leber's hereditary optic neuropathy. *Science* 1988; 242: 1427–30.
5. Man PYW, Griffiths PG, Brown DT, Howell N, Turnbull DM, Chinnery PF. The epidemiology of Leber hereditary optic neuropathy in the North East of England. *Am J Hum Genet* 2003; 72: 333–9.
6. Spruit L, Kolback DN, de Coo RF, Plomp AS, Bauer NJ, Smeets HJ, de Die-Smulders CEM. Influence of mutational type on clinical expression of Leber hereditary optic neuropathy. *Am J Ophthalmol* 2006; 141: 676–82.
7. Puomila A, Hamalainen P, Kiioja S, Savontaus ML, Koivumaki S, Huoponen K, Nikoskelainen E. Epidemiology and penetrance of Leber hereditary optic neuropathy in Finland. *Eur J Hum Genet* 2007; 20: 177–84.
8. Sadun AA, La Morgia C, Carelli V. Leber's hereditary optic neuropathy. *Curr Treat Options Neurol* 2011; 13: 109–17.
9. Man PYW, Griffiths PG, Hudson G, Chinnery PF. Inherited mitochondrial optic neuropathies. *J Med Genet* 2009; 46: 145–58.
10. Nikoskelainen EK. Clinical picture of LHON. *Clin Neurosci* 1994; 2: 115–20.
11. Riordan-Eva P, Sanders MD, Govan GG, Sweeney MG, DaCosta J, Harding AE. The clinical features of Leber's hereditary optic neuropathy defined by the presence of pathogenic mitochondrial DNA mutations. *Brain* 1995; 118: 319–37.
12. Kawasaki A, Herbst K, Sander B, Milea D. Selective wavelength pupillometry in Leber hereditary optic neuropathy. *Clin Experiment Ophthalmol* 2010; 38: 322–4.
13. LaMorgia C, Ross-Cisneros FN, Sadun AA, Hannibal J, Munarini A, Mantovani V. Melanopsin retinal ganglion cells are resistant to neurodegeneration in mitochondrial optic neuropathies. *Brain* 2010; 133: 2426–38.
14. Mashima Y, Kimura I, Yamamoto Y, Ohde H, Ohtake Y, Tanino T, Tomita G, Oguchi Y. Optic disc excavation in the atrophic stage of Leber's hereditary optic neuropathy. Comparison with normal tension glaucoma. *Graefes Arch Clin Exp Ophthalmol* 2003; 241: 75–80.
15. Nikoskelainen EK, Huoponen K, Juvonen V, Lamminen T, Nummelin K, Savontaus ML. Ophthalmic findings in Leber hereditary optic neuropathy, with special reference to mtDNA mutations. *Ophthalmology* 1996; 103: 504–14.
16. Vaphiades MS, Newman NJ. Optic nerve enhancement on orbital magnetic resonance imaging in Leber's hereditary optic neuropathy. *J Neuro-ophthalmol* 1999; 19: 238–9.
17. Phillips PH, Vaphiades MS, Glasier CM, Gray LG, Lee AG. Chiasmal enlargement and optic nerve enhancement on magnetic resonance imaging in Leber hereditary optic neuropathy. *Arch Ophthalmol* 2003; 121: 577–9.
18. Dorfman LJ, Nikoskelainen E, Rosenthal AR, Sogg RL. Visual evoked potentials in Leber's hereditary optic neuropathy. *Ann Neurol* 1977; 1: 565–8.
19. Nakamura M, Yamamoto M. Variable pattern of visual recovery of Leber's hereditary optic neuropathy. *Br J Ophthalmol* 2000; 84: 534–5.
20. Spruijt L, Smeets HJ, Hendrickx A, Bettink-Remeijer MW, Maat-Kievit A, Schoonderwoerd KC, Sluiter W, de Coo IF, Hintzen RQ. A MELAS-associated ND-1 mutation causing Leber hereditary optic neuropathy and spastic dystonia. *Arch Neurol* 2007; 64: 890–3.
21. LaMorgia C, Achilli A, Iommarini L, Barboni P, Pala M, Olivieri A. Rare mtDNA variants in Leber hereditary optic neuropathy families with recurrence of myoclonus. *Neurology* 2008; 70: 762–70.
22. Clarencon F, Touze E, Leroy-Willig A, Turmel H, Naggara O, Pavy S, Brezin A, Mas JL. Spastic paraparesis as a manifestation of Leber's disease. *J Neurol* 2006; 253; 525–6.
23. De Vries DD, Went LN, Bruyn GW, Scholte HR, Hofstra RM, Bolhuis PA. Genetic and biochemical impairment of mitochondrial complex I activity in a family with Leber hereditary optic neuropathy and hereditary spastic dystonia. *Am J Hum Genet* 1996; 58: 703–11.
24. Harding AE, Sweeney MG, Miller DH, Mumford CJ, Kellar-Wood H, Menard D, et al. Occurrence of a multiple sclerosis-like illness in women who have a Leber's hereditary optic neuropathy mitochondrial DNA mutation. *Brain* 1992; 115: 979–89.
25. Palace J. Multiple sclerosis associated with Leber's hereditary optic neuropathy. *J Neurol Sci* 2009; 286: 24–7.
26. Harding AE, Sweeney MG, Govan GG, Riordan-Eva P. Pedigree analysis in Leber hereditary optic neuropathy families with a pathogenic mtDNA mutation. *Am J Hum Genet* 1995; 57: 77–86.
27. Mackey DA, Oostra RJ, Rosenberg T, Nikoskelainen E, Bronte-Stewart J, Pulton J, Harding AE, Govan G, Bolhuis PA, Norby S. Primary pathogenic mtDNA mutations in multigeneration pedigrees with Leber hereditary optic neuropathy. *Am J Hum Genet* 1996; 59: 481–5.
28. Man PYW, Griffiths PG, Chinnery PF. Mitochondrial optic neuropathies – disease mechanisms and therapeutic strategies. *Progr Retin Eye Res* 2011; 30: 81–114.
29. Chinnery PF, Andrews RM, Turnbull DM, Howell NN. Leber hereditary optic neuropathy: does heteroplasmy influence the inheritance and expression of the G11778A mitochondrial DNA mutation? *Am J Med Genet* 2001; 98: 235–43.
30. Hudson G, Carelli V, Spruijt L, Gerards M, Mowbray C, Achilli A et al. Clinical expression of Leber hereditary optic neuropathy is affected by the mitochondrial DNA-haplotype background. *Am J Hum Genet* 2007; 81: 228–33.

31. Zanna C, Ghelli A, Porcelli AM, Martinuzzi A, Carelli V, Rugolo M. Caspase-independent death of Leber's hereditary optic neuropathy cybrids is driven by energetic failure and mediated by AIF and endonuclease G. *Apoptosis* 2005; 10: 997–1007.

32. Kirkman MA, Man PYU, Korsten A, Leonhardt M, Dimitriadis K, De Coo IF, Klopstock T, Chinnery PF. Gene-environment interactions in Leber hereditary optic neuropathy. *Brain* 2009; 132: 2317–26.

33. Sadun AA, LaMorgia C, Carelli V. Leber's hereditary optic neuropathy. *Curr Treat Options Neurol* 2011; 13: 109–11.

34. Klopstock T, Man PYW, Dimitiadis K, Rouleau J, Heck S, Bailie M et al. A randomised placebo-controlled trial of idebenone in Leber's hereditary optic neuropathy. *Brain* 2011; 134: 2677–86.

35. Newman NJ. Treatment of hereditary optic neuropathies. *Nat Rev Neurol* 2012; 8: 545–56.

36. Kjer P. Infantile optic atrophy with dominant mode of inheritance: a clinical and genetic study of 19 Danish families. *Acta Ophthalmol* **1959**: 1–146.

37. Kline LB, Glazer JS. Dominant optic atrophy – clinical profile. *Arch Ophthalmol* 1979; 97: 1680–6.

38. Man PYW, Griffiths PG, Burke A, Sellar PW, Clarke MP, Gnanaraj L, Ah Kine D, Hudson G, Szermin G, Taylor RW, Horvath R, Chinnery PJ. The prevalence and natural history of dominant optic atrophy due to OPA-1 mutations. *Ophthalmology* 2010; 117: 1538–46.

39. Lenaers G, Hamel CP, Lelettre C, Amati-Bonneau P, Procaccio V, Bonneau P, Milea D. Dominant optic atrophy. *Orphanet J Rare Dis* 2012; 7: 46.

40. Berninger TA, Jaeger W, Krastel H. Electrophysiology and colour perimetry in dominant infantile optic atrophy. *Br J Ophthalmol* 1991; 75: 49–52.

41. Milea D, Sander B, Wegener M, Jensen H, Kjer B, Jorgensen TM. Axonal loss occurs early in dominant optic atrophy. *Acta Ophthalmol* 2010; 88: 342–6.

42. Man PYW, Bailie M, Atawan A, Chinnery PF, Griffiths PG. Pattern of retinal ganglion cell loss in dominant optic atrophy due to OPA-1 mutations. *Eye (Lond)* 2011; 25: 596–602.

43. Man PYW, Shankar SP, Biousse V, Miller NR, Bean LJ, Coffee B, Heqde M, Newman NJ. Genetic screening for OPA1 and OPA3 mutations in patients with suspected inherited optic neuropathies. *Ophthalmology* 2011; 118: 558–63.

44. Katz BJ, Zhao Y, Warner JE, Tong Z, Yang Z, Zhang K. A family with X-linked optic atrophy linked to the OPA-2 locus Xp11.4-Xp11.2. *Am J Med Genet* 2006; 140: 2207–11.

45. Barbet F, Gerber S, Hakiki S, Perrault I, Hanein S, Ducroq D, et al. A first locus for isolated autosomal recessive optic atrophy (ROA1) maps to chromosome 8q. *Eur J Hum Genet* 2003; 11: 966–71.

46. Man PYW, Griffiths PG, Gorman GS, Lourenco CM, Wright AF, Auer-Grumbach M et al. Multi-system neurological disease is common in patients with OPA1 mutations. *Brain* 2010; 133: 771–86.

47. Chalmers RM, Bird AC, Harding AE. Autosomal dominant optic atrophy with asymptomatic peripheral neuropathy. *J Neurol Neurosurg Psychiatry* 1996; 60: 195–6.

48. Chalmers RM, Riordan-Eva P, Wood NW. Autosomal recessive inheritance of hereditary motor and sensory neuropathy with optic atrophy. *J Neurol Neurosurg Psychiatry* 1997; 62: 385–7.

49. Zuchner S, Mersiyanova IV, Muglia M, Bissar-Tadmouri N, Rochelle J, Daali EL et al. Mutations in the mitochondrial GTPase mitofusin 2 cause Charcot-Marie-Tooth neuropathy type 2A. *Nat Genet* 2004; 36: 449–51.

50. Chung KW, Kim SB, Park KD, Choi KG, Lee JH, Eun HW et al. Early onset severe and late-onset mild Charcot-Marie-Tooth disease with mitofusin 2 (MFN2) mutations. *Brain* 2006; 129: 2103–18.

51. Zuchner S, De Jonghe P, Jordanova A, Claeys KG, Guerguelteva V, Cherninkova S et al. Axonal neuropathy with optic atrophy (HMSN VI) is caused by mutations in mitofusin 2. *Ann Neurol* 2006; 59: 276–81.

52. Marmolino D. Friedreich's ataxia: past, present and future. *Brain Res Rev* 2011; 67: 311–30.

53. Fortuna F, Barboni P, Liquori R, Valentino ML, Savini G, Gellera C, Mariotti C, Rizzo G, Tonon C, Manners D, Lodi R, Sadun AA, Carelli V. Visual system involvement in Friedreich's ataxia. *Brain* 2009; 132: 116–23.

54. Stricker S, Oberwahrenbrock T, Zimmermann H, Schoeter J, Endres M, Brandt AU, Friedemann P. Temporal retinal nerve fiber loss in patients with spinocerebellar ataxia type 1. *PLoS One* 2011; 6: e23024.

55. Pula JH, Towle VL, Staszak VM, Cao D, Bernard JT, Gomez CM. Retinal nerve fibre layer and macular thinning in spinocerebellar ataxia and multiple system atrophy. *Neuroophthalmology* 2011; 35: 108–14.

56. Junck L, Fink JK. Machado-Joseph disease and SCA **3**: the genotype meets the phenotypes. *Neurology* 1996; 46: 4–8.

57. Wilkinson PA, Crosby AH, Turner C, Bradley LJ, Ginsberg L, Wood N, Schapira AH, Warner TT. A clinical, genetic and biochemical study of SPG7 mutations in hereditary spastic paraplegia. *Brain* 2004; 127: 973–80.

58. Hoffman S, Philbrook C, Gerbitz KD, Bauer MF. Wolfram syndrome: structural and functional analyses of mutant and wild type wolframin, the WSF1 gene product. *Hum Mol Genet* 2003; 12: 2003–12.

59. Rigoli L, Lombardo F, Di Bella C. Wolfram syndrome and WFS1 gene. *Clin Genet* 2011; 79: 103–17.

60. Mancuso M, Filosto M, Bellan M, Liguori R, Mantagna P, Baruzzi A, DiMauro S, Carelli V. POLG mutations causing ophthalmoplegia, sensorimotor polyneuropathy, ataxia, and deafness. *Neurology* 2004; 62: 316–8.

61. Carelli V, LaMorgia C, Valentino ML, Barboni P, Ross-Cisneros FN, Sadun AA. Retinal ganglion cell neurodegeneration in mitochondrial disorders. *Biochem Biophys Acta* 2009 1787: 518–28.

62. Tranebjaerg L, Scwartz C, Eriksen H, Anreasson S, Ponavic V, Dahl A, Stevenson RE, May M, Arena F, Barker D, et al. A new X linked recessive deafness syndrome with blindness, dystonia, fractures and mental deficiency is linked to Xq22. *J Med Genet* 1995; 32: 257–63.

63. Roesch K, Curran SP, Tranebjaerg L, Koehler CM. Human deafness dystonia syndrome is caused by a defect in assembly of the DDP1 / TIMM8A - TIMM13 complex. *Hum Mol Genet* 2002; 11: 477–86.

64. Binder J, Hoffman S, Kreisel S, Wohrle JC, Bazner H, Krauss JK, Hennerici MG, Bauer MF. Clinical and molecular findings in a patient with a novel mutation in the deafness-dystonia peptide (DDP1) gene. *Brain* 2003; 126: 1814–20.

65. Schapira AHV. Mitochondrial diseases. *Lancet* 2012; 379: 1825–34.

CHAPTER 19

Peripheral Nerve Neuropathies Including Charcot–Marie–Tooth Disease

Amelie Pandraud and Henry Houlden

Department of Molecular Neuroscience and MRC Centre for Neuromuscular Diseases, UCL Institute of Neurology, London, UK

Clinical definition, epidemiology, and causes of peripheral neuropathies

The peripheral nervous system

Peripheral nerves carry information from the brain and spinal cord located in the central nervous system (CNS) to all parts of the body, and relay this information back to the CNS. Nerve fibers may be myelinated or unmyelinated. In the peripheral nervous system (PNS), Schwann cells start to ensheath axons larger than 1 μm in diameter with their plasma membrane early on in development [1]. The myelin produced in this process nourishes the axon and facilitates saltatory conduction of action potentials at the nodes of Ranvier. In the PNS, compact myelin, which accounts for most of the myelin membrane, contains cholesterol and other lipids, as well as proteins such as myelin protein zero and peripheral myelin protein 22. The non-compact myelin contains proteins such as myelin-associated glycoprotein and connexin-32. The composition of the peripheral nerve is important to highlight because many of the structural proteins cause nerve dysfunction and a neuropathy when they are genetically defective.

Types and prevalence of peripheral neuropathies

Peripheral neuropathy can result from damage to sensory, motor, and/or autonomic nerves and may primarily affect the axon, cell body, or myelin sheath. Peripheral neuropathies may also be classified according to the number of nerves affected. Mononeuropathies such as carpal tunnel syndrome are damage of a single peripheral nerve; they usually have an acquired cause such as compression, but frequently the cause is idiopathic. A multiple mononeuropathy (or mononeuritis multiplex) affects two or more nerves in various body areas and may be caused by conditions such as infectious diseases and rheumatoid arthritis. Finally, polyneuropathies affect multiple nerves in all limbs, and include diseases such as Charcot–Marie–Tooth (CMT) disease and acute or chronic inflammatory demyelinating polyneuropathy [2].

Symmetrical polyneuropathy affects about 2.4% of the population and is more prevalent in the elderly [2]. Diabetic polyneuropathy affects about 50% of patients with a long history of diabetes [3]. In general, peripheral neuropathy may be the sole manifestation in an individual or be part of a more generalized disorder and may be acquired or inherited. We will focus on the neuropathy as a sole manifestation and concentrate our attention on the recent advances in inherited neuropathy.

Causes of peripheral neuropathy

Acquired peripheral neuropathies

There are many causes of acquired neuropathy: in developed countries the commonest cause is diabetes, whereas in developing countries leprosy is still the most prevalent cause of peripheral neuropathy. Other causes include traumatic injury to a nerve following an accident or compression due to body positioning or repetitive movements (e.g., carpal tunnel syndrome) and viral or bacterial infections such as Lyme disease, hepatitis B and C, HIV/AIDS, and varicella-zoster. A variety of autoimmune diseases are known to cause neuropathy, including vasculitis arising from rheumatoid arthritis or systemic lupus erythematosus, Guillain–Barré syndrome (GBS), chronic inflammatory demyelinating polyradiculoneuropathy (CIDP), sarcoidosis, celiac disease, multifocal motor neuropathy, and paraproteinemia (e.g., POEMS [polyneuropathy, organomegaly, endocrinopathy, monoclonal gammopathy, and skin changes], amyloidosis, and monoclonal gammopathy). Diabetes mellitus and chronic alcoholism are frequent causes of acquired peripheral neuropathy [4].

Exposure to toxic chemicals and heavy metals like lead or drugs such as vincristine in cancer treatment and some of the drug treatments used in HIV/AIDS may lead to a neuropathy. In some developing countries, this exposure can be pervasive. In Nigeria, mercury is used in the extraction of gold by small independent mines. In the event of heavy rains, as occurred in 2011, the mercury can seep into the water supply of villages close by and cause a large outbreak of poisoning with seizures and peripheral neuropathy in many individuals, usually children.

Other acquired causes of neuropathy include nutritional deficiencies in vitamins B_1, B_6, B_{12}, and E, underactive thyroid, kidney disease, and liver disease, among others. Excessive intake of vitamin B_6 also may lead to a sensory neuropathy. Tumors can also cause neuropathy by exerting pressure focally on a nerve.

Hereditary peripheral neuropathies

Hereditary peripheral neuropathies are generally less common than acquired peripheral neuropathies although this gap is closing with an aging population and the identification of genetic risk factors in the etiology of some of the acquired neuropathies. Examples of genetic disorders where peripheral neuropathy is part of the overall phenotype include hereditary spastic paraplegia, hereditary ataxia, neuroaxonal dystrophy, the genetic forms

Neurodegeneration, First Edition. Edited by Anthony Schapira, Zbigniew Wszolek, Ted M. Dawson and Nicholas Wood.
© 2017 John Wiley & Sons, Ltd. Published 2017 by John Wiley & Sons, Ltd.

of porphyrias, metachromatic leukodystrophy, Krabbe disease, Tangier disease, Fabry disease, and Refsum's disease [5].

We will focus here on the pure hereditary peripheral neuropathies including CMT, hereditary neuropathy with liability to pressure palsies (HNPP), distal hereditary motor neuropathy (dHMN), hereditary sensory and autonomic neuropathy (HSAN) or hereditary sensory neuropathy (HSN), hereditary brachial plexus neuropathy or hereditary neuralgic amyotrophy (HNA), and giant axonal neuropathy (GAN).

CMT disease, also known as hereditary motor and sensory neuropathy (HMSN), is the most common inherited neuromuscular disease with a prevalence of about 1/2500, although this prevalence varies in different populations [6, 7]. While autosomal dominant (AD) or X-linked inheritance accounts for 90% of CMT cases in European/UK and US populations, autosomal recessive (AR) inheritance accounts for about 40% of cases in populations where consanguineous marriage is frequent such as the Mediterranean basin [8]. CMT affects all ethnicities, although some recessive forms of CMT are more common in certain genetically isolated populations. For example, CMT associated with mutations in N-myc downstream regulated gene 1 (*NDRG1*), Src homology 3 domain and tetratricopeptide repeats 2 (*SH3TC2/KIAA1985*), and hexokinase 1 (*HK1*) is especially frequent in the Roma population.

Spectrum of peripheral neuropathy phenotypes

Peripheral neuropathy is generally length dependent, starting in the feet and then the hands in humans, but in other species such as horses the laryngeal nerve is the longest and therefore the first to be affected. Disease may be mild and detectable only by electrodiagnostic studies or severe enough to require ventilatory support. Symptoms will be dictated by which type of nerve is affected: damage to motor nerves leads to muscle weakness and fasciculations; damage to sensory nerves is associated with paresthesia (tingling, burning, and numbness), loss of sensation, and neuropathic pain; and involvement of autonomic nerve fibers leads to changes in blood pressure and perturbations of bladder or sexual functions [9]. In the case of a sensory neuropathy, small fiber involvement may result in pain, temperature alteration, and autonomic dysfunction while large fiber involvement leads to motor weakness and loss of reflexes. Pupillary abnormalities, tremor, muscle cramps, diaphragmatic weakness, and hearing loss may be part of the clinical picture of peripheral neuropathies.

The prognosis of peripheral neuropathies is variable. Disease may progress in a steady or fluctuating fashion, and may be acute, subacute, or chronic. Examples of neuropathies in which a relapsing course of disease is common include CIDP, GBS, HNPP, brachial plexopathy, porphyria, and Refsum's disease. Polyneuropathies are generally slowly progressive; CMT progresses by only 0.68 points on the CMT Neuropathy Score (CMTNS) scale per year [10]. Examples of acquired neuropathies with slow progression include paraproteinemic neuropathy and diabetic distal sensory neuropathy [9]. CMT is generally not life threatening, and patients rarely require the use of a wheelchair. However, early onset generally predicts a more severe disease. HNPP patients generally recover well, although long-term deficits are possible. Complications including ulceration and mutilation are common in HSN. HNA patients usually recover well after their attacks, and these tend to decrease over time. GAN patients are generally in a wheelchair or severely affected in the third decade, although cases with slower progression have been described.

CMT disease

Three physicians first described CMT in 1886: Jean-Marie Charcot, Pierre Marie, and Howard Henry Tooth [11, 12]. Initially thought to be one condition, over the years clinical and then genetic studies have revealed CMT to be one of the most heterogeneous conditions in neurology. Symptoms include symmetrical weakness, distal muscle wasting which may become proximal over time, loss of reflexes and sensation, and foot deformities such as pes cavus [13].

Before the 1.5-Mb duplication encompassing the peripheral myelin protein 22 (*PMP22*) gene on chromosome 17 was identified as the genetic cause of CMT1A [14, 15], major advances in the field of CMT were focused on the neurophysiology and pathology of peripheral nerves, leading to the classification of CMT into two main categories according to upper limb motor nerve conduction velocities (NCVs): CMT1 (previously HMSNI), the demyelinating form with abnormal myelin sheath and NCVs of less than 38 m/s; and CMT2 (previously HMSNII), the axonal form with NCVs greater than 38 m/s [13]. The intermediate forms of CMT have NCVs between 25 and 45 m/s and exhibit both axonal and demyelinating features. Importantly, NCVs in CMT1 are typically reduced before the disease manifests itself and the degree of reduction in NCV does not correlate with disease severity. In the case of a demyelinating neuropathy, symptoms result from the secondary axonal damage rather than from the primary damage to the myelin sheath. CMT is further categorized according to the inheritance pattern and mutated gene [8].

Onset of disease in CMT is generally in childhood or early adulthood, but may be later in CMT2. CMT has variable severity, from mild cases with symptoms of classic CMT to severe cases which tend to be typical of AR CMT. Severely affected children with early-onset demyelinating neuropathy may be classified as CMT3 (HMSNIII), congenital hypomyelinating neuropathy (CHN), or Dejerine–Sottas disease (DSD) [8]. The variable penetrance and great variability in disease severity both within and between families in many subtypes of CMT suggest that environmental factors, genetic modifiers, stochastic effects, and/or epigenetics may influence the degree to which a patient is affected. In fact, some patients may remain asymptomatic throughout their lives. Various cases of superimposed inflammatory neuropathy have been reported in CMT, which may explain some of the disease variability [16, 17].

Males and females are generally equally affected, although males are more impaired in CMT1X, which may be due to X-inactivation in females [8].

The specific phenotypes associated with each CMT subtype are summarized in Table 19.1.

Other inherited peripheral neuropathies: HNPP, dHMN, HSAN, HNA, and GAN

HNPP is characterized by recurrent, short episodes of sensory loss or focal weakness involving a single nerve, especially at areas susceptible to compression and entrapment. Onset is generally in early adulthood, and patients can be asymptomatic, although neurophysiology will still be abnormal [18]. NCVs show multifocal conduction slowing [8]. Some patients have pes cavus and decreased or lost tendon reflexes, and may therefore resemble CMT1. Some types of inherited neuropathy resemble CMT but are clinically entirely motor, such as dHMN. HSAN may be

Table 19.1 Classification of CMT, HNPP, and HNA and associated protein functions. Adapted from [8, 30].

Type	Gene/locus	Phenotype	Protein function
Autosomal dominant CMT – demyelinating			
CMT1A	PMP22 (Chr17p11.2 duplication)	Classic CMT1	Myelin structural component, myelin formation, Schwann cell differentiation
CMT1B	MPZ	CMT1/DSD/CHN/intermediate/CMT2	Myelin structural component, adhesion, compaction and maintenance of myelin
CMT1C	LITAF	Classic CMT1	Protein sorting at the early endosome
CMT1D	EGR2	Classic CMT1/DSD/CHN	Transcription factor, regulation of myelin program
CMT1E	PMP22 (point mutation)	Classic CMT1/DSD/CHN/HNPP	See CMT1A
CMT1F	NF-L	CMT2, may have early-onset severe disease with slow NCVs in CMT1 range	Organization and assembling of neurofilaments, mitochondrial dynamics
CMT1	FBLN5	CMT1, age-related macular degeneration and hyperextensible skin	Elastic fiber assembly
Autosomal recessive CMT – demyelinating			
CMT4A	GDAP1	Early-onset, severe, vocal cord and diaphragm paralysis	Glutathione transferase, mitochondrial fission
CMT4B1	MTMR2	Severe CMT1, facial, bulbar, focally folded myelin	Active phosphatase of P1(3,5)P2 and PI(3)P, membrane trafficking, endocytosis, and control of myelination
CMT4B2	MTMR13	Severe CMT1, glaucoma, focally folded myelin	Inactive phosphatase of P1(3,5)P2 and PI(3)P
CMT4C	SH3TC2	Severe CMT1, scoliosis, cytoplasmic expansions	Rab11 effector, endocytic recycling
CMT4D/HMSN-Lom	NDRG1	Severe CMT1, Roma, deafness, tongue atrophy	Unknown
CMT4E	EGR2	CMT1/CHN/DSD	See CMT1D
CMT4F	PRX	CMT1, severe sensory loss, focally folded myelin	Myelin structural component, membrane–protein interactions, extracellular matrix signaling during myelination
CMT4G/HMSN-R	HK1	Severe, early-onset CMT, significant sensory loss	Regulation of energy metabolism and cell survival
CMT4H	FGD4	CMT1	Guanine nucleotide exchange factor, regulation of GTPases of the Rho subfamily
CMT4J	FIG4	CMT1, mostly motor, progressive	P1(3,5)P2 5-phosphatase
CCFDN	CTDP1	CMT1, congenital cataracts, facial dysmorphism, Roma	Polymerase 11-mediated transcriptional regulation
AR CMT1	PMP22 (point mutation)	Classic CMT1/DSD/CHN	See CMT1A
AR CMT1	MPZ	CMT1/DSD/CHN/CMT2	See CMT1B
Autosomal dominant CMT – axonal			
CMT2A1	KIF1Bβ	Classic CMT2	Motor protein, vesicle trafficking
CMT2A2	MFN2	CMT2, severe, optic atrophy	GTPase, mitochondrial fusion and transport
CMT2B	RAB7	CMT2, ulcero-mutilation, foot ulcers, recurrent infections, and severe sensory loss	GTPase, vesicle trafficking between late endosomes and lysosomes
CMT2C	TRPV4	CMT2, vocal cord and diaphragm paralysis, allelic to scapuloperoneal spinal muscular atrophy	Cation channel, transduction of sensory inputs
CMT2D	GARS	CMT2, hand weakness, mostly motor, mild to moderate sensory involvement/dHMN type 5	T-RNA synthetase, protein synthesis
CMT2E	NF-L	CMT2, may have early-onset severe disease with slow NCVs in CMT1 range	See CMT1F
CMT2F	HSPB1/HSP27	Classic CMT2/dHMN type 2	Chaperone, protein folding/quality control, neurofilament network organization
CMT2G	12q12	Classic CMT2	N/A
CMT2I	MPZ	Classic CMT2	See CMT1B
CMT2J	MPZ	CMT2, hearing loss, pupillary abnormalities	See CMT1B
CMT2K	GDAP1	Late-onset CMT2	See CMT4A
CMT2L	HSPB8/HSP22 (allelic to dHMN2)	Classic CMT2/dHMN type 2	Chaperone, protein folding, stress response, and regulation of apoptosis
CMT2N	AARS	Classic CMT2	t-RNA synthetase, protein synthesis
CMT2O	DYNC1H1	Early-onset CMT2	Motor protein, retrograde axonal transport
CMT2 (HMSN-proximal)	3q13.1	CMT2, proximal involvement	N/A
CMT2	LRSAM1	Mild, slowly progressive CMT2	E3 ubiquitin ligase, receptor endocytosis
Autosomal recessive CMT – axonal			
AR-CMT2A/CMT2B1	Lamin A/C (LMNA)	CMT2, rapidly progressive, proximal involvement	Nuclear envelope structure, genomic stability, axonal survival and development
AR-CMT2B	MED25	Classic CMT2	Transcriptional co-activator
AR-CMT2/CMT2H	GDAP1	CMT2 with pyramidal signs	N/A
AR-CMT2	MFN2	Early-onset CMT2	See CMT2A2
AR-CMT2	LRSAM1	Classic CMT2	See CMT2A-associated LRSAM1
AR-CMT2	POLG1	CMT2, tremor, ataxia	Mitochondrial DNA polymerase

Continued

Table 19.1 *Continued*

X-linked CMT			
CMT1X	GJB1	Intermediate, males more severely affected	Myelin structural component, cell membrane channel, formation of intracellular gap junctions between the folds of the Schwann cell cytoplasm
CMT2X	PRPS1	CMT2, hearing impairment, optic atrophy	Metabolic enzyme, nucleotide biosynthesis, and purine metabolism
Autosomal dominant CMT – intermediate			
DI-CMTA	10q24.1-q25.1	Classic CMT	N/A
DI-CMTB	DNM2	Classic CMT	GTPase, cellular fusion and fission, vesicle trafficking, endocytosis
DI-CMTC	YARS	Classic CMT	t-RNA synthetase, protein synthesis
DI-CMTD	MPZ	Classic CMT	See CMT1B
DI-CMTE	INF2	CMT, glomerulopathy	Cytoskeleton remodeling
DI-CMT	3q28-q29	Classic CMT	N/A
Autosomal recessive CMT – intermediate			
RI-CMTA	GDAP1	Early-onset, severe CMT	See CMT4A
RI-CMTB	KARS	CMT, dysmorphic features, developmental delay	t-RNA synthetase, protein synthesis
Hereditary neuropathy with liability to pressure palsies (HNPP)			
HNPP	PMP22 (Chr17p11.2 deletion)	Classic HNPP	See CMT1A
	PMP22 (point mutation)	Classic HNPP	See CMT1A
Hereditary neuralgic amyotrophy (HNA)			
HNA	SEPT9	Recurrent neuralgic amyotrophy	Filament formation, cell division

CMT, Charcot–Marie–Tooth disease; HNA, hereditary neuralgic amyotrophy; HNPP, hereditary neuropathy with liability to pressure palsies; N/A, not applicable.

purely sensory or purely autonomic, or a combination of both, and may include some level of motor involvement. A nerve biopsy depicting lack of small myelinated fibers in a patient with HSAN resulting from an NTRK1 mutation is represented in Figure 19.1. dHMNs and HSANs show some clinical overlap with CMT [8]. HNA is a rare disease involving episodes of pain with multifocal paresis and sensory loss in the nerves of the brachial plexus. There are other types of neuropathy that equally involve the CNS and PNS. GAN, a distal sensorimotor neuropathy starting in childhood and often associated with skeletal abnormalities, kinky hair, and seizures [19], is a good example. GAN patients display axonal loss, axonal swellings, and secondary demyelination on nerve biopsy [20].

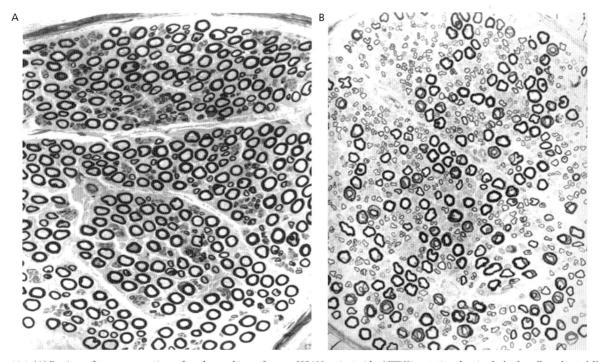

Figure 19.1 (A) Portions of transverse sections of sural nerve biopsy from an HSAN patient with a NTRK1 mutation showing lack of small myelinated fibers. (B) Biopsy of a post mortem specimen from an age-matched control. Thionin and acridine orange, × 400.

Molecular genetics of inherited peripheral neuropathies

CMT disease and HNPP

Demyelinating neuropathies result from defects in the development and functioning of Schwann cells and the myelin sheath they produce, leading to secondary axonal degeneration. In demyelinating neuropathies, muscle weakness is not the direct result of demyelination; the degree of axonal loss rather than the amount of demyelination is correlated to disease severity. Intermediate forms of CMT probably involve defects in both Schwann cells and axons. Mutations in genes associated with both axonal and demyelinating forms such as myelin protein zero (*MPZ*), neurofilament light polypeptide (*NF-L*), and ganglioside-induced differentiation-associated protein 1 (*GDAP1*) probably disturb the close interactions between Schwann cells and neurons.

Both CMT1 (demyelinating) and CMT2 (axonal) may be divided into dominant and recessive forms, where recessive forms of CMT1 are known as CMT4. Intermediate forms of CMT are also increasingly recognized. CMT is further divided according to the causative gene, of which more than 40 have been described to date [7, 8].

The genes found to be associated with CMT are expressed in Schwann cells and/or neurons, although many genes such as *FIG4*, dynamin 2 (*DNM2*), lamin A/C (*LMNA*), the t-RNA synthetases, myotubularin-related protein 2 (*MTMR2*), mitofusin 2 (*MFN2*), *RAB7*, heat shock protein beta-1 (*HSPB1*), and heat shock protein beta-8 (*HSPB8*) are ubiquitously expressed. To this day, how such widely expressed genes can selectively affect the PNS remains to be clarified. The identification of new CMT-associated genes and the functional studies carried out on disease-associated mutations are helping us improve our understanding of Schwann cell and peripheral nerve biology as well as that of neurodegenerative processes.

Myelin structural components

PMP22

Proteins coding for structural components of myelin were obvious candidates in the search for neuropathy-associated genes. However most other CMT genes are ubiquitously expressed and had no prior associated role in axons or Schwann cells.

Linkage of CMT1A to chromosome 17 [21, 22] was followed by the identification of a 1.5-Mb duplication on chromosome 17p11.2-12 [14, 15]. This duplication, the most important genetic discovery in CMT, results from unequal crossing over due to misalignment of repeat sequences termed CMT1A-REPs, which flank the duplicated region [15, 23]; however, different non-recurrent mechanisms have also been described [24]. The *PMP22* gene was subsequently found to map within this region, resulting in three copies of the gene instead of two [25–28]. However, the severity of disease is not entirely determined by the *PMP22* gene copy number [29]. CMT1A accounts for approximately 50% of all CMT [30].

Evidence that *PMP22* is the responsible gene included the discovery of the Trembler and Trembler-J mice with *Pmp22* mutations and a demyelinating phenotype modeling CMT1A [26]. A patient with the same PMP22 point mutation as that found in the Trembler-J mouse was subsequently identified, providing further proof that *PMP22* is the neuropathy-causing gene within the chromosome 17 duplication [31]. Point mutations in *PMP22* are classified as CMT1E.

The PMP22 protein is an integral membrane protein located in the compact portion of myelin, and accounts for 5% of peripheral myelin protein [32]. PMP22 is important for determination of myelin thickness and stability, Schwann cell differentiation, and maintenance of axons [33]. Knockout mice have delayed myelination, hypermyelination, and axonal loss [33] while *Pmp22* overexpressing mice show dysmyelination [34] and impaired Schwann cell differentiation into the myelinating stage [35].

CMT1A is thought to result from an increased gene dosage mechanism [36, 37]. In agreement with this hypothesis, elevated levels of PMP22 were found in nerve biopsies of patients. Furthermore, a patient with a duplication larger than, but completely encompassing, the CMT1A duplicated region was described and exhibited the same demyelinating phenotype [37]. Recently, copy number variations upstream of *PMP22* were found to cause CMT; *PMP22* expression must somehow be altered in these patients, potentially through the disruption of highly conserved regulatory sequences located in the upstream region [38, 39].

The mechanisms by which overexpression of *PMP22* leads to CMT1A are not yet fully understood. PMP22 is needed in very specific amounts in myelin and its expression levels must evidently be tightly controlled; alterations in its expression may destabilize the myelin sheath or disturb the complexes it forms with the MPZ protein [40]. The PMP22 protein is rapidly turned over but difficult to fold correctly: most newly synthesized PMP22 is rapidly degraded by the proteasome, and only a small portion is integrated into the plasma membrane. Not surprisingly, overexpression of *PMP22* in Schwann cell cultures slows protein turnover and impairs the proteasome, leading to the formation of aggregates [41]. These aggregates may interfere with intracellular protein sorting [41]. Such an accumulation of misfolded proteins is a common mechanism in neurodegenerative diseases.

Intra-axonal accumulation of mitochondria has also been reported in skin biopsies of CMT1A patients, which may suggest that impaired mitochondrial transport is also part of the pathogenic pathway in CMT1A [42].

PMP22 point mutations are also associated with CMT, although they are more rare and produce a more severe phenotype [31, 43]. The mutations in Trembler and Trembler-J mice are naturally occurring and cause a demyelinating neuropathy in these animals [26]. These mutations are not predicted to be loss of function because the phenotype is much more severe than is seen in HNPP where patients have a 50% decrease in PMP22 protein; the PMP22 protein must therefore gain a toxic function [30]. Accordingly, the Trembler mutant protein was found to exert a dominant-negative effect on wild-type Pmp22 in animal models by interfering with its intracellular trafficking [44, 45], possibly by forming homo- and heterodimers with the wild-type PMP22 and preventing it from reaching the cell membrane [46]. In fact, both the Trembler and Trembler-J mutants are retained in the endoplasmic reticulum (ER), most likely because of incorrect protein folding, while wild-type PMP22 is able to reach compact myelin at the plasma membrane [47]. The *Pmp22* mutation leads to reduced protein turnover in Trembler-J nerves and to the formation of aggregates and activation of autophagy, suggesting an impairment of the proteasome degradation pathway [48, 49]. This mechanism seems to be common to both *PMP22* overexpression and *PMP22* point mutations.

HNPP is due to a reciprocal 1.5-Mb deletion on chromosome 17 [50]. Although relatively rare, loss-of-function mutations in *PMP22* such as nonsense, splice site, or frameshift mutations may also cause HNPP [8]. Heterozygous *Pmp22*-null mice develop a progressive demyelinating tomaculous neuropathy [51]. *PMP22* expression is decreased in HNPP compared to control nerves [52], suggesting that HNPP results from underexpression of *PMP22*.

MPZ

MPZ mutations are responsible for CMT1B [53, 54]. MPZ, a structural protein located in the compact myelin of the PNS, is necessary for the adhesion, compaction, and maintenance of myelin [55]. MPZ accounts for over 50% of the total peripheral myelin protein composition [56]. Heterozygous null mice have a very mild phenotype, making a gain-of-function or dominant-negative mechanism highly likely [55, 57].

Generally, early-onset, severe demyelinating forms of *MPZ*-associated CMT are due to a compaction defect in the myelin sheath of mice due to disruption of the MPZ protein structure, thereby affecting myelination early on in development, whereas CMT1B-associated mutations do not reach the myelin sheath, cause protein misfolding, retention in the ER, induction of the unfolded protein response (UPR), and activation of the UPR mediator CHOP [57, 58]. In fact, demyelination is reduced when Chop is ablated in CMT1B mice [58]. CMT1B mutations also prevent wild-type Mpz from reaching the myelin sheath [59].

Mutations causing late-onset, axonal phenotypes may affect Schwann cell–axon interactions due to an abnormal myelin sheath; in this instance, the protein is transported to the cell membrane, but it exhibits reduced intercellular adhesion, evidence of a partial loss of function [60].

GJB1

Gap junction protein beta 1 *(GJB1),* the gene responsible for CMT1X [61], encodes connexin 32 (Cx32), a cell membrane channel found in uncompacted myelin and at the nodes of Ranvier and Schmidt-Lanterman incisures [62, 63]. Cx32 is responsible for the formation of intracellular gap junctions between the folds of the Schwann cell cytoplasm, which are needed for the transport of ions and signaling molecules through the myelin sheath [62]. In *GJB1*-associated CMT, the channel between the axon and myelin lamellae is disrupted, leading to an intermediate phenotype, which causes defects to both the axon and the Schwann cell.

GJB1 mutations are thought to act by a variety of mechanisms depending on the domain in which the mutation is located. Some mutations exhibit a dominant-negative effect of the mutant Cx32 protein on the normal Cx32 or other connexins, causing abnormal gap junctions, while others lead to loss of function whereby levels of the Cx32 protein are reduced and the resulting gap junctions are non-functional [63]. Early growth response 2 *(EGR2),* the causative gene in CMT1D, acts together with SRY (sex determining region Y)-box 10 (SOX10), a transcription factor necessary for PNS development, to activate the expression of *GJB1* by binding to its promoter. A *GJB1* mutation within the *SOX10* binding site of the nerve-specific promoter led to a significant decrease in *SOX10* activation of *GJB1*, indicating a defect in transcription of *GJB1* [64]. In this instance, the neuropathy may be a result of decreased Cx32 levels.

GJB1 mutations may also affect the physical properties of the channel such as the gating polarity [63]. Depending on the mutation, Cx32 may accumulate in the ER or Golgi, and may or may not be present on the cell surface [63].

CMT1X patients also display axonal pathology associated with increased neurofilament density and decreased number of microtubules, which may implicate defects in axonal transport in the pathomechanism of *GJB1* mutations [65].

PRX

Periaxin *(PRX),* associated with CMT4F [66, 67] is expressed by myelinating Schwann cells, encodes L- and S-periaxin and is part of a complex composed of the laminin receptor dystroglycan and dystroglycan–dystrophin-related protein 2 (DRP2) located at the plasma membrane [68, 69]. PRX is thought to be important for membrane–protein interactions and extracellular matrix signaling to the cytoskeleton during the myelination process [68]. Loss-of-function mutations in *PRX* result in a lack of L-periaxin in the myelin sheath [67]. *Prx*-null mice show evidence of demyelination due to unstable myelin [67, 70] followed by remyelination with dysregulated myelin thickness [71] and remodeling of motor nerve terminals [72]. DRP2 is mislocalized and depleted in nerves of *Prx*-null mice, indicating that *PRX* mutations may lead to destabilization of the complex and, possibly, disrupted signaling during myelination [69].

Transcription factors and regulation of gene expression

EGR2

CMT1D is caused by mutations in *EGR2*, which encodes a Cys_2His_2 type zinc-finger transcription factor that controls peripheral nerve myelination [73]. The mouse homolog *Krox-20* is necessary for the expression of late myelin genes in Schwann cells [74]. Schwann cells in *Krox-20* knockout mice are not able to differentiate fully and thus do not form compacted myelin [74]. *EGR2* acts in synergy with *SOX10* to regulate transcription of myelin genes such as *GJB1*, *PMP22*, and *MPZ*. Most *EGR2* mutations are located in the DNA-binding zinc-finger domain and act by a dominant-negative mechanism which inhibits wild-type EGR2, which agrees with the finding that heterozygous knockout mice are phenotypically normal [75, 76]. Dominant *Egr2* mutations cause a disruption in this transcriptional regulation by decreasing the affinity of *Sox10* to the binding site, leading to a disruption of the myelination program [77]. The degree of decrease in DNA binding that results from *EGR2* mutations correlates with disease severity [75].

LMNA

LMNA was the first gene found to be associated with autosomal recessive forms of CMT2 [78]. Mutations in different functional domains of LMNA are associated with other diseases such as autosomal dominant Emery–Dreifuss muscular dystrophy and limb-girdle muscular dystrophy type 1B [79]. LMNA, an intermediate filament protein, is important for the structure of the nuclear envelope, and may play a role in axonal survival and development [79]. A-type lamins have also been proposed to protect cells from physical damage, and to be important in the functioning of transcription factors needed for adult stem cell differentiation [80], as well as for genomic stability [81]. While *Lmna*-null mice display a similar phenotype to that of AR-CMT2 [82], heterozygous knockout mice do not have a neuropathy, therefore *LMNA* mutations are predicted to be loss of function [79].

MED25

Mediator of RNA polymerase II transcription subunit 25 *(MED25)* is mutated in AR CMT2B [83] and encodes a protein that is part of a family of transcriptional co-activator complexes. AR-CMT2 mutations in *MED25* may alter the specificity and levels of transcription of target genes downstream of *MED25* in peripheral nerves [84]. One of these downstream target genes may be *PMP22* as levels of *Pmp22* expression were found to correlate with *Med25* expression levels in transgenic animals [84].

Other rare genes

Congenital cataract, facial dysmorphism, and neuropathy syndrome (CCFDN) was found to be caused by mutations in carboxy-terminal domain, RNA polymerase II, polypeptide A phosphatase, subunit 1 (*CTDP1*) [85]. *CTDP1* encodes the phosphatase FCP1 and plays a role in polymerase II-mediated transcriptional regulation and mRNA processing. The mutation identified in *CTDP1* led to aberrant splicing. The mechanism of disease of *CTDP1* mutations is still unclear [85].

Protein synthesis

Thus far, four genes encoding t-RNA synthetases have been associated with CMT: glycyl t-RNA synthetase (*GARS*) [86, 87], tyrosyl t-RNA synthetase (*YARS*) [88, 89], alanyl t-RNA synthetase (*AARS*) [90], and lysyl t-RNA synthetase (*KARS*) [91].

t-RNA synthetases are housekeeping genes important for protein synthesis, specifically for the charging of t-RNAs with cognate amino acids during translation. A defect in their function may specifically affect peripheral nerves, which have high metabolic demands.

Impaired enzyme activity through loss of t-RNA charging function in yeast assays or altered cellular localization in some cell studies has been observed and has been suggested as a possible disease mechanism for all four CMT-associated t-RNA synthetases; however, it would imply that t-RNA synthetases play a specific function in peripheral nerves possibly unrelated to translation [89, 91–93]. Another potential mechanism that has been proposed is disturbed axonal transport of the mutant t-RNA synthetase during protein translation occurring in the axon [92].

Mischarging of amino acids, misfolding of proteins, insufficiency of protein synthesis, and altered subcellular localization were later discarded as mechanisms of neuropathy in a mouse model of CMT2D and yeast assays [94]. It is also unlikely that *Gars* mutations lead to a defect in an unknown function in the translation process, unless the protein has an unrecognized role in translation specifically in peripheral nerves [94]. This hypothesis of a defect in local protein synthesis has been proposed to explain the nerve-specific dominant-negative effect of *YARS* mutations: the normal function of the YARS protein, in part localized to neuronal endings, may be disrupted, thereby affecting synaptic plasticity or local metabolism [89]. *GARS* mutations may also act in a dominant-negative manner because haploinsufficiency does not lead to disease in a mouse model of Gars; a loss-of-function mechanism is therefore unlikely for *GARS* mutations [93, 95]. In fact, in mouse models of CMT2D, neuropathy is thought to arise from a toxic gain of function, which cannot be rescued by overexpression of wild-type Gars [96].

Mice carrying a homozygous *Aars* mutation in the editing domain have compromised proofreading activity, leading to mischarging of t-RNAs, accumulation of misfolded proteins, and induction of the UPR [97]. However, these mice do not exhibit a peripheral neuropathy [94].

It is still unclear whether CMT-associated mutations in t-RNA synthetases cause neuropathy through a loss of enzyme function, a toxic gain of function, or whether they are due to a defect in an as-of-yet unknown function of t-RNA synthetases.

Mitochondrial fusion and fission

Neurons have particularly high energy demands and are especially vulnerable, making the proper functioning of mitochondria essential to peripheral nerve function.

Mutations in *MFN2,* which encodes a protein located in the outer mitochondrial membrane, were identified in the CMT2A locus [98]. MFN2 is a mitofusin GTPase important for mitochondrial fusion: mouse embryonic fibroblasts lacking Mfn2 have fragmented mitochondria [99]. MFN2 is also necessary for axonal transport of mitochondria [100], for controlling ADP/ATP exchanges [101], and for signaling between the ER and the mitochondria by bridging the two organelles [102]. *Mfn2* mutations lead to defective mitochondrial movement via microtubules *in vitro* by slowing the rate of anterograde and retrograde transport; this dominant-negative effect was rescued by wild-type MFN2 [100]. Decreased mitochondrial transport may lead to depletion of the much-needed energy supply in long peripheral nerve axons. CMT2A2 patient fibroblasts had reduced mitochondrial membrane potential indicative of a coupling defect, further involving reduced energy sources in disease pathogenesis [101]. *MFN2* mutations are not likely to cause haploinsufficiency as carriers of heterozygous null alleles are unaffected [103].

GDAP1 mutations are associated with demyelinating, axonal, and intermediate forms of CMT, and exhibit both dominant and recessive inheritance [104, 105]. GDAP1 is a glutathione transferase located within the mitochondria with a role in mitochondrial fission. *GDAP1* is expressed in both neurons and Schwann cells. Recessively inherited mutations cause loss of its function in mitochondrial fragmentation [106]. As a result, the mitochondrial membrane potential, as well as the levels of the antioxidant glutathione, are reduced in CMT4A patient fibroblasts, indicating that oxidative stress may play a role in the etiology of CMT4A [106]. Dominantly inherited mutations perturb mitochondrial fusion and damage the mitochondria. Overall, a defect in mitochondrial dynamics is likely at the root of *GDAP1*-related CMT [107].

Cytoskeletal dynamics, axonal transport, and vesicular motility

Axonal transport is especially important for neurons with long, highly polarized axons that depend on mitochondrial transport for energy at the distal end of the axons [108]. As there is no protein synthesis machinery in axons and nerve endings, the transport via microtubules of organelles and proteins needed for survival is essential in neurons [109].

NF-L is mutated in CMT1F and CMT2E [110, 111]. NF-L, a component of intermediate filaments in the axon cytoskeleton, is one of three neurofilament proteins that are responsible for organizing and assembling neurofilaments and determining axonal diameter. NF-L is therefore important for axonal maintenance and structure, although it has recently been implicated in mitochondrial dynamics [112]. NF-L is known to regulate the expression of the other two neurofilament proteins, NF-M and NF-H [110]. *NF-L* mutations are mostly dominantly inherited and may cause axonal or demyelinating neuropathy. Heterozygous null mice do not develop neuropathy therefore a loss-of-function mechanism is unlikely for AD CMT-related *NF-L* mutations [113]. In cultured neurons, mutant NF-L prevents proper neurofilament assembly and axonal transport of neurofilaments [114, 115]. These defects were reversed and the neurofilament network was stabilized by expression of the wild-type HSPB1, a molecular chaperone mutated in CMT2F [115]. Accumulation of neurofilaments, which is also involved in *MTMR2-* and *HSPB1*-associated CMT and in other neurodegenerative diseases such as amyotrophic lateral sclerosis, Alzheimer's disease, Parkinson disease, and diabetic neuropathy, was present in nerve biopsies of patients with *NF-L* mutations [114–117]. Mutant NF-L neurons also exhibited mislocalized mitochondria, a decreased rate of fusion, and defective mitochondrial transport [112]. *NF-L* mutants associated with demyelinating phenotypes may result from impaired axon–Schwann cell signaling, which is essential in the myelination program. Alternatively, NF-L is known to interact with MTMR2, therefore *NF-L* mutations may disrupt the phosphatase activity of MTMR2 in Schwann cells [118].

Kinesin family member 1B beta (*KIF1Bβ*) mutations were identified in the CMT2A locus [109]; however *MFN2* mutations associated with CMT2A were later identified within this locus, and *MFN2* may be the primary gene causing CMT2 within the 1p36 locus. KIF1Bβ is a kinesin motor protein involved in transport of mitochondria and synaptic vesicle precursors. The phenotype of heterozygous Kif1bβ-knockout mice resembles that seen in CMT2A1 patients A mutation located in the ATP-binding domain resulted in decreased ATPase activity and impaired motor activity, which indicates that haploinsufficiency is the probable cause of neuropathy in CMT2A1 [109].

Dynein, cytoplasmic 1, heavy chain 1 (*DYNC1H1*) encodes the cytoplasmic dynein heavy chain 1, which is part of a motor protein complex and is needed for retrograde axonal transport [119], providing further evidence that effective axonal transport is crucial in peripheral nerves.

FGD1-related F-actin binding protein (*FGD4*) is mutated in CMT4H [120, 121]. FGD4 is a guanine nucleotide exchange factor responsible for regulating GTPases of the Rho subfamily, which play a role in cell growth, cell polarization, trafficking, and organization of the actin and microtubule cytoskeleton [121, 122]. FGD4 is able to induce changes in cell shape in transfected Schwann cells [123], pointing to a possible role in Schwann cell myelination [122]. CMT4H mutations are thought to prevent proper Rho GTPase signaling, leading to disrupted membrane transport in Schwann cells [123].

Inverted formin, FH2, and WH2 domain containing (*INF2*) mutations were identified in cases of focal segmental glomerulosclerosis (FSGS)-associated CMT [124]. INF2 is a formin protein involved in remodeling of the cytoskeleton. It interacts with the Rho GTPase CDC42 and with the myelin and lymphocyte protein (MAL), which are important for myelination. *INF2* mutations disturbed these interactions, leading to changes in subcellular localization and disturbed actin dynamics, possibly affecting intracellular protein transport and the formation of myelin [124].

Endocytosis, intracellular protein sorting, and quality control
A defect in the endocytic recycling of proteins or in the quality control system may have an impact on the tightly controlled myelination program in Schwann cells.

DNM2 mutations cause dominant intermediate CMT [125, 126]. DNM2 is a GTPase involved in cellular fusion and fission, centrosome cohesion, actin assembly, trafficking from the late endosome, and pinching of clathrin-coated vesicles during endocytosis [126]. *DNM2* mutations disturb the binding of the protein to the membrane and vesicles and cause disorganization of microtubules, thereby possibly affecting axonal transport [126]. In cell models, *DNM2* mutations led to decreased clathrin-mediated endocytosis [127].

The leucine rich repeat and sterile alpha motif 1 (*LRSAM1*) gene, also known as *TAL* (TSG101-associated ligase), is mutated in one type of axonal CMT [128]. The LRSAM1 protein is a predicted E3 ubiquitin ligase that regulates receptor endocytosis [128, 129]. In transfected cells, ubiquitin ligase activity was affected, as evidenced by increased levels of tumor suppressor gene 101 (TSG101), a target of LRSAM1 [130]. The authors proposed that *LRSAM1* mutations may act in a dominant-negative manner in AD CMT2; it remains unclear how loss-of-function AR CMT2-associated *LRSAM1* mutations cause a similar phenotype to the dominant forms [130]. Motor

neuron development was disturbed in zebrafish embryos injected with morpholino oligonucleotides against Lrsam1 [130].

CMT4B1 and CMT4B2 are both caused by mutations in myotubularin-related proteins. *MTMR2*[131, 132] encodes a dual specificity phosphatase that dephosphorylates phosphatidylinositol 3,5-bisphosphate (PI(3,5)P$_2$) and phosphatidylinositol 3-phosphate (PI(3)P), membrane-bound phosphoinositides with a role in signaling and intracellular trafficking of vesicles along the endosome–lysosome pathway [133]. MTMR2 may therefore play a role in membrane trafficking, endocytosis, and control of myelination [134, 135]. Disease-associated mutations in *MTMR2* cause a loss of phosphatase activity when assayed in the mouse ortholog *Mtmr2* [134]. *MTMR2* mutations also impair MTMR2 dimerization, which is needed for its phosphatase activity [117]. Perturbed homeostasis of PI(3,5)P$_2$ levels may lead to altered exocytosis or endocytosis/protein recycling and to loss of control over phospholipid metabolism; this provides one hypothesis for the excess membrane formation during myelination forming the myelin outfoldings seen in CMT4B1 [135] (Figure 19.2).

Mtmr2-null mice recapitulate the CMT4B1 phenotype [136]. Although loss of Mtmr2 in Schwann cells of mice is enough to cause CMT4B1 neuropathy, this is not the case when Mtmr2 is disrupted selectively in motor neurons [136]. However, MTMR2 was found to interact with FIG4 in Schwann cells and neurons, indicating a possible role of MTMR2 in neurons after all. In fact, loss of Mtmr2 activity is rescued by *Fig4* heterozygosity *in vivo* and *in vitro* [135]. The MTMR2 protein also interacts with NF-L, and CMT-associated mutations in *MTMR2* lead to NF-L aggregation [117].

Myotubularin-related protein 13 (*MTMR13*), mutated in CMT4B2 [137–139], is an inactive phosphatase of PI(3,5)P$_2$ and PI(3)P. *Mtmr13*-deficient mice develop a peripheral neuropathy mimicking CMT4B2. Mtmr2 and Mtmr13 associate to form a complex, leading to increased catalytic activity of Mtmr2 [140].

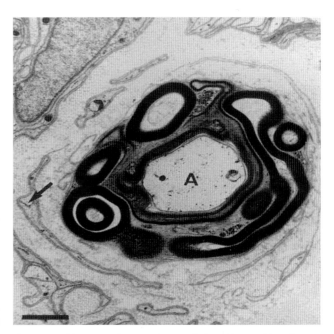

Figure 19.2 Transverse electron micrograph through a myelinated nerve fiber from a CMT4B1 patient showing multiple myelin outfoldings. Supernumerary Schwann cell processes (arrow) surround the fiber. A, axon. Bar = 1 μm.

Furthermore, *Mtmr2* levels are reduced in the nerves of these mice, indicating that Mtmr13 may regulate Mtmr2 [141].

FIG4, associated with CMT4J [108], is a PI(3,5)P$_2$ 5-phosphatase that is needed for PI(3,5)P$_2$ turnover. Fibroblasts from mice with a null mutation in *Fig4* (pale tremor mice) have reduced levels of PI(3,5)P$_2$; the reduced levels of PI(3,5)P$_2$ are unexpected but may be explained by the interaction of Fig4 with Fab1 and Vac14 which regulate the levels of PI(3,5)P$_2$ [133]. Given the peripheral neuropathy phenotype of the mutant *Fig4* mouse, *FIG4* was considered a candidate gene for CMT, and patients with mutations in *FIG4* leading to FIG4 deficiency were subsequently identified [142]. Vacuoles identified in affected patient fibroblasts in CMT4J, most likely representing dysfunctional late endosomes or lysosomes, obstructed the proper intracellular trafficking of organelles [108].

Pale tremor mice also contain vacuoles immunoreactive for lysosomal-associated membrane protein 2 (LAMP-2), evidence of disrupted membrane trafficking along the endosome–lysosome pathway [143]. Specifically, pale tremor mice have a defect in autophagy, which may ultimately lead to neuronal death due to decreased degradation of proteins in neurons [143]. These findings suggest that the degradation of membrane proteins is important for the functioning of cells of the nervous system [133]. The *FIG4* I41T mutation, usually found in combination with a null allele in patients, was found to destabilize FIG4 by affecting its interaction with VAC14, making I41T a hypomorphic allele. Increased expression of the mutant allele rescued this interaction and corrected the autophagy defect [144].

RAB7, the causative gene in CMT2B [145, 146], encodes a GTPase needed for transport between late endosomes and lysosomes [147]. Rab7 is important for growth factor signaling and for regulating endocytosis [148]. Mutant Rab7 is mostly in the GTP-bound form and has reduced GTPase activity, which causes the protein to bind more strongly to certain Rab7 effectors [147]. *Rab7* CMT2B mutants increased the phosphorylation of Trk-A, a nerve growth factor receptor that, together with Rab7, regulates neurite outgrowth [148]. Enhanced Trk-A phosphorylation led to increased phosphorylation of extracellular signal-regulated kinase 1/2 (Erk1/2), a signaling pathway downstream from Trk-A, on signaling endosomes. Activated Erk1/2 accumulated in the cytoplasm, which decreased its shuttling to the nucleus where it is needed for up-regulation of genes required for sensory neuron differentiation [148]. This mechanism may explain the inhibition of neurite outgrowth seen in cells transfected with CMT2B-associated mutations [149]. Alternatively, given its proposed functions, *RAB7* mutations may cause neuropathy through a defect in trafficking or protein degradation at the lysosome.

Lipopolysaccharide-induced TNF alpha factor/small integral membrane protein of lysosome/late endosome (*LITAF/SIMPLE*) mutations are associated with CMT1C [150–152]. LITAF is highly expressed in myelinating Schwann cells [153]. It is a membrane protein that regulates protein sorting at the early endosome [153]. LITAF binds to neural precursor cell expressed developmentally down-regulated protein 4 (Nedd4), an E3 ubiquitin ligase that regulates lysosomal degradation of plasma membrane proteins. LITAF also interacts with Itch, which induces the proteasomal degradation of a variety of substrates. Co-expression of LITAF and Itch causes Itch to relocalize from the *trans*-Golgi network to the lysosome [154]. In CMT1C, the mutant protein is mislocalized to the cytosol and is unstable, leading to degradation through the proteasome and aggresome–autophagy pathways. Therefore, *LITAF* mutations are thought to act by both loss- and gain-of-function mechanisms,

involving impaired trafficking of proteins such as myelin proteins, and protein aggregation, respectively [153].

SH3TC2 (also known as *KIAA1985*) encodes a protein located in the recycling endosome and expressed exclusively in Schwann cells in the PNS [155]. CMT4C-associated mutations [156, 157] prevent the binding of SH3TC2 to Rab11, a GTPase that regulates recycling of receptors and internalized membrane, leading to mistargeting of the protein away from the recycling endosome [158]. Accordingly, CMT4C may be due to defective membrane trafficking and sorting of myelin components, or to a problem with endocytic recycling of cargos essential for myelination [155, 158].

Two heat shock proteins have been associated with CMT, as well as dHMN. Heat shock proteins recognize and correct protein misfolding. *HSPB8,* which encodes the small heat shock protein 22 (HSP22), is associated with CMT2L [159, 160]. HSP22 is a chaperone protein with a role in protein folding, stress response, and regulation of apoptosis. In cell culture, mutant HSPB8 causes neurite degeneration selectively in motor neurons [161]. *HSPB8*-related CMT may be due to deficient protein quality control due to loss of its function as a chaperone. CMT2F is caused by mutations in *HSPB1,* which encodes the small heat shock protein 27 (HSP27) [162, 163]. HSP27 is a heat shock chaperone protein with a role in protein folding and quality control and in homeostasis of the neurofilament network [163]. *HSPB1* mutations lead to defects in neurofilament assembly and NF-L protein aggregation, thus affecting the cytoskeleton and axonal transport [115, 163]. Certain *HSPB1* mutations exhibit greater chaperone activity and increased affinity for tubulin and microtubules, which perturbs microtubule dynamics and affects axonal transport of proteins and vesicles [164]. Deficits in axonal transport, particularly that of mitochondria, were also found to result from decreased levels of acetylated α-tubulin in an *Hspb1* mouse model [165]. Acetylation serves as a guidance cue for axonal transport by motor proteins.

Ion channels

CMT has also been linked to mutations in a gene coding for a cation channel, transient receptor vanilloid 4 (TRPV4) [166–168], thus extending the range of functions of the proteins involved in CMT. The cation channel encoded by *TRPV4* is important for the transduction of sensory inputs. *TRPV4* mutations are associated with a variety of diseases, with neuropathy phenotypes resulting mainly from mutations in the ankyrin domain. CMT-associated mutations disturb calcium homeostasis; Ca^{2+} has many functions in neurons, including signaling, neurite outgrowth, and plasticity of synapses [168]. One hypothesis for the pathomechanism of neuropathy-associated *TRPV4* mutations involves decreased surface localization of mutant proteins and reduced calcium influx, indicating impaired ion channel assembly and trafficking [167]. In contrast, other functional studies have reported a loss of normal channel function, with increased calcium entry and toxicity due to increased channel conductance [168–170].

Miscellaneous

The role of some CMT-associated genes in the development of neuropathy remains to be discovered. For example, phosphoribosyl pyrophosphate synthetase (PRPS1) is a metabolic enzyme needed for nucleotide biosynthesis and purine metabolism. CMT2X [171] mutations cause a partial loss of function associated with decreased enzyme activity, which may damage the nervous system; however, the precise mechanism of disease is not yet elucidated [171].

Fibulin-5 (*FBLN5*) mutations have been identified in a CMT1 patient with age-related macular degeneration and hyperextensible skin [172]. FBLN5 is an extracellular matrix glycoprotein needed for elastic fiber assembly. *FBLN5* mutations may cause protein misfolding, leading to disrupted protein interactions at the extracellular matrix and impaired neuronal cell–cell interactions [172].

HMSN-Russe is a severe, early-onset form of demyelinating recessive CMT with significant sensory loss. *HK1* mutations were identified in an alternative untranslated exon of *HK1* [173]. HK1 is needed for the regulation of energy metabolism and cell survival. The functional mechanism causing neuropathy is still unknown [174].

POLG1 mutations were identified in an AR axonal CMT family with ataxia and tremor [175]. CMT-associated mutations in *POLG1*, which encodes mitochondrial DNA (mtDNA) polymerase γ, lead to impaired mtDNA maintenance [175].

Proteins of unknown function

The precise function of the gene associated with HMSN-Lom or CMT4D, *NDRG1* [176, 177] remains to be elucidated [178]. NDRG1 is highly expressed in Schwann cells [177] and has been postulated to play a role in various cell functions such as growth arrest, terminal differentiation, gene expression regulation, and proteasomal degradation [178]. *NDRG1* mutations have been postulated to cause neuropathy by impairment of Schwann cell trafficking needed for nerve growth [178].

Various loci have been linked to CMT, but the causative gene has not yet been identified. These include a locus at 12q12 in CMT2G [179] and a locus at 3q13.1 for HMSN-Proximal [180]. Two loci have been linked to dominant intermediate CMT: 10q24.1-q25.1, classified as DI-CMTA [181], and 3q28-q29 [182].

The environment may also play a role in modulating disease severity of inherited peripheral neuropathies. CMT1A patients display high intra- and inter-familial phenotypic variability, even between monozygotic twins [183], thus pointing to a role of the environment and epigenetics in influencing disease severity. Exposure to neurotoxins such as heavy metals and solvents, and medications such as vincristine may also exacerbate disease.

Distal hereditary motor neuropathy

dHMNs exhibit some overlap with axonal CMT, with some of the genes causing dHMN also associated with AD CMT2, such as *GARS, TRPV4, HSPB1,* and *HSPB8.* The genetic subtypes of dHMN and associated protein functions are summarized in Table 19.2. To date, about 80% of patients have no genetic diagnosis, therefore many dHMN genes remain to be discovered [184].

DNA/RNA processing

The function and potential pathogenic mechanisms of mutations in *GARS,* which encodes an amino acyl t-RNA synthetase, have been previously discussed since they are also associated with CMT2D [87]. *GARS* mutations may act via a toxic gain-of-function mechanism or may affect a non-canonical function of the protein [184]. Mutations in immunoglobulin μ binding protein 2 (*IGHMBP2*) are associated with spinal muscular atrophy with respiratory distress type 1 and classified as dHMN type 6 [185]. IGHMBP2 is a 5′-3′ helicase that unwinds RNA and DNA duplexes. *IGHMBP2* mutations impair helicase activity and may thus implicate impaired protein translation in disease pathogenesis [184]. Senataxin (*SETX*) mutations have been associated with dHMN and juvenile amyotrophic lateral sclerosis type 4

Table 19.2 Classification of dHMNs and associated protein functions.

Type	Phenotype	Gene/locus	Inheritance	Protein function
dHMN type 1	Early-onset, typical distal motor neuropathy beginning in lower limbs	HSPB1/HSP27	AD	Chaperone, protein folding/quality control, neurofilament network organization
		HSPB8/HSP22	AD	Chaperone, protein folding, stress response, and regulation of apoptosis
		GARS	AD	t-RNA synthetase, protein synthesis
		DYNC1H1	AD	Motor protein, retrograde axonal transport
dHMN type 2	Adult-onset, typical distal motor neuropathy beginning in lower limbs	HSPB1/HSP27	AD	See dHMN type 1
		HSPB8/HSP22	AD	See dHMN type 1
		BSCL2	AD	Unknown
		HSPB3	AD	Heat shock protein
dHMN type 3	Slow progression	11q13	AR	N/A
dHMN type 4	Slow progression with diaphragmatic palsy	11q13	AR	N/A
dHMN type 5	Upper limb predominance	BSCL2	AD	Unknown
		GARS	AD	See dHMN type 1
dHMN type 6	Spinal muscular atrophy with respiratory distress type 1, early-onset, distal weakness and respiratory failure	IGHMBP2	AR	DNA/RNA processing
dHMN type 7	Adult-onset, vocal cord paralysis	DCTN1	AD	Motor protein of microtubules, important for retrograde axonal transport
		TRPV4	AD	Cation channel, transduction of sensory inputs
		2q14	AD	N/A
X-linked dHMN	Distal-onset weakness and wasting	ATP7A	X-linked	Copper transport
dHMN with pyramidal features	Pyramidal signs	SETX	AD	Possibly DNA/RNA processing
		BSCL2	AD	Unknown
		4q34-35	AD	N/A
		7q34-q36	AD	N/A
HMN-J	Pyramidal signs, Jerash region of Jordan	9p21.1-p12	AR	N/A
Congenital distal spinal muscular atrophy	Congenital distal weakness, arthrogryposis	TRPV4	AD	See dHMN type 7

AD, autosomal dominant; AR, autosomal recessive; dHMN, distal hereditary motor neuropathy; N/A, not applicable.
Source: Rossor et al. 2011 [185]. Reproduced with permission of BMJ Publishing Group Ltd.

[184, 186]. SETX may be a DNA/RNA helicase with a role in mRNA splicing and transcription; dHMN probably results from a toxic gain of function in SETX [184].

Stress response and protein quality control
HSPB1 and *HSPB8*, which encode HSP27 and HSP22, respectively, were previously mentioned as heat shock chaperone proteins mutated in dominant axonal forms of CMT; however, they have also been associated with dHMN [163, 187]. These mutant proteins likely cause suboptimal protein quality control through the loss of their chaperone function. Mutant HSP22 may also lead to the formation of aggregates containing HSP27 in motor neurons [184]. The Berardinelli–Seip congenital lipodystrophy type 2 (*BSCL2*) gene encodes the protein seipin, an integral membrane protein of the ER with an unknown function. Mutations in *BSCL2* cause protein misfolding and result in aggregate formation [188] and activation of the UPR leading to increased apoptotic cell death [184].

The pathogenicity of the mutation in heat shock protein beta-3 (*HSPB3*) found in a dHMN patient remains to be confirmed. *HSPB3* codes for the heat shock protein HSPL27 [184, 189].

Axonal transport
As described above, *HSPB1* mutations caused defects in neurofilament assembly and led to NF-L protein aggregation, reduced acetylated α-tubulin, and disturbed axonal transport of mitochondria. The dynactin (DCTN1) protein forms part of a complex needed for dynein-mediated retrograde transport of organelles and vesicles. When mutated, the binding affinity of DCTN1 for microtubules is reduced, causing a motor neuron disease phenotype classified as dHMN type 7 [190]. A mutation in the motor protein DYNC1H1 was described to cause CMT2, however it may also fall under the category of dHMN as the sensory action potentials were normal in some affected individuals [119, 184].

Cation channels
ATP7A is an ATPase needed for the metalation of copper enzymes and for the inhibition of the toxic accumulation of copper [184]. The protein, usually translocated from the *trans*-Golgi network to the plasma membrane as part of its role in copper transport, accumulates at the plasma membrane in mutant cell lines, suggesting impaired endocytic recycling [184]. dHMN owing to *ATP7A* mutations may therefore result from disturbed copper homeostasis [191]. ATP7A has also been implicated in normal axonal outgrowth and synaptogenesis; disturbances in these functions may contribute to causing neuropathy [191]. In addition to CMT2C, *TRPV4* mutations may also cause dHMN [167]. As discussed previously, mutations in this cation channel often cause increased intracellular calcium and cytotoxicity, and may result from a gain-of-function mechanism [184].

Hereditary sensory and autonomic neuropathy
To date, 12 genes have been associated with HSAN, however the genetic cause of disease is unknown in approximately two-thirds of HSAN patients [192]. The genetic subtypes of HSANs and associated protein functions are summarized in Table 19.3.

Axonal transport
Kinesin family member 1A (KIF1A)/ATSV is a motor protein needed for the anterograde axonal transport of synaptic vesicle precursors [193]. Mutations in *KIF1A* are associated with HSAN type 2C. KIF1A interacts with WNK lysine deficient protein kinase 1 (WNK1); it may be that WNK1 is needed for the unloading of the KIF1A cargo at axonal tips [192, 193].

The inhibitor of kappa light polypeptide gene enhancer in B-cells, kinase complex-associated protein (*IKBKAP*) gene, encodes elongator complex protein 1 (ELP1), a scaffold protein needed for the assembly of the RNA polymerase II elongator complex. *IKBKAP* is mutated in HSAN3, also known as Riley–Day syndrome [194].

Table 19.3 Classification of HSAN and associated protein functions.

Type	Gene/locus	Phenotype	Inheritance	Protein function
HSAN1A	SPTLC1	Early adulthood-onset, acromutilation, neuropathic pain, loss of pain and temperature sensation, variable distal motor involvement, may be similar to CMT2B	AD	Sphingolipid metabolism
HSAN1B	3p24	Adult-onset, sensory loss, foot ulcerations, cough, gastroesophageal reflux	AD	N/A
HSAN1C	SPTLC2	Adult-onset, acromutilation, neuropathic pain, loss of pain and temperature sensation, variable distal motor involvement	AD	Sphingolipid metabolism
HSAN1D	ATL1	Adult-onset, severe distal sensory loss, ulcero-mutilations	AD	Endoplasmic reticulum tubulation
HSAN1E	DNMT1	Adult-onset, loss of sensation, neuropathic pain, ulcero-mutilations, dementia, sensorineural hearing loss	AD	DNA methylation, chromatin stability
CMT2B	RAB7	Adult-onset, loss of sensation, ulcero-mutilations, distal motor weakness	AD	GTPase, retrograde trafficking of vesicles
HSAN2	WNK1/HSN2	Early-onset, severe, sensory complications	AR	Ion channel regulation
HSAN2B	FAM134B	Early-onset, ulcero-mutilations, defective nociception, osteomyelitis	AR	Unknown
HSAN2C	ATSV (KIF1A)	Early-onset, ulcero-mutilations, loss of position and vibration sense, some distal weakness	AR	Transport of synaptic vesicle precursors
HSAN3 (Riley–Day)	IKBKAP	Ashkenazi Jewish population, neonatal-onset, predominant autonomic involvement, no pain and temperature sensation, fatal	AR	Cell migration, component of the RNA polymerase II elongator complex
HSAN4/congenital insensitivity to pain with anhidrosis (CIPA)	NTRK1	Congenital or early-onset, insensitivity to pain, anhidrosis, some mental retardation, joint deformities, unmyelinated fibers affected	AR	Nerve growth factor receptor, neuronal development and survival
HSAN5	NGFB	Israeli/Bedouins, similar to HSAN4 but no mental retardation, less anhidrosis	AR	Neuronal development and survival
HSAN5	NTRK1	Congenital insensitivity to pain, mild anhidrosis, no mental retardation, small myelinated fibers affected	AR	See HSAN4
Small fiber peripheral neuropathy	SCN9A	Congenital insensitivity to pain	AR	Voltage-gated sodium channel

AD, autosomal dominant; AR, autosomal recessive; HSAN, hereditary sensory and autonomic neuropathy; N/A, not applicable.
Source: Rotthier et al. 2012 [193]. Reproduced with permission of Nature Publishing Group.

Knockdown of IKBKAP is associated with defects in the integrity of this complex and causes impaired cell migration. The lack of a functional complex leads to down-regulation of genes related to cell motility, peripheral neurogenesis, and neuronal differentiation, as well as neuronal development and cerebral oligodendrocyte development and myelination [192]. The RNA polymerase II elongator complex is also important for the acetylation of α-tubulin; ELP1 knockdown leads to reduced acetylation of α-tubulin in microtubules and likely impacts the trafficking of various proteins. Disorganization of the actin cytoskeleton has been observed in migrating fibroblasts from HSAN3 patients [192].

Neurotrophin transport and signaling

Neurotrophic tyrosine kinase, receptor, type 1 (*NTRK1*) encodes the nerve growth factor receptor Trk-A, which is necessary for neurotrophin signaling. Mutations in NTRK1 are associated with two subtypes, HSAN4 and HSAN5 [195]. Trk-A binds to nerve growth factor beta (NGFB) and activates pathways involved in neurite outgrowth [192]. Activation of downstream signaling is impaired in Trk-A mutants [192]. *NGFB* mutations are also associated with HSAN [196]. Mutations in *NGFB*, which encodes a neurotrophin necessary for neuronal development and survival, disrupt the signaling pathway involving NGFB and Trk-A [192]. Sensory and autonomic ganglion neurons undergo apoptosis in the absence of neurotrophins [197]; it is therefore not surprising that mutations in NGFB, a neurotrophin, and its receptor Trk-A lead to HSAN.

RAB7, previously mentioned as being the CMT2B-associated gene, also comes under the umbrella of HSANs as mutations in this gene can cause significant sensory loss. RAB7 is responsible for retrograde transport of neurotrophins such as NGFB and its receptor Trk-A on signaling endosomes [148].

Neuronal membrane excitability

The *HSN2* gene was initially thought to be located within an intron of the *WNK1* gene [198]; however, *HSN2* is now recognized to be a nervous-tissue-specific exon of *WNK1* [192]. WNK1, a serine-threonine kinase important for sodium, chloride, and potassium homeostasis, decreases the expression of TrpV4 channels at the cell surface. Mutations in *WNK1* are predicted to cause loss of protein function, possibly causing increased expression of the TrpV4 channel and altered membrane excitability [192]. NGFB and Trk-A may also cause changes in membrane excitability as they are able to sensitize TrpV1 channels.

Sphingolipid metabolism

The two subunits of the serine palmitoyltransferase are mutated in HSAN1: serine palmitoyltransferase long chain base subunit-1 (*SPTLC1*) [199, 200] and serine palmitoyltransferase long chain base subunit-2 (*SPTLC2*) [201]. The enzyme is necessary for the biosynthesis of sphingolipids, which are components of lipid rafts, structures needed for signal transduction in the plasma membrane. Haploinsufficiency is not predicted to be the mechanism of disease; rather, mutations in both *SPTLC1* and *SPTLC2* lead to reduced enzyme activity and to production of deoxysphingoid bases, abnormal metabolites that accumulate in the cell and impair neurite outgrowth *in vitro* [192, 202]. The production of these deoxysphingoid bases may cause ER stress; alternatively, defects in the sphingolipid composition may affect endocytic recycling or sensory neuron excitability [192].

Mutations in atlastin-1 (*ATL1*), which encodes a dynamin-related GTPase previously known to be involved in early-onset hereditary spastic paraplegia (HSP), led to decreased GTPase activity and to defects in the ER network [203]. A dominant-negative effect was suggested in some of the HSP-associated *ATL1* mutations. It remains unknown how *ATL1* mutations can give rise to these two phenotypes [192].

Miscellaneous

DNA methyltransferase 1 (*DNMT1*) mutations cause an HSAN phenotype with dementia and hearing loss. DNMT1 is necessary for maintenance of methylation, chromatin stability, and gene regulation [204]. Mutations caused abnormal methylation through decreased enzyme activity and perturbed heterochromatin binding, thus implicating epigenetic mechanisms in neurodegenerative diseases [204].

The function of the FAM134B protein has not yet been fully elucidated, although it is involved in maintenance of the structure of the *cis*-Golgi matrix and is mainly expressed in sensory and autonomic ganglia. Mutations in *FAM134B* result in loss of protein function and *Fam134b* knockdown causes structural alterations in the *cis*-Golgi and apoptosis in dorsal root ganglion neurons [197].

Congenital inability to experience pain due to mutations in sodium channel, voltage-gated, type IX, alpha subunit (*SCN9A*) is also included in the HSAN group [205]. SCN9A encodes the α-subunit of the voltage-gated sodium channel, Nav1.7, which is highly expressed in nociceptive neurons. HSAN owing to *SCN9A* mutations leads to loss of function of the channel and reduction or loss of sensation of pain [205].

Similarly to some of the HSANs, familial amyloid polyneuropathy (FAP) involves damage to the autonomic nerve fibers. FAP is associated with amyloid fibril formation and protein aggregation. FAP is most commonly due to mutations in transthyretin (*TTR*), but is also associated with mutations in apolipoprotein A-1 and gelsolin [206].

Hereditary neuralgic amyotrophy

The genetic forms of HNA are associated with autosomal dominant mutations in septin 9 (*SEPT9*), which encodes a protein necessary for filament formation and cell division [207]. *SEPT9* mutations may cause disease by altering filament assembly. In addition to the genetic basis of the disease, immune-mediated mechanisms as well as a susceptibility to injury of the brachial plexus nerve are likely to be involved in the etiology of HNA [208].

Giant axonal neuropathy

GAN is an autosomal recessive disease caused by gigaxonin mutations in which axons are enlarged due to the accumulation of neurofilaments [209]. Gigaxonin is thought to be involved in axonal transport [210]. *GAN* mutations are associated with a loss of function of gigaxonin, causing defects in the organization of intermediate filaments in the cytoskeleton [209]. Although *Gan*-null mice exhibited relatively mild motor and sensory deficits, they showed severe dysregulation of neurofilaments as in the human neuropathy [210]. The exact pathomechanism of GAN remains to be elucidated.

Chronic inflammatory demyelinating polyradiculoneuropathy and Guillain–Barré syndrome: acquired inflammatory demyelinating neuropathies

CIDP is the most common acquired chronic autoimmune neuropathy [211]. CIDP causes multifocal demyelination of the spinal roots, plexuses, and proximal nerve trunks [211]. Electrophysiology reveals slowed NCV, conduction block with dispersion, and slowed latencies as well as axonal loss and denervation. Variants of CIDP include motor and sensory (this variant can be asymmetrical, unifocal, or multifocal), purely motor, purely sensory, or purely distal. GBS may be considered the acute form of CIDP based on their similar electrophysiological, histological, and immune descriptions [211].

The antigens targeted in CIDP have not been elucidated, although recent research has proposed that antigens in non-compact myelin and at the node, paranodal, and internodal axolemma might be attacked by the immune system in CIDP and GBS [211, 212]. Demyelination may result from a disturbance to the Schwann cell and axon integrity due to immune responses against adhesion molecules located in these structural areas [212].

Identification of biomarkers in peripheral neuropathies

As potential drugs are tested in future clinical trials, sensitive outcome measures will become necessary to measure amelioration over time, especially in slowly progressive neuropathies [8].

Magnetic resonance imaging (MRI) has recently been more extensively investigated as a possible method to measure disease severity and disease progression in neuropathies such as CMT, CIDP, and dHMN. Studies have used MRI to measure muscle atrophy and replacement of muscle by fat, as well as to establish denervation patterns. The longest nerves were more atrophied and showed greater fatty infiltration in CMT and dHMN [213]. MRI findings were found to correlate with disease severity in CMT1A, CIDP, and dHMN [213, 214]. Therefore, MRI could be used to detect disease before it manifests or in asymptomatic patients, and as an outcome measure in clinical trials [213].

The high phenotypic variability in CMT1A makes it difficult for clinicians to predict disease course in patients and their children. In the search for biomarkers, a study has identified lipid metabolism genes that are dysregulated in sciatic nerve transcriptomes of CMT1A rats; these may be modifiers of disease progression. Analysis of gene expression from skin biopsies of CMT1A patients in this study further showed that the mRNA levels of some lipid metabolism genes as well as the age of the patient together could explain 47% of the variance in disease severity defined by the CMTNS [215]. The development of disease severity markers would assist patients in planning their future with regards to treatment and family planning [8].

Biomarkers are also being investigated for immune-mediated neuropathies. Levels of neural protein such as glial fibrillary acidic protein in serum and cerebrospinal fluid are being considered for measuring axonal damage and predicting clinical outcome [216].

Investigation of peripheral neuropathies

An important part of the assessment of any patient with peripheral neuropathy is a careful history, assessment of acquired risk factors, family tree, and examination. The examination can often reveal diagnostic clues such as thickened peripheral nerves in CMT1A. The CMTNS is currently used to measure neuropathy progression and incorporates patient symptoms, signs, and neurophysiologic abnormalities [217]. Previously, impairment was measured using the 9-hole peg test, the ambulation index, and a Jamar® dynamometer to measure handgrip strength [217]. The CMTNS is important to document at each visit and in the assessment of any therapeutic trials.

Investigations may include blood tests to exclude acquired causes of neuropathy, including a test of glucose tolerance if a diabetic neuropathy is suspected and vitamin assays for nutritional deficiencies. Tests of liver function are used to exclude alcoholic neuropathy, and autoantibodies such as anti-MAG are measured to exclude monoclonal gammopathy [218]. Electromyography and nerve conduction studies (NCS) are essential in evaluating the velocities and amplitudes of sensory and motor nerves [218] and are useful in determining whether the neuropathy is symmetrical or asymmetrical and generalized, focal, or multifocal, as well as whether conduction block is present. NCS also assist clinicians in classifying CMT cases into demyelinating and axonal forms.

The advent of genetic testing has greatly reduced the need for sural nerve biopsies but biopsy can still be a helpful investigation of acquired and inflammatory neuropathies. Nerve biopsy may be particularly useful in the diagnosis of familial amyloid polyneuropathy and rare genetic conditions such as GAN that have pathognomonic biopsy features. Other investigations under development include skin biopsies, particularly in painful neuropathies, and peripheral nerve MRI.

Diagnosis of peripheral neuropathies

The clinician should first determine whether the neuropathy is motor, sensory and/or autonomic, symmetrical or asymmetrical, chronic or acute, and distal versus proximal. It is important that non-genetic causes are ruled out in the first instance. Clues that the neuropathy may be genetic include a positive family history; however, the lack of a positive family history does not necessarily preclude a patient from having a genetic form of neuropathy. Additional features that point towards a genetic neuropathy include early onset, foot deformities, and a slowly progressive disease course (except in HNPP [5]). A symmetrical rather than focal distribution (except HNPP) and the lack of conduction block and uniform NCV slowing are additional clues for a genetic etiology to the neuropathy [219]. A genetic cause is also likely in adults whose CMT involves sensory features but who present with no positive sensory symptoms [8].

Two decades after the discovery of the genetic cause of CMT1A, technological advances in genetics have allowed at least 40 additional causative genes to be linked to CMT. The diagnosis of CMT now involves a combination of neurophysiological studies, family history, and genetic testing as well as a consideration for the frequency of genetic subtypes in various ethnic backgrounds [8]. The clinician should decide whether the neuropathy is demyelinating or axonal using NCS, and should subsequently determine the inheritance pattern (dominant, recessive, X-linked).

Following a diagnostic algorithm that takes into consideration neurophysiology, inheritance patterns, and specific disease features is evidently useful in highly genetically heterogeneous neuropathies such as CMT (Figure 19.3), dHMN (Figure 19.4), and HSAN (Figure 19.5).

CMT1A, CMT1X, HNPP, CMT1B, and CMT2A are the most common subtypes of CMT, while other subtypes represent less than 1% of CMT patients [219]. Today, we are able to obtain a genetic diagnosis in 70% of patients with CMT [219], which is of great importance to patients despite there being no available treatments as it may help give a better prognosis and help patients and their families know how their disease is likely to progress [8]. Determining the genetic cause of disease is useful for genetic counseling as well as to rule out inflammatory forms of neuropathy that may be

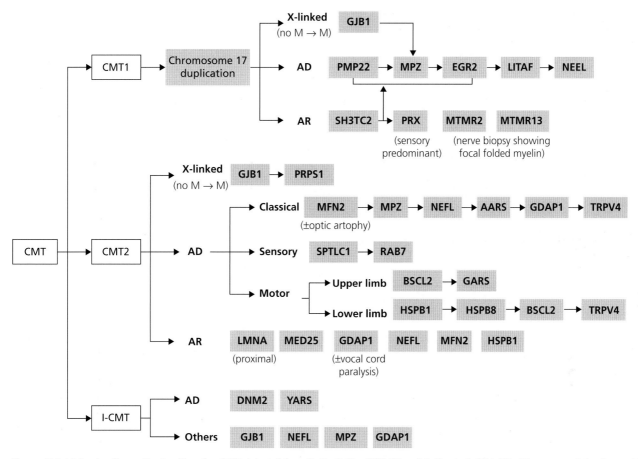

Figure 19.3 Molecular diagnostic algorithm for CMT. Adapted from Reilly & Shy 2009 [5] and Reilly et al. 2011 [8]. AD, autosomal dominant; AR, autosomal recessive.

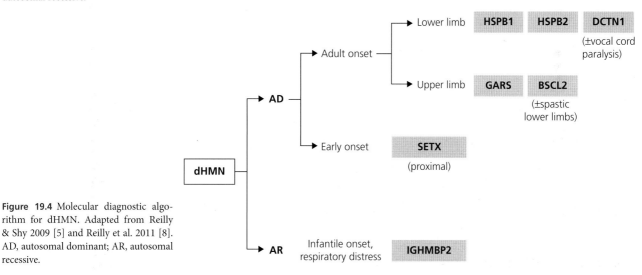

Figure 19.4 Molecular diagnostic algorithm for dHMN. Adapted from Reilly & Shy 2009 [5] and Reilly et al. 2011 [8]. AD, autosomal dominant; AR, autosomal recessive.

treatable such as CIDP and to avoid unnecessary interventions [8]. Reaching a genetic diagnosis is increasingly important for future treatments targeted to specific causative genes [5, 8].

Treatment options in peripheral neuropathies

Unfortunately, no effective treatment currently exists to reverse peripheral nerve damage. In acquired neuropathies, avoiding the cause, improving diabetes control, or treating infection are essential steps for prevention of neuropathy. Alcohol, toxins, or other drugs known to cause neuropathy such as vincristine should be avoided. Neuropathic pain may be relieved by the use of medication such as gabapentin, pregabalin, other anti-epileptics, and/or tricyclic antidepressants. CIDP patients benefit from treatment with corticosteroids, intravenous immunoglobulin (IVIg), and/or plasmapheresis [211].

High-dose ascorbic acid, which is needed for collagen synthesis and basal lamina formation, was shown to reduce levels of PMP22 and to improve the phenotype in a CMT1A mouse model [220],

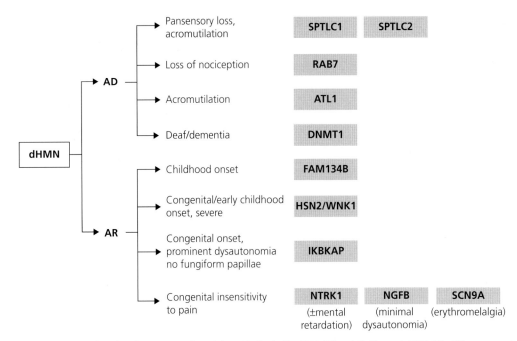

Figure 19.5 Molecular diagnostic algorithm for HSAN. Adapted from Reilly & Shy 2009 [5] and Reilly et al. 2011 [8]. AD, autosomal dominant; AR, autosomal recessive;

possibly by reducing cyclic adenosine monophosphate (cAMP) levels in Schwann cells [221, 222]. Clinical trials of ascorbic acid in CMT1A patients showed no efficacy; however, the outcome measures and length of the trial might be an issue as the disease progresses very slowly [223].

In some CMT cases, a superimposed inflammatory neuropathy may worsen symptoms over several weeks or months [16]. In this case, the use of immunosuppressive or immunomodulatory treatment may be beneficial. Physiotherapy and rehabilitation therapy including stretching, strength training, and gentle exercise to prevent contractures and foot deformities remain extremely valuable in managing the symptoms of neuropathies [221]. Orthotics, including ankle–foot orthoses, splints, insoles, braces, and adapted footwear, are useful for patients with foot drop or sprained ankles from weak muscles. Caring for feet, pressure sores, and skin problems that may arise from loss of sensation is also important [224]. Patients with HNPP should avoid trauma that may cause an episode, and should not keep one position for long periods of time. Nerve entrapment such as that occurring in HNPP may be resolved by the surgical release of ligaments or tendons, however this is not always helpful. Corrective surgery such as osteotomy, arthrodesis, and tendon transfer is used for foot deformities. Patients may benefit from help with everyday and occupational tasks from occupational therapists, as these tasks may be a source of fatigue. Weight control and a healthy diet should also be part of the long-term management of neuropathy patients.

Future developments in peripheral neuropathies

Next-generation sequencing
With the development of next-generation sequencing, we expect the diagnosis of inherited neuropathies to be more comprehensive, faster, and cheaper. New sequencing machines such as the Illumina® MiSeq and HiSeq will allow for targeted sequencing of inherited

neuropathy genes in customized gene panels. This technology, along with whole-genome and whole-exome sequencing, will lead to the identification of new genes for inherited neuropathy and modifier genes to explain variability in disease severity [225–229].

Experimental therapeutic treatments
Although ascorbic acid has not provided significant benefit to CMT1A patients in clinical trials thus far, this potential treatment should be re-assessed in trials over a longer time period and with more sensitive outcome measures.

CMT1A operates through a gene dosage mechanism therefore future therapies could aim to reduce levels of PMP22. However, it should be noted that PMP22 levels vary greatly between patients, therefore any such therapy would have to be adapted to individual patients [221]. Progesterone is a steroid that increases the expression of PMP22 both at the mRNA and protein level. Antagonists of progesterone receptors such as onapristone were beneficial in CMT1A rat models [230]. Unfortunately, these agents are too toxic to be used in humans [221, 230].

The commonly available spice curcumin promotes the translocation of misfolded proteins from the ER to the plasma membrane, thus reducing the cytotoxicity of aberrant proteins such as PMP22 and MPZ accumulating within the ER. Oral curcumin led to decreased apoptosis in cell lines expressing *PMP22* and *MPZ* mutants and an amelioration of the phenotype in Trembler-J mice [231]. A 12-month safety trial of oral curcumin in a DSD patient showed no adverse events but also no significant improvement in outcome measures such as muscle strength, pulmonary function, and neurophysiological studies [232].

Other potential drugs targeted to a specific disease mechanism include inhibitors of histone deacetylase 6 (HDAC6) which led to increased α-tubulin acetylation, improved axonal transport and amelioration of the neuropathy phenotype in mutant *Hspb1* mice [165]. Mitofusin 1 (MFN1) and MFN2 are both important for mitochondrial fusion, and wild-type MFN1 can form complexes with and complement mutant MFN2 [233]. Therefore molecules to increase expression of MFN1 in neurons may help repair mitochondrial fusion in CMT2A patients [233, 234]. Molecules that reduce channel conduction in patients with TRPV4 mutations might be of benefit [234]. Inducers of heat shock proteins helped to prevent neurofilament defects and mitochondrial abnormalities in a model of CMT2E; these may be good therapeutic candidates [221, 235].

Schwann cells produce trophic factors to provide support to axons; because the symptoms of disease in neuropathies are mainly due to the degeneration of axons, treatment with neurotrophic factors may be an effective therapy in CMT disease [221]. Neurotrophin-3 was tested in CMT1A mouse models and in a small cohort of CMT1A patients and showed promising results. However, problems with delivery methods and bioavailability may complicate the use of trophic factors in the treatment of neuropathies [221]. Potassium channel blockers to help maintain the charge separation in myelin and the depolarization at the nodes of Ranvier are also being investigated for demyelinating neuropathies, however preliminary trials have not shown any benefit [5]. Targeting Schwann cell–axon signaling pathways such as that responsible for the regulation of myelin thickness may improve neuropathies in which Schwann cell–axon interactions are defective [30].

In the future, treatment options will likely target specific pathogenic mechanisms, making accurate diagnosis even more essential. Gene replacement therapies may be used for loss-of-function or nonsense mutations. Gene silencing may be employed for regulating gene expression in CMT1A or for gain-of-function mutations [30]. Animal models in which a disease-causing gene has been knocked out are becoming increasingly available and will be of great value in further clarifying disease mechanisms and testing molecules for therapeutic treatment. Research is also currently focusing on the use of induced pluripotent stem cells from patients to produce neuronal lines on which to test new therapies [234]. These stem cells may also be used to generate new axons and treat peripheral neuropathies. However, differentiating stem cells into neurons and Schwann cells will likely prove to be a challenge [30].

References

1. Jessen KR, Mirsky R. Origin and early development of Schwann cells. *Microscope research and technique* 1998; 41:393–402.
2. Hughes R. Peripheral nerve diseases: the bare essentials. *Practical neurology* 2008; 8(6):396–405.
3. Shakher J, Stevens MJ. Update on the management of diabetic polyneuropathies. *Diabetes, metabolic syndrome and obesity: targets and therapy* 2011; 4:289–305.
4. Martin CN, Hughes RAC. Epidemiology of peripheral neuropathy. *Journal of neurology, neurosurgery, and psychiatry* 1997; 62:310–318.
5. Reilly MM, Shy ME. Diagnosis and new treatments in genetic neuropathies. *Journal of neurology, neurosurgery, and psychiatry* 2009; 80(12):1304–1314.
6. Skre H. Genetic and clinical aspects of Charcot-Marie-Tooth's disease. *Clinical genetics* 1974;6(2):98–118.
7. Braathen GJ, Sand JC, Lobato A, et al. Genetic epidemiology of Charcot-Marie-Tooth in the general population. *European journal of neurology* 2011; 18(1):39–48.
8. Reilly MM, Murphy M, Laura M. Charcot-Marie-Tooth disease. *Journal of the peripheral nervous system* 2011;14:1–14.
9. Asbury AK, Thomas PK. *Peripheral Nerve Disorders 2*. Butterworth-Heinemann: Oxford, 1995.
10. Shy ME, Chen L, Swan ER, et al. Neuropathy progression in Charcot-Marie-Tooth disease type 1A. *Neurology* 2008;70(5):378–383.
11. Charcot JM, Marie P. Sur une forme particulière d'atrophie musculaire progressive, souvent familiale débutant par les pieds et les jambes et atteignant plus tard les mains. *Revue de medecine* 1886; 6:97–138.
12. Tooth H. *The Peroneal Type of Progressive Muscular Atrophy*. H.K. Lewis and Co.: London, 1886.
13. Harding AE, Thomas PK. The clinical features of hereditary motor and sensory neuropathy types I and II. *Brain* 1980; 103:259–280.
14. Lupski JR, Oca-luna RMD, Slaugenhaupt S, et al. DNA duplication associated with Charcot-Marie-Tooth Disease Type 1A. *Cell* 1991; 66:219–32.
15. Rayemaekers P, Timmerman V, Nelis A, et al. Duplication in chromosome 17p11.2 in Charcot-Marie-Tooth Neuropathy Type 1a (CMT1a). *Neuromuscular disorders* 1991; 1(2):93-97.
16. Ginsberg L, Malik O, Kenton AR, et al. Coexistent hereditary and inflammatory neuropathy. *Brain* 2004; 127(Pt 1):193–202.
17. Vital A, Vital C, Lagueny A, et al. Inflammatory demyelination in a patient with CMT1A. *Muscle & nerve* 2003; 28(3):373–376.
18. Pareyson D, Scaioli V, Taroni F, et al. Phenotypic heterogeneity in hereditary neuropathy with liability to pressure palsies associated with chromosome 17p11.2-12 deletion. *Neurology* 1996; 46(4):1133–1137.
19. Ben Hamida C, Cavalier L, Belal S. Homozygosity mapping of giant axonal neuropathy gene to chromosome 16q24.1 *Neurogenetics* 1997; 1:129–133.
20. Houlden H, Groves M, Miedzybrodzka Z, et al. New mutations, genotype phenotype studies and manifesting carriers in giant axonal neuropathy. *Journal of neurology, neurosurgery, and psychiatry* 2007; 78(11):1267–1270.
21. Rayemaekers P, Timmerman V, De Jonghe P, et al. Localization of the mutation in an extended family with Charcot-Marie-Tooth neuropathy (HMSN1). *American journal of human genetics* 1989; 45:953–958.
22. Vance J, Nicholson G, Yamaoka L, et al. Linkage of Charcot-Marie-Tooth neuropathy type 1a to chromosome 17. *Experimental neurology* 1989; 104(2):186–189.
23. Pentao L, Wise CA, Chinault AC, et al. Charcot-Marie-Tooth type 1A appears to arise from recombination at repeat sequences flanking the 1.5Mb monomer unit. *Nature* 1992; 2:292–300.
24. Choi B-O, Kim NK, Park SW, et al. Inheritance of Charcot-Marie-Tooth disease 1A with rare nonrecurrent genomic rearrangement. *Neurogenetics* 2011; 12:51–58.
25. Matsunami N, Smith B, Ballard L, et al. Peripheral myelin protein-22 gene maps in the duplication in chromosome 17p11.2 associated Charcot-Marie-Tooth 1A. *Nature* 1992; 1:176–179.
26. Patel PI, Roa BB, Welcher AA, et al. The gene for the peripheral myelin protein PMP22 is a candidate for Charcot-Marie-Tooth Disease type 1A. *Nature* 1992; 1:159–165.
27. Timmerman V, Nelis E, Van Hul W, et al. The peripheral myelin protein gene PMP-22 is contained within the Charcot-Marie-Tooth disease type 1A duplication. *Nature* 1992; 1:171–175.
28. Valentijn LJ, Bolhuis PA, Zorn I, et al. The peripheral myelin gene PMP-22/GAS-3 is duplicated in Charcot-Marie-Tooth disease type 1A. *Nature* 1992; 1:166-170.
29. Leguern E, Tardieu S, Birouk N, et al. Patients homozygous for the 17p11.2 duplication in Charcot-Marie-Tooth type 1A disease. *Annals of neurology* 1997; 1:104–108.
30. Patzkó A, Shy ME. Update on Charcot-Marie-Tooth disease. *Current neurology and neuroscience reports* 2011; 11(1):78–88.
31. Valentijn LJ, Baas F, Wolterman RA, et al. Identical point mutations of PMP22 in Trembler-J mouse and Charcot-Marie-Tooth disease Type 1A. *Nature* 1992; 2:288–291.
32. Giambonini-Brugnoli G, Buchstaller J, Sommer L, et al. Distinct disease mechanisms in peripheral neuropathies due to altered peripheral myelin protein 22 gene dosage or a Pmp22 point mutation. *Neurobiology of disease* 2005; 18(3):656–668.
33. Adlkofer K, Martini R, Aguzzi A, et al. Hypermyelination and demyelinating peripheral neuropathy in Pmp22-deficient mice. *Nature genetics* 1995; 11(3):274–280.
34. Robaglia-Schlupp A, Pizant J, Norreel J-C, et al. PMP22 overexpression causes dysmyelination in mice. *Brain* 2002; 125(Pt 10):2213–2221.
35. Magyar JP, Martini R, Ruelicke T, et al. Impaired differentiation of Schwann cells in transgenic mice with increased PMP22 gene dosage. *Journal of Neuroscience* 1996; 16(17):5351–5360.
36. Lupski JR, Wise CA, Kuwano A, et al. Gene dosage is a mechanism for Charcot-Marie-Tooth disease Type 1A. *Nature* 1992; 1:29–33.
37. Roa BB, Luspki JR. Molecular basis of Charcot-Marie-Tooth disease type 1A: gene dosage as a novel mechanism for a common autosomal dominant condition. *Nature* 1993; 306:177–184.
38. Weterman MAJ, van Ruissen F, de Wissel M, et al. Copy number variation upstream of PMP22 in Charcot-Marie-Tooth disease. *European journal of human genetics* 2010; 18(4):421–428.
39. Zhang F, Seeman P, Liu P, et al. Mechanisms for nonrecurrent genomic rearrangements associated with CMT1A or HNPP: rare CNVs as a cause for missing heritability. *American journal of human genetics* 2010; 86(6):892–903.
40. D'Urso D, Ehrhardt P, Müller HW. Peripheral myelin protein 22 and protein zero: a novel association in peripheral nervous system myelin. *The Journal of neuroscience* 1999; 19(9):3396–3403.
41. Notterpek L, Ryan MC, Tobler AR, et al. PMP22 accumulation in aggresomes: implications for CMT1A pathology. *Neurobiology of disease* 1999; 6(5):450–460.

42. Saporta MA, Katona I, Lewis RA, *et al.* Shortened internodal length of dermal myelinated nerve fibres in Charcot-Marie-Tooth disease type 1A. *Brain* 2009; 132(Pt 12):3263–3273.

43. Roa BB, Garcia CA, Suter U, *et al.* Charcot-Marie-Tooth disease Type 1A: Association with a spontaneous point mutation in the PMP22 gene. *The New England journal of medicine* 1993; 329(2):96–100.

44. Naef R, Adlkofer K, Lescher B, *et al.* Aberrant protein trafficking in Trembler suggests a disease mechanism for hereditary human peripheral neuropathies. *Molecular and cellular neuroscience* 1997; 9:13–25.

45. Naef R, Suter U. Impaired intracellular trafficking is a common disease mechanism of PMP22 point mutations in peripheral neuropathies. *Neurobiology of disease* 1999; 6(1):1–14.

46. Tobler AR, Notterpek L, Naef R, *et al.* Transport of Trembler-J mutant peripheral myelin protein 22 is blocked in the intermediate compartment and affects the transport of the wild-type protein by direct interaction. *Journal of neuroscience* 1999; 19(6):2027–2036.

47. Colby J, Nicholson R, Dickson KM, *et al.* PMP22 carrying the trembler or trembler-J mutation is intracellularly retained in myelinating Schwann cells. *Neurobiology of disease* 2000; 7:561–573.

48. Fortun J, Li J, Go J, *et al.* Impaired proteasome activity and accumulation of ubiquitinated substrates in a hereditary neuropathy model. *Journal of neurochemistry* 2005; 92(6):1531–41.

49. Fortun J, Go JC, Li J, *et al.* Alterations in degradative pathways and protein aggregation in a neuropathy model based on PMP22 overexpression. *Neurobiology of disease* 2006; 22(1):153–164.

50. Chance PF, Alderson MK, Leppig KA, *et al.* DNA deletion associated with hereditary neuropathy with liability to pressure palsies. *Cell* 1993; 72:143–151.

51. Adlkofer K, Frei R, Neuberg DHH, *et al.* Heterozygous peripheral myelin protein 22-deficient mice are affected by a progressive demyelinating tomaculous neuropathy. *Journal of neuroscience* 1997; 17(12):4662–4671.

52. Schenone A, Nobbio L, Caponnetto C, *et al.* Correlation between PMP-22 messenger RNA expression and phenotype in hereditary neuropathy with liability to pressure palsies. *Annals of neurology* 1997; 42(6):866–872.

53. Bird TD, Ott J, Giblett ER. Evidence for linkage of Charcot-Marie-Tooth neuropathy to the Duffy locus on chromosome 1. *American journal of human genetics* 1982; 34:388–394.

54. Hayasaka K, Himoro M, Sato W, *et al.* Charcot-Marie-Tooth neuropathy type 1B is associated with mutations of the myelin P0 gene. *Nature* 1993; 5:31–34.

55. Giese KP, Martini R, Lemke G, *et al.* Mouse P0 gene disruption leads to hypomyelination, abnormal expression of recognition molecules, and degeneration of myelin and axons. *Cell* 1992; 71(4):565–576.

56. Kulkens T, Bolhuis PA, Wolterman RA, *et al.* Deletion of the serine 34 codon from the major peripheral myelin protein P0 gene in Charcot-Marie-Tooth disease type 1B. *Nature* 1993; 5:35–39.

57. Wrabetz L, D'Antonio M, Pennuto M, *et al.* Different intracellular pathomechanisms produce diverse myelin protein zero neuropathies in transgenic mice. *The Journal of neuroscience* 2006; 26(8):2358–2368.

58. Pennuto M, Tinelli E, Malaguti M, *et al.* Ablation of the UPR-mediator CHOP restores motor function and reduces demyelination in Charcot-Marie-Tooth 1B mice. *Neuron* 2008; 57(3):393–405.

59. Fratta P, Saveri P, Zambroni D, *et al.* P0S63del impedes the arrival of wild-type P0 glycoprotein to myelin in CMT1B mice. *Human molecular genetics* 2011; 20(11):2081–2090.

60. Grandis M, Vigo T, Passalacqua M, *et al.* Different cellular and molecular mechanisms for early and late-onset myelin protein zero mutations. *Human molecular genetics* 2008; 17(13):1877–1889.

61. Gal A, Mücke J, Theile H, *et al.* X-linked dominant Charcot-Marie-Tooth disease: suggestion of linkage with a cloned DNA sequence from the proximal Xq. *Human genetics* 1985; 70(1):38–42.

62. Bergoffen J, Scherer SS, Wang S, *et al.* Connexin mutations in X-linked Charcot-Marie-Tooth disease. *Science* 1993; 262:2039–2042.

63. Kleopa KA, Scherer SS. Molecular genetics of X-linked Charcot-Marie-Tooth disease. *Neuromolecular medicine* 2006; 8(1-2):107–122.

64. Houlden H, Girard M, Cockerell C, *et al.* Connexin 32 promoter P2 mutations: a mechanism of peripheral nerve dysfunction. *Annals of neurology* 2004; 56(5):730–734.

65. Kleopa KA. The role of gap junctions in Charcot-Marie-Tooth disease. *Journal of neuroscience* 2011; 31(49):17753–17760.

66. Delague V, Bareil C, Tuffery S, *et al.* Mapping of a new locus for autosomal recessive demyelinating Charcot-Marie-Tooth disease to 19q13.1-13.3 in a large consanguineous Lebanese family: exclusion of MAG as a candidate gene. *American journal of human genetics* 2000; 67:236–243.

67. Guilbot A, Williams A, Ravisé N, *et al.* A mutation in periaxin is responsible for CMT4F, an autosomal recessive form of Charcot-Marie-Tooth disease. *Human molecular genetics* 2001; 10(4):415–421.

68. Boerkoel CF, Takashima H, Stankiewicz P, *et al.* Periaxin mutations cause recessive Dejerine-Sottas neuropathy. *American journal of human genetics* 2001; 68:325–333.

69. Sherman DL, Fabrizi C, Gillespie CS, *et al.* Specific disruption of a schwann cell dystrophin-related protein complex in a demyelinating neuropathy. *Neuron* 2001; 30(3):677–687.

70. Gillespie CS, Sherman DL, Fleetwood-Walker SM, *et al.* Peripheral demyelination and neuropathic pain behavior in periaxin-deficient mice. *Neuron* 2000; 26(2):523–531.

71. Williams AC, Brophy PJ. The function of the Periaxin gene during nerve repair in a model of CMT4F. *Journal of anatomy* 2002; 200(4):323–330.

72. Court FA, Brophy PJ, Ribchester RR. Remodeling of motor nerve terminals in demyelinating axons of periaxin-null mice. *Glia* 2008; 56:471–479.

73. Warner LE, Mancias, P, Butler IJ, *et al.* Mutations in the early growth response 2 (EGR2) gene are associated with hereditary myelinopathies. *Nature* 1998; 18:382–384.

74. Topilko P, Schneider-Maunoury S, Levi G, *et al.* Krox-20 controls myelination in the peripheral nervous system. *Nature* 1994; 371:796–799.

75. Warner LE, Svaren J, Milbrandt J, *et al.* Functional consequences of mutations in the early growth response 2 gene (EGR2) correlate with severity of human myelinopathies. *Human molecular genetics* 1999; 8(7):1245–1251.

76. Nagarajan R, Svaren J, Le N, *et al.* EGR2 mutations in inherited neuropathies dominant-negatively inhibit myelin gene expression. *Neuron* 2001; 30(2): 355–368.

77. LeBlanc SE, Ward RM, Svaren J. Neuropathy-associated Egr2 mutants disrupt cooperative activation of myelin protein zero by Egr2 and Sox10. *Molecular and cellular biology* 2007; 27(9):3521–3529.

78. Bouhouche A, Benomar A, Birouk N, *et al.* A locus for an axonal form of autosomal recessive Charcot-Marie-Tooth disease maps to chromosome 1q21.2-q21.3. *American journal of human genetics* 1999; 65:722–727.

79. De Sandre-Giovannoli A, Chaouch M, Kozlov S, *et al.* Homozygous defects in LMNA, encoding lamin A/C nuclear-envelope proteins, cause autosomal recessive axonal neuropathy in human (Charcot-Marie-Tooth disorder type 2) and mouse. *American journal of human genetics* 2002; 70:726–736.

80. Hutchison CJ, Worman HJ. A-type lamins: guardians of the soma? *Nature cell biology* 2004; 6(11):1062–1067.

81. Gonzalez-Suarez I, Gonzalo S. A-type lamins preserve genomic stability. *Nucleus.* 2010; 1(2):129–135.

82. Sullivan T, Escalante-Alcalde D, Bhatt H, *et al.* Loss of A-type lamin expression compromises nuclear envelope integrity leading to muscular dystrophy. *Cell* 1999; 147(5):913–919.

83. Leal A, Morera B, Del Valle G, *et al.* A second locus for an axonal form of autosomal recessive Charcot-Marie-Tooth disease maps to chromosome 19q13.3. *American journal of human genetics* 2001; 68(1):269–274.

84. Leal A, Huehne K, Bauer F, *et al.* Identification of the variant Ala335Val of MED25 as responsible for CMT2B2: molecular data, functional studies of the SH3 recognition motif and correlation between wild-type MED25 and PMP22 RNA levels in CMT1A animal models. *Neurogenetics* 2009; 10(4):275–287.

85. Varon R, Gooding R, Steglich C, *et al.* Partial deficiency of the C-terminal-domain phosphatase of RNA polymerase II is associated with congenital cataracts facial dysmorphism neuropathy syndrome. *Nature genetics* 2003; 35(2):185–189.

86. Ionasescu V, Searby C, Sheffield VC, *et al.* Autosomal dominant Charcot-Marie-Tooth axonal neuropathy mapped on chromosome 7p (CMT2D). *Human molecular genetics* 1996; 5(9):1373–1375.

87. Antonellis A, Ellsworth RE, Sambuughin N, *et al.* Glycyl tRNA synthetase mutations in Charcot-Marie-Tooth disease Type 2D and distal spinal muscular atrophy type V. *American journal of human genetics* 2003; 72:1293–1299.

88. Jordanova A, Thomas FP, Guergueltcheva V, *et al.* Dominant intermediate Charcot-Marie-Tooth type C maps to chromosome 1p34-p35. *American journal of human genetics* 2003; 73(6):1423–1430.

89. Jordanova A, Irobi J, Thomas FP, *et al.* Disrupted function and axonal distribution of mutant tyrosyl-tRNA synthetase in dominant intermediate Charcot-Marie-Tooth neuropathy. *Nature genetics* 2006; 38(2):197–202.

90. Latour P, Thauvin-Robinet C, Baudelet-Mery C, *et al.* A major determinant for binding and aminoacylation of tRNA-Ala in cytoplasmic alanyl-tRNA synthetase is mutated in dominant axonal Charcot-Marie-Tooth Disease. *American journal of human genetics* 2010; 86:77–82.

91. McLaughlin HM, Sakaguchi R, Liu C, *et al.* Compound heterozygosity for loss-of-function lysyl-tRNA synthetase mutations in a patient with peripheral neuropathy. *American journal of human genetics* 2010; 87(4):560–566.

92. Antonellis A, Lee-Lin S-Q, Wasterlain A, *et al.* Functional analyses of glycyl-tRNA synthetase mutations suggest a key role for tRNA-charging enzymes in peripheral axons. *Journal of neuroscience* 2006;26(41):10397–10406.

93. McLaughlin HM, Sakaguchi R, Giblin W, *et al.* A recurrent loss-of-function alanyl-tRNA synthetase (AARS) mutation in patients with Charcot-Marie-Tooth disease type 2N (CMT2N). *Human mutation* 2012; 33(1):244–253.

94. Stum M, McLaughlin HM, Kleinbrink EL, *et al.* An assessment of mechanisms underlying peripheral axonal degeneration caused by aminoacyl-tRNA synthetase mutations. *Molecular and cellular neurosciences* 2010; 46(2):432–443.

95. Seburn KL, Nangle LA, Cox GA, *et al.* An active dominant mutation of glycyl-tRNA synthetase causes neuropathy in a Charcot-Marie-Tooth 2D mouse model. *Neuron* 2006; 51(6):715–726.

96. Motley WW, Seburn KL, Nawaz MH, *et al.* Charcot-Marie-Tooth-linked mutant GARS is toxic to peripheral neurons independent of wild-type GARS levels. *PLoS genetics* 2011; 7(12):e1002399.

97. Lee JW, Beebe K, Nangle LA, *et al.* Editing-defective tRNA synthetase causes protein misfolding and neurodegeneration. *Nature* 2006; 443(7107):50–55.

98. Züchner S, Mersiyanova IV, Muglia M, *et al.* Mutations in the mitochondrial GTPase mitofusin 2 cause Charcot-Marie-Tooth neuropathy type 2A. *Nature genetics* 2004; 36(5):449–451.

99. Chen, H, Detmer, SA, Ewald, AJ *et al.* Mitofusins Mfn1 and Mfn2 coordinately regulate mitochondrial fusion and are essential for embryonic development. *Journal of cell biology* 2003; 160(2):189–200.

100. Misko A, Jiang S, Wegorzewska I, *et al.* Mitofusin 2 is necessary for transport of axonal mitochondria and interacts with the Miro/Milton complex. *The Journal of neuroscience* 2010; 30(12):4232–4240.

101. Guillet V, Gueguen N, Verny C, *et al.* Adenine nucleotide translocase is involved in a mitochondrial coupling defect in MFN2-related Charcot-Marie-Tooth type 2A disease. *Neurogenetics* 2010; 11(1):127–133.

102. de Brito OM, Scorrano L. Mitofusin 2 tethers endoplasmic reticulum to mitochondria. *Nature* 2008; 456:605–610.

103. Polke JM, Laurá M, Pareyson D, *et al.* Recessive axonal Charcot-Marie-Tooth disease due to compound heterozygous mitofusin 2 mutations. *Neurology* 2011; 77(2):168–173.

104. Cuesta A, Pedrola L, Sevilla T, *et al.* The gene encoding ganglioside-induced differentiation-associated protein 1 is mutated in axonal Charcot-Marie-Tooth type 4A disease. *Nature genetics* 2002; 30:22–25.

105. Senderek J. Mutations in the ganglioside-induced differentiation-associated protein-1 (GDAP1) gene in intermediate type autosomal recessive Charcot-Marie-Tooth neuropathy. *Brain* 2003; 126(3):642–649.

106. Noack R, Frede S, Albrecht P, *et al.* Charcot-Marie-Tooth disease CMT4A: GDAP1 increases cellular glutathione and the mitochondrial membrane potential. *Human molecular genetics* 2012; 21(1):150–162.

107. Niemann A, Wagner KM, Ruegg M, *et al.* GDAP1 mutations differ in their effects on mitochondrial dynamics and apoptosis depending on the mode of inheritance. *Neurobiology of disease* 2009; 36(3):509–520.

108. Zhang X, Chow CY, Sahenk Z, *et al.* Mutation of FIG4 causes a rapidly progressive, asymmetric neuronal degeneration. *Brain* 2008; 131(Pt 8):1990–2001.

109. Zhao C, Takita J, Tanaka Y, *et al.* Charcot-Marie-Tooth disease type 2A caused by mutation in a microtubule motor KIF1Bbeta. *Cell* 2001; 105(5):587–597.

110. Mersiyanova IV, Perepelov AV, Polyakov AV, *et al.* A new variant of Charcot-Marie-Tooth disease type 2 is probably the result of a mutation in the neurofilament-light gene. *American journal of human genetics* 2000; 67(1):37–46.

111. Jordanova A, De Jonghe P, Boerkoel CF. Mutations in the neurofilament light chain gene (NEFL) cause early onset severe Charcot-Marie-Tooth disease. *Brain* 2003; 126(3):590–597.

112. Gentil BJ, Minotti S, Beange M, *et al.* Normal role of the low-molecular-weight neurofilament protein in mitochondrial dynamics and disruption in Charcot-Marie-Tooth disease. *The FASEB journal* 2011; 26:1–10.

113. Zhu Q, Couillard-Despres S, Julien JP. Delayed maturation of regenerating myelinated axons in mice lacking neurofilaments. *Experimental neurology* 1997; 148(1):299–316.

114. Brownlees J, Ackerley S, Grierson AJ, *et al.* Charcot–Marie–Tooth disease neurofilament mutations disrupt neurofilament assembly and axonal transport. *Human molecular genetics* 2002; 11(23):2837–2844.

115. Zhai J, Lin H, Julien J-P, *et al.* Disruption of neurofilament network with aggregation of light neurofilament protein: a common pathway leading to motor neuron degeneration due to Charcot-Marie-Tooth disease-linked mutations in NFL and HSPB1. *Human molecular genetics* 2007; 16(24):3103–3116.

116. Fabrizi GM, Cavallaro T, Angiari C, *et al.* Charcot-Marie-Tooth disease type 2E, a disorder of the cytoskeleton. *Brain* 2007; 130(Pt 2):394–403.

117. Goryunov D, Nightingale A, Bornfleth L, *et al.* Multiple disease-linked myotubularin mutations cause NFL assembly defects in cultured cells and disrupt myotubularin dimerization. *Journal of neurochemistry* 2008; 104(6):1536–1552.

118. Abe A, Numakura C, Saito K, *et al.* Neurofilament light chain polypeptide gene mutations in Charcot–Marie–Tooth disease: nonsense mutation probably causes a recessive phenotype. *Journal of human genetics* 2009; 54:94–97.

119. Weedon MN, Hastings R, Caswell R, *et al.* Exome sequencing identifies a DYNC1H1 mutation in a large pedigree with dominant axonal Charcot-Marie-Tooth Disease. *American journal of human genetics* 2011; 89:308–312.

120. De Sandre-Giovannoli A, Delague V, Hamadouche T, *et al.* Homozygosity mapping of autosomal recessive demyelinating Charcot-Marie-Tooth neuropathy (CMT4H) to a novel locus on chromosome 12p11.21-q13.11. *Journal of medical genetics* 2005; 42:260–265.

121. Delague V, Jacquier A, Hamadouche T, *et al.* Mutations in FGD4 encoding the Rho GDP/GTP exchange factor FRABIN cause autosomal recessive Charcot-Marie-Tooth type 4H. *American journal of human genetics* 2007; 81:1–16.

122. Fabrizi GM, Cavallaro T. Further evidence that mutations in FGD4/frabin cause Charcot-Marie-Tooth disease type 4H. *Neurology* 2009; 72:1160–1164.

123. Stendel C, Roos A, Deconinck T, *et al.* Peripheral nerve demyelination caused by a mutant Rho GTPase guanine nucleotide exchange factor, frabin/FGD4. *American journal of human genetics* 2007; 81(1):158–164.

124. Boyer O, Nevo F, Plaisier E, *et al.* INF2 mutations in Charcot-Marie-Tooth disease with glomerulopathy. *New England journal of medicine* 2011; 365(25):2377–2388.

125. Kennerson ML, Zhu D, Gardner RJ, *et al.* Dominant intermediate Charcot-Marie-Tooth neuropathy maps to chromosome 19p12-p13.2. *American journal of human genetics* 2001; 69(4):883–888.

126. Züchner S, Noureddine M, Kennerson M, *et al.* Mutations in the pleckstrin homology domain of dynamin 2 cause dominant intermediate Charcot-Marie-Tooth disease. *Nature genetics* 2005; 37(3):289–294.

127. Koutsopoulos OS, Koch C, Tosch V, *et al.* Mild functional differences of dynamin 2 mutations associated to centronuclear myopathy and Charcot-Marie-Tooth peripheral neuropathy. *PloS one* 2011; 6(11):e27498.

128. Guernsey DL, Jiang H, Bedard K, *et al.* Mutation in the gene encoding ubiquitin ligase LRSAM1 in patients with Charcot-Marie-Tooth disease. *PLoS genetics* 2010; 6(8):1–7.

129. Amit I, Yakir L, Katz M, *et al.* Tal, a Tsg101-specific E3 ubiquitin ligase, regulates receptor endocytosis and retrovirus budding. *Genes and development* 2004; 18:1737–1752.

130. Weterman MAJ, Sorrentino V, Kasher PR, *et al.* A frameshift mutation in LRSAM1 is responsible for a dominant hereditary polyneuropathy. *Human molecular genetics* 2012; 21(2):358–370.

131. Bolino A, Brancolini V, Bono F, *et al.* Localization of a gene responsible for autosomal recessive demyelinating neuropathy with focally folded myelin sheaths to chromosome 11q23 by homozygosity mapping and haplotype sharing. *Human molecular genetics* 1996; 5(7):1051–1054.

132. Bolino A, Muglia M, Conforti FL, *et al.* Charcot-Marie-Tooth type 4B is caused by mutations in the gene encoding myotubularin-related protein-2. *Nature genetics* 2000; 25:17–19.

133. Volpicelli-Daley L, De Camilli P. Phosphoinositides' link to neurodegeneration. *Nature medicine* 2007; 13(7):784–786.

134. Berger P, Bonneick S, Willi S, *et al.* Loss of phosphatase activity in myotubularin-related protein 2 is associated with Charcot–Marie–Tooth disease type 4B1. *Human molecular genetics* 2002; 11(13):1569–1579.

135. Vaccari I, Dina G, Tronchère H, *et al.* Genetic interaction between MTMR2 and FIG4 phospholipid phosphatases involved in Charcot-Marie-Tooth neuropathies. *PLoS genetics* 2011; 7(10):e1002319.

136. Bolis A, Coviello S, Bussini S, *et al.* Loss of Mtmr2 phosphatase in Schwann cells but not in motor neurons causes Charcot-Marie-Tooth type 4B1 neuropathy with myelin outfoldings. *Journal of neuroscience* 2005; 25(37):8567–8577.

137. Othmane KB, Johnson E, Menold M, *et al.* Identification of a new locus for autosomal recessive Charcot-Marie-Tooth disease with focally folded myelin on chromosome 11p15. *Genomics* 1999; 62(3):344–349.

138. Senderek J. Mutation of the SBF2 gene, encoding a novel member of the myotubularin family, in Charcot-Marie-Tooth neuropathy type 4B2/11p15. *Human Molecular Genetics* 2003; 12(3):349–356.

139. Azzedine H, Bolino A, Taïeb T, *et al.* Mutations in MTMR13, a new pseudophosphatase homologue of MTMR2 and Sbf1, in two families with an autosomal recessive demyelinating form of Charcot-Marie-Tooth disease associated with early-onset glaucoma. *American journal of human genetics* 2003; 72: 1141–1153.

140. Berger P, Berger I, Schaffitzel C, *et al.* Multi-level regulation of myotubularin-related protein-2 phosphatase activity by myotubularin- related protein-13/ set-binding factor-2. *Human molecular genetics* 2006; 15(4):569–579.

141. Robinson FL, Niesman IR, Beiswenger KK, *et al.* Loss of the inactive myotubularin-related phosphatase Mtmr13 leads to a Charcot–Marie–Tooth 4B2-like peripheral neuropathy in mice. *PNAS* 2008; 105(12):4916–4921.

142. Chow CY, Zhang Y, Dowling JJ, *et al.* Mutation of FIG4 causes neurodegeneration in the pale tremor mouse and patients with CMT4J. *Nature* 2007; 448:68–72.

143. Ferguson CJ, Lenk GM, Meisler MH. Defective autophagy in neurons and astrocytes from mice deficient in PI(3,5)P2. *Human molecular genetics* 2009; 18:4868–4878.

144. Lenk GM, Ferguson CJ, Chow CY, *et al.* Pathogenic mechanism of the FIG4 mutation responsible for Charcot-Marie-Tooth disease CMT4J. *PLoS genetics* 2011; 7(6):e1002104.

145. Kwon JM, Elliott JL, Yee W-Chee, *et al.* Assignment of a second Charcot-Marie Tooth locus to chromosome 3q. *American journal of human genetics* 1995; 57:853–858.

146. Verhoeven K, De Jonghe P, Coen K, *et al.* Mutations in the small GTP-ase late endosomal protein RAB7 cause Charcot-Marie-Tooth type 2B neuropathy. *American journal of human genetics* 2003; 72(3):722–727.

147. Spinoza MR, Progida C, De Luca A, *et al.* Functional characterization of Rab7 mutant proteins associated with Charcot-Marie-Tooth Type 2B disease. *Journal of neuroscience* 2008; 28(7):1649–1648.

148. Basuray S, Mukherjee S, Romero E, *et al.* Rab7 mutants associated with Charcot-Marie-Tooth disease exhibit enhanced NGF-stimulated signaling. *Plos One* 2010; 5(12): e15351.

149. Cogli L, Progida C, Lecci R, *et al.* CMT2B-associated Rab7 mutants inhibit neurite outgrowth. *Acta neuropathologica* 2010; 120:491–501.

150. Chance PF, Bird TD, O'Connell P, *et al.* Genetic linkage and heterogeneity in Type I Charcot-Marie-Tooth Disease (Hereditary Motor and Sensory Neuropathy Type I). *American journal of human genetics* 1990; 47:915–925.

151. Street VA, Goldy JD, Golden AS, *et al.* Mapping of Charcot-Marie-Tooth disease type 1C to chromosome 16p identifies a novel locus for demyelinating neuropathies. *American journal of human genetics* 2002; 70(1):244–250.

152. Street VA, Bennett CL, Goldy JD. Mutation of a putative protein degradation gene LITAF/SIMPLE in Charcot-Marie-Tooth disease 1C. *Neurology* 2003; 60:22–26.

153. Lee SM, Olzmann JA, Chin L-S, *et al.* Mutations associated with Charcot-Marie-Tooth disease cause SIMPLE protein mislocalization and degradation by the proteasome and aggresome-autophagy pathways. *Journal of cell science* 2011; 124:1–13.

154. Eaton HE, Desrochers G, Drory SB, *et al.* SIMPLE/LITAF expression induces the translocation of the ubiquitin ligase itch towards the lysosomal compartments. *PloS one* 2011; 6(2):e16873.

155. Stendel C, Roos A, Kleine H, *et al.* SH3TC2, a protein mutant in Charcot-Marie-Tooth neuropathy, links peripheral nerve myelination to endosomal recycling. *Brain* 2010; 133(Pt 8):2462–2474.

156. LeGuern E, Guilbot A, Kessali M, *et al.* Homozygosity mapping of an autosomal recessive form of demyelinating Charcot-Marie-Tooth disease to chromosome 5q23-q33. *Human molecular genetics* 1996; 5(10):1685–1688.

157. Senderek J, Bergmann C, Stendel C, *et al.* Mutations in a gene encoding a novel SH3/TPR domain protein cause autosomal recessive Charcot-Marie-Tooth type 4C neuropathy. *American journal of human genetics* 2003; 73(5):1106–1119.

158. Roberts RC, Peden AA, Buss F, *et al.* Mistargeting of SH3TC2 away from the recycling endosome causes Charcot-Marie-Tooth disease type 4C. *Human molecular genetics* 2010]; 19(6):1009–1018.

159. Tang B-S, Luo W, Xia K, *et al.* A new locus for autosomal dominant Charcot-Marie-Tooth disease type 2 (CMT2L) maps to chromosome 12q24. *Human genetics* 2004; 114(6):527–533.

160. Tang B-S, Zhao G-H Luo W, *et al.* Small heat-shock protein 22 mutated in autosomal dominant Charcot-Marie-Tooth disease type 2L. *Human genetics* 2005; 116(3):222–224.

161. Irobi J, Almeida-Souza L, Asselbergh B, *et al.* Mutant HSPB8 causes motor neuron-specific neurite degeneration. *Human molecular genetics* 2010; 19(16):3254–3265.

162. Ismailov SM, Fedotov VP, Dadali EL, *et al.* A new locus for autosomal dominant Charcot-Marie-Tooth disease type 2 (CMT2F) maps to chromosome 7q11-q21. *European Journal of Human Genetics* 2001; 9:646–650.

163. Evgrafov OV, Mersiyanova I, Irobi J, *et al.* Mutant small heat-shock protein 27 causes axonal Charcot-Marie-Tooth disease and distal hereditary motor neuropathy. *Nature genetics* 2004; 36(6):602–606.

164. Almeida-Souza L, Asselbergh B, D'Ydewalle C, *et al.* Small heat-shock protein HSPB1 mutants stabilize microtubules in Charcot-Marie-Tooth neuropathy. *Journal of neuroscience* 2011; 31(43):15328–15328.

165. d'Ydewalle C, Krishnan J, Chiheb DM, *et al.* HDAC6 inhibitors reverse axonal loss in a mouse model of mutant HSPB1-induced Charcot-Marie-Tooth disease. *Nature medicine* 2011; 17:968–974.

166. McEntagart ME, Reid SL, Irrthum A, *et al.* Confirmation of a hereditary motor and sensory neuropathy IIC locus at chromosome 12q23-q24. *Annals of neurology* 2005; 57(2):293–297.

167. Auer-Grumbach M, Olschewski A, Papic L, *et al.* Alterations in the ankyrin domain of TRPV4 cause congenital distal SMA, scapuloperoneal SMA and HMSN2C. *Nature genetics* 2010; 42(2):160–166.

168. Landoure G, Zdebik AA, Martinez TL, *et al.* Mutations in TRPV4 cause Charcot-Marie-Tooth disease type 2C. *Nature genetics* 2010;42(2):170–174.

169. Deng H-X, Klein CJ, Yan J, *et al.* Scapuloperoneal spinal muscular atrophy and CMT2C are allelic disorders caused by alterations in TRPV4. *Nature genetics* 2010; 42:165–169.

170. Klein CJ, Shi Y, Fecto F, *et al.* TRPV4 mutations and cytotoxic hypercalcemia in axonal Charcot-Marie-Tooth neuropathies. *Neurology* 2011; 76(10):887–894.

171. Kim H-J, Sohn K-M, Shy ME, *et al.* Mutations in PRPS1, which encodes the phosphoribosyl pyrophosphate synthetase enzyme critical for nucleotide biosynthesis, cause hereditary peripheral neuropathy with hearing loss and optic neuropathy (cmtx5). *American journal of human genetics* 2007;81(3):552–558.

172. Auer-Grumbach A, Weger M, Fink-Puches R, *et al.* Fibulin-5 mutations link inherited neuropathies, age-related macular degeneration and hyperelastic skin. *Brain* 2011; 134:1839–1852.

173. Rogers T, Chandler D, Angelicheva D, *et al.* A novel locus for autosomal recessive peripheral neuropathy in the EGR2 region on 10q23. *American journal of human genetics* 2000; 67(3):664–671.

174. Hantke J, Chandler D, King R, *et al.* A mutation in an alternative untranslated exon of hexokinase 1 associated with hereditary motor and sensory neuropathy – Russe (HMSNR). *European journal of human genetics* 2009; 17(12): 1606–1614.

175. Harrower T, Stewart JD, Hudson G, *et al.* POLG1 mutations manifesting as autosomal recessive axonal Charcot-Marie-Tooth disease. *Archives of neurology* 2008; 65(1):133–136.

176. Kalaydjieva L, Hallmayer K, Chandler D, *et al.* Gene mapping in Gypsies identifies a novel demyelinating neuropathy on chromosome 8q24. *Nature* 1996; 14:214–217.

177. Kalaydjieva L, Gresham D, Gooding R, *et al.* N-myc downstream-regulated gene 1 is mutated in hereditary motor and sensory neuropathy-Lom. *American journal of human genetics* 2000; 67(1):47–58.

178. King RHM, Chandler D, Lopaticki S, *et al.* Ndrg1 in development and maintenance of the myelin sheath. *Neurobiology of disease* 2011; 42(3):368–380.

179. Nelis E. Autosomal dominant axonal Charcot-Marie-Tooth disease type 2 (CMT2G) maps to chromosome 12q12-q13.3. *Journal of Medical Genetics* 2004; 41(3):193–197.

180. Takashima H, Nakagawa M, Suehara M, *et al.* Gene for hereditary motor and sensory neuropathy (proximal dominant form) mapped to 3q13.1. *Neuromuscular Disorders* 1999; 9(6-7):368–371.

181. Verhoeven K, Villanova M, Rossi A, *et al.* Localization of the gene for the intermediate form of Charcot-Marie-Tooth to chromosome 10q24.1-q25.1. *American journal of human genetics* 2001; 69(4):889–894.

182. Lee Y-C, Lee T-C, Lin K-P, *et al.* Clinical characterization and genetic analysis of a possible novel type of dominant Charcot-Marie-Tooth disease. *Neuromuscular disorders* 2010; 20(8):534–539.

183. Garcia CA, Malamut RE, England JD, *et al.* Clinical variability in two pairs of identical twins with the Charcot-Marie-Tooth disease type 1A duplication. *Neurology* 1995; 45(11):2090–2993.

184. Rossor AM, Kalmar B, Greensmith L, *et al.* The distal hereditary motor neuropathies. *Journal of neurology, neurosurgery, and psychiatry* 2011; 83:6–15.

185. Grohmann K, Schuelke M, Diers A, *et al.* Mutations in the gene encoding immunoglobulin mu-binding protein 2 cause spinal muscular atrophy with respiratory distress type 1. *Nature genetics* 2001; 29(1):75–77.

186. Chen Y-Z, Bennett CL, Huynh HM, *et al.* DNA/RNA helicase gene mutations in a form of juvenile Amyotrophic Lateral Sclerosis (ALS4). *American journal of human genetics* 2004; 74:1128–1135.

187. Irobi J, Van Impe K, Seeman P, *et al.* Hot-spot residue in small heat-shock protein 22 causes distal motor neuropathy. *Nature genetics* 2004; 36(6):597–601.

188. Windpassinger C, Auer-Grumbach M, Irobi J, *et al.* Heterozygous missense mutations in BSCL2 are associated with distal hereditary motor neuropathy and Silver syndrome. *Nature genetics* 2004; 36(3):271–276.

189. Kolb SJ, Snyder PJ, Poi EJ, *et al.* Mutant small heat shock protein B3 causes motor neuropathy: utility of a candidate gene approach. *Neurology* 2010; 74(6):502–506.

190. Puls I, Jonnakuty C, LaMonte BH, *et al.* Mutant dynactin in motor neuron disease. *Nature genetics* 2003; 33(4):455–456.

191. Kennerson ML, Nicholson GA, Kaler SG, *et al.* Missense mutations in the copper transporter gene ATP7A cause X-linked distal hereditary motor neuropathy. *American journal of human genetics* 2010; 86(3):343–352.

192. Rotthier A, Baets, J, Timmerman V, *et al.* Mechanisms of disease in hereditary sensory and autonomic neuropathies. *Nature reviews. Neurology* 2012;8(2):1–13.

193. Riviere JB, Ramalingam S, Lavastre V, *et al.* KIF1A, an axonal transporter of synaptic vesicles, is mutated in hereditary sensory and autonomic neuropathy type 2. *American journal of human genetics* 2011; 89:219–230.

194. Slaugenhaupt SA, Blumenfeld A, Gill SP, *et al.* Tissue-specific expression of a splicing mutation in the IKBKAP gene causes familial dysautonomia. *American journal of human genetics* 2001; 68(3):598–605.

195. Houlden H, King RHM, Hashemi-Nejad A, *et al.* A novel TRK A (NTRK1) mutation associated with hereditary sensory and autonomic neuropathy type V. *Annals of Neurology* 2001;41(4):521–525.

196. Einarsdottir E, Carlsson A, Minde J, *et al.* A mutation in the nerve growth factor beta gene (NGFB) causes loss of pain perception. *Human molecular genetics* 2004; 13(8):799–805.

197. Kurth I, Pamminger T, Hennings JC, *et al.* Mutations in FAM134B, encoding a newly identified Golgi protein, cause severe sensory and autonomic neuropathy. *Nature genetics* 2009; 41(11):1179–1181.

198. Lafreniere RG, MacDonald MLE, Dube M-P, *et al.* Identification of a novel gene (HSN2) causing hereditary sensory and autonomic neuropathy type II through the Study of Canadian Genetic Isolates. *American journal of human genetics* 2004; 74(5):1064–1073.

199. Bejaoui K, Wu C, Scheffler MD, *et al.* SPTLC1 is mutated in hereditary sensory neuropathy, type 1. *Nature genetics* 2001;27:261–262.

200. Dawkins JL, Hulme DJ, Brahmbhatt SB, *et al.* Mutations in SPTLC1, encoding serine palmitoyltransferase, long chain base subunit-1, cause hereditary sensory neuropathy type I. *Nature genetics* 2001; 27:309–312.

201. Rotthier A, Auer-Grumbach M, Janssens K, *et al.* Mutations in the SPTLC2 subunit of serine palmitoyltransferase cause hereditary sensory and autonomic neuropathy type I. *American journal of human genetics* 2010; 87(4):513–522.

202. Penno A, Reilly MM, Houlden H, *et al.* Hereditary sensory neuropathy type 1 is caused by the accumulation of two neurotoxic sphingolipids. *The Journal of biological chemistry* 2010; 285(15):11178–11187.

203. Guelly C, Zhu P-P, Leonardis L, *et al.* Targeted high-throughput sequencing identifies mutations in atlastin-1 as a cause of hereditary sensory neuropathy type I. *American journal of human genetics* 2011; 88(1):99–105.

204. Klein CJ, Botuyan M-V, Wu Y, *et al.* Mutations in DNMT1 cause hereditary sensory neuropathy with dementia and hearing loss. *Nature genetics* 2011; 43(6):595–600.

205. Cox JJ, Reimann F, Nicholas AK, *et al.* An SCN9A channelopathy causes congenital inability to experience pain. *Nature* 2006; 444:894–898.

206. Planté-Bordeneuve V, Said G. Familial amyloid polyneuropathy. *Lancet neurology* 2011; 10(12):1086–1097.

207. Kuhlenbäumer G, Hannibal MC, Nelis E, *et al.* Mutations in SEPT9 cause hereditary neuralgic amyotrophy. *Nature genetics* 2005; 37(10):1044–1046.

208. Van Alfen N. Clinical and pathophysiological concepts of neuralgic amyotrophy. *Nature reviews. Neurology* 2011; 7(6):315–322.

209. Bomont P, Cavalier L, Blondeau F, *et al.* The gene encoding gigaxonin, a new member of the cytoskeletal BTB/kelch repeat family, is mutated in giant axonal neuropathy. *Nature genetics* 2000; 26:370–374.

210. Ganay T, Boizot A, Burrer R, *et al.* Sensory-motor deficits and neurofilament disorganization in gigaxonin-null mice. *Molecular neurodegeneration* 2011; 6:1–11.

211. Dalakas MC. Advances in the diagnosis, pathogenesis and treatment of CIDP. *Nature reviews. Neurology* 2011; 7:507–517.

212. Pollard JD, Armati PJ. CIDP – the relevance of recent advances in Schwann cell / axonal neurobiology. *Journal of the peripheral nervous system* 2011; 23:15–23.

213. del Porto LA, Nicholson GA, Ketheswaren P. Correlation between muscle atrophy on MRI and manual strength testing in hereditary neuropathies. *Journal of clinical neuroscience* 2010; 17:874–878.

214. Sinclair CDJ, Morrow JM, Miranda MA, *et al.* Skeletal muscle MRI magnetisation transfer ratio reflects clinical severity in peripheral neuropathies. *Journal of neurology, neurosurgery, and psychiatry* 2012; 83(1):29–32.

215. Fledrich R, Schlotter-Weigel B, Schnizer TJ, *et al.* A rat model of Charcot-Marie-Tooth disease 1A recapitulates disease variability and supplies biomarkers of axonal loss in patients. *Brain* 2012; 135(Pt 1):72–87.

216. Jacobs BC, Willison HJ. Peripheral neuropathies: Biomarkers for axonal damage in immune-mediated neuropathy. *Nature reviews. Neurology* 2009;5(11):584–585.

217. Shy ME, Blake J, Krajewski K, *et al.* Reliability and validity of the CMT neuropathy score as a measure of disability. *Neurology* 2005; 64(7):1209–1124.

218. Warner TT and Hammans SR. *Practical Guide to Neurogenetics.* Saunders Elsevier: Philadelphia, 2009.

219. Pareyson D, Marchesi C. Diagnosis, natural history, and management of Charcot-Marie-Tooth disease. *Lancet neurology* 2009; 8(7):654–667.

220. Passage E, Norreel JC, Noack-Fraissignes P, *et al.* Ascorbic acid treatment corrects the phenotype of a mouse model of Charcot-Marie-Tooth disease. *Nature medicine* 2004; 10(4):396–401.

221. Schenone A, Nobbio L, Monti Bragadin M, *et al.* Inherited neuropathies. *Current treatment options in neurology* 2011;13(2):1–20.

222. Kaya F, Belin S, Bourgeois P, *et al.* Ascorbic acid inhibits PMP22 expression by reducing cAMP levels. *Neuromuscular disorders* 2007; 17(3):248–253.

223. Pareyson D, Reilly MM, Schenone A, *et al.* Ascorbic acid in Charcot-Marie-Tooth disease type 1A (CMT-TRIAAL and CMT-TRAUK): a double-blind randomised trial. *Lancet neurology* 2011; 10(4):320–328.

224. Houlden H, Charlton P, Singh D. Neurology and orthopaedics. *Journal of neurology, neurosurgery, and psychiatry* 2007;78(3):224–232.

225. Genin E, Feingold J, Clerget-Darpoux F. Identifying modifier genes of monogenic disease: strategies and difficulties. *Human genetics* 2008; 124(4):357–368.

226. Montenegro G, Powell E, Huang J, *et al.* Exome sequencing allows for rapid gene identification in a Charcot-Marie-Tooth family. *Annals of neurology* 2011; 69(3):464–470.

227. Singleton AB. Exome sequencing: a transformative technology. *The Lancet Neurology* 2011; 10(10):942–946.

228. Züchner S. Peripheral neuropathies: whole genome sequencing identifies causal variants in CMT. *Nature reviews. Neurology* 2010; 6(8):424–425.

229. Lupski JR, Reid JG, Gonzaga-Jauregui C, *et al.* Whole-genome sequencing in a patient with Charcot-Marie-Tooth neuropathy. *The New England journal of medicine* 2010;362(13):1181–1191.

230. Sereda MW, Meyer zu Hörste G, Suter U, *et al.* Therapeutic administration of progesterone antagonist in a model of Charcot-Marie-Tooth disease (CMT-1A). *Nature medicine* 2003; 9(12):1533–1537.

231. Khajavi M, Shiga K, Wiszniewski W, *et al.* Oral curcumin mitigates the clinical and neuropathologic phenotype of the Trembler-J mouse: a potential therapy for inherited neuropathy. *American journal of human genetics* 2007; 81(3):438–453.

232. Burns J, Joseph PD, Rose KJ *et al.* Effects of oral curcumin on Dejerine-Sottas disease. *Pediatric Neurology* 2009;41(4):306–308.

233. Detmer SA, Chan DC. Complementation between mouse Mfn1 and Mfn2 protects mitochondrial fusion defects caused by CMT2A disease mutations. *The Journal of cell biology* 2007; 176:405–414.

234. Shy ME, Patzkó A. Axonal Charcot-Marie-Tooth disease. *Current opinion in neurology* 2011;24:1–9.

235. Tradewell ML, Durham HD, Mushynski WE, *et al.* Mitochondrial and axonal abnormalities precede disruption of the neurofilament network in a model of charcot-marie-tooth disease type 2E and are prevented by heat shock proteins in a mutant-specific fashion. *Journal of neuropathology and experimental neurology* 2009; 68(6):642–652.

CHAPTER 20

Axonal Loss and Neurodegeneration in Multiple Sclerosis

Ranjan Dutta, Jacqueline Chen, Nobuhiko Ohno, Daniel Ontaneda, and Bruce D. Trapp

Department of Neurosciences, Lerner Research Institute, Cleveland Clinic, Cleveland, Ohio, USA

Clinical definition and epidemiology

Multiple sclerosis (MS) is the major cause of non-traumatic neurological disability in young adults in North America and Europe, where it affects over 2.5 million individuals [1, 2]. MS affects women twice as often as men, reduces the average lifespan by 7–8 years, and usually results in poor quality of life in later stages of the disease. The neurological disease course is variable and much of the disease process is clinically silent. MS usually manifests in the third or fourth decade of life and the uncertainty of disease progression impacts both personal and professional decisions of the patients. Variability in disease progression also influences MS clinical trials, which have to be powered with hundreds of patients to demonstrate efficacy of treatment. MS is a complex disease whose cause includes a genetic predisposition for susceptibility and environmental influences. A single gene, a DR2 haplotype in the class II region of the major histocompatibility complex (MHC) on chromosome 6, has a major influence on susceptibility (16–60%). Geographically, MS is more prevalent in northern Europe and North America than in Africa and Asia. Although incidences of MS have been documented worldwide, MS is most prevalent among people of European descent. While there have been reports of epidemics or clusters of increased MS incidence, causative agents have not been identified.

Spectrum of clinical phenotype

MS patients can be divided into two groups based upon their initial clinical presentation. Approximately 85% of MS patients begin with a course of recurrent and reversible neurological deficits. This phase of the disease is termed relapsing-remitting MS (RRMS). Brain imaging studies have established that rapid onset of neurological disability during RRMS is caused by focal inflammatory demyelinating lesions in white matter, which include massive influx of immune cells from the blood. The neurological disability depends upon the site of the lesion, and its rapid onset is likely due to breakdown of the blood–brain barrier (BBB). The edema associated with BBB breakdown causes axonal dysfunction via nerve conduction block at nodes of Ranvier prior to actual demyelination by infiltrating immune cells. Relapses usually last no more than a few months and the patient regains neurological function as the edema and inflammation resolve. Reorganization of axonal sodium channels on demyelinated axons and remyelination also facilitate the return

of axonal and neurological function. As discussed in detail in the section Axonal transection during inflammatory demyelination, axonal transection also occurs during active stages of demyelination, but remains clinically silent early in RRMS due to the compensatory capacity of the central nervous system (CNS). Functional magnetic resonance imaging (fMRI) studies have described reorganization of the cerebral cortex following demyelinating lesions in the white matter [3–6]. In a study using both fMRI and magnetic resonance spectroscopy (MRS), RRMS patients demonstrated a fivefold increase in sensorimotor cortex activation with simple hand movements compared to non-MS individuals [3]. In addition, brain imaging studies have shown that inflammatory brain lesions can outnumber relapses by as much as 10 to 1, supporting the concept that much of the disease process is clinically silent [7]. Disability associated with relapses, therefore, requires inflammatory demyelination in an articulate region of the brain. After 8–20 years, the majority of RRMS patients enter a secondary progressive disease phase (SPMS) characterized by continuous, irreversible neurological decline. The transition from RRMS to SPMS is thought to occur when axonal loss surpasses the compensatory capacity of the CNS. During SPMS, relapses and new gadolinium (GAD)-enhancing white matter lesions are rare or absent. Why the relapse rate declines during SPMS is unknown. Despite the lack of new inflammatory lesions, there is a steady progression of irreversible neurological disability during SPMS. During SPMS, MRI studies provide evidence for continuous brain atrophy [8, 9] while MRS studies measuring axon-specific N-acetyl aspartic acid support continuous axonal loss [10–12]. The transition from RRMS to SPMS is an ominous event because current therapeutics are ineffective for treating SPMS.

Primary progressive MS (PPMS) patients represent 15% of all MS cases. Relapses are rare or nonexistent in PPMS patients. Clinical disease onset occurs later in life for PPMS patients than for RRMS patients (39 years vs 29 years) and there is no gender predominance in PPMS. Similar human leukocyte antigen (HLA) associations have been reported in both PPMS and RRMS, and both subtypes are associated with the DR2 haplotype DRB1*1501 in the class II region of the MHC on chromosome 6 [13]. Pathologically, demyelinating lesions in PPMS patients contain fewer inflammatory cells compared to SPMS patients [14]. MRI studies have also shown that there are fewer focal white matter lesions in PPMS patients, suggesting that mechanisms other than inflammatory white matter demyelination

Neurodegeneration, First Edition. Edited by Anthony Schapira, Zbigniew Wszolek, Ted M. Dawson and Nicholas Wood.
© 2017 John Wiley & Sons, Ltd. Published 2017 by John Wiley & Sons, Ltd.

contribute to neurological disability in PPMS. Current anti-inflammatory disease-modifying therapies are approved for treatment of RRMS patients, but effective therapies are not available for SPMS or PPMS patients.

Genetic and environmental influences in MS

MS is a complex polygenic disease mediated by an interaction between modest inherited risk for disease susceptibility and environmental influences [15]. While individuals do not inherit MS, they can inherit a greater susceptibility to acquire the disease [16]. For example, the stated risk for MS in many parts of North America and Europe is 1/1000. For an offspring with a parent with MS, the risk increases to 20/1000, while having a monozygotic twin with MS raises the risk to 100/1000. The relationship between familial recurrence risk and genetic relatedness is non-linear, suggesting that the susceptibility to develop MS is determined by multiple risk alleles, each with modest individual effects. Genome-wide association studies (GWAS) have proven to be a powerful tool for identifying particular genetic variants associated with complex diseases and traits [15, 17]. For more than three decades, the only gene consistently associated with MS was the HLA-DRB1 gene on chromosome 6p21 [18], accounting for 16–60% of the genetic susceptibility in MS [19]. In a large multicenter study analyzing 9772 MS cases and 17,376 controls for 465,434 autosomal single nucleotide polymorphisms (SNPs), 29 additional MS loci were identified and the existing HLA locus was refined [20]. Pathway analysis of the candidate genes identified cytokine signaling (*CXCR5, IL2RA, IL7R, IL7, IL12RB1, IL22RA2, IL12A, IL12B, IRF8, TNFRSF1A, TNFRSF14, TNFSF14*), immune co-stimulation (*CD37, CD40, CD58, CD80, CD86, CLECL1*), and immune-related signal transduction (*CBLB, GPR65, MALT1, RGS1, STAT3, TAGAP, TYK2*). Addition genes included those related to the previously reported environmental risk factor, vitamin D (*CYP27B1, CYP24A1*), and those associated with MS therapies, including natalizumab (*VCAM1*) and daclizumab (*IL2RA*). Only a few genes relevant to potential pathways for neurodegeneration independent of inflammation (*GALC, KIF21B*) were found. The enrichment of SNPs in immune-related genes could be due to the use of blood as the starting material for these studies. There was no evidence of a genetic association with clinical course, severity of disease, or gender. How much these additional loci contribute to MS susceptibility remains to be determined. Meta-analysis of seven GWAS datasets combined with RNA expression data in peripheral blood mononuclear cells (PBMCs) detected three additional novel loci that reached genome-wide significance. These included regions close to the genes *EOMES*, (rs170934(T)), *MLANA* (rs2150702(G)), and *THADA* (rs6718520(A)) [21]. The functional effect of these genetic loci on the pathogenesis of MS is an active area of research.

Evidence for the involvement of environmental factors in MS etiology comes from prevalence and migration studies. The prevalence of MS varies geographically, with higher prevalence in polar regions compared to those near the equator. For example, MS incidence is below 5/100,000 in Africa, South America, and Asia and is over 100/100,000 in Scotland, Scandinavia, and Canada [22]. Possible environmental exposures include infections, nutritional factors, and toxins. Among non-infectious triggers of MS, vitamin D deficiency has received considerable attention. Epidemiological studies have shown an increase in MS frequency with increasing distance from the equator, which inversely correlates with duration and intensity of sunlight and vitamin D levels [23, 24]. Interestingly,

populations situated at high latitudes but having high consumption of vitamin D-rich food have reduced MS prevalence [24, 25]. Low serum levels of vitamin D are associated with increased risk of MS and correlate with increased disability and brain atrophy in MS patients [26]. Vitamin D appears to have immunomodulatory effects in experimental animal models, but the exact mechanism through which it acts in MS is unclear [16, 27].

Among the infectious environmental factors, viruses have received the most intense investigation. Much of this interest is based on the increased risk for acute disseminated encephalomyelitis following viral infections and vaccinations, the amino acid similarity of some viral antigens and myelin proteins, and the prevalence of seropositivity to certain viruses. Candidate viruses include measles, rubella, mumps, and the herpesviruses, including Epstein–Barr virus (EBV), herpes simplex virus 1 and 2, varicella zoster virus, and human herpesvirus 6 [28]. Serum measles antibody titers were higher in some MS patients compared to control patients, which led to the hypothesis of an association between the closely related CDV virus and MS pathogenesis [29]. Epstein–Barr virus is also a potential causative agent of MS [30]. The virus can be harbored in the immune cells and "reactivate" spontaneously from time to time. The link between EBV and MS has by far been the strongest, as MS patients have an increased incidence of infectious mononucleosis [31]. Furthermore, the presence of infectious mononucleosis correlates with a higher incidence of MS in low-risk geographical areas [24].

Neurodegeneration in MS

The pathological hallmarks of classic white matter MS lesions include demyelination, oligodendrocyte loss, the presence of blood-derived immune cells (mostly monocytes/macrophages with fewer T and B cells), breakdown of the BBB, and reactive gliosis [32]. Although a controversial subject, axonal pathology was mentioned in the early literature on MS (see the review by Kornek and Lassmann [33]) and included descriptions of axonal swellings, axonal transection, and Wallerian degeneration. In their classical works, both Charcot and Marburg described MS pathology in terms of demyelination, reactive gliosis, and relative sparing of axons in MS lesions [34, 35]. In 1936, Putnam [36] reported a 50% loss of axons in MS lesions from 11 patients. In the same year, Greenfield and King [37] reported normal axon densities in more than 90% of MS lesions from 13 patients. The differences between these works were suggested to result from the more sensitive axon staining used by Greenfield and King.

Axonal transection during inflammatory demyelination

Despite a significant literature describing axonal changes in brains of MS patients, the concept of axonal degeneration in MS was not widely accepted until the late 1990s, when a series of papers described a variety of axonal changes in actively demyelinating white matter lesions in post mortem MS brains. More importantly, these studies raised the possibility that axonal loss was the major cause of permanent neurological disability in MS and a major contributor to the transition from RRMS to SPMS [38]. Ferguson and colleagues reported accumulation of the amyloid precursor protein (APP) in axons within acute MS lesions [39]. Because APP is present at undetectable levels in normally myelinated axons, but accumulates to detectable levels following demyelination, this study supported altered fast axonal transport following demyelination and established that this axonal pathology correlated with the degree of inflammation within the lesion. It was subsequently shown that other proteins transported by fast axonal transport accumulate in acutely demyelinated axons, including the pore-forming subunit of N-type calcium channels [40] and metabotropic glutamate receptors [41]. If these proteins are inserted into the axolemma of demyelinated axons, they may contribute to axonal dysfunction and/or degeneration. The distribution and shape of APP staining in acute white matter lesions raised the possibility that demyelinated axons may be transected. This possibility was confirmed and extended by identification and quantification of terminal axonal ovoids in acute MS lesions [42]. Identified by a marked reduction in the phosphorylation states of neurofilament proteins, many acutely demyelinated axonal profiles had ovoid shapes. Three-dimensional reconstructions using confocal microscopy located most of these ovoids at the transected end of demyelinated axons [42] (Figure 20.1A). Transected axons in acute MS lesions from patients with clinical disease durations ranging from 2 weeks to 27 years were abundant and exceeded 11,000 per mm^3 of lesion area [42]. The identification of significant axonal transection in patients with a 2-week clinical disease course supported the concept that axonal transection occurs at disease onset in MS. The number of transected axons was decreased in the core of chronic active lesions (875/ mm^{3}tissue) and only occasionally detected in chronic inactive or aged-matched control brains. This and other studies correlated consistent and abundant axonal transection with the inflammatory activity of the acutely demyelinating lesion [38, 40–46]. In addition to postmortem studies, progressive brain atrophy [9] and reductions in the neuronal-specific marker, *N*-acetyl aspartic acid [10, 47–49], as measured by brain imaging of living patients, also supported axonal loss in MS brains.

Mechanisms of axonal transection in acute MS lesions

Axonal transection in acute MS lesions is thought to occur due to the vulnerability of demyelinated axons to inflammation (Figure 20.1B). The inflammatory microenvironment contains a variety of substances

that could injure axons, including proteolytic enzymes, cytokines, oxidative products, and free radicals produced by activated immune and glial cells [50]. Cytotoxic CD8+ T cells may mediate axonal transection in active MS lesions [51], as described in EAE mice [52] and *in vitro* [53]. iNOS, one of the key enzymes involved in the synthesis of nitric oxide (NO), is up-regulated in acute inflammatory MS lesions [54] and has a detrimental effect on axonal survival [55]. Glutamate-mediated excitotoxicity is observed in many acute and chronic neurodegenerative conditions [56] and may also be involved in axonal transection in MS [57–59]. It has also been proposed that inflammatory intermediates inhibit mitochondria function [60–62] and that local inflammatory edema may interfere with blood supply and induce an ischemic mechanism of axonal degeneration.

The identification of extensive axonal transection in acute MS lesions had important clinical and therapeutic implications. Reports of axonal loss in MS paralleled the availability of anti-inflammatory therapies. Confirmation of early but clinically silent axonal transection provided a rationale for early and continuous anti-inflammatory treatment for MS patients. While not primarily neuroprotective, anti-inflammatory treatments indirectly reduce axonal transection, which is abundant in areas of inflammatory demyelination.

Degeneration of chronically demyelinated axons

Despite the large number of transected axons in acute MS lesions, most demyelinated axons survive and alterations of axonal transport and axonal cytoskeleton are reversed. Progressive clinical disability associated with severe brain atrophy, however, provides evidence for continuous and irreversible neurodegeneration in the chronic MS brain. Because this neurodegeneration occurs when new inflammatory lesions are rare, mechanisms other than inflammatory demyelination must contribute to axon loss in chronic MS brains. Degeneration of chronically demyelinated axons is considered a major mechanism for axonal loss in the progressive stages of MS. While the most compelling experiments of counting axons within individual lesions at progressive time points cannot be performed, evidence for the degeneration of chronically demyelinated

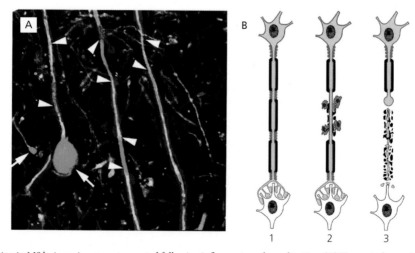

Figure 20.1 Axonal transection in MS lesions. Axons are transected following inflammatory demyelination. (A) Transected axon (arrow) in confocal images of an actively demyelinating MS lesion stained for myelin (red) and axons (green). The three vertically oriented axons have areas of demyelination (arrowheads). The axon on the left in (A) ends in a large swelling (arrow), or axonal retraction bulb, which is the hallmark of the proximal end of a transected axon. (B) Schematic summary of axonal response during and following transection. 1. Normal appearing axon. 2. Immune-mediated demyelination. 3. Axonal transection leads to rapid degeneration of the distal end, while the proximal end connected to the neuronal cell body survives. Following transection, the neuronal cell body continues to transport organelles down the axon, resulting in swellings or "axonal retraction bulbs". (A) Source: Trapp et al. 1998 [42]. Reproduced with permission of the New England Journal of Medicine. (B) Source: Trapp et al. 2008 [60]. Reproduced with permission of Annual Reviews.

axons comes from brain imaging, pathological studies of MS brains and studies of animal models with altered myelin protein expression [60, 63].

Proof of principle for degeneration of chronically demyelinated axons comes from several lines of transgenic mice that have null mutations in myelin proteins [61, 63, 64]. While initially designed to study the role of these proteins in myelination, these studies established that myelin proteins have essential roles in maintaining long-term axonal integrity. Surprisingly, myelin in mice null for the myelin-associated glycoprotein (MAG) and 2′,3′-cyclic nucleotide 3′-phosphodiesterase (CNP) appeared normal [65, 66]. Mice null for proteolipid protein (PLP), the major structural protein of CNS myelin, had altered compaction of CNS myelin, but all axons appeared to be ensheathed by oligodendrocyte membranes [67]. In all three lines of mice, a late-onset axonal degeneration developed [61, 64]. These studies established that, in addition to their insulating role, oligodendrocytes provide trophic support that is essential for axonal survival. MAG- and CNP-dependent trophic support appears to be independent of any role in myelination. If removal of minor components of myelin can cause axonal degeneration without affecting myelin internode integrity, loss of large segments of myelin over decades should result in axonal degeneration in MS.

Identification of terminal axonal ovoids in chronic inactive MS lesions provided direct support for transection of chronically demyelinated axons. While only a few axonal retraction bulbs were detected at autopsy, the total loss of chronically demyelinated axons over decades can be substantial. Estimates of total axonal loss in spinal cord lesions and corpus callosum of severely disabled MS patients approach 70% [68–70]. While not specific for axonal degeneration, the degree of brain atrophy seen in many MS patients must include significant axonal loss. Axonal loss and not axonal dysfunction due to demyelination, therefore, is the major cause of permanent neurological disability in MS.

Mechanisms of chronically demyelinated axonal degeneration

There has been considerable speculation regarding the mechanisms by which chronically demyelinated axons degenerate. The most popular mechanisms include of axonal degeneration following ischemic/hypoxic insults and involve an imbalance between axonal energy demand and limited energy supply [71–73]. Myelination concentrates voltage-gated Na^+ channels at nodes of Ranvier [61, 74]. The nerve impulse jumps from node to node by a process called saltatory conduction. As soon as Na^+ enters the nodal axon, it is rapidly pumped out in an energy-dependent manner by the Na^+/K^+-ATPases. This repolarizes the axolemma and permits rapid and repetitive axon firing. Following demyelination, Na^+ channels are diffusely distributed along the demyelinated axon [75–77]. While this redistribution restores nerve conduction, it does so at the expense of increased energy demand to operate the Na^+/K^+-ATPase during axolemma repolarization. The chronically demyelinated axon, therefore, is vulnerable to reduced axoplasmic ATP production. If the demyelinated axon cannot meet the increased energy demand of non-saltatory conduction, the Na^+/K^+-ATPase will not exchange axoplasmic Na^+ for extracellular K^+. If axonal Na^+ concentrations increase above 20mmol, the Na^+/Ca^{2+} exchanger, an energy-independent antiporter, is reversed and axoplasmic Na^+ will be exchanged for extracellular Ca^{2+}[72, 78]. Elevated axoplasmic Ca^{2+} will eventually activate degradative enzymes, impair mitochondrial function, reduce ATP production, and compromise axonal transport (Figure 20.2). Studies of post mortem MS brains support the concept that the mitochondria in chronically demyelinated axoplasm are compromised and have a reduced capacity for ATP production. In microarray comparisons of control and MS motor cortex, 26 nuclear-encoded mitochondrial genes were decreased in MS cortex and the function of mitochondrial complexes I and III was reduced by 40–50%

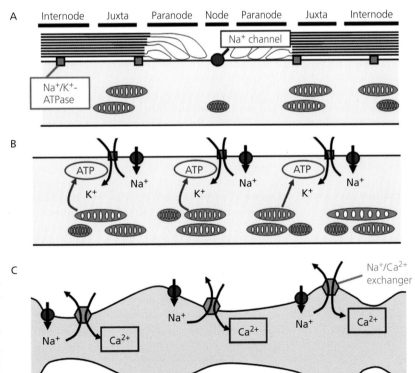

Figure 20.2 Ionic imbalance and axonal degeneration. (A) In myelinated axons, voltage-gated Na^+ channels are exclusively located at nodes of Ranvier whereas Na^+/K^+-ATPases are enriched in juxtaparanodal (Juxta) and internodal regions. (B) Upon demyelination, mitochondrial volume/numbers are increased throughout axons, where Na^+ channels redistribute diffusely and energy demand for Na^+ exclusion after nerve conduction is increased. (C) When axons fail to exclude Na^+ from demyelinated axons due to dysfunction of Na^+/K^+-ATPases and/or insufficient energy production, an increase of axonal Na^+ reverses Na^+/Ca^{2+} exchangers, increases axonal Ca^{2+}, and leads to axonal damage through activation of Ca^{2+}-dependent proteases.

in mitochondrial-enriched preparations from MS cortex [79]. These mitochondrial gene changes are restricted to neurons and are not detected in glia. Neurons in chronic MS cortex, therefore, are likely to be sending defective mitochondria into chronically demyelinated axons. Demyelinated axons in chronic MS lesions and following acute demyelination *in vitro* contain increased mitochondria [62, 80–82]. Many of the mitochondria in MS lesions have defective function of complex 2, and neuronal peri-karya in chronic MS brains contain clonally expanded deletions of mitochondria DNA [83]. These mutations are heterogeneous within a brain region and it remains to be determined if the increased heteroplasmy is also maintained in the axon projecting from these neurons. In any event, neuronal and axonal mitochondrial pathology may play a prominent role in axonal and neuronal degeneration. In addition, live imaging of mouse spinal cord during immune-mediated demyelination has documented fragmentation of axonal mitochondria that preceded axonal swelling and degeneration [84]. Reactive oxygen species (ROS) released from activated microglia/macrophages were proposed as mediators of mitochondrial damage and axonal degeneration, as suggested in previous studies using nitric oxide [55, 85].

Chronically demyelinated axons may eventually sustain an additional and probably fatal insult as the $\alpha 1$ and $\alpha 3$ Na$^+$/K$^+$-ATPase subunits, which are present in internodal axolemma of myelinated and acutely demyelinated axons, become virtually undetectable in many chronically demyelinated MS lesions [86]. Thus, these axons are chronically depolarized, unexcitable, and unable to sustain a number of critical homeostatic functions that depend on a healthy transaxolemmal Na$^+$ gradient. Loss of the Na$^+$/K$^+$-ATPase protein may be a key component of the vicious circle of impaired energy production and Ca^{2+} accumulation and suggests that many chronically demyelinated axons are functionally dead before they degenerate.

Cortical and deep gray matter demyelination in MS

Historically, cortical involvement in MS has received little attention, even though cortical demyelination is extensive in most MS brains that come to autopsy [60]. A major reason for this is that cortical demyelination is not detected macroscopically in brain slices or by standard pathological or brain imaging methods. When demyelinated, the cerebral cortex or deep gray matter does not change color like white matter lesions. Cortical myelin is not readily detected following routine staining with Luxol Fast Blue, the preferred stain for myelin by pathologists. Cortical lesions are not hypercellular and therefore are not obvious in hematoxylin and eosin-stained sections. Most importantly, cortical lesions are not routinely detected by MRI procedures [87]. Therefore, we do not know the extent and dynamics of cortical demyelination or whether cortical lesion load correlates with clinical disabilities or disease course. Although most MS researchers until the late 1990s or early 2000s were not focused on cortical demyelination, earlier reports had described it in post mortem MS brains. Brownell and Hughes reported that 26% of the brain lesions in MS involved the gray matter [88]. A study of 60 MS brains detected cortical lesions in 93% of the cases, and 59% of the cerebral lesions were in the cortex [89]. A significant expansion in studies describing cortical demyelination closely followed the renewed interest in axonal degeneration. Three patterns of cortical lesions were described [90]. Type I, or leukocortical lesions, are areas of demyelination that contiguously include both cerebral cortex and subcortical white matter (Figure 20.3A). These are informative lesions to study because the white and gray matter

portions are of a similar age, thus any differences detected are due to the environment in which demyelination is occurring. Type II cortical lesions are small perivascular areas of demyelination that do not contribute significantly to cortical lesion load (Figure 20.3B). Type III, or subpial lesions, are bands of demyelination that extend from the pial surface, often stop at cortical layer 3 or 4, and can occupy several gyri (Figure 20.3C). Subpial lesions occasionally extend through layer 6 of the cortex but rarely, if ever, invade subcortical white matter. Subpial lesions are the most abundant pattern of cortical demyelination. Total cortical lesion load cannot be determined because the only reliable means of detecting cortical demyelination is by immunocytochemical detection of myelin in post mortem tissue. Estimates of cortical demyelination have been limited to small samples of cortical tissues because it is impossible to sample the whole brain. Despite these limitations, current estimates raise the possibility that cortical lesion load exceeds that of white matter lesion load in many MS patients [91]. Confirmation of this possibility awaits the development of imaging modalities that reliably detect cortical and deep gray matter demyelination. It also appears that not all cortical areas are equally demyelinated. Cortical areas associated with deep sulci have a higher incidence of subpial demyelination than other cortical areas [91]. Deep sulci have expanded Virchow–Robin spaces, which can contain abundant immune cells. These Virchow–Robin spaces are contiguous with the CSF space that covers the brain surface. The possibility has been raised that immune cells in the Virchow–Robin or other CSF spaces secrete molecules that diffuse to the brain surface, penetrate the pial surface, and mediate or induce subpial demyelination [92, 93]. B cell-like follicles have also been identified in the CSF space of post mortem MS brains and were reported to correlate with the extent of cortical lesions [94, 95]. The possibility has also been raised that these B cells may be harboring EBV [96]. While there is a significant association between EBV and MS [97], the infection of B cell-like follicles by EBV is a controversial issue [98]. Attempts to identify immunoglobulin, complement, or other molecules that may diffuse into the brain surface have not been successful.

Why are cortical lesions not seen by routine brain imaging? The major reason is that cortical demyelination occurs without significant breakdown of the BBB or influx of immune cells from the blood. Therefore, GAD-enhancing cortical lesions are rarely seen. This is also the case for leukocortical lesions, where GAD is restricted to the white matter portion of the lesion. Pathologically, the white matter portions of active Type I lesions are filled with parenchymal monocytes/macrophages and perivascular cuffs, while the cortical portions contain few monocytes/macrophages and no perivascular cuffs, but do contain reactive microglia at the lesion border. Because myelin density is low in cortex compared to white matter, its absence does not alter T1 or T2 signals.

Cortical demyelination does cause neuronal pathology and degeneration. In cortical portions of acute Type I lesions, transected neurites (axons and dendrites) averaged 3000 per mm^3 lesion area, which is about one-third of the transected axons found in acute white matter lesions (Figure 20.3D) [90]. Apoptotic neurons were also increased in cortical lesions when compared to normally myelinated cortex from the same brains (Figure 20.3E) [90]. Gray matter demyelination may provide pathological correlates of fatigue, depression, and the decreased cognitive function that are common in individuals with MS [99]. Of special interest has been the possibility that hippocampal demyelination causes cognitive dysfunction in MS patients. Cognitive dysfunction occurs in more than 50% of MS patients, affecting episodic learning and memory,

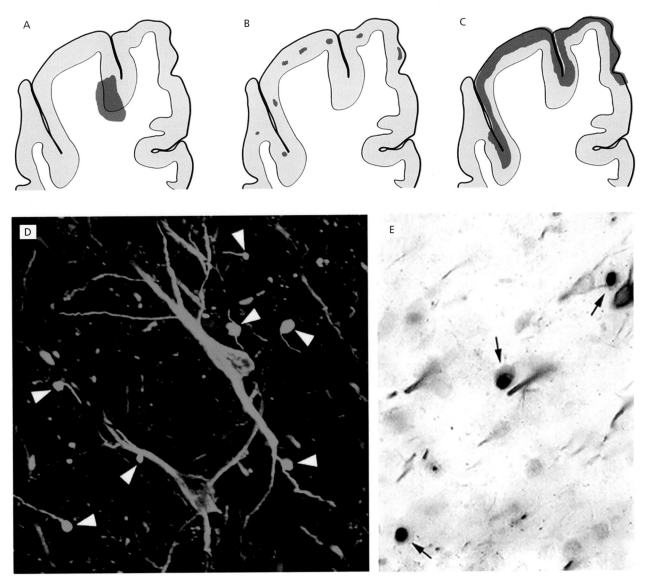

Figure 20.3 Cortical demyelination and neuronal pathology. Three patterns of cortical demyelination (orange) occur in MS brains. (A) Type I, or leuko-cortical lesions, demyelinate both subcortical white matter and cortex. (B) Type II lesions are small perivascular lesions. (C) Type III lesions extend into the cortex from the pial surface and often involve multiple gyri. (D) Axons and dendrites are transected (arrowheads) during cortical demyelination. (E) Apoptotic neurons (arrows), identified by TUNEL staining, are increased in demyelinated cortex. (A–C) Source: Peterson et al. 2001 [90]. Reproduced with permission of John Wiley and Sons. (D, E) Source: Peterson 2005 [149]. Reproduced with permission of Elsevier.

information processing speed, and working memory [100–104]. Neuropsychological decline is a better predictor of occupational and social impairment than physical disability. Cognitive decline has a major impact on the quality of life of MS patients. There is little correlation between physical disability on the Expanded Disability Status Scale (EDSS) and cognitive dysfunction in MS patients [105]. On average, cognitively impaired MS patients have significantly more white matter lesions and greater atrophy than cognitively intact MS patients. However, many cognitively impaired MS patients have white matter lesion loads that are comparable to those of cognitively intact MS patients [106, 107]. Imaging and pathological studies support the possibility that hippocampal demyelination contributes to cognitive decline in MS patients. Hippocampal demyelination is a prominent feature of post mortem MS brains, with 50–80% of hippocampi showing some degree of demyelination [108, 109, 110]. An encouraging observation

was the retention of 80% or more of neurons in demyelinated hippocampi [110]. This identifies the demyelinated hippocampal neuron as a promising therapeutic target. Despite the minimal neuronal loss, demyelinated hippocampi had a 40% decrease in synaptic densities and decreased expression of neuronal proteins associated with axonal transport, glutamate neurotransmission, glutamate homeostasis, and memory and learning [110]. Changes in genes associated with glutamate function or memory and learning were not found in demyelinated motor cortices from MS patients. These data support the concept that demyelination alters neuronal gene expression and synaptic connectivity. Furthermore, the neuronal genes altered by demyelination vary and depend upon the function of the neuron. If reduced synaptic densities are a general consequence of demyelination, this could contribute to cortical atrophy and to the continuous neurological decline seen in progressive stages of MS.

Diagnosis and disease progression

There is no single test to diagnose MS. Diagnosis is best confirmed based upon a combination of neurological examination and MRI of the brain. In 2001, 2005, and then again in 2011, the consensus diagnostic criteria for MS were updated [111–113]. Diagnosis of MS can be made without MRI being performed (e.g., two or more neurological attacks typical of MS with either objective clinical evidence of two or more lesions or objective clinical evidence of one lesion with reasonable historical evidence of a prior attack). MRI can support, supplement, or replace some clinical criteria [113] and it has been previously suggested that extreme caution should be exercised if MRI does not show lesions typical of MS [111]. The consensus MRI criteria for brain abnormality consistent with MS are based on the presence of T2-weighted (T2w) hyperintense white matter lesions and GAD-enhancing lesions of the CNS.

T2w lesions are white matter lesions that are hyperintense relative to the surrounding white matter on T2w MRI. In MS patients, T2w lesions on MRI include demyelinated lesions with variable degrees of axonal loss [114] and myelinated regions of white matter that are not macroscopically visible on post mortem brain slices but have an altered BBB and microglial activation [114–116]. T2w lesions are nonspecific and may include such pathological features as edema, demyelination, axonal loss, and gliosis.

GAD lesions are focal white matter areas that are enhanced (significantly brighter) compared to most cerebral white matter on T1-weighted (T1w) MRI following the intravenous injection of a GAD contrast agent. Under normal conditions, an intact BBB will confine the GAD contrast agent to the circulation. In MS white matter regions featuring acute increases in the permeability of the BBB, local extravasations of GAD contrast agent will occur. MS white matter lesions that enhance on post-GAD T1w MRI are new lesions exhibiting demyelination and intense inflammatory activity. Lesion enhancement has been shown to persist for an average of 4 weeks, and usually not longer than 8 weeks [117–119]. Older chronic active or chronic inactive white matter lesions do not enhance [120]. GAD enhancement is an indication of active disease activity. In RRMS, GAD lesions along with relapses have been valuable readouts for the efficacy of anti-inflammatory therapies in Phase III clinical trials.

An important aspect in the diagnosis of MS is that lesions should be disseminated in both space and time. The 2010 McDonald MRI criteria for demonstration of dissemination in space are: at least one T2w lesion in at least two of the four areas characteristic for MS (i.e., periventricular, juxtacortical, infratentorial, spinal cord) [113]. The 2010 McDonald MRI criteria for demonstration of dissemination in time are: at least one new T2w and/or GAD lesion on follow-up MRI with reference to a baseline scan, or the simultaneous presence of asymptomatic GAD lesions and T2w lesions at any time [113].

Total T2w lesion loads weakly correlate with MS disease progression. There are likely to be many reasons for this, including the variety of brain changes that can cause T2w signals and the inability of current imaging modalities to detect most cortical lesions (see section Cortical and deep gray matter demyelination in MS). One of the best predictors of disability progression in MS patients is brain atrophy [116, 121, 122]. In addition, patients with high rates of brain atrophy during initial stages of MS reach disability milestones faster than patients with initially slower atrophy rates [122–125]. Imaging studies also raise the possibility that cortical atrophy is a major and possibly very early component of MS pathogenesis that is at least partially independent of white matter lesion load. Cortical thinning appears to be most prominent in regions with cortico-cortical connections (cingulate gyrus, insular, frontal, parietal, and temporal cortices) compared to cortical regions that extend or receive long projection axons (motor, sensory, and occipital cortices) [126]. Because we cannot reliably detect cortical demyelination, the relationship between cortical atrophy and cortical demyelination is currently unknown. A major advance for MS clinical research would be the development of noninvasive imaging methods that would routinely and reliably detect myelin in cortical lesions. With such technology it could be established if total demyelination lesion load (white and gray matter) correlates with disability progression. MRI-based techniques shown to be sensitive to myelin pathology in MS include: detection of the protons associated with the water in the myelin bilayers (short T2 imaging [127]; detection of myelin phospholipids (phosphorus and proton spectroscopy [47, 128]; detection of restricted water diffusion (DTI) [129]; and detection of magnetization transfer (MT) from myelin-associated protons (quantitative MT and MT ratio [129, 130]).

Treatment options

Over the past 30 years, significant progress has been made in the treatment of MS. Several disease-modifying treatments (DMTs) are approved for treatment of relapsing forms of MS. The clinical efficacy of these agents has been demonstrated in multiple large Phase III trials [131, 132], many of which have included secondary MRI endpoints that measure brain atrophy and T1 black hole conversion. Although the control of relapses and inflammatory brain activity contributes to a decreasing burden of disability, the demonstration of a therapy that halts or slows the accumulation of disability in progressive forms of MS remains elusive. Several injectable agents are available for MS treatment and these include three formulations of interferon β and glatiramer acetate, an amino acid mimic of myelin basic protein. All are given by frequent intramuscular or subcutaneous injections and have a moderate effect on relapses with a favorable safety profile [133–135]. Natalizumab (Tysabri) is a humanized monoclonal antibody specific for α4 integrin and suppresses binding of leukocytes to vascular endothelia, a critical step for the entry of immune cells into the CNS. Natalizumab shows a significant reduction in GAD-enhancing lesions, with a two-thirds reduction in the relapse rate.

Three oral agents are now available for the treatment of MS: fingolimod, teriflunomide, and dimethyl fumarate. Fingolimod is a sphingosine 1-phosphate receptor modulator that sequesters lymphocytes in lymph nodes, preventing them from contributing to an autoimmune reaction. Dimethyl fumarate is a fumaric acid ester that is thought to exert its anti-inflammatory effects through several mechanisms including activation of nuclear factor E2 related factor 2 [136]. Teriflunomide is the active metabolite of leflunomide and is an inhibitor of dihydroorotate dehydrogenase. It shows efficacy similar to injectable agents [137]. Dimethyl fumarate and fingolimod show a one-half reduction of the relapse rate, while teriflunomide has shown an efficacy profile considered to be similar to injectable agents.

The more aggressive anti-inflammatory drugs carry potential side effects that have limited their more widespread use [138–140]. The occurrence of progressive multifocal leukoencephalopathy (PML), a rare but usually fatal CNS infection caused by JC virus, was reported in MS patients receiving Tysabri [141]. Mitoxantrone is a chemotherapeutic agent that is approved to treat worsening relapsing MS but carries significant risk of cardiac disease and potential malignancy and is seldom used [142].

The potential role of natalizumab and fingolimod is currently being studied in Phase III trials of secondary progressive and primary progressive MS, respectively. Fingolimod has shown a very robust and dose-dependent effect on brain atrophy, which is encouraging for its role in progressive forms of MS.

Several therapies that are thought to have either primary neuroprotective or neurorestorative effects are currently being studied. Mesenchymal stem cell transplantation has the potential to offer immunomodulatory effects as well as to promote neural repair and is currently being studied in Phase I/II trials [143, 144]. Blockade of sodium channels has also been proposed as a possible strategy to promote axonal integrity [145]. A small Phase II trial of lamotrigine showed no effect on brain atrophy measures in secondary progressive MS [146]; however, more sensitive measures of gray matter atrophy and advanced imaging metrics were not used. Medications that may potentially promote myelin repair by inhibiting the Nogo receptor interacting protein 1 (Lingo1) are currently in early clinical testing [147]. Ibudilast, a phosphodiesterase inhibitor, is being studied both in Europe and North America in large multicenter Phase II trials in progressive MS after it showed a significant effect on atrophy, but not inflammatory measures, in RRMS [148]. The success of therapies that promote neural repair and protection will depend not only on identification of adequate compounds in preclinical studies, but also on the adequate design of Phase II and Phase III trials in progressive MS. Novel clinical and MRI measures that are validated with meaningful patient outcomes are clearly needed to achieve this goal.

Future developments

Anti-inflammatory MS therapies have dramatically slowed disease progression and improved the quality of life of many MS patients. It is probable, however, that we have hit a ceiling in the effectiveness of immune suppression, as more unacceptable adverse side effects may be inevitable with more aggressive treatment. The future of MS therapeutics will include a search for additional targets. Because neurodegeneration is responsible for the irreversible neurological disability that most MS patients endure, neuroprotective therapies for MS patients are high on the list of future developments. There are two possible approaches: remyelination and neuroprotection. MS may be the most appropriate CNS disease in which to study neuroprotective therapies. Patients are diagnosed at an early stage of disease progression when little permanent or irreversible damage has occurred. This is in contrast to other neurodegenerative diseases that have a prolonged and undiagnosed, clinically silent neurodegeneration. Remyelination is the best documented neuroprotective therapy for MS patients. Some MS lesions spontaneously remyelinate, so endogenous remyelination should be a viable target. Future studies need to delineate why MS lesions fail to repair. The field desperately needs noninvasive imaging methods that can detect cortical and deep gray matter demyelination, remyelination, and axonal loss. When neuroprotective or remyelinating therapies enter clinical trials, we will need the means to measure their efficacy. Recent studies have also questioned whether inflammatory demyelination is a primary or secondary event in the MS disease process [60]. There is no question that the immune system plays an important and therapeutically treatable role in the pathogenesis of MS. It is possible, however, that the immune response is triggered by a primary CNS deficit. The challenge is to design studies that will address the primary role of the immune system in MS pathogenesis. An unequivocal answer to this question is at the heart of discovering the cause of MS.

Acknowledgments

Work performed in the authors' laboratories is supported by grants from the National Institutes of Health, NINDS (NS096148 to RD; R01NS091683 to BDT), and the National Multiple Sclerosis Society, USA (RG 5298 to RD). The authors would like to thank Dr. Christopher Nelson for editorial assistance. Dr. Ohno was supported by a Fellowship from the NMSS, USA, and Dr. Chen was supported by a Fellowship from the Canadian MS Society.

References

1. Noseworthy JH, Lucchinetti C, Rodriguez M, et al. Multiple sclerosis. *N Engl J Med* 2000; 343: 938–952.
2. Weinshenker BG. Epidemiology of multiple sclerosis. *Neurol Clin* 1996; 14: 291–308.
3. Reddy H, Narayanan S, Arnoutelis R, et al. Evidence for adaptive functional changes in the cerebral cortex with axonal injury from multiple sclerosis. *Brain* 2000; 123 (**Pt 11**): 2314–2320.
4. Pantano P, Iannetti GD, Caramia F, et al. Cortical motor reorganization after a single clinical attack of multiple sclerosis. *Brain* 2002; 125: 1607–1615.
5. Rocca MA, Mezzapesa DM, Falini A, et al. Evidence for axonal pathology and adaptive cortical reorganization in patients at presentation with clinically isolated syndromes suggestive of multiple sclerosis. *Neuroimage* 2003; 18: 847–855.
6. Parry AM, Scott RB, Palace J, et al. Potentially adaptive functional changes in cognitive processing for patients with multiple sclerosis and their acute modulation by rivastigmine. *Brain* 2003; 126: 2750–2760.
7. Mews I, Bergmann M, Bunkowski S, et al. Oligodendrocyte and axon pathology in clinically silent multiple sclerosis lesions. *Multiple Sclerosis* 1998; 4: 55–62.
8. Rudick RA, Fisher E, Lee JC, et al. Use of the brain parenchymal fraction to measure whole brain atrophy in relapsing-remitting MS. Multiple Sclerosis Collaborative Research Group. *Neurology* 1999; 53: 1698–1704.
9. Miller DH, Barkhof F, Frank JA, et al. Measurement of atrophy in multiple sclerosis: pathological basis, methodological aspects and clinical relevance. *Brain* 2002; 125: 1676–1695.
10. De Stefano N, Matthews PM, Fu L, et al. Axonal damage correlates with disability in patients with relapsing-remitting multiple sclerosis. Results of a longitudinal magnetic resonance spectroscopy study. *Brain* 1998; 121: 1469–1477.
11. Matthews PM, De Stefano N, Narayanan S, et al. Putting magnetic resonance spectroscopy studies in context: axonal damage and disability in multiple sclerosis. *Semin Neurol* 1998; 18: 327–336.
12. Gonen O, Catalaa I, Babb JS, et al. Total brain N-acetylaspartate: a new measure of disease load in MS. *Neurology* 2000; 54: 15–19.
13. McDonnell GV, Mawhinney H, Graham CA, et al. A study of the HLA-DR region in clinical subgroups of multiple sclerosis and its influence on prognosis. *J Neurol Sci* 1999; 165: 77–83.
14. Revesz T, Kidd D, Thompson AJ, et al. A comparison of the pathology of primary and secondary progressive multiple sclerosis. *Brain* 1994; 117: 759–765.
15. Hauser SL, Oksenberg JR. The neurobiology of multiple sclerosis: genes, inflammation, and neurodegeneration. *Neuron* 2006; 52: 61–76.
16. Ramagopalan SV, Dyment DA, Ebers GC. Genetic epidemiology: the use of old and new tools for multiple sclerosis. *Trends Neurosci* 2008; 31: 645–652.
17. Oksenberg JR, Baranzini SE. Multiple sclerosis genetics—is the glass half full, or half empty? *Nat Rev Neurol* 2010; 6: 429–437.
18. Oksenberg JR, Barcellos LF, Cree BA, et al. Mapping multiple sclerosis susceptibility to the HLA-DR locus in African Americans. *Am J Hum Genet* 2004; 74: 160–167.
19. Haines JL, Terwedow HA, Burgess K, et al. Linkage of the MHC to familial multiple sclerosis suggests genetic heterogeneity. The Multiple Sclerosis Genetics Group. *Hum Mol Genet* 1998; 7: 1229–1234.
20. Sawcer S, Hellenthal G, Pirinen M, et al. Genetic risk and a primary role for cell-mediated immune mechanisms in multiple sclerosis. *Nature* 2011; 476: 214–219.
21. Patsopoulos NA, Esposito F, Reischl J, et al. Genome-wide meta-analysis identifies novel multiple sclerosis susceptibility loci. *Ann Neurol* 2011; 70: 897–912.
22. Rosati G. The prevalence of multiple sclerosis in the world: an update. *Neurol Sci* 2001; 22: 117–139.
23. Kurtzke JF, Beebe GW, Norman JE, Jr. Epidemiology of multiple sclerosis in U.S. veterans: 1. Race, sex, and geographic distribution. *Neurology* 1979; 29: 1228–1235.
24. Kakalacheva K, Lunemann JD. Environmental triggers of multiple sclerosis. *FEBS Lett* 2011; 585: 3724–3729.
25. Swank RL, Lerstad O, Strom A, et al. Multiple sclerosis in rural Norway its geographic and occupational incidence in relation to nutrition. *N Engl J Med* 1952; 246: 722–728.

26. Weinstock-Guttman B, Zivadinov R, Qu J, et al. Vitamin D metabolites are associated with clinical and MRI outcomes in multiple sclerosis patients. *J Neurol Neurosurg Psychiatry* 2011; 82: 189–195.

27. Berlanga-Taylor AJ, Disanto G, Ebers GC, Ramagopalan SV. Vitamin D-gene interactions in multiple sclerosis. *J Neurol Sci* 2011; 311: 32–36.

28. Tselis A. Evidence for viral etiology of multiple sclerosis. *Semin Neurol* 2011; 31: 307–316.

29. Adams JM, Brooks MB, Fisher ED, Tyler CS. Measles antibodies in patients with multiple sclerosis and with other neurological and nonneurological diseases. *Neurology* 1970; 20: 1039–1042.

30. Ascherio A, Munger KL. Epstein-barr virus infection and multiple sclerosis: a review. *J Neuroimmune Pharmacol* 2010; 5: 271–277.

31. Warner HB, Carp RI. Multiple sclerosis and Epstein-Barr virus. *Lancet* 1981; 2: 1290.

32. Prineas J. Pathology of multiple sclerosis. In: CookS (editor). *Handbook of Multiple Sclerosis*. Marcel Dekker, New York, 2001; 289–324.

33. Kornek B, Lassmann H. Axonal pathology in multiple sclerosis. A historical note. *Brain Pathol* 1999; 9: 651–656.

34. Charcot M. Histologie de la sclerose en plaques. *Gaz Hosp* 1868; 141: 554–555.

35. Marburg O. Die sogenannte "akute multiple sklerose" (Encephalomyelitis peraxialis scleroticans). *Jahrb Neurol Psych* 1906; 27: 211–312.

36. Putnam TJ. Studies in multiple sclerosis. *Arch Neurol Psych* 1936; 35: 1289–1308.

37. Greenfield JG, King LS. Observations on the histopathology of the cerebral lesions in disseminated sclerosis. *Brain* 1936; 59: 445–458.

38. Trapp BD, Ransohoff RM, Fisher E, Rudick RA. Neurodegeneration in multiple sclerosis: Relationship to neurological disability. *The Neuroscientist* 1999; 5: 48–57.

39. Ferguson B, Matyszak MK, Esiri MM, Perry VH. Axonal damage in acute multiple sclerosis lesions. *Brain* 1997; 120: 393–399.

40. Kornek B, Storch MK, Bauer J, et al. Distribution of a calcium channel subunit in dystrophic axons in multiple sclerosis and experimental autoimmune encephalomyelitis. *Brain* 2001; 124: 1114–1124.

41. Geurts JJ, Wolswijk G, Bo L, et al. Altered expression patterns of group I and II metabotropic glutamate receptors in multiple sclerosis. *Brain* 2003; 126: 1755–1766.

42. Trapp BD, Peterson J, Ransohoff RM, Rudick R, Mork S, Bo L. Axonal transection in the lesions of multiple sclerosis. *N Engl J Med* 1998; 338: 278–285.

43. Trapp BD, Ransohoff R, Rudick R. Axonal pathology in multiple sclerosis: relationship to neurologic disability. *Curr Opin Neurol* 1999; 12: 295–302.

44. Geurts JJ, Stys PK, Minagar A, et al. Gray matter pathology in (chronic) MS: modern views on an early observation. *J Neurol Sci* 2009; 282: 12–20.

45. Kornek B, Storch MK, Weissert R, et al. Multiple sclerosis and chronic autoimmune encephalomyelitis: a comparative quantitative study of axonal injury in active, inactive, and remyelinated lesions. *Am J Pathol* 2000; 157: 267–276.

46. Bitsch A, Schuchardt J, Bunkowski S, et al. Acute axonal injury in multiple sclerosis. Correlation with demyelination and inflammation. *Brain* 2000; 123: 1174–1183.

47. Arnold DL, Riess GT, Matthews PM, et al. Use of proton magnetic resonance spectroscopy for monitoring disease progression in multiple sclerosis. *Ann Neurol* 1994; 36: 76–82.

48. Matthews PM, Pioro E, Narayanan S, et al. Assessment of lesion pathology in multiple sclerosis using quantitative MRI morphometry and magnetic resonance spectroscopy. *Brain* 1996; 119: 715–722.

49. Bjartmar C, Kinkel RP, Kidd G, et al. Axonal loss in normal-appearing white matter in a patient with acute MS. *Neurology* 2001; 57: 1248–1252.

50. Hohlfeld R. Biotechnological agents for the immunotherapy of multiple sclerosis. Principles, problems and perspectives (invited review). *Brain* 1997; 120: 865–916.

51. Babbe H, Roers A, Waisman A, et al. Clonal expansions of CD8(+) T cells dominate the T cell infiltrate in active multiple sclerosis lesions as shown by micromanipulation and single cell polymerase chain reaction. *J Exp Med* 2000; 192: 393–404.

52. Huseby ES, Liggitt D, Brabb T, et al. A pathogenic role for myelin-specific CD8(+) T cells in a model for multiple sclerosis. *J Exp Med* 2001; 194: 669–676.

53. Medana I, Martinic MA, Wekerle H, Neumann H. Transection of major histocompatibility complex class I-induced neurites by cytotoxic T lymphocytes. *Am J Pathol* 2001; 159: 809–815.

54. Bo L, Dawson TM, Wesselingh S, Mork S, et al. Induction of nitric oxide synthase in demyelinating regions of multiple sclerosis brains. *Ann Neurol* 1994; 36: 778–786.

55. Smith KJ, Lassmann H. The role of nitric oxide in multiple sclerosis. *Lancet Neurol* 2002; 1: 232–241.

56. Lipton SA, Rosenberg PA. Excitatory amino acids as a final common pathway for neurologic disorders. *N Engl J Med* 1994; 330: 613–622.

57. Pitt D, Werner P, Raine CS. Glutamate excitotoxity in a model of multiple sclerosis. *Nat Med* 2000; 6: 67–70.

58. Smith T, Groom A, Zhu B, Turski L. Autoimmune encephalomyelitis ameliorated by AMPA antagonists. *Nat Med* 2000; 6: 62–66.

59. Groom AJ, Smith T, Turski L. Multiple sclerosis and glutamate. *Ann N Y Acad Sci* 2003; 993: 229–275.

60. Trapp BD, Nave KA. Multiple sclerosis: an immune or neurodegenerative disorder? *Annu Rev Neurosci* 2008; 31: 247–269.

61. Trapp BD, Stys PK. Virtual hypoxia and chronic necrosis of demyelinated axons in multiple sclerosis. *Lancet Neurol* 2009; 8: 280–291.

62. Mahad D, Ziabreva I, Lassmann H, Turnbull D. Mitochondrial defects in acute multiple sclerosis lesions. *Brain* 2008; 131: 1722–1735.

63. Nave KA, Trapp BD. Axon-glial signaling and the glial support of axon function. *Annu Rev Neurosci* 2008; 31: 535–561.

64. Nave KA. Myelination and the trophic support of long axons. *Nat Rev Neurosci* 2010; 11: 275–283.

65. Yin X, Crawford TO, Griffin JW, et al. Myelin-associated glycoprotein is a myelin signal that modulates the caliber of myelinated axons. *J Neurosci* 1998; 18: 1953–1962.

66. Lappe-Siefke C, Goebbels S, Gravel M, et al. Disruption of Cnp1 uncouples oligodendroglial functions in axonal support and myelination. *Nat Genet* 2003; 33: 366–374.

67. Griffiths I, Klugmann M, Anderson T, et al. Axonal swellings and degeneration in mice lacking the major proteolipid of myelin. *Science* 1998; 280: 1610–1613.

68. Bjartmar C, Kidd G, Mork S, et al. Neurological disability correlates with spinal cord axonal loss and reduce *N*-acetyl aspartate in chronic multiple sclerosis patients. *Ann Neurol* 2000; 48: 893–901.

69. Ganter P, Prince C, Esiri MM. Spinal cord axonal loss in multiple sclerosis: a postmortem study. *Neuropathol Appl Neurobiol* 1999; 25: 459–467.

70. Lovas G, Szilagyi N, Majtenyi K, et al. Axonal changes in chronic demyelinated cervical spinal cord plaques. *Brain* 2000; 123: 308–317.

71. Waxman SG. Axonal conduction and injury in multiple sclerosis: the role of sodium channels. *Nat Rev Neurosci* 2006; 7: 932–941.

72. Stys PK. General mechanisms of axonal damage and its prevention. *J Neurol* 2005; 223: 3–13.

73. Stys PK. The axo-myelinic synapse. *Trends Neurosci* 2011; 34: 393–400.

74. Trapp BD, Kidd GJ. Structure of the myelinated axon. In: Lazzarini R (editor). *Myelin Biology and Disorders*. Elsevier, San Diego, 2004; 3–25.

75. Bostock H, Sears TA. The internodal axon membrane: Electrical excitability and continuous conduction in segmental demyelination. *J Physiol* 1978; 280: 273–301.

76. Bostock H, Sherratt RM, Sears TA. Overcoming conduction failure in demyelinated nerve fibers by prolonging action potentials. *Nature* 1978; 274: 385–387.

77. Felts PA, Baker TA, Smith KJ. Conduction in segmentally demyelinated mammalian central axons. *J Neurosci* 1997; 17: 7267–7277.

78. Stys PK. Axonal degeneration in multiple sclerosis: Is it time for neuroprotective strategies? *Ann Neurol* 2004; 55: 601–603.

79. Dutta R, McDonough J, Yin X, et al. Mitochondrial dysfunction as a cause of axonal degeneration in multiple sclerosis patients. *Ann Neurol* 2006; 59: 478–489.

80. Mahad DJ, Ziabreva I, Campbell G, et al. Mitochondrial changes within axons in multiple sclerosis. *Brain* 2009; 132: 1161–1174.

81. Zambonin JL, Zhao C, Ohno N, et al. Increased mitochondrial content in remyelinated axons: implications for multiple sclerosis. *Brain* 2011; 134: 1901–1913.

82. Kiryu-Seo S, Ohno N, Kidd GJ, et al. Demyelination increases axonal stationary mitochondrial size and the speed of axonal mitochondrial transport. *J Neurosci* 2010; 30: 6658–6666.

83. Campbell GR, Ziabreva I, Reeve AK, et al. Mitochondrial DNA deletions and neurodegeneration in multiple sclerosis. *Ann Neurol* 2011; 69: 481–492.

84. Nikic I, Merkler D, Sorbara C, et al. A reversible form of axon damage in experimental autoimmune encephalomyelitis and multiple sclerosis. *Nat Med* 2011; 17: 495–499.

85. Smith KJ. Sodium channels and multiple sclerosis: roles in symptom production, damage and therapy. *Brain Pathol* 2007; 17: 230–242.

86. Young EA, Fowler CD, Kidd GJ, et al. Imaging correlates of decreased axonal Na+/K+ ATPase in chronic multiple sclerosis lesions. *Ann Neurol* 2008; 63: 428–435.

87. Calabrese M, Filippi M, Gallo P. Cortical lesions in multiple sclerosis. *Nat Rev Neurol* 2010; 6: 438–444.

88. Brownell B, Hughes JT. Distribution of plaques in the cerebrum in multiple sclerosis. *J Neurol Neurosurg Psychiatry* 1962; 25: 315–320.

89. Lumsden CE. The neuropathology of multiple sclerosis. In: Vinken PJ, Bruyn GW (editors). *Handbook of Clinical Neurology*. Amsterdam: 1970; 217–309.

90. Peterson JW, Bo L, Mork S, et al. Transected neurites, apoptotic neurons and reduced inflammation in cortical MS lesions. *Ann Neurol* 2001; 50: 389–400.

91. Bo L, Vedeler CA, Nyland HI, et al. Subpial demyelination in the cerebral cortex of multiple sclerosis patients. *J NeuropatholExp Neurol* 2003; 62: 723–732.

92. Howell OW, Reeves CA, Nicholas R, et al. Meningeal inflammation is widespread and linked to cortical pathology in multiple sclerosis. *Brain* 2011; 134: 2755–2771.

93. Lucchinetti CF, Popescu BF, Bunyan RF, et al. Inflammatory cortical demyelination in early multiple sclerosis. *N Engl J Med* 2011; 365: 2188–2197.

94. Disanto G, Morahan JM, Barnett MH, et al. The evidence for a role of B cells in multiple sclerosis. *Neurology* 2012; 78: 823–832.

95. Magliozzi R, Howell O, Vora A, et al. Meningeal B-cell follicles in secondary progressive multiple sclerosis associated with early onset of disease and severe cortical pathology. *Brain* 2007; 130: 1089–1104.

96. Serafini B, Rosicarelli B, Franciotta D, et al. Dysregulated Epstein-Barr virus infection in the multiple sclerosis brain. *J Exp Med* 2007; 204: 2899–2912.

97. Giovannoni G. Epstein-Barr virus and MS. *Int MS J* 2011; 17: 44–49.

98. Lassmann H, Niedobitek G, Aloisi F, Middeldorp JM. Epstein-Barr virus in the multiple sclerosis brain: a controversial issue—report on a focused workshop held in the Centre for Brain Research of the Medical University of Vienna, Austria. *Brain* 2011; 134: 2772–2786.

99. Calabrese M, Rinaldi F, Grossi P, Gallo P. Cortical pathology and cognitive impairment in multiple sclerosis. *Expert Rev Neurother* 2011; 11: 425–432.

100. Rao S, Grafman J, DiGiulio D, et al. Memory dysfunction in multiple sclerosis: Its relation to working memory, semantic encoding, and implicit learning. *Neuropsychology* 1993; 7: 364–374.

101. Rao SM, Leo GJ, Bernardin L, Unverzagt F. Cognitive dysfunction in multiple sclerosis. I. Frequency, patterns, and prediction. *Neurology* 1991; 41: 685–691.

102. Ron MA, Callanan MM, Warrington EK. Cognitive abnormalities in multiple sclerosis: a psychometric and MRI study. *Psychol Med* 1991; 21: 59–68.

103. Beatty WW, Paul RH, Wilbanks SL, et al. Identifying multiple sclerosis patients with mild or global cognitive impairment using the Screening Examination for Cognitive Impairment (SEFCI). *Neurology* 1995; 45: 718–723.

104. Foong J, Rozewicz L, Davie CA, et al. Correlates of executive function in multiple sclerosis: the use of magnetic resonance spectroscopy as an index of focal pathology. *J Neuropsychiatry Clin Neurosci* 1999; 11: 45–50.

105. Benedict RH, Zivadinov R. Risk factors for and management of cognitive dysfunction in multiple sclerosis. *Nat Rev Neurol* 2011; 7: 332–342.

106. Benedict RH, Carone DA, Bakshi R. Correlating brain atrophy with cognitive dysfunction, mood disturbances, and personality disorder in multiple sclerosis. *J Neuroimaging* 2004; 14: 36S–45S.

107. Rao SM, St Aubin-Faubert P, Leo GJ. Information processing speed in patients with multiple sclerosis. *J Clin Exp Neuropsychol* 1989; 11: 471–477.

108. Papadopoulos D, Dukes S, Patel R, et al. Substantial archaeocortical atrophy and neuronal loss in multiple sclerosis. *Brain Pathol* 2009; 19: 238–253.

109. Geurts JJ, Bo L, Roosendaal SD, et al. Extensive hippocampal demyelination in multiple sclerosis. *J Neuropathol Exp Neurol* 2007; 66: 819–827.

110. Dutta R, Chang A, Doud MK, et al. Demyelination causes synaptic alterations in hippocampi from multiple sclerosis patients. *Ann Neurol* 2011; 69: 445–454.

111. McDonald WI, Compston A, Edan G, et al. Recommended diagnostic criteria for multiple sclerosis: guidelines from the International Panel on the diagnosis of multiple sclerosis. *Ann Neurol* 2001; 50: 121–127.

112. Polman CH, Wolinsky JS, Reingold SC. Multiple sclerosis diagnostic criteria: three years later. *Mult Scler* 2005; 11: 5–12.

113. Polman CH, Reingold SC, Banwell B, et al. Diagnostic criteria for multiple sclerosis: 2010 revisions to the McDonald criteria. *Ann Neurol* 2011; 69: 292–302.

114. van Waesberghe JH, Kamphorst W, De Groot CJ, et al. Axonal loss in multiple sclerosis lesions: magnetic resonance imaging insights into substrates of disability. *Ann Neurol* 1999; 46: 747–754.

115. Newcombe J, Hawkins CP, Henderson CL, et al. Histopathology of multiple sclerosis lesions detected by magnetic resonance imaging in unfixed postmortem central nervous system tissue. *Brain* 1991; 114: 1013–1023.

116. Fisher E, Chang A, Fox RJ, et al. Imaging correlates of axonal swelling in chronic multiple sclerosis brains. *Ann Neurol* 2007; 62: 219–228.

117. Harris JO, Frank JA, Patronas N, et al. Serial gadolinium-enhanced magnetic resonance imaging scans in patients with early, relapsing-remitting multiple sclerosis: implications for clinical trials and natural history. *Ann Neurol* 1991; 29: 548–555.

118. Miller DH, Rudge P, Johnson G, et al. Serial gadolinium enhanced magnetic resonance imaging in multiple sclerosis. *Brain* 1988; 111 (Pt 4): 927–939.

119. Silver NC, Lai M, Symms MR, et al. Serial magnetization transfer imaging to characterize the early evolution of new MS lesions. *Neurology* 1998; 51: 758–764.

120. Katz D, Taubenberger JK, Cannella B, et al. Correlation between magnetic resonance imaging findings and lesion development in chronic, active multiple sclerosis. *Ann Neurol* 1993; 34: 661–669.

121. Fazekas F, Soelberg-Sorensen P, Comi G, Filippi M. MRI to monitor treatment efficacy in multiple sclerosis. *J Neuroimaging* 2007; 17 **Suppl 1**: 50S–55S.

122. Filippi M, Rocca MA, Comi G. The use of quantitative magnetic-resonance-based techniques to monitor the evolution of multiple sclerosis. *Lancet Neurol* 2003; 2: 337–346.

123. Fisher E, Rudick RA, Cutter G, et al. Relationship between brain atrophy and disability: an 8-year follow-up study of multiple sclerosis patients. *Mult Scler* 2000; 6: 373–377.

124. Bakshi R. Magnetic resonance imaging advances in multiple sclerosis. *J Neuroimaging* 2005; 15: 5S–9S.

125. Bakshi R, Thompson AJ, Rocca MA, et al. MRI in multiple sclerosis: current status and future prospects. *Lancet Neurol* 2008; 7: 615–625.

126. Charil A, Dagher A, Lerch JP, et al. Focal cortical atrophy in multiple sclerosis: relation to lesion load and disability. *Neuroimage* 2007; 34: 509–517.

127. MacKay A, Whittall K, Adler J, et al. In vivo visualization of myelin water in brain by magnetic resonance. *Magn Reson Med* 1994; 31: 673–677.

128. Kilby PM, Bolas NM, Radda GK. 31P-NMR study of brain phospholipid structures in vivo. *Biochim Biophys Acta* 1991; 1085: 257–264.

129. Schmierer K, Wheeler-Kingshott CA, Boulby PA, et al. Diffusion tensor imaging of post mortem multiple sclerosis brain. *Neuroimage* 2007; 35: 467–477.

130. Barkhof F, Bruck W, De Groot CJ, et al. Remyelinated lesions in multiple sclerosis: magnetic resonance image appearance. *Arch Neurol* 2003; 60: 1073–1081.

131. Miller AE, Rhoades RW. Treatment of relapsing-remitting multiple sclerosis: current approaches and unmet needs. *Curr Opin Neurol* 2012; 25 **Suppl**: S4–10.

132. Kita M. FDA-approved preventative therapies for MS: first-line agents. *Neurol Clin* 2011; 29: 401–409.

133. Miller A, Spada V, Beerkircher D, Kreitman RR. Long-term (up to 22 years), open-label, compassionate-use study of glatiramer acetate in relapsing-remitting multiple sclerosis. *Mult Scler* 2008; 14: 494–499.

134. Reder AT, Ebers GC, Traboulsee A, et al. Cross-sectional study assessing long-term safety of interferon-beta-1b for relapsing-remitting MS. *Neurology* 2010; 74: 1877–1885.

135. Gold R, Rieckmann P, Chang P, Abdalla J. The long-term safety and tolerability of high-dose interferon beta-1a in relapsing-remitting multiple sclerosis: 4-year data from the PRISMS study. *Eur J Neurol* 2005; 12: 649–656.

136. Linker RA, Gold R. Dimethyl fumarate for treatment of multiple sclerosis: mechanism of action, effectiveness, and side effects. *Curr Neurol Neurosci Rep* 2013;13(**11**):394.

137. Bar-Or A, Pachner A, Menguy-Vacheron F, Kaplan J, Wiendl H. Teriflunomide and its mechanism of action in multiple sclerosis. *Drugs* 2014; 74(**6**): 659–674.

138. Clifford DB, De Luca A, Simpson DM, et al. Natalizumab-associated progressive multifocal leukoencephalopathy in patients with multiple sclerosis: lessons from 28 cases. *Lancet Neurol* 2010; 9: 438–446.

139. Yousry TA, Major EO, Ryschkewitsch C, et al. Evaluation of patients treated with natalizumab for progressive multifocal leukoencephalopathy. *N Engl J Med* 2006; 354: 924–933.

140. Cohen JA, Chun J. Mechanisms of fingolimod's efficacy and adverse effects in multiple sclerosis. *Ann Neurol* 2011; 69: 759–777.

141. Kleinschmidt-DeMasters BK, Tyler KL. Progressive multifocal leukoencephalopathy complicating treatment with natalizumab and interferon beta-1a for multiple sclerosis. *N Engl J Med* 2005; 353: 369–374.

142. Martinelli V, Radaelli M, Straffi L, Rodegher M, Comi G. Mitoxantrone: benefits and risks in multiple sclerosis patients. *Neurol Sci* 2009; 30 **Suppl 2**: S167–S170.

143. Saidha S, Eckstein C, Calabresi PA. New and emerging disease modifying therapies for multiple sclerosis. *Ann N Y Acad Sci* 2012; 1247: 117–137.

144. Freedman MS, Bar-Or A, Atkins HL, et al. The therapeutic potential of mesenchymal stem cell transplantation as a treatment for multiple sclerosis: consensus report of the International MSCT Study Group. *Mult Scler* 2010; 16: 503–510.

145. Waxman SG. Mechanisms of disease: sodium channels and neuroprotection in multiple sclerosis—current status. *Nat Clin Pract Neurol* 2008; 4: 159–169.

146. Kapoor R, Furby J, Hayton T, et al. Lamotrigine for neuroprotection in secondary progressive multiple sclerosis: a randomised, double-blind, placebo-controlled, parallel-group trial. *Lancet Neurol* 2010; 9: 681–688.

147. Mi S, Hu B, Hahm K, et al. LINGO-1 antagonist promotes spinal cord remyelination and axonal integrity in MOG-induced experimental autoimmune encephalomyelitis. *Nat Med* 2007; 13: 1228–1233.

148. Barkhof F, Hulst HE, Drulovic J, et al. Ibudilast in relapsing-remitting multiple sclerosis: a neuroprotectant? *Neurology* 2010; 74(**13**):1033–1040.

149. Peterson JW, Kidd GJ, Trapp BD. Axonal degeneration in multiple sclerosis: the histopathological evidence. In: Waxman S (editor). *Multiple Sclerosis as a Neuronal Disease.* Elsevier, San Diego, 2005; 165–168.

CHAPTER 21

Huntington's Disease and Other Choreas

Salman Haider[1], Edward Wild[2], and Sarah J. Tabrizi[2]

[1] London Deanery, Barking, Havering and Redbridge University Hospitals NHS Trust, Essex, UK
[2] Department of Neurodegenerative Disease, UCL Institute of Neurology and National Hospital for Neurology and Neurosurgery, London, UK

Huntington's disease

Introduction

History of the movement disorder

Chorea is derived from the Greek *"choreia"* meaning "to dance", and employed as a descriptor for the rapid, irregular, and jerky movements that are universally accepted as the most obvious outward sign of the disease. Historical commentaries date back as far as the 14th century, when Paracelsus first introduced the term to describe the movements as part of an organic medical disease. In the 17th century English colonists first coined the term "San Vitus' dance", which was formalized by Sydenham's description of childhood chorea in 1686. The association of this with rheumatic fever was not made until the advent of the 20th century.

Milestones in Huntington's disease

Originally termed Huntington's chorea, the nomenclature of Huntington's disease changed relatively recently to its current form in order to better represent the plethora of clinical features beyond the movement disorder. The first definite description of Huntington's disease (HD) was given by Charles Oscar Waters in 1841, who gave a clear account of the natural history of the disease. On 15 February 1872, George Huntington, aged 21 and a recent graduate from Columbia University, presented the earliest most complete description of HD before the Meigs and Mason Academy of Medicine at Middleport, Ohio. It was published two months later in the *Medical and Surgical Reporter of Philadelphia* [1]. The comprehensive nature of the description is likely attributable to the fact that from a young age Huntington observed patients while accompanying his father's family practice rounds in East Hampton, Long Island, New York [2].

By far the most important milestone of modern times was the herculean collaborative effort, driven notably by affected families, that galvanized doctors and scientists and culminated in the identification of a mutation in the IT15 ("interesting transcript 15") or *Huntingtin (HTT)* gene in 1993 [3]. The gene is located on the short arm of chromosome 4 (4p 16.3) and in HD it contains a CAG repeat expansion in exon 1, which results in an abnormal polyglutamine tract in the protein, huntingtin (HTT) (Figure 21.1).

Clinical features of Huntington's disease

Epidemiology

In the Western hemisphere prevalence reaches 7–10/100,000. In the United Kingdom (UK), incidence estimates range from 0.44 to 0.78 per 100,000 person-years, and prevalence ranges from 5.96 to 6.54 per 100,000 of the population. From a primary care based study, a figure of at least 12.4/100,000 was produced and even this may be an underestimate [4, 5]. This makes HD one of the more common inherited neurological diseases in the UK after neurofibromatosis type 1, Charcot–Marie–Tooth disease, and Duchenne muscular dystrophy [6] (Figure 21.2).

It is likely that some HD patients have an ancestral origin from healthy carriers of intermediate alleles and there has been some suggestion of a northern European origin to the gene. Although this is not rigorously established, it is based on the finding that the gene is 10 times more common in North Americans of European origin than in those of pure African or Asian descent or in Native Americans. This could be explained by the fact that the majority of HD chromosomes in Europe are found on haplogroup A. In contrast, an association to haplogroup C is seen in China and Japan, with the highest-risk haplotypes (A1 and A2) absent from the general and HD populations. Thus geographical variations in the haplotype may underlie differing prevalence rates [7, 11].

The highest prevalence in the world is in Venezuela at the edge of Lake Maracaibo with 700 cases per 100,000 persons. The region is relatively isolated, both socially and geographically, which has led to the high gene frequency in this small population. It was the systematic study of this small Venezuelan community in 1979 that was crucial in the linkage and cloning of the HD gene. In the UK there are regions of higher prevalence in South Wales, Northern Ireland, East Anglia, and parts of Scotland. Conversely, in Finland, Norway, and Japan, a significantly reduced prevalence is noted [2, 6]. A sub-Saharan African study showed considerable variation between population-based prevalence of 3.5 cases per 100,000, and hospital-based studies, where it ranged from 0.2 to 46 cases per 100,000 although clearly diagnostic accuracy and undercoverage were obvious limitations [12].

Neurodegeneration, First Edition. Edited by Anthony Schapira, Zbigniew Wszolek, Ted M. Dawson and Nicholas Wood.
© 2017 John Wiley & Sons, Ltd. Published 2017 by John Wiley & Sons, Ltd.

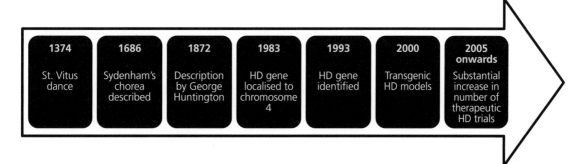

Figure 21.1 Milestones in Huntington's disease.

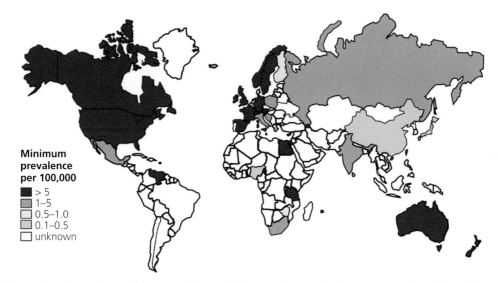

Figure 21.2 World map of prevalence estimates in Huntington's disease [7]. Worldwide estimates of the prevalence of HD. Overall, the prevalence of HD is much higher in European populations than in East Asia. Average minimum prevalence on the basis of several studies is shown. Note that prevalence studies occurring before the discovery of the HD gene in 1993 could underestimate the true prevalence of HD by as much as 14–24% [8, 9]. In particular, many of the studies in Africa have small sample sizes and the HD diagnosis has not confirmed by molecular testing. As HD phenocopy disorders are relatively common in Africa [10], these studies could have significantly overestimated the HD prevalence in these regions. Source: Warby et al. 2011 [7]. Reproduced with permission of Nature Publishing Group.

Clinical features

Overview

Huntington's disease is a monogenic, autosomal dominant, neurodegenerative condition. Due to relatively early loss of function and productivity and the chronic, slowly progressive nature of the disease with its increasing requirements for medication and social and multidisciplinary care, HD carries a substantial resource burden [13]. In an address to the New York Medical Society in 1909, Huntington summarized some important features we recognize today as being part of the disease, alongside the classical description of chorea, "... two women, mother and daughter, both tall, thin, almost cadaverous, both bowing, twisting, grimacing".

Disease onset

The onset of disease is currently defined as the point at which characteristic motor signs develop, when a patient moves from being a *premanifest gene carrier* to having *manifest* disease [14]. This distinction is somewhat arbitrary because most patients develop cognitive or psychiatric symptoms (or both) during the premanifest period, often many years before any motor signs are seen (Figure 21.3). The range

of clinical features reported in HD is extensive and expanding and covers multiple domains (Table 21.1). Although other phenotypes do exist, the most common is the classical adult-onset disease, with symptoms usually manifesting between the ages of 30 and 50 and progressing over 15–20 years. Here we find the classical triad of motor, cognitive, and psychiatric features. However, even within the same family, there can be a striking difference in the relative manifestation and severity of these features.

Neurological

Motor Despite the motor symptoms of HD being among its most recognized features, a detailed breakdown of the prevalence of individual or indeed groups of motor symptoms is lacking. The importance of motor impairment is evident in that it correlates with functional limitation in HD, predicts need for nursing home placement and falls risk, and defines clinical diagnosis [16, 17].

Falls are a significant cause of morbidity in HD. Although the management of recurrent falls is well established in geriatric practice, data in HD are limited. A recent observational study showed

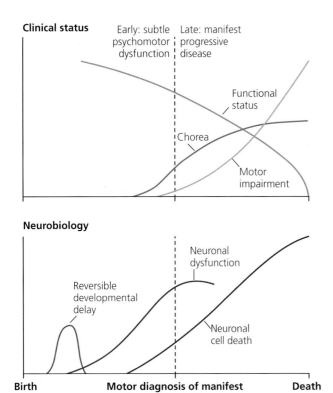

Figure 21.3 Outline of clinico-pathological progression in Huntington's disease [15]. Subtle signs and symptoms of Huntington's disease begin years before a motor diagnosis can be made, and correlate with neurobiological changes such as striatal atrophy, giving rise to the concept of a premanifest phase of Huntington's disease. Early in the disease course, neuronal dysfunction is likely to be important, but later, neuronal cell death in vulnerable regions of the brain is predominant and correlates with motor impairment and functional disability. Source: Ross 2011 [15]. Reproduced with permission of Elsevier.

Table 21.1 Clinical features of Huntington's disease.

Neurological
Motor:
• Chorea, dystonia, bradykinesia, rigidity, spasticity, myoclonus, tics, motor impersistence
• Loss of postural reflexes, poor balance, and impairment of voluntary motor control, e.g., walking, manual dexterity
• Dysphagia and dysarthria
Non-motor:
• Urge incontinence
• Sleep disturbance including sleep-wake cycle reversal, insomnia, periodic leg movements, REM sleep behavior disorders and sleep disordered breathing
Cognitive
• Perseveration, impulsivity, perceptual difficulties, impaired insight, distractibility, impairment in learning novel tasks
• Difficulties with planning, initiating, and organizing thoughts, activities, and communication
Psychiatric
• Depression, obsessive-compulsive disorders, anxiety, bipolar disorder, irritability, apathy, hypersexuality, psychosis
• Verbal and/or physical aggression
Other
• Weight loss, muscle wasting

that 58.3% of attenders to an outpatient HD clinic had sustained up two falls in the last year, while a retrospective study in 45 early- to mid-stage HD patients produced comparable figures with 60% reporting two or more falls in the last year [18, 19].

Although there are a legion of motor signs in HD, they can be reasonably divided into those representative of impairment of *voluntary* motor control (e.g., limb incoordination or loss of fine motor control of fingers), those in keeping with loss of *involuntary* motor control (e.g., loss of balance and postural reflexes), and finally those that indicate the presence of involuntary movements (hyperkinetic features, e.g., chorea, tics, and dystonia). There can evidently be overlap of features, for example where chorea or dystonia of the trunk is superimposed upon impairment of postural reflexes, impacting additively on balance and mobility.

Intriguingly, even quite marked chorea often remains unnoticed by the patient. It can also be passed over initially by relatives as nervousness but it is usually the persistence of these movements that prompts the first medical consultation. Alternatively, in those with a clear family history, partners or relatives can comment on similarities of behavior or movements between generations. Descriptions such as "twitchy", "fidgety", or "restless" can be applied, and subjects themselves can report symptoms of akathisia. Typically, there are minor movements of the hands or toes, although there can be much larger amplitude movements of a whole body part where they are termed "ballistic". Subtle deterioration in fine motor control can be suggested by a change in handwriting or loss of dexterity in the use of a computer, mobile phone, or cutlery.

A common motor complaint is of walking difficulty, which is related to composite loss of voluntary motor control, excess involuntary movements, and impaired coordination and balance. It can produce a gait that is often difficult to classify, with varying amounts of ataxia, chorea, and dystonia. Early mild swallowing impairment or dysarthria can also be seen. However, it is clear that the motor features can vary significantly in their relative predominance and location – chorea itself can be seen extra-axially in the face, mouth, and tongue.

Generally, mild amounts of dystonia, bradykinesia, and rigidity of limbs coexist with relatively more prominent chorea, which itself reaches a peak in mid-stage disease, after which this balance reverses as disease progresses. In moderate and advanced stages, loss of both involuntary and voluntary movement occurs with abnormal fixed postures, especially of the trunk or neck, which are usually dystonic in origin. Flexion contractures can ensue reflecting overriding spasticity and rigidity and representing more florid degeneration of corticospinal tracts.

The exception is the Westphal, akinetic-rigid variant, where rigidity and bradykinesia prevail and tremor and chorea are rarely seen. This is the characteristic presentation of juvenile HD although it also occurs in around 10% of adult cases. Axial rigidity appears to be more significantly associated with disability and loss of ambulation than chorea [20].

Motor impersistence is also seen in HD, characterized by an inability to maintain muscle contraction at a fixed level, which has given rise to the term "milkmaid's grip" because the patient is unable to apply a constant force during the handshake [21]. Motor impersistence can also be elicited by asking the patient to maintain a fully protruded tongue for 10 seconds.

Balance and posture Balance impairment can occur early on in concert with the above motor features, but may only be noticed when the patient is in an environment that presents a greater motor challenge (at night or on getting onto or off an escalator or while walking on uneven ground). Formal quantitative analysis using an obstacle test, sit-to-stand test, and a step and turn test using kinematic and kinetic variables has shown that HD patients perform slower in all three tests, produce less rising force, and have greater sway velocity of the center of gravity. Patients display significant postural control deficits when replicating motor skills employed in activities of daily living, emphasizing the functional impairment these symptoms confer [22]. At advanced stages of disease, fixed dystonic posturing of head, trunk, or limbs can occur, necessitating appropriate secondary preventative measures.

Eye movements The broken pursuit movements and slowed saccades (vertical worse than horizontal) seen early on the disease worsen, requiring head movements or eye blinking to initiate, and at the advanced stages a complete supranuclear gaze palsy is possible [23]. A characteristic sign is gaze impersistence with difficulty fixating on an object. These oculomotor abnormalities are likely to represent disruption to the fronto-striatal control of eye movements [24].

Dysphagia The swallowing difficulties seen in HD likely reflect several processes: lack of coordination between the oral and pharyngeal stage; tachyphagia, or rapid uncontrolled swallowing secondary to impaired sensory and corticobulbar function; buccolingual chorea resulting in food being transferred inadvertently; failure of the normal respiratory–deglutition cycle; and esophageal dysmotility [25]. Patients report difficulty in swallowing solid and liquids and can also choke occasionally, emphasizing the importance of speech and language therapists, dieticians, and judicious investigation in the form of videofluoroscopy. In the later stages, progressive swallowing and speaking impairment gives way to anarthria and mutism.

Continence Urge incontinence with associated frequency and urgency is probably the most commonly reported complaint, usually occurring in mid-stage disease. In advanced stages patients become doubly incontinent. A study of six patients revealed four with detrusor instability while two had a normal study suggesting a non-organic disturbance. A characteristic urodynamic pattern consisting of choreiform movements of the pelvic floor musculature during filling with selective suppression of choreiform contractions in the perineum during detrusor contraction was observed although this has never been followed up [26]. In a more recent study, cystometry performed in 12 manifest patients and 1 premanifest patient demonstrated detrusor–sphincter dyssynergia, detrusor overactivity, and reduced detrusor capacity [27].

In a large study of autonomic symptomatology in HD, using a clinical questionnaire rather than formal urological investigation, urgency, urinary incontinence, frequency, nocturia, incomplete emptying, and straining on defecation were all found in both manifest and premanifest subjects [28].

Sleep disturbance The etiology of sleeping difficulties in HD is likely to be multifactorial as patients have a profound circadian rhythm disturbance which mirrors that seen in transgenic mice where diminished gene expression in the suprachiasmatic nucleus is noted [29, 30]. Hypothalamic-pituitary dysfunction does undoubtedly play a role leading to sleep fragmentation and sleep-wake cycle reversal. Depression and apathy may contribute also through a loss of daytime stimulation and activity. Involuntary movements can hinder getting off to sleep as well as contribute to middle-of-the-night insomnia. Clinical research has shown that sleep disturbance in HD includes insomnia, advanced sleep phase, periodic leg movements, REM sleep behavior disorders, and reduced REM

sleep [31]. There is also emerging evidence that sleep-disordered breathing can impact on HD patients due to medication-related weight gain and potentially uncharacterized central and/or peripherally driven neuromuscular disease.

Dysautonomia This is a relatively new clinical entity in the HD phenotype although research has shown that patients with HD commonly have impairment of the autonomic nervous system [32, 33]. In a recent study, the most prevalent symptoms in 63 patients with HD and 21 premanifest mutation carriers were dysphagia, erectile and ejaculatory dysfunction, sialorrhea (although xerostomia can also be seen), early abdominal fullness, and light-headedness while standing [28].

Cognition

A global dementia is not seen in HD until the later stages; instead specific domains and their connections are affected by a focal frontal-subcortical dementia, manifesting typically as a dysexecutive syndrome where patients complain of mental slowing, difficulty multitasking, and failure to initiate, plan, and organize tasks or maintain concentration, and rigid thinking. Occasionally this may manifest or indeed be supplemented with a prominent behavioral change such as aggression or alternatively withdrawal and change of personality.

Symptoms may be present from the premanifest stage, with one study showing that 38% of patients in the premanifest stage had mild cognitive impairment [34]. Deficits in processing speed, visuospatial processing, time estimation and timekeeping, learning, and working memory are also seen in this group. Correspondingly, they report difficulty in picking up new tasks but retrieval of task-specific memories is also affected. There is also reliable evidence of olfactory impairment in both premanifest and manifest patients [35, 36]. It is clear also that cognitive and behavioral symptoms place the greatest burden on carers and correlate with functional decline and institutionalization [37].

Language is markedly spared until the advanced stages where there is undoubtedly a mixed component of both dysphasia and dysarthria. However comprehension is believed to be well preserved even in late stages of the disease. Communication, however, can be impacted upon by diminished processing speed and loss of coordinated oro-motor function with respiration [36].

Characterization of the cognitive impairment seen in HD has been driven largely by clinical research. Although there is substantial evidence of cognitive impairment in HD, there is no accepted cognitive battery for clinical testing in premanifest HD. Current practice may include the Verbal Fluency, Symbol Digit, Stroop, and Category fluency as well as Trails A and B and the Hopkins Verbal Learning Test, as derived from several years of observational data [36, 38, 39].

Neuropsychiatric features (Table 21.2)

The lifetime prevalence of psychiatric disease in HD ranges between 33% and 76%. It encompasses low mood, anxiety, irri-

Table 21.2 Prevalence of neuropsychiatric symptomatology in Huntington's disease (adapted from van Duijn et al. 2007 [40]).

Symptom	Prevalence (%)
Irritability [41]	38–73%
Apathy [41]	34–76%
Anxiety [41]	34–61%
Depressed mood [41]	33–69%
Obsessive and compulsive [41]	10–52%
Bipolar symptoms [42]	5–10%
Psychotic [41]	3–11%

tability, apathy, obsessive-compulsive symptoms, psychosis, and substance abuse among others. Similarly, in premanifest sufferers, psychiatric features are noted on scales of depression, obsessive-compulsiveness, anxiety, and psychosis, although often not enough to meet established diagnostic criteria. There are no robust data on the incidence or indeed prevalence of rarer behavioral disorders such as hypersexuality, eating disorders, and excessive gambling or spending. Over a 2-year follow-up of mutation carriers, 15% of patients without a pre-existing psychiatric disease at baseline developed a disorder, most frequently depression, which was seen in 64% of subjects [40, 42].

It is apparent in clinical practice that individual, so-called "subsyndromic" aspects of several psychiatric diseases can be present in the same subject. Patients with obsessive and compulsive symptoms show a higher prevalence of depression, suicidal ideation, and psychotic phenomena, while others have isolated low mood or obsessive, repetitive behaviors without the accompanying compulsions, rendering their clinical management challenging [43]. Obsessive-compulsive disorder according to DSM-IV criteria is rare in HD. Repetitive behaviors, verbal and motor tics, and perseveration are common in HD but are more likely to be related to frontal dysexecutive syndrome [44].

Depression Depression is one of the most frequent findings in the HD population at all stages. However, it is clear that this group is subject to significant stressors throughout the disease, beginning with deciding when to get tested and dealing with expectation surrounding the test result. This is notwithstanding experiencing the loss of family members from HD as well as seeing their own future morbidity reflected in their family members. Further on, transitioning from premanifest to manifest disease, followed most poignantly by progressive loss of function, status, and independence, has the potential to aggravate or indeed unmask psychopathology.

In a survey of 2835 sufferers, 40% had symptoms consistent with depression, while 50% had previously received treatment for depression [45]. The diagnosis can also be confounded as biological symptoms such as weight loss and sleep disturbance also occur in HD, as well as apathy and loss of motivation.

Suicidality In Huntington's original description he notes "the tendency to insanity and sometimes to that form of insanity which leads to suicide is marked" [1]. Although statistics on suicide rates have been somewhat conflicting, patients have a lifetime risk 4–6 times greater than the general population. A meta-analysis of mortality associated with mental health disorders which included 4171 gene carriers revealed that 17.5% displayed suicidal ideation at or around the time of assessment, while 10% had made at least one suicide attempt in the past [46]. The risk appeared greatest in those who were perimanifest, experiencing the first, significant losses in function, and suffering with depression and impulsivity [2].

Irritability Alongside depressive symptoms, irritability is commonly encountered either as an isolated presentation or as part of depression and occasionally psychosis. A working definition of irritability is loss of temper at a much reduced threshold compared to the general population, at seemingly innocuous stimuli. This can be complicated by aggressive outbursts, which can range from verbal aggression with cursing, to verbal threats of physical violence, and finally to physically injury itself.

Irritability results from a multitude of factors, including frustration at declining function and cognitive overload in the setting of diminished psychomotor ability and planning. Some correlation with anxiety and depression is seen but is unrelated to cognitive and motor features of HD [47]. Irritability appears to be as frequent as depression, if not more so, and occurs throughout. Indeed, in retrospect, it is often noted as the first sign of disease.

Bipolar symptoms Bipolar symptoms are more common in HD than in the general population, and can be the presenting feature. Differentiation of certain aspects of the presentation such as disinhibition, irritability, or hypersexuality, from frontal symptomatology may be difficult. Moreover, the classic triad of altered fluctuating mood, a grandiose thought content, and overactivity is frequently lacking in these patients. In more severe forms, delusions and hallucinations can occur, while at the other end of the spectrum, rapid cycling of mood without other overt bipolar signs can be seen.

Psychosis A 9% lifetime prevalence of schizophrenia has been reported in HD. Delusions and hallucinations are reported using dedicated questionnaires. The usual psychotic presentation comprises paranoid and fixed ideas with accompanying aggression, irritability, and poor impulse control [48].

Delusional and schizophrenia-like psychotic states are infrequent but can feature delusions centered on erotomania, bodily decay, parasitosis, and third-party auditory hallucinations. Psychosis can also present in the later stages of the disease, where it can be masked by the concomitant cognitive decline.

Obsessions and compulsions Obsessive-compulsive disorder that meets diagnostic criteria is a relative rarity in HD. However, repetitive and perseverative behaviors and speech content are often seen as part of the frontal dysexecutive syndrome.

In a large study, 22.3% of HD patients were found to show signs of obsessive or compulsive symptoms but it is unlikely that this reflects true obsessive-compulsive disorder, rather aspects of its composite features [49]. In a pragmatic sense, these can affect the patient's quality of life and lead to verbal and even physical conflict with carers.

Anxiety This is present throughout the disease but understandably there is particular clustering around the time of conversion to manifest disease. In a 2-year follow-up of an HD cohort, generalized anxiety disorder was the most commonly occurring psychiatric disease [42]. Situational anxiety can also be seen in HD.

Apathy A loss of interest and increasingly passive behavior is seen in HD, and although it can be difficult to separate from depressive withdrawal, it does represent a distinct entity. In support, following a cross-sectional study, lack of energy and apathy was found to affect more than 75% of patients. Correlation was noted with the length of illness and although there was coexistence of irritability and depression, a subsequent study demonstrated that apathy was independent of depressive pathology [44, 50].

In a separate, comparative study, 32% of HD patients showed apathy versus controls. When depressed patients were excluded, male sex, diminished global performance, and greater neuroleptic and benzodiazepine burden were independently correlated with apathy [51].

Metabolic/endocrine

The hypothalamus, pituitary gland, pancreatic islets, and adrenal glands all seem to be affected by mutant HTT in patients and animal models of HD [52–54]. HD is a catabolic disease as a result of a combination of endocrine dysfunction, altered fat metabolism, and intracellular bioenergetic pathology. Melatonin deficiency, recently described in HD, is a likely contributor to sleep problems [55].

Weight loss Unintended weight loss despite increased appetite and calorie intake, at least in early disease, culminates in the cachexia of advanced stages. In certain patients startling weight loss can be seen because of a combination of dysphagia and physical difficulties in using cutlery and going out to purchase food. Weight loss can be exacerbated by neuropsychiatric aspects such as depression and loss of motivation and desire to eat, in addition to the known catabolic nature of the disease.

Increased levels of the orexigenic hormone ghrelin and low levels of the adipocyte hormone leptin suggest that the balance of hunger and satiety hormones may be altered in HD [56]. This may be compounded by loss of hypothalamic somatostatin and orexin neurons [57]. Xerostomia, together with loss of lingual dexterity and swallowing difficulties, may also contribute to mechanistic impairment of the feeding process [58]. Sedentary energy expenditure is also higher in HD patients [59]. Importantly, it has been noted that patients with a higher body mass index have a slower rate of progression, and accordingly clinical practice recommends weight maintenance with high-calorie diets [60].

Glucose intolerance In both rodent models and patients with HD, pancreatic dysfunction is evidenced by glucose intolerance, reduced insulin secretion, and sensitivity [61–63]. However, a recent study has called this into question; despite the finding of insulin resistance in a mouse model, oral glucose tolerance testing of 14 HD patients failed to show any difference from controls [64].

Musculoskeletal
Skeletal muscle atrophy is another hallmark of HD; it is probably the result of corticospinal tract degeneration, although evidence of cumulative toxicity of mutant HTT to myocytes as well as mitochondrial dysfunction is emerging [65]. *In vivo* studies using magnetic resonance spectroscopy (MRI) have also demonstrated abnormal muscle energy utilization [66].

Bone densitometry data indicate that osteoporosis may be a feature in HD, resulting most likely from immobility, skeletal muscle atrophy, or other endocrine effects although recent research failed to identify any hormonal alteration versus controls, suggesting an alternate mechanism [67]. Further research is needed to identify any evidence of reduced osteoblastic activity, potentially mediated by mutant HTT.

Cardiac disease
There is a clear increase in the incidence of heart failure in HD patients: approximately 30% in patients with HD, compared with 2% in age-matched controls [68]. There may be some contribution from disruption of the autonomic nervous system. In a large retrospective study, heart disease was the second leading cause of death [69]. This aspect has not been well studied in human HD patients, however [70, 71].

Reproductive pathology
Reduced libido and inhibited orgasm have been reported as the most common symptoms of sexual dysfunction in HD, occurring in 63% and 56% of men, and 75% and 42% of women [72].

Males with HD have reduced levels of testosterone as well as testicular pathology with reduced numbers of germ cells and abnormal seminiferous tubule morphology [73, 74]. There seems to be no effect on fertility however. Rodent data seem to suggest that this results from a direct effect of mutant HTT rather than hypothalamic deficiency.

General medical complications of Huntington's disease
Delirium is not unusual in HD. Multiple contributory factors including the disease itself, its complications, and the medications employed in its management are implicated. Any sudden change in behavior or diminution in cognitive performance should prompt clinical exploration of secondary causes because HD itself is slowly progressive over years. In this setting, occult subdural hematomas from unwitnessed falls and head injuries should always be considered, as should cerebrovascular disease. Poor nutritional intake can result in volume depletion and metabolic disturbances; urogenital dysfunction may predispose to urinary tract infections, and oromotor dysfunction to pneumonia.

It should be noted that, as with other neurological diseases, in the presence of generalized sepsis even previously intermittent chorea can appear florid and any subclinical features such as cognitive impairment, neuropsychiatric disease, and balance difficulties may be magnified.

The cumulative effects of diminished saliva production, poor food clearance, and reduced ability to brush teeth mean that oral hygiene may be compromised and therefore dental health must be rigorously maintained as disease advances.

In advanced stages the following are essential: prevention of pressure sores, flexion contractures, and self-injury; good skin and nail care; padded wheelchair provision; and prevention of deep vein thrombosis.

Finally, although a wide range of symptoms exist, clinicians must guard against automatically attributing any new symptom to disease progression, as other common medical conditions can and do occur in this population.

Premanifest phase of disease
Classically, diagnosis has relied heavily on the presence of motor symptoms. It is only relatively recently that large multicenter observational studies have formally confirmed what clinicians have long suspected – the existence of a premanifest phase, characterized variably by evolving subtle motor deficits, and at times significant cognitive or psychiatric symptoms and signs, occurring well before overt onset of motor symptoms and signs. This period has been variously termed pre-symptomatic, pre-disease, or prodromal; a universally agreed taxonomy is lacking, although here we use the term premanifest.

In terms of presenting symptoms, subtle motor features such as slight chorea can be present. Early instability of balance and posture can also be considered a premanifest motor sign as balance and posture have been objectively demonstrated to be impaired in premanifest subjects versus controls [75].

Abnormalities in smooth pursuit and saccadic eye movements are arguably one of the most reliable early motor signs. Alongside the abnormalities on the Luria test and presence of chorea, they appear to correlate most closely with an escalating probability of clinical diagnosis. It is equally clear, however, that the majority of premanifest patients have either normal or very low motor scores on the Unified HD Rating Scale (UHDRS), indicating that clinical assessment alone does not adequately define this group.

Consequently there has been great interest in finding other measures – cognitive, imaging, and quantitative motor –to quantitatively define this period. PREDICT-HD aimed to determine the genetic, neurobiological, and clinical features that demonstrated progression of HD in 438 premanifest individuals. Elevated total motor scores at baseline were associated with higher genetic probability of disease diagnosis in the near future and smaller striatal volumes [76, 77]. In a longitudinal sub-study, 29 premanifest subjects and 43 non-carrier controls underwent clinical testing and an extensive neuropsychological test battery addressing global cognitive function, memory, language, and executive function. Premanifest subjects fared consistently worse on tests of executive function: the symbol digit modalities test (SDMT), Stroop test, trail making test (TMT), and Wechsler adult intelligence scale–revised (WAIS-R) arithmetic. They also showed a decline in memory and concentration function on the Wechsler Memory Scale (WMS) and in motor function (UHDRS motor scale). Premanifest subjects also showed subtle cognitive abnormalities in executive tasks, however a decline over time could not be proven [78].

In symptomatic terms, patients may display change in behavior such as aggression, apathy, and loss of interest or report poor performance at work, particularly during multitasking. Emotional recognition, which requires interpretation of facial expressions and verbal intonations as well as body language representative of fear, sadness, or disgust, was also shown to be impaired in premanifest subjects [79].

Although there were initially confounding results in the literature, methodological improvements have shown increased frequency of psychiatric symptoms in premanifest subjects suggestive of depression, anxiety, and obsessive-compulsive disorder in comparison with gene-negative individuals. Indeed, those with higher motor scores appeared to have greater levels of psychiatric morbidity, despite the fact that the majority of subjects were estimated to be more than 10 years from predicted diagnosis [80]. Moreover, current evidence suggests that in the case of affective disorders, this greater morbidity is not solely explained by the psychological sequelae of a positive predictive genetic test and impending onset of HD or indeed the HD environment, implicating the disease itself as the pathogenic culprit, in part at least [41, 81].

TRACK-HD was a longitudinal, multicenter clinical and imaging biomarker project, carried out at baseline and at 12, 24, and 36 months; 116 control individuals, 117 premanifest gene carriers, and 116 participants with early HD completed the study. Significantly greater progressive gray-matter, white-matter, whole-brain, and regional atrophy was recorded in the premanifest and early HD groups than in the control group, with largest effect sizes for atrophy rates noted in the caudate and white matter. In the premanifest group, despite significant declines in regional and overall brain volumes, few functional variables showed significant 24-month change compared with controls; total motor score, emotion recognition, and speeded tapping were exceptions. Premanifest individuals with progression exhibited higher rates of brain atrophy and deterioration on some quantitative motor tasks compared with other premanifest participants [38, 39, 82]. The study has created a potential series of outcome measures for clinical trials in early HD, although for premanifest subjects reliable detection of change over time has proved much more challenging.

As a result of TRACK-HD and other observational studies the nomenclature has expanded further to include a *perimanifest* phase, where individuals may be described as at the cusp of a clinical diagnosis, with clear evidence of dysfunction in at least one domain: neurological, psychiatric, or behavioral [39, 83, 84]. A new observational study, Track-On HD, utilizing state of the art functional and structural brain imaging in combination with a battery of cognitive and motor assessments, aims to further characterize the premanifest group, including this perimanifest subset.

Stages of Huntington's disease

Clinical staging (Table 21.3)

A working classification of HD denotes early, middle, and late stages while the most commonly used, the Shoulson and Fahn Total Functional Capacity Rating Scale, rates the person's functional abilities over five domains [25].

The early stage represents the point at which patients have minimal limitation, are usually able to maintain employment without compromise, and continue to live independently. Minor involuntary movements, psychiatric disease, and some difficulty when multitasking may be reported.

The major difference at the middle stage is the loss of employment while still maintaining activities of daily living. Chorea is usually at its peak at this stage, with loss of fine motor control, increasing falls, and abnormal mobility and gait. Mental inflexibility manifests more prominently.

At the late disease stage, complete immobility is present as individuals are bedbound and require assistance in all activities of daily living. Profound dysarthria also occurs to the point of severe communication difficulties. Chorea gives way to rigidity, dystonia, and bradykinesia. There is a high risk of medical complications.

Clinical variants

Late-onset Huntington's disease

This has been variously termed senile chorea or late-onset HD, describing a subset of HD patients who present over the age of 75.

Table 21.3 Clinical staging of Huntington's disease, the Total Functional Capacity rating scale (adapted with permission from [14]).

Domain	Ability	Score
Occupation	Unable	0
	Marginal work only	1
	Reduced capacity for usual job	2
	Normal	3
Finances	Unable	0
	Major assistance	1
	Slight assistance	2
	Normal	3
Domestic chores	Unable	0
	Impaired	1
	Normal	2
Activities of daily living	Total care	0
	Gross tasks only	1
	Minimal impairment	2
	Normal	3
Care level	Full-time nursing care	0
	Home or chronic care	1
	Home	2
Total	Range 0–13	

TFC total score	Stage
11–13	I
7–10	II
3–6	III
1–2	IV
0	V

Of all known HD patients, approximately 25% present over the age of 50. Although other causes of chorea should be looked for in this age group, the most likely cause remains HD. Chorea is almost universal but the course is milder and slower with mild cognitive and psychiatric disease. Gait disturbance and dysphagia are also seen but are not severe. Late-onset disease is usually associated with repeat sizes of 40, although lengths of up to 48 have been recorded. Often a family history can be lacking, which may reflect expansion of an intermediate range allele [85, 86].

Juvenile-onset Huntington's disease

Although Lyon is credited with the first description of juvenile HD in 1863, closer examination reveals this cohort as more likely to have had benign hereditary chorea, given the absence of significant disease progression [2, 87]. Juvenile HD is defined as HD with age of onset prior to the age of 20. It accounts for 5–10% of all HD presentations and is paternally transmitted in 90% of cases. The number of CAG repeat expansions is almost always greater than 55.

In the largest case series of juvenile patients, over half experienced symptom onset under the age of 14 while 1 in 10 cases occurred before the age of 1 year. Under the age of 10, developmental delay specifically in speech and language may be prominent and may manifest as failure to progress at school. Behavioral changes, learning difficulties, rapid cognitive decline, psychiatric disease, and parkinsonian motor features with predominating rigidity and bradykinesia were seen in 50% of cases, as well as dystonia and ataxia. The range of psychiatric disease can include drug and alcohol abuse as well as eating disorders [88].

In a multi-sourced survey of prescribing practices in juvenile HD, the most commonly prescribed agents were anti-psychotics, anti-depressants, anti-parkinsonian medications and anti-epileptics, of which valproic acid was the most commonly used. Polypharmacy was an issue in a minority of cases. The most common symptoms reported by the families were speech difficulties, dysphagia, stiffness/spasticity, sleeping difficulty, pain, and behavioral problems [89].

In contrast to the adult form, chorea itself is rare and early oropharyngeal dysfunction appears more commonly in juvenile cases. Seizures occur in around 25–50% of juvenile HD cases. They are usually generalized or myoclonic in nature although absence seizures have also been noted and occasionally seizures prove intractable [90].

Akinetic-rigid or Westphal variant

Westphal described an 18-year-old patient with prominent rigidity, a variant that later became known as the akinetic-rigid Westphal variant [91] and is most typically associated with juvenile HD. However, this variant has also been noted rarely in young adult populations with much lower CAG repeat sizes. In one case series of three patients no significant eye movement or cognitive abnormalities were seen although mild cardiovascular dysautonomia was present [92, 93]. Pathologically, the Westphal variant may be different, with studies demonstrating loss of both direct and indirect striatopallidal pathways [94, 95].

Clinical diagnosis of Huntington's disease

Classically, diagnosis has been based on the well-established triad of symptoms – motor, psychiatric, and cognitive, although only motor symptomatology could be deemed as all but essential – alongside a family member who is a proven gene carrier. In this setting, the most commonly clinically encountered scenario, there is no need for imaging or other ancillary tests beyond diagnostic genetic testing.

The other frequent referral seen in specialist clinics is an asymptomatic patient, with a known family history, who wishes to consider genetic testing. A detailed family history should be a key focus of the consultation.

Even in the absence of a genetic test, if there is early dementia in combination with psychiatric disease or institutionalization with a consistent clinical presentation, a diagnosis can usually be made. Medical records of deceased family members can be requested if feasible to aid in this determination. However, in up to 25% of new HD cases presenting to specialist clinics, a family history may either not be available or be confounding, with nonspecific clinical features [96]. It is worth noting additionally that if the parent has died of another cause prior to manifesting symptoms, family history can be falsely reassuring. Rarely, cases of non-paternity emerge. A de novo mutation via expansion of an intermediate allele, usually transmitted from the male line, should also be borne in mind if the clinical presentation is conducive.

Examination

The motor part of the Unified HD Rating Scale (UHDRS) provides a template for a directed examination to identify the motor features of the disease [14]. Accordingly, with an appropriate clinical history, the combination, in the early stage of the illness, of broken smooth pursuits, slowed saccades, impaired tongue protrusion, mild chorea of the distal extremities, incoordinate finger taps, and alternating hand movements with impaired tandem gait and postural reflexes, is highly suggestive of HD. Finger tapping (index finger on thumb) should be rapid, regular, and of equivalent speed to the examiner (25 taps in 5 seconds); slowing and irregular tempo are characteristically seen in HD. Head movements and eye blinking to initiate saccades, which are unable to be suppressed, as well as overaction of frontalis in upward gaze can be seen in the later stages of disease.

Mild or even debatable chorea can be brought out by walking and maintaining elevated hand position with a simultaneous cognitive challenge such as serial sevens or counting backwards. A "milkmaid's grip" with variation in the intensity of a requested squeeze may be elicited. In addition facial tics and bucco-oro-lingual chorea may be misinterpreted as odd facial expressions. Tandem walking may bring out chorea, imbalance, or other problems.

Red flags in examination

In practice, the presence of prominent cognitive dysfunction, hemichorea, pyramidal signs, especially if unilateral, established supranuclear gaze palsy and/or early incontinence should prompt exclusion of alternate possibilities. Rigidity and orofacial dyskinesia should remind the clinician to look for neuroleptic use and neuroacanthocytosis, although the Westphal akinetic-rigid variant should be considered. A preponderance of cerebellar signs would also be unexpected.

Investigations

Genetic testing

Genetic testing is diagnostic and is usually the only test that needs to be carried out in clear-cut cases. Adequate genetic counseling must be undertaken and informed consent obtained. In some instances there may be no previous known family history of HD, so the diagnosis comes as a huge shock to the person and their family. In these situations it is ideal to involve partners and other family members early in the diagnostic counseling process, as a confirmatory result has profound implications for siblings and offspring. In patients with a negative gene test, the clinical approach is as follows.

Imaging
Brain imaging may show atrophy of the caudate even prior to clinical symptoms but this is not validated for clinical practice. Similarly, unless exceptional features are present, sampling of cerebrospinal fluid is not indicated.

Cognitive assessment
In clinical settings, the mini mental state examination is unlikely to be sensitive enough to pick up deficits. Neuropsychometry is not essential but can be utilized in specific situations, where defining cognitive performance gives an indicator towards continuing working life or differentiating an affective disorder from disease onset.

Neurophysiology
There is no indication for neurophysiology in the routine investigation of HD unless clinically indicated, for example in the investigation of epilepsy in juvenile subjects or as part of a sleep study. As a research tool it has been studied, but to a limited extent given the effort required by both subject and operator in this population. Nonetheless, in a 2-year longitudinal study of 20 patients, a significant deterioration with time was found for blink reflex latency, long latency reflexes, and various somatosensory evoked potential parameters with some correlation with functional decline and motor score [97].

Management
The majority of the management of HD is non-drug based. Moreover, current pharmacological management of HD is symptomatic as no disease-modifying therapy has yet been identified [98]. A primary care based research study found that 44% of prescriptions for HD patients targeted the central nervous system (nearly half of which were anti-depressants), over 40% were analgesics, and 15% comprised nutritional supplements [99].

Chorea

Non-pharmacological based intervention Devices such as padded chairs or wrist and ankle weights to reduce the amplitude of chorea may be helpful. Shoes with non-slip soles and grab rails around the home can improve safety, and assessment of the home by an occupational therapist may be useful. Physiotherapy can also help to optimize mobility and preserve independence for as long as possible. Like most involuntary movements, chorea is worsened by stress, anxiety, and depression, so screening and treatment for these conditions should be attempted before anti-chorea drug therapy.

Pharmacological intervention Most patients do not notice and are not troubled by chorea and therefore, as anti-chorea medications possess a strong side effect profile, initiation of therapy must be weighed carefully. Treatment of chorea that is affecting daily tasks such as walking and feeding or is socially disabling may provide an improvement in functional ability and in these circumstances is worth serious consideration. As disease advances, chorea may lessen and medication may no longer be necessary.

Tetrabenazine is the only drug used in HD that has met current evidence-based standards [100]. The mode of action is via reversible inhibition of the vesicular monoamine transporter 2 (VMAT2), causing depletion of presynaptic dopamine with lesser reductions

in norepinephrine and serotonin. A randomized placebo-controlled clinical study demonstrated significant reduction of chorea and improvement in motor scores compared to controls, which was sustained for over a year; most patients were on a total dose of 50–75 mg. Adverse effects included suicide, depression, anxiety, sedation, parkinsonism and akathisia, and cognitive diminution [101, 102]. In the absence of active psychiatric disease, tetrabenazine is probably the drug of choice for chorea, although it requires around 6 weeks to reliably determine response, and efficacy can decline over time.

It is important to note that tetrabenazine is metabolized by the hepatic isoenzyme CYP2D6, which has variable activity between individuals. In patients receiving greater than 50 mg, genotyping for CYPD26 activity is recommended; interaction with the selective serotonin reuptake inhibitors (SSRIs) paroxetine and fluoxetine necessitates a halving of the tetrabenazine dose. Co-prescribing of tricyclic anti-depressants is not recommended due to the potential augmentation of adverse effects [103, 104].

Second-line therapies are anti-psychotics, which mediate post-synaptic dopamine D2 receptor blockage. Atypical anti-psychotics are preferred because of the reduced incidence of extra-pyramidal side effects. Olanzapine is the mainstay of this class as it is useful for mood stabilization and augments anti-depressant effect. Higher doses of olanzapine (i.e. >10 mg/day) carry a greater risk of dyslipidemia and hyperglycemia. There is some evidence that long-term, high-dose use can promote apathy. Tardive dyskinesia, acute dyskinesia, drug-induced parkinsonism, and neuroleptic malignant syndrome are important adverse events to consider at each follow-up consultation. A strong evidence base for use of anti-psychotics in HD is lacking. Tiapride, which is licensed in the USA and Europe, at 3 g/day dosing, ameliorated chorea versus placebo over a 9-week period in a double-blind, placebo-controlled trial, although sedation and extra-pyramidal effects were noted [105].

Sulpiride and tiapride are substituted benzamide anti-psychotics with selectivity for dopamine D2 receptors and have shown some subjective improvement in chorea scores. A double-blind, randomized, crossover trial of 11 HD patients and a case series advocate the use of sulpiride [106–108]. Sulpiride has an alerting and anti-depressant effect in addition, which may be useful or disadvantageous depending on the clinical circumstance. Riluzole and clozapine have been studied in randomized controlled clinical trials but have not met required efficacy standards; the latter had an unfavorable effect on self-rated function and well-being [109, 110].

Amantadine, a non-competitive N-methyl-D-aspartate receptor antagonist, has demonstrated efficacy in one double-blind, placebo-controlled study, but a similar study failed to show any benefit. It may have a role in management of the akinetic-rigid variant [111].

Clonazepam can be extremely useful to treat chorea, especially occurring in combination with situational anxiety, where it can be used prophylactically or to treat coexisting myoclonus, spasticity, or rigidity.

Ridigity/parkinsonism
The akinetic-rigid, parkinsonian phenotype can be treated as for Parkinson disease with levodopa; pramipexole, amantadine, and cabergoline have also been used. Bruxism can occur in HD and responds to botulinum toxin.

Dystonia (Table 21.4)
Their use has not been studied directly but current clinical practice would support the use of tetrabenazine or olanzapine and employing botulinum toxin for fixed dystonias. The dopamine stabilizer

Table 21.4 Drug management of movement disorder

Symptom	Drug class	Medication	Main adverse effects and treatment notes
Chorea	Atypical neuroleptics	Olanzapine	Sedation, parkinsonism, tardive dyskinesias but less risk than with older neuroleptics; raised triglycerides; weight gain from increased appetite, which may be beneficial in HD. Caution should be exercised in patients with diabetes and blood glucose monitored. May rarely cause prolonged QT interval. Useful if also significant agitation, irritability, and anxiety
	Atypical neuroleptics	Risperidone	As above but less effect on increasing appetite
	Atypical neuroleptics	Quetiapine	As above, less effect on lipids and glucose
	Older neuroleptics	Sulpiride	Agitation, dystonia, akathisia, sedation, hypotension, dry mouth, constipation
		Haloperidol	Sedation, more parkinsonism, dystonia, akathisia, hypotension, constipation, dry mouth, weight gain, higher risk of neuroleptic malignant syndrome than atypical neuroleptics
	Dopamine-depleting agents	Tetrabenazine	Depression and sedation
Myoclonus Chorea Dystonia Rigidity Spasticity	Benzodiazepines	Clonazepam	Sedation, ataxia, apathy. Cognitive impairment may be exacerbated. Withdrawal seizures
Myoclonus	Anticonvulsant	Sodium valproate	Gastrointestinal disturbance, weight gain, blood dyscrasia, hyperammonemia
		Levetiracetam	Gastrointestinal disturbance, rash, mood changes, myalgia
Rigidity (particularly associated with juvenile HD or young adult-onset parkinsonian phenotype)	Amino acid precursor of dopamine	Levodopa	Gastrointestinal disturbance, postural hypotension, insomnia, agitation, psychiatric symptoms
Rigidity Spasticity	Skeletal muscle relaxants	Baclofen Tizanidine	Sedation, drowsiness, confusion, gastrointestinal disturbances, hypotension
Bruxism Dystonia	Inhibits acetylcholine release at neuromuscular junction to cause muscle paralysis	Botulinum toxin	May paralyze nearby muscles

Source: Novak & Tabrizi 2010 [114]. Reproduced with permission of BMJ Publishing Group Ltd.

pridopidine showed a significant reduction of dystonia following a secondary analysis [112, 113].

Cognitive impairment

Premanifest cognitive change is not uncommon and takes the form of a subcortical frontal dysexecutive dementia. There is currently no proven effective therapy for this in HD; management takes the form of patient and relative education.

There is no proven efficacy for acetylcholinesterase inhibitors in HD. In a placebo-controlled trial of 30 patients with HD, donepezil showed no positive effect on motor or cognitive dysfunction [115]. A trial of rivastigmine found improvement in motor scores and a trend towards gain in cognitive function [116]. Memantine, an N-methyl-D-aspartate receptor (NMDAR) antagonist, has also created interest due to its potentially pathologically relevant mode of action and promising mouse model data [117].

Neuropsychiatric disease (Table 21.5)

Great attention must be paid to psychotropic, particularly neuroleptic and benzodiazepine, usage as missed doses or sudden dose changes can lead to altered behavior.

Irritability and aggressive behavior Although behavior modification may have some effect, medication will be necessary for most patients. Most commonly an SSRI is initiated, but if there is an element of verbal or physical aggression, atypical anti-psychotics such as olanzapine, risperidone, and quetiapine can have a role. Sertraline, lithium (in combination with haloperidol), and buspirone have also been used to manage aggressive behavior in HD.

Depression First-line management is SSRI therapy. If this is ineffectual, move to second-line therapy with venlafaxine, which, while demonstrating significant efficacy, can frequently provoke adverse effects such as nausea and irritability. The noradrenergic

and specific serotonergic antidepressant (NaSSA) mirtazapine and the serotonin antagonist and reuptake inhibitor (SARI) trazodone have found a niche in the management of coexisting insomnia and depression. Mirtazapine also has an anxiolytic action. Refractory depression has also responded to electroconvulsive therapy.

Psychosis No studies exist to outline evidence-based recommendations but current clinical practice is to use olanzapine or other antipsychotic agents, thus broadly following the standard psychiatric management of psychosis.

Obsessive-compulsive disorder Isolated case reports suggest the use of standard SSRI therapy with fluoxetine or sertraline. Clomipramine can be helpful for fixed or perseverative thoughts or negative ruminations.

Apathy Cholinesterase inhibitors, the dopaminergic antidepressant bupropion, amantadine, levodopa, bromocriptine, methylphenidate, and atypical antipsychotics have all been tried in other neurodegenerative disorders, but not in HD. A bupropion trial for apathy is under way.

Psychological treatments Psychological treatments such as cognitive behavioral therapy (CBT) can also be helpful in selected patients and may be a useful way for people with premanifest disease to learn cognitive strategies that will be useful once they develop cognitive and psychiatric symptoms. One case study has reported benefit from CBT for a patient with premanifest disease [118]. Support from local community mental health teams is invaluable.

Sleep disturbance

Unless used in short courses and in combination with a program of day activities to restore the patient to a normal sleep pattern, benzodiazepines and other hypnotics almost always lose their efficacy

Table 21.5 Drug management of neuropsychiatric disease.

Symptom	Drug class	Medication	Main adverse effects and treatment notes
Psychosis	Atypical neuroleptics	Olanzapine, Risperidone, Quetiapine	See Table 21.4. Careful use in the elderly where there is increased risk of stroke with olanzapine and risperidone
Treatment-resistant psychosis	Neuroleptics	Clozapine	As for the other neuroleptics, plus agranulocytosis, myocarditis, and cardiomyopathy. Requires blood monitoring
Psychosis with prominent negative symptoms	Neuroleptics	Aripiprazole	Parkinsonism, akathisia, drowsiness, gastrointestinal disturbance, tremor, blurred vision
Depression, anxiety, OCD, irritability, aggression	Selective serotonin reuptake inhibitors (SSRIs)	Citalopram	Gastrointestinal disturbance, hypersensitivity reactions, drowsiness, syndrome of inappropriate antidiuretic hormone secretion (SIADH), postural hypotension
		Fluoxetine	As for citalopram, sleep disturbances
		Paroxetine	As for other SSRIs, raised cholesterol
		Sertraline	As for other SSRIs
	Presynaptic α_2-antagonist, increases central noradrenaline and serotonin activity	Mirtazapine	Weight gain, edema, sedation, headache, dizziness, tremor. Useful when insomnia is a problem as it is sedating
	Serotonin and noradrenaline reuptake inhibitor	Venlafaxine	Hypertension, gastrointestinal disturbance, hypersensitivity reactions, drowsiness, agitation, SIADH, palpitations
Irritability, aggression	Neuroleptics	Olanzapine Risperidone Quetiapine	See above
Altered sleep-wake cycle	Hypnotics	Zopiclone Zolpidem	Drowsiness, confusion, memory disturbance, gastrointestinal disturbance
Mood stabilizers	Anticonvulsants	Sodium valproate	See above
		Lamotrigine	Hypersensitivity reactions, blood dyscrasias, dizziness, gastrointestinal disturbance, depression
		Carbamazepine	Hypersensitivity reactions, drowsiness, blood dyscrasias, hepatitis, hyponatremia, dizziness, gastrointestinal disturbance

Source: Novak & Tabrizi 2010 [114]. Reproduced with permission of BMJ Publishing Group Ltd.

over time, although they remain first-line management. Melatonin has emerged as a potential alternative in re-establishing sleep cycles but has yet to be tested in a randomized clinical trial.

Encouraging good sleep hygiene, managing any night-time chorea, and screening for sleep behavior disorders as well as obstructive sleep apnea should also be pursued, especially if weight gain is occurring in association with medication use.

Urological symptoms
Management of urge incontinence and frequency is along standard lines with oxybutynin and other detrusor-stabilizing agents, but consideration should be given to the degree of central action of anti-cholinergic therapy as it may augment cognitive impairment and slowing.

Multidisciplinary (Table 21.6)
The complex nature of the disease necessitates a multidisciplinary team. In the outpatient setting this means neurologists, psychiatrists, psychologists, genetic counsellors, and specialist nurses with support group representation; comprehensive advice and guidelines have been published [119]. Family members and caregivers often suffer from fatigue, loneliness, and stress-related illnesses and they should be included in the support offered by the multidisciplinary team.

Advanced Huntington's disease
The nature of the disease necessitates that careful planning for end-of-life care be discussed openly and sensitively with patients. By moderate stage HD, the ability of patients to understand, determine, and, crucially, communicate their wishes can be impaired. Advance decisions (previously known as advance directives) should, where appropriate, be discussed earlier on in the disease when capacity is not an issue. This can then inform clinicians about how far to take medical interventions in advanced stages. An independent capacity advocate can be helpful if a patient does not have capacity and his

or her next of kin is unable or unwilling to make decisions on the patient's behalf.

Similarly, raising the possibility of a trusted person to assume power of attorney, to manage the finances and estate of the patient, only when he or she is no longer able, can be extremely helpful and avoid considerable angst, especially if made while the patient still holds capacity.

As HD progresses, it often becomes increasingly difficult to provide care at home, and a nursing home may be the best option. Early involvement of a palliative care team at this stage can be beneficial,

Table 21.6 Non-drug based management of Huntington's disease.

Domain	Examples of management measures
Gait disturbance and chorea	Physiotherapy to optimize and strengthen gait and balance, and to assess for walking aids; occupational therapy assessment to modify home environment to improve safety; weighted wrist bands to combat limb chorea
Cognitive symptoms	Ensure every day has a structure to overcome apathy and difficulty in initiating activities (occupational therapy can advise on this); maintain routines to reduce need for flexibility
Social support	Carers to help at home; residential or nursing home care; day centers to maintain social interactions
Communication	Speech and language therapy to optimize speech, and later in disease to assess for communication aids; ensure patient has time to comprehend and respond to speech, and that information is presented simply
Nutrition	Speech and language therapy to advise on safest food consistencies at different stages of disease, and, in later disease, to advise on need to consider enteral nutrition; dietician to optimize nutritional intake, especially adequate calorie intake; minimize distractions to optimize swallowing safety
Psychological problems	Develop strategies to deal with cognitive and/or emotional challenges of disease using counseling or cognitive behavioral therapy

Source: Novak & Tabrizi 2010 [114]. Reproduced with permission of BMJ Publishing Group Ltd.

principally in facilitating access to respite or indeed hospice care, as well as symptom control.

Insertion of a gastrostomy tube can be considered if nutrition is impaired; again, if this is discussed in advance, the opinion of the patient proves invaluable. Planning for PEG feeding in the mid stages of the disease is more desirable if the patient is beginning to experience signs of dysphagia with or without weight loss and aspiration pneumonia. However, as is the case with other neuro-degenerative conditions, it is not clear if this specific intervention improves quality of life.

Careful attention to mouth care is important at all stages, given that patients often have xerostomia that can exacerbate dysphagia and dysarthria, and may neglect or be unable to attend to their own mouth care, particularly in the later stages of disease.

Nursing homes and hospices with a specialist interest in HD are the gold standard. HD patients face similar issues to patients with other late-stage dementias: sleep-wake cycle disruption, severe psychiatric and behavioral problems including delusions, and screaming, which can represent a response to physical or psychological injury. Pain may arise from hyperkinetic movements and injury, or hypokinesis, dystonia, and spasticity, and these abnormalities of movement and muscle tone, as well as good pain control, should be addressed. Obviously, pain should also prompt examination for reversible causes such as occult fractures, ulcers, constipation, urinary retention, and infection, among others.

Death in HD is usually a consequence of respiratory complications, the most common cause being pneumonia [68, 69]. In a 2012 study, this was further refined to aspiration pneumonia in 86.8% of cases examined [120].

Genetics of Huntington's disease

Molecular genetics

The HD locus was one of the first disease-associated loci to be mapped using restriction fragment length polymorphisms [121]. This finding allowed presymptomatic detection of HD allele carriers. It was 10 years later in 1993 that the gene responsible was discovered [3]. Exon amplification of cosmids in the chromosome 4p16.3 interval yielded "interesting transcript 15" (IT15) from a novel gene in which an expanded CAG repeat within the predicted open reading frame was associated with HD. The protein product was termed huntingtin (HTT). The polyglutamine expansion is located in exon 1 and starts at residue 18. Other than the poly CAG tract, the gene lacked homology to any known gene. Genomic sequencing of the exon-intron boundaries indicated that IT15 (now called the *HTT* gene) spans 180 kb and contains 67 exons [122]. The predicted open reading frame yields a protein containing 3144 amino acid residues, with a predicted molecular mass of 348 kDa [123]. Studies have shown that there is significant sequence homology of *HTT* across a wide variety of mammalian species [124] and this high degree of conservation across species suggests that normal huntingtin is an essential protein. Indeed, homozygous huntingtin knockout in mice is embryonic lethal [125]. The codon CAG encodes the amino acid glutamine.

Anticipation and parent of origin effect

CAG repeat lengths can vary from generation to generation, with both expansion and contraction of the number, but with a tendency for repeat lengths to increase. The sex of the transmitting parent was found to be important in terms of repeat length expansion. When transmitted from the mother, repeat length increases or decreases up to seven CAG repeat lengths with an overall mean change of zero. When transmission occurs from the father, there is a tendency towards much larger expansions, with up to a doubling of paternal repeat length and expansions occurring much more than contractions, resulting in a mean intergenerational increase of four CAG repeats from paternal transmission [126–128]. This is caused by genetic instability of the CAG repeat during spermatogenesis, perhaps from slippage of the DNA replication apparatus along CAG tracts [126, 129]. The tendency of the CAG expansion to expand during transmission underlies the phenomenon of anticipation. Genetic anticipation describes the increasing severity of an inherited disease during intergenerational transmission and is a hallmark of HD and the other trinucleotide repeat disorders. The CAG repeat instability during paternal transmission is important in the development of large expansions associated with juvenile HD, and approximately 80% of patients with large CAG repeat lengths inherited the HD gene from their father [6].

Intermediate repeat alleles and new mutations

New mutations in HD were originally thought to be very rare but it is now known that intermediate alleles with CAG repeat lengths between 27 and 35 may expand into the pathogenic range when transmitted through the paternal line. This has important implications for the molecular epidemiology of HD, because the frequency of intermediate allele carriers is between 1.5 and 1.9% in the general population in Europe and the USA [130]. It also explains two clinical phenomena, first genetic anticipation, where successive generations have earlier ages of onset, and second, the predominant paternal transmission of juvenile-onset HD, where the CAG repeat size is almost always greater than 55. However, the vast majority of gene carriers, around 90% or so, have CAG repeat lengths in the 40–55 range and follow the typical pattern of disease, with onset in adulthood.

Correlation between CAG length and disease (Table 21.7)

In a study of 178 patients worldwide with HD, the researchers found 7 patients with 36 repeats (found no cases with a lower number), as well as individuals with 36, 37, 38, and 39 repeats who did not have any signs of the disease (all aged >69 years old). They described a 95-year-old man with 39 repeats who did not have the disease, which suggests the gene may not be fully penetrant in rare cases [131]. Reports of individuals with manifest HD and repeat lengths below 36 remain controversial [132, 133].

There is a direct correlation between the CAG repeat size and the age of onset, such that the larger the size of the repeat, the earlier the disease onset (Figure 21.4) [134, 135]. Most individuals with greater than 50 repeats develop the disease before the age of 30. The size of the CAG repeat itself allows some estimate of the age of onset in premanifest individuals [136]. However this can be variable, and generally such estimates are confined to the research setting when estimating years to onset in premanifest gene carriers. It has also been found that the CAG repeat number appears to govern directly the development rate of neuropathological changes [137]

Table 21.7 Relationship of CAG size to phenotype.

CAG repeat length	Phenotype
<27	Normal
27–35	Normal, intermediate allele
36–40	Abnormal, reduced penetrance
>40	Abnormal – HD

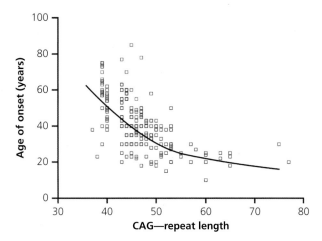

Figure 21.4 Correlation of CAG repeat size and age of onset. Data from the Welsh HD population showing the inverse correlation of CAG repeat length with age of onset. Source: Bates, Harper, & Jones 2002 [2]. Reproduced with permission of Oxford University Press.

with more rapid degenerative changes seen with longer CAG repeat lengths. This may explain the earlier onset with longer CAG repeats. However, it is now known that the CAG repeat accounts for only 50–70% of variation of age of onset [138], not the clinical phenotype or the rate of clinical disease progression. Thus there is interest in modifying genes that affect age of onset and these other factors. This is supported by the finding that identical twins do show similar ages of disease onset but intriguingly can have different clinical phenotypes, while homozygosity largely eliminates any significant differences in age of onset [139–141].

A study of the Venezuelan kindred revealed that both genetic and environmental factors modulate the age of onset of disease [142]. A genome scan of 629 affected sib-pairs found linkage at 4p16 (logarithm of the odds to the base 10 [LOD] = 1.93), 6p21-23 (LOD = 2.29), and 6q24-26 (LOD = 2.28) [138]. Only a few linkage and association studies have been done to date, in which several candidate modifier genes were identified, including *HAP1*, *GRIK2* (formerly *GLUR6*), and *TCERG1* (formerly *CA150*) [143–145]. However, publications involving re-analyses of a large combined dataset have not found evidence for any association with these candidate modifier genes [146, 147].

There was some interest in exploring the contribution of the size of the normal allele in influencing the age of onset, however a linear regression based analysis refuted an interaction between expanded and normal alleles, or indeed a second expanded allele [148].

Genetic diagnosis

In clinical practice, genetic testing would be considered in three circumstances: (i) a confirmatory or diagnostic test, (ii) predictive testing of an asymptomatic individual known to be at risk, and (iii) prenatal testing.

A diagnosis of manifest HD delivers the emotional and psychological impact that the patient has a slowly progressive incurable disease. In addition, a positive predictive test places the extra burden of uncertainty over the timing of disease onset. Most people who have predictive genetic testing for HD will have watched a parent develop the disease.

Therefore, genetic testing for any disease should not be performed without detailed counseling. Most clinicians are aware of the need for counseling of at-risk individuals for predictive testing, but the fact that a patient is symptomatic does not remove the need to provide detailed counseling. There are internationally agreed guidelines for testing of asymptomatic individuals at risk for HD, and testing should be performed in a specialist genetics setting [149].

Principles of genetic counseling

The discovery of the gene in 1993 allowed the accurate genetic diagnosis of HD and also paved the way for predictive testing of healthy persons at risk of inheriting the disorder. This risk is dependent on the at-risk subject's age; for a person in early adult life with an affected parent the risk is 50%, but by the time the person reaches the age of 65 and is still asymptomatic, the risk of a positive test has dropped considerably to about 13% (see Table 21.8).

The risk for a healthy subject at 50% prior risk of inheriting the HD gene at different ages has been calculated based on the life-table analysis of South Wales data (Table 21.8) [150]. Issues can arise when an at-risk person has an allele with a reduced penetrance CAG repeat size between 36 and 39 (reduced penetrance allele).

Genetic counseling

Genetic counseling is necessary whenever genetic testing is being undertaken, regardless of whether a predictive or a diagnostic test is being contemplated.

In broad terms, an initial consultation would involve determination of the level of risk of the individual through evaluation of the family history, clinical history, and neurological examination. The presence of a family member or spouse/partner is strongly recommended. A psychological assessment would be undertaken also to identify any patient with active, untreated psychiatric disease such as depression or anxiety, to assess suicide risk as well as establish the level of emotional support available. Following this would be an explanation in simple terms of the inheritance and nature of HD together with the limitations of the test including the possibility of an intermediate range result and that uncertainty over onset of symptoms would remain in the case of a predictive test.

Each of the possible results and ensuing implications for the person, family including children, employment, driving, and life

Table 21.8 Risk for a healthy individual at 50% prior risk of Huntington's disease carrying the HD gene at different ages.

Age (years)	Risk of an HD mutation (%)
20	49.6
22.5	49.3
25	49
27.5	48.4
30	47.6
32.5	46.6
35	45.5
37.5	44.2
40	42.5
42.5	40.3
45	37.8
47.5	34.8
50	31.5
52.5	27.8
55	24.8
57.5	22.1
60	18.7
62.5	15.2
65	12.8
67.5	10.8
70	6.2
72.5	4.6

Source: Harper & Newcombe 1992 [150]. Reproduced with permission of BMJ Publishing Group Ltd.

insurance would also be covered. Strict confidentiality must be practised and permission must be obtained to discuss medical history with other family members, whose right to confidentiality and appropriate genetic counseling must equally be respected.

A second consultation would then be arranged after at least a month to allow sufficient time for the patient to adequately consider the information given. Once the patient has confirmed their understanding of the test and its scope, genetic testing would be undertaken following written, informed consent. The result would be given at a third consultation, after which a follow-up should also be carried out to assess how the patient is dealing with the result.

Studies indicate that despite understandable concerns about reactive psychiatric disease following a positive test, this is not necessarily the case [151]. In those with a negative gene test, improvement in psychological well-being is noted, although paradoxically around 10% have difficulty adjusting to an uncertain future free from disease rather than a clearer future afflicted with disease [152].

Diagnostic genetic testing

Diagnostic testing is undertaken to confirm or exclude a diagnosis in an individual with symptoms suggestive of HD. Reasons commonly cited for having predictive testing include wishing to relieve uncertainty, to inform decisions about reproduction, and to plan for the future. Adequate genetic counseling and informed consent in these situations is equally important.

Predictive genetic testing

Prior to the availability of the genetic test, surveys suggested that 80% of those with a family history of the disease would take up predictive testing, but the demand has been lower than expected. The reasons most commonly given for desiring a test were to relieve uncertainty, plan for the future, plan a family, and inform children [153]. The HD predictive testing guidelines recommend that individuals at risk are seen for two to four counseling sessions spread over a 3-month period, before disclosure of the test results. This is to allow the person to consider all possible benefits and harms, for them personally and for others close to them. What is absolutely clear from the extensive research that has been carried out in this area is the importance of providing accurate information and pre- and post-test counseling and support, and for mechanisms to be in place to ensure adequate safeguards against discrimination and breaches of confidentiality. These guidelines were updated in 2012 [154].

An informed, competent adult should be free to make his or her own decision, but in certain circumstances, such as when the patient is depressed, testing should be delayed. It is generally agreed that it is unethical to perform presymptomatic testing on children below the age of 18 (or age of majority in the respective country) for an adult-onset, untreatable neurodegenerative condition such as HD [155].

The test is able to determine if the genetic mutation has been transmitted and therefore that the person will develop HD, assuming they live long enough to manifest symptoms. It gives no indication of what age they will be when they develop symptoms or what type of symptoms they will have. Following counseling, around 5–20% of those at risk in the UK undertake predictive testing [156].

Prenatal testing

It is recommended that individuals with HD or those who are at risk undergo genetic counseling prior to getting pregnant, as the nature of the tests and potential options carry different implications. Chorionic villus sampling can be performed at 8–10 weeks or alternatively amniocentesis can be undertaken at 15–18 weeks.

At the outset it is important to make explicitly clear that the procedure is embarked upon with the explicit intention of ending the pregnancy if the embryo is gene positive. If, after careful consideration, termination of pregnancy is not a viable option then prenatal testing cannot be offered.

Another approach where one parent is gene positive or at risk is pre-implantation diagnosis, which uses *in vitro* fertilization (IVF) technology to make a genetic diagnosis at the embryonic stage, facilitating the implantation of embryos that have a less than 1% chance of carrying the expanded HTT gene. A live birth can be expected to occur in about one out of five cycles.

If the individual does not wish to know their own result, an exclusion test can be offered. This uses linkage analysis to compares the genotype of the embryo with its grandparents, such that the result is either 0% risk for the fetus or 50% risk, whereby the fetus has received a chromosome from the affected grandparent. However, the probability of the parent being positive remains unaltered by the act of testing and therefore his or her result is undisclosed (Figure 21.5).

In a European study looking at outcomes following prenatal testing carried out over a 5- year period, 43% were high risk for HD, and of these pregnancies 6% were continued [157].

Practical implications: insurance, employment, and driving

Insurance In general, insurers will weight applicants who have a family history of HD but cannot require them to take a predictive genetic test. People at risk of HD can apply for a certain amount of life insurance, critical illness insurance, and income protection without disclosing the results of any predictive genetic test. In the UK, HD is, however, the one disease that is exempt from a total ban on disclosure; applicants must disclose HD predictive test results if they apply for life insurance over £500,000. A negative predictive test result will bring insurance premiums back in line with those of people without a family history of HD. A positive predictive test does not need to be declared when applying for travel insurance in the UK, but manifest disease does.

Employment Under the 1995 Disability Discrimination Act in the UK, it is illegal for employers to discriminate against someone who is disabled by dismissing them or treating them differently. We recommend that patients with HD who feel that their ability to work is deteriorating inform their employers about their diagnosis to ensure that their job is legally protected. Once the diagnosis is revealed, regular assessment should take place according to occupational risk. The legal situation for people at risk of HD because of their family history is less clear cut, and there is currently no law in the UK to prevent discrimination against those with a genetic diagnosis (in employment, or elsewhere). Research on genetic discrimination in HD is limited, but a recent survey of 233 tested and untested people at risk of HD in Canada found that 6.4% reported genetic discrimination related to employment. Anecdotal evidence also suggests that some premanifest gene carriers have been discriminated against in the UK.

Driving In the UK, HD patients are under legal obligation to notify the regulatory driving authority of their condition when they are aware of a "relevant" or "prospective" disability that could affect their ability to drive. If they have a positive predictive test but have no disease signs then they are excused from notification. It is prudent for them to inform their insurance company as failure to disclose may invalidate their cover.

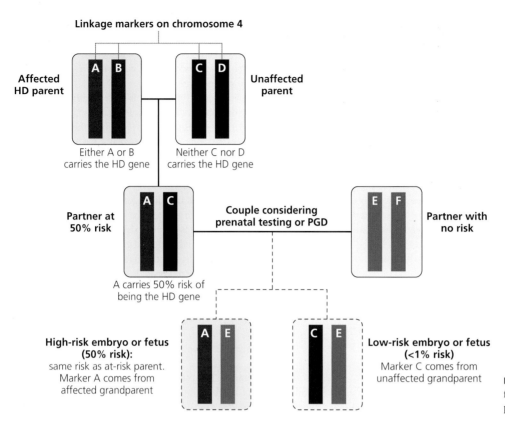

Linkage markers on chromosome 4

Affected
HD parent

A B

C D

Unaffected
parent

Either A or B
carries the HD gene

Neither C nor D
carries the HD gene

Partner at
50% risk

A C

**Couple considering
prenatal testing or PGD**

E F

Partner with
no risk

A carries 50% risk of
being the HD gene

**High-risk embryo or fetus
(50% risk):**
same risk as at-risk parent.
Marker A comes from
affected grandparent

A E

C E

**Low-risk embryo or fetus
(<1% risk)**
Marker C comes from
unaffected grandparent

Figure 21.5 Use of linkage analysis for prenatal testing. PDG, preimplantation genetic diagnosis.

Driving can present an increasing challenge to patients because of a combination of impaired voluntary motor control and psychomotor processing, and diminished reaction times. Clinical research has suggested that global cognitive performance and UHDRS Total Functional Capacity scores provide the best estimate of when driving should cease [158].

Generally, if concern is voiced by either the patient themselves or a partner or relative, or if clinical examination indicates significant incoordination, bradykinesia, or perseveration, or judgment is called into question, the patient should be told to stop driving and inform the relevant driver licensing authority. Often a fitness to drive test can be arranged at the discretion of the licensing authority.

Pathology

Neuropathology

Huntingtin (HTT) is ubiquitously expressed throughout the body but is found in particularly high concentration in the brain (in neurons more than glia) and testes and to a moderate extent in the lungs, liver, and heart. It is predominantly a cytoplasmic protein, which is amenable to cleavage by proteases.

In specific terms, neuronal loss and atrophy occur particularly in the neostriatum – the caudate and putamen – although the former is affected to a greater extent. As the disease progresses, generalized brain atrophy ensues such that at post mortem the brain is between 300 and 400 g lighter than the average adult brain weight for patient age [159]. Interneurons are generally spared; in contrast, the striatal medium spiny neurons, which comprise 90% of the striatal neuronal population, are selectively lost. These are predominantly the encephalin-containing projections to the external globus pallidus rather than the substance P neurons that connect to the internal globus pallidus. From a functional neuroanatomical perspective, the occurrence of chorea early in disease may reflect preferential damage to the indirect pathway of basal ganglia-thalamocortical circuitry [160]. In later disease the direct pathway is affected as well as cortical neurons, which may contribute to the loss of motor control, abnormalities of eye movements, and neuropsychiatric symptomatology.

The substantia nigra, distinct cortical layers, the hippocampus, angular gyrus in the parietal lobe, Purkinje cells of the cerebellum, hypothalamus, and thalamus are all also affected in HD [161–166]. At 15 years prior to calculated disease onset, there is demonstrable striatal, thalamic, and cortical white matter loss and whole brain atrophy on brain MRI [167–169].

At a microscopic level, cortical neurons show decreased staining of nerve fibers, neurofilaments, tubulin, and microtubule-associated protein 2 and diminished complexin 2 concentrations, suggesting impairment of synaptic function, cytoskeleton, and axonal transport [170, 171]. Nuclear, cytoplasmic, and neuritic HTT inclusions are seen even in the premanifest stage of disease and are the pathological hallmark of HD. Ubiquinated HTT aggregates are found throughout vulnerable and seemingly more preserved regions [172]. Accordingly, a direct toxic effect is not supported by current research, indeed it may represent an attempt by the neurons to sequester toxic protein fragments and render them biologically inert [173]. The most widely recognized neuropathological classification is the Vonsattel grade. There are five grades, from grade 0, in which HD brains show no gross or generalized microscopic abnormalities consistent with HD, despite pre mortem symptomatology and positive family history, to grade 4, in which there is extreme atrophy [174].

Principles of pathogenesis

HTT is a very large protein of approximately 350 kDa whose structure is predicted to consist mainly of repeated units of about 50 amino acids. These repeats are composed of two antiparallel α-helices with a helical hairpin configuration [175], which assemble into a superhelical structure with a continuous hydrophobic core. HTT bears many points of interaction, particularly at its N-terminus [176], suggesting that it serves as a scaffold to coordinate complexes of other proteins. HTT also undergoes extensive post-translational modification including palmitoylation, acetylation, and phosphorylation.

The cellular functions of HTT are still not completely understood [177–179]. The protein is mostly cytoplasmic, with membrane attachment via palmitoylation at cysteine 214 [180]. A putative nuclear export signal is present near the C-terminus but a classical nuclear localization signal has not been identified. HTT shuttles into the nucleus, has a role in vesicle transport, and can regulate gene transcription [176, 181]. It might also regulate RNA trafficking [182].

Most available evidence, including dominant genetic transmission, the presence of abnormal aggregated proteins, and findings of biochemical, cell, and mouse model studies, suggests that HD arises predominantly from gain of a toxic function from an abnormal conformation of mutant HTT [183, 184]. The HTT RNA might also have toxic properties, and loss of function of HTT could also contribute to disease pathogenesis, perhaps entailing antisense RNA [177]. Furthermore, HTT is necessary for early embryonic development. Transgenic expression of mutant HTT can complement loss of function of HTT, via knockout, during development, consistent with the idea that the HD phenotype does not arise predominantly from loss of HTT function. Findings of recent studies have suggested that the presence of the mutant protein in a knockin mouse model with 111 CAG repeats leads to transient early developmental abnormalities, which the researchers suggest compromise neuronal homeostasis and subsequently render medium spiny neurons more vulnerable to late life stressors [185]. Homozygous subjects appear to be normal developmentally but may have an earlier disease onset and more severe phenotype, although at a microscopic level their early neuronal biology and circuitry remains unstudied. This in turn has led to the question as to whether HD patients are developmentally normal.

Key features of HD pathogenesis have been described consistently. First, mutant HTT has the propensity to form abnormal conformations, including β-sheet structures, although HTT in large inclusions is not the primary pathogenic species in HD. Second, systems for handling abnormal proteins are impaired in cells and tissues from HD patients or models. Third, HTT is truncated and gives rise to potentially toxic N-terminal fragments. Fourth, post-translational modifications of HTT influence toxicity, via conformational changes, aggregation propensity, cellular localization, and clearance. Fifth, nuclear translocation of mutant HTT enhances toxic effects of the protein, in part via transcription-related effects. Finally, cellular metabolic pathways are impaired in samples from HD patients and models (Figure 21.6).

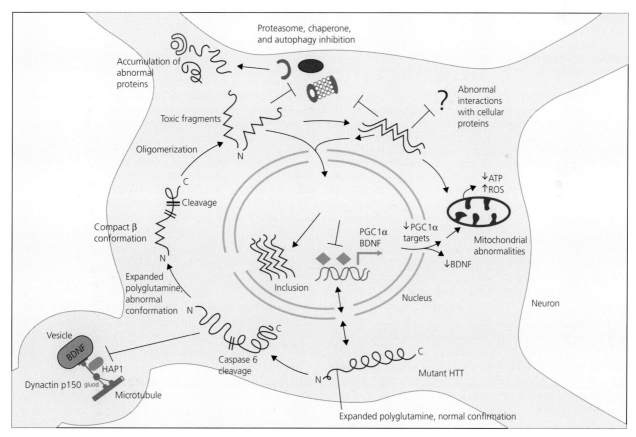

Figure 21.6 Postulated intracellular pathogenesis of Huntington's disease. Mutant HTT (shown as a blue helical structure) with an expanded polyglutamine repeat (shown in red) undergoes a conformational change and interferes with cellular trafficking, especially of BDNF. Mutant HTT is cleaved at several points to generate toxic fragments with abnormal compact β conformation. Pathogenic species can be monomeric or, more likely (and as shown), form small oligomers. Toxic effects in the cytoplasm include inhibition of chaperones, proteasomes, and autophagy, which can cause accumulation of abnormally folded proteins and other cellular constituents. There may be direct interactions between mutant HTT and mitochondria. Other interactions between mutant HTT and cellular proteins in the cytoplasm are still poorly understood. Pathognomonic inclusion bodies are found in the nucleus (and small inclusions are also found in cytoplasmic regions). However, inclusions are not the primary pathogenic species. A major action of mutant HTT is interference with gene transcription, in part via PGC1α, leading to decreased transcription of BDNF and nuclear-encoded mitochondrial proteins. ROS, reactive oxygen species. Source: Reproduced from Ross & Tabrizi, 2011 [15], with permission from Elsevier.

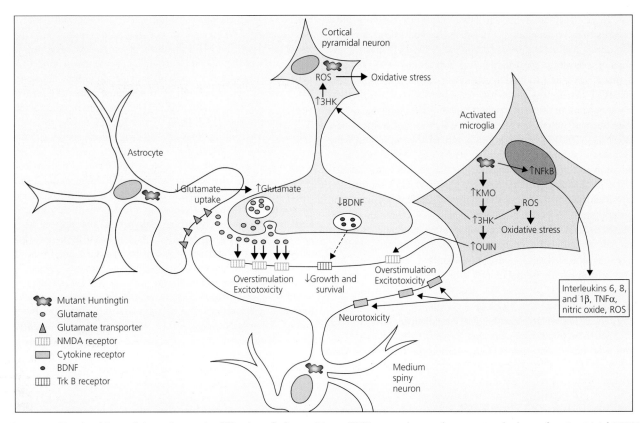

Figure 21.7 Postulated intercellular pathogenesis of Huntington's disease. Mutant HTT causes decreased transport and release of corticostriatal BDNF. Increased stimulation of extrasynaptic glutamate receptors takes place, and reuptake of glutamate by glia is diminished, leading to excitotoxicity and enhanced susceptibility to metabolic toxic effects. Activated microglia produce increased inflammatory activity. Mutant HTT itself might also be transmitted cell to cell. 3HK, 3 hydroxykynurenine; KMO, kynurenine 3 monooxygenase; NMDA, *N*-methyl-D-aspartic acid; QUIN, quinolinic acd; ROS, reactive oxygen species; Trk B, tyrosine kinase B receptor. Source: Reproduced from Ross & Tabrizi, 2011 [15], with permission from Elsevier.

In addition to cell autonomous processes arising within vulnerable neurons, cell interactions likely play a part in pathogenesis, including both interneuronal interactions and interactions between glial cells and neurons (Figure 21.7). For instance, findings of neuronal glial co-culture experiments showed that expression of mutant HTT in glia triggered the death of neurons not expressing mutant HTT and that mutant HTT in glia contributed to neuronal excitotoxicity [186]. Similarly, transgenic expression of mutant HTT in astrocytes in mice causes an HD-like phenotype on its own, or exacerbates the neuronal phenotype in the N171-82Q mouse model [187].

Protein misfolding and proteolysis
The presence of an expanded polyglutamine repeat in the HTT protein (either full-length or truncated) causes a conformational change, which is believed to trigger a pathogenic cascade (Figure 21.6). The abnormal configuration results in the formation of aggregates and fibrillar structures and shows clear parallels with other neurodegenerative diseases such as Alzheimer's disease, Parkinson disease, and prion disorders. Structural evidence suggests that the expanded polyglutamine tail undergoes cleavage, from monomeric aggregates to oligomers, in a process that is dependent on reaching a threshold of protein concentration and a minimum of 37 glutamine residues, providing a pathological basis for the delay in onset and CAG repeat length association [188].Whether the aggregates are toxic, protective, or neutral is debated, but the soluble, oligomeric mutant HTT seems likely to be the most toxic species.

Proteolytic cleavage of HTT may play an important role in pathogenesis as inclusions contain truncated HTT species. Cleavage is mediated by specific enzymes including caspases, which are primarily associated with apoptosis, and where experimental paradigms in mice have demonstrated amelioration of phenotype if cleavage is pharmacologically or genetically prevented. Later work however has cast doubt on caspase activity generating fragment toxicity although it may have a role in clearance [189]. Calpains, which are calcium-dependent proteases, have also been implicated in proteolysis of HTT and may contribute to a pathological cycle in which excitotoxic cell death leads to intracellular calcium release, calpain activation, toxic cleavage of HTT, and further cell death. Calpains may also act pathologically by inhibiting lysosomal mediated removal of intracellular aggregates [190, 191].

Post-translational modifications of Huntingtin
Post-translational modifications of HTT are vital early steps in modulating the protein's toxic effects, although evidently they are also part of its normal, physiological processing. Phosphorylation at threonine 3 influences toxicity, and phosphorylation at serines 13 and 16 has mostly protective effects *in vivo* [192]. Most phosphorylation events seem to be protective [193–196]. HTT can undergo palmitoylation at cysteine 214, enhancing membrane association. Expansion of the polyglutamine tract diminishes this modification, which then contributes to enhanced neuronal toxicity [180]. HTT can also be acetylated at lysine 444, augmenting its clearance [197].

Clearance of mutant Huntingtin

There are two major mechanisms by which misfolded proteins are removed: the ubiquitin-proteasome system (UPS), and autophagy. Researchers have postulated that a toxic effect of mutant HTT could be to compromise ubiquitin-proteasome activity [198]. Changes in the ubiquitin system, observed in both an HD mouse model and human post mortem brain tissue, might represent cellular anomalies or an appropriate cellular response to the abnormal protein [198–200]. Mutant HTT can interfere with target recognition and compromise autophagic clearance [201]. Application of UPS and autophagy inhibitors in a cellular HD model resulted in accumulation of N-terminal mutant HTT fragments [202]. In a *Drosophila* HD model, the use of histone deacetylase inhibitors prevented neuronal degeneration in *Drosophila*, through acetylation which marks the protein for degradation [197, 203]. It is postulated that in this compromised state, the UPS and autophagic systems are overwhelmed, which in turn leads to accumulation of increasing amounts of mutant HTT and other toxic proteins and finally to cell death.

Huntingtin and transcriptional dysregulation

Many transcription factors with key roles in neuronal function and survival interact with both wild-type and mutant HTT [204]. Huntingtin also binds directly to DNA, altering the function of gene promoters in a polyglutamine-dependent manner [205]. Gene expression studies in mouse and cellular models and post mortem tissues have revealed widespread transcriptional alterations in HD. The distribution of these alterations echoes the neuropathological damage, with the caudate, motor cortex, and to a lesser extent the cerebellum showing the most significant changes [206].

It is postulated that truncated fragments of mutant HTT gain access to the nucleus and interact with transcription factors and possibly the DNA itself, altering transcription. Huntingtin aggregates also compete for transcription factors and thereby levels of mRNA and corresponding proteins are reduced. cAMP response element binding protein (CBP) is a transcriptional co-activator that regulates histone acetylation/deacetylation and is sequestered by mutant HTT in the cytoplasm in aggregates. Through this histone gatekeeper role, access to DNA is prevented and transcription down-regulated. Histone deacetylase inhibitors are an important potential therapeutic under investigation and have shown some ability to modify the disease in mouse models [203]. Transcriptional dysregulation is thought to be one mechanism underlying deficits in synaptic transmission, signal transduction, and calcium homeostasis in HD [207–209]. Brain-derived neurotrophic factor (BDNF) has a key role in neuronal maintenance but in the presence of mutant HTT its expression is reduced through failure to bind a transcription repressor, neuron-restrictive silencer element (NRSE) [210].

Metabolism

Mutant HTT could have effects on cellular metabolism in several different ways. First, the cell must deal with the unfolded and abnormal protein, via mechanisms such as the ubiquitin-proteasome pathway, autophagy, and molecular chaperones that require energy. Second, mutant HTT could have direct or indirect effects on mitochondria, compromising energy metabolism and increasing oxidative damage [211, 212]. Third, calorie restriction can ameliorate the HD phenotype in mouse models [213], indicating that pathways related to aging and cell metabolism can modify the disease's pathogenesis. Fourth, transcription of *PPARGC1A* (formerly *PGC1A*) is altered by mutant HTT [214, 215]. The encoded protein, PGC-1α, is itself a transcription factor, which in turn controls transcription of many nuclear-encoded proteins necessary for mitochondrial function and cellular energy metabolism.

Vesicular trafficking and cytoskeleton signaling

Huntingtin appears to have a role in cytoskeletal motor functions, including vesicle transport and recycling, which is disturbed in the presence of mutant HTT. Cell culture and HTT knockout mice show deficiencies in axonal transport and vesicular and mitochondrial trafficking with accompanying neurodegeneration [216]. Huntingtin facilitates vesicular transport of BDNF along microtubules, implying that loss of this function might contribute to pathogenesis [217].

Mitochondrial pathology

Deficits of the electron transport chain and of cellular respiration are seen in mitochondria in HD muscle samples [218]. Mutant HTT has been shown to affect mitochondrial morphology and the bioenergetics status [219, 220].

Mitochondria may play a role in aberrant excitotoxic pathways central to pathogenesis due to loss of calcium buffering. Indeed, human HD lymphoblasts exhibit an impaired calcium-buffering ability and develop increased permeability at lower thresholds [221].

Mutant HTT is proposed to inhibit expression of PGC-1α, a transcription co-activator that plays a role in mitochondrial biogenesis and cellular metabolism, through a promoter interaction and disruption of its transcriptional pathway. In the CNS, PGC-1α is reduced exclusively in the medium spiny neurons that are preferentially affected in HD striatum, as well as muscle and adipose tissue of subjects. Its involvement across several tissues marks it out as a key target for further study [215, 222, 223].

Inflammation

There is evidence suggesting simultaneous dysfunction of CNS and peripheral inflammatory pathways in HD. A pattern of pro-inflammatory cytokine elevation has been observed in plasma in HD: IL-6 was significantly elevated in a group of subjects predicted to be, on average, 16 years from disease, with a parallel post mortem cytokine expression profile seen in the striatum. Furthermore, lipopolysaccharide stimulation of monocytes from HD patients reveals inherent hyperreactivity similar to that seen in microglia on positron emission tomography (PET) studies, suggesting a cell-autonomous effect of mutant HTT in peripheral myeloid cells as well as in the CNS, where microglial activation has been shown to correlate with disease severity and striatal loss [83, 84].

Excitotoxicity

Since the 1970s excitotoxicity has been proposed as a non-cell-autonomous mechanism with a role in pathogenesis of HD, after the discovery that neuronal degeneration was seen following intrastriatal injection of kainic acid [224, 225]. Similarly, many years later, quinolinic acid (QA) injection reproduced selective striatal loss via NMDARs activation. An inhibitor of mitochondrial function, 3-nitropropionic acid, produced a similar neurodegenerative pattern that could be abrogated by pretreatment with an NMDAR antagonist. Radioligand-binding studies in post mortem brain samples demonstrated a greater than expected reduction in NMDARs from the striatum of both premanifest and early HD subjects [226, 227], which supports the hypothesis of selective vulnerability of striatal neurons with high NMDAR expression. Specifically, the GluN2B subunits that make up part of the NMDAR have been highlighted. Compared to other NMDAR subtypes they are highly expressed in mature striatal medium spiny neurons [228–231], as well as occupying a key role in the initiation of cell death signaling pathways [232, 233].

From a broader perspective, current opinion favors time- and region-dependent alterations in synaptic and receptor function, with early synaptic dysfunction characterized by aberrant glutamate release in striatum followed by progressive deafferentation between cortex and striatum [234].

Kynurenine pathway

Several studies have shown elevated levels of neurotoxic metabolites of the kynurenine pathway. This pathway regulates tryptophan metabolism and is implicated in reactive oxygen species generation and excitotoxicity. Genetic deletion of one of the enzymes in the pathway, kynurenine 3-monooxygenase (KMO), which is primarily found on microglia, was found to suppress mutant HTT toxicity in yeast, supporting non-cell-autonomous mediated damage in HD and suggesting a role for the immune cells in the CNS [235, 236] (Figure 21.7).

Models of Huntington's disease

Cell models

Cell models have improved our understanding of the molecular pathogenesis of HD. Biochemical analyses are facilitated using this method but their major drawback is clear in that they might not capture the complete neurobiology of the disease. They are useful for transient, stable, or inducible expression paradigms. Primary neurons reproduce many characteristics of neurons *in vivo*, but not all the complexities of neuronal circuits. Induced pluripotent stem cells are currently being derived from patients with HD for study of disease pathogenesis and for therapeutic screening [237].

The available models can be divided into neuronal and non-neuronal groupings. The former include the mouse neuron teratoma hybrid stably transfected with polyglutamine-containing peptides and immortalized mouse striatal neurons. The latter comprises the inducible PC12 models of HD expressing wild-type and mutant HTT, either in the context of an exon 1 fragment or the full-length protein. PC12 cells show normal morphology and aggregate formation, in both the nucleus and cytoplasm. Rat embryonic striatum

derived ST14A cells have also been used to produce inducible cell lines expressing the N-terminal fragment of HTT [238, 239].

Invertebrate models (*Drosophila melanogaster* and *Caenorhabditis elegans*)

Invertebrate models provide the ability to perform forward genetic screens to detect disease-influencing genes. They enable rapid production and analysis of transgenic lines expressing variants of disease-associated proteins [240]. However, as they lack an immune system and myelin, the contribution of these key pathogenic components cannot be determined. Moreover, they provide a limited series of experimental outcomes and as they are far removed from the human disease the relevance of acquired data can always be called into question [241].

Expression of truncated wild-type and mutant HTT in a *Drosophila* model showed that increased polyglutamine expansion led to more severe degeneration, age-dependent degeneration, and repeat length-dependent nuclear aggregation [242]. The model has also been used to study the mechanisms of disease and effect of potential therapies [243].

As *Caenorhabditis elegans* does not contain an *HTT* homolog or long polyglutamine tracts, transgenic phenotypes in worms can be attributed to expression of transgenes. Mild nose touch abnormalities, perinuclear protein accumulation, and cell death in sensory neurons have been observed in several studies [244, 245].

Mouse models

Although mouse models in HD do provide reproducible and important experimental results, subtle differences exist between the *Htt* gene and its promoters and the human ortholog. In comparison to invertebrate models mouse models have a considerably wider phenotype to interrogate, however the representation of the human disease is clearly incomplete.

In broad terms models can be divided into those that incorporate the full length of the gene, or a fragment, or alternatively a knockin or conditional model. Additionally, they differ in length of the CAG repeat, age of phenotype onset, rate of disease progression, extent of neuronal death, and their ability to reproduce the human behavioral (cognitive, psychiatric, and motor) phenotype (Table 21.9).

Table 21.9 Mouse models of Huntington's disease.

Strain name	Transgenic or knockin	Gene characteristics	Repeat length	Motor symptom onset	Lifespan
R6/2	Transgenic fragment	Exon 1 of human *HTT* gene	~150	6 weeks	10–13 weeks
R6/1	Transgenic fragment	Exon 1 of human *HTT* gene	116	18 weeks	32–40 weeks
N171-82Q	Transgenic fragment	First 171 AA of human *HTT* (exons 1, 2, part of 3)	82	3 months	16–22 weeks
Tg100	Transgenic fragment	First ~3 kb of human *HTT* cDNA	100	3 months (nonspecific)	Normal
HD94	Transgenic fragment	Chimeric human/mouse *HTT* exon 1	94	4–8 weeks (clasping)	Normal
YAC72	Transgenic full-length	Full-length human *HTT* gene	72	16 months	Normal
YAC128	Transgenic full-length	Full-length human *HTT* gene	120	6 months	Normal
BACHD	Transgenic full-length	Full-length human *HTT* gene (floxed exon 1)	97 (mixed)	2 months	Normal
HdhQ72,Q80	Knockin	Endogenous murine *Htt* gene, expanded CAG inserted	72, 80	12 months	Normal
HdhQ111	Knockin	Endogenous murine *Htt* gene, chimeric human/mouse exon 1	109	24 months (gait)	Normal
HdhQ94	Knockin	Endogenous murine *Htt* gene, chimeric human/mouse exon 1	94	2 months (rearing)	Normal
HdhQ140	Knockin	Endogenous murine *Htt* gene, chimeric human/mouse exon 1	140	4 months	Normal
HdhQ150	Knockin	Endogenous murine *Htt* gene, expanded CAG inserted	150	100 weeks	Normal

Source: Crook 2011 [246]. Reproduced with permission of Elsevier.

Mouse models expressing N-terminal fragments of HTT (e.g., the exon-1 or 90 amino acid N-terminal fragment of the R6/2 model, the 171 amino acid fragment of the N171-82Q model, or the caspase 6 fragment or 586 amino acid N-terminal fragment of the N586-82Q model) seem to have the most robust and rapidly progressive phenotypes, including incoordination, hindlimb clasping when suspended by the tail, gait instability on rotarod apparatus, cognitive and other behavioral abnormalities, and weight loss, progressing to early death, and thus have frequently been used for therapeutic trials [247].

Indeed, intranuclear inclusions were discovered in the fragment R6/2 mouse model before their discovery in human post mortem brain. The R6/2 model expressing the 90 amino acid N-terminal fragment of HTT recapitulates some of the post mortem findings, including inclusion formation, some striatal and cortical neuronal death (although not to the same degree), ventricular enlargement, widespread white matter atrophy, and similar patterns of transcriptional dysregulation [207, 248–250].

Mice overexpressing full-length HTT generally present more subtle phenotypes than those mentioned above but may have somewhat more selective neurodegeneration; models incorporating the entire *HTT* gene using transgenic insertion via bacterial/yeast artificial chromosomes (BACs/YACs) have been used for studies of pathogenesis. The BAC, YAC, and knockin models are especially valuable for studies where the entire HTT protein is needed, such as studies of cleavage of full-length HTT, or studies of stages before overt behavioral and pathological phenotypes [247]. YAC72 mice demonstrate abnormal behavior at 7 months and medium spiny neuron degeneration in the lateral striatum by 12 months [251, 252]. However, because the phenotypes develop so slowly, these studies require substantial commitment of time and resources. Behavioral tests need to be standardized to allow comparability across laboratories.

As well as the standard neuropathological analyses, high-field-strength micro MRI studies are a relatively recent development and provide quantitative disease progression data [253].

Large mammalian models

Pigs, sheep, or monkeys could have advantages for studies of behavior and in tests of whether gene therapy agents such as viral expression vectors or antisense nucleotides can penetrate throughout all the relevant regions of the brain, including cortex, subcortical white matter, and subcortical gray matter nuclei. Owing to the physiological and genetic similarities between humans and higher primates, monkeys can serve as very useful models for understanding human physiology and diseases. A transgenic rhesus macaque that expresses polyglutamine-expanded HTT showed classical neuropathological and clinical features of HD, including nuclear inclusions and neuropil aggregates, chorea and dystonia respectively [254].

Development of disease-modifying therapies for Huntington's disease

Challenges in Huntington's disease

Although many compounds have demonstrated promise in animal studies, they fail to make the transition to the bedside. This can be explained in part at least by the lack of animal models that faithfully replicate human pathology, an incomplete understanding of the pathways through which drugs mediate their effect, and an inability to meet safety, tolerability, and drug delivery challenges.

The monogenic nature of HD allows identification of the at-risk population many years before onset of symptoms. In this premanifest phase the early pathogenesis of disease can be studied and therapy may be able to prevent the transition from neuronal dysfunction to neuronal death.

Given the slowly progressive and varied nature of the HD phenotype, there is currently no biomarker that is sensitive enough to detect disease progression over the sort of time frames that would be required for cost-effective clinical trials in premanifest HD. In early HD there are emerging measures over a 24-month period. It is likely that no single modality will be sufficient to assess the effect of a treatment and that a range of functional measures will be needed.

Biomarkers in Huntington's disease

Current rating scales used to measure disease progression are often too insensitive to detect subtle changes occurring in mutation carriers, particularly during the premanifest period, before clinical diagnosis, emphasizing the need for sensitive markers. An ideal state biomarker is a measurable marker that would correlate linearly (in a negative or in a positive way) with the state of disease progression before diagnosis and through the five clinical stages after phenoconversion (the stages are categorized using the UHDRS total functional capacity scores: early [score of 11–13], mid [7–10], moderate [3–6], late [1–2], and severe [0]). Development of robust state biomarkers for HD to track disease progression could yield targets on which treatments could be based and could also offer a scale against which the efficacy of a particular therapeutic intervention could be measured. Asymptomatic mutation carriers can be differentiated on the basis of the probability of disease onset within 5 years or the predicted time until clinical diagnosis, calculated using mathematical modeling based on age and CAG repeat length, which has led to classification of Pre-HD A (far from predicted diagnosis) and Pre-HD B (near to predicted diagnosis) (Figure 21.8).

Observational studies

Several large, multinational, longitudinal, observational studies such as PREDICT-HD, TRACK-HD, COHORT, and REGISTRY have examined clinical markers [82, 256–258]. The Enroll-HD study combines volunteers from the COHORT and REGISTRY studies and includes additional volunteers from Central and South America in the largest natural history study of HD [259].

The European HD Network's (EHDN) Registry study is the largest study of HD to date and is an observational, prospective, multicenter cohort study of HD that aims to establish a well-characterized European-based HD population to facilitate high-quality research. It collects phenotypical data and biospecimens from individuals who are at risk of, premanifest, or manifest for HD, and includes age- and gender-matched control participants [260].

The HDClarity study is the first multi-site collection of cerebrospinal fluid to study HD [261].

Unified Huntington's Disease Rating Scale

The UHDRS is a comprehensive tool for the clinical assessment of HD patients developed first in 1996 and refined in 1999, comprising motor, behavioral, cognitive, functional, and historical domains. It remains the most utilized assessment in observational and clinical trials. The Total Functional Capacity (TFC) subscale of the UHDRS represents the rate of functional decline in Huntington's disease patients [14, 262] but limited reliability and sensitivity of this 13-point scale may diminish its usefulness in clinical trials.

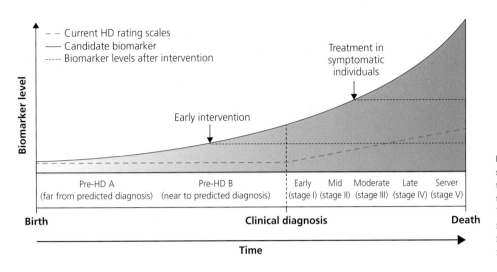

Figure 21.8 Potential role of an ideal state marker of progression in Huntington's disease in a therapeutic intervention. HD, Huntington's disease; UHDRS, unified Huntington's disease rating scale. Source: Reproduced from Weir et al., 2011 [255], with permission from Elsevier.

Progression of UHDRS item scores was assessed in a longitudinal study of 379 patients suffering from early HD. Linear progression was found for all three functional measure and specific motor features including chorea, finger tapping and pronation/supination, gait, tongue protrusion, and tandem walking, suggesting a potential role for an abbreviated version [263]. However the timeframes necessary in which to see a reliable change are not feasible for clinical trials, which are usually designed with 6-month to 1-year efficacy intervals in mind. They are also subject to bias and intra-rater and inter-rater variability [264].

PREDICT-HD
This study aimed to identify biological predictors of disease onset and progression in premanifest subjects. Psychomotor processing, emotion recognition, and working memory were the most sensitive measures in distinguishing individuals according to time to predicted disease onset [35].

TRACK-HD
TRACK-HD was a multisite international study aimed at determining what assessments are suitable as outcome measures in clinical trials. It had a unique, novel objective quantitative motor assessment battery, assessing finger tapping, tongue protrusion, and postural control, which was able to differentiate patients according to disease stage [82]. However, only the indirect circle tracing task changed significantly over 1 year in premanifest individuals [38]. In the early HD group, the largest effect size was seen in the symbol digit modality test, a test of cognitive and motor processing [39].

Longitudinal imaging data have also been acquired and analyzed as part of TRACK-HD. Significantly greater progressive gray-matter, white-matter, whole-brain, and regional atrophy was seen in the premanifest and early HD groups, with the caudate and white matter most affected (Figure 21.9). However, no significant effects over 24 months were seen in the premanifest group [39]. Thus a series of validated assessments can be recommended as sensitive outcome measures for use in disease-modifying trials in early HD subjects.

Functional MRI
In premanifest subjects with normal cognitive scores, fMRI revealed enhanced activation in selective cortical regions, which may be explained by a compensatory response to ongoing primary striatal or localized cortical dysfunction [265]. Alternatively, these unexpected activation patterns might be markers of neuronal dysfunction [266]. However, results have been inconsistent using this modality and although its potential to interrogate specific neural networks is evident, further technical advancements need to be made.

Magnetic resonance spectroscopy (MRS)
Confirming earlier studies, lower concentrations of putaminal N-acetyl aspartate were seen in HD subjects following an MRS study, suggestive of striatal pathology [267]. MRS can also provide a means of assessing striatal glutamate and glutamine and therefore a way of modeling excitotoxicity in HD.

Positron emission tomography (PET)
PET has been employed to assess regional patterns of glucose uptake and dopaminergic signaling as potential disease markers in HD. Accordingly, striatal and cortical glucose reductions have been recorded. In patients with HD and in premanifest gene carriers, longitudinal PET imaging revealed a rate of deteriorating striatal metabolism that seemed more aggressive in manifest than in premanifest individuals. Reduced D1 and D2 receptors, which are highly expressed in vulnerable medium spiny neurons, have been observed, correlating with disease duration, cognitive impairment, and motor deficits [268–271].

24S-hydroxycholesterol
24S-hydroxycholesterol (24OHC) is a product of brain oxidative cholesterol metabolism and is thought to be important for CNS development and function. Lowered concentrations of plasma 24OHC have been reported in patients and premanifest individuals, and they correlated with caudate atrophy and probability of onset of motor symptoms [272]. A previously reported plasma marker, 8-hydroxydeoxyguanosine (8OHdG), was carefully studied and found not to be a biomarker of disease state or progression in HD [273].

Novel biomarkers
Genomic profiling This approach has significant potential but a limited number of studies have been done, one of which found transcriptional alterations in HD patients sensitive enough to distinguish between controls and premanifest individuals [274].

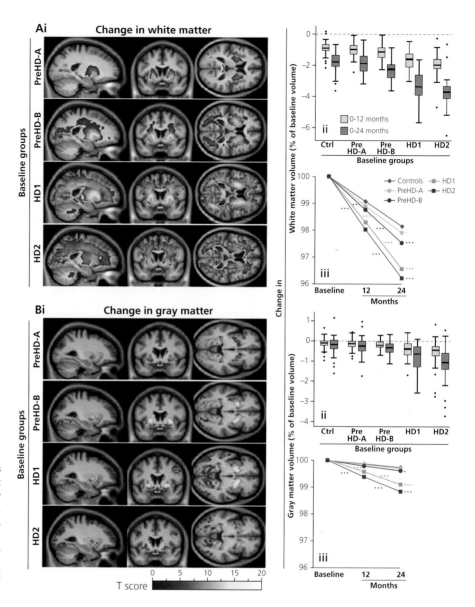

Figure 21.9 Statistical parametric maps showing regions with statistically significant atrophy in (Ai), white matter, and (Bi), gray matter over 24 months, relative to controls. Source: Reproduced from Tabrizi et al., 2012 [39], with permission from Elsevier. Results were adjusted for age, sex, study site, and scan interval and are corrected for multiple comparisons with family-wise error at the P <.05 level.

Huntingtin quantification A novel soluble mutant HTT assay, using a technique known as Förster resonance energy transfer (FRET), has been used and others are in development [275]. This and next-generation assays will allow quantification from a variety of sources and will be essential for mutant HTT reduction based therapies.

Immune biology Elevated cytokine levels have been found in post mortem brain and plasma samples of patients with HD. Concentrations of IL-6 were increased in premanifest subjects 16 years from predicted phenoconversion, the earliest biochemical abnormality recognized in gene carriers [276].Clinical trials in HD (Table 21.10)

Clinical trials in HD (Table 21.10)
At the time of writing, no drug has been shown to delay disease progression in HD. The vast majority of clinical trials to date in HD have used drugs that were not developed specifically for the treatment of HD.

Studies with vitamin E, idebenone, baclofen, lamotrigine, creatine, coenzyme Q10, remacemide, riluzole, latrepirdine, (Dimebon), and ethyl-eicosapentanoic acid have shown no effect. More recently, minocycline failed to show convincing therapeutic potential in a futility study. Selisistat, a sirtuin inhibitor, with supportive preclinical data, has undergone Phase 1 and 2 trials. Reversible liver dysfunction was noted in the latter, but there was no change in clinical endpoints [278, 279].

In the coming years, many disease-modifying trials are planned, including human trials of novel gene-silencing techniques.

Therapeutic approaches in Huntington's disease
Deriving from our understanding of the diverse effects of the HD mutation, there are many potentially viable treatments that may reach clinical trials in the foreseeable future (Figure 21.10).

Enhancing clearance of mutant huntingtin
Being monogenic and fully penetrant, Huntington's disease is an ideal candidate for the therapeutic approach of gene silencing. Gene

Table 21.10 Completed clinical trials in Huntington's disease.

Study	Trial drug and dose	Mechanism of action	No. of individuals participating	Disease severity	Study duration	Outcome and outcome measures
DOMINO	Minocycline 200 mg/day	Caspase (-1 and -3) inhibitor	114	Early HD	18 months	No significant change; measure: UHDRS-TFC
TREND-HD	Ethyl-EPA 2 g/day	Unknown, possible neuronal membrane stabilizer	316 (N. America) 290 (Europe)	Early HD	6 months	No significant change; measure: UHDRS-TMS
TETRA-HD	Tetrabenazine 100 mg/day	Central monoamine depletion	84	Early and mid-stage HD	12 weeks	Improved chorea score; measure: UHDRS-chorea score
CARE-HD	Coenzyme Q10 and remacemide; CoQ10 600 mg/day, remacemide 600 mg/day	CoQ10, antioxidant and cofactor in mitochondrial electron transfer; remacemide, NMDA receptor antagonist	347	Early HD	30 months	CoQ10: nonsignificant trend to slowing of TFC decline; measure: UHDRS-TFC
Riluzole in HD	Riluzole 100 mg/day	Anti-excitotoxic (modulator of glutamate release)	537	Early HD	36 months	No significant change; measure: combined UHDRS-TFC and TMS
DIMOND	Dimebon (latrepirdine) 60 mg/day	Improved mitochondrial stabilization and function	91	Early and mid-stage HD	90 days	Improved MMSE; measures: tolerability, UHDRS score, MMSE, ADAS-Cog
HORIZON	Dimebon (latrepirdine) 60 mg/day	Improved mitochondrial stabilization and function	403	Early and mid-stage HD	26 weeks	Study ongoing; measures: MMSE, CIBIC-Plus, NPI, ADCS-ADL, UHDRS-TMS
HART MermaiHD (in Europe)	ACR16 (pridopidine) 45 mg/day; 90 mg/day	Dopamine stabilizer	437	Early and mid-stage HD	16 weeks 26 weeks	No change in modified motor score (mMS). Improvement in dystonia (MermaiHD results). Measures: UHDRS-TMS, mMS
PADDINGTON Phase 1B	Selisistat 10 mg/d and 100 mg/d	SirT1 Inhibitor	55	Early HD	14 days	Safe and well tolerated; no change in motor, cognitive, or psychiatric domains
*Phase 2a	Selisistat 50 mg/d and 200 mg/d	SirT1 Inhibitor	125	Early and mid-stage HD	12 weeks	No change in UHRDS; reversible liver dysfunction

Source: Sturrock 2010 [277]. Reproduced with permission of Sage Journals.
*Awaiting full publication.
ADAS-Cog, Alzheimer Disease Assessment Scale Cognitive subscore; ADCS-ADL, Alzheimer's Disease Cooperative Study Activities of Daily Living; CIBIC-Plus, Clinician's Interview-Based Impression of Change, plus caregiver input; HD, Huntington's disease; MMSE, mini mental status exam; NMDA, N-methyl-D-aspartate; NPI, Neuropsychiatric Inventory; UHDRS, Unified Huntington's Disease Rating Scale (UHDRS-TFC, Total Functional Capacity, UHDRS-TMS, Total Motor Score).

silencing is an experimental approach to selectively modify protein expression. Custom designed nucleotide-based molecules are introduced into cells to target specific messenger RNA transcripts for removal, resulting in reduced levels of the corresponding protein [281]. The most prominent technique for gene silencing is RNA interference (RNAi), in which the silencing molecules are small interfering RNAs. Other gene-silencing approaches use different nucleotide chemistries such as antisense oligonucleotides (ASOs) but share the same basic principles. Different silencing molecule chemistries may alter tolerability, distribution, uptake, silencing efficacy, and duration of effect [282].

Several groups have now reported success using different techniques to reduce production of the HTT protein. Intracranial delivery of either RNAi or ASOs is capable of significantly reducing HTT production, and ameliorates both motor and neuropathological phenotypes in Huntington's disease model rodents [283–285]. The first application of HTT RNA interference in primates demonstrated effective partial knockdown 6 weeks after treatment [286]. A 6-month non-human primate safety trial used stereotactic neurosurgery to inject adeno-associated virus to deliver small interfering RNA (siRNA) into five sites in the caudate and putamen of four healthy, wild-type rhesus macaques. Four further animals received injections of a placebo comparator with a scrambled RNA sequence. After this one-off treatment,

the animals' general health and motor function were monitored for 6 months before neuropathological inspection. Quantitative polymerase chain reaction demonstrated expression of the silencing and scrambled RNA encoded by the viral vector. The level of HTT RNA was reduced in actively treated animals by 28% compared with placebo treatment. HTT protein expression was also significantly reduced. The transgene was expressed over a diameter of 12 mm, while a 10 mm rostral–caudal section of the striatum showed reduced total HTT protein levels. This represents an increase from the least optimistic extrapolations from rodent trials, but whether it will translate into a clinically meaningful improvement in patients remains unknown [287].

Significant questions remain before gene-silencing therapeutics can be taken into trials in human patients with Huntington's disease. First, the best means of drug delivery is not clear. Second, the penetration of RNA interference compounds is incomplete even in the mouse brain, although ASO drugs have much more widespread penetration. Third, the degree to which RNA interference can be translated to the human brain remains unresolved. Importantly, however, it is fundamental to establish whether it is safe to silence wild-type HTT. Silencing both *HTT* alleles could produce harmful effects as the function of wild-type HTT in the adult brain is unclear. Significant loss of wild-type HTT is harmful in both developmental and adult contexts [288, 289] and results in decreased

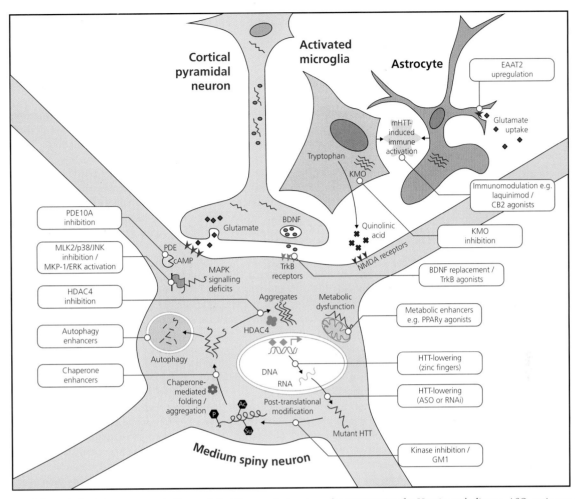

Figure 21.10 Schematic depicting current priority preclinical therapeutic targets under investigation for Huntington's disease. ASO, antisense oligonucleotide; EAAT2, excitatory amino acid transporter 2; HTT, huntingtin; KMO, kynurenine monooxygenase; MLK2, mixed lineage kinase 2; NMDA, *N*-methyl-D-aspartate; PDE, phosphodiesterase; BDNF, brain-derived neurotrophic factor; HDAC, histone deacetylase; Trk, Tyrosine receptor kinase. Adapted from Ross et al. 2014 [280].

levels of brain-derived neurotrophic factor (BDNF), together with impaired axonal trafficking and endosomal recycling, leading to accumulation of toxic reactive oxygen species [282]. Complete HTT knockout is lethal for embryos [290]. However, huntingtin-lowering drugs are unlikely to achieve such profound reductions in HTT.

It may be desirable to target the expanded CAG tract directly, or identify individuals heterozygous for small nucleotide polymorphisms (SNPs) that enable mutant HTT messenger RNA to be targeted selectively by allele-specific silencing. However, this approach would limit treatment to those patients with Huntington's disease who carry such SNPs, and each different SNP-targeting drug would have to be tested and licensed independently [282].

Some insights into these questions have already been provided by recent work showing that transient ASO infusion into the CSF of non-human primates reduced HTT levels in multiple brain regions known to be affected in HD and led to partial phenotypic improvement. This was sustained for up to 3 months after infusion, lending weight to the hypothesis that even temporary reductions in mutant HTT may be enough to produce significant and maintained clinical

benefit [291]. Similarly, convection-enhanced delivery is already in use to increase tissue penetration of chemotherapy drugs for CNS tumors and is likely to be advanced to a clinical trial in patients with Huntington's disease [292]. Exosomes have emerged as another potentially exciting delivery method. They are endogenously occurring vesicles that transport RNAs and proteins and deliver therapeutics. They have been used to reduce expression of the BACE1 gene in an Alzheimer's mouse model [293].

Other approaches to gene silencing include using mismatch-containing duplex RNA that targets mutant HTT. *In vitro*, this has been shown to alter mutant HTT production and reduce generation of toxic HTT fragments [294].

Genomic editing via zinc-finger nuclease is a novel, potentially promising approach for Huntington's disease that has been successfully applied to treat liver cells from mice with hemophilia B [295].

In 2013 the first Phase 1 human trial of an intrathecally delivered ASO, targeting SOD1 in familial amyotrophic lateral sclerosis, completed without significant safety issues being reported, paving the way for such trials with such agents in HD [296].

Other approaches to enhancing clearance of mutant huntingtin

Studies have shown that acetylation of HTT targets the mutant protein for degradation. Acetylation at a single lysine (K444) facilitates trafficking of mutant HTT into autophagosomes and improves clearance of the mutant protein by macroautophagy [197].

Sirtuins are NAD-dependent histone deacetylators (HDACs) that regulate transcription, cell survival, and metabolism. They govern many pathogenetically relevant pathways: both activation and inhibition of SirT1 have been shown as beneficial in HD models. Sirtuin inhibitors may act beyond their histone targets by promoting acetylation of mutant HTT and thereby promoting its clearance. Early Phase 1B studies of the SirT1 inhibitor selisistat have shown tolerability and safety in human HD patients. Phase 2a studies have been completed but are yet to be published.

Pharmacological activation of mTOR (mammalian target of rapamycin)-dependent autophagy with rapamycin attenuated the toxic effects of mutant HTT in fly and mouse models of HD. Small-molecule enhancers of autophagy, including mTOR-independent pathways such as autophagy inducers, are in preliminary development and being tested in cell models [297]. Inhibition of farnesyl transferase, a protein responsible for the farnesylation, or lipid modification, of a number of proteins has been suggested as a possible means of influencing autophagy [298]. This is complicated by the fact that a knockin mouse HD model suggests that HD-specific alterations in autophagy block the trafficking or degradation of HTT, necessitating a precise understanding and targeting of the autophagic process [299]. HD-derived lymphoblasts may provide a good cell model in which to study potential therapeutic compounds as autophagic deficits are established in this cell type. The important issues to address are: (i) whether peripheral change can have a central effect, and (ii) significant side effects of peripheral inhibition of mTOR signaling including ulcerative mucositis, anemia, and neutropenia, which will need to be avoided as new compounds are developed [300].

A screen of 253 approved drugs identified several candidates that appear to down-regulate huntingtin through autophagy, although this has not been definitely confirmed. They include L-type calcium channel blockers such as nimodipine, the α2 agonist clonidine, and the antihypertensive minoxidil [301].

Restoring connectivity

In HD mouse models, researchers have found that the levels of 3′-5′-cyclic adenosine monophosphate (cAMP) in the striatum are lower than in normal mice. Mutant huntingtin disables cAMP signaling and transcription mediated by the cAMP response element binding protein (CREB) [204, 302, 303]. Enhancing synaptic function by preventing breakdown of cAMP and cyclic guanosine monophosphate (cGMP) is a potential mechanism that is currently being explored. A phosphodiesterase (PDE) 10a inhibitor improves striatal and cortical pathology in the R6/2 HD mouse model, and human trials are planned in the next two years [304]. Clinical trials of PDE10A inhibition in HD patients are already under way, with motor and functional MRI endpoints [305].

Restoring healthy gene regulation

Mutant HTT mediated transcriptional dysregulation has been well established as a pathogenic mechanism in HD. Rolipram, a PDE4 inhibitor, may be able to exert influence on transcriptional processes via modulation of CREB signaling; efficacy has been demonstrated in the R6/2 mouse model [306, 307].

Genetic and pharmacological reduction of Sir2, the ortholog of human SirT1, in *Drosophila*, rescued neurodegeneration and promoted survival [243]. The success of non-selective HDAC inhibitors such as suberoylanilide hydroxamic acid (SAHA) in ameliorating HD phenotypes in the R6/2 mouse [308] prompted investigation of other individual HDACs, with class II HDAC-selective inhibitors in preclinical development. Development of histone deacetylase 4 inhibitors is also planned after promising knockdown results in HD mice, although the mechanism of action is not yet clear [309].

Other approaches include up-regulation of SirT1. Genetic over-expression confers survival and neuropathological benefits as well as increased expression of brain-derived neurotrophic factor (BDNF) [310]. In another separate study, genetic SirT1 overexpression improves motor function, reduces brain atrophy, and attenuates metabolic abnormalities by maintaining BDNF concentrations and the signaling of its receptor, TrkB [311]. However no small molecule activator- of SirT1 currently exists.

Transglutaminase inhibitors were suggested to have a role in preventing HTT aggregation. Cystamine, a transglutaminase inhibitor, prolonged survival and improved motor features in an animal model of HD, although aggregation load was not altered [312, 313]. Its effect may be explained by up-regulation of neuroprotective genes, including perhaps *BDNF*, which has been seen in *Drosophila* models [314]. An aspartyl protease has a key role in the cleavage of HTT, raising the potential for the development of specifically targeted inhibitors [295].

Reducing peripheral and central inflammation

Intrastriatal injection of quinolinic acid (QUIN), an NMDA receptor agonist, in rats was shown to recapitulate many features of HD [315]. Glutamate receptor-mediated excitotoxicity and free radical formation have been correlated with decreased levels of the neuroprotective metabolite kynurenic acid in HD mouse models. Genetic deletion of kynurenine 3-monooxygenase (KMO) was found to suppress toxicity in a HD model [235]. KMO is largely expressed in microglial cells and not found in neurons [236, 316], suggesting a non-cell- autonomous mechanism in HD.

The enzyme kynurenine mono-oxygenase (KMO) is a key branchpoint in this pathway, and its activity determines the balance of quinolinic acid and the neuroprotectant metabolites kynurenic acid (KA) and kynurenine. In the CNS, the kynurenine pathway is confined to microglial cells. In a transgenic HD mouse model, a peripherally administered KMO3 inhibitor, JM6, prevents formation of the neurotoxic QUIN and ameliorates neurodegeneration [317]. The implied promise of this approach, which is yet to be validated in HD, is that by applying a compound peripherally a meaningful central effect can be achieved. Interestingly, it was observed that neither JM6 nor its metabolites cross the blood–brain barrier, suggesting that its beneficial effects are mediated by peripheral KMO inhibition producing beneficial effects for the CNS via the transit of an intermediate compound, possibly kynurenine [318]. Subsequent work by Beconi and colleagues has questioned the status of JM6 as a KMO inhibitor, suggesting that the observed effects were likely a result of contamination by the known KMO inhibitor Ro-61-8048 [318]; however, the status of KMO inhibition, peripherally and/or centrally, as a therapeutic target remains strong.

Neurotrophic support

The neurotrophic factor BDNF mediates neural development and neuroprotection, and is up-regulated by normal huntingtin. A few studies have used adeno-associated virus (AAV) to introduce

BDNF expression into the subventricular zone, increasing striatal neuron survival in mouse models [319, 320].

Ampakines have been shown to up-regulate the production of BDNF, which in turn leads to a proliferation of neural stem cells in the striatum. Reduced degeneration and improvements in cognitive function were seen in an HD transgenic mouse model [321]. Research is being directed toward identifying TrKB receptor agonists to increase BDNF levels.

Cell transplantation

Most cell implant concepts for HD have focused on the striatum; while this could be relevant to motor symptoms, the cognitive deterioration is unlikely to be affected. Surgically delivered striatal cell replacement therapy for HD has been attempted in small studies for over two decades, with the majority using human fetal tissue for cell harvesting. Although modest motor improvements have been seen, no sustained improvement has been achieved thus far and, importantly, deterioration of grafted cells was seen at autopsy in three patients [322–324]. Lack of integration with host neural architecture and early degeneration through microglial activation are arguably the most significant difficulties to overcome. This approach appears to offer a temporary symptomatic benefit only. Autologous cell sourcing may be a viable alternative but needs to be developed.

Mitochondrial protection/antioxidants

Mitochondrial pathology has been strongly implicated in HD leading directly to free radical production and accelerated apoptosis. A 5-year coenzyme Q10 study was terminated early on the grounds of futility. A large, 650-patient creatine study in HD will finish in 2016.

Post-translational modification

In a murine model, intraventricular infusions of ganglioside GM-1, a natural component of "lipid rafts", which serve myriad cell-signaling support roles in the brain, resulted in phosphorylation of mutant HTT, neutralizing its toxic effects and improving motor function [325]. This was associated with post-translational modification alterations to mHTT. The striking result requires replication.

Other degenerative choreas

Huntington's disease phenocopy syndromes

Following the discovery of the mutation that causes HD, it emerged that around 1% of patients clinically suspected to have HD in fact lacked the mutation. Such cases are variously referred to as HD-like

syndromes, phenocopies, or look-alikes [326]. HD phenocopy syndromes are rare – probably of the order of 1 per million, although this has not been studied formally.

The clinical heterogeneity of HD is such that many conditions may overlap sufficiently with one or more aspects of it to be considered phenocopies. Thus we have proposed, *a posteriori*, a broad definition of HD phenocopies that encompasses this clinical heterogeneity [327, 328]:

1 A movement disorder consistent with HD as determined by an experienced neurologist; *and*
2 A negative test for the pathogenic CAG repeat expansion in the *HTT* gene; *and*
3 At least one of the following:
   • family history suggestive of autosomal dominant inheritance;
   • cognitive impairment;
   • behavioral or psychiatric symptoms.

Note that we do not consider autosomal dominant inheritance to be essential because many cases of HD lack such a history.

Several large cohorts of HD phenocopy patients have been studied in different centers in an attempt to establish causative mutations (reviewed in [327]). Unfortunately, the central message to emerge from such studies is that the vast majority of phenocopy patients, around 94%, will remain undiagnosed (Figure 21.11).

Some conditions that can mimic HD are treatable, such as Wilson disease. Although the majority are not, seeking a genetic diagnosis is nonetheless a worthwhile endeavor because it can provide certainty around care and family planning. It is also worth pointing out that some conditions that can produce an HD-like phenotype are sufficiently common and distinctive that they are generally diagnosed rapidly, so are probably under-represented in the described phenocopy cohorts.

Major syndromes

The differential diagnosis of HD-like syndromes is summarized in Table 21.11. The major causes are discussed individually in the following sections.

HD-like syndrome 1

HD-like syndrome 1, or HDL1, is so called because it was the first novel genetic cause of an HD-like picture with ataxia. It is caused by a specific 8-octapeptide insertion in the prion protein encoded by *PRNP* [329]. HDL1 itself is rare, but more generally, *PRNP* mutations can cause a broad spectrum of neurological symptoms and the common 6-octapeptide repeat insertion is a described cause of an HD-like presentation with rigidity and ataxia. Thus, familial prion

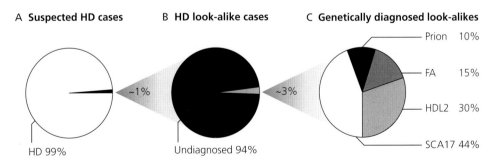

Figure 21.11 Relative frequencies of (A) Huntington's disease and look-alike cases, (B) undiagnosed and genetically diagnosed look-alikes, and (C) individual look-alike cases. FA, Friedreich's ataxia; HDL2, Huntington's disease like syndrome 2; SCA17, spinocerebellar ataxia 17. Source: Wild & Tabrizi 2007 [327]. Reproduced with permission of Wolters Kluwer Health, Inc.

Table 21.11 Principal causes of Huntington's disease look-alike cases [2].

Condition	Gene	Protein	Inheritance	Notes
Familial prion disease	PRNP	Prion	AD	Includes HDL1
HDL2	JPH3	Junctophilin 3	AD	African ancestry
HDL3	Unknown	Unknown	AR	Two pedigrees only
C9orf72 mutation	C9orf72	C9ORF72	AD	Commonest cause of HD phenocopy syndromes
SCA17	TBP	TATA-binding protein	AD	Cerebellar atrophy and ataxia
SCA1	ATXN1	Ataxin 1	AD	
SCA2	ATXN2	Ataxin 2	AD	
SCA3	ATXN3	Ataxin 3	AD	
DRPLA	ATN1	Atrophin 1	AD	Myoclonic epilepsy
PKAN (NBIA1)	PANK2	Pantothenate kinase	AR	MRI "eye-of-the tiger sign"; pigmentary retinopathy
Neuroferritinopathy	FTL	Ferritin light chain	AD	Early dysarthria and persistent asymmetry
Chorea–acanthocytosis	CHAC	Chorein	AR	Mutilating orofacial dystonia
Macleod syndrome	XK	Krell antigen	XR	Systemic features
Wilson disease	ATP7B	Copper-transporting ATPase	AR	Kayser–Fleischer rings, etc.
Friedreich's ataxia	FRDA	Frataxin	AR	Rarely resembles HD
Mitochondrial disease	mtDNA or nuclear mitochondrial genes			
Benign hereditary chorea	TITF1	Thyroid transcription factor 1	AD	Non-choreic features rare
Acquired causes	e.g., Sydenham's chorea, anti-basal ganglia antibodies, neuro-SLE, thyrotoxicosis, vascular disease, and medications			

AD, autosomal dominant; AR, autosomal recessive; XR, X-linked recessive. For other abbreviations, see text.

disease in general should be considered in HD phenocopy cases, and if genetic testing is undertaken it should consist of screening the entire gene rather than simply the HDL1 mutation [330].

HD-like syndrome 2

HDL2, caused by GTC/CAG triplet expansions in the *JPH3* gene encoding junctophilin-3, is a relatively common cause of HD phenocopy syndrome. HDL2 is almost exclusively seen in individuals with African ancestry and in some black African populations is more common than HD itself. HDL2 tends to produce a combination of extrapyramidal rigidity alongside chorea and a psychiatric and cognitive phenotype similar to HD. Overall it resembles the Westphal variant of HD. It has autosomal dominant inheritance but, unusually, the protein product of the *JPH3* gene is not toxic; rather, as in myotonic dystrophy type 1, the pathology in HDL2 appears to be driven by toxic triplet-expanded RNA [331].

Although immortalized as HDL3, the autosomal recessive disorder linked to chromosome 4p15.3 remains obscure and only two pedigrees are known [332].

C9orf72 expansions

After screening our 514-patient cohort, we recently reported that hexanucleotide expansions in *C9orf72*, originally described in familial and sporadic frontotemporal lobar degeneration and amyotrophic lateral sclerosis, were in fact the commonest genetic cause of HD phenocopies, accounting for around 2% of cases overall. The presence of disproportionate cognitive and psychiatric features, and some movement disorder features (dystonia, bradykinesia/rigidity, tremor, myoclonus, and upper motor neuron features), were significantly associated with a positive *C9orf72* test. We now advise testing for *C9orf72* expansions as a first-line investigation [333].

Spinocerebellar ataxia

Several of the spinocerebellar ataxias (SCAs) can produce syndromes that resemble HD, with varying degrees of closeness. Undoubtedly the most accurate mimic is SCA17, which is produced by CAG or CAA repeat expansions in *TBP*, encoding a variant of the TATA-binding protein with an expanded polyglutamine tract. On the basis of SCA17 patients resembling HD remarkably closely,

it has been suggested that SCA17 should be renamed HDL4, but we feel this would be a disservice to the majority (80%) of SCA17 patients who lack chorea. The psychiatric and cognitive features of SCA17 with chorea can be indistinguishable from HD, but the degree of cerebellar ataxia and atrophy is more prominent than that generally witnessed in HD. Putaminal enhancement on MRI has also been reported but is not typical. That *TBP* encodes a crucial transcription factor evokes the transcriptional dysregulation seen in HD; the diseases are also similar pathologically. SCA1, 2, and 3 can also cause HD like syndromes, typically with chorea and ataxia but less cognitive impairment [334].

Dentato-pallido-rubro-luysian atrophy

Like HD, dentato-pallido-rubro-luysian atrophy (DRPLA or Naito-Oyanagi disease) is a polyglutamine disease caused by CAG repeat expansion, this time in the atrophin-1 gene (*ATN1*). DRPLA is phenotypically diverse but the disease course of 15–20 years and the combination of dementia, ataxia, and choreoathetosis are reminiscent of HD. Typically, though, DRPLA has younger onset in the teens or twenties, and the prominence of myoclonic epilepsy, which can be difficult to treat or intractable, is a key feature not seen in HD. MRI in DRPLA shows volume loss in the brainstem and cerebellum, and sometimes white matter lesions on T2 sequences [335].

Neurodegeneration with brain iron accumulation

The conditions collectively classified as neurodegeneration with brain iron accumulation (NBIA) are characterized by the abnormal deposition of iron in brain tissues, usually favoring the basal ganglia, accompanied by progressive neurological syndromes, typically extrapyramidal syndromes with dementia and behavioral features. There are several such conditions, of which only two are potential HD phenocopies. MRI with susceptibility-weighted or gradient-echo sequences can detect abnormal iron deposition in these conditions.

NBIA1

NBIA1, synonymous with PKAN (pantothenate kinase-associated neurodegeneration) and caused by mutations in *PANK2*, is the commonest of these syndromes. It is autosomal recessive, usually presents in early childhood, and is dominated by dystonia and spasticity without chorea, but can resemble juvenile HD clinically. Atypical, late-onset cases may have a more slowly progressive phenotype and simulate minimally choreic HD. The "eye-of-the-tiger" sign on MRI (Figure 21.12A), caused by iron deposition in the globus pallidus, is characteristic of PKAN [336].

NBIA2

NBIA2, or neuroferritinopathy, is a rarer condition but it features chorea prominently and may mimic HD closely. It is autosomal dominant, caused by mutations in the *FTL* gene encoding ferritin light chain, and produces a combination of chorea, dystonia, progressive cognitive impairment, and psychiatric problems. One useful clue is that the chorea may be strikingly asymmetrical or even strictly unilateral, and this asymmetry may persist well into the disease course. In HD, mild asymmetry is common but unilaterality rare, and the chorea usually becomes generalized soon after its appearance. Task-specific orofacial dystonia triggered by speech is another clue to the diagnosis of neuroferritinopathy. As expected, MRI (Figure 21.12B) reveals iron deposition in the basal ganglia, even in asymptomatic mutation carriers [337].

Neuroacanthocytosis

The neuroacanthocytosis syndromes are a group of disorders in which neurological symptoms are accompanied by the presence of acanthocytes – red cells with thorn-like deformities – in peripheral blood. It should be noted that although the presence of acanthocytes may be informative, their absence does not exclude these disorders. Two of these syndromes, chorea–acanthocytosis and Macleod syndrome, are associated with chorea and neurodegeneration.

Chorea–acanthocytosis

Chorea–acanthocytosis, which is autosomal recessive, results from mutations in the *CHAC* gene encoding chorein. Although onset is typically at an earlier age, it resembles HD, with chorea, dystonia,

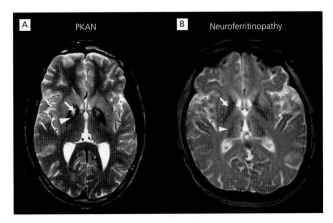

Figure 21.12 MR imaging in brain iron-accumulation disorders. (A) Axial T2-weighted brain MRI in PKAN demonstrating "eye-of-the-tiger sign", due to globus pallidus hypointensity (arrowhead) containing a high-intensity focus (arrow). Source: Reproduced from Hartig et al., 2006 [336], with permission of Wiley. (B) T2* MRI scan in neuroferritinopathy, showing reduced signal in the basal ganglia (arrow) and thalamus (white arrowhead). Source: Reproduced from Chinnery et al., 2007 [337], with permission of Oxford University Press.

and tics. The distinguishing features are prominent orofacial dystonia, which can be mutilating in cases, and a "rubber man" appearance caused by truncal instability and loss of axial tone. In addition, it can be associated with peripheral neuropathy, seizures, and elevated creatine kinase. Because of the size of the *CHAC* gene and diversity of mutations, western blotting for the chorein protein may be needed to make the diagnosis [338].

Macleod syndrome

Macleod syndrome, caused by mutations in the Kell erythrocyte antigen encoded by *XK*, is distinguished by X-linked recessive inheritance and the presence of neuropathy, hepatosplenomegaly, cardiomyopathy, and hemolytic anemia. In other respects, the combination of chorea, tics, dementia, and behavioral symptoms may mimic HD [338].

Wilson disease

Wilson disease, described fully in Chapter 26, can produce an array of hyper- and hypokinetic movement disorders, including chorea, choreoathetosis, and dystonia. In addition, mood and cognitive disturbances can be seen. Wilson disease can present as an HD phenocopy syndrome, perhaps mimicking dystonic juvenile HD with an absent family history. It is crucial to exclude the diagnosis through ocular examination for Kayser–Fleischer rings and biochemical and genetic testing as required, because copper chelation therapy can treat the condition effectively [339].

Benign hereditary chorea

Benign hereditary chorea is probably not strictly a neurodegenerative illness because it typically produces mild chorea in early life that does not progress. The condition is caused by *TITF1* mutations and can present as part of the brain–thyroid–lung syndrome. Intellectual impairment and dystonia have been described, but the condition rarely mimics HD closely, especially after longitudinal observation [340].

Other causes of chorea

Other genetic causes of chorea are rare. Friedreich's ataxia can occasionally produce generalized chorea, and this genetic diagnosis has been detected in association with cognitive and oculomotor abnormalities in one patient in a large HD phenocopy cohort [329]. Chorea is one of the myriad of symptoms that can be produced by mitochondrial disease [341].

Finally, any acquired cause of chorea, such as drug toxicity or small vessel ischemic disease, may produce a progressive picture mimicking neurodegeneration if the cause is not remedied.

Management

Huntington's disease is overwhelmingly the commonest degenerative cause of chorea, and the availability of a reliable genetic test for HD makes the diagnosis easy to attain, at least in theory, avoiding the need for protracted and expensive clinical investigations. In other hereditary cases where a dominant family history of a known disorder exists, the diagnosis may be equally straightforward. But in sporadic cases or pedigrees with no known diagnosis, the most likely outcome is that a definitive cause will not be found, even after exhaustive testing.

With this in mind, three principles underlie our approach to such patients. The first is to manage expectations realistically, preparing the patient and their family for a low probability of reaching a diagnosis, less still a treatable one, despite a potentially lengthy diagnostic process. Second, although genetic testing can be invaluable and should not be avoided where a diagnosis is suspected, its results – whether positive or negative – can have far-reaching and sometimes devastating consequences for the patient and other family members, so must always be accompanied by expert neurogenetic counseling with sufficient time to ask questions, reflect, and consider whether to proceed. Third, we suggest a rational, evidence-based approach beginning with careful history-taking and examination, followed by systematic genetic and other investigation guided by the context in which chorea is seen [328].

As summarized, we suggest that *C9orf72* expansions and SCA17 are sufficiently common that they should be tested for whenever HD is suspected but not found (Figure 21.13). Next-line testing depends on the associated features. If ataxia or peripheral neuropathy is present, SCA1–3 and Friedreich's ataxia testing should be considered. In the presence of myoclonus or dementia, consider testing for prion and mitochondrial disease. In patients with African descent, testing for HDL2 should be the first resort. If myoclonic seizures are present, DRPLA should be suspected. If the blood film reveals acanthocytes, genetic testing or western blotting for neuroacanthocytosis would be the next step, bearing in mind that these may be necessary in the presence of a normal film in suggestive cases. Brain MRI can also help to guide further testing, by revealing the presence of pathological iron deposits, or focal atrophy of, for instance, the cerebellum [328].

Except in rare cases where a diagnosis with a potential disease-modifying treatment is reached, such as Wilson disease, multidisciplinary management and symptomatic care are inevitably the mainstay of treatment for patients with HD phenocopy syndromes. In many cases, the burden of physical, behavioral, and cognitive symptoms is no less onerous for patients and family members than for HD, combined with the additional worry arising from the lack of a clear diagnosis and unknown risk to relatives. The high rate of non-diagnosis implies that there are many more as yet unknown genetic causes of such syndromes. One potential source of comfort to patients and family members is offering their DNA and time to ongoing research efforts to shed light on those causes, with the ultimate aim of moving them into the realm of the treatable.

Conclusions and the future

In almost 20 years since the gene mutation for Huntington's disease was identified, important advances have been made, but much is still unknown and fundamental questions remain. Of all

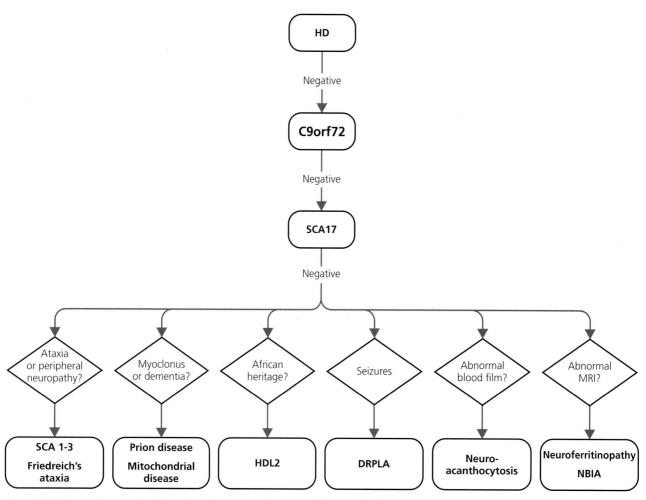

Figure 21.13 Suggested approach to directed genetic testing in Huntington's disease look-alike cases. Source: Hensman et al. 2014 [334]. Reproduced with permission of Wolters Kluwer Health, Inc.

the protein interactions of mutant HTT, which are most important for pathogenesis? Which of the post-translational modifications of HTT will yield the best therapeutic targets? To what extent does loss of HTT function contribute to pathogenesis or modify the effects of gain of function? Therapeutic strategies focusing on mutant HTT expression – such as lowering HTT mRNA – seem promising, but it is not clear how much of a decline in normal or mutant HTT can be tolerated without cellular dysfunction or death. Moreover, effects of mutant HTT that seem to be fairly distal, such as metabolic effects, might feed back to alter cellular ability to deal with misfolded proteins [15].

In terms of disease modeling, several issues remain unresolved. Why do current animal models replicate so poorly the massive selective striatal cell death of human Huntington's disease and what can be done to improve them? Enhanced disease models – both *in vivo* and cellular models, such as induced pluripotent stem cells or other patient-derived cell models – will be vital. What biomarkers will be most suitable for tracking disease progression and response to treatments, particularly in gene carriers who are clinically well? Can we identify functional disease-related markers that will be responsive to therapeutics in the short term, or will we need to use structural imaging measures, which are fairly slow to change? Formal validation of these approaches will not be forthcoming without both positive and definitive negative results from well-designed human therapeutic trials [15].

Although no cure for the disease exists, in the last few years there has been an exponential rise in the number of publications delineating its basic and clinical science, and therapeutic trials. Furthermore, as the disease is fully penetrant, a positive predictive HD gene test results in development of disease at some point. The *premanifest* phase therefore creates an invaluable window of opportunity, both to study the disease in its earliest stages, and a unique point at which to intervene therapeutically.

Finally, there is evidence of shared mechanisms between HD and other neurodegenerative diseases such as Alzheimer's disease, where synaptic dysfunction, protein misfolding, and aggregation are also found. This highlights a potentially pivotal role in developing both a pathophysiological understanding of the preclinical phase of neurodegeneration using HD as a model disease, as well as therapies for neurodegenerative diseases as a whole [342].

References

1. Huntington G. On Chorea. *Med Surg Reporter* 1872;26:320–1.
2. Bates G, Harper PS, Jones L. Huntington's Disease. Third ed. Oxford: Oxford University Press; 2002.
3. The Huntington's Disease Collaborative Research Group. A novel gene containing a trinucleotide repeat that is expanded and unstable on Huntington's disease chromosomes. *Cell* 1993 Mar 26;72(6):971–83.
4. Hoppitt T, Pall H, Calvert M, Gill P, Yao G, Ramsay J, et al. A systematic review of the incidence and prevalence of long-term neurological conditions in the UK. *Neuroepidemiology* 2011;36(1):19–28.
5. Rawlins M. Huntington's disease out of the closet? *Lancet* 2010 Oct 23;376(9750):1372–3.
6. Harper PS. The epidemiology of Huntington's disease. *Hum Genet* 1992 Jun;89(4):365–76.
7. Warby SC, Visscher H, Collins JA, Doty CN, Carter C, Butland SL, et al. HTT haplotypes contribute to differences in Huntington disease prevalence between Europe and East Asia. *Eur J Hum Genet* 2011 May;19(5):561–6.
8. Siesling S, Vegter-van de Vlis M, Losekoot M, Belfroid RD, Maat-Kievit JA, Kremer HP, et al. Family history and DNA analysis in patients with suspected Huntington's disease. *J Neurol Neurosurg Psychiatry* 2000 Jul;69(1):54–9.
9. Almqvist EW, Elterman DS, MacLeod PM, Hayden MR. High incidence rate and absent family histories in one quarter of patients newly diagnosed with Huntington disease in British Columbia. *Clin Genet* 2001 Sep;60(3):198–205.
10. Margolis RL, Rudnicki DD, Holmes SE. Huntington's disease like-2: review and update. *Acta Neurol Taiwan* 2005 Mar;14(1):1–8.
11. Warby SC, Montpetit A, Hayden AR, Carroll JB, Butland SL, Visscher H, et al. CAG expansion in the Huntington disease gene is associated with a specific and targetable predisposing haplogroup. *Am J Hum Genet* 2009 Mar;84(3):351–66.
12. Lekoubou A, Echouffo-Tcheugui JB, Kengne AP. Epidemiology of neurodegenerative diseases in sub-Saharan Africa: a systematic review. *BMC Public Health* 2014;14:653.
13. Aubeeluck A, Moskowitz CB. Huntington's disease. *Part 3: family aspects of HD. Br J Nurs* 2008 Mar 13;17(5):328–31.
14. Huntington Study Group. Unified Huntington's Disease Rating Scale: reliability and consistency. *Mov Disord* 1996 Mar;11(2):136–42.
15. Ross CA, Tabrizi SJ. Huntington's disease: from molecular pathogenesis to clinical treatment. *Lancet Neurol* 2011 Jan;10(1):83–98.
16. Mahant N, McCusker EA, Byth K, Graham S. Huntington's disease: clinical correlates of disability and progression. *Neurology* 2003;61(8):1085–92.
17. Wheelock VL, Tempkin T, Marder K, Nance M, Myers RH, Zhao H, et al. Predictors of nursing home placement in Huntington disease. *Neurology* 2003 Mar 25;60(6):998–1001.
18. Busse ME, Wiles CM, Rosser AE. Mobility and falls in people with Huntington's disease. *J Neurol Neurosurg Psychiatry* 2009 Jan;80(1):88–90.
19. Grimbergen YA, Knol MJ, Bloem BR, Kremer BP, Roos RA, Munneke M. Falls and gait disturbances in Huntington's disease. *Mov Disord* 2008 May 15;23(7):970–6.
20. Nance MA. Huntington disease: clinical, genetic, and social aspects. *J Geriatr Psychiatry Neurol* 1998;11(2):61–70.
21. Gordon AM, Quinn L, Reilmann R, Marder K. Coordination of prehensile forces during precision grip in Huntington's disease. *Exp Neurol* 2000;163(1):136–48.
22. Panzera R, Salomonczyk D, Pirogovsky E, Simmons R, Goldstein J, Corey-Bloom J, et al. Postural deficits in Huntington's disease when performing motor skills involved in daily living. *Gait Posture* 2011 Mar;33(3):457–61.
23. Quinn N, Schrag A. Huntington's disease and other choreas. *J Neurol* 1998 Nov;245(11):709–16.
24. Lasker AG, Zee DS. Ocular motor abnormalities in Huntington's disease. *Vision Res* 1997 Dec;37(24):3639–45.
25. Shoulson I, Fahn S. Huntington disease: clinical care and evaluation. *Neurology* 1979;29(1):1–3.
26. Wheeler JS, Sax DS, Krane RJ, Siroky MB. Vesico-urethral function in Huntington's chorea. *Br J Urol* 1985 Feb;57(1):63–6.
27. Kolenc M, Moharic M, Kobal J, Podnar S. Bladder dysfunction in presymptomatic gene carriers and patients with Huntington's disease. *J Neurol* 2014 Dec;261(12):2360–9.
28. Aziz NA, Anguelova GV, Marinus J, Van Dijk JG, Roos RA. Autonomic symptoms in patients and pre-manifest mutation carriers of Huntington's disease. *Eur J Neurol* 2010 Aug;17(8):1068–74.
29. Morton AJ, Wood NI, Hastings MH, Hurelbrink C, Barker RA, Maywood ES. Disintegration of the sleep-wake cycle and circadian timing in Huntington's disease. *J Neurosci* 2005;25(1):157–63.
30. Maywood ES, Fraenkel E, McAllister CJ, Wood N, Reddy AB, Hastings MH, et al. Disruption of peripheral circadian timekeeping in a mouse model of Huntington's disease and its restoration by temporally scheduled feeding. *J Neurosci* 2010 Jul 28;30(30):10199–204.
31. Arnulf I, Nielsen J, Lohmann E, Schieffer J, Wild E, Jennum P, et al. Rapid eye movement sleep disturbances in Huntington disease. *Arch Neurol* 2008;65(4):482–8.
32. Kobal J, Meglic B, Mesec A, Peterlin B. Early sympathetic hyperactivity in Huntington's disease. *Eur J Neurol* 2004 Dec;11(12):842–8.
33. Bar KJ, Boettger MK, Andrich J, Epplen JT, Fischer F, Cordes J, et al. Cardiovagal modulation upon postural change is altered in Huntington's disease. *Eur J Neurol* 2008 Aug;15(8):869–71.
34. Duff K, Beglinger LJ, Theriault D, Allison J, Paulsen JS. Cognitive deficits in Huntington's disease on the Repeatable Battery for the Assessment of Neuropsychological Status. *J Clin Exp Neuropsychol* 2010 Mar;32(3):231–8.
35. Stout JC, Paulsen JS, Queller S, Solomon AC, Whitlock KB, Campbell JC, et al. Neurocognitive signs in prodromal Huntington disease. *Neuropsychology* 2011 Jan;25(1):1–14.
36. Paulsen JS. Cognitive impairment in Huntington disease: diagnosis and treatment. *Curr Neurol Neurosci Rep* 2011 Oct;11(5):474–83.
37. Hamilton JM, Salmon DP, Corey-Bloom J, Gamst A, Paulsen JS, Jerkins S, et al. Behavioural abnormalities contribute to functional decline in Huntington's disease. *J Neurol Neurosurg Psychiatry* 2003 Jan;74(1):120–2.
38. Tabrizi SJ, Scahill RI, Durr A, Roos RA, Leavitt BR, Jones R, et al. Biological and clinical changes in premanifest and early stage Huntington's disease in the TRACK-HD study: the 12-month longitudinal analysis. *Lancet Neurol* 2011 Jan;10(1):31–42.

39. Tabrizi SJ, Reilmann R, Roos RA, Durr A, Leavitt B, Owen G, et al. Potential endpoints for clinical trials in premanifest and early Huntington's disease in the TRACK-HD study: analysis of 24 month observational data. *Lancet Neurol* 2012 Jan;11(1):42–53.

40. van Duijn E, Kingma EM, van der Mast RC. Psychopathology in verified Huntington's disease gene carriers. *J Neuropsychiatry Clin Neurosci* 2007;19(4):441–8.

41. van Duijn E, Kingma EM, Timman R, Zitman FG, Tibben A, Roos RA, et al. Cross-sectional study on prevalences of psychiatric disorders in mutation carriers of Huntington's disease compared with mutation-negative first-degree relatives. *J Clin Psychiatry* 2008 Nov;69(11):1804–10.

42. Reedeker W, van der Mast RC, Giltay EJ, Kooistra TA, Roos RA, van Duijn E. Psychiatric disorders in Huntington's disease: a 2-year follow-up study. *Psychosomatics* 2012 May;53(3):220–9.

43. Anderson KE, Gehl CR, Marder KS, Beglinger LJ, Paulsen JS. Comorbidities of obsessive and compulsive symptoms in Huntington's disease. *J Nerv Ment Dis* 2010 May;198(5):334–8.

44. Craufurd D, Thompson JC, Snowden JS. Behavioral changes in Huntington Disease. *Neuropsychiatry Neuropsychol Behav Neurol* 2001;14(4):219–26.

45. Paulsen JS, Nehl C, Hoth KF, Kanz JE, Benjamin M, Conybeare R, et al. Depression and stages of Huntington's disease. *J Neuropsychiatry Clin Neurosci* 2005;17(4):496–502.

46. Harris EC, Barraclough B. Suicide as an outcome for mental disorders. A meta-analysis. *Br J Psychiatry* 1997 Mar;170:205–28.

47. Nimmagadda SR, Agrawal N, Worrall-Davies A, Markova I, Rickards H. Determinants of irritability in Huntington's disease.

48. Guttman M, Alpay M, Chouinard. Clinical management of psychosis and mood disorders in Huntington's disease. In: Be´dard M-A AYCSFSKA, editor. *Mental and Behavioral Dysfunction in Movement Disorders.Totawa*, New Jersey: Humana; 2002. p. 409–26.

49. Marder K, Zhao H, Myers RH, Cudkowicz M, Kayson E, Kieburtz K, et al. Rate of functional decline in Huntington's disease. *Huntington Study Group. Neurology* 2000 Jan 25;54(2):452–8.

50. Naarding P, Janzing JG, Eling P, van der Werf S, Kremer B. Apathy is not depression in Huntington's disease. *J Neuropsychiatry Clin Neurosci* 2009;21(3):266–70.

51. van Duijn E, Reedeker N, Giltay EJ, Roos RA, van der Mast RC. Correlates of apathy in Huntington's disease. *J Neuropsychiatry Clin Neurosci* 2010;22(3):287–94.

52. Bjorkqvist M, Fex M, Renstrom E, Wierup N, Petersen A, Gil J, et al. The R6/2 transgenic mouse model of Huntington's disease develops diabetes due to deficient beta-cell mass and exocytosis. *Hum Mol Genet* 2005 Mar 1;14(5):565–74.

53. Petersen A, Bjorkqvist M. Hypothalamic-endocrine aspects in Huntington's disease. *Eur J Neurosci* 2006;24(4):961–7.

54. Sathasivam K, Hobbs C, Turmaine M, Mangiarini L, Mahal A, Bertaux F, et al. Formation of polyglutamine inclusions in non-CNS tissue. *Hum Mol Genet* 1999 May;8(5):813–22.

55. Kalliolia E, Silajdzic E, Nambron R, Hill NR, Doshi A, Frost C, et al. Plasma melatonin is reduced in Huntington's disease. *Mov Disord* 2014 Oct;29(12):1511–5.

56. Popovic V, Svetel M, Djurovic M, Petrovic S, Doknic M, Pekic S, et al. Circulating and cerebrospinal fluid ghrelin and leptin: potential role in altered body weight in Huntington's disease. *Eur J Endocrinol* 2004;151(4):451–5.

57. Petersen A, Bjorkqvist M. Hypothalamic-endocrine aspects in Huntington's disease. *Eur J Neurosci* 2006 Aug;24(4):961–7.

58. Wood NI, Goodman AO, van der Burg JM, Gazeau V, Brundin P, Bjorkqvist M, et al. Increased thirst and drinking in Huntington's disease and the R6/2 mouse. *Brain Res Bull* 2008 May 15;76(1-2):70–9.

59. Pratley RE, Salbe AD, Ravussin E, Caviness JN. Higher sedentary energy expenditure in patients with Huntington's disease. *Ann Neurol* 2000 Jan;47(1):64–70.

60. Myers RH, Sax DS, Koroshetz WJ, Mastromauro C, Cupples LA, Kiely DK, et al. Factors associated with slow progression in Huntington's disease. *Arch Neurol* 1991;48(8):800–4.

61. Lalic NM, Maric J, Svetel M, Jotic A, Stefanova E, Lalic K, et al. Glucose homeostasis in Huntington disease: abnormalities in insulin sensitivity and early-phase insulin secretion. *Arch Neurol* 2008 Apr;65(4):476–80.

62. Farrer LA. Diabetes mellitus in Huntington disease. *Clin Genet* 1985 Jan;27(1):62–7.

63. Podolsky S, Leopold NA, Sax DS. Increased frequency of diabetes mellitus in patients with Huntington's chorea. *Lancet* 1972 Jun 24;1(7765):1356–8.

64. Boesgaard TW, Nielsen TT, Josefsen K, Hansen T, Jorgensen T, Pedersen O, et al. Huntington's disease does not appear to increase the risk of diabetes mellitus. *J Neuroendocrinol* 2009 Sep;21(9):770–6.

65. Farrer LA, Meaney FJ. An anthropometric assessment of Huntington's disease patients and families. *Am J Phys Anthropol* 1985 Jul;67(3):185–94.

66. Lodi R, Schapira AHV, Manners D, Styles P, Wood NW, Taylor DJ, et al. Abnormal in vivo skeletal muscle energy metabolism in Huntington's disease and dentatorubropallidoluysian atrophy. *Ann Neurol* 2000;48(1):72–6.

67. Goodman AO, Barker RA. Body composition in premanifest Huntington's disease reveals lower bone density compared to controls. *PLoS Curr* 2011;3:RRN1214.

68. Lanska DJ, Lanska MJ, Lavine L, Schoenberg BS. Conditions associated with Huntington's disease at death. *A case-control study. Arch Neurol* 1988 Aug;45(8):878–80.

69. Lanska DJ, Lavine L, Lanska MJ, Schoenberg BS. Huntington's disease mortality in the United States. *Neurology* 1988;38(5):769.

70. Kiriazis H, Jennings NL, Davern P, Lambert G, Su Y, Pang T, et al. Neurocardiac dysregulation and neurogenic arrhythmias in a transgenic mouse model of Huntington's disease. *J Physiol* 2012 Nov 15;590(Pt 22):5845–60.

71. Mihm MJ, Amann DM, Schanbacher BL, Altschuld RA, Bauer JA, Hoyt KR. Cardiac dysfunction in the R6/2 mouse model of Huntington's disease. *Neurobiol Dis* 2007 Feb;25(2):297–308.

72. Fedoroff JP, Peyser C, Franz ML, Folstein SE. Sexual disorders in Huntington's disease. *J Neuropsychiatry Clin Neurosci* 1994;6(2):147–53.

73. Markianos M, Panas M, Kalfakis N, Vassilopoulos D. Plasma testosterone in male patients with Huntington's disease: relations to severity of illness and dementia. *Ann Neurol* 2005 Apr;57(4):520–5.

74. Van Raamsdonk JM, Murphy Z, Selva DM, Hamidizadeh R, Pearson J, Petersen A, et al. Testicular degeneration in Huntington disease. *Neurobiol Dis* 2007 Jun;26(3):512–20.

75. Salomonczyk D, Panzera R, Pirogovsky E, Goldstein J, Corey-Bloom J, Simmons R, et al. Impaired postural stability as a marker of premanifest Huntington's disease. *Mov Disord* 2010 Oct 30;25(14):2428–33.

76. Biglan KM, Ross CA, Langbehn DR, Aylward EH, Stout JC, Queller S, et al. Motor abnormalities in premanifest persons with Huntington's disease: the PREDICT-HD study. *Mov Disord* 2009 Sep 15;24(12):1763–72.

77. Paulsen JS, Hayden M, Stout JC, Langbehn DR, Aylward E, Ross CA, et al. Preparing for preventive clinical trials: the Predict-HD study. *Arch Neurol* 2006;63(6):883–90.

78. Hart E, Middelkoop H, Jurgens CK, Witjes-Ane MN, Roos RA. Seven-year clinical follow-up of premanifest carriers of Huntington's disease. *PLoS Curr* 2011;3:RRN1288.

79. Henley SM, Novak MJ, Frost C, King J, Tabrizi SJ, Warren JD. Emotion recognition in Huntington's disease: a systematic review. *Neurosci Biobehav Rev* 2012 Jan;36(1):237–53.

80. Duff K, Paulsen JS, Beglinger LJ, Langbehn DR, Stout JC. Psychiatric symptoms in Huntington's disease before diagnosis: the predict-HD study. *Biol Psychiatry* 2007 Dec 15;62(12):1341–6.

81. Julien CL, Thompson JC, Wild S, Yardumian P, Snowden JS, Turner G, et al. Psychiatric disorders in preclinical Huntington's disease. *J Neurol Neurosurg Psychiatry* 2007 Sep;78(9):939–43.

82. Tabrizi SJ, Langbehn DR, Leavitt BR, Roos RA, Durr A, Craufurd D, et al. Biological and clinical manifestations of Huntington's disease in the longitudinal TRACK-HD study: cross-sectional analysis of baseline data. *Lancet Neurol* 2009 Sep;8(9):791–801.

83. Bjorkqvist M, Wild EJ, Thiele J, Silvestroni A, Andre R, Lahiri N, et al. A novel pathogenic pathway of immune activation detectable before clinical onset in Huntington's disease. *J Exp Med* 2008 Aug 4;205(8):1869–77.

84. Tai YF, Pavese N, Gerhard A, Tabrizi SJ, Barker RA, Brooks DJ, et al. Microglial activation in presymptomatic Huntington's disease gene carriers. *Brain* 2007 Jul;130(Pt 7):1759–66.

85. James CM, Houlihan GD, Snell RG, Cheadle JP, Harper PS. Late-onset Huntington's disease: a clinical and molecular study. *Age Ageing* 1994 Nov;23(6):445–8.

86. Kremer B, Squitieri F, Telenius H, Andrew SE, Theilmann J, Spence N, et al. Molecular analysis of late onset Huntington's disease. *J Med Genet* 1993 Dec;30(12):991–5.

87. Lyon JW. Chronic Hereditary Chorea. America Medical Times 1863;7:289–90.

88. Ribai P, Nguyen K, Hahn-Barma V, Gourfinkel-An I, Vidailhet M, Legout A, et al. Psychiatric and cognitive difficulties as indicators of juvenile huntington disease onset in 29 patients. *Arch Neurol* 2007 Jun;64(6):813–9.

89. Robertson L, Santini H, O'Donovan KL, Squitieri F, Barker RA, Rakowicz M, et al. Current pharmacological management in juvenile Huntington's disease. *PLoS Curr* 2012;4:RRN1304.

90. Gonzalez-Alegre P, Afifi AK. Clinical characteristics of childhood-onset (juvenile) Huntington disease: report of 12 patients and review of the literature. *J Child Neurol* 2006 Mar;21(3):223–9.

91. Westphal C. Ueber eine dem Bilde der cerebrospinalen grauen Degeneration Ahnliche Erkrankung des centralen Nervensystems ohne anatomischen Befund, nebst einigen Bemerkungen über paradoxe Contraction. *Arch Psychiatr Nervenkr* 1883;14(1):87–134.

92. Reuter I, Hu MT, Andrews TC, Brooks DJ, Clough C, Chaudhuri KR. Late onset levodopa responsive Huntington's disease with minimal chorea masquerading as Parkinson plus syndrome. *J Neurol Neurosurg Psychiatry* 2000 Feb;68(2):238–41.

93. Racette BA, Perlmutter JS. Levodopa responsive parkinsonism in an adult with Huntington's disease. *J Neurol Neurosurg Psychiatry* 1998 Oct;65(4):577–9.

94. Albin RL, Reiner A, Anderson KD, Penney JB, Young AB. Striatal and nigral neuron subpopulations in rigid Huntington's disease: implications for the functional anatomy of chorea and rigidity-akinesia. *Ann Neurol* 1990 Apr;27(4):357–65.

95. Bugiani O, Tabaton M, Cammarata S. Huntington's disease: survival of large striatal neurons in the rigid variant. *Ann Neurol* 1984 Feb;15(2):154–6.

96. Almqvist EW, Elterman DS, MacLeod PM, Hayden MR. High incidence rate and absent family histories in one quarter of patients newly diagnosed with Huntington disease in British Columbia. *Clin Genet* 2001 Sep;60(3):198–205.

97. Lefaucheur JP, Menard-Lefaucheur I, Maison P, Baudic S, Cesaro P, Peschanski M, et al. Electrophysiological deterioration over time in patients with Huntington's disease. *Mov Disord* 2006 Sep;21(9):1350–4.

98. Mestre T, Ferreira J, Coelho MM, Rosa M, Sampaio C. Therapeutic interventions for disease progression in Huntington's disease. *Cochrane Database Syst Rev* 2009;(3):CD006455.

99. Sackley C, Hoppitt TJ, Calvert M, Gill P, Eaton B, Yao G, et al. Huntington's disease: current epidemiology and pharmacological management in UK primary care. *Neuroepidemiology* 2011;37(3-4):216–21.

100. Mestre T, Ferreira J, Coelho MM, Rosa M, Sampaio C. Therapeutic interventions for symptomatic treatment in Huntington's disease. *Cochrane Database Syst Rev* 2009;(3):CD006456.

101. Huntington Study Group. Tetrabenazine as antichorea therapy in Huntington disease: a randomized controlled trial. *Neurology* 2006 Feb 14;66(3):366–72.

102. Frank S. Tetrabenazine as anti-chorea therapy in Huntington disease: an open-label continuation study. *Huntington Study Group/TETRA-HD Investigators. BMC Neurol* 2009;9:62.

103. Droll K, Bruce-Mensah K, Otton SV, Gaedigk A, Sellers EM, Tyndale RF. Comparison of three CYP2D6 probe substrates and genotype in Ghanaians, Chinese and Caucasians. *Pharmacogenetics* 1998 Aug;8(4):325–33.

104. Xenazine (tetrabenazine) package insert, Deerfield,IL: Lundbeck,Inc. 2009.

105. Deroover J, Baro F, Bourguignon RP, Smets P. Tiapride versus placebo: a double-blind comparative study in the management of Huntington's chorea. *Curr Med Res Opin* 1984;9(5):329–38.

106. Reveley MA, Dursun SM, Andrews H. Improvement of abnormal saccadic eye movements in Huntington's disease by sulpiride: a case study. *J Psychopharmacol* 1994 Jan;8(4):262–5.

107. Reveley MA, Dursun SM, Andrews H. A comparative trial use of sulpiride and risperidone in Huntington's disease: a pilot study. *J Psychopharmacol* 1996 Jan;10(2):162–5.

108. Quinn N, Marsden CD. A double blind trial of sulpiride in Huntington's disease and tardive dyskinesia. *J Neurol Neurosurg Psychiatry* 1984 Aug;47(8):844–7.

109. van Vugt JP, Siesling S, Vergeer M, van der Velde EA, Roos RA. Clozapine versus placebo in Huntington's disease: a double blind randomised comparative study. *J Neurol Neurosurg Psychiatry* 1997 Jul;63(1):35–9.

110. Landwehrmeyer GB, Dubois B, de Yebenes JG, Kremer B, Gaus W, Kraus PH, et al. Riluzole in Huntington's disease: a 3-year, randomized controlled study. *Ann Neurol* 2007 Sep;62(3):262–72.

111. Magnet MK, Bonelli RM, Kapfhammer HP. Amantadine in the akinetic-rigid variant of Huntington's disease. *Ann Pharmacother* 2004 Jul;38(7-8):1194–6.

112. Dahlen P, Hofman-Bang T. The HART study with Huntexil shows significant effect on total motor function in patients with Huntington's disease although it did not meet the primary endpoint after 12 weeks of treatment. *Neurosearch, editor.* 2012. 14-10-2010.

113. de Yebenes JG, Landwehrmeyer B, Squitieri F, Reilmann R, Rosser A, Barker RA, et al. Pridopidine for the treatment of motor function in patients with Huntington's disease (MermaiHD): a phase 3, randomised, double-blind, placebo-controlled trial. *Lancet Neurol* 2011 Dec 1;10(12):1049–57.

114. Novak MJ, Tabrizi SJ. Huntington's disease. *Bmj* 2010;340:c3109.

115. Cubo E, Shannon KM, Tracy D, Jaglin JA, Bernard BA, Wuu J, et al. Effect of donepezil on motor and cognitive function in Huntington disease. *Neurology* 2006 Oct10;67(7):1268–71.

116. de Tommaso M, Difruscolo O, Sciruicchio V, Specchio N, Livrea P. Two years' follow-up of rivastigmine treatment in Huntington disease. *Clin Neuropharmacol* 2007 Jan;30(1):43–6.

117. Milnerwood AJ, Gladding CM, Pouladi MA, Kaufman AM, Hines RM, Boyd JD, et al. Early increase in extrasynaptic NMDA receptor signaling and expression contributes to phenotype onset in Huntington's disease mice. *Neuron* 2010 Jan 28;65(2):178–90.

118. Silver A. Cognitive-behavioural therapy with a Huntington's gene positive patient. *Patient Educ Couns* 2003 Feb;49(2):133–8.

119. Special Focus: A standard of care for Huntington's disease. *Neurodegenerative Disease Management* 2012;2(1):1–87.

120. Heemskerk AW, Roos RA. Aspiration pneumonia and death in Huntington's disease. *PLoS Curr* 2012;4:RRN1293.

121. Gusella JF, Wexler NS, Conneally PM, Naylor SL, Anderson MA, Tanzi RE, et al. A polymorphic DNA marker genetically linked to Huntington's disease. *Nature* 1983 Nov 17;306(5940):234–8.

122. Ambrose CM, Duyao MP, Barnes G, Bates GP, Lin CS, Srinidhi J, et al. Structure and expression of the Huntington's disease gene: evidence against simple inactivation due to an expanded CAG repeat 1. *Somat Cell Mol Genet* 1994 Jan;20(1):27–38.

123. Hoogeveen AT, Willemsen R, Meyer N, de Rooij KE, Roos RA, van Ommen GJ, et al. Characterization and localization of the Huntington disease gene product. *Hum Mol Genet* 1993 Dec;2(12):2069–73.

124. Rubinsztein DC, Amos W, Leggo J, Goodburn S, Ramesar RS, Old J, et al. Mutational bias provides a model for the evolution of Huntington's disease and predicts a general increase in disease prevalence. *Nat Genet* 1994 Aug;7(4):525–30.

125. Duyao MP, Auerbach AB, Ryan A, Persichetti F, Barnes GT, McNeil SM, et al. Inactivation of the mouse Huntington's disease gene homolog Hdh. *Science* 1995;269(5222):407–10.

126. Kremer B, Almqvist E, Theilmann J, Spence N, Telenius H, Goldberg YP, et al. Sex-dependent mechanisms for expansions and contractions of the CAG repeat on affected Huntington disease chromosomes. *Am J Hum Genet* 1995;57(2):343–50.

127. Ranen NG, Stine OC, Abbott MH, Sherr M, Codori AM, Franz ML, et al. Anticipation and instability of IT-15 (CAG)n repeats in parent-offspring pairs with Huntington disease. *Am J Hum Genet* 1995;57(3):593–602.

128. Zuhlke C, Riess O, Bockel B, Lange H, Thies U. Mitotic stability and meiotic variability of the (CAG)n repeat in the Huntington disease gene. *Hum Mol Genet* 1993;2(12):2063–7.

129. Pearson CE. Slipping while sleeping? Trinucleotide repeat expansions in germ cells. *Trends Mol Med* 2003;9(11):490–5.

130. Goldberg YP, McMurray CT, Zeisler J, Almqvist E, Sillence D, Richards F, et al. Increased instability of intermediate alleles in families with sporadic Huntington disease compared to similar sized intermediate alleles in the general population 1. *Hum Mol Genet* 1995 Oct;4(10):1911–8.

131. Rubinsztein DC, Leggo J, Coles R, Almqvist E, Biancalana V, Cassiman JJ, et al. Phenotypic characterization of individuals with 30-40 CAG repeats in the Huntington disease (HD) gene reveals HD cases with 36 repeats and apparently normal elderly individuals with 36-39 repeats. *Am J Hum Genet* 1996;59(1):16–22.

132. Semaka A, Warby S, Leavitt BR, Hayden MR. Re: Autopsy-proven Huntington's disease with 29 trinucleotide repeats. *Mov Disord* 2008;23(12):1794–5.

133. Kenney C, Powell S, Jankovic J. Autopsy-proven Huntington's disease with 29 trinucleotide repeats. *Mov Disord* 2007;22(1):127–30.

134. Duyao M, Ambrose C, Myers R, Novelletto A, Persichetti F, Frontali M, et al. Trinucleotide repeat length instability and age of onset in Huntington's disease. *Nat Genet* 1993;4(4):387–92.

135. Snell RG, Macmillan JC, Cheadle JP, Fenton I, Lazarou LP, Davies P, et al. Relationship between trinucleotide repeat expansion and phenotypic variation in Huntington's disease. *Nat Genet* 1993;4(4):393–7.

136. Langbehn DR, Brinkman RR, Falush D, Paulsen JS, Hayden MR. A new model for prediction of the age of onset and penetrance for Huntington's disease based on CAG length. *Clin Genet* 2004;65(4):267–77.

137. Penney JB, Jr., Vonsattel JP, MacDonald ME, Gusella JF, Myers RH. CAG repeat number governs the development rate of pathology in Huntington's disease. *Ann Neurol* 1997;41(5):689–92.

138. Li JL, Hayden MR, Warby SC, Durr A, Morrison PJ, Nance M, et al. Genome-wide significance for a modifier of age at neurological onset in Huntington's disease at 6q23-24: the HD MAPS study. *BMC Med Genet* 2006;7:71.

139. Anca MH, Gazit E, Loewenthal R, Ostrovsky O, Frydman M, Giladi N. Different phenotypic expression in monozygotic twins with Huntington disease. *Am J Med Genet A* 2004 Jan 1;124A(1):89–91.

140. Georgiou N, Bradshaw JL, Chiu E, Tudor A, O'Gorman L, Phillips JG. Differential clinical and motor control function in a pair of monozygotic twins with Huntington's disease. *Mov Disord* 1999 Mar;14(2):320–5.

141. Wexler NS, Young AB, Tanzi RE, Travers H, Starosta-Rubinstein S, Penney JB, et al. Homozygotes for Huntington's disease. *Nature* 1987;326(6109):194–7.

142. Wexler NS. Venezuelan kindreds reveal that genetic and environmental factors modulate Huntington's disease age of onset. *Proc Natl Acad Sci USA* 2004 Mar 9;101(10):3498–503.

143. Taherzadeh-Fard E, Saft C, Andrich J, Wieczorek S, Arning L. PGC-1alpha as modifier of onset age in Huntington disease. *Mol Neurodegener* 2009;4:10.

144. Metzger S, Rong J, Nguyen HP, Cape A, Tomiuk J, Soehn AS, et al. Huntingtin-associated protein-1 is a modifier of the age-at-onset of Huntington's disease. *Hum Mol Genet* 2008 Apr 15;17(8):1137–46.

145. Li XJ, Friedman M, Li S. Interacting proteins as genetic modifiers of Huntington disease. *Trends Genet* 2007 Nov;23(11):531–3.

146. Lee JH, Lee JM, Ramos EM, Gillis T, Mysore JS, Kishikawa S, et al. TAA repeat variation in the GRIK2 gene does not influence age at onset in Huntington's disease. *Biochem Biophys Res Commun* 2012 Aug;424(3):404–8.

147. Lee JM, Gillis T, Mysore JS, Ramos EM, Myers RH, Hayden MR, et al. Common SNP-based haplotype analysis of the 4p16.3 Huntington disease gene region. *Am J Hum Genet* 2012 Mar 9;90(3):434–44.

148. Lee JM, Ramos EM, Lee JH, Gillis T, Mysore JS, Hayden MR, et al. CAG repeat expansion in Huntington disease determines age at onset in a fully dominant fashion. *Neurology* 2012 Mar 6;78(10):690–5.

149. International Huntington Association (IHA) and the WorldFederation of Neurology (WFN) Research Group on Huntington's Chorea. *Guidelines for the molecular genetics predictive test in Huntington's disease. Neurology* 1994 Aug;44(8):1533–6.

150. Harper PS, Newcombe RG. Age at onset and life table risks in genetic counselling for Huntington's disease. *J Med Genet* 1992 Apr;29(4):239–42.

151. Bloch M, Adam S, Wiggins S, Huggins M, Hayden MR. Predictive testing for Huntington disease in Canada: the experience of those receiving an increased risk. *Am J Med Genet* 1992 Feb 15;42(4):499–507.

152. Hayden MR, Bloch M, Wiggins S. Psychological effects of predictive testing for Huntington's disease. *Adv Neurol* 1995;65:201–10.

153. Meiser B, Dunn S. Psychological impact of genetic testing for Huntington's disease: an update of the literature. *J Neurol Neurosurg Psychiatry* 2000 Nov;69(5):574–8.

154. Macleod R, Tibben A, Frontali M, Evers-Kiebooms G, Jones A, Martinez-Descales A, et al. Recommendations for the predictive genetic test in Huntington's disease. *Clin Genet* 2013;83:221–31.

155. British Medical Association. Human Genetics: Choice and Responsibility.Oxford: Oxford University Press; 2012. p. 236.

156. Harper PS, Lim C, Craufurd D. Ten years of presymptomatic testing for Huntington's disease: the experience of the UK Huntington's Disease Prediction Consortium 1. *J Med Genet* 2000 Aug;37(8):567–71.

157. Simpson SA, Zoeteweij MW, Nys K, Harper P, Durr A, Jacopini G, et al. Prenatal testing for Huntington's disease: a European collaborative study. *Eur J Hum Genet* 2002 Nov;10(11):689–93.

158. Beglinger LJ, Prest L, Mills JA, Paulsen JS, Smith MM, Gonzalez-Alegre P, et al. Clinical predictors of driving status in Huntington's disease. *Mov Disord* 2012 Aug;27(9):1146–52.

159. Mann DM, Oliver R, Snowden JS. The topographic distribution of brain atrophy in Huntington's disease and progressive supranuclear palsy. *Acta Neuropathol* 1993;85(5):553–9.

160. Paulsen JS, Hoth KF, Nehl C, Stierman L. Critical periods of suicide risk in Huntington's disease. *Am J Psychiatry* 2005 Apr;162(4):725–31.

161. Jeste DV, Barban L, Parisi J. Reduced Purkinje cell density in Huntington's disease. *Exp Neurol* 1984;85(1):78–86.

162. Kremer HP, Roos RA, Dingjan GM, Bots GT, Bruyn GW, Hofman MA. The hypothalamic lateral tuberal nucleus and the characteristics of neuronal loss in Huntington's disease. *Neurosci Lett* 1991;132(1):101–4.

163. Spargo E, Everall IP, Lantos PL. Neuronal loss in the hippocampus in Huntington's disease: a comparison with HIV infection. *J Neurol Neurosurg Psychiatry* 1993;56:487–91.

164. Macdonald V, Halliday GM, Trent RJ, McCusker EA. Significant loss of pyramidal neurons in the angular gyrus of patients with Huntington's disease. *Neuropathol Appl Neurobiol* 1997 Dec;23(6):492–5.

165. Macdonald V, Halliday G. Pyramidal cell loss in motor cortices in Huntington's disease. *Neurobiol Dis* 2002 Aug;10(3):378–86.

166. Heinsen H, Rub U, Bauer M, Ulmar G, Bethke B, Schuler M, et al. Nerve cell loss in the thalamic mediodorsal nucleus in Huntington's disease. *Acta Neuropathol* 1999 Jun;97(6):613–22.

167. Tabrizi SJ, Reilmann R, Roos RA, Durr A, Leavitt B, Owen G, et al. Potential endpoints for clinical trials in premanifest and early Huntington's disease in the TRACK-HD study: analysis of 24 month observational data. *Lancet Neurol* 2012 Jan;11(1):42–53.

168. Paulsen JS, Nopoulos PC, Aylward E, Ross CA, Johnson H, Magnotta VA, et al. Striatal and white matter predictors of estimated diagnosis for Huntington disease. *Brain Res Bull* 2010 May 31;82(3-4):201–7.

169. Rosas HD, Hevelone ND, Zaleta AK, Greve DN, Salat DH, Fischl B. Regional cortical thinning in preclinical Huntington disease and its relationship to cognition. *Neurology* 2005;65(5):745–7.

170. DiProspero NA, Chen EY, Charles V, Plomann M, Kordower JH, Tagle DA. Early changes in Huntington's disease patient brains involve alterations in cytoskeletal and synaptic elements. *J Neurocytol* 2004 Sep;33(5):517–33.

171. Modregger J, DiProspero NA, Charles V, Tagle DA, Plomann M. PACSIN 1 interacts with huntingtin and is absent from synaptic varicosities in presymptomatic Huntington's disease brains. *Hum Mol Genet* 2002 Oct 1;11(21):2547–58.

172. DiFiglia M, Sapp E, Chase KO, Davies SW, Bates GP, Vonsattel JP, et al. Aggregation of huntingtin in neuronal intranuclear inclusions and dystrophic neurites in brain. *Science* 1997 Sep 26;277(5334):1990–3.

173. Saudou F, Finkbeiner S, Devys D, Greenberg ME. Huntingtin acts in the nucleus to induce apoptosis but death does not correlate with the formation of intranuclear inclusions. *Cell* 1998 Oct 2;95(1):55–66.

174. Vonsattel JP, Myers RH, Stevens TJ, Ferrante RJ, Bird ED, Richardson EP, Jr. Neuropathological classification of Huntington's disease. *J Neuropathol Exp Neurol* 1985;44(6):559–77.

175. Li W, Serpell LC, Carter WJ, Rubinsztein DC, Huntington JA. Expression and characterization of full-length human huntingtin, an elongated HEAT repeat protein. *J Biol Chem* 2006 Jun 9;281(23):15916–22.

176. Li SH, Li XJ. Huntingtin-protein interactions and the pathogenesis of Huntington's disease. *Trends Genet* 2004 Mar;20(3):146–54.

177. Cattaneo E, Zuccato C, Tartari M. Normal huntingtin function: an alternative approach to Huntington's disease. *Nat Rev Neurosci* 2005 Dec;6(12):919–30.

178. Walker FO. Huntington's disease. *Lancet* 2007 Jan 20;369(9557):218–28.

179. Young AB. Huntingtin in health and disease. *J Clin Invest* 2003 Feb;111(3): 299–302.

180. Yanai A, Huang K, Kang R, Singaraja RR, Arstikaitis P, Gan L, et al. Palmitoylation of huntingtin by HIP14 is essential for its trafficking and function. *Nat Neurosci* 2006 Jun;9(6):824–31.

181. Sadri-Vakili G, Cha JH. Mechanisms of disease: Histone modifications in Huntington's disease. *Nat Clin Pract Neurol* 2006 Jun;2(6):330–8.

182. Savas JN, Ma B, Deinhardt K, Culver BP, Restituito S, Wu L, et al. A role for huntington disease protein in dendritic RNA granules. *J Biol Chem* 2010 Apr 23;285(17):13142–53.

183. Tobin AJ, Signer ER. Huntington's disease: the challenge for cell biologists. *Trends Cell Biol* 2000 Dec;10(12):531–6.

184. Shao J, Diamond MI. Polyglutamine diseases: emerging concepts in pathogenesis and therapy. *Hum Mol Genet* 2007 Oct 15;16 Spec No. 2:R115–R123.

185. Molero AE, Gokhan S, Gonzalez S, Feig JL, Alexandre LC, Mehler MF. Impairment of developmental stem cell-mediated striatal neurogenesis and pluripotency genes in a knock-in model of Huntington's disease. *Proc Natl Acad Sci U S A* 2009 Dec 22;106(51):21900–5.

186. Shin JY, Fang ZH, Yu ZX, Wang CE, Li SH, Li XJ. Expression of mutant huntingtin in glial cells contributes to neuronal excitotoxicity. *J Cell Biol* 2005;171(6):1001–12.

187. Bradford J, Shin JY, Roberts M, Wang CE, Sheng G, Li S, et al. Mutant huntingtin in glial cells exacerbates neurological symptoms of Huntington disease mice. *J Biol Chem* 2010 Apr 2;285(14):10653–61.

188. Wanker E, Droge R. Structural biology of Huntington's disease. In: Bates G, Harper PS, Jones L, editors. *Huntington's Disease*. Third ed. Oxford: Oxford University Press; 2002. p. 327–47.

189. Gafni J, Papanikolaou T, Degiacomo F, Holcomb J, Chen S, Menalled L, et al. Caspase-6 activity in a BACHD mouse modulates steady-state levels of mutant huntingtin protein but is not necessary for production of a 586 amino acid proteolytic fragment. *J Neurosci* 2012 May30;32(22):7454–65.

190. Cowan CM, Fan MM, Fan J, Shehadeh J, Zhang LY, Graham RK, et al. Polyglutamine-modulated striatal calpain activity in YAC transgenic huntington disease mouse model: impact on NMDA receptor function and toxicity. *J Neurosci* 2008 Nov 26;28(48):12725–35.

191. Williams A, Sarkar S, Cuddon P, Ttofi EK, Saiki S, Siddiqi FH, et al. Novel targets for Huntington's disease in an mTOR-independent autophagy pathway. *Nat Chem Biol* 2008;4(5):295–305.

192. Gu X, Greiner ER, Mishra R, Kodali R, Osmand A, Finkbeiner S, et al. Serines 13 and 16 are critical determinants of full-length human mutant huntingtin induced disease pathogenesis in HD mice. *Neuron* 2009 Dec 24;64(6):828–40.

193. Aiken CT, Steffan JS, Guerrero CM, Khashwji H, Lukacsovich T, Simmons D, et al. Phosphorylation of threonine 3: implications for Huntingtin aggregation and neurotoxicity. *J Biol Chem* 2009 Oct 23;284(43):29427–36.

194. Thompson LM, Aiken CT, Kaltenbach LS, Agrawal N, Illes K, Khoshnan A, et al. IKK phosphorylates Huntingtin and targets it for degradation by the proteasome and lysosome. *J Cell Biol* 2009 Dec 28;187(7):1083–99.

195. Wang Y, Lin F, Qin ZH. The role of post-translational modifications of huntingtin in the pathogenesis of Huntington's disease. *Neurosci Bull* 2010 Apr;26(2):153–62.

196. Warby SC, Doty CN, Graham RK, Shively J, Singaraja RR, Hayden MR. Phosphorylation of huntingtin reduces the accumulation of its nuclear fragments. *Mol Cell Neurosci* 2009 Feb;40(2):121–7.

197. Jeong H, Then F, Melia TJ, Jr., Mazzulli JR, Cui L, Savas JN, et al. Acetylation targets mutant huntingtin to autophagosomes for degradation. *Cell* 2009 Apr 3;137(1):60–72.

198. Bennett EJ, Bence NF, Jayakumar R, Kopito RR. Global impairment of the ubiquitin-proteasome system by nuclear or cytoplasmic protein aggregates precedes inclusion body formation. *Mol Cell* 2005 Feb 4;17(3):351–65.

199. Bennett EJ, Shaler TA, Woodman B, Ryu KY, Zaitseva TS, Becker CH, et al. Global changes to the ubiquitin system in Huntington's disease. *Nature* 2007 Aug 9;448(7154):704–8.

200. Kaganovich D, Kopito R, Frydman J. Misfolded proteins partition between two distinct quality control compartments. *Nature* 2008 Aug 28;454(7208):1088–95.

201. Martinez-Vicente M, Talloczy Z, Wong E, Tang G, Koga H, Kaushik S, et al. Cargo recognition failure is responsible for inefficient autophagy in Huntington's disease. *Nat Neurosci* 2010 May;13(5):567–76.

202. Li X, Wang CE, Huang S, Xu X, Li XJ, Li H, et al. Inhibiting the ubiquitin-proteasome system leads to preferential accumulation of toxic N-terminal mutant huntingtin fragments. *Hum Mol Genet* 2010 Jun 15;19(12):2445–55.

203. Steffan JS, Bodai L, Pallos J, Poelman M, McCampbell A, Apostol BL, et al. Histone deacetylase inhibitors arrest polyglutamine-dependent neurodegeneration in Drosophila. *Nature* 2001 Oct 18;413(6857):739–43.

204. Sugars KL, Rubinsztein DC. Transcriptional abnormalities in Huntington disease. *Trends Genet* 2003;19(5):233–8.

205. Benn CL, Sun T, Sadri-Vakili G, McFarland KN, DiRocco DP, Yohrling GJ, et al. Huntingtin modulates transcription, occupies gene promoters in vivo, and binds directly to DNA in a polyglutamine-dependent manner. *J Neurosci* 2008;28(42):10720–33.

206. Hodges A, Strand AD, Aragaki AK, Kuhn A, Sengstag T, Hughes G, et al. Regional and cellular gene expression changes in human Huntington's disease brain. *Hum Mol Genet* 2006;15(6):965–77.

207. Luthi-Carter R, Strand A, Peters NL, Solano SM, Hollingsworth ZR, Menon AS, et al. Decreased expression of striatal signaling genes in a mouse model of Huntington's disease. *Hum Mol Genet* 2000 May 22;9(9):1259–71.

208. Cha JH, Frey AS, Alsdorf SA, Kerner JA, Kosinski CM, Mangiarini L, et al. Altered brain neurotransmitter receptor expression in transgenic mouse models of Huntington's disease. *Philos Trans R Soc Lond B Biol Sci* 1999 Jun 29;354(1386):981–9.

209. Cha JH. Transcriptional dysregulation in Huntington's disease. *Trends Neurosci* 2000;23(9):387–92.

210. Zuccato C, Ciammola A, Rigamonti D, Leavitt BR, Goffredo D, Conti L, et al. Loss of huntingtin-mediated BDNF gene transcription in Huntington's disease. *Science* 2001 Jul 20;293(5529):493–8.

211. Browne SE. Mitochondria and Huntington's disease pathogenesis: insight from genetic and chemical models. *Ann N Y Acad Sci* 2008 Dec;1147:358–82.

212. Imarisio S, Carmichael J, Korolchuk V, Chen CW, Saiki S, Rose C, et al. Huntington's disease: from pathology and genetics to potential therapies. *Biochem J* 2008 Jun 1;412(2):191–209.

213. Duan W, Guo Z, Jiang H, Ware M, Li XJ, Mattson MP. Dietary restriction normalizes glucose metabolism and BDNF levels, slows disease progression, and increases survival in huntingtin mutant mice. *PNAS* 2003;100(5):2911–6.

214. Weydt P, Pineda VV, Torrence AE, Libby RT, Satterfield TF, Lazarowski ER, et al. Thermoregulatory and metabolic defects in Huntington's disease transgenic mice implicate PGC-1alpha in Huntington's disease neurodegeneration. *Cell Metab* 2006 Nov;4(5):349–62.

215. Cui L, Jeong H, Borovecki F, Parkhurst CN, Tanese N, Krainc D. Transcriptional repression of PGC-1alpha by mutant huntingtin leads to mitochondrial dysfunction and neurodegeneration. *Cell* 2006 Oct 6;127(1):59–69.

216. Trushina E, Dyer RB, Badger JD, Ure D, Eide L, Tran DD, et al. Mutant huntingtin impairs axonal trafficking in mammalian neurons in vivo and in vitro. *Mol Cell Biol* 2004 Sep;24(18):8195–209.

217. Gauthier LR, Charrin BC, Borrell-Pages M, Dompierre JP, Rangone H, Cordelieres FP, et al. Huntingtin controls neurotrophic support and survival of neurons by enhancing BDNF vesicular transport along microtubules. *Cell* 2004 Jul 9;118(1):127–38.

218. Arenas J, Campos Y, Ribacoba R, Martin MA, Rubio JC, Ablanedo P, et al. Complex I defect in muscle from patients with Huntington's disease. *Ann Neurol* 1998 Mar;43(3):397–400.

219. Costa V, Giacomello M, Hudec R, Lopreiato R, Ermak G, Lim D, et al. Mitochondrial fission and cristae disruption increase the response of cell models of Huntington's disease to apoptotic stimuli. *EMBO Mol Med* 2010 Dec;2(12):490–503.

220. Song W, Chen J, Petrilli A, Liot G, Klinglmayr E, Zhou Y, et al. Mutant huntingtin binds the mitochondrial fission GTPase dynamin-related protein-1 and increases its enzymatic activity. *Nat Med* 2011 Mar;17(3):377–82.

221. Panov AV, Gutekunst CA, Leavitt BR, Hayden MR, Burke JR, Strittmatter WJ, et al. Early mitochondrial calcium defects in Huntington's disease are a direct effect of polyglutamines. *Nat Neurosci* 2002;5(8):731–6.

222. Chaturvedi RK, Adhihetty P, Shukla S, Hennessy T, Calingasan N, Yang L, et al. Impaired PGC-1 alpha function in muscle in Huntington's disease. *Hum Mol Genet* 2009 Aug 15;18(16):3048–65.

223. Phan J, Hickey MA, Zhang P, Chesselet MF, Reue K. Adipose tissue dysfunction tracks disease progression in two Huntington's disease mouse models. *Hum Mol Genet* 2009 Mar 15;18(6):1006–16.

224. Coyle JT, Schwarcz R. Lesion of striatal neurones with kainic acid provides a model for Huntington's chorea. *Nature* 1976 Sep 16;263(5574):244–6.

225. McGeer EG, McGeer PL. Duplication of biochemical changes of Huntington's chorea by intrastriatal injections of glutamic and kainic acids. *Nature* 1976 Oct 7;263(5577):517–9.

226. Albin RL, Young AB, Penney JB, Handelin B, Balfour R, Anderson KD, et al. Abnormalities of striatal projection neurons and N-methyl-D-aspartate receptors in presymptomatic Huntington's disease. *N Engl J Med* 1990 May 3;322(18):1293–8.

227. Young AB, Greenamyre JT, Hollingsworth Z, Albin R, D'Amato C, Shoulson I, et al. NMDA receptor losses in putamen from patients with Huntington's disease. *Science* 1988 Aug 19;241(4868):981–3.

228. Standaert DG, Friberg IK, Landwehrmeyer GB, Young AB, Penney JB, Jr. Expression of NMDA glutamate receptor subunit mRNAs in neurochemically identified projection and interneurons in the striatum of the rat. *Brain Res Mol Brain Res* 1999 Jan 22;64(1):11–23.

229. Rigby M, Le Bourdelles B, Heavens RP, Kelly S, Smith D, Butler A, et al. The messenger RNAs for the N-methyl-D-aspartate receptor subunits show region-specific expression of different subunit composition in the human brain. *Neuroscience* 1996 Jul;73(2):429–47.

230. Landwehrmeyer GB, McNeil SM, Dure LS, Ge P, Aizawa H, Huang Q, et al. Huntington's disease gene: regional and cellular expression in brain of normal and affected individuals. *Ann Neurol* 1995 Feb;37(2):218–30.

231. Ghasemzadeh MB, Sharma S, Surmeier DJ, Eberwine JH, Chesselet MF. Multiplicity of glutamate receptor subunits in single striatal neurons: an RNA amplification study. *Mol Pharmacol* 1996 May;49(5):852–9.

232. Liu Y, Wong TP, Aarts M, Rooyakkers A, Liu L, Lai TW, et al. NMDA receptor subunits have differential roles in mediating excitotoxic neuronal death both in vitro and in vivo. *J Neurosci* 2007 Mar 14;27(11):2846–57.

233. Kim MJ, Dunah AW, Wang YT, Sheng M. Differential roles of NR2A- and NR2B-containing NMDA receptors in Ras-ERK signaling and AMPA receptor trafficking. *Neuron* 2005 Jun 2;46(5):745–60.

234. Raymond LA, Andre VM, Cepeda C, Gladding CM, Milnerwood AJ, Levine MS. Pathophysiology of Huntington's disease: time-dependent alterations in synaptic and receptor function. *Neuroscience* 2011 Dec 15;198:252–73.

235. Giorgini F, Guidetti P, Nguyen Q, Bennett SC, Muchowski PJ. A genomic screen in yeast implicates kynurenine 3-monooxygenase as a therapeutic target for Huntington disease. *Nat Genet* 2005;37(5):526–31.

236. Giorgini F, Moller T, Kwan W, Zwilling D, Wacker JL, Hong S, et al. Histone deacetylase inhibition modulates kynurenine pathway activation in yeast, microglia, and mice expressing a mutant huntingtin fragment. *J Biol Chem* 2008 Mar 21;283(12):7390–400.

237. Park IH, Arora N, Huo H, Maherali N, Ahfeldt T, Shimamura A, et al. Disease-specific induced pluripotent stem cells. *Cell* 2008 Sep 5;134(5):877–86.

238. Kim M, Lee HS, LaForet G, McIntyre C, Martin EJ, Chang P, et al. Mutant huntingtin expression in clonal striatal cells: dissociation of inclusion formation and neuronal survival by caspase inhibition. *J Neurosci* 1999 Feb 1;19(3):964–73.

239. Rigamonti D, Bauer JH, De Fraja C, Conti L, Sipione S, Sciorati C, et al. Wild-type huntingtin protects from apoptosis upstream of caspase-3. *J Neurosci* 2000;20(10):3705–13.

240. Link CD. Transgenic invertebrate models of age-associated neurodegenerative diseases. *Mech Ageing Dev* 2001 Sep 30;122(14):1639–49.

241. Gama Sosa MA, De Gasperi R, Elder GA. Modeling human neurodegenerative diseases in transgenic systems. *Hum Genet* 2012 Apr;131(4):535–63.

242. Jackson GR, Salecker I, Dong X, Yao X, Arnheim N, Faber PW, et al. Polyglutamine-expanded human huntingtin transgenes induce degeneration of Drosophila photoreceptor neurons. *Neuron* 1998 Sep;21(3):633–42.

243. Pallos J, Bodai L, Lukacsovich T, Purcell JM, Steffan JS, Thompson LM, et al. Inhibition of specific HDACs and sirtuins suppresses pathogenesis in a Drosophila model of Huntington's disease. *Hum Mol Genet* 2008 Dec 1;17(23):3767–75.

244. Parker JA, Connolly JB, Wellington C, Hayden M, Dausset J, Neri C. Expanded polyglutamines in Caenorhabditis elegans cause axonal abnormalities and severe dysfunction of PLM mechanosensory neurons without cell death. *Proc Natl Acad Sci U S A* 2001 Nov 6;98(23):13318–23.

245. Faber PW, Alter JR, MacDonald ME, Hart AC. Polyglutamine-mediated dysfunction and apoptotic death of a Caenorhabditis elegans sensory neuron. *Proc Natl Acad Sci U S A* 1999 Jan 5;96(1):179–84.

246. Crook ZR, Housman D. Huntington's disease: can mice lead the way to treatment? Neuron 2011 Feb 10;69(3):423–35.

247. Heng MY, Detloff PJ, Albin RL. Rodent genetic models of Huntington disease. *Neurobiol Dis* 2008;32(1):1–9.

248. Johnson MA, Rajan V, Miller CE, Wightman RM. Dopamine release is severely compromised in the R6/2 mouse model of Huntington's disease. *J Neurochem* 2006 May;97(3):737–46.

249. Strand AD, Baquet ZC, Aragaki AK, Holmans P, Yang L, Cleren C, et al. Expression profiling of Huntington's disease models suggests that brain-derived neurotrophic factor depletion plays a major role in striatal degeneration. *J Neurosci* 2007 Oct 24;27(43):11758–68.

250. Tabrizi S, Workman J, Hart PE, Mangiarini L, Mahal A, Bates G, et al. Mitochondrial dysfunction and free radical damage in the Huntington R6/2 transgenic mouse. *Ann Neurol* 2000 Jan;47(1):80–6.

251. Hodgson JG, Agopyan N, Gutekunst CA, Leavitt BR, LePiane F, Singaraja R, et al. A YAC mouse model for Huntington's disease with full-length mutant huntingtin, cytoplasmic toxicity, and selective striatal neurodegeneration. *Neuron* 1999 May;23(1):181–92.

252. Slow EJ, van Raamsdonk J, Rogers D, Coleman SH, Graham RK, Deng Y, et al. Selective striatal neuronal loss in a YAC128 mouse model of Huntington disease. *Hum Mol Genet* 2003;12(13):1555–67.

253. Zhang J, Peng Q, Li Q, Jahanshad N, Hou Z, Jiang M, et al. Longitudinal characterization of brain atrophy of a Huntington's disease mouse model by automated morphological analyses of magnetic resonance images. *Neuroimage* 2010 Feb 1;49(3):2340–51.

254. Yang SH, Cheng PH, Banta H, Piotrowska-Nitsche K, Yang JJ, Cheng EC, et al. Towards a transgenic model of Huntington's disease in a non-human primate. *Nature* 2008 Jun 12;453(7197):921–4.

255. Weir DW, Sturrock A, Leavitt BR. Development of biomarkers for Huntington's disease. *Lancet Neurol* 2011 Jun;10(6):573–90. (see also http://www.sciencedirect.com/science/article/pii/S1474442211700709 and http://dx.doi.org/10.1016/S1474-4422(11)70070-9)

256. Huntington Study Group. Cooperative Huntington's Observational Research Trial (COHORT). 2012. (see also http://huntingtonstudygroup.org/all-hsg-trials-and-studies/)

257. Paulsen JS, Langbehn DR, Stout JC, Aylward E, Ross CA, Nance M, et al. Detection of Huntington's disease decades before diagnosis: the Predict-HD study. *J Neurol Neurosurg Psychiatry* 2008;79(8):874–80.

258. Euro-HD Network REGISTRY Steering Committee. EHDN REGISTRY Study (in progress). 2003 [cited 2007 Oct 3]; Available from: URL: http://www.euro-hd.net

259. Enroll-HD. A prospective registry study in a global HD cohort. (www.enroll-hd.org). 2012.

260. Orth M, Handley OJ, Schwenke C, Dunnett SB, Craufurd D, Ho AK, et al. Observing Huntington's Disease: the European Huntington's Disease Network's REGISTRY. *PLoS Curr* 2010;2:RRN1184.

261. http://hdclarity.net

262. Huntington Study Group. Unified Huntington's Disease Rating Scale-99. Huntington Study Group: 1999.

263. Meyer C, Landwehrmeyer B, Schwenke C, Doble A, Orth M, Ludolph AC. Rate of change in early Huntington's disease: a clinicometric analysis. *Mov Disord* 2012 Jan;27(1):118–24.

264. Henley SM, Bates GP, Tabrizi SJ. Biomarkers for neurodegenerative diseases. *Curr Opin Neurol* 2005;18(6):698–705.

265. Paulsen JS. Functional imaging in Huntington's disease. *Exp Neurol* 2009 Apr;216(2):272–7.

266. Georgiou-Karistianis N.A peek inside the Huntington's brain: will functional imaging take us one step closer in solving the puzzle? *Exp Neurol* 2009 Nov;220(1):5–8.

267. Sturrock A, Laule C, Decolongon J, Dar SR, Coleman AJ, Creighton S, et al. Magnetic resonance spectroscopy biomarkers in premanifest and early Huntington disease. *Neurology* 2010 Nov 9;75(19):1702–10.

268. Young AB, Penney JB, Starosta-Rubinstein S, Markel DS, Berent S, Giordani B, et al. PET scan investigations of Huntington's disease: cerebral metabolic correlates of neurological features and functional decline. *Ann Neurol* 1986 Sep;20(3):296–303.

269. Kuwert T, Lange HW, Langen KJ, Herzog H, Aulich A, Feinendegen LE. Cortical and subcortical glucose consumption measured by PET in patients with Huntington's disease. *Brain* 1990 Oct;113 (Pt 5):1405–23.

270. Ciarmiello A, Cannella M, Lastoria S, Simonelli M, Frati L, Rubinsztein DC, et al. Brain white-matter volume loss and glucose hypometabolism precede the clinical symptoms of Huntington's disease. *J Nucl Med* 2006 Feb;47(2):215–22.

271. Berent S, Giordani B, Lehtinen S, Markel D, Penney JB, Buchtel HA, et al. Positron emission tomographic scan investigations of Huntington's disease: cerebral metabolic correlates of cognitive function. *Ann Neurol* 1988 Jun;23(6):541–6.

272. Leoni V, Mariotti C, Tabrizi SJ, Valenza M, Wild EJ, Henley SM, et al. Plasma 24S-hydroxycholesterol and caudate MRI in pre-manifest and early Huntington's disease. *Brain* 2008;131(Pt 11):2851–9.

273. Borowsky B. 8OHdG is not a biomarker for Huntington disease state or progression. 2013 May 21.

274. Borovecki F, Lovrecic L, Zhou J, Jeong H, Then F, Rosas HD, et al. Genome-wide expression profiling of human blood reveals biomarkers for Huntington's disease. *Proc Natl Acad Sci USA* 2005;102(31):11023–8.

275. Weiss A, Abramowski D, Bibel M, Bodner R, Chopra V, Difiglia M, et al. Single-step detection of mutant huntingtin in animal and human tissues: a bioassay for Huntington's disease. *Anal Biochem* 2009 Dec 1;395(1):8–15.

276. Björkqvist M, Wild EJ, Thiele J, Silvestroni A, Andre R, Lahiri N, et al. A novel pathogenic pathway of immune activation detectable before clinical onset in Huntington's disease. *J Exp Med* 2008;205:1869–77.

277. Sturrock A, Leavitt BR. The clinical and genetic features of Huntington disease. *J Geriatr Psychiatry Neurol* 2010 Dec;23(4):243–59.

278. Reilmann R, Squitieri F, Priller J. Safety and Tolerability of Selisistat for the Treatment of Huntington's Disease: Results from a Randomized, Double-Blind, Placebo-Controlled Phase II Trial. *Neurology* 2014;82:S47.004.

279. Sussmuth SD, Haider S, Landwehrmeyer GB, Farmer R, Frost C, Tripepi G, et al. An exploratory double blind, randomised clinical trial with selisistat, a SirT1 inhibitor, in patients with Huntington's disease. *Br J Clin Pharmacol* 2015 Mar;79(3):465–76.

280. Ross CA, Aylward EH, Wild EJ, Langbehn DR, Long JD, Warner JH, et al. Huntington disease: natural history, biomarkers and prospects for therapeutics. *Nat Rev Neurol* 2014 Apr; 10(4):204–16.

281. Andre R, Wild EJ, Tabrizi SJ. Huntington's disease: fighting on many fronts. *Brain* 2012 Apr;135(Pt 4):998–1001.

282. Sah DW, Aronin N. Oligonucleotide therapeutic approaches for Huntington disease. *J Clin Invest* 2011 Feb;121(2):500–7.

283. Harper SQ, Staber PD, He X, Eliason SL, Martins IH, Mao Q, et al. RNA interference improves motor and neuropathological abnormalities in a Huntington's disease mouse model. *Proc Natl Acad Sci U S A* 2005 Apr 19;102(16):5820–5.

284. Franich NR, Fitzsimons HL, Fong DM, Klugmann M, During MJ, Young D. AAV vector-mediated RNAi of mutant huntingtin expression is neuroprotective in a novel genetic rat model of Huntington's disease. *Mol Ther* 2008 May;16(5):947–56.

285. Carroll JB, Warby SC, Southwell AL, Doty CN, Greenlee S, Skotte N, et al. Potent and selective antisense oligonucleotides targeting single-nucleotide polymorphisms in the Huntington disease gene / allele-specific silencing of mutant huntingtin. *Mol Ther* 2011 Dec;19(12):2178–85.

286. McBride JL, Pitzer MR, Boudreau RL, Dufour B, Hobbs T, Ojeda SR, et al. Preclinical safety of RNAi-mediated HTT suppression in the rhesus macaque as a potential therapy for Huntington's disease. *Mol Ther* 2011 Dec;19(12):2152–62.

287. Grondin R, Kaytor MD, Ai Y, Nelson PT, Thakker DR, Heisel J, et al. Six month partial suppression of Huntingtin is well tolerated in the adult rhesus striatum. *Brain* 2012 Apr;135(Pt 4):1197–209.

288. Reiner A, Dragatsis I, Zeitlin S, Goldowitz D. Wild-type huntingtin plays a role in brain development and neuronal survival. *Mol Neurobiol* 2003 Dec;28(3):259–76.

289. Auerbach W, Hurlbert MS, Hilditch-Maguire P, Wadghiri YZ, Wheeler VC, Cohen SI, et al. The HD mutation causes progressive lethal neurological disease in mice expressing reduced levels of huntingtin. *Hum Mol Genet* 2001 Oct 15;10(22):2515–23.

290. Nasir J, Floresco SB, O'Kusky JR, Diewert VM, Richman JM, Zeisler J, et al. Targeted disruption of the Huntington's disease gene results in embryonic lethality and behavioral and morphological changes in heterozygotes. *Cell* 1995 Jun 2;81(5):811–23.

291. Kordasiewicz HB, Stanek LM, Wancewicz EV, Mazur C, McAlonis MM, Pytel KA, et al. Sustained therapeutic reversal of Huntington's disease by transient repression of huntingtin synthesis. *Neuron* 2012 Jun 21;7(6):1031–44.

292. Stiles DK, Zhang Z, Ge P, Nelson B, Grondin R, Ai Y, et al. Widespread suppression of huntingtin with convection-enhanced delivery of siRNA. *Exp Neurol* 2012 Jan;233(1):463–71.

293. Alvarez-Erviti L, Seow Y, Yin H, Betts C, Lakhal S, Wood MJ. Delivery of siRNA to the mouse brain by systemic injection of targeted exosomes. *Nat Biotechnol* 2011 Apr;29(4):341–5.

294. NeuroPerspective. Neuroperspective 2012 Apr 1;(201). (see http://www.niresearch.com/?page_id=14)

295. Li H, Haurigot V, Doyon Y, Li T, Wong SY, Bhagwat AS, et al. In vivo genome editing restores haemostasis in a mouse model of haemophilia. *Nature* 2011 Jul 14;475(7355):217–21.

296. Miller TM. An antisense oligonucleotide against SOD1 delivered intrathecally for patients with SOD1 familial amyotrophic lateral sclerosis: a phase 1, randomised, first-in-man study. 2013 May;12(5):435–42.

297. Pan J, Song E, Cheng C, Lee MH, Yeung SC. Farnesyltransferase inhibitors-induced autophagy: alternative mechanisms? *Autophagy* 2009 Jan;5(1):129–31.

298. Pan T, Rawal P, Wu Y, Xie W, Jankovic J, Le W. Rapamycin protects against rotenone-induced apoptosis through autophagy induction. *Neuroscience* 2009 Dec 1;164(2):541–51.

299. Martinez-Vicente M, Talloczy Z, Wong E, Tang G, Koga H, Kaushik S, et al. Cargo recognition failure is responsible for inefficient autophagy in Huntington's disease. *Nat Neurosci* 2010 May;13(5):567–76.

300. Mesa RA. Tipifarnib: farnesyl transferase inhibition at a crossroads. *Expert Rev Anticancer Ther* 2006 Mar;6(3):313–9.

301. Williams A, Sarkar S, Cuddon P, Ttofi EK, Saiki S, Siddiqi FH, et al. Novel targets for Huntington's disease in an mTOR-independent autophagy pathway. *Nat Chem Biol* 2008 May;4(5):295–305.

302. Sugars KL, Brown R, Cook LJ, Swartz J, Rubinsztein DC. Decreased cAMP response element-mediated transcription: an early event in exon 1 and full-length cell models of Huntington's disease that contributes to polyglutamine pathogenesis. *J Biol Chem* 2004 Feb 6;279(6):4988–99.

303. Gines S, Seong IS, Fossale E, Ivanova E, Trettel F, Gusella JF, et al. Specific progressive cAMP reduction implicates energy deficit in presymptomatic Huntington's disease knock-in mice. *Hum Mol Genet* 2003 Mar 1;12(5):497–508.

304. Giampa C, Laurenti D, Anzilotti S, Bernardi G, Menniti FS, Fusco FR. Inhibition of the striatal specific phosphodiesterase PDE10A ameliorates striatal and cortical pathology in R6/2 mouse model of Huntington's disease. *PLoS One* 2010;5(10):e13417.

305. Pfizer. National Institutes of Health: Study Evaluating The Safety, Tolerability And Brain Function Of 2 Doses Of PF-0254920 In Subjects With Early Huntington's Disease. 2014. 29-9-2014. (https://clinicaltrials.gov/ct2/show/NCT01806896)

306. DeMarch Z, Giampa C, Patassini S, Bernardi G, Fusco FR. Beneficial effects of rolipram in the R6/2 mouse model of Huntington's disease. *Neurobiol Dis* 2008 Jun;30(3):375–87.

307. Giampa C, Middei S, Patassini S, Borreca A, Marullo F, Laurenti D, et al. Phosphodiesterase type IV inhibition prevents sequestration of CREB binding protein, protects striatal parvalbumin interneurons and rescues motor deficits in the R6/2 mouse model of Huntington's disease. *Eur J Neurosci* 2009 Mar;29(5):902–10.

308. Hockly E, Richon VM, Woodman B, Smith DL, Zhou X, Rosa E, et al. Suberoylanilide hydroxamic acid, a histone deacetylase inhibitor, ameliorates motor deficits in a mouse model of Huntington's disease. *Proc Natl Acad Sci U S A* 2003;100(4):2041–6.

309. Cronk D, Aziz O, Vann J, Pett HWM, Gowers I, Martin R, et al. Selective HDAC4 inhibitors as potential therapeutics for Huntington's disease (M155). Biofocus, editor. 2012.

310. Jeong H, Cohen DE, Cui L, Supinski A, Savas JN, Mazzulli JR, et al. Sirt1 mediates neuroprotection from mutant huntingtin by activation of the TORC1 and CREB transcriptional pathway. *Nat Med* 2012 Jan;18(1):159–65.

311. Jiang M, Wang J, Fu J, Du L, Jeong H, West T, et al. Neuroprotective role of Sirt1 in mammalian models of Huntington's disease through activation of multiple Sirt1 targets. *Nat Med* 2012 Jan;18(1):153–8.

312. Dedeoglu A, Kubilus JK, Jeitner TM, Matson SA, Bogdanov M, Kowall NW, et al. Therapeutic effects of cystamine in a murine model of Huntington's disease. *J Neurosci* 2002 Oct 15;22(20):8942–50.

313. Bailey CD, Johnson GV. The protective effects of cystamine in the R6/2 Huntington's disease mouse involve mechanisms other than the inhibition of tissue transglutaminase. *Neurobiol Aging* 2006 Jun;27(6):871–9.

314. Borrell-Pages M, Canals JM, Cordelieres FP, Parker JA, Pineda JR, Grange G, et al. Cystamine and cysteamine increase brain levels of BDNF in Huntington disease via HSJ1b and transglutaminase. *J Clin Invest* 2006 May;116(5):1410–24.

315. Schwarcz R, Whetsell WO, Jr., Mangano RM. Quinolinic acid: an endogenous metabolite that produces axon-sparing lesions in rat brain. *Science* 1983 Jan 21;219(4582):316–8.

316. Guillemin GJ, Croitoru-Lamoury J, Dormont D, Armati PJ, Brew BJ. Quinolinic acid upregulates chemokine production and chemokine receptor expression in astrocytes. *Glia* 2003 Mar;41(4):371–81.

317. Zwilling D, Huang SY, Sathyasaikumar KV, Notarangelo FM, Guidetti P, Wu HQ, et al. Kynurenine 3-monooxygenase inhibition in blood ameliorates neurodegeneration. *Cell* 2011 Jun 10;145(6):863–74.

318. Beconi MG, Yates D, Lyons K, Matthews K, Clifton S, Mead T, et al. Metabolism and pharmacokinetics of JM6 in mice: JM6 is not a prodrug for Ro-61-8048. *Drug Metab Dispos* 2012 Dec;40(12):2297–306.

319. Kells AP, Fong DM, Dragunow M, During MJ, Young D, Connor B. AAV-mediated gene delivery of BDNF or GDNF is neuroprotective in a model of Huntington disease. *Mol Ther* 2004 May;9(5):682–8.

320. Bemelmans AP, Horellou P, Pradier L, Brunet I, Colin P, Mallet J. Brain-derived neurotrophic factor-mediated protection of striatal neurons in an excitotoxic rat model of Huntington's disease, as demonstrated by adenoviral gene transfer. *Hum Gene Ther* 1999 Dec 10;10(18):2987–97.

321. Simmons DA, Rex CS, Palmer L, Pandyarajan V, Fedulov V, Gall CM, et al. Up-regulating BDNF with an ampakine rescues synaptic plasticity and memory in Huntington's disease knockin mice. *Proc Natl Acad Sci U S A* 2009 Mar 24;106(12):4906–11.

322. Cicchetti F, Saporta S, Hauser RA, Parent M, Saint-Pierre M, Sanberg PR, et al. Neural transplants in patients with Huntington's disease undergo disease-like neuronal degeneration. *Proc Natl Acad Sci U S A* 2009 Jul 28;106(30):12483–8.

323. Bachoud-Levi AC, Remy P, Nguyen JP, Brugieres P, Lefaucheur JP, Bourdet C, et al. Motor and cognitive improvements in patients with Huntington's disease after neural transplantation. *Lancet* 2000 Dec 9;356(9246):1975–9.

324. Bachoud-Levi AC, Gaura V, Brugieres P, Lefaucheur JP, Boisse MF, Maison P, et al. Effect of fetal neural transplants in patients with Huntington's disease 6 years after surgery: a long-term follow-up study. *Lancet Neurol* 2006 Apr;5(4):303–9.

325. Di Pardo A, Maglione V, Alpaugh M, Horkey M, Atwal RS, Sassone J, et al. Ganglioside GM1 induces phosphorylation of mutant huntingtin and restores normal motor behavior in Huntington disease mice. *Proc Natl Acad Sci U S A* 2012 Feb 28;109(9):3528–33.

326. Kremer B, Goldberg P, Andrew SE, Theilmann J, Telenius H, Zeisler J, et al. A worldwide study of the Huntington's disease mutation. *The sensitivity and specificity of measuring CAG repeats. N Engl J Med* 1994 May 19;330(20):1401–6.

327. Wild EJ, Tabrizi S. Huntington's disease phenocopy syndromes. *Curr Opin Neurol* 2007 Dec;20(6):681–7.

328. Wild EJ, Mudanohwo EE, Sweeney MG, Schneider SA, Beck J, Bhatia KP, et al. Huntington's disease phenocopies are clinically and genetically heterogeneous. *Mov Disord* 2008;23 (5):716–20.

329. Moore RC, Xiang FQ, Monaghan J, Han D, Zhang ZP, Edström L, et al. Huntington disease phenocopy is a familial prion disease. *Am J Hum Genet* 2001 Dec;69(6):1385–8.

330. Mead S, Poulter M, Beck J, Webb TE, Campbell TA, Linehan JM, et al. Inherited prion disease with six octapeptide repeat insertional mutation–molecular analysis of phenotypic heterogeneity. *Brain* 2006;129(Pt 9):2297–317.

331. Krause A, Hetem C, Holmes SE, Margolis RL. HDL2 mutations are an important cause of Huntington's disease in patients with African ancestry. *J Neurol Neurosurg Psychiatry* 2005;76(suppl 4):A16–A26.

332. Kambouris M, Bohlega S, Al Tahan A, Meyer BF. Localization of the gene for a novel autosomal recessive neurodegenerative Huntington-like disorder to 4p15.3. *Am J Hum Genet* 2000;66(2):445–52.

333. Hensman Moss DJ, Poulter M, Beck J, Hehir J, Polke JM, Campbell T, et al. C9orf72 expansions are the most common genetic cause of Huntington disease phenocopies. *Neurology* 2014 Jan 28;82(4):292–9.

334. Schneider SA, van de Warrenburg BPC, Hughes TD, Davis M, Sweeney M, Wood N, et al. Phenotypic homogeneity of the Huntington disease-like presentation in a SCA17 family. *Neurology* 2006;67(9):1701–3.

335. Yamada M. Dentatorubral-pallidoluysian atrophy (DRPLA): The 50th Anniversary of Japanese Society of Neuropathology. *Neuropathology* 2010 Oct;30(5):453–7.

336. Hartig MB, Hörtnagel K, Garavaglia B, Zorzi G, Kmiec T, Klopstock T, et al. Genotypic and phenotypic spectrum of PANK2 mutations in patients with neurodegeneration with brain iron accumulation. *Ann Neurol* 2006 Feb;59(2):248–56.

337. Chinnery PF, Crompton DE, Birchall D, Jackson MJ, Coulthard A, Lombes A, et al. Clinical features and natural history of neuroferritinopathy caused by the FTL1 460InsA mutation. *Brain* 2007;130(1):110–9.

338. Danek A, Walker RH. Neuroacanthocytosis. *Curr Opin Neurol* 2005;18(4):386–92.

339. Ferenci P. Review article: diagnosis and current therapy of Wilson's disease. *Aliment Pharmacol Ther* 2004 Jan 15;19(2):157–65.

340. Kleiner-Fisman G, Rogaeva E, Halliday W, Houle S, Kawarai T, Sato C, et al. Benign hereditary chorea: Clinical, genetic, and pathological findings. *Ann Neurol* 2003;54(2):244–7.

341. Caer M, Viala K, Levy R, Maisonobe T, Chochon F, Lombes A, et al. Adult-onset chorea and mitochondrial cytopathy. *Mov Disord* 2005;20(4):490–2.

342. Ehrnhoefer DE, Wong BK, Hayden MR. Convergent pathogenic pathways in Alzheimer's and Huntington's diseases: shared targets for drug development. *Nat Rev Drug Discov* 2011 Nov;10(11):853–67.

CHAPTER 22

Spinocerebellar Ataxias

H. Brent Clark[1] and Harry T. Orr[1,2]

[1] Department of Laboratory Medicine and Pathology, University of Minnesota Medical School, Minneapolis, Minnesota, USA
[2] Institute for Translational Neuroscience, University of Minnesota Medical School, Minneapolis, Minnesota, USA

Clinical definition and epidemiology

Spinocerebellar ataxias (SCA) are rare, dominantly inherited neurodegenerative diseases that present clinically with ataxia as the major feature in most patients. Ataxia typically includes loss of coordination involving balance, gait, speech, and finer motor movements to varying degrees. Oculomotor disturbances such as nystagmus, irregular gaze pursuit, and even gaze palsy are frequent associated findings in many types of SCA. Although ataxia is the defining clinical feature of this group of diseases, there are variant presentations in some types of SCA in which other neurological abnormalities such as extrapyramidal, pyramidal, or sensory deficits may be early or dominant findings, and in others these latter features and others such as cognitive problems may be variably present later in the course. A hallmark of SCA is that there is considerable heterogeneity in the clinical features, sometimes even within disease categories, but there is much overlap among different conditions as well. Therefore, with a few exceptions, it is difficult to specifically identify distinct forms of SCA based on the clinical phenotype.

As a guide to sorting out the variable features of the dominantly inherited ataxias, Harding [1] introduced a clinically based classification system. Patients with significant other neurological findings in addition to ataxia were classified as having autosomal dominant cerebellar ataxia (ADCA) type I. An infrequent category, ADCA II, was composed of patients with ataxia and progressive visual loss. These patients are now known to have SCA7. The third category, ADCA III, features patients with "pure" cerebellar ataxia although pathological studies have shown that their abnormalities are not always confined to the cerebellum.

The prevalence of SCA is estimated to be somewhere between 1 and 5 per 100,000 persons [2–4]. Incidence and prevalence of SCA differ among ethnic groups and geographic areas [5–7]. Because of founder effects, there may be geographic "hotspots" of prevalence. The most common forms of SCA in Europe and North America are SCA3, SCA2, SCA1, SCA7, and SCA6, which account for roughly 75% of affected families [8, 9]. In Japan SCA1 and SCA2 are uncommon while SCA31 and dentato-rubro-pallido-luysian atrophy, conditions rarely seen elsewhere, are common. Rarer forms of SCA have been reported only in isolated ethnic groups to date.

With autosomal dominant inheritance, SCA affects men and women equally. Ages of onset typically range from early to late adult life although pediatric onset is seen in some forms. Many of the common autosomal dominant ataxias have abnormally expanded CAG repeats in the mutant genes, in which case the age of onset is inversely correlated with the size of repeat expansion [10]. Late onset is characteristic of SCA 6 (age 50) and SCA31 (age 60) but can also occur within the clinical spectrum of many other forms of SCA.

Spectrum of clinical and pathological phenotypes

Clinical features

The clinical findings in SCA are often common to the different forms but may vary within the same disease entity where there may be heterogeneity of the age of onset, involvement of different neurological systems, and rate of clinical progression. All of these factors make clinical diagnosis of these conditions extremely challenging. As mentioned above, the Harding classification separates the autosomal dominant cerebellar ataxias into three major categories: ADCA I, with ataxia plus other significant neurological problems; ADCA II, with ataxia and retinal degeneration; and ADCA III, with more or less pure ataxia.

Although not typical of most types of SCA, there are several forms in which the clinical presentation is distinctive and narrows the differential diagnosis. SCA7, ataxia with progressive visual loss (ADCA II), in particular, has a unique phenotype. SCA17 presents with ataxia and psychiatric or cognitive impairment early in the course of the disease. SCA20 presents with ataxia and palatal myoclonus and there is dense calcification of the dentate nucleus on CT imaging.

The most common SCAs in populations of developed countries are SCA3, SCA2, SCA1, SCA7, and SCA6 – all of which are caused by CAG repeat expansions resulting in extended polyglutamine tracts in the mutant protein [11]. Except in SCA6, variations in the length of the repeat expansion appear to have an effect on the phenotype, with longer repeats resulting in earlier onset, rapid progression, and more severe or diverse pathology. The clinical presentations of these five types of SCA are discussed; findings seen in other types are listed in Tables 22.1 and 22.2

Neurodegeneration, First Edition. Edited by Anthony Schapira, Zbigniew Wszolek, Ted M. Dawson and Nicholas Wood.
© 2017 John Wiley & Sons, Ltd. Published 2017 by John Wiley & Sons, Ltd.

Table 22.1 Aid to differential diagnosis by clinical presentation in SCA.

Feature	Differential diagnosis
Pure cerebellar ataxia	SCA5, SCA6, SCA11, SCA15/16, SCA22, SCA26
Ataxia with:	
Amyotrophy	SCA36
Chorea	SCA17, SCA1 (only late in course), SCA14
Cognitive impairment	SCA17 (early), SCA2, SCA13, SCA19, SCA21 (mild), SCA27, SCA32 (developmental)
Dystonia	SCA3, SCA17, SCA29
Hearing loss	SCA31
Myoclonus	SCA2, SCA14. SCA19
Ophthalmoplegia	SCA3, SCA2. SCA1, SCA28
Parkinsonism	SCA3, SCA2, SCA21
Psychiatric symptoms	SCA17, SCA27
Pyramidal signs	SCA3, SCA1, SCA7, SCA8, SCA23
Retinal degeneration	SCA7
Seizures	SCA10, SCA12, SCA17
Sensory neuropathy	SCA3, SCA4, SCA1, SCA18, SCA25
Slow saccades	SCA2, SCA1, SCA3, SCA7, SCA17, SCA28
Tremor	SCA2, SCA12, SCA14, SCA27

SCA3

SCA3 is the most common form of SCA worldwide and also is known as Machado–Joseph disease (MJD), which was once thought to be a separate entity but is caused by the same mutation, a polyglutamine expansion in the ataxin-3 protein. Common presenting signs are ataxia of gait, dysarthria, spasticity, and nystagmus. Supranuclear gaze paralysis, bulbar and milder limb amyotrophy, and areflexia subsequently appear in most cases. The age of onset is variable and often correlates with the clinical features. The entity of MJD was originally described in patients of Portuguese-Azorean ancestry and was subdivided into different clinical types [12]. Type 1, the rarest, has early onset, at 5–30 years of age, and presents with extrapyramidal signs including rigidity, bradykinesia, and dystonia with spasticity, but minimal ataxia. Tongue and facial fasciculation and bulging of the eyes are often present. There are abnormalities of gaze with horizontal nystagmus and restriction of upward gaze. Type 2, the most common form, usually has onset in the third or fourth decade with progressive ataxia, dystonia, and

Table 22.2 Spinocerebellar ataxias (the most common forms are in bold type).

Type	OMIM No.*	Locus/mutation	Clinical (Harding [1]) pathological features
SCA1	164400	6q23/ataxin 1 CAG repeat expansion	ADCA I, cerebellar cortex and dentate nuclei affected
SCA2	183090	12q24/ataxin 2 CAG repeat expansion	ADCA I, dentate sparing
SCA3/Machado–Joseph disease	109150	14q24–q32/ataxin 3 CAG repeat expansion	ADCA I, cerebellar cortical sparing
SCA4	600223	16q22/unknown	Ataxia with sensory neuropathy
SCA5	600224	11p11–q11/beta-II-spectrin	ADCA III
SCA6	183086	19p13/CACNA1A CAG repeat expansion	ADCA III
SCA7	164500	3p21–p12/ataxin 7 CAG repeat expansion	ADCA II with retinal degeneration
SCA8	608768	13q21/SCA8 Untranslated CTG repeat expansion	Ataxia, sensory neuropathy, spasticity
SCA10	603516	22q13/ataxin 10 Intronic ATTCT repeat	Seizures are common
SCA11	604432	15q14–q21/TTBK2	ADCA III, mild, late onset
SCA12	604326	5q21–q33/PPP2R2B 5' untranslated CAG repeat expansion	ADCA I, tremor
SCA13	605259	19q13.3–q13.4/KCNC3	Early onset, cognitive delay
SCA14	605361	19q3.4/PKC-gamma	ADCA I or ACDA III depending on age of onset, myoclonus, dystonia if ADCA I
SCA15/SCA16	606658	3p26.2-p25.3/ITPB1	ADCA III, slow progression
SCA17	607136	6q27/TBP CAG repeat expansion	ADCA I with cognitive/psychiatric features
SCA18	607458	7q22–q32/IFRD1 is a candidate gene	Sensorimotor neuropathy
SCA19/SCA22	607346	1p21–q21/unknown	Cognitive impairment in SCA19; SCA22 locus is the same but without cognitive features
SCA20	608687	11p13–q11/unknown	Maps near SCA5, palatal myoclonus, dysphonia, and calcification of dentate nuclei
SCA21	607454	7p21.3–p15.1/unknown	Extrapyramidal involvement is common
SCA23	610245	20p13–p12.3/ prodynorphin	Hyperreflexia, reduced vibration
SCA25	608703	2p21–p13/unknown	Early onset, sensory neuropathy
SCA26	609306	19p13.3/unknown	ADCA III
SCA27	609307	13q34/FGF-14 Fibroblast growth factor 14	Early onset with tremor, later ataxia and cognitive changes
SCA28	610246	18p11.22–q11.2/AFG3L2	Early onset, slow progression, pyramidal signs, oculomotor weakness
SCA29	117360	3p26/see SCA15/16	Dystonia, cognitive changes
SCA30	613371	4q34.3–q35.1/unknown	Late onset, mild ataxia, mild spasticity
SCA31	117210	16q21/BEAN Intronic TGAAA repeat expansion	Late onset, pure ataxia with hearing loss, common in Japan
SCA32	613909	7q32-q33/unknown	Variable cognitive impairment, male infertility
SCA34	133190	6p12.3–q16.2/unknown	Infantile onset, erythrokeratodermia, hyporeflexia
SCA35	613908	20p13/TGM6	Tremor, hyperreflexia, decreased proprioception
SCA36	614153	20p13/NOP56 Intronic GGCCTG repeat expansion,	Late onset, cranial and spinal motor neuron involvement with amyotrophy

*OMIM, Online Mendelian Inheritance in Man.

spasticity. Nystagmus is prominent. Type 3 usually presents in the fifth decade with ataxia accompanied by sensorimotor neuropathy with amyotrophy and areflexia. Parkinsonism is the major finding in some patients categorized as MJD and is sometimes referred to as type 4. Restless leg syndrome also may be present in close to half of patients with SCA3. The prognosis is highly dependent upon the size of the repeat expansion, with shorter expansions typically presenting with later onset and a more protracted progression. Milder forms of SCA3 do not necessarily shorten life.

SCA2

SCA2, the second most common form, features ataxia, tremor, myoclonus, diminished deep tendon reflexes, and decreased vibration sense in most cases. Slow saccadic eye movements are a particularly characteristic feature of SCA2. Extrapyramidal features including parkinsonism or chorea may be present as well as variable manifestations of oculomotor paresis, dysphagia, amyotrophy, and cognitive dysfunction. As is the case for most of the polyglutamine diseases, the age of onset is determined largely by the length of the repeat expansion and ranges from infancy to later adulthood, but most cases present prior to the fourth decade. Infantile SCA2 is seen with hyperexpansions in the range of several hundred glutamine repeats and does not always present with ataxia. Prognosis is somewhat similar to SCA3 but milder forms are less common.

SCA1

SCA1 also has widely variable clinical findings with onset ranging from childhood to late adult life, most commonly presenting in the fourth decade. The earliest features are truncal and limb ataxia with dysarthria with subsequent slowing or loss of saccadic eye movements. Ataxic ocular disturbances are prominent and include gaze nystagmus, reduced opticokinetic nystagmus, and disruption of smooth pursuit. Supranuclear or nuclear ophthalmoparesis, bulbar paresis with dysphagia, spasticity, and decreased vibration sense are also frequently present. Cognitive impairment is occasionally seen as are parkinsonism and dystonia. Most patients are significantly disabled within 5–10 years and die 10–20 years after onset.

SCA7

SCA7 was originally classified as ADCA II because of the association of ataxia with retinal macular degeneration. The age of onset is widely variable and ranges from infancy to the eighth decade of life, with an average age of 30 years at presentation. The visual findings appear early in the course in infantile-onset cases but may lag behind the ataxia by several decades in patients with late-onset SCA7; however most patients develop visual loss. Typical patients present with truncal and limb ataxia and dysarthria. Hyperreflexia and supranuclear ophthalmoplegia with slow saccades also are frequently seen. Cognitive deficits, peripheral neuropathy, and extrapyramidal features sometimes are present as well. Patients with later onset and shorter repeat expansions can have a normal life expectancy.

SCA6

SCA6 usually presents in the fifth to sixth decade or later and has a slowly progressive course. The disease may start with episodic ataxia progressing to persistence. Patients with SCA6 have truncal and limb ataxia, dysarthria, and oculomotor disturbances including vertical nystagmus, oscillopsia, and an abnormal vestibulo-ocular reflex. Increased reflexes have been described in some patients as

have extrapyramidal signs. SCA6 usually is a late-onset disease and despite the severe cerebellar atrophy it does not typically alter the life expectancy of affected individuals.

Overview of the neuropathology of spinocerebellar ataxias

Pathological classifications of ataxias historically have been separated into three patterns of neurodegeneration.

1 **Cerebellar cortical degeneration:** This pattern corresponds to the ADCA III category of Harding and is the most frequent among the forms of SCA. There is atrophy of the cerebellar folia with sulcal widening secondary to loss of Purkinje cells. Granular cells and cortical interneurons typically are less affected or unaffected and there is no involvement of the neurons of the deep cerebellar nuclei, although there is frequently gliosis caused by loss of Purkinje cell terminals. Inferior olivary neurons may be reduced in number, although gross atrophy is not always appreciated.

2 **Olivo-ponto-cerebellar degeneration or atrophy (OPCA):** This pattern is seen in many patients within the ADCA I category. The basis pontis and its projections in the middle cerebellar peduncles and cerebellar hemispheric white matter are often severely atrophic with significant loss of basal pontine neurons and transverse fibers on microscopy. There is also gross atrophy of the cerebellar folia and more severely the inferior olives. Cortical changes include loss of Purkinje cells with variable severity. The middle cerebellar peduncles and cerebellar white matter are gliotic and atrophic. Although known as OPCA, in many of the conditions with this pattern there are other structures that also may be affected including cranial nerve nuclei, deep cerebellar nuclei, spinal cord neurons and tracts, striatum, substantia nigra (which may be depigmented grossly), or red nuclei. Recent studies using more anatomically detailed methodology have detected even more extensive involvement of brainstem and cerebral deep gray matter as well as cerebral cortical structures [13–15].

3 **Spinocerebellar degeneration:** Despite the name, only a few forms of SCA have this pattern of alterations, which is characterized by selective degeneration of proprioceptive afferent pathways including sensory peripheral nerves, the posterior columns, and spinocerebellar tracts. There may be involvement of the pyramidal tracts but there is usually minimal involvement of the cerebellar cortex with little or no loss of Purkinje cells. The deep cerebellar nuclei are affected in some conditions with this pattern, such as SCA3 and the common recessively inherited Friedreich's ataxia (see Chapter 18).

These three basic patterns serve as a framework for pathological classification, but there are different combinations of degeneration in SCA that overlap these categories.

In keeping with the difficulty of the clinical diagnosis of the different forms of SCA, neuropathological diagnosis is subject to the same types of problems. Many of the SCAs have overlap of pathological features among them, but to add further complexity there is pathological variability within individual entities, particularly those mediated by polyglutamine expansions in the mutant gene. Thus, patients sharing the same genetic disease can have quite different clinical and pathological phenotypes while patients who share clinical and pathological features often have different forms of SCA. Most types of SCA, with a few exceptions that will be noted, cannot be distinguished from one another solely on the neuropathological findings. Because of the variability in the findings, the discussion of pathological features focuses on the more common presentations of some of the better characterized disorders.

Pathological features

SCA3

SCA3 is one of the most distinctive forms of SCA neuropathologically in that the disease largely spares the cerebellar cortex and inferior olivary nuclei. Principal neuropathological targets include the cerebellar afferent and efferent pathways, as well as extrapyramidal structures and lower motor neurons [12]. Of note, cerebellar afferents including spinocerebellar, pontocerebellar, and vestibulocerebellar along with their neurons of origin in Clarke's nuclei, basal pontine nuclei, and vestibular nuclei are major targets of the disease. The deep cerebellar nuclei also have extensive neuronal loss with atrophy of the superior cerebellar peduncles. Other affected areas may include the red nuclei, the dorsal root ganglia, and posterior columns of the spinal cord as well as the substantia nigra, the subthalamic nuclei, and less severely the globus pallidus. The caudate, putamen, and cerebral cortex are not obviously affected. Motor neurons in the cranial nerve nuclei and anterior horns degenerate, but even though there often is clinical spasticity, corticospinal tract atrophy is not conspicuous. Thick-section studies have found more extensive involvement of brainstem nuclei [13]. A cytological change seen in SCA3 and some of the other polyglutamine-mediated diseases is the presence of intranuclear neuronal inclusions that stain with antibodies against the disease-specific protein (ataxin-3 in SCA3), ubiquitin, or a monoclonal antibody, 1C2, that detects expanded polyglutamine tracts [16]. As is the case for other polyglutamine diseases, the pathological patterns seen in SCA3 tend to correlate with the length of the expanded CAG repeat.

SCA2

SCA2 typically has olivo-ponto-cerebellar atrophy but with relative sparing of the deep cerebellar nuclei and more involvement of the striatonigral system. Purkinje cells are significantly depleted. The substantia nigra has loss of dopaminergic neurons, and the caudate, putamen, and globus pallidus typically have neuronal loss. There is neuronal loss in Clarke's nuclei, with atrophy of the spinocerebellar tracts and dorsal columns, but little or no involvement of the corticospinal tracts. Thick-section techniques have found more widespread involvement of the brainstem and cerebral deep gray structures [15, 17]. Cytoplasmic and nuclear inclusions, immunoreactive for ubiquitin and expanded ataxin-2, have been described, but are not as reliably present as in some other polyglutamine diseases. Infantile cases with CAG repeat lengths numbering in the hundreds have variable neuropathology that does not mimic what is seen in the adult-onset disease.

SCA1

SCA1 most frequently is pathologically characterized as an olivo-ponto-cerebellar atrophy [18]. The cerebellum shows loss of Purkinje cells, but unlike SCA2 there is significant neuronal loss in the dentate nuclei. Olivary neuronal loss is extensive and may be disproportionately greater than the loss of Purkinje cells. Loss of neurons in the basal pontine nuclei often is severe, but can be less so in some cases. Of clinical importance there is usually significant involvement of cranial nerve motor nuclei, particularly the vagal and hypoglossal. Other brainstem targets include the red nuclei and oculomotor complex. The anterior horns, posterior columns, and spinocerebellar tracts also have atrophy. The substantia nigra usually is spared, but the pallidum and, to a lesser extent, the neostriatum are mildly affected in some cases. Cerebral cortex and hippocampus may have mild neuronal loss including motor cor-

tex. Intranuclear inclusions immunoreactive for ataxin-1, ubiquitin, and 1C2 antibody can be found in brains from SCA1 patients, but not typically in Purkinje cells. A recent study using thick-section techniques has identified more extensive involvement in the brainstem, deep gray nuclei, and cerebral cortex [14].

SCA7

Neuropathological changes in SCA7 also have an olivo-ponto-cerebellar pattern [19, 20], although the basal pontine atrophy is usually less severe than in SCA1 and SCA2. The cerebellar cortex has severe loss of Purkinje cells, milder loss of granule cells, and variable loss of neurons in the dentate nuclei. The inferior olives typically have severe gliosis and neuronal loss. The spinocerebellar and corticospinal tracts have loss of axons, but the posterior columns usually are largely intact. Variably, there is degeneration of cranial nerve and anterior horn motor neurons. Extrapyramidal sites include the subthalamic nuclei, the globus pallidus, and substantia nigra, which are typically less affected than in SCA2. The ocular pathology is characterized by severe loss of retinal photoreceptors and ganglion cells. Neuronal intranuclear inclusions can be identified immunohistochemically using antibodies against ataxin-7 and ubiquitin.

SCA6

Neuropathological studies in SCA6 have shown cerebellar cortical atrophy with severe loss of Purkinje cells that is more pronounced in the vermis and the superior portions of the cerebellar hemispheres. Purkinje cells that remain have been described as having heterotopic, irregularly shaped nuclei and swollen dendrites with spiny protrusions [21]. The basal pons is spared and although there is gliosis in the dentate nuclei, neuronal loss is not conspicuous. Despite reports of extrapyramidal symptoms in some patients, pathological studies to date have not confirmed significant involvement of the substantia nigra and basal ganglia [22]. Neuronal intranuclear inclusions are not present in SCA6, but cytoplasmic inclusions in Purkinje cells that stain with antibodies against the mutant protein, CACNA1A, have been reported [23].

Diagnostic examination and investigations

The clinical presentations of SCA are quite variable but there are some features of different types that are more distinctive. Table 22.1 lists a number of features that may coexist with ataxia, which could direct the clinician toward a specific diagnosis. Table 22.2 provides a more comprehensive listing of the different forms of SCA including what is known about their genetic causes and pertinent clinical or pathological features. A comprehensive neurological history and examination is paramount for establishing a differential diagnosis. Because of the autosomal dominant inheritance pattern, patients with SCA usually have an obvious family history and careful historical characterization of the disease process in affected family members can be beneficial in determining a diagnosis.

Neuroimaging

Neuroimaging studies also can be helpful although many of the forms of SCA have similar findings. Magnetic resonance imaging (MRI) is valuable for distinguishing simple cerebellar atrophy from cases with brainstem involvement (Figure 22.1). SCA3 often has pontine atrophy without significant cerebellar cortical atrophy, while SCA2, SCA1, and SCA7 usually have both. A number of the forms of SCA, particularly those with the ADCA III clinical patterns, which

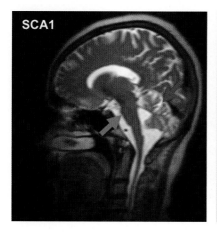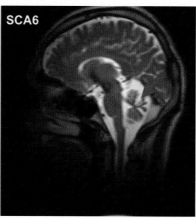

Figure 22.1 Midsagittal T2 (4T magnet)-weighted MR images showing the atrophy characteristic of a "pure" cerebellar SCA (SCA6) and a "mixed" SCA (SCA1). Cerebellar atrophy (red arrow) is present in both while only in SCA1 is there brainstem/pons atrophy (green arrow). MRI images generated and provided by Dr. Gülin Öz, University of Minnesota.

includes SCA6, have only cerebellar atrophy on MRI. Involvement of other brain regions such as the striatonigral pathways is less reliably detectable by neuroimaging.

Non-conventional MR techniques, including spectroscopy (MRS), and functional MR have been used in patients with chronic ataxia. Such approaches are being investigated as potential tools to monitor progression of neurodegeneration in chronic ataxia and to serve as "surrogate markers" in clinical trials. In SCA1, changes in certain neurochemical markers detected by MRS differentiated patients from controls and correlated with severity of ataxia as assessed by the Scale for the Assessment and Rating of Ataxia (SARA scale) [24, 25]. More recently, the detection of neurochemical markers by MRS was found to distinguish SCA1, SCA2, and SCA6 patients from one another [26]. In a mouse model of SCA1, changes in neurochemical markers were detectable prior to onset of neurological symptoms and progressed with disease [27].

Traditional laboratory testing of blood or CSF is nonspecific and of no value in determining a diagnosis of SCA. There are no specific biomarkers of these diseases other than identification of the genetic mutations.

The current system of classification and diagnosis of SCA is based entirely on genetic linkages and identification of specific mutations within families. The most widely available diagnostic genetic tests are for the CAG repeat diseases, in particular SCA1, SCA2, SCA3, SCA6, SCA7, and SCA17. Identification of many of the other identified mutations associated with SCA depends upon specialized testing in research laboratories and is not routinely performed in hospital-based or commercial diagnostic laboratories. Many families with dominantly inherited ataxias have mutations that still have not been characterized genetically. Conversely, patients with apparently sporadic ataxias may have genetically characterized forms of SCA that are not appreciated by family history [8, 28, 29]. The polyglutamine-mediated diseases may present in a child of an unaffected parent as the result of an increase in the repeat length from a non-pathogenic to a pathogenic size, or in other forms of SCA there may be spontaneous mutations. Other circumstances such as premature death of a parent carrying the mutant gene (SCA6 often has a late onset and an affected parent might die prior to symptomatic disease) or non-paternity also hinder the detection of a genetic pattern.

Clinical assessment scales have been developed to determine the degree of impairment in patients with ataxia. These scales include the International Cooperative Ataxia Rating Scale (ICARS) [30], the Scale for the Assessment and Rating of Ataxia (SARA) [25],

and the Brief Ataxia Rating Scale (BARS) [31]. These rating systems allow for ascertainment of the stage of disease a patient has attained and can be utilized to evaluate progression of disease, and perhaps in the future, response of disease to therapeutic intervention.

SCA genetics and pathogenesis

Typically, SCAs are the ataxias that are inherited in an autosomal dominant manner, sometimes alternatively designated as the autosomal dominant cerebellar ataxias (ADCA). Of the approximately 50% of SCAs for which the mutation is known, about 6% are due to conventional mutations (e.g., point mutations) and 45% are due to nucleotide repeat expansions. In most instances the nucleotide expansions are CAG repeat expansions resulting in expansion of a glutamine tract within the affected protein – the so-called "polyglutamine repeat ataxias" [11].

An intriguing aspect of SCA pathogenesis is that as a group they are caused by mutations in genes that encode proteins that function in seemingly disparate cellular pathways (Table 22.2). For example, among the pathways impacted by mutations causing a form of SCA are: transcription (SCA1, SCA7, and SCA17); RNA processing (SCA1, SCA2, and SCA31); protein phosphorylation (SCA11, SCA12, and SCA14); ion channels (SCA6 and SCA13); a growth factor (SCA27); and intracellular protein trafficking (SCA5).

The cellular and molecular mechanisms responsible for pathogenesis of the polyglutamine neurodegenerative diseases in general are a matter of considerable debate, largely between the extent to which the polyglutamine tract alone drives pathogenesis, perhaps through the tendency of mutant polyglutamine proteins to aggregate, or whether it is a polyglutamine alteration of the native/normal functions of the polyglutamine proteins that is required for development of disease. While polyglutamine expansion does render proteins more prone to aggregate and form inclusion bodies that are a pathological hallmark of these polyglutamine disorders [32], the extent to which these inclusions cause disease continues to be a complex issue. There are several studies demonstrating that in mouse models disease severity can be disassociated from presence of inclusions [33–35]. Moreover, there are data indicating that inclusions may be protective, perhaps by sequestrating the mutant protein [35–37]. More recent studies support the concept that the native/normal functions of the polyglutamine proteins are required for development of disease [38–42], suggesting that understanding the polyglutamine SCA diseases requires knowledge of the role the protein has in basic cellular processes [43] (Figure 22.2).

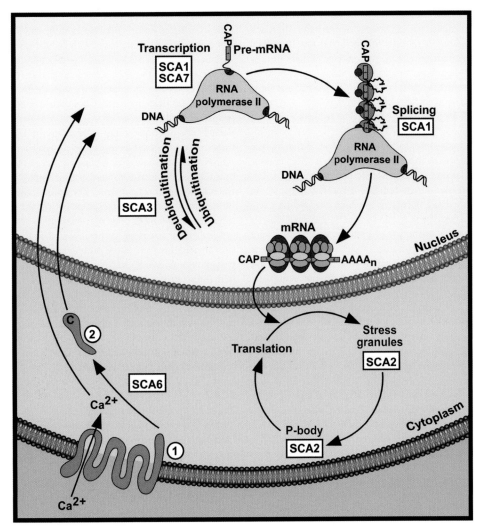

Figure 22.2 Proposed functional targets of the more prevalent polyglutamine *SCA*-encoded proteins. In the nucleus, *SCA1*, *SCA7*, and *SCA17* all have a role in transcription regulation with the *SCA1* protein postulated to have an additional role in splicing through its interaction with RBM17 and U2AF65. By virtue of its deubiquitinating activity and transport to the nucleus with stress, the *SCA3* protein may impact transcription. SCA6 is caused by a CAG expansion in a bicistronic mRNA that encodes two proteins. Thus, disease is due to alterations at the membrane in calcium transport, protein 1, and/or changes in gene expression due to mutant transcription factor protein 2. In the cytoplasm, the *SCA2* encoded protein is postulated as having a role in mRNA metabolism by virtue of it being a component of cytoplasmic stress granules and P-bodies.

An important approach to understanding pathogenesis of the SCAs is to utilize a variety of strategies to model these diseases in mice (Table 22.3). Because SCAs are neurodegenerative diseases that may take decades to manifest in patients, it cannot be certain that the genetic changes found in affected patients will be manifest during the short lifespan of mice carrying those exact changes. Two approaches used to create a readily discernable clinical phenotype in mice are either to overexpress the SCA transgene or to express an SCA transgene with a CAG repeat expansion even longer than the maximum repeat length seen in human mutant alleles. These manipulations create a potential for results unrelated to the human disease and thus require careful controls, such as lines with matched overexpression of normal allelic transgenes. Another tactical issue is whether to express the mutant transgene in all neurons or cells of the CNS, or to target critical populations such as the Purkinje cell. The advantage of the former approach is that it more closely

Table 22.3 Manipulations of SCA transgenic models to evaluate pathogenesis and potential therapy.

Disease	Manipulations of transgenic models of SCA
SCA1	Conditional reversal of transgene [104, 110]
	Cross-breeding with other transgenic mice [111–113]
	Drug therapy [114]
	Gene therapy [105, 115]
	Modification of mutant gene to alter its function [33, 40, 41, 86]
	Transplantation of precursor cells [116]
SCA2	Drug therapy [101]
	Transplantation of stem cells [117]
SCA3	Conditional reversal of transgene [118]
	Cross-breeding with other transgenic mice [119]
	Drug therapy [102, 120, 121]
	Gene therapy [122]
	Modification of mutant gene to alter its function [123, 124]
SCA6	None
SCA7	Cross-breeding with other transgenic mice [88]

models the human disease, but in turn it makes interpretation of mechanisms more complex. The advantage of the latter approach is that Purkinje cells are critical cells for cerebellar function, they are affected in nearly all forms of SCA, and damage to them usually creates a behavioral phenotype. In addition, Purkinje cells have an elaborate dendritic structure that can be readily studied for morphological alterations.

SCA3

Also known as Machado–Joseph disease, SCA3 is caused by the expansion of a polyQ stretch in ataxin-3 (ATXN3). ATXN3 is associated with two cellular processes: transcription repression [44, 45], and protein homeostasis [46]. It remains unclear whether these two processes are linked and the extent to which one or both drive SCA3 pathogenesis.

Supporting the nucleus as the site of pathogenesis in SCA3 are studies using cell [47, 48] and mouse models [49], which show that ATXN3 is more toxic in the nucleus than in the cytoplasm. In addition, ATXN3 interacts with several transcription regulators including TAFII130 [50], CBP [51], RAD23 [52], NCoR, HDAC3, and HDAC6 [45]. More recently, heat shock and oxidative stress were found to increase the nuclear localization of wild-type and mutant ATXN3 [46]. This observation raises an interesting question regarding the nuclear function of ATXN3; perhaps it functions to regulate expression of genes that encode components of the cellular stress response.

In addition to modulating the cellular stress response by regulating gene expression, ATXN3 likely regulates the ubiquitin–proteasome system directly. Considerable data show that ATXN3 can function as a deubiquitinating (DUB) enzyme [53, 54]. ATXN3 contains at its N-terminus a Josephin domain (JD) that has ubiquitin protease activity and up to three ubiquitin-interacting motifs (UIM) that bind ubiquitin [53]. The number of UIMs varies due to alternative splicing, with the three UIM isoforms predominating in the brain [55]. Both the JD and UIMs of ATXN3 are critical for its ability in *Drosophila* to protect neurons from the toxicity of other mutant polyQ proteins [56]. ATXN3 selectively edits Lys63 linkages in mixed ubiquitin chains [54]. In contrast to the role of Lys48-linked chains in targeting proteins to the proteasome for degradation, Lys63-linked chains are thought to convey regulatory information to the proteins. Lastly, the three-dimensional structure of the JD from ATXN3 demonstrates a tight connection between polyubiquitin binding and the DUB activity of ATXN3 [57, 58].

A 2011 study showed that ATXN3, along with the initiator E2 Ube2w, regulates the ability of the E3 ligase C-terminus of Hsc70-interacting protein (CHIP) to ubiquitinate its substrates [59]. Monoubiquitination of CHIP by Ube2w promotes the interaction of CHIP with ATXN3, which in turn through its DUB activity restricts the length of ubiquitin chains attached to CHIP substrates. Once substrate ubiquitination is completed, ATXN3 deubiquitinates CHIP, thereby stopping the reaction. In terms of the role such a pathway might play in SCA3/MJD pathogenesis, this study showed that polyQ expansion in ATXN3 increases its affinity for CHIP, and that could underlie the decreased activity of this neuroprotective E3 seen in a mouse model of SCA3.

Thus, a substantial body of data supports a role for ATXN3 in regulating the ubiquitin–proteasome system, most likely in editing polyubiquitin chains. It is worth noting that the ubiquitin–proteasome system, besides dealing with misfolded proteins, has a role in transcription by regulating the assembly and disassembly of transcription complexes that accompany each cycle of promoter activation/inactivation. Because nuclear localization of wild-type and mutant ATXN3 increases with cellular stress, it is tempting to speculate that the nuclear and cytoplasmic functions of ATXN3 are variations on the same molecular theme. That is, the ability of ATXN3 to remove monoubiquitin side-chains from yet to be identified nuclear proteins – as it does with CHIP [59] – is critical for proper ubiquitin-dependent regulation of gene expression in the nucleus. Through its ability to regulate the Ube2w/CHIP ubiquitination cycle as well as its ability to function as a DUB enzyme, ATXN3 can associate with E2 ligases to regulate gene expression to promote a ubiquitination/deubiquitination cycle on yet to be identified transcription factors. ATXN3 might also regulate the ubiquitination of transcription factors critical for setting up a proper assembly/disassembly cycle of transcription complexes.

While most attention has been placed on the CAG repeat expansion altering function at the protein level for ATXN3 and the other polyglutamine SCAs, ATXN3 studies in *Drosophila* have shown that interrupting the CAG repeat with a CAA glutamine codon increases the protein to RNA ratio over that seen with a pure CAG repeat [60]. This finding raises the possibility that aspects of the mRNA with an expanded repeat also contribute to toxicity. Along the same lines, for SCA2, individuals with mutant-length CAG repeats that are interrupted with a CAA seem to present with parkinsonism rather than ataxia [61].

SCA2

The polyQ protein affected in SCA2, ATXN2, as well as its closely related homologs, is implicated in range of biological functions, including cell specification, actin filament formation, receptor-mediated signaling, and secretion [62–64]. Evidence indicates that ATXN2 is involved in this diverse group of functions by virtue of it having a role in cytoplasmic RNA-related functions, in particular the regulation of translation of RNA to protein. First of all, the primary sequence of ATXN2 contains Lsm (like-Sm) motifs known to function in RNA splicing and mRNA decay in the cytoplasm [65]. In addition, the ATXN2 sequence contains a polyA-binding protein (PABP) interacting motif, PAM2 [66]. Consequently, ATXN2 interacts with PABP and also with a putative RNA protein called ataxin-2-binding protein [67]. Studies further indicate that important subcellular sites for the regulation of translation by ATXN2 are stress granules and P-bodies, the main cellular compartments for regulating mRNA degradation and translation. Another stress granule and P-body component with which ATXN2 also interacts, is the DEAD/H-box RNA helicase DDX6 [68]. This study also found that ATXN2 has a role in assembly of stress granules and P-bodies. In *Drosophila* Atx2 is required for repression of several miRNA target mRNAs, suggesting that ATXN2 also functions in miRNA pathways [69].

Data linking ATXN2 to regulation of translation also come from studies on the homologs of *ATXN2* in other model organisms. In yeast there is a genetic interaction between *Pab1*, a gene that promotes translation, and the yeast ATXN2 homolog *Pbp1* [70]. Furthermore, overexpression of Pbp1 in yeast results in the same phenotype as does inhibiting translation with cycloheximide [71]. In *C. elegans*, partial loss of function of the ATXN2 homolog, ATX-2, alters the abundance of certain proteins without altering the level of their mRNAs, indicating that ATX-2 functions in the regulation of translation in *C. elegans*. More direct evidence that ATXN2 functions in translation comes from the *Drosophila* homolog of ATXN2, ATX2. By sucrose gradient centrifugation, ATX2 assembles with polyribosomes in a manner dependent on the Lsm and PAM2 motifs [72]. This study also found that ATXN2 in transfected human HEK293 cells co-sediments with polyribosomes.

Thus, there are considerable data indicating that ATXN2 interacts with various components of the cellular machinery involved in the regulation of mRNA translation. ATXN2's association with components of translational active polysomes as well as translational silent RNA granules suggests a role in the regulated trafficking of mRNA between these structures that allows a cell to tailor translation to meet the needs of changes in its environment. Intriguingly, in a *Drosophila* model of synaptic plasticity, long-term olfactory habituation (LTH), Atx2 functions along with the miRNA-pathway components Me31B and Ago1 to generate the synaptic plasticity associated with LTH that is linked to translational repression [69].

While there are few data indicating whether and at what points in the cellular translational pathway SCA2-associated polyQ expansion alters ATXN2 function, there is a suggestion that the polyQ tract length in ATXN2 affects risk for another neurodegenerative disorder, amyotrophic lateral sclerosis (ALS). This observation provides additional evidence linking ATXN2 to RNA metabolism because mutations in the gene encoding 43-kDa TAR DNA-binding protein (TDP-43) are associated with some sporadic and familial forms of ALS [73]. TDP-43 is a heterogeneous nuclear riboprotein (hnRNP) that associates with single-stranded nucleic acids and is implicated in several aspects of RNA metabolism, including transcription, alternative splicing, and RNA stability. In an unbiased screen for modifiers of TDP-43 toxicity in yeast, the yeast ATXN2 homolog, Pbp1, enhanced TDP-43 toxicity. Atx2 was also found to modify TDP-43 toxicity in *Drosophila*. In yeast and mammalian cells, TDP-43 and ATXN2 interact in a fashion dependent on RNA [74]. Further linking ATXN2 with TDP-43 is the observation that ATXN2 is mislocalized in ALS motor neurons. Taking the functional relationship between ATXN2 and TDP-43 one step further, Elden et al. [74] showed that intermediate expansions (27–33 glutamines) are significantly higher in ALS patients than in neurologically normal controls. The association between longer wild-type SCA2 repeat alleles and an increased risk for ALS is supported by a study by Van Damme et al. [75]. This association is interesting in two respects. First, it indicates that *ATXN2* is a relatively common susceptibility gene for ALS. In addition, this relationship between risk for ALS and intermediate alleles of *ATXN2* suggests that variation in the polyQ tract, within the wild-type range, affects its function – perhaps through some aspect of RNA metabolism impacted by both ATXN2 and TDP-43.

SCA1

SCA1 is caused by the expansion of a polyglutamine tract within the ataxin-1 (ATXN1) protein [76]. ATXN1 is located in the cytoplasm and nucleus. The dynamics of ataxin-1 within the nucleus are altered by expansion of the polyglutamine tract. Although mutant ATXN1 with an expanded polyglutamine tract is able to enter the nucleus, its ability to be transported back into the cytoplasm is dramatically reduced [77]. Also, the length of the polyglutamine tract negatively affects SUMOylation of ATXN1, which occurs when ATXN1 is transported to the nucleus [78].

While ATXN1 normally interacts with a variety of cellular molecules including RNA, several regulators of transcription, and RNA splicing factors, the two cellular interactions that are major drivers of pathogenesis are with the transcriptional regulator Capicua (Cic) [79] and the RNA splicing factor RBM17 [40]. ATXN1's interaction with these two proteins involves two evolutionarily conserved regions within ATXN1: (i) the 120 amino acid AXH domain [80], which interacts with Cic; and (ii) a 12 amino acid segment, residues 768–780 towards the C-terminus of ATXN1, that contains a UHM ligand motif (ULM), amino acids 771–776, with which RBM17 interacts [40, 81]. Besides the ULM, this C-terminal segment contains two overlapping functional motifs: (i) a nuclear localization sequence (NLS), amino acids 771–774, and a 14-3-3 binding motif, amino acids 774–778; and (ii) an endogenous site of phosphorylation at Ser776 (S776).

The biological effect on Cic of ATXN1 polyglutamine expansion is complex. First, overexpression of Cic was protective in a fly model of SCA1 [79], whereas partial loss of Cic prolonged lifespan in mice [82]. It seems that for some Cic gene targets expanded ATXN1 causes a loss of function while at other targets polyglutamine-expanded ATXN1 enhances Cic binding, inducing a state of hyper-repression. In the mouse, it is postulated that the hyper-repressive effect of expanded polyglutamine ATXN1 is toxic. Intriguingly, mild exercise, perhaps involving the Cic pathway in the brainstem, improves survival in a mouse model of SCA1 in absence of improving the cerebellar motor dysfunction. While more vigorous motor activity that engages the cerebellum might restore motor function, one also needs to consider that distinct ATXN1 complexes, that is, cellular pathways, contribute to disease in different regions of the CNS. Such a hypothesis is supported by the ability of a partial loss of 14-3-3 to improve cerebellar phenotypes and not brainstem phenotypes [83].

The C-terminal region of ATXN1, encompassing residues 771–778, also plays a key role in SCA1. First, inactivation of the NLS in ATXN1, which prevents mutant ATXN1 from entering the nucleus of neurons, blocks the ability of ATXN1 with an expanded polyglutamine tract to cause neurodegeneration *in vivo* [33]. Second, phosphorylation of S776, immediately adjacent to the NLS, stabilizes ATXN1 because the phospho-resistant Ala776 (A776) ATXN1 is far less stable than either S776 or a potentially phospho-mimicking Asp776 (D776) ATXN1 [84, 85]. In a mouse model of SCA1, ATXN1[82Q]-A776 is not pathogenic when expressed in Purkinje cells [86]. Moreover, expression of ATXN1 with a wild-type 30Q polyglutamine tract but with an Asp amino acid at position 776, ATXN1[30Q]-D776, in Purkinje neurons of transgenic mice results in a disease similar to that seen with ATXN1[82Q]-S776 [41].

Importantly, the interaction of ATXN1 with the RNA splicing factor RBM17 also is impacted by the length of the polyQ tract as well as the amino acid residue at position 776. The ATXN1/RBM17 interaction increases with increasing length of the polyglutamine tract and when there is an Asp at residue 776 regardless of polyQ tract length. Moreover, the interaction of RBM17 with ATXN1-A776 is decreased dramatically regardless of polyglutamine tract length [40]. Together the data indicate a direct link between pathogenicity of mutant ATXN1 and the strength of its interaction with RBM17 in a manner suggesting a cellular pathway that involves its phosphorylation at S776 as a critical aspect of SCA1 pathogenesis.

SCA7

Besides progressive cerebellar degeneration, patients with SCA7 uniquely display retinal degeneration. ATXN7 functions as a component of the SAGA (**S**pt–**A**da–**G**cn5 **a**cetyltransferase) complex [87]. SAGA regulates transcription via its two histone-modifying activities, the Gcn5 histone acetyltransferase and the Usp22 deubiquitinase. Although ATXN7 has no enzymatic activity, it is reported to anchor the Usp22 component to the SAGA complex. It is the Gcn5 histone acetyltransferase (HAT) activity of SAGA that seems to be affected by the presence of ATXN7 with an expanded polyQ tract. Whether mutant ATXN7 decreases or increases HAT activity remains unclear. The reported increase in HAT activity with mutant ATXN7 is based on an *in vivo* analysis in the retina while the studies showing a loss of activity either used human ATXN7 in yeast or transfected 293T cells. Perhaps differences between model systems and/or tissue underlie the discrepancies regarding the effect that mutant ATXN7 has on Gcn5 HAT activity. It is worth noting that a mutant ATXN7-induced gain in Gcn5 HAT activity is in line with the autosomal dominant inheritance pattern of SCA7.

Using an elegant conditional inactivation approach, Furrer and colleagues showed that cerebellar disease in mice involves the action of mutant ATXN7 in both neurons and glia [88]. This study was also able to demonstrate that dysfunction of inferior olivary neurons, whose axons (i.e., climbing fibers) are one of the two major excitatory inputs to Purkinje cells, also contributes to SCA7 pathogenesis. These findings nicely illustrate the complexity of disease in SCA7, and likely other SCAs.

SCA6

This disease is caused by an expansion of a polyglutamine tract in the C-terminus of the α1A transmembrane subunit of the P/Q-type voltage-gated calcium channel *CACNA1A* [89, 90]. Thus, at first, the pathogenesis of SCA6 seemed to be a relatively straightforward channelopathy. This channel is known to be abundant in Purkinje cells of the cerebellum and is the mutational target in several other inherited neurological disorders [91].

Although initial studies indicated that SCA6 was a disorder resulting from P/Q channel dysfunction [92–94], two additional findings complicate this concept. Electrophysiological analysis of $Sca6^{84Q}$ knockin mice failed to find a change in the intrinsic properties of Purkinje cells [95]. Noting earlier evidence that the polyQ containing cytoplasmic C-terminus is cleaved to form a stable peptide, Kordasiewicz et al. examined the α1A C-terminus in more detail [96]. They found that the α1A C-terminal peptide localizes to Purkinje cell nuclei in wild-type mice and humans. Moreover, the C-terminal peptide with an expanded polyglutamine tract is toxic to tissue culture cells, with toxicity being dependent on its nuclear localization. Subsequently, Du et al. [97] showed that the *CACNA1A* gene encodes a bicistronic mRNA with an internal ribosomal entry site (IRES) that is translated into two proteins (Figure 22.2). One protein is the α1A subunit of the P/Q-type Ca^{+2} channel. The second protein is the transcription factor α1ACT. Data indicate that pathogenesis is largely driven by alterations in gene expression due to α1ACT with an expanded polyQ. Moreover, blocking the IRES-driven translation of α1ACT rescues SCA6-like phenotypes in a mouse model of SCA6 [98].

Nevertheless, one should be cautious in discarding SCA6 as a calcium channelopathy given the vast amount of data implicating altered calcium signaling in the SCAs. Evidence for alterations in calcium signaling and/or handling is reported for SCA1 [99, 100], SCA2 [101], and SCA3 [102]. In addition, recent data show that SCA15, a non-polyQ SCA, is caused by to a mutation in the InsP3 receptor 1 gene encoding a receptor that functions in the release of Ca^{2+} from intracellular stores [103].

Approaches to therapy

Clearly, for the more prevalent polyglutamine SCAs there remains much to learn before a targeted approach to treatment, one based on correcting an altered function that drives pathology, is in

hand. However, several studies have been performed to evaluate potential therapies using the mouse models of SCA (Table 22.3). Moreover, there are a couple of encouraging points worth noting regarding treatments for the SCAs. First, there is evidence, at least for SCA1, that pathology and neurological deficits can be reversed even after disease is underway [104]. In the case of SCA1, the data indicate that the ability to recover normal function decreases with age and progression of disease. This provides support for the widely held notion that the sooner one intervenes therapeutically, the better the chance of having a positive impact. The second key point is that for these SCAs – regardless of the mechanism by which disease develops – pathogenesis requires the presence of the mutant protein. Thus, decreasing the amount of mutant protein becomes a viable approach to therapy even in the absence of an understanding of the downstream effects that lead to disease.

One approach shown to be effective in reducing expression of mutant ATXN1 *in vivo* is using RNA interference (RNAi) expressing adeno-associated viruses injected into the deep cerebellar nuclei [105–107]. Mutant ATXN1 expression was reduced such that motor function was significantly improved and Purkinje cell morphology was normalized in transduced cells. While this SCA1 study utilized an shRNA that would target both wild-type and mutant ATXN1, allele-specific strategies where the mutant allele would be preferentially targeted are under development for several of the polyglutamine disorders including SCA3 [108].

That these diseases require expression of the mutant protein for disease to manifest itself has an additional implication in terms of a potential approach to therapy. The term proteostasis is applied to the protein homeostatic network of cellular pathways that regulate the overall quality control of proteins that normally make up the proteome of each cell. In numerous instances the ability of this system to adapt to normal metabolic demands becomes compromised with aging and with the presence of misfolded mutant proteins such as those associated with many of the inherited neurodegenerative diseases [109, 110]. One can anticipate that as these pathways and the ways in which they are compromised in neurodegenerative diseases like the SCAs are defined, regulators of protein homeostasis could become novel therapeutic agents in the polyglutamine ataxias.

References

1. Harding AE. The clinical features and classification of the late onset autosomal dominant cerebellar ataxias. A study of 11 families, including descendants of the Drew family of Walworth. *Brain* 1982; **105**: 1–28.
2. Plaitakis A. Classification and epidemiology of cerebellar degenerations. In: PlaitakisA (ed.) *Cerebellar Degenerations: Clinical Neurobiology*. Kluwer Academic Press: Boston, 1992: 185–204.
3. Silva MC, Coutinho P, Pinheiro CD, *et al.* Hereditary ataxias and spastic paraplegias: methodological aspects of a prevalence study in Portugal. *J Clin Epidemiol* 1997; **50**: 1377–1384.
4. van de Warrenburg BP, Sinke RJ, Verschuuren-Bemelmans CC, *et al.* Spinocerebellar ataxias in the Netherlands: prevalence and age at onset variance analysis. *Neurology* 2002; **58**: 702–708.
5. Ranum LP, Lundgren JK, Schut LJ, *et al.* Spinocerebellar ataxia type 1 and Machado-Joseph disease: incidence of CAG expansions among adult-onset ataxia patients from 311 families with dominant, recessive, or sporadic ataxia. *Am J Hum Genet* 1995; **57**: 603–608.
6. Sasaki H, Fukazawa T, Yanagihara T, *et al.* Clinical features and natural history of spinocerebellar ataxia type 1. *Acta Neurol Scand* 1996; **93**: 64–71.
7. Filla A, Mariotti, C, Caruso G, *et al.* Relative frequencies of CAG expansions in spinocerebellar ataxia and dentatorubropallidoluysian atrophy in 116 Italian families. *Eur Neurol* 2000; **44**: 31–36.

8. Moseley ML, Benzow, KA. Schut LJ, *et al*. Incidence of dominant spinocerebellar and Friedreich triplet repeats among 361 ataxia families. *Neurology* 1998; **51**: 1666–1671.

9. Schols L, Kruger R, Amoiridis G, *et al*. Spinocerebellar ataxia type 6: genotype and phenotype in German kindreds. *J Neurol Neurosurg Psychiatry* 1998; **64**: 67–73.

10. Zoghbi HY. The expanding world of ataxins. *Nat Genet* 1996; **14**: 237–238.

11. Durr A. Autosomal dominant cerebellar ataxias: polyglutamine expansions and beyond. *Lancet Neurol* 2010; **9**: 885–894.

12. Sesqueiros J, Coutinho P. *Epidemiology and Clinical Aspects of Machado-Joseph Disease*. Raven Press: New York, 1993.

13. Rub U, Brunt ER, Petrasch-Parwez E, *et al*. Degeneration of ingestion-related brainstem nuclei in spinocerebellar ataxia type 2, 3, 6 and 7. *Neuropathol Appl Neurobiol* 2006; **32**: 635–649.

14. Rub U, Burk K, Timmann D, *et al*. Spinocerebellar ataxia type 1 (SCA1): New pathoanatomical and clinico-pathological insights. *Neuropathol Appl Neurobiol* 2012; **38**: 665–680.

15. Rub U, Del Turco D, Burk K, *et al*. Extended pathoanatomical studies point to a consistent affection of the thalamus in spinocerebellar ataxia type 2. *Neuropathol Appl Neurobiol* 2005; **31**: 127–140.

16. Paulson H L, Perez MK, Trottier Y, *et al*. Intranuclear inclusions of expanded polyglutamine protein in spinocerebellar ataxia type 3. *Neuron* 1997; **19**: 333–344.

17. Gierga K, Burk K, Bauer M, *et al*. Involvement of the cranial nerves and their nuclei in spinocerebellar ataxia type 2 (SCA2). *Acta Neuropathol* 2005; **109**: 617–631.

18. Robitaille Y, Schut L, Kish SJ. Structural and immunocytochemical features of olivopontocerebellar atrophy caused by the spinocerebellar ataxia type 1 (SCA-1) mutation define a unique phenotype. *Acta Neuropathol* 1995; **90**: 572–581.

19. Gouw LG, Digre KB, Harris CP, *et al*. Autosomal dominant cerebellar ataxia with retinal degeneration: clinical, neuropathologic, and genetic analysis of a large kindred. *Neurology* 1994; **44**: 1441–1447.

20. Martin JJ, Van Regemorter N, Krols L, *et al*. On an autosomal dominant form of retinal-cerebellar degeneration: an autopsy study of five patients in one family. *Acta Neuropathol* 1994; **88**: 277–286.

21. Yang Q, Hashizume Y, Yoshida M, *et al*. Morphological Purkinje cell changes in spinocerebellar ataxia type 6. *Acta Neuropathol (Berl)* 2000; **100**: 371–376.

22. Gomez CM. Thompson RM, Gammack JT, *et al*. Spinocerebellar ataxia type 6: gaze- evoked and vertical nystagmus, Purkinje cell degeneration, and variable age of onset. *Ann Neurol* 1997; **42**: 933–950.

23. Ishikawa K, Fujigasaki H, Saegusa H, *et al*. Abundant expression and cytoplasmic aggregations of [alpha]1A voltage-dependent calcium channel protein associated with neurodegeneration in spinocerebellar ataxia type 6. *Hum Mol Genet* 1999; **8**: 1185–1193.

24. Öz G, Hutter D, Tkác I, *et al*. Neurochemical alterations in spinocerebellar ataxia type 1 and their correlations with clinical status. *Mov Disorder* 2010; **25**: 1253–1261.

25. Schmitz-Hubsch T, du Montcel ST, Baliko L, *et al*. Scale for the assessment and rating of ataxia: development of a new clinical scale. *Neurology* 2006; **66**: 1717–1720.

26. Öz G, Ilis, I, Hutter D, *et al*. Distinct neurochemical profiles of spinocerebellar ataxias 1, 2, 6, and cerebellar multiple system atrophy. *Cerebellum* 2011; **10**: 208–217.

27. Öz G, Nelson CD, Koski DM, *et al*. Noninvasive detection of pre-symptomatic and progressive neurodegeneration in a mouse model of spinocerebellar ataxia type 1. *J Neuroscience* 2010; **30**: 3831–3838.

28. Pujana MA, Corral J, Gratacos M, *et al*. Spinocerebellar ataxias in Spanish patients: genetic analysis of familial and sporadic cases. The Ataxia Study Group. *Hum Genet* 1999; **104**: 516–522.

29. Schols L, Szymanski, Peters S, *et al*. Genetic background of apparently idiopathic sporadic cerebellar ataxia. *Hum Genet* 2000; **107**: 132–137.

30. Trouillas P, Takayanagi T, Hallett M, *et al*. International Cooperative Ataxia Rating Scale for pharmacological assessment of the cerebellar syndrome. The Ataxia Neuropharmacology Committee of the World Federation of Neurology. *J Neurol Sci* 1997; **145**: 205–211.

31. Schmahmann JD, Gardner R, MacMore J, *et al*. Development of a brief ataxia rating scale (BARS) based on a modified form of the ICARS. *Mov Disord* 2009; **24**: 1820–1828.

32. Orr HT, Zoghbi HY. Trinucleotide repeat disorders. *Ann Rev Neurosci* 2007; **30**: 575–621.

33. Klement IA, Skinner, PJ, Kaytor MD, *et al*. Ataxin-1 nuclear localization and aggregation: Role in polyglutamine-induced disease in *SCA1* transgenic mice. *Cell* 1998; **95**: 41–53.

34. Saudou F, Finkbeiner S, Devys D, Greenberg ME. Huntingtin acts in the nucleus to induce apoptosis but death does not correlate with the formation of intranuclear inclusions. *Cell* 1998; **95**:55–66.

35. Cummings CJ, Reinstein E, Sun Y, *et al*. Mutation of the E6-AP ubiquitin ligase reduces nuclear inclusion frequency while accelerating polyglutamine-induced pathology in SCA1 transgenic mice. *Neuron* 1999; **24**:879–892.

36. Arrasate M, Mitra S, Schweitzer ES, Segal MR, Finkbeiner S. Inclusion body formation reduces levels of mutant huntingtin and the risk of neuronal death. *Nature* 2004; **431**: 805–810.

37. Bowman AB, Lam YC, Jafar-Nejad P, *et al*. Duplication of *Ataxin-1B/Boat* suppresses SCA1 neuropathology by decreasing incorporation of polyglutamine-expanded ATAXIN-1 into its native complexes. *Nat Genet* 2007; **39**: 373–379.

38. Katsuno M, Adachi H, Kume M, *et al*. Testosterone reduction prevents phenotypic expression in a transgenic mouse model of spinal and bulbar muscular atrophy. *Neuron* 2002; **35**: 843–854.

39. Takeyama K, Ito S, Yamamoto A, *et al*. Androgen-dependent neurodegeneration by polyglutamine-expanded human androgen receptor in *Drosophila*. *Neuron* 2002; **35**: 855–864.

40. Lim J, Crespo-Barreto J, Jafar-Nejad P, *et al*. Opposing effects of polyglutamine expansion on native protein complexes contribute to SCA1. *Nature* 2008; **452**: 713–719.

41. Duvick L, Barnes J, Ebner B, *et al*. SCA1-like disease in mice expressing wild type ataxin-1 with a serine to aspartic acid replacement at residue 776. *Neuron* 2010; **67**: 929–935.

42. Nedelsky NB, Pennuto M, Smith RB, *et al*. Native functions of the androgen receptor are essential to pathogenesis in a Drosophila model of spinobulbar muscular atrophy. *Neuron* 2010; **67**:936–952.

43. Orr HT. Beyond the Qs in the polyglutamine diseases. *Genes Dev* 2001; **15**: 925–932.

44. Li F, Macfarlan T, Pittman RH, Chakravarti. Ataxin-3 is a histone-binding protein with two independent transcriptional corepressor activities. *J Biol Chem* 2002; **277**: 45004–45012.

45. Evert BO, Araujo J, Vieira-Saeker AM, *et al*. Ataxin-3 represses transcription via chromatin binding, interaction with histone deacetylase 3, and histone deacetylation. *J Neurosci* 2006; **26**: 11474–11486.

46. Reina CP, Zhong X, Pittman RN. Proteotoxic stress increases nuclear localization of ataxin-3. *Hum Mol Genet* 2009; **9**: 235–249.

47. Chai Y, Koppenhafer SL, Shoesmith SJ, *et al*. Evidence for proteasome involvement in polyglutamine disease: localization to nuclear inclusions in SCA3/MJD and suppression of polyglutamine aggregation *in vivo*. *Hum Mol Genet* 1999; **8**: 673–682.

48. Fujigaski H, Uschihara T, Koyano S, *et al*. Ataxin-3 is translocated into the nucleus for the formation of intranuclear inclusions in normal and Machado-Joseph disease brains. *Exp Neurol* 2000; **165**: 248–256.

49. Bichelmeier U, Schmidt T, Hubener J, *et al*. Nuclear localization of ataxin-3 is required for the manifestations of symptoms in SCA3; *in vivo* evidence. *J Neurosci* 2007; **27**: 7418–7428.

50. Shimohata T, Nakajima T, Yamada M, *et al*. Expanded polyglutamine stretches interact with TAFII130, interfering with CREB-dependent transcription. *Nat Genet* 2000; **26**: 29–36.

51. McCampbell A, Taylor JP, Taye AA, *et al*. CREB-binding protein sequestration by expanded polyglutamine. *Hum Mol Genet* 2000; **9**: 2197–2202.

52. Wang G, Swai N, Kotliarova S, Kanazawa I, Nukina N. Ataxin-3, the MJD1 gene product, interacts with the two human homologs of yeast DNA repair protein RAD23, HHR23A, and HHR23B. *Hum Mol Genet* 2000; **9**: 1795–1803.

53. Burnett BG, Pittman RN. The polyglutamine neurodegenerative protein ataxin-3 binds polyubiquitylated proteins and has ubiquitin protease activity. *Hum Mol Genet* 2003; **12**: 3195–3205.

54. Winborn BJ, Travis SM, Todi SV, *et al*. The deubiquitinating enzyme ataxin-3, a polyglutamine disease protein, edits Lys[63] linkages in mixed linkage ubiquitin chains. *J Biol Chem* 2008; **283**: 26436–26443.

55. Harris GM, Dodelzon K, Gong L, *et al*. Splice isoforms of the polyglutamine disease proteins ataxin-3 exhibit similar enzymatic yet different aggregation properties. *PLoS ONE* 2010; **5**: e13695.

56. Warrick JM, Morabito LM, Bilen J, *et al*. Ataxin-3 suppresses polyglutamine neurodegeneration in Drosophila by a ubiquitin-associated mechanism. *Mol Cell* 2005; **18**: 37–48.

57. Mao Y, Senic-Maruglia F, DiFiore PP, *et al*. Deubiquitinating function of ataxin-3: insights from the solution structure of the Josephin domain. *Proc Natl Acad Sci USA* 2005; **102**: 12700–12705.

58. Nicastro G, Menon RP, Masino L, *et al*. The solution structure of the Josephin domain of ataxin-3: structural determinants for molecular recognition. *Proc Natl Acad Sci USA* 2005; **102**: 10493–10498.

59. Scaglione KM, Zavodszky E, Todi SV, *et al*. Ube2w and ataxin-3 coordinately regulate the ubiquitin ligase CHIP. *Mol Cell* 2011; **43**: 599–612.

60. Li L-B, Yu Z, Teng X, Bonini NM. RNA toxicity is a component of ataxin-3 degeneration in Drosophila. *Nature* 2008; **453**: 1107–1111.

61. Furtado S, Payami H, Lockhart PJ, *et al*. Profile of families with parkinsonism-predominant spinocerebellar ataxia type 2 (SCA2). *Mov Disord* 2004; **19**: 622–629.

62. Huynh DP, Yang HT, Vakharia H, Nguyen D, Pulst SM. Expansion of the polyQ repeat in ataxin-3 alters its Golgi localization, disrupts the Golgi complex and causes cell death. *Hum Mol Genet* 2003; **12**: 1485–1496.

63. Satterfield TF, Jackson SM, Pallanck LJ. A Drosophila homolog of the polyglutamine disease gene SCA2 is a dosage-sensitive regulator of actin filament formation. *Genetics* 2003; **162**:1687–1702.

64. Wiedemeyer R, Westermann F, Wittke I, *et al*. Ataxin-2 promotes apoptosis of human neuroblastoma cells. *Oncogene* 2003; **22**:401–411.

65. Neuwald AF, Koonin EV. Ataxin-2, global regulators of bacterial gene expression and spliceosomal snRNP proteins share a conserved domain. *J Mol Med* 1998; **76**: 3–5.

66. Kozlov G, Trempe JF, Khaleghpour K, *et al*. Structure and function of the C-terminal PABC domain of human poly(A)-binding protein. *Proc Natl Acad Sci USA* 2001; **98**: 4409–4413.

67. Shibata H, Huynh DP, Pulst SM. A novel protein with RNA-binding motifs interacts with ataxin-2. *Hum Mol Genet* 2000; **9**: 1303–1313.

68. Nonhoff U, Ralser M, Welzel F, *et al*. Ataxin-2 interacts with the DEAD/H-box RNA helicase DDX6 and interferes with P-bodies and stress granules. *Mol Biol Cell* 2007; **18**: 1385–1396.

69. McCann C, Holohan EE, Das S, *et al*. The Ataxin-2 protein is required for micro-RNA function and synapse-specific long-term olfactory habituation. *Proc Natl Acad Sci USA* 2011; **108**: E655–E662.

70. Mangue DA, Amrani N, Jacobson A. Pbp1p, a factor interacting with Saccharomyces cerevisiae poly(A)-binding protein, regulates polyadenylation. *Mol Cell Biol* 1998; **18**: 7383–7396.

71. Dunn CD, Jensen RE. 2003. Suppression of a deficit in mitochondrial protein import identifies cytosolic proteins required for viability of yeast cells lacking mitochondrial DNA. *Genetics* 2003; **165**: 35–45.

72. Satterfield TF, Pallanck LJ. Ataxin-2 and its *Drosophila* homolog, ATX2, physically assemble with polyribosomes. *Hum Mol Genet* 2006; **15**: 2523–2532.

73. Lagier-Tourenne C, Cleveland DC. Rethinking ALS: the FUS about TDP-43. *Cell* 2009; **136**: 1001–1004.

74. Elden AC, Kim H-J, Hart MP, *et al*. Ataxin-2 intermediate-length polyglutamine expansions are associated with increased risk of ALS. *Nature* 2010; **466**: 1069–1075.

75. Van Damme P, Veldink JH, van Blitterswijk, *et al*. Expanded *ATXN2* CAG repeat size in ALS identifies genetic overlap between ALS and SCA2. *Neurology* 2011; **76**: 2066–2072.

76. Orr HT, Chung MY, Banfi S, *et al*. Expansion of an unstable trinucleotide CAG repeat in spinocerebellar ataxia type 1. *Nat Genet* 1993; **4**: 221–226.

77. Irwin S, Vandelft M, Howell JL, *et al*. RNA association and nucleocytoplasmic shuttling by ataxin-1. *J Cell Sci* 2005; **118**: 233–242.

78. Riley BE, Zoghbi HY, Orr HT. SUMOylation of the polyglutamine protein, ataxin-1 is dependent on a functional nuclear localization signal. *J Biol Chem* 2005; **280**: 21942–21948.

79. Lam YC, Bowman AB, Jafar-Nejad P, *et al*. Mutant ATAXIN-1 interacts with the repressor Capicua in its native complex to cause SCA1 neuropathology. *Cell* 2006; **127**: 1335–1347.

80. de Chiara C, Giannini C, Adinolfi S, *et al*. The AXH module: an independently folded domain common to ataxin-1 and HBP. *FEBS Lett* 2003; **551**: 107–112.

81. de Chiara C, Menon RP, Strom M, *et al*. Phosphorylation of S776 and 14-3-3 binding modulate ataxin-1 interaction with splicing factors. *PLoS One* 2009; **4**: e8372.

82. Fryer JD, Yu P, Kang H, *et al*. Exercise and genetic rescue of SCA1 via the transcriptional repressor Capicua. *Science* 2011; **334**: 690–693.

83. Jafar-Nejad P, Ward CS, Richman R, *et al*. Regional rescue of spinocerebellar ataxia type 1 phenotypes by 14-3-3epsilon haploinsufficiency in mice underscores complex pathogenicity in neurodegeneration. *Proc Natl Acad Sci USA* 2011; **108**: 2142–2147.

84. Jorgensen ND, Andresen JM, Lagalwar S, *et al*. Phosphorylation of ATXN1 at Ser776 in the cerebellum. *J Neurochem* 2009; **110**: 675–686.

85. Lai S, O'Callaghan B, Zoghbi HY, Orr HT. 14-3-3 binding to ataxin-1(ATXN1) regulates its dephosphorylation at S776 and transport to the nucleus. *J Biol Chem* 2011; **286**: 34606–34616.

86. Emamian ES, Kaytor MD, Duvick LA, *et al*. Serine 776 of ataxin-1 is critical for polyglutamine-induced disease in *SCA1* transgenic mice. *Neuron* 2003; **38**: 375–387.

87. Helmlinger D, Hardy S, Eberlin A, Devys D, Tora L. Both normal and polyglutamine-expanded ataxin-7 are components of TFTc-type GCN5 histone acetyltransferase-containing complexes. *Biochem Soc Symp* 2006; **73**: 155–163.

88. Furrer SA, Mohanachandran MS, Waldherr SM, *et al*. Spinocerebellar ataxia type 7 cerebellar disease requires the coordinated action of mutant ataxin-7 in neurons and glia, and displays non-cell-autonomous Bergmann glia degeneration. *J Neurosci* 2011; **31**: 16269–16278.

89. Riess O, Schols L, Bottger H, *et al*. SCA6 is caused by moderate CAG expansion in the alpha 1A-voltage-dependent calcium channel gene. *Hum Mol Genet* 1997; **6**: 1289–1293.

90. Zhuchenko O, Bailey J, Bonnen P, *et al*. Autosomal dominant cerebellar ataxia (SCA6) associated with small polyglutamine expansions in the alpha 1A-voltage-dependent calcium channel. *Nat Genet* 1997; **15**: 62–69.

91. Pietrobon D. Calcium channels and channelopathies of the central nervous system. *Mol Neurobiol* 2002; **25**: 31–50.

92. Matsuyama Z, Wakamori M, Mori Y, *et al*. Direct alteration of the P/Q-type Ca^{2+} channel property by polyglutamine expansion in spinocerebellar ataxia 6. *J Neurosci* 1999; **19**: RC14(1–5).

93. Restituito S, Thompson RM, Eliet J, *et al*. The polyglutamine expansion in spinocerebellar ataxia type 6 causes a beta subunit-specific enhanced activation of P/Q-type calcium channels in Xenopus oocytes. *J Neurosci* 2000; **20**: 6394–6403.

94. Toru S, Murakoshi T, Ishikawa K, *et al*. Spinocerebellar ataxia type 6 mutation alters P-type calcium channel function. *J Biol Chem* 2000; **275**: 10893–10898.

95. Watase K, Barrett CF, Miyazaki T, *et al*. Spinocerebellar ataxia type 6 knockin mice develop a progressive neuronal dysfunction with age-dependent accumulation of mutant C2.1 channels. *Proc Natl Acad Sci USA* 2008; **105**: 11987–11992.

96. Kordasiewicz HB, Thompson RM, Clark HB, Gomez GM. C-termini of P/Q-type Ca^{2+} channel a1a subunits translocate to nuclei and promote polyglutamine-mediated toxicity. *Hum Mol Genet* 2006; **15**: 1587–1599.

97. Du X, Wang J, Zhu H, Rinaldo L, Lamar K-M, Palmenberg AC, Hansel C, Gomez CM. Second cistron in CACNA1A gene encodes a transcription factor mediating cerebellar development and SCA6. *Cell* 2013; **154**: 118–133.

98. Miyazaki Y, Du X, Muramatsu S-I, Gomez CM. An miRNA-mediated therapy for SCA6 blocks IRES-driven translation of the CACNA1A second cistron. *Sci Trans Med* 2016; **8**: 347ra94.

99. Vig PJ, Subramony SH, McDaniel DO. Calcium homeostasis and spinocerebellar ataxia type 1 (SCA-1). *Brain Res Bull* 2001; **56**: 221–225.

100. Serra HG, Byam CE, Lande JD, *et al*. Gene profiling links SCA1 pathophysiology to glutamate signaling in Purkinje cells of transgenic mice. *Hum Mol Genet* 2004; **13**: 2535–2543.

101. Liu J, Tang TS, Tu H, *et al*. Deranged calcium signaling and neurodegeneration in spinocerebellar ataxia type 2. *J Neurosci* 2009; **29**: 9148–9162.

102. Chen X, Tang T-S, Tu H, *et al*. Deranged calcium signaling and neurodegeneration in spinocerebellar ataxia type 3. *J Neurosci* 2008; **28**: 12713–12724.

103. van de Leemput J, Chandran J, Knight MA, *et al*. Deletion at ITPR1 underlies ataxia in mice and spinocerebellar ataxia type 15 in humans. *PLoS Genet* 2007; **3**: e108.

104. Zu T, Duvick LA, Kaytor MD, *et al*. Recovery from polyglutamine-induced neurodegeneration in conditional *SCA1* transgenic mice. *J Neurosci* 2004; **24**: 8853–8861.

105. Xia H, Mao O, Eliason SI, *et al*. RNAi suppresses polyglutamine-induced neurodegeneration in a model of spinocerebellar ataxia. *Nat Med* 2004; **10**: 816–820.

106. Keiser MS, Geoghegan JC, Boudreau RL, Lennox KA, Davidson BL. RNAi or overexpression; alternative therapies for Spinocerebellar Ataxia Type 1. *Neurobiol Dis* 2013; **56**: 6–13.

107. Keiser MS, Boudreau RL, Davidson BL. Broad therapeutic benefit after RNAi expression vector delivery to deep cerebellar nuclei: implications for spinocerebellar ataxia type 1 therapy. *Mol Ther* 2014; **22**: 588–595.

108. Alves S, Nascimento-Ferrira I, Auregan G, *et al*. Allele-specific RNA silencing of mutant ataxin-3 mediates neuroprotection in a rat model of Machado-Joseph disease. *PLoS ONE* 2008; **3**: e3341.

109. Voisine C, Pedersen JS, Morimoto RI. 2010. Chaperone networks: tipping the balance in protein folding diseases. *Neurobiol Dis* 2010; **40**: 12–20.

110. Balch WE, Mormoto RI, Dillin A, Kelly JW. Adapting proteostasis for disease intervention. *Science* 2008; **319**: 916–919.

111. Cummings CJ, Sun Y, Opal P, *et al*. Over-expression of inducible HSP70 chaperone suppresses neuropathology and improves motor function in SCA1 mice. *Hum Mol Genet* 2001; **10**: 1511 1518.

112. Gehrking KM, Andresen JM, Duvick L, *et al*. Partial loss of Tip60 slows mid-stage neurodegeneration in a spinocerebellar ataxia type 1 (SCA1) mouse model. *Hum Mol Genet* 2011; **20**: 2204–2212.

113. Serra HG, Duvick L, Zu T, *et al*. RORalpha-mediated Purkinje cell development determines disease severity in adult SCA1 mice. *Cell* 2006; **127**: 697–708.

114. Watase K, Gatchel JR, Sun Y, *et al*. Lithium therapy improves neurological function and hippocampal dendritic arborization in a spinocerebellar ataxia type 1 mouse model. *PLoS Med* 2007; **4**: –e182.

115. Chen KA, Cruz PE, Lanuto DJ, *et al.* Cellular fusion for gene delivery to SCA1 affected Purkinje neurons. *Mol Cell Neurosci* 2011; **47**: 61–70.

116. Chintawar S, Hourez R, Ravella A, *et al.* Grafting neural precursor cells promotes functional recovery in an SCA1 mouse model. *J Neurosci* 2009; **29**: 13126–13135.

117. Chang YK, Chen MH, Chiang YH, *et al.* Mesenchymal stem cell transplantation ameliorates motor function deterioration of spinocerebellar ataxia by rescuing cerebellar Purkinje cells. *J Biomed Sci* 2011; **18**: 54.

118. Boy J, Schmidt T, Wolburg H, *et al.* Reversibility of symptoms in a conditional mouse model of spinocerebellar ataxia type 3. *Hum Mol Genet* 2009; **18**: 4282–4295.

119. Williams AJ, Knutson TM, Colomer Gould VF, Paulson HL. In vivo suppression of polyglutamine neurotoxicity by C-terminus of Hsp70-interacting protein (CHIP) supports an aggregation model of pathogenesis. *Neurobiol Dis* 2009; **33**: 342–353.

120. Chou AH, Chen SY, Yeh TH, Weng YH, Wang HL. HDAC inhibitor sodium butyrate reverses transcriptional downregulation and ameliorates ataxic symptoms in a transgenic mouse model of SCA3. *Neurobiol Dis* 2011; **41**: 481–488.

121. Menzies FM, Huebener J, Renna M, *et al.* Autophagy induction reduces mutant ataxin-3 levels and toxicity in a mouse model of spinocerebellar ataxia type 3. *Brain* 2010; **133**: 93–104.

122. Qin Q, Inatome R, Hotta A, *et al.* A novel GTPase, CRAG, mediates promyelocytic leukemia protein-associated nuclear body formation and degradation of expanded polyglutamine protein. *J Cell Biol* 2006; **172**: 497–504.

123. Bichelmeier U, Schmidt T, Hubener J, *et al.* Nuclear localization of ataxin-3 is required for the manifestation of symptoms in SCA3: in vivo evidence. *J Neurosci* 2007; **27**: 7418–7428.

124. Ikeda H, Yamaguchi M, Sugai S, *et al.* Expanded polyglutamine in the Machado-Joseph disease protein induces cell death in vitro and in vivo. *Nat Genet* 1996; **13**: 196–202.

CHAPTER 23

Ataxia Telangiectasia

Malcolm Taylor

Institute of Cancer and Genomic Sciences, University of Birmingham, Edgbaston, Birmingham, UK

Clinical definition and epidemiology

Ataxia telangiectasia (A-T) is an autosomal recessive cerebellar ataxia caused, in its classical form, by biallelic inactivation of the *ATM* gene. Boder and Sedgwick [1] first identified A-T as the only predominantly cerebellar degeneration of infancy and childhood. Their review is still an excellent description of A-T although we now know about important genotype–phenotype correlations in A-T.

Ataxia of gait and posture is almost always the presenting feature of classical A-T in childhood, consisting of swaying of the head and trunk and the ataxia becoming obvious at the time when the child starts to walk. Inevitable progression of the ataxia may be masked temporarily by the rate of normal development during young school age [1]. Dysarthria and drooling are also early features. There are also progressive oculomotor abnormalities, including an abnormal oculokinetic nystagmus, saccades, pursuits, and strabismus. The eye movement defects are multiple and complex [2–4]. However, although early features may be principally cerebellar in origin, extrapyramidal features such as choreoathetosis are also usually present from a young age in classical A-T [1, 5].

By the age of 8–12 years the progressive ataxia leads to the requirement of a wheelchair for mobility [1, 5]. With increasing age, children develop a characteristic seated posture with hypotonia. Characteristics of the middle and late teens include neuromuscular features such as weakness, atrophy, a sensory deficit, absent deep reflexes, and development of peripheral neuropathy.

Non-neurological aspects of presentation almost always include bulbar telangiectasia, from which the disorder gets its name, although this has nothing to do with the movement disorder of the eyes. Telangiectasias may also be seen elsewhere, such as on the head, trunk, or arms. Other non-neurological features include frequent small size and an immune deficiency. Some patients may develop serious chest infections. Cutaneous granulomas, refractory to treatment, are a feature of A-T [6] seen in approximately10% of patients. The unusual sensitivity to therapeutic doses of ionizing radiation (IR) and predisposition to lymphoid malignancies are described in the section on Pathology/pathophysiology.

Nowadays the majority of cases of A-T present in early childhood and have the classical form. Conversely, the final diagnosis of some A-T patients with a milder and different presentation may not be made until their 30s, 40s, or even older (see section Spectrum of clinical phenotype and genetics).

The prevalence of A-T in those aged 50 years or under was approximately 1/500,000 and the birth frequency 1/300,000 in 1990 [7]. Our estimate is that in the British Isles (UK and Ireland) there are currently approximately 132 families with approximately 150 cases of A-T, giving a prevalence of around 1/430,000. The carrier frequency would therefore be of the order of 0.3%.

Spectrum of clinical phenotype and genetics

Ataxia telangiectasia is a progressive neurological disorder [8] caused by mutations in the *ATM* gene which encodes ATM, a 370-kDa serine/threonine protein kinase. ATM is activated by autophosphorylation in response to DNA double strand breaks [8] and phosphorylates many downstream substrates leading to activation of cell cycle checkpoints and either DNA repair or apoptosis [8]. Therefore, ATM deficiency leads to inappropriate progression through the cell cycle and retention of cells with damaged DNA. In the brain, damaged cells may become incorporated into neuronal tissues and lead to neurodegeneration, possibly as a result of failure of apoptosis [8].

The classical form of A-T results from biallelic loss of ATM function and has its clinical presentation in toddlerhood. However, a significant proportion of A-T patients show a different combination of age of onset and/or rate of progress, resulting in a spectrum of clinical phenotypes. Patients may be diagnosed as having ataxia telangiectasia in their fifth decade and only as a consequence of another non-neurological feature of A-T. With rare exceptions, there is a good genotype–phenotype correlation in A-T that appears to result from the degree of ATM protein activity in the patient's cells; the absence of activity is associated with the most severe form of the disorder and the presence of some activity is associated with a less severe form. Therefore A-T patients can be subdivided into six subgroups based on a combination of age of onset and rate of progress of the neurodegeneration. There are two distinguishable subgroups of onset in childhood, the typical or classical form and a later-onset milder form, two subgroups of distinguishable adult onset (early and later age of onset), a subgroup with disparity between the cellular and clinical phenotypes, and finally A-T caused by a completely different gene, *MRE11*.

These subgroups and the mutational basis of the different clinical phenotypes are as follows.

(i) Childhood onset – young age of onset (~2 years), typical/classical

This form of A-T is associated with biallelic mutation of *ATM* that results in instability and total loss of the ATM protein. Cells from

Neurodegeneration, First Edition. Edited by Anthony Schapira, Zbigniew Wszolek, Ted M. Dawson and Nicholas Wood.
© 2017 John Wiley & Sons, Ltd. Published 2017 by John Wiley & Sons, Ltd.

such patients will, therefore, show no ATM protein activity (thus far only the kinase activity – an ability to phosphorylate other proteins – has been identified as an ATM activity that can be readily measured in patients' cells). A-T patients with either two *ATM* null mutations or other mutation types that result in protein but without activity should all have a similar presentation, with a similar age of onset. This class of A-T can arise from different combinations of *ATM* mutation types that include substitution resulting in a stop codon, an insertion or deletion resulting in a frameshift mutation and downstream stop codon, small in frame deletions, missense mutations producing protein without activity, etc. [9]. These mutations have in common absence of ATM kinase activity; indeed, 75% of A-T patients in the UK and Netherlands have no ATM kinase activity and can therefore be described as having classical or typical forms of A-T. Even within this group of A-T patients with the "classical" form of the disorder, there is some variation in presentation. Crawford et al. [10] described a quantitative neurological assessment of A-T that included an assessment of eye movement, standing and sitting ability, gait, head movements, adventitious movements, neuropathy, feeding skills, and swallowing. They reported that although there was good intrafamilial similarity between patients there was interfamilial variation when patients of the same age were compared. This suggested that there were some modifying factors at work in what might, otherwise, be considered a genetically homogeneous group.

(ii) Childhood onset – atypical, slower rate of progress

This neurologically measurably milder form of A-T results from the expression of some ATM protein with residual activity. Approximately 25% of patients in the UK and the Netherlands have some retained kinase activity and therefore have an atypical presentation [9].

This activity can be derived either from normal ATM protein, expressed at a low level, or mutant ATM. The single largest proportion of these patients in the UK population result from the expression of a low level of normal ATM with normal activity, and this is associated with the leaky splice site mutation c.5763-1050A>G (p.Pro1922fs) [9, 11, 12]. This mutation results in a slightly older age of onset of A-T, a slower progression, and greater longevity. Parents noted a later mean age of onset of 3 years (12 patients) compared with 1.5 years in 31 consecutive classical A-T patients [11]; the median age of this group of 22 A-T patients in the UK is 35 years at the time of writing.

A low level of normal ATM with normal activity is also associated with another, less frequently observed, leaky splice site mutation, c.1066-6T>G (p.Val356fs) [13].

A different cause of a milder clinical presentation in A-T is the expression of mutant ATM protein, expressed from a missense allele that has some activity (see Table 23.1 for examples). Some of these patients also have a different presentation to classical A-T. An example of this is an atypical case of slowly progressing A-T but with a prominent and striking oromandibular dystonia [14] although there was normal gait at age 18 years. Interestingly, although this patient showed no bulbar telangiectasia, a leash of telangiectasia was detected on the pharyngeal wall. The patient was homozygous for the p.Gly197Glu mutant ATM protein (c.590G>A mutation) with kinase activity.

Saunders-Pullman et al. [15] described 12 Canadian Mennonite A-T patients with primary appearing dystonia. Median age of onset of neck dystonia was 12 years, and generalized dystonia eventually affected approximately 60% of these patients. All had preserved but

Table 23.1 Types of ataxia telangiectasia caused by *ATM* mutation and identified mutations associated with them.

(i) Typical or classical A-T – onset at age of ~2 years	
Biallelic mutation resulting in absence of any ATM kinase activity	
A combination of different types of truncating ATM mutations and/or missense mutations expressing either a low or high level (e.g., 9022C>T; p.Arg3008Cys and 8293G>A; p.Gly2765Ser) of ATM protein without activity	[9]
(ii) Atypical A-T – childhood onset, slower rate of progress	
Leaky splice site mutations – allowing some ATM kinase activity	
c.5763-1050A>G; p.Pro1922fs	[9, 11–13]
c.1066-6T>G;p.Val356fs	
Missense mutations – allowing some ATM kinase activity	
c.590 G>A; p.Gly197Glu	[14]
c.6115G>A; p.Glu2039Lys	
ªc.6200C>A; p.Ala2067Asp	[15]
c.7271T>G; p.Val2424Gly	[16]
c.8480T>G;p.Phe2827Cys	[17]
c.8494C>T; p.Arg2832Cys	[17]
(iii) Early adult-onset A-T and slower rate of progress	
Leaky splice site mutations – allowing some ATM kinase activity	
Homozygosity for c.5763-1050A>G; p.Pro1922fs	[18]
Missense mutations – allowing some ATM kinase activity	
c.7184A>T; p.Asp2395Val	
(iv) Late adult-onset A-T	
Missense mutations – allowing some ATM kinase activity	
c.8147T>C; p.Val2716Ala	[19, 20]
c.8672G>A; p.Gly2891Asp	[21]
?c.3136 C>T; p.Leu1046Phe	[19]
?c.7622 T>G; p.Leu2541Arg	
c.7271T>G; p.Val2424Gly	[16]
(v) Disparity of cellular and clinical phenotype	[22]

ª Kinase activity not established.

clumsy or lumbering gait but not ataxia; longevity (median age 51.5 years) was a feature of this group of 12 patients. All patients were homozygous for the mutant protein p.Ala2067Asp (c.6200C>A) and in one of two patients tested a "trace" of ATM protein was detected although no data were presented on kinase assays carried out on cells from these patients. The homozygous missense mutation present resulted in the milder clinical phenotype and the authors could not exclude the possibility that this was due to expression of a low level of ATM with activity.

(iii) Adult onset – early, slow rate of progress

There are, probably, some genuine early adult onset cases of A-T. An example of this is homozygosity for the c.5763-1050A>G (p.Pro1922fs) mutation, as described for subgroup (ii), in two brothers [18]. One brother was 22 years of age when he first noted problems with balance; the second was examined at age 17 years (following diagnosis of a peptic ulcer) and showed ocular telangiectasia and mild ataxia. At ages 28 years and 29 years they were both fully independent in all aspects of daily living and walked unaided, although some abnormalities of eye movement were noted as well as some incoordination, pes cavus, very mild muscle weakness, and some reduction in reflexes. Overall, however, they scored the unusually high scores of 82% and 72%, at these ages respectively, in a quantitative neurological assessment of A-T [10, 18].

Hiel et al. [19] also described three brothers (with missense mutations 7622T>G p.Leu2541Arg and 3136C>T p.Leu1046Phe) and a further patient in a second family (with missense mutation 8147T>C; p.Val2716Ala) with distal spinal muscular atrophy as a major feature of adult-onset A-T in all four cases. More recently Verhagen et al. [5, 23] described Dutch patients with adult onset of A-T.

(iv) Adult onset – later age

In rare instances, A-T is not recognized through a neurological deficiency but through another feature of the disease. Most striking are four examples where each patient received a therapeutic dose of IR, as part of the treatment for breast cancer, which resulted in a severe radiation reaction that subsequently was investigated; in three of the patients a definite diagnosis of A-T was made. Because severe early and late radiation reaction to radiotherapy is extremely rare in breast cancer patients, such a reaction prompted an investigation into a 44-year-old mother who was normally ambulant with no ataxia and minimal other neurological features. T lymphocytes and skin fibroblasts were unusually radiosensitive, although less sensitive than in classical ataxia telangiectasia (A-T). A lymphoblastoid cell line and skin fibroblasts expressed ATM protein with some retained kinase activity. A missense *ATM* mutation c.8672G>A (p.Gly2891Asp) and a c.1A>G substitution were identified, with the p.Gly2891Asp mutant protein shown to have the residual ATM kinase activity [21].

Stankovic et al. [16] previously described a woman who experienced a severe reaction of the breast and skin tissues after receiving adjuvant radiotherapy following resection of her breast cancer. This woman and two siblings, including a sister who also developed breast cancer, were homozygous for the *ATM* mutation c.7271T>G (p.Val2424Gly). In a further case, a 42-year-old breast cancer patient showed extreme radiosensitivity in response to adjuvant radiotherapy following mastectomy [20]. Only one *ATM* mutation c.8147T>C (p.Val2716Ala) – which also has some ATM kinase activity [23] was identified and the patient was subsequently diagnosed with A-T. In the final case, a 50-year-old breast cancer patient had a severe, late, adverse normal tissue reaction to radiotherapy [24]. Nucleotide sequence analysis identified two non-allelic *ATM* mutations in novel premature termination mutation – c.1918A>T (Lys640Stop) and a c.1066- 6T>G (IVS10-6T>G) – described above [13]. Although the patient was not described as having A-T, this must be a possible diagnosis.

All four of these patients carried an *ATM* mutation (either a missense mutation or leaky splice site mutation) that allowed survival to an age when breast cancer occurred. The nature of the underlying *ATM* mutation, which on the one hand allows expression of ATM with sufficient activity to protect against early neurodegeneration but on the other does not protect against radiation damage or breast cancer development, is not understood. It is possible that other genes (modifying genes) may affect these cellular and clinical responses.

(v) Disparity of cellular and clinical phenotypes

In the i–iv subgroups of A-T, the severity of the clinical presentation can be related to the amount of ATM kinase activity present in the patients' cells, with absence of activity found in most severe, classical forms of A-T, and with the presence of some kinase activity in the milder forms.

Interestingly, there are one or two exceptions to this general pattern where there the relationship is not apparent. Alterman et al. [22] described two siblings homozygous for a truncating *ATM* mutation 5653delA that did not allow expression of ATM protein, however both brothers showed a relatively mild phenotype. These observations raise the possibility that modifying genes may be influencing the clinical phenotype in the absence of any ATM protein.

(vi) Ataxia telangiectasia caused by mutation of the *MRE11* gene

The much rarer A-T-like disorder (ATLD) caused by mutation of the *MRE11* gene results in an early onset but slower progression of neurodegeneration. Indeed, two brothers were initially described as having benign hereditary chorea (generalized chorea with additional mild distal dystonia in the absence of other neurological signs in early childhood). In one, at age 11, both dystonia and gait ataxia were more obvious. At age 16, abnormalities of eye movement were present, as were cerebellar dysarthria and mild dystonic posturing of hands and feet; there was no ocular or skin telangiectasia although a CT scan showed cerebellar atrophy. Alpha-fetoprotein (AFP) level was normal and there was moderately increased chromosomal radiosensitivity [25].

There was the appearance, therefore, of a milder form of ataxia telangiectasia.

Only around 20 cases have been published: 4 from the UK [26–29], 2 from Italy [30], 10 from Saudi Arabia [31], and 4 from Japan [32, 33]. ATLD patients also show normal levels of total IgM, IgA, and IgG, although there may be reduced levels of specific functional antibodies. hMre11 is a component of a complex containing the Nbs1 protein. It might be expected therefore, that deficiency of hMre11 would result in a clinical phenotype more like Nijmegen breakage syndrome in which there is deficiency of Nbs1 protein [34–36]. Why this is not the case is not understood. The function of the Mre11 complex is required for full ATM activation and so loss of Mre11 might explain the A-T-like phenotype. Radiosensitivity of ATLD cells by survival is intermediate between A-T and normal, and the same is true for G2 chromosomal radiosensitivity [26, 30, 33].

Other related disorders – RIDDLE syndrome

Two patients with radiosensitivity, immunodeficiency, dysmorphic features, and learning difficulty (RIDDLE) have so far been described with biallelic mutations in the *ATM* pathway gene, *RNF168*. In the first, an individual with absence of IgG, and requiring IgG, also showed stunted growth and a slight ataxic gait. The patient's cultured skin fibroblasts could be shown to be unusually radiosensitive by colony forming assay, and an increased level of unrepaired chromatid type damage following G2 irradiation of his blood lymphocytes could be demonstrated [37, 38]. The RNF168 deficient cells showed a defect in the G2M checkpoint and a mild intra S phase checkpoint (RDS) defect following exposure to IR. Compared with ataxia telangiectasia the increased radiosensitivity is mild, as measured by both colony forming assay and G2 irradiation. Another patient has been described [39] who showed some clinical similarities to the first. A small increased radiosensitivity was demonstrated in lymphoblastoid cells in suspension from the patient.

Cerebellar versus extrapyramidal symptoms in ataxia telangiectasia

Alterman et al. [22] and others [18, 40] have pointed out that the severity of the neurological phenotype in A-T may be dissociated from the extent of cerebellar atrophy. The relationship between the degree of cerebellar atrophy and its effect on the ability of the patient to walk is unclear. This may be because although the cerebellum is almost universally affected in A-T, the integrity of other systems such as the basal ganglia, anterior horn cells, dorsal columns, and peripheral nerves which also determine walking ability can be affected by the disease process to differing degrees [18, 40]. Neither does cerebellar disease explain all the abnormal oculomotor abnormalities in A-T. Saccade abnormalities similar to those found in A-T patients are seen in disorders of the basal ganglia [3].

Overall, cerebellar ataxia has been shown to be absent in some patients with milder A-T [15] and patients with some retained cellular ATM kinase activity [5]. The presence of residual kinase activity mainly resulted in extrapyramidal instead of cerebellar signs, milder or absent neuropathy, and predominance of anterior horn cell degeneration [5].

The finding that all A-T patients show an extrapyramidal movement disorder during the course of the disease [1, 5], while cerebellar ataxia was found only in the most severely affected patients, suggests that the basal ganglia are more sensitive to the pathological mechanism associated with ATM deficiency and that cerebellar signs are the consequence of a more severe ATM deficiency.

Pathology/pathophysiology specific to the disease

In their important review of 1991 [1], Sedgwick and Boder summarized autopsy findings in 60 A-T patients. They described the basic neuropathological hallmark of A-T as diffuse, cortical cerebellar degeneration involving mainly Purkinje and granular layer cells.

A more recent publication on autopsies of three cases of A-T (two of which were genetically confirmed) [41] made the important point that very few autopsies had been reported on genetically confirmed cases of A-T. The hallmark of A-T as a primary cerebellar cortical degeneration with severe loss of Purkinje cells was confirmed although the oldest patient, with milder A-T, showed a more moderate to severe loss of Purkinje cells and also granular cells.

The main neuropathological changes are, therefore, cerebellar atrophy, degeneration of the posterior columns, and an axonal sensorimotor polyneuropathy [1, 41]. With increasing age of the patient, these changes progress and other changes occur in the cerebrum, basal ganglia, and brainstem. Dystrophic and degenerative changes in the anterior horns were also noted [41].

Clinical biomarkers

A-T patients show a high serum AFP level [42]; interestingly, a raised level of serum AFP is also a feature of patients with ataxia oculomotor apraxia type 2, where diagnosis is usually made at an older age compared with A-T. Therefore, a raised level of serum AFP will in all likelihood be an indication of either A-T or AOA2. While AFP level is usually determined (for A-T) in cerebellar degeneration of early childhood, it is also a very useful test to indicate either milder or later onset A-T as well as AOA2.

Chromosomal translocations, principally involving chromosomes 7 and 14, with breakpoints in immune system genes, in approximately 2–10% of stimulated T lymphocytes and occasionally in a much larger proportion, have been a consistent feature of A-T lymphocytes, providing a widely available test.

An increased sensitivity to IR is a feature of A-T, and although this can have fatal consequences for the patient exposed to therapeutic doses of IR, it is widely used for laboratory confirmation of the diagnosis, either by chromosomal radiosensitivity on blood lymphocytes or colony forming assay on skin fibroblasts exposed to IR [43]. However, there are A-T patients, such as those with the leaky splice site mutation c.5763-1050A>G (p.Pro1922fs), whose cells are not significantly more radiosensitive than normal by the chromosomal assay; therefore radiosensitivity should be just one of the laboratory confirmations of the diagnosis.

A-T is also classified as an immunodeficiency disorder. A consequence of the immunodeficiency is recurrent sinopulmonary infection and common warts although serious opportunistic infections are uncommon. Patients may have reduced levels of serum IgA and IgG and an increased level of IgM (possibly indicating a defect in class switching, at least in some patients) [44, 45]. Most A-T patients are lymphopenic due to reduced numbers of both T and B lymphocytes [46], including reduced proportions of both naïve B and T cells [47–49], and so the immunodeficiency affects both humoral and cellular immunity. There is restriction of both TCRV-beta usage and the B cell repertoire [47]. Classical A-T patients with no ATM kinase activity have a more severe immunological phenotype than those expressing low levels of activity [48, 50]. A-T patients expressing a low level of normal ATM protein from the leaky splice site mutation c.5763-1050A>G (p.Pro1922fs) show a premature age associated deficiency of immune system function [48] and there is evidence that classical A-T patients have a congenitally aged immune system [49]. One of the mysteries of A-T is that not all "classical A-T patients" (without any ATM activity) are clinically immunodeficient and that not all patients with laboratory markers of immunodeficiency have an excess of infection [50].

Micol et al. [51] defined A-T clinically as ataxia with two of the following: oculocutaneous telangiectasia, recurrent infections, low serum level of IgA, high serum level of AFP, chromosomal abnormalities (≥4% of lymphocyte metaphases with translocations at 7p14, 7q35, 14q11, 14q32, 2p12, or 22q11).

Examination and investigations (including imaging)

A standard neurological assessment will show the consequences of cerebellar ataxia (ataxia, dysarthria, abnormal eye movements, and also a movement disorder) and MRI will reveal cerebellar atrophy. A neurological assessment specifically for ataxia telangiectasia has been published [10] and this continues to be further developed based on standing and sitting postures, head alignment, the presence of adventitious movements, neuropathy, weight for height, feeding independence, and swallowing. Such a rating scale for A-T is required for reliable measurement of responses to potential future treatments.

Diagnosis and prognosis

A clinical diagnosis of ataxia telangiectasia in early childhood can be made based on the presence of ataxia of both upper and lower limbs, ocular telangiectasia, and abnormal eye movements. The laboratory confirmation of the clinical diagnosis is now quite straightforward. It can be based on a combination of results from a single blood test. The following is carried out on a sample of blood in lithium heparin:

1 DNA should be extracted from the original patient blood sample and the coding region screened for *ATM* mutations. The identification of two pathogenic *ATM* mutations is the gold standard for confirmation of the clinical diagnosis. In the vast majority of cases both *ATM* mutations will be identified quite quickly. In a few instances a more complex mutation will be present. The identification of both *ATM* mutations is not absolutely required for confirmation of the diagnosis of A-T, as long as there is increased radiosensitivity and decrease/absence of ATM protein or its activity as shown by western blotting (see item **5**). An important

advantage of knowing the identity of both *ATM* mutations is their utility in prenatal diagnosis.

2 An examination of the chromosomal radiosensitivity in a 72-hour blood culture. Typical A-T patients show a 5- to 10-fold increased level of chromosomal damage following exposure of the whole blood to 1 Gy gamma rays in the G2 phase of the cell cycle. It should be noted, however, that some A-T patients will not show a significantly increased chromosomal radiosensitivity because they express some ATM with retained function. Part of the blood can be used to carry out a normal blood culture and the frequency of translocations and inversions, involving chromosomes 7 and 14, estimated. In 100 metaphases from an A-T patient, up to 10% of the spreads may show the presence of such rearrangements.

3 A lymphoblastoid cell line (LCL) can be made from the blood; this can be used as a source of RNA and DNA and also to examine the level of ATM (or Mre11) protein in the patient's cells. Typical A-T patients show total absence of ATM protein. Where there is absence of ATM protein, there will be absence of ATM kinase activity and this can be tested for. For those patients whose cells show expression of some ATM protein, the LCL can be used to determine whether the ATM protein has any kinase activity using phosphospecific antibodies to detect phosphorylation of targets of normal ATM. Generally speaking, patients who show the presence of some ATM activity will have a milder form of A-T, to a lesser or greater extent.

The patient with classical A-T will show unambiguous increased chromosomal radiosensitivity, partial or total loss of ATM protein, total loss of ATM kinase activity (despite the presence of any ATM protein), and the presence of two pathogenic mutations that, most often, will be clear truncating mutations leading to instability and loss of ATM protein from both alleles.

4 For ATLD caused by *MRE11* mutation, the laboratory confirmation can be made on the basis of an increased chromosomal radiosensitivity using blood lymphocytes, a reduction in the level of the Mre11 protein and consequently also Rad50 and Nbs1 proteins which are part of the same complex, and reduction in ATM kinase activity as this is dependent on Mre11. Finally, identifying both allelic *MRE11* mutations is important. Interestingly, unlike *ATM*, *MRE11* is an essential gene and so all *MRE11* patients carry at least one *MRE11* mutation that allows expression of either full-length or truncated protein with some residual activity/function.

5 A-T and ataxia oculomotor apraxias types 1 and 2 all share some neurological features, although AOA1 has a later age of onset in childhood and AOA2 in teenage. Neither AOA1 nor AOA2 has the non-neurological features of A-T; there is no increased radiosensitivity, immunodeficiency, or predisposition to cancer. They are much more pure neurological disorders. AOA1 is rarer than A-T, but curiously, as in A-T, AOA2 patients show an elevated level of serum AFP and probably have a similar prevalence. The presence of an increase in serum AFP, therefore, is an important indicator of A-T or AOA2. In the laboratory, these can be quickly distinguished on the basis of loss/reduction in level of ATM and senataxin respectively by western blotting and particularly by identifying pathogenic mutations in either *ATM* or *SETX*.

Prognosis for ataxia telangiectasia

Cancer predisposition

The cancer predisposition in A-T was noted soon after the description of the disorder by Boder and Sedgwick in 1958. In a study of 296 consecutive, genetically confirmed cases of A-T from the British Isles and the Netherlands, 66 patients were identified with a tumor – 47 of lymphoid origin and 19 non-lymphoid – giving an overall cancer risk of 66/296 (~22%). Non-lymphoid tumors included brain tumors, hepatocellular carcinoma, endocrine tumors, breast cancer, and myeloid leukemia. In 187 patients with classical A-T (as defined by absence of ATM kinase activity in their cells) we found 51 tumors (40 lymphoid and 11 non-lymphoid) – a risk of 51/187 (27%). We were able to show that the development of childhood tumors (lymphoid and brain) in A-T patients is associated almost exclusively with absence of ATM kinase activity. We could also show that expression of some residual ATM kinase activity had a strong protective effect against tumor development in A-T children. Surviving female A-T patients also showed a substantial increased risk of breast cancer with the risk at age 50 being 45% [9]. By definition the majority of these patients had a milder form of A-T and survived longer. A-T patients carrying the c.7271T>G mutation may be at particular risk of breast cancer.

The c.7271T>G mutation was also identified in a second A-T family where breast cancer occurred in carriers of the mutation. The authors computed a relative risk of 12.7 associated with carrying this *ATM* mutation, compared with a relative risk of 74.1 in homozygotes, of developing breast cancer [16]. This is consistent with the increased risk of breast cancer also observed in female carriers of *ATM* mutations [52–54], with the risk being larger in women under 50 [54].

The major causes of increased mortality in A-T, therefore, are lymphoid malignancies in children and non-lymphoid malignancies in adult A-T patients, but also infection and complications of treatment including surgery, where for example three A-T patients with severe restrictive lung function died following complications of ventilatory treatment [55]. Crawford et al. [56] reported a median survival for a prospective and a retrospective cohort of 25 and 19 years, respectively. These authors also pointed out that most deaths should be considered to be the result of a complication of A-T rather than the inevitable consequence of severe neurological debilitation [56].

Interestingly, however, the presence of particular founder missense mutations or leaky splice site mutations in some populations can result in a much extended lifespan for a significant group. For example the median age of the group of 22 A-T patients in the UK with the leaky splice site mutation c.5763-1050A>G (p.Pro1922fs) is currently 35 (range 16–51) and the median age for 12 Canadian Mennonite A-T patients homozygous for c.6200C>A; p.Ala2067Asp was 51.5 (range 12–64). It is likely that retention of some ATM kinase activity protects against lymphoid tumor development in childhood but possibly not against non-lymphoid tumours in adulthood [9, 15]. In addition, it is likely that retained activity protects against immunodeficiency and severe lung disease. It is important, therefore, that mutation analysis is available to patients. While improving the survival of classical patients remains a challenge, Crawford et al. [56] suggested that there was a trend toward improving survival in more recent years with advances in care.

Treatment options

There is no treatment at present for A-T. The management of the immunodeficiency [46, 48, 57], pulmonary function [55, 58, 59], feeding and swallowing [60, 61] in A-T have all been discussed. There have been reports on treatment of motor impairment and there are ongoing trials with betamethasone [62–64]. Treatment with amantidine has also been reported [65].

References

1. Sedgwick RP, Boder E. Ataxia telangiectasia. In: de Jong JMBV, editor. *Handbook of Clinical Neurology: Hereditary Neuropathies and Spinocerebellar Atrophies*. Elsevier Science Publishers BV, Oxford; 1991. 347–342.

2. Shaikh AG, Marti S, Tarnutzer AA, Palla A, Crawford TO, Straumann D, Taylor AM, Zee DS. Gaze fixation deficits and their implication in ataxia-telangiectasia. *J Neurol Neurosurg Psychiatry*. 2009; 80(8): 858–864.

3. Farr AK, Shalev B, Crawford TO, Lederman HM, Winkelstein JA, Repka MX. Ocular manifestations of ataxia-telangiectasia. *Am J Ophthalmol*. 2002; 134: 891–896.

4. Lewis RF, Crawford TO. Slow target-directed eye movements in ataxia-telangiectasia. *Invest Ophthalmol Vis Sci*. 2002; 43: 686–691.

5. Verhagen MM, Last JI, Hogervorst FBL, Smeets DF, Roeleveld N, Verheijen F, Catsman-Berrevoets CE, Wulffraat NM, Cobben JM, Hiel J, Brunt ER, Peeters EA, Gómez Garcia EB, van der Knaap MS, Lincke CR, Laan LA, Tijssen MA, van Rijn MA, Majoor-Krakauer D, Visser M, van't Veer LJ, Kleijer WJ, van de Warrenburg BP, Warris A, de Groot IJ, de Groot R, Broeks A, Preijers F, Kremer BH, Weemaes CM, Taylor MA, van Deuren M, Willemsen MA. Presence of ATM protein and residual kinase activity correlates with the phenotype in ataxia-telangiectasia: a genotype-phenotype study. *Hum Mutat*. 2012; 33: 561–571.

6. Chiam LY, Verhagen MM, Haraldsson A, Wulffraat N, Driessen GJ, Netea MG, Weemaes CM, Seyger MM, van Deuren M. Cutaneous granulomas in ataxia telangiectasia and other primary immunodeficiencies: reflection of inappropriate immune regulation? *Dermatology*. 2011;223(1):13–19.

7. Woods CG, Bundey SE, Taylor AM. Unusual features in the inheritance of ataxia telangiectasia. *Hum Genet*. 1990; 84(6): 555–562.

8. Lavin MF. Ataxia-telangiectasia: from a rare disorder to a paradigm for cell signalling and cancer. *Nat Rev Mol Cell Biol*. 2008 Oct; 9(10): 759–69. Erratum in Nat Rev Mol Cell Biol. 2008 Dec; 9(12).

9. Reiman A, Srinivasan V, Barone G, Last JI, Wootton LL, Davies EG, Verhagen MM, Willemsen MA, Weemaes CM, Byrd PJ, Izatt L, Easton DF, Thompson DJ, Taylor AM. Lymphoid tumours and breast cancer in ataxia telangiectasia; substantial protective effect of residual ATM kinase activity against childhood tumours. *Br J Cancer*. 2011; 105(4): 586–591.

10. Crawford TO, Mandir AS, Lefton-Greif MA, et al. Quantitative neurologic assessment of ataxia telangiectasia. *Neurology*. 2000; 54: 1505–1509.

11. McConville CM, Stankovic T, Byrd PJ, McGuire GM, Yao QY, Lennox GG, Taylor MR. Mutations associated with variant phenotypes in ataxia-telangiectasia. *Am J Hum Genet*. 1996; 59(2): 320–330.

12. Stewart GS, Last JI, Stankovic T, et al. Residual ataxia telangiectasia mutated protein function in cells from ataxia telangiectasia patients, with 5762ins137 and 7271T→G mutations, showing a less severe phenotype. *J Biol Chem*. 2001; 276: 30133–30141.

13. Austen B, Barone G, Reiman A, Byrd PJ, Baker C, Starczynski J, Murphy RP, Enright H, Chaila E, Quinn J, Stankovic T, Pratt G, Taylor AMR. Pathogenic ATM mutations occur at a low frequency in multiple myeloma. *Brit J Haematol*. 2008; 142: 925–933.

14. Carrillo F, Schneider SA, Taylor AM, Srinivasan V, Kapoor R, Bhatia KP. Prominent oromandibular dystonia and pharyngeal telangiectasia in atypical ataxia telangiectasia. *Cerebellum*. 2009; 8(1): 22–27.

15. Saunders-Pullman R, Raymond D, Stoessl AJ, Hobson D, Nakamura K, Pullman S, Lefton D, Okun MS, Uitti R, Sachdev S, Stanley K, San Luciano M, Hagenah J, Gatti R, Ozelius LJ, Bressman SB. Variant ataxia-telangiectasia presenting as primary-appearing dystonia in Canadian Mennonites. *Neurology*. 2012; 78(9): 649–657.

16. Stankovic T, Kidd AM, Sutcliffe A, McGuire GM, Robinson P, Weber P, Bedenham T, Bradwell AR, Easton DF, Lennox GG, Haites N, Byrd PJ, Taylor AM. ATM mutations and phenotypes in ataxia-telangiectasia families in the British Isles: expression of mutant ATM and the risk of leukemia, lymphoma, and breast cancer. *Am J Hum Genet*. 1998; 62(2): 334–345.

17. Barone G, Groom A, Reiman A, Srinivasan V, Byrd PJ, Taylor AM. Modeling ATM mutant proteins from missense changes confirms retained kinase activity. *Hum Mutat*. 2009; 30: 1222–1230.

18. Sutton IJ, Last JI, Ritchie SJ, Harrington HJ, Byrd PJ, Taylor AM. Adult-onset ataxia telangiectasia due to ATM 5762ins137 mutation homozygosity. *Ann Neurol*. 2004; 55(6): 891–895.

19. Hiel JA, van Engelen BG, Weemaes CM, Broeks A, Verrips A, ter Laak H, Vingerhoets HM, van den Heuvel LP, Lammens M, Gabreëls FJ, Last JI, Taylor AM. Distal spinal muscular atrophy as a major feature in adult-onset ataxia telangiectasia. *Neurology*. 2006; 67(2): 346–349.

20. Mandigers CM, van de Warrenburg BP, Strobbe LJ, Kluijt I, Molenaar AH, Schinagl DA. Ataxia telangiectasia: the consequences of a delayed diagnosis. *Radiother Oncol*. 2011; 99(1): 97–98.

21. Byrd PJ, Srinivasan V, Last JI, Smith A, Biggs P, Carney EF, Exley A, Abson C, Stewart GS, Izatt L, Taylor AM. Severe reaction to radiotherapy for breast cancer as the presenting feature of ataxia telangiectasia. *Br J Cancer*. 2012; 106(2): 262–268.

22. Alterman N, Fattal-Valevski A, Moyal L, et al. Ataxia-telangiectasia: mild neurological presentation despite null ATM mutation and severe cellular phenotype. *Am J Med Genet A*. 2007; 143A: 1827–1834.

23. Verhagen MM, Abdo WF, Willemsen MA, Hogervorst FB, Smeets DF, Hiel JA, Brunt ER, van Rijn MA, Majoor Krakauer D, Oldenburg RA, Broeks A, Last JI, van't Veer LJ, Tijssen MA, Dubois AM, Kremer HP, Weemaes CM, Taylor AM, van Deuren M. Clinical spectrum of ataxia-telangiectasia in adulthood. *Neurology*. 2009; 73(6): 430–437.

24. Fang Z, Kozlov S, McKay MJ, Woods R, Birrell G, Sprung CN, Murrell DF, Wangoo K, Teng L, Kearsley JH, Lavin MF, Graham PH, Clarke RA. Low levels of ATM in breast cancer patients with clinical radiosensitivity. *Genome Integr*. 2010; 1(1): 9.

25. Klein C, Wenning GK, Quinn NP, Marsden CD. Ataxia without telangiectasia masquerading as benign hereditary chorea. *Mov Disord*. 1996; 11(2): 217–220.

26. Stewart GS, Maser RS, Stankovic T, et al. The DNA double-strand break repair gene hMRE11 is mutated in individuals with an ataxia-telangiectasia-like disorder. *Cell*. 1999; 99: 577–587.

27. Hernandez D, McConville CM, Stacey M, Woods CG, Brown MM, Shutt P, Rysiecki G, Taylor AM. A family showing no evidence of linkage between the ataxia telangiectasia gene and chromosome 11q22-23. *J Med Genet*. 1993; 30(2): 135–140.

28. Pitts SA1, Kullar HS, Stankovic T, Stewart GS, Last JI, Bedenham T, Armstrong SJ, Piane M, Chessa L, Taylor AM, Byrd PJ. hMRE11: genomic structure and a null mutation identified in a transcript protected from nonsense-mediated mRNA decay. *Hum Mol Genet*. 2001; 10(11): 1155–1162.

29. Taylor AM, Groom A, Byrd PJ. Ataxia-telangiectasia-like disorder (ATLD)-its clinical presentation and molecular basis. *DNA Repair (Amst)*. 2004; 3(8-9): 1219–1225. Review.

30. Delia D, Piane M, Buscemi G, et al. MRE11 mutations and impaired ATM-dependent responses in an Italian family with ataxia-telangiectasia-like disorder. *Hum Mol Genet*. 2004; 13: 2155–2163.

31. Fernet M, Gribaa M, Salih MA, Seidahmed MZ, Hall J, Koenig M. Identification and functional consequences of a novel MRE11 mutation affecting 10 Saudi Arabian patients with the ataxia telangiectasia-like disorder. *Hum Mol Genet*. 2005; 14: 307–318.

32. Uchisaka N, Takahashi N, Sato M, Kikuchi A, Mochizuki S, Imai K, Nonoyama S, Ohara O, Watanabe F, Mizutani S, Hanada R, Morio T. Two brothers with ataxia-telangiectasia-like disorder with lung adenocarcinoma. *J Pediatr*. 2009; 155(3): 435–438.

33. Matsumoto Y, Miyamoto T, Sakamoto H, Izumi H, Nakazawa Y, Ogi T, Tahara H, Oku S, Hiramoto A, Shiiki T, Fujisawa Y, Ohashi H, Sakemi Y, Matsuura S. Two unrelated patients with MRE11A mutations and Nijmegen breakage syndrome-like severe microcephaly. *DNA Repair (Amst)*. 2011; 10(3): 314–321.

34. Taalman RD, Jaspers NG, Scheres JM, de Wit J, Hustinx TW. Hypersensitivity to ionizing radiation, in vitro, in a new chromosomal breakage disorder, the Nijmegen Breakage Syndrome. *Mutat Res*. 1983; 112(1): 23–32.

35. Varon R, Vissinga C, Platzer M, Cerosaletti KM, Chrzanowska KH, Saar K, Beckmann G, Seemanová E, Cooper PR, Nowak NJ, Stumm M, Weemaes CM, Gatti RA, Wilson RK, Digweed M, Rosenthal A, Sperling K, Concannon P, Reis A. Nibrin, a novel DNA double-strand break repair protein, is mutated in Nijmegen breakage syndrome. *Cell*. 1998; 93(3): 467–476.

36. Carney JP, Maser RS, Olivares H, Davis EM, Le Beau M, Yates JR 3rd, Hays L, Morgan WF, Petrini JH. The hMre11/hRad50 protein complex and Nijmegen breakage syndrome: linkage of double-strand break repair to the cellular DNA damage response. *Cell*. 1998; 93(3): 477–486.

37. Stewart GS, Stankovic T, Byrd PJ, Wechsler T, Miller ES, Huissoon A, Drayson MT, West SC, Elledge SJ, Taylor AMR. RIDDLE immunodeficiency syndrome is linked to defects in 53BP1-mediated DNA damage signaling Proc Natl Acad Sci USA. 2007; 104: 16910–16915.

38. Stewart GS, Panier S, Townsend K, Al-Hakim AK, Kolas NK, Miller ES, Nakada S, Ylanko J, Olivarius S, Mendez M, Oldreive C, Wildenhain J, Tagliaferro A, Pelletier L, Taubenheim N, Durandy A, Byrd PJ, Stankovic T, Taylor AM, Durocher D. The RIDDLE syndrome protein mediates a ubiquitin-dependent signaling cascade at sites of DNA damage. *Cell*. 2009; 136(3): 420–434.

39. Devgan SS, Sanal O, Doil C, Nakamura K, Nahas SA, Pettijohn K, Bartek J, Lukas C, Lukas J, Gatti RA. Homozygous deficiency of ubiquitin-ligase ring-finger protein RNF168 mimics the radiosensitivity syndrome of ataxia-telangiectasia. *Cell Death Differ*. 2011; 18(9): 1500–1506.

40. Tavani F, Zimmerman RA, Berry GT, Sullivan K, Gatti R, Bingham P. Ataxia-telangiectasia: the pattern of cerebellar atrophy on MRI. *Neuroradiology*. 2003; 45(5): 315–319.

41. Verhagen MM, Martin JJ, van Deuren M, Ceuterick-de Groote C, Weemaes CM, Kremer BH, Taylor MA, Willemsen MA, Lammens M. Neuropathology in classical and variant ataxia-telangiectasia. *Neuropathology*. 2012; 32(3): 234–244.

42. Woods CG, Taylor AMR. Ataxia telangiectasia in the British Isles: the clinical and laboratory features of 70 affected individuals. *Q J Med*. 1992; 82(298): 169–179.

43. Taylor AM, Byrd PJ. Molecular pathology of ataxia telangiectasia. *J Clin Pathol*. 2005; 58: 1009–1015.

44. Pan-Hammarström Q, Lähdesmäki A, Zhao Y, Du L, Zhao Z, Wen S, Ruiz-Perez VL, Dunn-Walters DK, Goodship JA, Hammarström L. Disparate roles of ATR and ATM in immunoglobulin class switch recombination and somatic hypermutation. *J Exp Med*. 2006; 203(1): 99–110. Erratum in: J Exp Med. 2006; 203(1): 251.

45. Pan-Hammarström Q, Dai S, Zhao Y, van Dijk-Härd IF, Gatti RA, Børresen-Dale AL, Hammarström L. ATM is not required in somatic hypermutation of VH, but is involved in the introduction of mutations in the switch mu region. *J Immunol*. 2003; 170(7): 3707–3716.

46. Nowak-Wegrzyn A, Crawford TO, Winkelstein JA, Carson KA, Lederman HM. Immunodeficiency and infections in ataxia-telangiectasia. *J Pediatr*. 2004; 144: 505–511.

47. Giovannetti A, Mazzetta F, Caprini E, Aiuti A, Marziali M, Pierdominici M, Cossarizza A, Chessa L, Scala E, Quinti I, Russo G, Fiorilli M. Skewed T-cell receptor repertoire, decreased thymic output, and predominance of terminally differentiated T cells in ataxia telangiectasia. *Blood*. 2002; 100(12): 4082–4089.

48. Exley AR, Buckenham S, Hodges E, Hallam R, Byrd P, Last J, Trinder C, Harris S, Screaton N, Williams AP, Taylor AM, Shneerson JM. Premature ageing of the immune system underlies immunodeficiency in ataxia telangiectasia. *Clin Immunol*. 2011; 140(1): 26–36.

49. Carney EF, Srinivasan, V, Moss PA, Taylor AM. Classical ataxia telangiectasia patients have a congenitally aged immune system with high expression of CD95. *J Immunol*. 2012; 189(1): 261–8.

50. Staples ER, McDermott EM, Reiman A, Byrd PJ, Ritchie S, Taylor AMR, Davies EG. Immunodeficiency in ataxia telangiectasia is strongly correlated with the presence of two null mutations in the ATM gene. *Clin Exp Immunol*. 2008; 153: 214–220.

51. Micol R, Ben Slama L, Suarez F, Le Mignot L, Beauté J, Mahlaoui N, Dubois d'Enghien C, Laugé A, Hall J, Couturier J, Vallée L, Delobel B, Rivier F, Nguyen K, Billette de Villemeur T, Stephan JL, Bordigoni P, Bertrand Y, Aladjidi N, Pedespan JM, Thomas C, Pellier I, Koenig M, Hermine O, Picard C, Moshous D, Neven B, Lanternier F, Blanche S, Tardieu M, Debré M, Fischer A, Stoppa-Lyonnet D; CEREDIH Network Investigators. Morbidity and mortality from ataxia-telangiectasia are associated with ATM genotype. *J Allergy Clin Immunol*. 2011; 128(2): 382–389.

52. Geoffroy-Perez B, Janin N, Ossian K, Laug A, Croquette MF, Griscelli C et al. Cancer risk in heterozygotes for ataxia-telangiectasia. *Int J Cancer*. 2001;; 93: 288–293.

53. Olsen JH, Hahnemann JM, Borresen-Dale AL, Brondum-Nielsen K, Hammarstrom L, Kleinerman R et al. Cancer in patients with ataxia-telangiectasia and in their relatives in the nordic countries. *J Natl Cancer Inst*. 2001; 93: 121–127.

54. Thompson D, Duedal S, Kirner J, McGuffog L, Last J, Reiman A, Byrd P, Taylor M, Easton DF. Cancer risks and mortality in heterozygous ATM mutation carriers. *J Natl Cancer Inst*. 2005; 97(11): 813–822.

55. Verhagen MMM, van Deuren M, Willemsen MAAP, Van der Hoeven HJ, Heijdra YF, Yntema JB, Weemaes CMR, Neeleman C. Ataxia telangiectasia and mechanical ventilation: a word of caution. *Netherlands Journal of Critical Care*. 2009; 13: 90–93.

56. Crawford TO, Skolasky RL, Fernandez R, Rosquist KJ, Lederman HM. Survival probability in ataxia telangiectasia. *Arch Dis Child*. 2006; 91: 610–611.

57. Davies EG. Update on the management of the immunodeficiency in ataxia-telangiectasia. *Expert Rev Clin Immunol*. 2009; 5(5): 565–575.

58. McGrath-Morrow S, Lefton-Greif M, Rosquist K, Crawford T, Kelly A, Zeitlin P, Carson KA, Lederman HM. Pulmonary function in adolescents with ataxia telangiectasia. *Pediatr Pulmonol*. 2008; 43(1): 59–66.

59. McGrath-Morrow SA, Gower WA, Rothblum-Oviatt C, Brody AS, Langston C, Fan LL, Lefton-Greif MA, Crawford TO, Troche M, Sandlund JT, Auwaerter PG, Easley B, Loughlin GM, Carroll JL, Lederman HM. Evaluation and management of pulmonary disease in ataxia-telangiectasia. *Pediatr Pulmonol*. 2010; 45(9): 847–859.

60. Lefton-Greif MA, Crawford TO, Winkelstein JA, Loughlin GM, Koerner CB, Zahurak M, Lederman HM. Oropharyngeal dysphagia and aspiration in patients with ataxia-telangiectasia. *J Pediatr*. 2000; 136(2): 225–231.

61. Lefton-Greif MA, Crawford TO, McGrath-Morrow S, Carson KA, Lederman HM. Safety and caregiver satisfaction with gastrostomy in patients with ataxia telangiectasia. *Orphanet J Rare Dis*. 2011; 6: 23.

62. Broccoletti T, Del Giudice E, Cirillo E, Vigliano I, Giardino G, Ginocchio VM, Bruscoli S, Riccardi C, Pignata C. Efficacy of very-low-dose betamethasone on neurological symptoms in ataxia-telangiectasia. *Eur J Neurol*. 2011; 18(4): 564–570.

63. Broccoletti T, Del Giudice E, Amorosi S, Russo I, Di Bonito M, Imperati F, Romano A, Pignata C. Steroid-induced improvement of neurological signs in ataxia-telangiectasia patients. *Eur J Neurol*. 2008; 15(3): 223–228.

64. Russo I, Cosentino C, Del Giudice E, Broccoletti T, Amorosi S, Cirillo E, Aloj G, Fusco A, Costanzo V, Pignata C. In ataxia-telangiectasia betamethasone response is inversely correlated to cerebellar atrophy and directly to antioxidative capacity. *Eur J Neurol*. 2009; 16(6): 755–759.

65. Nissenkorn A, Hassin-Baer S, Lerman SF, Banet Levi Y, Tzadok M, Ben-Zeev B. Movement disorder in ataxia-telangiectasia: treatment with amantadine sulfate. *J Child Neurol*. 2013; 28(2): 155–160.

CHAPTER 24

Niemann–Pick Disease

Marc C. Patterson

Departments of Neurology, Pediatrics, and Medical Genetics, Mayo Clinic Children's Center, Rochester, Minnesota, USA

Introduction

The term Niemann–Pick disease embraces a family of two genetically distinct disorders. The first subgroup comprises those disorders originally described by Niemann in 1914 and then later by Pick in 1927 that are associated with primary deficiency of acid sphingomyelinase (ASM) [1], which leads to progressive deposition of sphingomyelin, mainly in the reticuloendothelial cells. This subgroup is traditionally subdivided into types A and B that are allelic disorders. The former is characterized by rapid neurodegeneration and organomegaly (neuronopathic form) [2], the latter by organomegaly without primary neurologic involvement (non-neuronopathic form) [3]. It is now known that these phenotypes represent ends of a wide spectrum and that intermediate forms exist in a continuum of neurological findings [4].

The second subgroup within the Niemann–Pick family is classified as Niemann–Pick disease, type C. Through historical accident, this disorder, which is a result of mutations in two separate genes that regulate endosomal-lysosomal trafficking, was grouped together with the primary sphingomyelinase deficiencies [5, 6]. Older literature uses terms such as juvenile dystonic idiocy, juvenile dystonic lipidosis [7], sea blue histiocyte syndrome [8, 9], neurovisceral lipidosis with vertical supranuclear gaze palsy, and DAF (downgaze paralysis, ataxia, foam cells) syndrome to describe this disease [10]. All forms of Niemann–Pick disease, type C, are characterized by neurodegeneration, apart from the perinatal forms in which visceromegaly, ascites, pulmonary infiltrates, and often early death are characteristic [11].

Primary acid sphingomyelinase deficiencies– Niemann–Pick diseases type A and B

Clinical definition and epidemiology

The primary acid sphingomyelinase deficiencies (Niemann–Pick diseases, type A and B) are lysosomal storage diseases defined by deficient activity of acid sphingomyelinase (ASM), typically less than 10% of control values, with corresponding mutations in each copy of the gene [2]. *SMPD1* is the only gene known to be associated with acid sphingomyelinase deficiency [12]. These autosomal recessive disorders are rare with an incidence estimated at between 0.5 and 1.0 per 100,000 [13]. Niemann–Pick disease (NPD), type A is more frequent in the Ashkenazi Jewish population and targeted mutation analysis for common population-specific mutations is

available for individuals of Ashkenazi Jewish background with NPD type A. Type B disease does not have an Ashkenazi predilection [14].

Spectrum of clinical phenotypes

Classic NPD type A is a neurodegenerative disorder characterized by infantile onset (usually within the first three months of life) with marked hepatosplenomegaly causing abdominal distension, failure to thrive, interstitial lung disease, cherry red spot on funduscopic examination, and progressive neurodegeneration and regression of milestones with a rapid course to death, typically in the second year of life [2].

NPD type B is characterized by hepatosplenomegaly, pulmonary infiltrates, and skeletal dysostosis accompanied by a slowly progressive course in most cases [3]. These patients were originally thought to have no neurologic manifestations, but more recent studies have demonstrated neurological involvement in the form of cerebellar signs, and intellectual disability in addition to the presence of cherry red spots at the macula in a substantial proportion of patients. Other patients have a distinct fundal abnormality – the macular halo syndrome [15]. The absence of significant brain involvement likely reflects higher residual enzyme activity compared to NPD type A.

It is now known that there is a spectrum of phenotypes between NPD types A and B, and that acid sphingomyelinase deficiency can thus present at any age [2].

Pathology, pathophysiology specific to the disease

Genetics

The acid sphingomyelinase deficiencies are autosomal recessive disorders. *SMPD1* is the only gene known to be associated with acid sphingomyelinase deficiency. A large number of mutations have been defined, although some specific mutations causing NPD type A are more common in the Ashkenazi Jewish population. Combined carrier frequency for the three common mutations in Ashkenazi Jewish population is between 1:80 and 1:100 [16]. Three mutations (p.Arg498Leu, p.Leu304Pro, p.Phe333SerfsX52) account for approximately 90% of NPD type A disease-causing alleles in the Ashkenazi Jewish population. NPD type B is a more panethnic disorder [14]. Targeted mutation analysis is the first step in genetic diagnosis. Sequence analysis of the coding region of the *SMPD1* gene is commercially available and detects mutations in 95% of individuals with enzymatically confirmed ASM deficiency.

Neurodegeneration, First Edition. Edited by Anthony Schapira, Zbigniew Wszolek, Ted M. Dawson and Nicholas Wood.
© 2017 John Wiley & Sons, Ltd. Published 2017 by John Wiley & Sons, Ltd.

Environment

There are no well-defined environmental factors that influence the course of this disease, although dietary factors are potential modifiers in patients with NPD types A and B, who typically have hyperlipidemia [17].

Clinical prodrome and biomarkers

The acid sphingomyelinase deficiencies typically declare themselves through neurologic presentations such as developmental delay and regression accompanied by hepatosplenomegaly (enlargement of the liver typically being more marked that that of the spleen). Hyperlipidemia is characteristic of NPD type B (although it is also seen in type A disease), but there are no well-established biomarkers for the neurological manifestations of these diseases [17]. Neuroimaging studies, in particular magnetic resonance imaging (MRI) of the brain, do not show consistent abnormalities until late in the course of the illness.

Examination and investigations

The most prominent physical finding in all forms of acid sphingomyelinase deficiency is hepatosplenomegaly, the liver typically being more markedly enlarged than the spleen [3]. Those with significant organomegaly have hypersplenism with secondary thrombocytopenia. Infarction of the spleen can cause acute abdominal pain. Pulmonary infiltrates are often apparent on X-rays of the chest, although the examination of the chest may be relatively unremarkable. On high-resolution chest CT, ground glass attenuation representing interstitial lung disease can be seen clearly [18–20]. On many occasions patients may have intercurrent viral infections, and when chest X-rays are obtained these are interpreted as showing signs of infection, although the findings may simply reflect infiltrates unrelated to the more acute event. Some patients may be oxygen dependent because of interstitial lung disease [21]. Imaging of bones may reveal evidence of dysostosis, reflecting bone marrow displacement and bone remodeling secondary to accumulation of foam cells [22]. This may affect linear growth and result in significant growth restriction in children [23] and short stature and fractures in adults [24]. Bone marrow examination (although rarely performed for diagnosis) reveals lipid-laden foamy histiocytes with a soap bubble appearance; sea blue histiocytes may also be found [25]. MRI of the brain is usually unremarkable or nonspecifically abnormal until late in the course of the illness [20].

Diagnosis

Diagnosis is made primarily by demonstrated deficiency of acid sphingomyelinase (less than 10% of controls) in cultured skin fibroblasts; peripheral blood lymphocytes can also be used for this purpose. Genetic analysis of the acid sphingomyelinase gene is commercially available and is typically used to confirm the biochemical diagnosis and to provide information for genetic counseling.

Treatment options

Medical

Stem cell transplantation has been tried without success in a few patients with NPD type A [26]. There are isolated case reports of initially successful bone marrow transplantation for NPD type B [27, 28], but the long-term results were mixed [29]. The acid sphingomyelinase enzyme has been purified and is currently in clinical trial for patients with NPD type B. This treatment is not currently under investigation in the predominantly neurological, infantile-onset form of the disease, although intracerebroventricular delivery of recombinant acid sphingomyelinase has shown benefit in the murine model of NPD type A [30]. Medical treatment is available for complications of the disease:

- *Hematologic complications*: Transfusion can be used to manage life-threatening bleeding due to thrombocytopenia.
- *Pulmonary complications*: Supplemental oxygen and whole lung lavage may be employed for symptomatic pulmonary disease [31].
- *Hyperlipidemia*: Standard treatments may be employed – there have been no systematic studies. Fenofibrate has been reported to be effective in one child with NPD type B [32].

Surgical

Surgical treatment is not generally applicable to the acid sphingomyelinase deficiencies.

Social

Support for individuals affected by acid sphingomyelinase deficiency is available through lay groups in a number of countries, including the National Niemann–Pick Disease Foundation in the United States, Niemann–Pick UK in the United Kingdom, and a number of other organizations worldwide.

Future developments

A clinical trial of enzyme replacement therapy for NPD type B is currently in progress. Investigations of enzyme replacement therapy [30] and gene transfer [33] have been undertaken in the murine models of NPD type A. It is conceivable that these approaches may be employed in humans in the future.

Endosomal/lysosomal trafficking deficiency – Niemann–Pick disease, type C

Clinical definition and epidemiology

Niemann–Pick disease, type C, is a neurovisceral disorder of late endosomal/lysosomal trafficking of cholesterol and glycosphingolipids [11]. The disorder results from mutations in either of two genes, *NPC1* (the majority of the cases) or *NPC2* (4% of the cases), that are both inherited in autosomal recessive fashion. The phenotypes caused by mutations in the two genes are clinically indistinguishable, but the forms of the disease are sometimes designated as NPC1 and NPC2 to denote the underlying mutation. The incidence of the disorder has been calculated as 1:120,000 [11]. It is likely that this is roughly correct for most developed countries, although there are individual variations in specific populations. The carrier frequency in Yarmouth County, Nova Scotia, where ancestors of Jean Amirault settled beginning in the late 17th century, has been estimated at 1:26 [34]. The disease in this population was originally designated Niemann–Pick disease, type D, by Crocker [6]. Following cloning of the *NPC1* gene, these patients were found to carry a specific *NPC1* mutation (G3097>T), confirming that NPD type D is a genetic isolate of NPD type C [35]. Genetic isolates have also been described in New Mexico and Colorado [36] and among Bedouin groups [37].

Spectrum of clinical phenotype

The most severe forms of NPD type C present in the perinatal period, either as fetal ascites with organomegaly [38], or at birth with marked hepatosplenomegaly, ascites, pulmonary infiltrates, and jaundice accompanied by hepatic failure. There is a high mortality rate among such affected neonates [11]. Ultrasound in pregnancy may reveal fetal hepatosplenomegaly, ascites, or growth retardation [38]. Overall, about 50% of children with NPD type C have prolonged jaundice in the perinatal period [39, 40], which may be misdiagnosed as biliary atresia on hepatobiliary iminodiacetic acid (HIDA) scans. Pulmonary infiltrates with foam cells may be the presenting sign in neonates or may accompany neonatal liver disease [21]. Pulmonary alveolar proteinosis has been described in NPD type C2 [41, 42]. The NPC pathway modulates cholesterol efflux from lamellar bodies of type II pneumocytes, and may thus influence surfactant function [43]. More commonly, the disease is detected after the infantile period as developmental delay associated with hypotonia [44], or in childhood with the insidious onset of ataxia, vertical supranuclear gaze palsy, and school failure proceeding to progressive dementia [45]. A substantial proportion of children experience seizures, which can be of any type, and about one-third of cases have gelastic cataplexy. In some children cataplexy can occur many times a day and cause injuries. Sleep disturbances and variable reduction in hypocretin levels in CSF have been described [46–48]. Spasticity and dystonia are also frequent findings. Later-onset forms of the disease first manifesting in adolescence or adulthood may be dominated by psychiatric manifestations, typically associated with an insidiously progressive dementia [49–52]. In the experience of the author, all patients beyond infancy with neurologic manifestations exhibit vertical supranuclear gaze palsy, which is often complete at the time of diagnosis. This is succeeded by horizontal supranuclear gaze palsy, and in patients who survive long enough, the end result is complete saccadic paralysis [53, 54]. A suspicion index has been developed that allows appropriate selection of patients beyond infancy for laboratory investigation [55].

Pathology, pathophysiology specific to the disease

Genetics

Niemann–Pick disease, type C (NPC), results from mutations in either the *NPC1* gene (accounting for approximately 95% of cases) or the *NPC2* gene [56]. Most individuals are compound heterozygotes with mutations unique to their family. Currently, there are a few percent of patients with biochemically and clinically proven NPC in whom either one or, rarely, two mutations cannot be detected in either gene. This is thought to be likely the result of technical challenges in sequencing the *NPC1* gene, in which as many as 300 mutations, most of them private, have already been described [11, 57]. The *NPC2* gene is much smaller [58] and complete sequencing is not as technically challenging. Both the gene products are believed to function in a coordinated fashion [59]; the biochemical phenotype associated with both *NPC1* and *NPC2* mutations is indistinguishable, showing accumulation of unesterified cholesterol and glycolipids in the lysosome–late endosome.

Environment

There are no well-described or recognized environmental factors that influence the expression or outcome of NPC.

Clinical prodrome and biomarkers

Except for the infantile period, the onset of this disease is typically insidious and children are often misdiagnosed as having learning disabilities, dyspraxias, or nonspecific clumsiness. Variable reduction in hypocretin levels in CSF have been described [46–48]. Recently, elevated oxysterols have been described as a biomarker of this disease. Current data suggest that this is the most sensitive means of detecting the disorder, even in patients with minimal symptoms [60, 61]. Oxysterol assays may prove to be a valuable test for following the progression of disease, although a great deal more data will be required to establish this. Early and rapid Purkinje cell loss in the cerebellum has been demonstrated in animal models of NPC [62], accompanied by activation of microglial cells and elevation of inflammatory markers. Potential biomarkers are being investigated in humans and animal models of NPD type C and a number of candidates have been identified. Galectin-3 (LGALS3), a pro-inflammatory molecule, and cathepsin D (CTSD), a lysosomal aspartic protease, are elevated in NPC subjects compared to controls [63]. Studies of CSF in humans and cats with NPC show subtle abnormalities of the amyloid β pathway [64, 65]. Brain histology has shown neurofibrillary tangles similar to those seen in Alzheimer's disease [66]. There was no accompanying amyloid β deposition, except in NPC patients who were homozygous for apolipoprotein E epsilon 4 [67], and in whom the disease process appeared to be accelerated.

Examination

The physical examination in infants is usually dominated by hepatosplenomegaly with or without jaundice. Later in life, hepatomegaly is typically absent and splenomegaly is frequently, but not invariably present. Its absence does not rule out this diagnosis. The most characteristic finding on examination is vertical supranuclear gaze palsy [53, 54]. This may be apparent initially as increased saccadic latency before slowing and eventual complete saccadic paralysis is appreciated. Horizontal saccadic paralysis also occurs, but at a slower rate and with later onset than the vertical gaze palsy. Patients exhibit axial, gait, and appendicular ataxia, and eventually cerebellar dysarthria and dysphagia. There is often dystonia, present initially only when stressed, but subsequently at rest. Dystonia can initially be focal; later, as disease progresses, it becomes generalized. Spasticity occurs in the course of the illness, although it is generally not markedly disabling [39, 40, 68].

Investigations

The diagnosis has traditionally been made by obtaining a skin biopsy, culturing the fibroblasts in lipid-deficient serum, and then exposing them to a pulse of LDL-derived cholesterol. Control cells rapidly down-regulate the expression of LDL receptors and HMG-CoA reductase and up-regulate ACAT2 (whose role in this circumstance is to re-esterify free cholesterol, which is toxic within cells). These homeostatic responses are all delayed and diminished in NPC cells. The most marked biochemical difference between mutant and control cells occurs in cholesterol re-esterification and this was initially selected as the primary biochemical diagnostic test [69]. This finding is confirmed by staining the cultured fibroblasts with filipin, an antibiotic which binds strongly to unesterified cholesterol, and which autofluoresces when exposed to appropriate wavelengths of light [70]. It has become apparent in recent years that this is a difficult test to perform outside of a few reference laboratories; even there, filipin staining appears to be more sensitive than cholesterol esterification, which has considerable variability [45]. Filipin staining produces a characteristic pattern of intense perinuclear fluorescence in classic cases. The availability of molecular testing has been very helpful in confirming the diagnosis in most patients, but as noted above, there are still a number of cases in which the diagnosis is biochemically clear cut but in which at least one mutation cannot be identified. The recent description of elevated oxysterols in this disease now adds a valuable tool to the diagnostic armamentarium and we expect that this will become the first-line diagnostic test in the near future [60, 61].

It seems prudent when obtaining a skin biopsy to secure a portion for electron microscopic examination. The demonstration of polymorphous cytoplastic bodies is specific for this disease and can confirm the diagnosis rapidly in many cases where an experienced pathologist is available to interpret the images [7, 45].

Routine CT and MR imaging of the brain is usually normal until late in the course of the illness. Volume loss in the cerebellar vermis is usually the first structural abnormality, followed by progressive atrophy of the cerebellar and cerebral hemispheres. Cerebellar and cerebral atrophy may progress rapidly in aggressive disease [71]. Preliminary studies suggest that magnetization transfer techniques may permit more sensitive and quantifiable assessment of brain involvement in NPC [72], and one study of nine adults with NPC has correlated clinical status with structure and size of the corpus callosum [73].

Prognosis

The prognosis of this disease is one of inexorable neurologic progression to loss of mobility and of the ability to speak or swallow, accompanied by dementia. Dysphagia appears to be a predictor of mortality [74]. Patients may survive for prolonged periods with suitable nutritional and physical support. Some patients with late onset of the disease are alive in the seventh decade, but most individuals with early-onset disease succumb in the second to fourth decade [11, 40, 50, 68].

Treatment options

Medical

The only disease-modifying therapy that has been approved for treating the neurologic manifestations of NPC, is miglustat [75]. This agent is an inhibitor of glucosylceramide synthase, although it likely has many modes of action, and substrate inhibition may not be the primary mechanism of its effect in NPC [76]. Experiments in the animal model of NPC, showed that the onset of the disease and the longevity of these mice could be prolonged by about 25% by the administration of this agent in their chow, beginning at weaning [77]. Subsequently, prospective [78–81] and retrospective human studies [82] have provided supportive evidence for a beneficial effect of this agent in at least temporarily stabilizing the disease. It should be noted that as this is a very rare disorder, studies have generally been underpowered and have been subject to a number of criticisms. These reservations notwithstanding, miglustat has been approved by regulators in the European Union, Canada, Australia, Brazil, Taiwan, and several other countries. It has not received approval for this purpose by the Food and Drug Administration in the United States. There are no other disease-modifying therapies approved at present, although a number of other agents have shown promise in the animal models of this disease. Most recently, cyclodextrin has shown the most dramatic effects in delaying onset and extending lifespan in the murine [83] and feline models of NPC [84].

Although the options for disease-modifying therapy are limited, patients with NPC, benefit from treatment of common medical problems that occur in this and other neurodegenerative disorders [45]. Active treatment of constipation, intercurrent infections, cataplexy [85], seizures, and dystonia should be pursued. Although no prospective data are available, it is likely that lifespan may be increased and quality of life improved if general medical and pediatric care is vigorously pursued. In addition, physical therapy to maintain mobility, joint flexibility, and pulmonary function appears to be beneficial.

Surgical

In general, there are no surgical options for the management of NPC.

Social

Support from social workers to help families navigate aid systems is essential to providing the best possible care. In addition, lay groups such as the National Niemann–Pick Disease Foundation in the United States, the Niemann–Pick Disease Group in the United Kingdom, and other groups in Europe and elsewhere in the world are extremely valuable resources for patient support.

Future developments

Cyclodextrin is under active investigation as a potential disease-modifying therapy for NPC, based on promising results in the animal models of the disease [83, 84]. A clinical trial is currently (2016) in progress. Vorinostat, a histone deacetylase (HDAC) inhibitor, and arimoclomol, which stimulates the expression of heat shock proteins, have shown promise in cell-based and animal models of NPC respectively, and are also being studied in clinical trials in 2016 [86, 87]. Studies of gene therapy have been pursued in animal models, but there are many challenges to be overcome before this would be applicable in NPC [88]. Similarly, the possibility of stem cell therapy has been entertained, but because NPC1 is a cell autonomous disorder, the likelihood of benefit from this intervention is thought to be small. In contrast, the gene product in NPC2 is a small, potentially transducible protein, and thus hematopoietic stem cell transplantation is a rational therapy. Promising results have been reported in one child who survived the procedure [89]. Inflammation has been shown to play an important part in the pathology of NPC [90, 91], and anti-inflammatory agents may prove to be useful adjuvants in combination therapeutic approaches.

References

1. Brady RO, Kanfer JN, Mock MB, Fredrickson DS. The metabolism of sphingomyelin. II. Evidence of an enzymatic deficiency in Niemann-Pick diseae. *Proc Natl Acad Sci U S A* 1966;55:366–9.
2. McGovern MM, Aron A, Brodie SE, Desnick RJ, Wasserstein MP. Natural history of Type A Niemann-Pick disease: possible endpoints for therapeutic trials. *Neurology* 2006;66:228–32.
3. McGovern MM, Wasserstein MP, Giugliani R, et al. A prospective, cross-sectional survey study of the natural history of Niemann-Pick disease type B. *Pediatrics* 2008;122:e341–9.
4. Wasserstein MP, Aron A, Brodie SE, Simonaro C, Desnick RJ, McGovern MM. Acid sphingomyelinase deficiency: prevalence and characterization of an intermediate phenotype of Niemann-Pick disease. *J Pediatr* 2006;149:554–9.
5. Crocker AC, Farber S. Niemann-Pick disease: a review of eighteen patients. *Medicine (Baltimore)* 1958;37:1–95.
6. Crocker AC. The cerebral defect in Tay-Sachs disease and Niemann-Pick disease. *J Neurochem* 1961;7:69–80.
7. Martin JJ, Lowenthal A, Ceuterick C, Vanier MT. Juvenile dystonic lipidosis (variant of Niemann-Pick disease type C). *J Neurol Sci* 1984;66:33–45.
8. Long RG, Lake BD, Pettit JE, Scheuer PJ, Sherlock S. Adult Niemann-Pick disease: its relationship to the syndrome of the sea-blue histiocyte. *Am J Med* 1977;62:627–35.
9. Viana MB, Leite VH, Giugliani R, Fensom A. Sea-blue histiocytosis in a family with Niemann-Pick disease. *A clinical, morphological and biochemical study. Sangre (Barc)* 1992;37:59–67.
10. Cogan DG, Chu FC, Reingold D, Barranger J. Ocular motor signs in some metabolic diseases. *Arch Ophthalmol* 1981;99:1802–8.
11. Vanier MT. Niemann-Pick disease type C. *Orphanet J Rare Dis* 2010;5:16.
12. Jones I, He X, Katouzian F, Darroch PI, Schuchman EH. Characterization of common SMPD1 mutations causing types A and B Niemann-Pick disease and generation of mutation-specific mouse models. *Mol Genet Metab* 2008;95:152–62.

13. Schuchman EH. The pathogenesis and treatment of acid sphingomyelinase-deficient Niemann-Pick disease. *Int J Clin Pharmacol Ther* 2009;47 Suppl 1:S48–57.
14. Simonaro CM, Desnick RJ, McGovern MM, Wasserstein MP, Schuchman EH. The demographics and distribution of type B Niemann-Pick disease: novel mutations lead to new genotype/phenotype correlations. *Am J Hum Genet* 2002;71:1413–9.
15. McGovern MM, Wasserstein MP, Aron A, Desnick RJ, Schuchman EH, Brodie SE. Ocular manifestations of Niemann-Pick disease type B. *Ophthalmology* 2004;111:1424–7.
16. Levran O, Desnick RJ, Schuchman EH. Type A Niemann-Pick disease: a frameshift mutation in the acid sphingomyelinase gene (fsP330) occurs in Ashkenazi Jewish patients. *Hum Mutat* 1993;2:317–9.
17. McGovern MM, Pohl-Worgall T, Deckelbaum RJ, et al. Lipid abnormalities in children with types A and B Niemann Pick disease. *J Pediatr* 2004;145:77–81.
18. Nicholson AG, Florio R, Hansell DM, et al. Pulmonary involvement by Niemann-Pick disease. *A report of six cases. Histopathology* 2006;48:596–603.
19. Mendelson DS, Wasserstein MP, Desnick RJ, et al. Type B Niemann-Pick disease: findings at chest radiography, thin-section CT, and pulmonary function testing. *Radiology* 2006;238:339–45.
20. Simpson WL, Jr., Mendelson D, Wasserstein MP, McGovern MM. Imaging manifestations of Niemann-Pick disease type B. *AJR Am J Roentgenol* 2010;194:W12–9.
21. Guillemot N, Troadec C, de Villemeur TB, Clement A, Fauroux B. Lung disease in Niemann-Pick disease. *Pediatr Pulmonol* 2007;42:1207–14.
22. Wasserstein M, Godbold J, McGovern MM. Skeletal manifestations in pediatric and adult patients with Niemann Pick disease type B. *J Inherit Metab Dis* 2012.
23. Wasserstein MP, Larkin AE, Glass RB, Schuchman EH, Desnick RJ, McGovern MM. Growth restriction in children with type B Niemann-Pick disease. *J Pediatr* 2003;142:424–8.
24. Volders P, Van Hove J, Lories RJ, et al. Niemann-Pick disease type B: an unusual clinical presentation with multiple vertebral fractures. *Am J Med Genet* 2002;109:42–51.
25. Suzuki O, Abe M. Secondary sea-blue histiocytosis derived from Niemann-Pick disease. *J Clin Exp Hematop* 2007;47:19–21.
26. Morel CF, Gassas A, Doyle J, Clarke JT. Unsuccessful treatment attempt: cord blood stem cell transplantation in a patient with Niemann-Pick disease type A. *J Inherit Metab Dis* 2007;30:987.
27. Vellodi A, Hobbs JR, O'Donnell NM, Coulter BS, Hugh-Jones K. Treatment of Niemann-Pick disease type B by allogeneic bone marrow transplantation. *Br Med J (Clin Res Ed)* 1987;295:1375–6.
28. Schneiderman J, Thormann K, Charrow J, Kletzel M. Correction of enzyme levels with allogeneic hematopoietic progenitor cell transplantation in Niemann-Pick type B. *Pediatr Blood Cancer* 2007;49:987–9.
29. Victor S, Coulter JB, Besley GT, et al. Niemann-Pick disease: sixteen-year follow-up of allogeneic bone marrow transplantation in a type B variant. *J Inherit Metab Dis* 2003;26:775–85.
30. Dodge JC, Clarke J, Treleaven CM, et al. Intracerebroventricular infusion of acid sphingomyelinase corrects CNS manifestations in a mouse model of Niemann-Pick A disease. *Exp Neurol* 2009;215:349–57.
31. Nicholson AG, Wells AU, Hooper J, Hansell DM, Kelleher A, Morgan C. Successful treatment of endogenous lipid pneumonia due to Niemann-Pick Type B disease with whole-lung lavage. *Am J Respir Crit Care Med* 2002;165:128–31.
32. Choi JH, Shin YL, Kim GH, Hong SJ, Yoo HW. Treatment of hyperlipidemia associated with Niemann-Pick disease type B by fenofibrate. *Eur J Pediatr* 2006;165:138–9.
33. Bu J, Ashe KM, Bringas J, et al. Merits of combination cortical, subcortical, and cerebellar injections for the treatment of niemann-pick disease type a. *Mol Ther* 2012;20:1893–901.
34. Winsor EJ, Welch JP. Genetic and demographic aspects of Nova Scotia Niemann-Pick disease (type D). *Am J Hum Genet* 1978;30:530–8.
35. Greer WL, Riddell DC, Gillan TL, et al. The Nova Scotia (type D) form of Niemann-Pick disease is caused by a G3097→T transversion in NPC1. *Am J Hum Genet* 1998;63:52–4.
36. Wenger DA, Barth G, Githens JH. Nine cases of sphingomyelin lipidosis, a new variant in Spanish-American Children. *Juvenile variant of Niemann-Pick Disease with foamy and sea-blue histiocytes. Am J Dis Child* 1977;131:955–61.
37. Patterson MC. A riddle wrapped in a mystery: understanding Niemann-Pick disease, type C. *Neurologist* 2003;9:301–10.
38. Spiegel R, Raas-Rothschild A, Reish O, et al. The clinical spectrum of fetal Niemann-Pick type C. *Am J Med Genet A* 2009;149A:446–50.
39. Garver WS, Francis GA, Jelinek D, et al. The National Niemann-Pick C1 disease database: report of clinical features and health problems. *Am J Med Genet A* 2007;143A:1204–11.
40. Imrie J, Dasgupta S, Besley GT, et al. The natural history of Niemann-Pick disease type C in the UK. *J Inherit Metab Dis* 2007;30:51–9.
41. Bjurulf B, Spetalen S, Erichsen A, Vanier MT, Strom EH, Stromme P. Niemann-Pick disease type C2 presenting as fatal pulmonary alveolar lipoproteinosis: morphological findings in lung and nervous tissue. *Med Sci Monit* 2008;14:CS71–5.
42. Griese M, Brasch F, Aldana VR, et al. Respiratory disease in Niemann-Pick type C2 is caused by pulmonary alveolar proteinosis. *Clin Genet* 2010;77:119–30.
43. Roszell BR, Tao JQ, Yu KJ, Huang S, Bates SR. Characterization of the Niemann-Pick C pathway in alveolar type II cells and lamellar bodies of the lung. *Am J Physiol Lung Cell Mol Physiol* 2012;302:L919–32.
44. Iturriaga C, Pineda M, Fernandez-Valero EM, Vanier MT, Coll MJ. Niemann-Pick C disease in Spain: clinical spectrum and development of a disability scale. *J Neurol Sci* 2006;249:1–6.
45. Patterson MC, Hendriksz CJ, Walterfang M, Sedel F, Vanier MT, Wijburg F. Recommendations for the diagnosis and management of Niemann-Pick disease type C: an update. *Mol Genet Metab* 2012;106:330–44.
46. Vankova J, Stepanova I, Jech R, et al. Sleep disturbances and hypocretin deficiency in Niemann-Pick disease type C. *Sleep* 2003;26:427–30.
47. Kanbayashi T, Abe M, Fujimoto S, et al. Hypocretin deficiency in niemann-pick type C with cataplexy. *Neuropediatrics* 2003;34:52–3.
48. Oyama K, Takahashi T, Shoji Y, et al. Niemann-Pick disease type C: cataplexy and hypocretin in cerebrospinal fluid. *Tohoku J Exp Med* 2006;209:263–7.
49. Walterfang M, Fietz M, Fahey M, et al. The neuropsychiatry of Niemann-Pick type C disease in adulthood. *J Neuropsychiatry Clin Neurosci* 2006;18:158–70.
50. Sevin M, Lesca G, Baumann N, et al. The adult form of Niemann-Pick disease type C. *Brain* 2007;130:120–33.
51. Klarner B, Klunemann HH, Lurding R, Aslanidis C, Rupprecht R. Neuropsychological profile of adult patients with Niemann-Pick C1 (NPC1) mutations. *J Inherit Metab Dis* 2007;30:60–7.
52. Klunemann HH, Santosh PJ, Sedel F. Treatable metabolic psychoses that go undetected: what Niemann-Pick type C can teach us. *Int J Psychiatry Clin Pract* 2012;16:162–9.
53. Salsano E, Umeh C, Rufa A, Pareyson D, Zee DS. Vertical supranuclear gaze palsy in Niemann-Pick type C disease. *Neurol Sci* 2012;33:1225–32.
54. Abel LA, Bowman EA, Velakoulis D, et al. Saccadic eye movement characteristics in adult niemann-pick type C disease: relationships with disease severity and brain structural measures. *PLoS One* 2012;7:e50947.
55. Wijburg FA, Sedel F, Pineda M, et al. Development of a suspicion index to aid diagnosis of Niemann-Pick disease type C. *Neurology* 2012;78:1560–7.
56. Rosenbaum AI, Maxfield FR. Niemann-Pick type C disease: molecular mechanisms and potential therapeutic approaches. *J Neurochem* 2011;116:789–95.
57. Park WD, O'Brien JF, Lundquist PA, et al. Identification of 58 novel mutations in Niemann-Pick disease type C: correlation with biochemical phenotype and importance of PTC1-like domains in NPC1. *Hum Mutat* 2003;22:313–25.
58. Naureckiene S, Sleat DE, Lackland H, et al. Identification of HE1 as the second gene of Niemann-Pick C disease. *Science* 2000;290:2298–301.
59. Wang ML, Motamed M, Infante RE, et al. Identification of surface residues on Niemann-Pick C2 essential for hydrophobic handoff of cholesterol to NPC1 in lysosomes. *Cell Metab* 2010;12:166–73.
60. Porter FD, Scherrer DE, Lanier MH, et al. Cholesterol oxidation products are sensitive and specific blood-based biomarkers for Niemann-Pick C1 disease. *Sci Transl Med* 2010;2:56ra81.
61. Jiang X, Sidhu R, Porter FD, et al. A sensitive and specific LC-MS/MS method for rapid diagnosis of Niemann-Pick C1 disease from human plasma. *J Lipid Res* 2011;52(7):1435–45.
62. Li H, Repa JJ, Valasek MA, et al. Molecular, anatomical, and biochemical events associated with neurodegeneration in mice with Niemann-Pick type C disease. *J Neuropathol Exp Neurol* 2005;64:323–33.
63. Cluzeau CV, Watkins-Chow DE, Fu R, et al. Microarray expression analysis and identification of serum biomarkers for Niemann-Pick disease, type C1. *Hum Mol Genet* 2012;21:3632–46.
64. Mattsson N, Zetterberg H, Bianconi S, et al. Gamma-secretase-dependent amyloid-beta is increased in Niemann-Pick type C: a cross-sectional study. *Neurology* 2011;76:366–72.
65. Mattsson N, Olsson M, Gustavsson MK, et al. Amyloid-beta metabolism in Niemann-Pick C disease models and patients. *Metab Brain Dis* 2012;27:573–85.
66. Suzuki K, Parker CC, Pentchev PG, et al. Neurofibrillary tangles in Niemann-Pick disease type C. *Acta Neuropathol* 1995;89:227–38.
67. Saito Y, Suzuki K, Nanba E, Yamamoto T, Ohno K, Murayama S. Niemann-Pick type C disease: accelerated neurofibrillary tangle formation and amyloid beta deposition associated with apolipoprotein E epsilon 4 homozygosity. *Ann Neurol* 2002;52:351–5.
68. Wraith JE, Guffon N, Rohrbach M, et al. Natural history of Niemann-Pick disease type C in a multicentre observational retrospective cohort study. *Mol Genet Metab* 2009;98:250–4.

69. Pentchev PG, Comly ME, Kruth HS, et al. A defect in cholesterol esterification in Niemann-Pick disease (type C) patients. *Proc Natl Acad Sci U S A* 1985;82:8247–51.

70. Vanier MT, Rodriguez-Lafrasse C, Rousson R, et al. Type C Niemann-Pick disease: biochemical aspects and phenotypic heterogeneity. *Dev Neurosci* 1991;13:307–14.

71. Fusco C, Russo A, Galla D, Hladnik U, Frattini D, Giustina ED. New Niemann-Pick Type C1 Gene Mutation Associated With Very Severe Disease Course and Marked Early Cerebellar Vermis Atrophy. *J Child Neurol* 2012.2013;28:1694–7.

72. Zaaraoui W, Crespy L, Rico A, et al. In vivo quantification of brain injury in adult Niemann-Pick Disease Type C. *Mol Genet Metab* 2011;103:138–41.

73. Walterfang M, Fahey M, Abel L, et al. Size and shape of the corpus callosum in adult Niemann-Pick type C reflects state and trait illness variables. *AJNR Am J Neuroradiol* 2011;32:1340–6.

74. Walterfang M, Yu-Chien C, Imrie J, Rushton D, Schubiger D, Patterson MC. Dysphagia as a risk factor for mortality in Niemann-Pick disease type C: systematic literature review and evidence from studies with miglustat. *Orphanet J Rare Dis* 2012;7:76.

75. Wraith JE, Imrie J. New therapies in the management of Niemann-Pick type C disease: clinical utility of miglustat. *Ther Clin Risk Manag* 2009;5:877–87.

76. Nietupski JB, Pacheco JJ, Chuang WL, et al. Iminosugar-based inhibitors of glucosylceramide synthase prolong survival but paradoxically increase brain glucosylceramide levels in Niemann-Pick C mice. *Mol Genet Metab* 2012;105:621–8.

77. Zervas M, Somers KL, Thrall MA, Walkley SU. Critical role for glycosphingolipids in Niemann-Pick disease type C. *Curr Biol* 2001;11:1283–7.

78. Patterson MC, Vecchio D, Prady H, Abel L, Wraith JE. Miglustat for treatment of Niemann-Pick C disease: a randomised controlled study. *Lancet Neurol* 2007;6:765–72.

79. Wraith JE, Vecchio D, Jacklin E, et al. Miglustat in adult and juvenile patients with Niemann-Pick disease type C: long-term data from a clinical trial. *Mol Genet Metab* 2010;99:351–7.

80. Patterson MC, Vecchio D, Jacklin E, et al. Long-term miglustat therapy in children with Niemann-Pick disease type C. *J Child Neurol* 2010;25:300–5.

81. Pineda M, Perez-Poyato MS, O'Callaghan M, et al. Clinical experience with miglustat therapy in pediatric patients with Niemann-Pick disease type C: a case series. *Mol Genet Metab* 2010;99:358–66.

82. Pineda M, Wraith JE, Mengel E, et al. Miglustat in patients with Niemann-Pick disease Type C (NP-C): a multicenter observational retrospective cohort study. *Mol Genet Metab* 2009;98:243–9.

83. Ramirez CM, Liu B, Taylor AM, et al. Weekly cyclodextrin administration normalizes cholesterol metabolism in nearly every organ of the Niemann-Pick type C1 mouse and markedly prolongs life. *Pediatr Res* 2010;68:309–15.

84. Stein VM, Crooks A, Ding W, et al. Miglustat improves purkinje cell survival and alters microglial phenotype in feline Niemann-Pick disease type C. *J Neuropathol Exp Neurol* 2012;71:434–48.

85. Zarowski M, Steinborn B, Gurda B, Dvorakova L, Vlaskova H, Kothare SV. Treatment of cataplexy in Niemann-Pick disease type C with the use of miglustat. *Eur J Paediatr Neurol* 2011;15:84–7.

86. Pipalia NH, Cosner CC, Huang A, et al. Histone deacetylase inhibitor treatment dramatically reduces cholesterol accumulation in Niemann-Pick type C1 mutant human fibroblasts. *Proc Natl Acad Sci U S A.* 2011;108(14):5620–5.

87. Kirkegaard T, Gray J, Priestman DA, et al. Heat shock protein-based therapy as a potential candidate for treating the sphingolipidoses. *Sci Transl Med.* 2016;8(355):355ra118.

88. Patterson MC, Platt F. Therapy of Niemann-Pick disease, type C. *Biochim Biophys Acta* 2004;1685:77–82.

89. Breen C, Wynn RF, O'Meara A, et al. Developmental outcome post allogenic bone marrow transplant for Niemann Pick Type C2. *Mol Genet Metab* 2012. 2013;108:82–4.

90. Lee H, Bae JS, Jin HK. Human umbilical cord blood-derived mesenchymal stem cells improve neurological abnormalities of Niemann-Pick type C mouse by modulation of neuroinflammatory condition. *J Vet Med Sci* 2010;72:709–17.

91. Lopez ME, Klein AD, Hong J, Dimbil UJ, Scott MP. Neuronal and epithelial cell rescue resolves chronic systemic inflammation in the lipid storage disorder Niemann-Pick C. *Hum Mol Genet* 2012;21:2946–60.

CHAPTER 25

X-linked Adrenoleukodystrophy

Deborah L. Renaud

Departments of Neurology and Pediatrics, Mayo Clinic, Rochester, Minnesota, USA

Clinical definition and epidemiology

X-linked adrenoleukodystrophy (X-ALD) is a peroxisomal disorder characterized by primary adrenal insufficiency and neurological manifestations. The inheritance is X-linked, affecting males more severely than females; however the clinical manifestations are variable, even within families with the same underlying genetic mutation. The primary defect is caused by a mutation in the *ABCD1* gene, located on chromosome Xq28, resulting in an elevation of very long chain fatty acids (VLCFAs).

The minimum frequency of X-ALD in the United States has been estimated at 1:21,000 males (hemizygous). The minimum frequency of heterozygous females who are carriers of X-ALD was estimated at 1:14,000, giving an overall minimum frequency of 1:16,800 [1]. The minimal incidence in Brazil [2] has been estimated at 1:35,000 males and in Japan [3] at 1:30,000 to 1:50,000. All ethnic groups are affected.

Spectrum of clinical phenotype (Table 25.1)

Childhood cerebral adrenoleukodystrophy (CCALD)

Early developmental milestones are usually normal. Boys with CCALD initially present between the ages of 3 and 10 years with symptoms of attention deficit hyperactivity disorder and learning problems. Once neurological symptoms become clinically apparent, the disease progression can be quite rapid with development of spastic quadriplegia, cortical blindness, loss of auditory processing, and cognitive decline over 12 months or less. Seizures often occur and may be the initial presenting sign. The natural course of this form without early intervention leads to complete disability and early death [4, 5].

Table 25.1 Clinical phenotypes in males with X-ALD [4, 5].

Phenotype	Age of onset	Estimated relative frequency
Childhood cerebral	3–10 years	31–35%
Adolescent cerebral	11–19 years	4–7%
Adult cerebral	Adulthood	2–5%
Adrenomyeloneuropathy	28 ± 9 years	40–46%
Addison's disease only	Any age	Varies with age
Spinocerebellar variant	Adulthood	Rare
Asymptomatic	–	Diminishes with age

Adolescent cerebral adrenoleukodystrophy

The symptoms in adolescents with cerebral disease are similar to CCALD but with slower progression [4, 5].

Adult cerebral adrenoleukodystrophy

Adults presenting with cerebral disease without preceding adrenomyeloneuropathy (AMN) comprise a small group. The men usually present with dementia and behavioral change. Progression is similar to childhood cerebral disease. Approximately 20–40% of men with AMN will present with cerebral involvement during the course of their neurological disease [4–6].

Adrenomyeloneuropathy

Unlike the inflammatory cerebral leukodystrophy forms, AMN is a primary axonopathy affecting adults. Symptoms result from a combination of myelopathy and peripheral neuropathy. Men in their twenties and thirties present with slowly progressive spastic paraparesis, sensory loss, and bowel and bladder dysfunction. Unless cerebral disease develops, intellectual abilities are not affected in pure AMN [4, 5].

Addison's disease only

X-linked adrenoleukodystrophy is the most common cause of idiopathic Addison's disease. Primary adrenal insufficiency can occur at any age and does not correlate with the development of neurological symptoms. The proportion of males with Addison's disease alone decreases with age as more boys and men develop neurological symptoms. Approximately 85% of boys with the childhood cerebral form and 65% of men with AMN have primary adrenal insufficiency. Once primary adrenal insufficiency develops, the treatment should be lifelong. Both glucocorticoid and mineralocorticoid function can be affected. Unrecognized adrenal insufficiency in asymptomatic boys with X-ALD can result in significant morbidity and therefore all at-risk boys should be monitored for the possible development of subclinical adrenal insufficiency. Boys and men with idiopathic Addison's disease should be screened for X-ALD with VLCFAs because early diagnosis of X-ALD in this population may improve neurological outcome [4, 7–9].

Spinocerebellar variant

The spinocerebellar variant of X-ALD is rare. Progressive gait unsteadiness is accompanied by dysarthria and tremulousness. Symptoms of ataxia may be followed by the development of

Neurodegeneration, First Edition. Edited by Anthony Schapira, Zbigniew Wszolek, Ted M. Dawson and Nicholas Wood.
© 2017 John Wiley & Sons, Ltd. Published 2017 by John Wiley & Sons, Ltd.

progressive spastic paraparesis. Bladder and bowel dysfunction may be present. Addison's disease may precede the onset of neurological symptoms [10–12].

Asymptomatic boys and men

Males with X-ALD confirmed by elevated VLCFAs and/or mutation analysis who do not have adrenal or neurological involvement have been described at all ages. The prevalence of this group decreases with age as men develop evidence of adrenal insufficiency or symptoms of AMN. Close monitoring of asymptomatic boys and men is important.

Symptomatic female heterozygote

Approximately 50% of female heterozygote carriers of X-ALD will develop neurological symptoms in adulthood. They generally present in a similar fashion to men with AMN but with milder symptoms and later age of onset. Women with neurological symptoms may be the first member of the family diagnosed with X-ALD and are often misdiagnosed as having multiple sclerosis or hereditary spastic paraparesis. The severity of symptoms is variable, ranging from hyperreflexia with impaired vibratory sense to severe spastic paraparesis. Bowel and bladder dysfunction may also be present [13, 14]. Adrenal insufficiency occurs in approximately 1.4% of female heterozygotes although subclinical glucocorticoid and mineralocorticoid dysfunction is more commonly seen. Women with subclinical adrenal dysfunction should be closely monitored for adrenal insufficiency [15].

Pathology/pathophysiology specific to the disease

Neuropathology

Cerebral X-ALD [16]

Gray matter of the cerebral and cerebellar cortex, deep cerebral nuclei, and brainstem are spared. White matter demyelination is confluent and symmetric, affecting the parieto-occipital region more frequently than the frontal region. Demyelination is also seen in the corpus callosum, optic pathways, and posterior limb of the internal capsule (in occipital form) but with sparing of the U fibers. Cerebellar white matter is less commonly affected.

Three histopathological zones have been described within the demyelinating lesions of cerebral X-ALD. (i) The peripheral edge demonstrates destruction of myelin with PAS-positive and sudanophilic macrophages and sparing of axons. (ii) The second zone has lipid-laden macrophages with lamellar inclusions and some surviving myelinated axons. (iii) The central zone consists of dense glial fibrils with absence of oligodendrocytes and myelin. Axons may be absent and advanced lesions show cavitation and calcification.

Loss of myelin and axons is associated with perivascular and infiltrating macrophages containing PAS-positive granular and lamellar inclusions. This site of active degeneration is between the first and second zone, corresponding with the active inflammatory edge of demyelination. Reactive microglia are present in the active zone of demyelination with infiltrating B and T lymphocytes. There is a loss of oligodendrocytes and astrocytes in demyelinating regions of white matter.

Adrenomyeloneuropathy [16, 17]

Gray matter of the cerebral and cerebellar cortex, deep cerebral nuclei, and brainstem are spared. Men with pure AMN and heterozygous

women usually do not have visible white matter lesions but may have microscopic demyelinating foci with relative axonal and oligodendrocyte sparing. Confluent changes can be seen in the cerebral white matter, and less frequently in the cerebellar white matter, without associated inflammation. Active inflammatory demyelinating lesions with axonal loss, similar to CCALD, can be seen in up to 20–40% of men with AMN and represent secondary cerebral involvement.

The spinal cord pathology predominates in patients with AMN. Bilateral, symmetric degeneration of the long ascending and descending tracts occurs with both axon and myelin loss. The degeneration of the ascending tracts and the gracile and dorsal spinocerebellar tracts is more prominent in the upper spinal cord. The descending pyramidal tract is most affected in the lower spinal cord. The gray matter of the spinal cord is unaffected. Axonal loss predominates with secondary myelin loss and a dying back type of axonopathy. There is no associated inflammation and gliosis is prominent.

Schwann cells in peripheral nerves contain lamellar inclusions. The pathology is suggestive of an axonopathy with secondary demyelination although nerve conduction studies may be suggestive of a demyelinating neuropathy. Loss of large myelinated fibers corresponds with the clinical loss of vibration and position sense. Optic nerve involvement with optic atrophy may be seen.

Non-inflammatory atrophy of the adrenal gland and testis is common in men with AMN. Atrophy of the zona reticularis and inner zona fasciculata leads to primary hypocortisolism. Lamellar lipid inclusions are seen in the cytoplasm of ballooned, striated adrenocortical cells. Similar lamellae in the Leydig cells result in incompetent Sertoli cells and atrophy of the seminiferous tubules, explaining the infertility seen in many men with AMN.

Genetics

X-linked adrenoleukodystrophy is caused by mutations in the *ABCD1* gene at Xq28. ABCD1 is a member of the D subfamily of ATP-binding cassette (ABC) transporters. There are 49 ABC transporters, which use energy released by ATP hydrolysis to move substrates across membranes. The D subfamily consists of four half-transporters: ABCD1, ABCD2, ABCD3 (PMP70), and ABCD4 (PMP69). The first three are located in the peroxisomal membrane and the fourth has been shown to be in the membrane of the endoplasmic reticulum. *ABCD1* encodes ALDP (adrenoleukodystrophy protein) which transports very long chain fatty acyl-CoA esters across the peroxisomal membrane for B-oxidation within the peroxisome. Mutations in *ABCD1* result in impairment of peroxisomal B-oxidation and accumulation of VLCFAs. ABCD2 may be involved in DHA synthesis but appears to have some overlap in function with ABCD1 since overexpression of ABCD2 results in a decrease in VLCFA accumulation. ABCD1 has very low expression in cortex and is primarily expressed in astrocytes, oligodendrocytes, and microglia in the brain, whereas ABCD2 is expressed mostly in the cortex and cerebellar Purkinje cells [18–21].

More than 1200 mutations have been described. Approximately 61% are missense mutations, 22% are frameshift mutations, 10% are nonsense, and 7% other types of mutations. There is no clear genotype to phenotype correlation [20]. X-ALD families with mutations in *ABCD1* show significant clinical heterogeneity: there can be CCALD boys, AMN men and women, and Addison's disease alone patients within the same family despite sharing a common mutation. Modifier genes have been proposed to explain this heterogeneity although no specific modifier gene has been found to date. An evaluation of single nucleotide polymorphisms in the *ABCD2*, *ABCD3*, and *ABCD4* genes failed to show any significant association with clinical phenotype [22]. An evaluation of the effect of genetic variants of methionine metabolism suggested that the c.776C>G variant of transcobalamin 2 may predispose to CNS demyelination [23, 24].

Pathophysiology

The pathophysiology underlying the various clinical phenotypes of X-ALD is unclear. A three-hit hypothesis has been proposed: (i) the metabolic derangement associated with mutations in *ABCD1* results in an elevation of VLCFAs, decreased plasmalogens, and resulting oxidative stress with axonal damage; (ii) as yet undefined genetic, epigenetic, and environmental triggers initiate the inflammatory cascade resulting in neuroinflammation; and (iii) cytokine- and chemokine-mediated inflammation causes generalized loss of peroxisomal functions resulting in cell loss and progressive inflammatory demyelination with associated neurodegeneration [25]. Research is underway to evaluate each component of this hypothesis including the effects of elevated VLCFAs on various cell types and cellular processes, oxidative stress models, cholesterol metabolism and its interplay with inflammatory processes, cell-mediated inflammatory processes, and other mechanisms. Genetic, epigenetic, and environmental triggers that may play a role in the pathophysiology of X-ALD are currently being explored. An improved understanding of the pathophysiology of the various clinical phenotypes of X-ALD will help design specific treatments to modify the clinical course for patients with X-ALD.

Environment

Although environmental factors may play a role in determining the clinical phenotype, few specific environmental influences have been found. Head trauma can precipitate the onset of cerebral inflammatory disease and rapid deterioration in at-risk boys with presymptomatic X-ALD and men with AMN [26].

Clinical prodrome and biomarkers

Males and female carriers with X-ALD usually have normal intelligence and neurological function prior to the onset of neurological symptoms of cerebral disease or AMN. It is not currently possible to predict which clinical phenotype will occur for any individual, because a wide range of clinical phenotypes can be seen within the same family. Boys or men who develop idiopathic Addison's disease should be tested for X-ALD. Addison's disease may precede, coexist with, or follow the neurological symptoms and is not predictive of the neurological phenotype. Prospective evaluation of boys and men at risk with X-ALD for subclinical adrenal insufficiency and early clinical or neuroradiological evidence of evolving cerebral disease is essential to providing appropriate and timely medical care.

Specific biomarkers to predict which clinical phenotype a specific patient with X-ALD will develop are lacking. Chitotriosidase, an enzyme produced by activated monocytes and macrophages, has been shown to be increased in the plasma and cerebrospinal fluid of boys with CCALD [27]. It is unclear whether this biomarker is able to predict clinical phenotype in presymptomatic males.

Examination, investigations (including imaging)

Neurological examination

At the time of presentation, boys and men with cerebral X-ALD may have subtle changes in personality and cognitive function by history, which are difficult to detect clinically without formal neuropsychological testing. Once neurological symptoms develop, boys and men with untreated cerebral X-ALD usually present with progressive spasticity, seizures, cognitive decline, and severe disability.

Hyperreflexia may be an early sign of spasticity in men and women with AMN. An assessment of gait and ability to drive safely can be performed by the physical medicine team. Sensory deficits, particularly impaired vibratory sense, may be present.

Boys and men with untreated cerebral X-ALD have progressive loss of visual acuity associated with demyelination of central visual tracts followed by optic nerve atrophy [28]. Despite successful hematopoietic stem cell transplantation (HSCT), progressive visual loss can still be seen in some patients. The predictive factors for visual loss are pretransplant magnetic resonance imaging (MRI) severity score greater than 11, performance IQ less than 76, and parieto-occipital distribution of inflammatory demyelination. These factors are indicative of more aggressive/advanced disease and may indicate that it is too late to stabilize the demyelination in the visual pathways to prevent visual loss [29].

Neurogenic bladder and erectile dysfunction can be significant problems for men with AMN. Referral to an urologist for appropriate evaluation and treatment is indicated. Bowel dysfunction may require the attention of a gastroenterologist.

Endocrine evaluation

Presenting symptoms of subclinical adrenal insufficiency may include fatigue/weakness, poor growth, recurrent abdominal pain, and decrease in school performance. Adrenal crisis may be the initial presenting symptom, particularly in the setting of an acute infection. Clinical examination may reveal bronze pigmentation of the skin. Hypoglycemia and electrolyte imbalance may suggest adrenal insufficiency. Serum adrenocorticotropic hormone (ACTH) and cortisol should be monitored regularly in boys and men with X-ALD to detect subclinical and overt adrenal insufficiency early so that appropriate treatment is not delayed. ACTH stimulation testing may be necessary to detect subclinical adrenal insufficiency in symptomatic patients or those preparing for HSCT. A plasma ACTH level between 70 pg/mL and 500 pg/mL is rated as borderline if the ACTH stimulation test shows a normal cortisol response. The adrenal function is rated as abnormal if the plasma ACTH level is greater than 500 pg/mL or the cortical response to ACTH stimulation is suboptimal. Mineralocorticoid deficiency is considered to be present if the aldosterone level is less than 5 ng/dL [9, 30, 31].

Neuropsychological testing

Overall cognitive function based on neuropsychological testing is normal in asymptomatic boys with X-ALD who have normal findings on conventional brain MRI [32]. Asymptomatic boys with X-ALD but early changes on MRI demonstrate deficits in naming and verbal fluency despite normal IQ testing [33]. Boys with neurological symptoms associated with MRI changes consistent with CCALD have significantly impaired neuropsychological profiles. The performance IQ is disproportionately affected compared to the verbal IQ. Executive function, naming, visual perception, and visual short-term sequential memory are impaired. Most neuropsychological scores correlate with the Loes MRI severity score indicating the degree of white matter involvement. Boys with CCALD receiving bone marrow or HSCT early in the course of their disease show a stabilization or improvement in neuropsychological scores post transplant, unless severe graft-versus-host disease is present [33,

34]. Neuropsychological testing is recommended every 6 months for boys at risk of developing CCALD.

Neuroimaging

MRI

An MRI severity score for patients with X-ALD was developed by Loes and colleagues [35] based on location and extent of disease. This scoring system has been helpful to study the natural progression of MRI changes in cerebral disease for individual patients and for the pretransplant evaluation of boys with CCALD. Three patterns of brain involvement were described. The posterior white matter pattern (Figure 25.1), present in 80%, involved the parieto-occipital white matter, splenium of the corpus callosum, visual and auditory pathways, and occasionally the corticospinal tracts. The anterior white matter pattern, present in 15%, involved the frontal white matter, genu of the corpus callosum, and frontopontine tract. The remaining 5% had isolated projection fiber abnormalities [35]. Contrast enhancement on T1-weighted images is predictive of clinical and MRI disease progression. This enhancement, when present, is limited to the leading edge of the affected white matter [36]. Fluid attenuated inversion recovery (FLAIR) imaging clearly distinguishes the central necrotic zone of the affected white matter from the more peripheral zones [37, 38]. Analysis of MRI patterns is useful for the prediction of progression. Five patterns of MRI abnormalities are described (pattern 1: parieto-occipital white matter; pattern 2: frontal white matter; pattern 3: isolated corticospinal; pattern 4: cerebellar white matter; and pattern 5: concomitant parieto-occipital and frontal white matter). Patterns 1 and 2 demonstrate a rapid rate of progression, particularly if accompanied by contrast enhancement and early age of onset. Pattern 5 shows the most rapid progression while patterns 3 and 4 are slowest in rate of progression. Patterns 1 and 5 were seen primarily in children, patterns 2 and 4 in adolescents, and pattern 3 in adults [39].

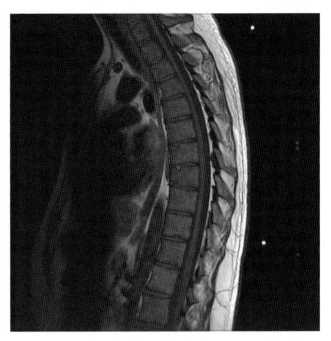

Figure 25.2 Sagittal fast spin echo T1-weighted MR image of the spine from a man with adrenomyeloneuropathy demonstrating mild diffuse spinal cord atrophy.

Men with AMN without evidence of cerebral disease may present with evidence of spinal cord atrophy on MRI (Figure 25.2).

MRI in patients with the spinocerebellar variant demonstrates T2 signal hyperintensity in the posterior limb of the internal capsule (Figure 25.3) and cerebral peduncles with atrophy of the cerebellum (especially the vermis), brainstem, and cervical spinal cord [10–12].

Overt cerebral disease is rare in women but MRI may detect subtle symmetric hyperintensity of the white matter in the parieto-occipital lobes [13, 14, 40].

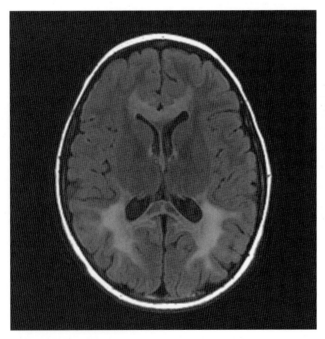

Figure 25.1 T2-weighted FLAIR axial MR image of a patient with X-linked adrenoleukodystrophy demonstrating confluent symmetric signal abnormality in the parieto-occipital regions.

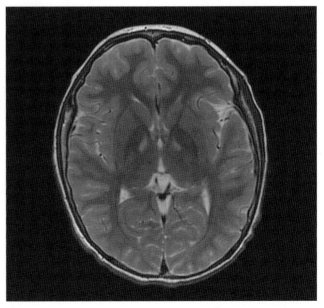

Figure 25.3 MR image from an adolescent with mild spinocerebellar variant demonstrating T2 signal hyperintensity in the posterior limb of the internal capsule.

Magnetic resonance spectroscopy (MRS)

In boys with untreated CCALD, MRS reveals abnormalities in metabolite ratios within the affected white matter. *N*-acetyl-aspartate (NAA): creatine and NAA: choline ratios are decreased and the choline: creatine ratio is increased in comparison to white matter from normal controls [41–43]. MRS changes may show improvement following HSCT when clinical status has stabilized [42, 44].

Specialized MRI sequences

Conventional diffusion-weighted imaging can demonstrate the three different lesion zones with the burnt-out central zone appearing hypointense, the intermediate inflammatory zone appearing moderately hyperintense, and the most peripheral demyelinating zone appearing faintly hyperintense [45, 46]. The value of diffusion tensor imaging in cerebral forms of X-ALD is yet to be determined. Diffusion tensor imaging may be useful for determining the extent of corticospinal tract involvement in AMN [7, 47]. Magnetization transfer-weighted imaging may also be a useful tool for evaluating spinal cord pathology in men with AMN [48, 49].

Nuclear imaging techniques

A 5.5-year-old boy with CCALD with abnormal MRI signal in a bilaterally symmetric pattern involving the occipital, parietal, and posterior temporal white matter as well as the splenium of the corpus callosum, posterolateral thalamus, posterior limbs of the external and internal capsules, and the corticospinal tract was studied with ^{11}C-[R]-PK11195 positron emission tomography (PET). The distribution of neuroinflammation on PET was concordant with the regions of abnormal signal on MRI with the most prominent signal corresponding to the intermediate inflammatory zone behind the leading edge of demyelination where contrast enhancement occurs [50].

Diagnosis and prognosis

Diagnosis

Plasma VLCFAs are elevated in male hemizygotes with X-ALD. The parameters measured are the concentration of C26:0, the ratio of C26:0 to C22:0, and the ratio of C24:0 to C22:0. In approximately 15–20% of female carriers of X-ALD, VLCFAs are normal resulting in a false negative test. A computerized discriminant factor is helpful in detecting X-ALD hemizygotes and heterozygotes but does not eliminate the false negative tests for female carriers. Mutation analysis of the *ABCD1* gene is useful for detecting carriers and can also be used for extended-family testing once the mutation in the proband has been determined. Greater than 1200 mutations have been described in the X-ALD mutation database (www.x-ald.nl). The majority of these are private mutations. There is no genotype–phenotype correlation between the mutations described and the clinical phenotype [4, 51–53].

VLCFAs are elevated at birth. A high-throughput screening method using combined liquid chromatography–tandem mass spectrometry to detect X-ALD in newborn blood spots has been developed. Detection of boys with X-ALD at birth will decrease morbidity and mortality by prospectively monitoring for evidence of adrenal insufficiency and early detection of childhood cerebral disease [4, 54, 55].

Prognosis

The prognosis for X-ALD depends on the clinical phenotype. Boys and men with untreated cerebral disease have rapidly progressive neurological symptoms and a significantly reduced lifespan. In these patients successful HSCT early in the course of cerebral disease can arrest disease progression and stabilize the neurological disease. Men and women with AMN have a slowly progressive neurological course over many years. Boys and men with unrecognized adrenal insufficiency are at risk of death or morbidity as a result of unanticipated adrenal crisis, particularly at a time of illness.

Treatment options (including comorbid conditions)

Medical

Lorenzo's oil

Lorenzo's oil is a 4:1 mixture of glyceryl trioleate and glyceryl trierucate. This is administered as part of a fat-modified diet with Lorenzo's oil comprising 20% of dietary calories with 5% essential fatty acids and 10–15% fat from other sources. The overall fat content of the diet is limited to approximately 35%. This requires close monitoring by a dietician and multidisciplinary team. Multiple studies have shown that administration of Lorenzo's oil decreases plasma VLCFAs [4, 56, 57]. Side effects related to Lorenzo's oil are frequent and include thrombocytopenia in 40–55%, elevated liver enzymes, gastrointestinal symptoms, and gingivitis [56–58]. Lorenzo's oil does not alter the natural course of neurological symptoms in boys with symptomatic cerebral disease or adults with AMN [4, 57–59]. Lorenzo's oil, when administered to asymptomatic boys with X-ALD, may prevent or delay the onset of CCALD [56].

Lovastatin

Lovastatin is an inhibitor of 3-hydroxy-3-methylglutarylcoenzyme A reductase and is used primarily for the treatment of hypercholesterolemia. Studies evaluating the effect of lovastatin on VLCFA levels have shown mixed results. Decreased plasma VLCFAs were seen in patients within 1–3 months of initiation of lovastatin therapy, associated with a decrease in the percentage of VLCFAs in red blood cell membrane fatty composition after 6 months of therapy [60]. Lovastatin lowered the cellular VLCFA content of X-ALD fibroblasts to normal levels *in vitro* [61]. Other clinical studies have not shown any significant lowering of VLCFA levels during treatment with either simvastatin or lovastatin [62, 63]. Although the aim of treatment has historically been the lowering of VLCFAs, the effect of lovastatin on pro-inflammatory cytokines may be important for the prevention of cerebral inflammatory disease. The potential preventative effect of lovastatin is currently being investigated.

Hematopoietic stem cell transplantation (HSCT)

Bone marrow transplantation (BMT) and HSCT have been shown to be beneficial for boys with early cerebral disease. Survival is improved by BMT/HSCT in the group with early findings compared with the natural history of boys not receiving transplantation and those receiving transplantation at an advanced stage. When performed early, BMT/HSCT results in stabilization or improvement of MRI findings, stabilization of neurological findings, and improvement or stabilization of cognitive function, especially performance IQ, in most boys. VLCFA levels decrease following transplantation. Boys with more advanced cerebral disease at the time of transplantation tend to have further progression of their MRI and clinical findings following transplantation. Death in these patients is frequently due to progression of their underlying X-ALD. Early cerebral disease has been defined as minimal or absent neurological symptoms, performance IQ greater than or equal to 80, and MRI score less than 9. Currently, HSCT is recommended for boys who fulfill the criteria for early disease. Boys with more advanced disease are considered high risk and have poorer outcomes. HSCT is not currently recommended for men with AMN or asymptomatic boys with no evidence of cerebral disease [64–67].

Umbilical cord blood transplantation from unrelated donors has been performed in boys with CCALD who do not have a bone marrow/hematopoietic stem cell donor match [68, 69]. Unfortunately, neurological outcome was not described in these studies. A more recent study demonstrated stabilization of MRI and neurological status following cord blood transplantation with reduced-intensity conditioning [70]. Cord blood transplantation may have the advantage of a lower rate of graft-versus-host disease but engraftment rates may also be lower than with BMT or HSCT.

Improvement in motor function and stabilization of MRI findings was described in a 20-year-old man following HSCT [71]. An adult male with more severe cerebral disease at the time of HSCT died due to severe graft-versus-host disease but demonstrated progression of his neurological symptoms following transplant [72]. Recent unpublished trials of HSCT in adult males with early cerebral disease have shown some promise (personal communication). These studies highlight the importance of continued monitoring of adults with X-ALD for MRI changes consistent with early cerebral disease.

Gene therapy

The first gene therapy trial for X-ALD included two boys with CCALD without a matched donor. CD34+ cells were removed from both patients, genetically corrected with a lentiviral vector encoding wild-type ABCD1, and then re-infused following myeloablative therapy. Progressive cerebral demyelination stabilized in both boys by 14–16 months after the procedure, a result similar to HSCT [73]. Additional boys have been enrolled in the ongoing trial. Gene therapy provides an alternative for boys without a matched donor and may be beneficial for adults with cerebral disease whose risk is greater with allogenic HSCT. The potential long-term risks of gene therapy have not yet been determined.

Treatment of Addison's disease

Acute management of adrenal crisis consists of normal saline rehydration and intravenous corticosteroids. Chronic management of adrenal insufficiency includes oral glucocorticoid replacement in the form of hydrocortisone and mineralocorticoid replacement given as fludrocortisone. Additional stress steroid dosing should be given at times of illness [9, 30, 31].

Symptomatic treatment

For a significant proportion of patients, definitive treatment for the underlying disease is not possible and therefore symptomatic treatment is provided in order to improve the quality of life. Anticonvulsant medications for seizures and nutritional support are provided as indicated. Physical therapy and pharmacological treatments for spasticity may improve the quality of life for men and women with AMN in particular because issues related to mobility and driving are central to their quality of life. Referral as needed for bowel and bladder dysfunction is particularly important for patients with AMN. Psychological support for patients and their families also plays an important role in the treatment of X-ALD.

Surgical

In later stages of CCALD and later onset forms of cerebral disease, the insertion of a gastrostomy tube may be necessary in order to maintain adequate nutrition. When severe spasticity is present, orthopedic intervention may be indicated.

"Social" – family-based or third-party care

Surveys of families affected by CCALD and AMN indicate a high level of support for presymptomatic testing for both males at risk and female carriers (88–95%). The majority felt that testing should be performed prenatally or shortly after birth. Newborn screening for X-ALD for both males and females was supported by 90% of survey respondents in the more recent study [74, 75]. Parents of boys with CCALD have been shown to have increased risk for depression and anxiety [76].

Future developments

N-acetyl-L-cysteine, an anti-oxidant, is currently used as an adjunct to HSCT in one center and may improve survival in boys with advanced cerebral disease [67]. Valproic acid has been shown to decrease oxidative damage of proteins by inducing the expression of ABCD2, a peroxisomal transporter with similarities to ABCD1, in a mouse model of X-ALD and may warrant clinical trials [77]. 4-Phenylbutyrate treatment of cells from X-ALD patients and X-ALD knockout mice resulted in decreased VLCFA level and increased levels of ALDP. These observations have not extended to clinical changes in patients treated with 4-phenylbutyrate [78]. Clinical trials utilizing a combination of anti-oxidant agents have been proposed and are underway [78].

The induction of pluripotential stem cells from X-ALD patient fibroblasts to produce patient-specific neural cells and oligodendrocytes may provide a useful model for X-ALD pathogenesis [79].

References

1. Bezman L, Moser AB, Raymond GV, Rinaldo P, Watkins PA, Smith KD, et al. Adrenoleukodystrophy: incidence, new mutation rate, and results of extended family screening. *Ann Neurol.* 2001 Apr;49(4):512–7.
2. Jardim LB, da Silva AC, Blank D, Villanueva MM, Renck L, Costa ML, et al. X-linked adrenoleukodystrophy: clinical course and minimal incidence in South Brazil. *Brain Dev.* 2010 Mar;32(3):180–90.
3. Takemoto Y, Suzuki Y, Tamakoshi A, Onodera O, Tsuji S, Hashimoto T, et al. Epidemiology of X-linked adrenoleukodystrophy in Japan. *J Hum Genet.* 2002;47(11):590–3.
4. Raymond GV. X-linked adrenoleukodystrophy. In: Raymond G, Eichler F, Fatemi A, Naidu S, editors. *Leukodystrophies.* London, UK: Mac Keith Press; 2011. p. 75–89.
5. Moser HW, Mahmood A, Raymond GV. X-linked adrenoleukodystrophy. *Nat Clin Pract Neurol.* 2007 Mar;3(3):140–51.
6. Sutovsky S, Petrovic R, Chandoga J, Turcani P. Adult onset cerebral form of X-linked adrenoleukodystrophy with dementia of frontal lobe type with new L160P mutation in ABCD1 gene. *J Neurol Sci.* 2007 Dec 15;263(1–2):149–53.
7. Dubey P, Fatemi A, Huang H, Nagae-Poetscher L, Wakana S, Barker PB, et al. Diffusion tensor-based imaging reveals occult abnormalities in adrenomyeloneuropathy. *Ann Neurol.* 2005 Nov;58(5):758–66.
8. Aubourg P, Chaussain JL. Adrenoleukodystrophy: the most frequent genetic cause of Addison's disease. *Horm Res.* 2003;59 Suppl 1:104–5.
9. Polgreen LE, Chahla S, Miller W, Rothman S, Tolar J, Kivisto T, et al. Early diagnosis of cerebral X-linked adrenoleukodystrophy in boys with Addison's disease improves survival and neurological outcomes. *Eur J Pediatr.* 2011 Aug;170(8):1049–54.
10. Li JY, Hsu CC, Tsai CR. Spinocerebellar variant of adrenoleukodystrophy with a novel ABCD1 gene mutation. *J Neurol Sci.* 2010 Mar 15;290(1–2):163–5.
11. Vianello M, Manara R, Betterle C, Tavolato B, Mariniello B, Giometto B. X-linked adrenoleukodystrophy with olivopontocerebellar atrophy. *Eur J Neurol.* 2005 Nov;12(11):912-4.

12. Mishra S, Modi M, Das CP, Prabhakar S. Adrenoleukodystrophy manifesting as spinocerebellar degeneration. *Neurol India*. 2006 Jun;54(2):195–6.

13. Jangouk P, Zackowski KM, Naidu S, Raymond GV. Adrenoleukodystrophy in female heterozygotes: Underrecognized and undertreated. *Mol Genet Metab*. 2012 Feb;105(2):180–5.

14. Schmidt S, Traber F, Block W, Keller E, Pohl C, von Oertzen J, et al. Phenotype assignment in symptomatic female carriers of X-linked adrenoleukodystrophy. *J Neurol*. 2001 Jan;248(1):36–44.

15. el-Deiry SS, Naidu S, Blevins LS, Ladenson PW. Assessment of adrenal function in women heterozygous for adrenoleukodystrophy. *J Clin Endocrinol Metab*. 1997 Mar;82(3):856–60.

16. Ferrer I, Aubourg P, Pujol A. General aspects and neuropathology of X-linked adrenoleukodystrophy. *Brain Pathol*. 2010 Jul;20(4):817–30.

17. Powers JM, DeCiero DP, Ito M, Moser AB, Moser HW. Adrenomyeloneuropathy: a neuropathologic review featuring its noninflammatory myelopathy. *J Neuropathol Exp Neurol*. 2000 Feb;59(2):89–102.

18. Wanders RJ, Visser WF, van Roermund CW, Kemp S, Waterham HR. The peroxisomal ABC transporter family. *Pflugers Arch*. 2007 Feb;453(5):719–34.

19. Kim WS, Weickert CS, Garner B. Role of ATP-binding cassette transporters in brain lipid transport and neurological disease. *J Neurochem*. 2008 Mar;104(5):1145–84.

20. Kemp S, Theodoulou FL, Wanders RJ. Mammalian peroxisomal ABC transporters: from endogenous substrates to pathology and clinical significance. *Br J Pharmacol*. 2011 Dec;164(7):1753–66.

21. Genin EC, Geillon F, Gondcaille C, Athias A, Gambert P, Trompier D, et al. Substrate specificity overlap and interaction between adrenoleukodystrophy protein (ALDP/ABCD1) and adrenoleukodystrophy-related protein (ALDRP/ABCD2). *J Biol Chem*. 2011 Mar 11;286(10):8075–84.

22. Matsukawa T, Asheuer M, Takahashi Y, Goto J, Suzuki Y, Shimozawa N, et al. Identification of novel SNPs of ABCD1, ABCD2, ABCD3, and ABCD4 genes in patients with X-linked adrenoleukodystrophy (ALD) based on comprehensive resequencing and association studies with ALD phenotypes. *Neurogenetics*. 2011 Feb;12(1):41–50.

Linnebank M, Kemp S, Wanders RJ, Kleijer WJ, van der Sterre ML, Gartner J, et al. Methionine metabolism and phenotypic variability in X-linked adrenoleukodystrophy. *Neurology*. 2006 Feb 14;66(3):442–3.

23. Semmler A, Bao X, Cao G, Kohler W, Weller M, Aubourg P, et al. Genetic variants of methionine metabolism and X-ALD phenotype generation: results of a new study sample. *J Neurol*. 2009 Aug;256(8):1277–80.

24. Singh I, Pujol A. Pathomechanisms underlying X-adrenoleukodystrophy: a three-hit hypothesis. *Brain Pathol*. 2010 Jul;20(4):838–44.

25. Raymond GV, Seidman R, Monteith TS, Kolodny E, Sathe S, Mahmood A, et al. Head trauma can initiate the onset of adreno-leukodystrophy. *J Neurol Sci*. 2010 Mar 15;290(1-2):70–4.

26. Orchard PJ, Lund T, Miller W, Rothman SM, Raymond G, Nascene D, et al. Chitotriosidase as a biomarker of cerebral adrenoleukodystrophy. *J Neuroinflammation*. 2011 Oct 20;8(1):144.

27. Traboulsi EI, Maumenee IH. Ophthalmologic manifestations of X-linked childhood adrenoleukodystrophy. *Ophthalmology*. 1987 Jan;94(1):47–52.

28. Gess A, Christiansen SP, Pond D, Peters C. Predictive factors for vision loss after hematopoietic cell transplant for X-linked adrenoleukodystrophy. *J AAPOS*. 2008 Jun;12(3):273–6.

29. Simm PJ, McDonnell CM, Zacharin MR. Primary adrenal insufficiency in childhood and adolescence: advances in diagnosis and management. *J Paediatr Child Health*. 2004 Nov;40(11):596–9.

30. Dubey P, Raymond GV, Moser AB, Kharkar S, Bezman L, Moser HW. Adrenal insufficiency in asymptomatic adrenoleukodystrophy patients identified by very long-chain fatty acid screening. *J Pediatr*. 2005 Apr;146(4):528–32.

31. Cox CS, Dubey P, Raymond GV, Mahmood A, Moser AB, Moser HW. Cognitive evaluation of neurologically asymptomatic boys with X-linked adrenoleukodystrophy. *Arch Neurol*. 2006 Jan;63(1):69–73.

32. Riva D, Bova SM, Bruzzone MG. Neuropsychological testing may predict early progression of asymptomatic adrenoleukodystrophy. *Neurology*. 2000 Apr 25;54(8):1651–5.

33. Shapiro EG, Lockman LA, Balthazor M, Krivit W. Neuropsychological outcomes of several storage diseases with and without bone marrow transplantation. *J Inherit Metab Dis*. 1995;18(4):413–29.

34. Loes DJ, Hite S, Moser H, Stillman AE, Shapiro E, Lockman L, et al. Adrenoleukodystrophy: a scoring method for brain MR observations. *AJNR Am J Neuroradiol*. 1994 Oct;15(9):1761–6.

35. Melhem ER, Loes DJ, Georgiades CS, Raymond GV, Moser HW. X-linked adrenoleukodystrophy: the role of contrast-enhanced MR imaging in predicting disease progression. *AJNR Am J Neuroradiol*. 2000 May;21(5):839–44.

36. Melhem ER, Gotwald TF, Itoh R, Zinreich SJ, Moser HW. T2 relaxation measurements in X-linked adrenoleukodystrophy performed using dual-echo fast fluid-attenuated inversion recovery MR imaging. *AJNR Am J Neuroradiol*. 2001 Apr;22(4):773–6.

37. Sener RN. Atypical X-linked adrenoleukodystrophy: new MRI observations with FLAIR, magnetization transfer contrast, diffusion MRI, and proton spectroscopy. *Magn Reson Imaging*. 2002 Feb;20(2):215–9.

38. Loes DJ, Fatemi A, Melhem ER, Gupte N, Bezman L, Moser HW, et al. Analysis of MRI patterns aids prediction of progression in X-linked adrenoleukodystrophy. *Neurology*. 2003 Aug 12;61(3):369–74.

39. Di Filippo M, Luchetti E, Prontera P, Donti E, Floridi P, Di Gregorio M, et al. Heterozygous X-linked adrenoleukodystrophy-associated myelopathy mimicking primary progressive multiple sclerosis. *J Neurol*. 2011 Feb;258(2):323–4.

40. Tzika AA, Ball WS, Jr., Vigneron DB, Dunn RS, Nelson SJ, Kirks DR. Childhood adrenoleukodystrophy: assessment with proton MR spectroscopy. *Radiology*. 1993 Nov;189(2):467–80.

41. Rajanayagam V, Grad J, Krivit W, Loes DJ, Lockman L, Shapiro E, et al. Proton MR spectroscopy of childhood adrenoleukodystrophy. *AJNR Am J Neuroradiol*. 1996 Jun-Jul;17(6):1013–24.

42. Rajanayagam V, Balthazor M, Shapiro EG, Krivit W, Lockman L, Stillman AE. Proton MR spectroscopy and neuropsychological testing in adrenoleukodystrophy. *AJNR Am J Neuroradiol*. 1997 Nov-Dec;18(10):1909–14.

43. Warren DJ, Connolly DJ, Wilkinson ID, Sharrard MJ, Griffiths PD. Magnetic resonance spectroscopy changes following haemopoietic stem cell transplantation in children with cerebral adrenoleukodystrophy. *Dev Med Child Neurol*. 2007 Feb;49(2):135–9.

44. Ito R, Melhem ER, Mori S, Eichler FS, Raymond GV, Moser HW. Diffusion tensor brain MR imaging in X-linked cerebral adrenoleukodystrophy. *Neurology*. 2001 Feb 27;56(4):544–7.

45. Patay Z. Diffusion-weighted MR imaging in leukodystrophies. *Eur Radiol*. 2005 Nov;15(11):2284–303.

46. Zackowski KM, Dubey P, Raymond GV, Mori S, Bastian AJ, Moser HW. Sensorimotor function and axonal integrity in adrenomyeloneuropathy. *Arch Neurol*. 2006 Jan;63(1):74–80.

47. Fatemi A, Smith SA, Dubey P, Zackowski KM, Bastian AJ, van Zijl PC, et al. Magnetization transfer MRI demonstrates spinal cord abnormalities in adrenomyeloneuropathy. *Neurology*. 2005 May 24;64(10):1739–45.

48. Smith SA, Golay X, Fatemi A, Mahmood A, Raymond GV, Moser HW, et al. Quantitative magnetization transfer characteristics of the human cervical spinal cord in vivo: application to adrenomyeloneuropathy. *Magn Reson Med*. 2009 Jan;61(1):22–7.

49. Kumar A, Chugani HT, Chakraborty P, Huq AH. Evaluation of neuroinflammation in X-linked adrenoleukodystrophy. *Pediatr Neurol*. 2011 Feb;44(2):143–6.

50. Moser AB, Kreiter N, Bezman L, Lu S, Raymond GV, Naidu S, et al. Plasma very long chain fatty acids in 3,000 peroxisome disease patients and 29,000 controls. *Ann Neurol*. 1999 Jan;45(1):100–10.

51. Kemp S, Pujol A, Waterham HR, van Geel BM, Boehm CD, Raymond GV, et al. ABCD1 mutations and the X-linked adrenoleukodystrophy mutation database: role in diagnosis and clinical correlations. *Hum Mutat*. 2001 Dec;18(6):499–515.

52. Kemp S, Wanders R. Biochemical aspects of X-linked adrenoleukodystrophy. *Brain Pathol*. 2010 Jul;20(4):831–7.

53. Hubbard WC, Moser AB, Tortorelli S, Liu A, Jones D, Moser H. Combined liquid chromatography-tandem mass spectrometry as an analytical method for high throughput screening for X-linked adrenoleukodystrophy and other peroxisomal disorders: preliminary findings. *Mol Genet Metab*. 2006 Sep-Oct;89(1–2):185–7.

54. Hubbard WC, Moser AB, Liu AC, Jones RO, Steinberg SJ, Lorey F, et al. Newborn screening for X-linked adrenoleukodystrophy (X-ALD): validation of a combined liquid chromatography-tandem mass spectrometric (LC-MS/MS) method. *Mol Genet Metab.*. 2009 Jul;97(3):212–20.

55. Moser HW, Raymond GV, Lu SE, Muenz LR, Moser AB, Xu J, et al. Follow-up of 89 asymptomatic patients with adrenoleukodystrophy treated with Lorenzo's oil. *Arch Neurol*. 2005 Jul;62(7):1073–80.

56. Moser HW, Moser AB, Hollandsworth K, Brereton NH, Raymond GV. "Lorenzo's oil" therapy for X-linked adrenoleukodystrophy: rationale and current assessment of efficacy. *J Mol Neurosci*. 2007 Sep;33(1):105–13.

57. van Geel BM, Assies J, Haverkort EB, Koelman JH, Verbeeten B, Jr., Wanders RJ, et al. Progression of abnormalities in adrenomyeloneuropathy and neurologically asymptomatic X-linked adrenoleukodystrophy despite treatment with "Lorenzo's oil". *J Neurol Neurosurg Psychiatry*. 1999 Sep;67(3):290–9.

58. Restuccia D, Di Lazzaro V, Valeriani M, Oliviero A, Le Pera D, Barba C, et al. Neurophysiologic follow-up of long-term dietary treatment in adult-onset adrenoleukodystrophy. *Neurology*. 1999 Mar 10;52(4):810–6.

59. Pai GS, Khan M, Barbosa E, Key LL, Craver JR, Cure JK, et al. Lovastatin therapy for X-linked adrenoleukodystrophy: clinical and biochemical observations on 12 patients. *Mol Genet Metab*. 2000 Apr;69(4):312–22.

60. Singh I, Pahan K, Khan M. Lovastatin and sodium phenylacetate normalize the levels of very long chain fatty acids in skin fibroblasts of X-adrenoleukodystrophy. *FEBS Lett*. 1998 Apr 24;426(3):342–6.

61. Verrips A, Willemsen MA, Rubio-Gozalbo E, De Jong J, Smeitink JA. Simvastatin and plasma very-long-chain fatty acids in X-linked adrenoleukodystrophy. *Ann Neurol.* 2000 Apr;47(4):552–3.

62. Engelen M, Ofman R, Dijkgraaf MG, Hijzen M, van der Wardt LA, van Geel BM, et al. Lovastatin in X-linked adrenoleukodystrophy. *N Engl J Med.* 2010 Jan 21;362(3):276–7.

63. Shapiro E, Krivit W, Lockman L, Jambaque I, Peters C, Cowan M, et al. Long-term effect of bone-marrow transplantation for childhood-onset cerebral X-linked adrenoleukodystrophy. *Lancet.* 2000 Aug 26;356(9231):713–8.

64. Baumann M, Korenke GC, Weddige-Diedrichs A, Wilichowski E, Hunneman DH, Wilken B, et al. Haematopoietic stem cell transplantation in 12 patients with cerebral X-linked adrenoleukodystrophy. *Eur J Pediatr.* 2003 Jan;162(1):6–14.

65. Peters C, Charnas LR, Tan Y, Ziegler RS, Shapiro EG, DeFor T, et al. Cerebral X-linked adrenoleukodystrophy: the international hematopoietic cell transplantation experience from 1982 to 1999. *Blood.* 2004 Aug 1;104(3):881–8.

66. Miller WP, Rothman SM, Nascene D, Kivisto T, DeFor TE, Ziegler RS, et al. Outcomes after allogeneic hematopoietic cell transplantation for childhood cerebral adrenoleukodystrophy: the largest single-institution cohort report. *Blood.* 2011 Aug 18;118(7):1971–8.

67. Martin PL, Carter SL, Kernan NA, Sahdev I, Wall D, Pietryga D, et al. Results of the cord blood transplantation study (COBLT): outcomes of unrelated donor umbilical cord blood transplantation in pediatric patients with lysosomal and peroxisomal storage diseases. *Biol Blood Marrow Transplant.* 2006 Feb;12(2):184–94.

68. Tokimasa S, Ohta H, Takizawa S, Kusuki S, Hashii Y, Sakai N, et al. Umbilical cord-blood transplantations from unrelated donors in patients with inherited metabolic diseases: Single-institute experience. *Pediatr Transplant.* 2008 Sep;12(6):672–6.

69. Niizuma H, Uematsu M, Sakamoto O, Uchiyama T, Horino S, Onuma M, et al. Successful cord blood transplantation with reduced-intensity conditioning for childhood cerebral X-linked adrenoleukodystrophy at advanced and early stages. *Pediatr Transplant.* 2012 Mar;16(2):E63–70.

70. Hitomi T, Mezaki T, Tomimoto H, Ikeda A, Shimohama S, Okazaki T, et al. Long-term effect of bone marrow transplantation in adult-onset adrenoleukodystrophy. *Eur J Neurol.* 2005 Oct;12(10):807–10.

71. Fitzpatrick AS, Loughrey CM, Johnston P, McKee S, Spence W, Flynn P, et al. Haematopoietic stem-cell transplant for adult cerebral adrenoleukodystrophy. *Eur J Neurol.* 2008 Mar;15(3):e21–2.

72. Cartier N, Hacein-Bey-Abina S, Bartholomae CC, Veres G, Schmidt M, Kutschera I, et al. Hematopoietic stem cell gene therapy with a lentiviral vector in X-linked adrenoleukodystrophy. *Science.* 2009 Nov 6;326(5954):818–23.

73. Costakos D, Abramson RK, Edwards JG, Rizzo WB, Best RG. Attitudes toward presymptomatic testing and prenatal diagnosis for adrenoleukodystrophy among affected families. *Am J Med Genet.* 1991 Dec 1;41(3):295–300.

74. Schaller J, Moser H, Begleiter ML, Edwards J. Attitudes of families affected by adrenoleukodystrophy toward prenatal diagnosis, presymptomatic and carrier testing, and newborn screening. *Genet Test.* 2007 Fall;11(3):296–302.

75. Kuratsubo I, Suzuki Y, Shimozawa N, Kondo N. Parents of childhood X-linked adrenoleukodystrophy: high risk for depression and neurosis. *Brain Dev.* 2008 Aug;30(7):477–82.

76. Fourcade S, Ruiz M, Guilera C, Hahnen E, Brichta L, Naudi A, et al. Valproic acid induces antioxidant effects in X-linked adrenoleukodystrophy. *Hum Mol Genet.* May 15;19(10):2005–14.

77. Berger J, Pujol A, Aubourg P, Forss-Petter S. Current and future pharmacological treatment strategies in X-linked adrenoleukodystrophy. *Brain Pathol.* 2010 Jul;20(4):845–56.

78. Parent JM. Turning skin into brain: using patient-derived cells to model X-linked adrenoleukodystrophy. *Ann Neurol.* 2011 Sep;70(3):350–2.

CHAPTER 26

Neurodegeneration with Brain Iron Accumulation, Wilson Disease, and Manganism

Alisdair McNeill

Sheffield Institute of Translational Neuroscience, Sheffield, South Yorkshire, UK

Neurodegenerative disorders with brain iron accumulation (NBIA)

Clinical definition and epidemiology

NBIA are a clinically and genetically heterogeneous group of disorders, defined by the presence of elevated levels of cerebral iron on neuroimaging or at pathological examination [1]. Five main genotypes are recognized, with about 50% of all cases having no identifiable mutation [2]. In childhood, recessive forms of NBIA are caused by *PANK2* mutations (pantothenate kinase associated neurodegeneration, PKAN) [3] or *PLA2G6* mutations (PLA2G6 associated neurodegeneration, PLAN) [4]. In adults, recessive NBIA is caused by ceruloplasmin mutations (aceruloplasminemia) [5] or *FA2H* mutations [6]; the only dominant NBIA subtype is associated with mutations in the ferritin light chain gene (neuroferritinopathy) [7]. Brain iron deposition has been reported in some cases of Kufor Rakeb syndrome (*ATP13A2* mutations) [8], but it is not a consistent feature [9] and it is unclear if this should be included within the NBIA family. Brain iron accumulation has been identified in Woodhouse–Sakati syndrome (WSS) [10] and the newly described mitochondrial protein associated neurodegeneration (MPAN) [11]. All of the genetic subtypes of NBIA are rare disorders, with several dozen families affected by PKAN, PLAN, *FA2H*, MPAN, WSS, neuroferritinopathy, and aceruloplasminemia worldwide. Each of the genetic diagnoses is discussed in turn.

Neuroferritinopathy

Spectrum of clinical phenotype

Neuroferritinopathy was first recognized as a dominantly inherited choreiform disorder in the Cumbrian region of England, being distinguished from Huntington's disease by preserved cognition [7]. In 2001 the 460insA mutation in the ferritin light chain (*FTL*) was identified in the original Cumbrian pedigrees [7]. The phenotype of the 460insA *FTL* mutation has been extensively defined by a European cohort study [12]. The mean age of onset was 39.4 years (SD = 13.3, range 13–63 years), the majority presenting with focal onset chorea (50%) or dystonia (43%) in a leg or arm. Seven percent of individuals presented initially with parkinsonism. With disease progression the majority develop a complicated movement disorder with chorea and dystonia. A characteristic oro-mandibular dystonia develops in some. Up to one-third were reported to develop bradykinesia. Patients remained ambulant up to 20 years from disease onset with minimal cognitive involvement [12]. Abnormalities of gait, some caused by dystonia, have been reported in neuroferritinopathy resulting from the 460insA mutation [13, 14]. Neither cranial nerve palsies nor upper motor neuron signs have been reported. Neuroferritinopathy cases caused by the 460insA mutation have been reported in Australia [15] and America [16].

Several different *FTL* mutations have been reported worldwide. In a French family, 458dupA closely resembled 460insA but resulted in a predominantly parkinsonian phenotype with cerebellar ataxia, more marked cognitive involvement, and central sleep apnea in two patients [17]. In a Japanese family, a duplication of the 469–484 sequence of exon 4 (c.469_484dup16nt) has been associated with neuroferritinopathy [18]. The proband presented with hand tremor in his teenage years; on examination at age 42 he was hypotonic with aphonia, micrographia, and an abnormal gait. His tremor was mainly postural. He did not have the typical extrapyramidal features associated with neuroferritinopathy. In a French-Canadian neuroferritinopathy kindred, a 498–499insTC exon 4 *FTL* mutation has been reported [19]. The proband presented in her twenties with hand tremor, which was predominantly postural but which progressed to an action tremor that was disabling by her late forties. She developed a severe cerebellar syndrome in her late forties and fifties. She was also noted to have cogwheel rigidity, facial dyskinesia, and severe cognitive impairment. The marked tremor, cerebellar ataxia, and dementia differ from the 460insA phenotype. The 646insC exon 4 *FTL* mutation was reported in a large French-Canadian/Dutch kindred [20]. The proband presented aged 63 with cerebellar ataxia, pseudobulbar affect, and chorea. The proband's sister presented at age 49 with festinant gait, emotional lability, oro-mandibular and cervical dystonia, and mild proximal leg weakness. There was no parkinsonism or dementia in either case. It is intriguing that the presentation of two individuals an identical mutation should differ so substantially, and the explanation is unclear. The 474G>A exon 4 mutation has been reported in a Spanish teenager and his mother [21]. The 13-year-old proband developed acute psychosis and gait disturbance with an akinetic-rigid syndrome following neuroleptic medication. It is not totally clear how much of this phenotype was iatrogenic and how much was caused by the *FTL* mutation.

Neurodegeneration, First Edition. Edited by Anthony Schapira, Zbigniew Wszolek, Ted M. Dawson and Nicholas Wood.
© 2017 John Wiley & Sons, Ltd. Published 2017 by John Wiley & Sons, Ltd.

Pathophysiology

Ferritin is a hollow shell composed of a polymer of ferritin light chains (FTL) and ferritin heavy chains (FTH) [7]. FTL offers acidic residues to aid iron nucleation around the ferritin molecule while FTH acts as a ferroxidase. The 460insA, 646insC, 498-499insTC, and 458dupA mutations all extend the carboxy-terminus of FTL, disrupting the dodecahedron structure of ferritin and interfering with its ability to transport iron [1]. This is proposed to lead to neuronal injury by depositing redox active iron in neurological tissue. There is histological evidence of iron and ferritin deposition in brain tissue from neuroferritinopathy patients with the 460insA, 646insC, and 498-499insTC mutations [7, 19, 20]. Moreover, analysis of fresh frozen brains from neuroferritinopathy patients has confirmed the presence of grossly elevated nanocrystalline iron oxide (magnetite) [22]. In the 646insC case there was histological evidence of hem-oxygenase-1 and 4-hydroxynonenal accumulation, both of which are markers of oxidative damage [23]. Fibroblasts from neuroferritinopathy patients and cell lines overexpressing *FTL* mutations also demonstrated oxidative stress [24, 25]. A mouse model of neuroferritinopathy was generated by expressing 499insTC in a transgene [26]. The transgenic mice had a reduced lifespan and abnormal posturing. Histologically, there was neuronal and glial ferritin accumulation accompanied by Perls-positive staining of cytoplasm. Interestingly, ubiquitin and proteosome staining was observed at sites of ferritin accumulation, suggesting a role for disrupted protein folding in this disease [26]. Oxidative damage to mitochondrial DNA was demonstrated in this mouse model using long-range polymerase chain reaction (PCR) [27], and loss of staining for mitochondrial proteins has been described in brain tissue from the 499insTC patient [19], implicating mitochondrial dysfunction in the pathogenesis of neuroferritinopathy. Together these results suggest a model whereby iron deposition leads to oxidative stress, mitochondrial dysfunction, and cell death.

Investigations

Serum ferritin is low in most men and postmenopausal women, but only a quarter of premenopausal women with neuroferritinopathy have this finding [12]. Hemoglobin and serum iron are normal [12]. Neurophysiological tests are unremarkable. The most useful investigation is brain magnetic resonance imaging (MRI). In early disease (460insA *FTL* mutation) there is hypointensity of the red nucleus, caudate, globus pallidus, putamen, thalamus, substantia nigra, and cerebral cortex on T2-weighted scans [28]. This probably represents iron deposition. With disease progression and tissue damage there is the development of areas of hyperintensity within the globus pallidus and caudate heads on T2-weighted scans [29]. This probably represents tissue edema and correlates with fluid-filled cysts found in the globus pallidus at autopsy. In two neuroferritinopathy cases an "eye-of-the-tiger" sign has been observed [28]. In the c.469_484dup16nt case there was marked cerebellar atrophy on brain imaging (Ohta, personal communication). The most sensitive MRI sequence for detection of brain iron is gradient echo imaging (T2*) and the earliest imaging changes in presymptomatic carriers are hypointensity of the globus pallidus and substantia nigra. MRI evidence of brain iron deposition (T2 signal hypointensity in the basal ganglia) precedes onset of clinical disease and can occur in childhood, providing evidence that iron accumulation may play a primary role in pathogenesis [30].

Diagnosis and prognosis

A diagnosis of neuroferritinopathy depends upon molecular genetic testing demonstrating a mutation of *FTL*. Brain iron deposition is evident on brain MRI in all reported cases of neuroferritinopathy,

and in presymptomatic carriers, and the decision to undertake molecular genetic testing of *FTL* should be taken only when the appropriate imaging features and clinical context are present. Sufficient data on prognosis in neuroferritinopathy are available only for the 460insA mutation. These individuals are reported to remain ambulant for up to 20 years after diagnosis with relatively mild cognitive involvement [12].

Treatment options

There is currently no effective treatment; iron chelation has not been shown to be effective. It is important to note that levodopa is generally not effective for parkinsonian syndromes in neuroferritinopathy [12].

Aceruloplasminemia

Spectrum of clinical phenotype

Aceruloplasminemia is an autosomal recessive disorder caused by mutations in ceruloplasmin and is almost exclusively found in people of Japanese extraction [31]. Both biallelic [32] and heterozygous [33] ceruloplasmin gene mutations produce a distinctive phenotype. In biallelic disease, compound heterozygous mutations are associated with diabetes, retinopathy, and a neurological disorder. The diabetes can precede the neurological disorder by decades [32]. The most common neurological phenotype is dementia with craniocervical dyskinesia and cerebellar tremor. Chorea and parkinsonism have been reported. Presentation is at a mean age of 51 years (range 15–71 years) with no gender predominance. Only five heterozygous cases have been described [33]. Three patients from the same family presented with cerebellar ataxia. Of two isolated cases, one presented with postural tremor and one with chorea–athetosis. The patients were not diabetic. Interestingly, there are no reports of neurological disease in obligate carriers from families with probands who carried two ceruloplasmin mutations.

Pathophysiology

Ceruloplasmin acts as a free radical scavenger and a ferroxidase, liberating iron from tissue, and its absence results in tissue iron accumulation. More than 50 different ceruloplasmin mutations have been reported [32]. Brain iron levels are 2- to 5-fold greater in brain tissue from aceruloplasminemia patients, especially in the globus pallidus [34]. Neuronal loss and intracellular iron accumulation are most prominent in the basal ganglia [35]. Iron accumulation is more prominent in astroglia than in neurons [35]. There is strong evidence of oxidative stress in brains of aceruloplasminemia patients, with increased levels of 4-hydroxynonenal and malondialdehyde demonstrated on quantitative assays of homogenized brain tissue and immunohistology [35]. Assays of mitochondrial function reveal loss of complex I and IV activity [35]. These data support a model of iron accumulation inducing oxidative stress and leading to mitochondrial dysfunction and cell death.

Investigations

In homozygous cases, serum ceruloplasmin is absent and ferritin elevated (mean 12 times the upper limit of normal) [32]. Serum ferroxidase activity is absent and most homozygous cases have a microcytic anemia [32]. Heterozygous cases have a serum ceruloplasmin level approximately half the level found in healthy control subjects. The most useful investigation is brain MRI [28]. In homozygous cases, T2 MRI sequences demonstrate hypointensity of cerebral and cerebellar cortex, globus pallidus, caudate nucleus, putamen, thalamus, red nucleus, and substantia nigra. There are no hyperintense lesions. Functional neuroimaging with [¹⁸F]fluoro-deoxyglucose positron emission tomography (FDG-PET) demonstrates hypometabolism in caudate heads early in disease, with more widespread basal ganglia and cortical hypometabolism later in disease. In heterozygotes with cerebellar ataxia MRI demonstrates cerebellar atrophy only [33].

Diagnosis and prognosis

The clinical phenotype of aceruloplasminemia overlaps with that of common sporadic neurological conditions. The diagnosis should be suspected when the MRI features are compatible and serum ceruloplasmin is absent. Given the potential implications for treatment, diagnosis should be confirmed with molecular genetic testing.

Treatment options

There are no large studies of iron chelation or iron depletion therapy for aceruloplasminemia, but multiple case reports provide evidence of its efficacy. Oral deferasirox (an oral iron chelator) was used to treat a 59-year-old Belgian woman [36]. Over a 6-month period orofacial dyskinesia and cerebellar ataxia improved, there was an improvement of putaminal hypometabolism on FDG-PET, and serum ferritin fell from 555 to 283 ng/L. A 53-year-old American woman also responded to oral deferasirox, with improved clinical features and a reduction in serum ferritin [37]. A 52-year-old Japanese woman responded to treatment with intravenous desferrioxamine [38]. Her blepharospasm and rigidity improved, as did electromyographic evidence of dystonia, and MRI demonstrated reduced iron deposition. A 16-year-old German girl heterozygote did not respond to iron chelation, but treatment with oral zinc sulfate prevented further neurological deterioration and led to improvements on her FDG-PET scan [39]. The lack of robust trials of treatment of aceruloplasminemia is unsurprising given the rarity of the condition. Iron chelation is not successful in all cases and long-term outcome is unclear [40].

Pantothenate kinase associated neurodegeneration (PKAN)

Spectrum of clinical phenotype

PKAN is a rare disorder that accounts for approximately half of all cases of NBIA, has a proposed prevalence rate of between 1 and 3 per million population, and shows no male or female preponderance [2]. The clinical features of PKAN have been defined by large cohort studies of patients from North America [41] and Western Europe [42]. PKAN can be classified into classical and atypical phenotypes.

In Hayflick's study, two-thirds of PKAN cases had a classical phenotype [41]. Classical PKAN develops in childhood, with 88% presenting before age 6 (range 6 months to 12 years). The presentation is usually with gait or postural problems, with an extrapyramidal syndrome (dystonia in 87%, rigidity and chorea in others) developing later. Corticospinal tract signs are also common. The majority also have retinitis pigmentosa, which can lead to significant visual impairment. The natural history of classical PKAN is stepwise deterioration, with periods of clinical stability interspersed with 1–2 months of neurological deterioration [41]. There is no correlation of neurological deterioration with periods of catabolic stress such as intercurrent infection. The majority of patients (85%) become wheelchair bound within 15 years after diagnosis.

Atypical PKAN presents later in life, at a mean age of 14 years (range 1–28) [41]. Non-motor phenotypes are more prominent in atypical PKAN than in the classical form. For example, in almost 40%, palilalia or dysarthria was the presenting feature rather than a movement disorder. Most atypical PKAN patients develop an extrapyramidal syndrome, although the dystonia was considered to be less severe than that seen in classical disease by Hayflick et al. Corticospinal tract signs and freezing of gait were also prevalent. Almost one-third of patients with atypical disease manifest psychiatric problems or a frontotemporal type dementia early in their disease. Atypical PKAN is less aggressive than classical disease, and most patients remain ambulant into adulthood. Hayflick et al. [41] found that null mutations were associated with classical PKAN while only two null mutations were found in atypical PKAN cases.

Hartig et al. [42] described a series of European PKAN cases. Similarly to Hayflick et al.'s study the patients fell broadly into classical or atypical PKAN phenotypes with the most common presentation being gait disturbance or dystonia. The atypical cases presented with behavioral or psychiatric disturbances and had a less marked movement disorder than the classical cases. The almost universal presence of oro-mandibular dystonia and dysarthria in PKAN patients was highlighted in this series.

An intermediate phenotype of PKAN, in which the patients do not have the characteristics of the classical or atypical group, has been described by Pellecchia et al. [43]. These patients either presented early but had slow disease progression or presented in the second decade with an aggressive disease. These investigators also identified a unique presentation of PKAN as two of their cases had motor tics and obsessions suggestive of Tourette syndrome. Several other rare motor presentations of PKAN have been identified. Vasconcelos et al. [44] described a 36-year-old man who developed dysarthria with an atrophic tongue. Electromyography suggested a diagnosis of bulbar amyotrophic lateral sclerosis, but MRI demonstrated an "eye-of-the-tiger" sign and *PANK2* mutations were confirmed. An adult-onset pure akinesia [45], adult-onset psychosis [46], freezing of gait in childhood [47], early-onset parkinsonism [3], focal hand dystonia, and intermittent severe dystonia [3] have also been reported. The HARP (hypoprebetalipoproteinemia, acanthocytosis, retinitis pigmentosa, and pallidal degeneration) syndrome is caused by *PANK2* mutations and is part of the PKAN spectrum [48].

Although a movement disorder is the most prominent manifestation of PKAN, both visual impairment and cognitive dysfunction contribute to the burden of disability. Clinical evidence of retinitis pigmentosa occurs in 68% of PKAN patients [41] and Egan et al. (2005) demonstrated electroretinographic evidence of subclinical retinopathy in half of the PKAN patients examined [49]. Optic nerve atrophy has not been reported in PKAN but cataracts can develop as a consequence of retinitis pigmentosa. Patients with PKAN have a wide range of cognitive abilities [50], but tests of both IQ and adaptive behavior indicate that cognition declines with disease progression.

Pathophysiology

PKAN is caused by biallelic mutations in pantothenate kinase 2 (PANK2) [41]. Mutations have been identified in all seven exons of the *PANK2* gene. Hartig et al. [42] sequenced the entire coding sequence of *PANK2* from the 5′ mitochondrial targeting sequence to the 3′ catalytic domain in 72 patients with suspected PKAN. They identified 96 mutated alleles, with 33 different missense mutations and 4 exon deletions, the most common being c.1583C-T ($n = 11$), c.573delC ($n = 10$), and c.1561G-A ($n = 10$). The c.573delC mutation was found exclusively in Polish patients. Hartig et al. identified seven small deletions causing frameshifts and one splice mutation. The point mutations observed were evenly distributed across the conserved domains of *PANK2*. Hayflick et al. [41] sequenced a shorter transcript of the *PANK2* gene, using a transcription start site 330 nucleotides downstream from the start site used by Hartig et al. (2006). In this series, the c.1231G-A (designated 1561G-A by Hartig et al. 2006) mutation accounted for 31/123 disease-associated alleles and c.1253C-T (designated 1583C-T by Hartig et al. 2006) for 10/123 disease-associated alleles. The c.1231G-A mutation (designated 1561G-A by Hartig et al. 2006) was seen on a background of a shared haplotype, suggesting a founder effect. Hayflick et al. [41] identified 17 frameshifts and 8 mutations causing aberrant splicing. Globally the c.1231G-A mutation is the most common cause of PKAN, and homozygotes have classic disease. In about 10% of cases only one mutated allele can be detected by current methodology and it is believed that intragenic deletions and duplications account for these cases. Several rare mutations have been reported in individual families.

The *PANK2* gene codes for an enzyme, pantothenate kinase 2, which phosphorylates pantothenate, the initial and rate-limiting step in coenzyme A (CoA) biosynthesis [51]. CoA has a vital role in ATP synthesis and fatty acid and neurotransmitter metabolism [51]. In *Drosophila* PKAN models, loss of CoA results in decreased histone and tubulin acetylation, associated with impaired DNA repair and reduced survival [52]. This phenotype was rescued by histone deacetylase (HDAC) inhibitors. The potential central role of coenzyme A deficiency in PKAN is reinforced by studies in the *Drosophila* PKAN model showing that pantethine restores CoA synthesis via a pathway independent of PANK2 which results in phenotypic rescue [51]. The PANK2 enzyme has a mitochondrial targeting sequence and is localized to mitochondria in human brain [53]. Mitochondrial dysfunction is proposed to result from *PANK2* mutations, leading to neurodegeneration. The neurotoxic metabolites cysteine and pantetheine are substrates for PANK2, and mutation of *PANK2* will lead to their accumulation. Cysteine is a potent iron chelator and it is proposed that high local cysteine levels lead to secondary iron accumulation. Iron accumulation will exacerbate neuronal injury by inducing oxidative stress. Silencing of *PANK2* in HeLa cells resulted in up-regulation of ferroporin mRNA, which provides a further mechanism by which iron might enter neurons [54]. The amount of residual activity in the mutated PANK2 enzyme influences disease severity, with earlier disease onset in patients with homozygous null mutations and later disease onset in patients with mutations that allow residual enzyme activity [41, 42].

The neuropathology of PKAN has been described in a series of six genetically confirmed cases [55]. Pathological changes were almost completely restricted to the globus pallidus. Iron accumulation was seen as hemosiderin in a mainly perivascular distribution in the globus pallidus and not in other brain regions. Ferritin accumulation was observed in pallidal neurons by immunohistochemistry. Neuronal loss was extensive in the globus pallidus and was accompanied by reactive astrogliosis. Two populations of eosinophilic spheroids were observed: one composed of degenerating neurons, and the other true, amyloid precursor protein positive, neuroaxonal spheroids. Notably, no α-synuclein staining/Lewy body pathology was observed. This work provides a histopathological correlate of the "eye-of-the-tiger" sign – the hypointensity being related to iron deposition and the hyperintensity related to astrogliosis.

Investigations

Definitive diagnosis of PKAN rests upon molecular genetic testing, but routine clinical tests can help define the patient's phenotype. Electroretinography can demonstrate subclinical retinopathy [41, 42], and a full blood count will reveal acanthocytosis in 8%.

The most useful investigation is brain MRI [28]. The characteristic imaging feature is the "eye-of-the-tiger" sign, defined as a medial area of hyperintensity within a hypointense globus pallidus. Cases of PKAN may also have hypointensity of the substantia nigra. Hayflick and colleagues [41] noted that all patients with a *PANK2* mutation have this radiological sign. However, Hartig et al. (2006) described seven patients with an NBIA phenotype and an "eye-of-the-tiger" sign who were *PANK2* mutation negative [42]. Moreover, there are multiple reports of the occurrence of this sign in conditions other than PKAN and neuroferritinopathy [28]. Thus, whilst diagnostically useful, this sign must be interpreted in the clinical context.

Diagnosis and prognosis

Definitive diagnosis rests upon molecular genetic confirmation of biallelic *PANK2* mutations.

Clinical progression is described in the section above.

Treatment options

There is currently no curative treatment for PKAN, and management is aimed at palliation of symptoms. Dystonia and spasticity can managed with trihexyphenidyl and baclofen [41, 42]. In specialist settings botulinum toxin injection may be especially effective in managing focal dystonia. Levodopa therapy is not helpful for parkinsonism caused by *PANK2* mutations. An intrathecal baclofen pump may be considered if oral treatment of the movement disorder fails. Recently deep brain stimulation targeting the pallidum has been shown to be effective, reducing dystonia severity scores at up to 15 months post implantation [56]. In addition to medical treatment of the movement disorder, good nursing care is vital for patients with PKAN, with special attention to bowel management, nutrition, and bulbar function. It should not be forgotten that diagnosis of an inherited neurodegenerative disease will have implications for other family members and their offspring, and genetic counseling should be offered as appropriate.

Phospholipase A2 (*PLA2G6*) mutation associated neurodegeneration (PLAN)

Spectrum of clinical phenotype

PLAN consists of two broad phenotypes: infantile neuroaxonal dystrophy (INAD) [4], and dystonia–parkinsonism [57]. INAD is a severe psychomotor disorder with progressive hypotonia, hyperreflexia, and tetraparesis [58]. The phenotype of INAD has been defined by the multinational study of Gregory and colleagues [58]. The majority (79%) of cases in this series had a mutation in the *PLA2G6* gene. A classical and an atypical INAD phenotype were recognized. In classical INAD the mean age at onset was 1 year (range 5 months to 2.5 years), with a presentation of psychomotor regression with truncal hypotonia progressing to tetraparesis in almost all cases. In the majority the weakness was spastic but in one-third there was areflexic weakness. Most patients lost ambulation within 5 years of onset. Nearly 50% had ataxia or gait problems and the majority developed ocular signs (optic atrophy, strabismus, nystagmus). One-third developed generalized seizures. The average age at death was 9.4 years. The atypical INAD phenotype had a later onset with a mean age of 4.4 years (range 1.5–6.5). The main presentation was gait instability or ataxia, and speech delay and abnormal social interaction were common. The frequency of optic atrophy, nystagmus, and seizures was similar to the classical

INAD group. However, truncal hypotonia was not seen in the atypical INAD group.

PLA2G6 mutations have been recognized as a recessive cause of dystonia–parkinsonism [57]. Paisan-Ruiz reported three individuals from two unrelated families with early-onset levodopa-responsive parkinsonism, dystonia, cognitive dysfunction, and pyramidal signs. *PLA2G6* mutation was confirmed as a cause of dystonia–parkinsonism in small Japanese cohort who showed the presence of dementia and frontotemporal atrophy on brain MRI [59]. None of the patients had brain iron accumulation.

Pathophysiology

The causative gene for INAD was established as being *PLA2G6* by Morgan et al. [60]. They identified 44 unique mutations: 32 missense, 5 frameshift, 3 nonsense, 2 deletions, 1 splice site mutation, and 1 large deletion. A *PLA2G6* mutation was found in 79% of INAD cases by Gregory and colleagues [58], who identified a wide spectrum of missense mutations and deletions. No common mutations were identified in either study, with no allele accounting for more than 10% of cases.

There are several neuropathological descriptions of PLAN. Gregory et al. [58] described a patient who presented at age 3 with leg spasticity, developed dystonia and dysarthria, and was wheelchair bound by age 5; she died aged 23. There was gross atrophy of cerebral cortex and cerebellum, with brown discoloration of globus pallidus and substantia nigra. There was widespread neuronal loss and gliosis in cerebral cortex and basal ganglia with loss of both cerebellar Purkinje and granule cell layers. Axonal swellings and spheroids were found throughout the cortex, basal ganglia, cerebellum, brainstem, and spinal cord. Spheroids appeared as rounded eosinophilic swellings 30–100 μm across; they stained positively with antibodies to neurofilament proteins. There were brown, granular iron deposits in a perivascular distribution within the globus pallidus and substantia nigra. Perls Prussian blue stain revealed iron in large extracellular deposits and in perivascular spaces. Neuropathological features of Parkinson disease and Alzheimer's disease were also noted. In most pigmented neurons of the substantia nigra classic Lewy bodies were observed; these stained for α-synuclein. Many regions of the cerebral cortex and basal ganglia contained α-synuclein-positive Lewy bodies. Neurofibrillary tangles, composed of hyperphosphorylated tau, were observed in the temporal and mid-frontal cortex. The mechanism leading to formation of axonal spheroids, Lewy bodies, and neurofibrillary tangles in INAD is unclear. It is possible that their formation reflects oxidative damage to the cytoskeleton. Paisan-Ruiz et al. [61] confirmed widespread α-synuclein and tau pathologies in a series of five pathological examinations of INAD patients. These findings are given added pertinence by the description of *PLA2G6* mutations in adult dystonia–parkinsonism [57].

Murine models of PLAN have suggested roles for mitochondrial dysfunction, oxidative stress, and defective lipid metabolism. *PLA2G6* null mice demonstrate reduced numbers of muscle mitochondria on electron microscopy and induction of oxidative stress associated genes [62]. In support of these findings, *PLA2G6* null mice have been shown to accumulate 4-hydroxynonenal and structurally abnormal mitochondria in their anterior horn cells [63]. Neuropathological studies of human NBIA resulting from *PLA2G6* mutations demonstrated accumulation of α-synuclein-positive Lewy bodies and tau, showing a link between brain iron accumulation and pathological mechanisms of Parkinson disease and other late-onset sporadic neurodegenerative disorders [61].

Investigations

In *PLA2G6* mutation positive INAD 87% of patients have axonal spheroids on peripheral nerve biopsy (skin, conjunctiva, rectum, or sural nerve) [4, 58]. However, with the advent of molecular genetic testing for the *PLA2G6* gene, biopsy should be a second-line investigation. Most classical INAD patients have denervation on EMG and fast rhythms on EEG, but only one-third have decreased nerve conduction velocity [4, 58]. Brain MRI is valuable in diagnosis of INAD. Ninety-five percent of mutation-positive classical INAD cases have cerebellar atrophy and 50% have high brain iron in the globus pallidus and substantia nigra [58]. Cerebellar gliosis, manifested by high cerebellar signal on T2, is also frequent. Atypical INAD cases are significantly less likely to have cerebellar atrophy (83%) but more likely to have high iron in the pallidum and substantia nigra (100%) [58].

Treatment

Treatment of INAD is limited to palliation. Dystonia may be managed with baclofen or trihexyphenidyl. Seizures may need treatment with anti-epileptic medication. Attention to nutrition and bulbar function, and good nursing care are crucial [58].

Mitochondrial membrane protein associated neurodegeneration (MPAN)

Spectrum of clinical phenotype

Recessive *c19orf12* mutations have been identified in childhood-onset NBIA and a single case of juvenile Parkinson disease in a German and Polish cohort [11]. Age of onset of NBIA was at a mean of 9 years (range 4–20 years). The most common presentation was with speech or gait difficulties; almost all had dystonia (general or oro-mandibular) and developed pyramidal signs with disease progression. Forty-four percent had neurophysiological evidence of axonal neuropathy and all had optic atrophy.

Pathophysiology

c19orf12 NBIA is caused most commonly by an 11 base pair deletion (c.204_214del11) either in homozygosity or compound heterozygosity with a missense mutation [11]. Patients with missense mutations seem to have a more benign clinical course, but studies of larger cohorts are required to confirm genotype–phenotype correlations. The c19orf12 protein is expressed in mitochondria and missing in patient-derived fibroblasts. The gene regulates proteins involved in fatty acid metabolism, but detailed biochemical characterization is required before firm conclusions on its physiological role can be reached. Neuropathological examination in a single case identified iron deposits in the basal ganglia and abundant α-synuclein-positive Lewy bodies and tau-positive neurites.

Investigations

Brain MRI in MPAN demonstrates T2 hypointensity of the substantia nigra and globus pallidus.

One case had an "eye-of-the-tiger" sign [11].

Neurophysiology may demonstrate an axonal neuropathy and ophthalmological examination optic atrophy but no retinitis pigmentosa (in contrast to PKAN). There are no reports of acanthocytosis in MPAN.

Diagnosis and prognosis

Definitive diagnosis depends upon molecular genetic testing of the *c19orf12* gene. Numbers of reported cases are small, but MPAN caused by missense mutations seems to cause a relatively mild phenotype with minimal disability. Longitudinal studies are required to define the prognosis of MPAN.

Treatment

There is no disease-modifying treatment for MPAN. A single case of MPAN presenting as Parkinson disease responded well to levodopa [11].

Kufor Rakeb syndrome (KRS, *ATP13A2* mutations)

Spectrum of clinical phenotypes

KRS is characterized by juvenile-onset parkinsonism and dementia [64]. Patients with biallelic and heterozygous mutations may both develop neurodegeneration [65]. Supranuclear gaze palsy and facial–faucial–finger minimyoclonus are characteristic. A study of the initial Chilean kindred documented onset of the motor syndrome at age 10–12 [66].

Pathophysiology

KRS is caused by biallelic mutations in the *ATP13A2* gene [64]. *ATP13A2* is localized to acidic intracellular vesicles (lysosomes) and expressed in human cortical and nigral neurons, being expressed at higher levels in sporadic Parkinson disease than control brain [67]. Recent evidence suggests that defective mitophagy may lead to mitochondrial dysfunction and neuronal loss [68]. In patient fibroblasts there was reduction of ATP generation, increased oxygen consumption, and increased markers of mitochondrial DNA damage and fragmentation of the mitochondrial network. This implicates defective mitochondrial quality control in neurodegeneration in KRS. Cell biology studies have demonstrated endoplasmic reticulum retention and proteasomal degradation of mutant ATP13A2 proteins, which sensitizes cells to endoplasmic reticulum stress associated cell death [69].

Investigations

Dopamine transporter (DAT) imaging demonstrates loss of nigral dopaminergic neurons. Cranial MRI frequently shows global atrophy, but in a subset reveals caudate and globus pallidus hypointensity, leading some to classify KRS as a member of the NBIA family. There is lack of substantia nigra hyperechogenicity in KRS, leading some to propose that this implies that KRS has a different pathophysiology to other forms of genetic parkinsonism.

Diagnosis and prognosis

Definitive diagnosis depends upon molecular genetic testing demonstrating *ATP13A2* mutations.

The reports of the initial Chilean family indicate potential for a prolonged disease course with progressive motor and cognitive disability.

Treatment

There is no specific or disease-modifying treatment for KRS. The parkinsonism in KRS is variably reported to be levodopa responsive [64–66].

Woodhouse–Sakati syndrome (WSS)

Spectrum of clinical phenotype

WSS is a rare recessive disorder caused by mutations in *c2orf37* [10]. This is a multisystem syndrome with mental retardation, facial dysmorphism, alopecia, hypogonadism, and diabetes mellitus. The neurological syndrome is predominantly focal or generalized dystonia or chorea. Additional features include sensorineural deafness, peripheral neuropathy, seizures, and T2 white matter hyperintensities.

Pathophysiology

WSS is caused by biallelic mutations in *c2orf37*, most commonly a 1-bp deletion c.436delC [10]. Three nonsense mutations and a splice site mutation have been identified in *c2orf37* in families of various ethnic origins. The function of this gene has not been fully elucidated, but it is thought to encode a nucleolar protein. A muscle biopsy from a single case demonstrated increased lipid storage, but the pathological significance of this is unclear [70].

Investigations

T2 MRI demonstrates basal ganglia hypointensity and white matter hyperintensities in some cases. The hypointensity is proposed to be due to iron deposition.

Diagnosis and prognosis

Definitive diagnosis rests upon molecular genetic testing, which may be available on a research basis.

Treatment

There are no reports in the literature that address management of WSS.

FA2H associated NBIA

Spectrum of clinical phenotype

In two families recessive *FA2H* mutations were found to cause a neurodegenerative syndrome associated with hypointensity of the globus pallidus on MRI accompanied by confluent white matter hypointensity and profound pontocerebellar atrophy [6]. There was no pathological proof of brain iron deposition, but the iron was considered to be the most likely cause of T2 hypointensities in these patients. The first family was consanguineous and Italian. Three brothers developed gait ataxia aged 4 with mild spastic paraparesis, and this developed into severe spastic quadriparesis accompanied by ataxia. Two of the brothers died in their late twenties from aspiration pneumonia. Cognition was relatively spared even late in the disease. Electromyography and nerve conduction studies were normal in all three. The second family was Albanian and non-consanguineous. Two brothers developed gait ataxia around the age of 4 years accompanied by a spastic paraparesis which then developed into spastic quadriparesis accompanied by ataxia. The first brother had seizures from age 2. Prominent dystonia and pyramidal tract signs were also observed in all affected individuals. The authors suggest that pontocerebellar atrophy and absence of peripheral neuropathy distinguish *FA2H* associated NBIA from *PLA2G6* mutation associated NBIA.

Pathophysiology

Fatty acid hydroxylase (FA2H) is an enzyme that produces 2-hydroxylated fatty acids for incorporation into ceramide species, which serve as precursors for myelin synthesis. A murine model of FA2H disease showed significant demyelination and axonal loss throughout the brain with deteriorating cerebellar function on behavioral tests from 7 months of age [71]. If loss of FA2H was restricted to Schwann cells and oligodendrocytes then the cerebellar phenotype was identical to that of germline *FA2H* silencing but learning defects present with germline gene deletion were absent.

Investigations

MRI demonstrates white matter hypointensities, basal ganglia hypointensity (presumed to be iron deposition), and characteristic pontocerebellar hypoplasia [6]. Nerve conduction studies are normal.

Diagnosis and prognosis

Definitive diagnosis requires molecular genetic testing of *FA2H*, which may be available on a research basis. Given the rarity of the disorder there are no studies systematically defining prognosis, but based on the reported families it is a disorder associated with progressive neurological disability and death.

Beta-propeller protein associated neurodegeneration (BPAN)

Spectrum of clinical phenotype

Individuals with this subtype of NBIA present with global developmental delay in childhood, with slow acquisition of skills until adolescence [72, 73]. A movement disorder with dystonia and parkinsonism then develops. Seizures, spasticity, and disordered sleep are common. This disorder was previously dubbed static encephalopathy with neurological deterioration in adulthood (SENDA) syndrome. De novo inactivating mutations in the *WDR45* gene are causative [72, 73]. Inheritance is X-linked. Male and female patients have a similar phenotype. Affected male cases are thought to harbor post-zygotic somatic *WDR45* mutations with germline mutations likely lethal in males.

Pathophysiology

In BPAN, substantia nigra iron deposition is greater than that seen in the globus pallidus. No Lewy bodies were observed (unlike in MPAN and PLAN) but neuroaxonal spheroids were prominent. Numerous tau-positive tangles were observed. Mutations in *WDR45* are proposed to result in defective autophagy.

Investigations

Brain MRI reveals a characteristic pattern in the substantia nigra with central hypointensity and peripheral hyperintensity [72, 73]. There is progressive cerebral atrophy when dementia supervenes.

CoA synthase protein-associated neurodegeneration (CoPAN)

Spectrum of clinical phenotype

Recessive, loss-of-function mutations in CoA synthase were initially reported as a cause of NBIA in two unrelated individuals [74]. The phenotype consisted of spasticity with dystonia and cognitive impairment. Formal eye examination was normal. One patient had evidence of an axonal neuropathy on nerve conduction studies. This is the second disorder of CoA synthesis to result in NBIA, alongside PKAN. CoPAN seems to be a very rare cause of NBIA as it has only been reported in two cases thus far.

Pathophysiology

CoA synthase is crucial for the final steps in the generation of CoA. It is postulated that deficiency of CoA synthase may thus lead to mitochondrial dysfunction.

Manganism

Spectrum of clinical phenotype

Acute, high-level exposure to manganese leads to a severe parkinsonian disorder termed manganism, while chronic low-level exposure is proposed by some to be a risk factor for late-onset Parkinson

disease (PD) and others have identified subtle neurological deficits in those chronically exposed [75]. Manganism was first described in five Scottish men working as ore grinders in 1837 by James Couper; these individuals had parkinsonian features and in three of them recovery occurred after cessation of exposure. The key exposure for manganism is inhalation of fumes from manganese dioxide ores [76]. The onset of symptoms can occur acutely (weeks to months after exposure) to decades later. In general, psychiatric disturbances occur in the early phase with neurological signs predominating later on. The parkinsonism of manganism is distinct from sporadic PD in that rest tremor is less prominent (action or postural tremor being more common), but there is the "cock-walk" gait in which there is foot dystonia and the patient walks on the balls of their feet, the tendency to fall backwards, and more widespread dystonia [75–77]. Welders exposed to manganese have been shown to have an increased risk of developing typical PD with loss of dopaminergic neurons on DAT imaging [78–80]. Thus manganese exposure has been linked to both typical and atypical PD. Manganese toxicity has also been reported in drug abusers exposed to ephedra, patients on parenteral nutrition, and patients with chronic liver disease [75, 78].

More controversial are the health effects of chronic exposure to low levels of manganese. Epidemiological studies provide some evidence that chronic low-level exposure can lead to increased risk of late-onset PD. In Sauda (Norway), where the world's largest ferroalloy plant operated until 1923, the crude prevalence of Parkinson disease was 10-fold greater than the crude prevalence for the general Scandinavian population [81]. Similar results were found for an Italian population living in the vicinity of a ferroalloy plant [82].

Pathophysiology

Manganese deposition selectively occurs in the globus pallidus with sparing of the substantia nigra, partly because the dopamine transporter facilitates internalization into neurons [83]. Manganism is proposed to occur with high levels of exposure ($1\,mg/m^3$ in inhalable particles), whereas manganese-related parkinsonism may occur after lifetime exposure to much lower levels, possibly around $100\,ng/m^3$ of manganese in respirable particles [84]. The pathology of manganese-related PD differs from sporadic PD in that the substantia nigra is spared with pathology focusing on the globus pallidus internus with absence of Lewy bodies, the cardinal histological finding being loss of neurons [83]. Evidence from neurochemical studies of brain tissue from patients with liver disease and parkinsonism indicates that there is loss of D2 dopamine receptors and no observed decrease in dopamine levels [83]. There is emerging evidence from primate studies that manganese exposure may somehow inhibit release of dopamine [83]. These observations fit with the lack of response to levodopa in manganese-induced parkinsonism.

Investigations

Most patients with manganism have normal nigrostriatal function on DAT scans, although a subset have dopaminergic deficiency (e.g., welders with a clinical phenotype of sporadic PD) [80]. Manganese deposition correlates with T1-weighted hyperintensity in the globus pallidus on MRI. However these MRI findings can reverse despite ongoing clinical symptoms, and asymptomatic welders can have MRI appearances identical to those of patients with clinical manganism.

Diagnosis and prognosis

Prognostic data are limited. In a Taiwanese cohort, clinical deterioration continued for up to 10 years after cessation of exposure with a stabilization of clinical progression thereafter [85].

Treatment

Cessation of exposure to manganese is mandated. However, several studies indicate that ongoing clinical deterioration can occur even after exposure has stopped. Parkinsonism associated with manganese exposure is generally not responsive to levodopa but there are some reports of an excellent response in welders [79, 80].

Wilson disease

Spectrum of clinical phenotype

Wilson disease (WD, hepatolenticular degeneration) is a recessive disorder caused by mutations in *ATP7B* [86]. Wilson disease can present from age 3 to age 60 with neurological, psychiatric, or hepatic features. The clinical phenotype varies widely.

The movement disorder in Wilson disease includes tremor, poor coordination of fine finger movements, chorea, or athetosis [87]. Dystonia is also common. Pseudobulbar involvement with dysarthria and dysphagia is common, particularly in older patients. Depression and personality change are common psychiatric accompaniments. Seizures occur in up to 8% of cases of WD [88].

Pathophysiology

WD is caused by biallelic mutations in *ATP7B*. Heterozygous carriers are clinically normal. More than 260 different *ATP7B* mutations have been identified [89]. The most common mutation in Europeans is H1069Q. The product of *ATP7B* is copper-transporting ATPase-2 [90]. This copper transporter incorporates copper in ceruloplasmin and excretes it into bile. In the *ATP7B* null mouse, copper was shown to accumulate in the striatum and corpus callosum but not the cortex or hippocampus [91]. There was no neuronal loss in any of the studied brain regions. *ATP7B* null mice have evidence of cerebral oxidative stress, with reduced aconitase activity and up-regulation of superoxide dismutase, and mitochondrial dysfunction with reduction of complex II–IV activity [92].

Investigations

See Diagnosis and prognosis. In neurologically symptomatic (but not asymptomatic) WD patients T2* hypointensities have been observed in the caudate, globus pallidus, and substantia nigra. In addition, tectal plate hyperintensity, "central pontine myelinolysis like" lesions, and simultaneous lesions of basal ganglia and brainstem are claimed to be MRI features that are diagnostic of WD [93].

Diagnosis and prognosis

Diagnosis can be made based upon biochemical analysis of blood and urine [86]. Two out of three of the following support a diagnosis of WD: (i) low serum ceruloplasmin; (ii) 24-hour urine copper excretion greater than 0.6 μmol; and (iii) increased hepatic copper concentration (>250 μg/g). Diagnosis can be confirmed by molecular genetic testing of the *ATP7B* gene. With treatment, lifespan in WD is normal. However, a German study found that among treated WD patients 50.5% had ongoing neurological symptoms such as tremor and dystonia [94]. A prospective clinical study has demonstrated that tremor is most likely to improve with treatment whilst dystonia is more likely to be resistant [95].

Treatment

The mainstay of treatment is lifelong copper chelation [86]. D-penicillamine tablets increase urinary copper excretion, but patients must be monitored with full blood counts and urinalysis as blood dyscrasias and proteinuria/nephritic syndrome can occur as side effects. Trientine is an alternative copper chelator. Oral zinc reduces gastrointestinal copper absorption by inducing enterocyte metallothionein which binds copper; the enterocytes are shed into the feces carrying excess copper with them. Zinc treatment is usually used in conjunction with a chelator.

References

1. McNeill A, Chinnery PF. Neurodegeneration with brain iron accumulation. *Handb Clin Neurol* 2011; 100: 161–72.
2. Gregory A, Hayflick SJ. Genetics of neurodegeneration with brain iron accumulation. *Curr Neurol Neurosci Rep* 2011; 11: 254–61.
3. Zhou B, Westaway SK, Levinson B, et al. A novel pantothenate kinase gene (PANK2) is defective in Hallervorden–Spatz syndrome. *Nat Genet* 2001; 28: 345–9.
4. Gregory A, Hayflick SJ. Infantile neuroaxonal dystrophy. In: Pagon RA, Bird TD, Dolan CR, Stephens K, editors. GeneReviews [Internet]. Seattle (WA): University of Washington, Seattle; 1993-.2008 Jun 19 [updated 2009 Sep 1].
5. Morita H, Ikeda S, Yamamoto Y, et al. Hereditary ceruloplasmin deficiency with hemosiderosis: a clinicopathological study of a Japanese family. *Ann Neurol* 1995; 37: 646–56.
6. Kruer MC, Paisán-Ruiz C, Boddaert N, et al. Defective FA2H leads to a novel form of neurodegeneration with brain iron accumulation (NBIA). *Ann Neurol* 2010; 68: 611–18.
7. Curtis AR, Fey C, Morris CM, et al. Mutation in the gene encoding ferritin light chain polypeptide causes adult onset basal ganglia disease. *Nat Genet* 2001; 28: 350–4.
8. Schneider SA, Paisan-Ruiz C, Quinn NP, et al. ATP13A2 mutations cause neurodegeneration with brain iron accumulation. *Mov Disord* 2010; 25: 979–84.
9. Chien HF, Bonifati V, Barbosa ER. ATP13A2 related neurodegeneration without evidence of brain iron accumulation. *Mov Disord* 2011; 26: 1364.
10. Alazami AM, Al-Saif A, Al-Semari A, et al. Mutations in c2orf37, encoding a nucleolar protein, cause hypogonadism, alopecia, diabetes mellitus, mental retardation and extrapyramidal syndrome. *Am J Hum Genet* 2008; 83: 684–91.
11. Hartig MB, Iuso A, Haack T, et al. Absence of an orphan mitochondrial protein c19orf12 causes a distinct clinical subtype of neurodegeneration with brain iron accumulation. *Am J Hum Genet* 2011; 89: 543–50.
12. Chinnery PF, Crompton DE, Birchall D, et al. The clinical features and natural history of neuroferritinopathy caused by the *FTL1* 460insA mutation. *Brain* 2007; 130: 110–19.
13. Keogh MJ, Khan A, Gorman G, et al. An unusual gait following the discovery of a new disease. *Pract Neurol* 2011; 11: 81–4.
14. Cassidy AJ, Williams ER, Goldsmith P, Baker SN, Baker MR. The man who could not walk backwards: an unusual presentation of neuroferritinopathy. *Mov Disord* 2011; 26: 362–4.
15. Lehn A, Mellick G, Boyle R. Teaching neuroimages: Neuroferritinopathy. *Neurology* 2011; 77: e107.
16. Ondo WG, Adam OR, Jankovic J, Chinnery PF. Dramatic response of facial stereotype/tic to tetrabenazine in the first reported cases of neuroferritinopathy in the United States. *Mov Disord* 2010; 25: 2470–2.
17. Devos D, Tchofo J, Vuillaume, et al. Clinical features and natural history of neuroferritinopathy caused by the 458dupA FTL mutation. *Brain* 2009; 132: e109.
18. Ohta E, Nagasaka T, Shindo K, et al. Neuroferritinopathy in a Japanese family with a duplication in the ferritin light chain gene. *Neurology* 2008; 70: 1493–4.
19. Ory-Magne F, Brefel-Courbon C, Payoux P, et al. Clinical phenotype and neuroimaging findings in a French family with hereditary ferritinopathy (FTL498-499insTC). *Mov Disord* 2009; 24: 1676–83.
20. Vidal R, Ghetti B, Takao M, et al. Intracellular ferritin accumulation in neuronal and extra-neuronal tissues characterises a neurodegenerative disorder associated with a mutation in the ferritin light polypeptide gene. *J Neuropath Exp Neurol* 2004; 63: 363–80.
21. Maciel P, Cruz VT, Constante M, et al. Neuroferritinopathy: missense mutation in FTL causing early-onset bilateral pallidal involvement. *Neurology* 2005; 65: 603–5.
22. Hautot D, Pankhurst QA, Morris CM, et al. Preliminary observation of elevated levels of nanocrystalline iron oxide in the basal ganglia of neuroferritinopathy patients. *Biochim Biophys Acta* 2007; 1772: 21–5.

23. Powers JM. P53-mediated apoptosis, neuroglobulin overexpression, and globin deposits in a patient with hereditary ferritinopathy. *J Neuropathol Exp Neurol* 2006; 65: 716–21.

24. Barbeito A, Levade T, Delisle M Ghetti B, Vidal R. Abnormal iron metabolism in fibroblasts from a patient with the neurodegenerative disease hereditary ferritinopathy. *Mol Neurodegen* 2010; 5: 50–60.

25. Cozzi A, Rovelli E, Frizzale G, et al. Oxidative stress and cell death in cells expressing L-ferritin variants causing neuroferritinopathy. *Neurobiol Dis* 2010; 37: 77–85.

26. Vidal R, Miravalle L, Gao X, et al. Expression of a mutant form of the ferritin light chain gene induces neurodegeneration and iron overload in transgenic mice. *J Neurosci* 2008; 28: 60–7.

27. Deng X, Vidal R, Englander EW. Accumulation of oxidative damage in brain mitochondria in mouse model of hereditary ferritinopathy. *Neurosci Lett* 2010; 479: 44–8.

28. McNeill A, Birchall D, Hayflick SJ, et al. T2* and FSE MRI distinguishes 4 subtypes of neurodegeneration with brain iron accumulation. *Neurology* 2008; 70: 1614–9.

29. McNeill A, Gorman G, Khan A, Horvath R, Burn J, Blamire A, Chinnery PF. Progressive iron accumulation in neuroferritinopathy measured by thalamic R2*. *Am J Neuradiol* 2012; 33: 1810–3.

30. Keogh MJ, Jonas P, Coulthard A, Chinnery PF, Burn J. Neuroferritinopathy: a new inborn error of iron metabolism. *Neurogenetics* 2012; 13: 93–6.

31. Miyajima H, Ikeda S, Yamamoto K, et al. Hereditary ceruloplasmin deficiency: a clinicopathological study of a Japanese family. *Ann Neurol* 1995; 36: 646–56.

32. McNeill A, Pandolfo M, Shang H, et al. The neurological presentation of ceruloplasmin gene mutations. *Eur Neurol* 2008; 60: 200–6.

33. Miyajima H, Kono S, Takahashi Y, et al. Cerebellar ataxia associated with heteroallelic ceruloplasmin gene mutation. *Neurology* 2001; 57: 2205–10.

34. Miyajima H, Adachi J, Kohno S, et al. Increased oxysterols associated with iron accumulation in the brains and visceral organs of aceruloplasminemia patients. *QJM* 2001; 94: 417–22.

35. Miyajima H, Takahashi Y, Kono S. Aceruloplasminemia, an inherited disorder of iron metabolism. *Biometals* 2003; 16: 205–13.

36. Haemers I, Kono S, Goldman S, et al. Clinical, molecular and PET study of a case of aceruloplasminemia presenting with focal cranial dyskinesia. *J Neurol Neurosurg Psych* 2004; 75: 334–7.

37. Skidmore FM, Drago V, Foster P, et al. Aceruloplasminemia with progressive atrophy without brain iron overload: treatment with oral chelation. *J Neurol Neurosurg Psych* 2007; 79: 467–70.

38. Miyajima H, Takahashi Y, Kamata T, Shimizu H, Sakai N, Gitlin JD. Use of desferrioxamine in the treatment of aceruloplasminemia. *Ann Neurol* 1997; 41: 404–7.

39. Kuhn J, Bewermeyer H, Miyajima H, et al. Treatment of symptomatic heterozygous aceruloplasminemia with oral zinc sulphate. *Brain Dev* 2007; 29: 450–3.

40. Pan PL, Tang HH, Chen Q, Song W, Shang HF. Desferrioxamine treatment of aceruloplasminemia: long term follow up. *Mov Disord* 2011; 26: 2142–4.

41. Hayflick SJ, Westaway SK, Levinson B, et al. Genetic, clinical, and radiographic delineation of Hallervordern–Spatz syndrome. *N Engl J Med* 2003; 348: 33–40.

42. Hartig MB, Hortnagel K, Garavaglia B, et al. Genotypic and phenotypic spectrum of PANK2 mutations in patients with neurodegeneration with brain iron accumulation. *Ann Neurol* 2006; 59: 248–56.

43. Pellecchia MT, Valente EM, Cif L, et al. The diverse phenotype and genotype of pantothenate-kinase associated neurodegeneration. *Neurology* 2005; 64: 1810–2.

44. Vasconcelos OM, Harter DH, Duffy C, et al. Adult Hallervorden–Spatz simulating amyotrophic lateral sclerosis. *Muscle Nerve* 2003; 28: 118–22.

45. Molinuevo JL, Martí MJ, Blesa R, Tolosa E. Pure akinesia: an unusual phenotype of Hallervorden-Spatz syndrome. *Mov Disord* 2003; 18: 1351–3.

46. del Valle-López P, Pérez-García R, Sanguino-Andrés R, González-Pablos E. Adult onset Hallervorden-Spatz with psychotic symptoms. *Actas Esp Psiquiatr* 2011; 39: 260–2.

47. Kuo SH, Greene P. A 16-year old boy with freezing of gait. *Neurology* 2010; 75: e23–7.

48. Ching KH, Westaway SK, Gitschier J, Higgins JJ, Hayflick SJ. HARP syndrome is allelic with Hallervorden-Spatz syndrome. *Neurology* 2002; 58: 1673–4.

49. Egan R, Weber RG, Hogarth P, et al. Neuro-ophthalmologic and electroretinographic findings in pantothenate kinase-associated neurodegeneration (formerly Hallervorden-Spatz syndrome). *Am J Ophthalmol* 2005; 140: 267–74.

50. Freeman K, Gregory A, Turner A, et al. Intellectual and adaptive behaviour functioning in pantothenate kinase-associated neurodegeneration. *J Intellect Disabil Res* 2007; 51: 417–26.

51. Rana A, Seinen E, Siudeja K, et al. Pantethine rescues a Drosophila model for Pantothenate kinase associated neurodegeneration. *Proc Nat Acad Sci USA* 2010; 107: 6988–93.

52. Siudeja K, Srinivasan B, Xu L, et al. Impaired Coenzyme A metabolism affects histone and tubulin acetylation in Drosophila and human cell models of pantothenate kinase associated neurodegeneration. *EMBO Mol Med* 2011; 3: 755–66.

53. Kotzbauer PT, Truax AC, Trojanowski JQ, et al. Altered neuronal mitochondrial coenzyme A synthesis in neurodegeneration with brain iron accumulation caused by abnormal processing, stability, and catalytic activity of mutant pantothenate kinase-2. *J Neurosci* 2005; 19: 689–98.

54. Poli M, Derosas M, Luscieti S, et al. PANK2 silencing causes cell growth reduction, cell specific ferroportin upregulation and iron deregulation. *Neurobiol Dis* 2010; 39: 204–10.

55. Kruer MC, Hiken M, Gregory A, et al. Novel histopathologic findings in molecularly confirmed Pantothenate Kinase Associated Neurodegeneration. *Brain* 2011; 134: 947–58.

56. Timmermann L, Pauls KA, Wieland K, et al. Dystonia in neurodegeneration with brain iron accumulation: outcome of deep brain stimulation. *Brain* 2011; 133: 701–12.

57. Paisan-Ruiz C, Bhatia KP, Li A, et al. Characterization of PLA2G6 as a locus for dystonia-parkinsonism. *Ann Neurol* 2009; 65: 19–23.

58. Gregory A, Westaway SK, Holm IE, et al. Neurodegeneration associated with genetic defects in phospholipase A2. *Neurology* 2008; 71:1402–9.

59. Yoshino H, Tomiyama H, Tachibana N, et al. Phenotypic spectrum of patients with PLA2G6 mutation and PARK14 linked Parkinsonism. *Neurology* 2010; 75: 1356–61.

60. Morgan NV, Westawat SK, Morton JE, et al. PLA2G6, encoding a phospholipase A2, is mutated in neurodegenerative disorders with high brain iron. *Nat Genet* 2006; 38: 752–4.

61. Paisán-Ruiz C, Li A, Schneider SA, et al. Widespread Lewy body and tau accumulation in childhood and adult onset dystonia-parkinsonism cases with PLA2G6 mutations. *Neurobiol Aging* 2012; 33: 814–23.

62. Yoda E, Hachisu K, Taketomi Y, et al. Mitochondrial dysfunction and reduced prostaglandin synthesis in skeletal muscle of Group VIB Ca2+-independent phospholipase A2gamma-deficient mice. *J Lipid Res* 2010; 51: 3003–15.

63. Beck G, Sugiura Y, Shinzawa K, et al. Neuroaxonal dystrophy in calcium independent phospholipase A2β deficiency results from insufficient remodeling and degeneration of mitochondrial and presynaptic membranes. *J Neurosci* 2011; 31: 11411–20.

64. Ramirez A, Heimbach A, Gründemann J, et al. Hereditary parkinsonism with dementia is caused by mutations in ATP13A2, encoding a lysosomal type 5 P-type ATPase. *Nat Genet* 2006; 38:1184–91.

65. Brüggemann N, Hagenah J, Reetz K, et al. Recessively inherited parkinsonism: effect of ATP13A2 mutations on the clinical and neuroimaging phenotype. *Arch Neurol* 2010; 67: 1357–63.

66. Behrens MI, Brüggemann N, Chana P, et al. Clinical spectrum of Kufor-Rakeb syndrome in the Chilean kindred with ATP13A2 mutations. *Mov Disord* 2010; 15: 1929–37.

67. Ramonet D, Podhajska A, Stafa K, et al. PARK9 associated ATP13A2 localises to intracellular acidic vesicles and regulates cation homeostasis and neuronal integrity. *Hum Mol Genet* 2012; 21: 1725–43.

68. Grünewald A, Arns B, Seibler P, et al. ATP13A2 mutations impair mitochondrial function in fibroblasts from patients with Kufor-Rakeb syndrome. *Neurobiol Aging* 2012; 33: 1843.

69. Ugolino J, Fang S, Kubisch C, Monteiro MJ. Mutant ATP12A2 mutations involved in parkinsonism are degraded by ER-associated degradation and sensitise cells to ER-stress induced cell death. *Hum Mol Genet* 2011; 20: 3565–77.

70. Schneider SA, Bhatia KP. Dystonia in Woodhouse-Sakati syndrome. *Mov Disord* 2008; 23: 592–6.

71. Potter KA, Kern MJ, Fullbright G, et al. Central nervous system dysfunction in a mouse model of FA2H deficiency. *Glia* 2011; 59: 1009–21.

72. Hayflick SJ, Kruer MC, Gregory A, et al. Beta-propeller protein associated neurodegeneration: a new X-linked dominant disorder with brain iron accumulation. *Brain* 2013; 136:1708–17.

73. Haack TB, Hogarth P, Kruer MC, et al. Exome sequencing reveals de novo WDR45 mutations causing a phenotypically distinct, X-linked dominant form of NBIA. *Am J Hum Genet* 2012; 91: 1144–9.

74. Dusi S, Valletta L, Hack TB, et al. Exome sequence reveals mutations in CoA synthase as a cause of neurodegeneration with brain iron accumulation. *Am J Hum Genet* 2014; 94: 11–22.

75. Guilarte TR. Manganese and Parkinson's disease: a critical review and new findings. *Env Health Perspect* 2010; 8: 1071–1080.

76. Couper J. On the effects of black oxide of manganese when inhaled in the lungs. *Br Ann Med Pharmacol* 1837; 1: 42.

77. Kessler KR, Wunderlich G, Hefter H, Seitz RJ. Secondary progressive chronic manganism associated with markedly decreased striatal dopamine D2 receptor. *Mov Disord* 2003; 18: 217–8.

78. Colosimo C, Guidi M. Parkinsonism due to ephedrine neurotoxicity: a case report. *Eur J Neurol* 2009; 16: e114.

79. Racette BA, McGee-Minnich L, Moerlein SM, et al. Welding related Parkinsonism: clinical features, treatment and pathophysiology. *Neurology* 2001; 56: 8–13.

80. Criswell SR, Perlmutter JS, Videen TO, et al. Reduced uptake of [¹⁸F]FDOPA PET in asymptomatic welders with occupational manganese exposure. *Neurology* 2011; 76: 1296–301.

81. Oygard K, Riise T, Moen B, Engelsen BA. Occurrence of Parkinson's disease (PD) and Parkinsonism (P) in Sauda community. *Proceedings of the Symposium on Manganese Toxicity* **1992**: 179–182.

82. Lucchini R, Albini E, Benedetti L, et al. High prevalence of parkinsonian disorders associated to manganese exposure in the vicinities of ferroalloy industries. *Am J Indust Med* 2007; 50: 788–800.

83. Perl DP, Onalow CW. The neuropathology of manganese induced Parkinsonism. *J Neuropathol Exper Neurol* 2007; 66: 675–82.

84. Lucchini RG, Martin CJ, Doney BC. From manganism to manganese induced Parkinsonism: a conceptual model based on the evolution of exposure. *Neuromol Med* 2009; 11: 311–321.

85. Huang CC, Chu NS, Lu CS, et al. The natural history of neurological manganism over 18 years. *Parkinsonism Relat Disord* 2007; 13: 143–5.

86. Cox DW, Roberts E. Wilson Disease. GeneReviews. Bookshelf ID: NBK1512P-MID: 20301685.

87. Westermark K, Tedroff J, Thuomas KA. Neurological Wilson's disease studied with magnetic resonance imaging and with positron emission tomography using dopaminergic markers. *Mov Disord* 1995; 10: 596–603.

88. Prashanth LK, Sinha S, Taly AB, et al. Spectrum of epilepsy in Wilson's disease with electroencephalographic, MR imaging and pathological correlates. *J Neurol Sci* 2010; 291: 44–51.

89. Coffey AJ, Durkie M, Hague S, et al. A genetic study of Wilson disease in the United Kingdom. *Brain* 2013; 136: 1476–87.

90. Hercend C, Bauvais C, Bollot G, et al. Elucidation of the *ATP7B* N-domain Mg2+-ATP coordination site and its allosteric regulation. *PLoS One* 2011; 6: e26245.

91. Terwel D, Löschmann YN, Schmidt HH, Schöler HR, Cantz T, Heneka MT. Neuroinflammatory and behavioural changes in the Atp7B mutant mouse model of Wilson's disease. *J Neurochem* 2011; 118: 105–12.

92. Sauer SW, Merle U, Opp S, et al. Severe dysfunction of respiratory chain and cholesterol metabolism in Atp7b(-/-) mice as a model for Wilson disease. *Biochim Biophys Acta* 2011; 1812: 1607–15.

93. Prashanth LK, Sinha S, Taly AB, Vasudev MK. Do MRI features distinguish Wilson's disease from other early onset extrapyramidal disorders? *Mov Disord* 2010; 25: 672–8.

94. Hölscher S, Leinweber B, Hefter H, et al. Evaluation of the symptomatic treatment of residual symptoms in neurological Wilson's disease. *Eur Neurol* 2010; 64: 83–7.

95. Burke JF, Dayalu P, Nan B, Askari F, Brewer GJ, Lorincz MT. Prognostic significance of neurologic examination findings in Wilson's disease. *Parkinsonism Relat Disord* 2011; 17: 551–6.

Index

Page numbers in *italics* refer to illustrations; those in **bold** refer to tables

Neurodegeneration, First Edition. Edited by Anthony Schapira, Zbigniew Wszolek, Ted M. Dawson and Nicholas Wood.
© 2017 John Wiley & Sons, Ltd. Published 2017 by John Wiley & Sons, Ltd.